Orthopaedic Knowledge Update®

OKU® 6

Pediatrics

Orthopaedic Knowledge Update®

OKU®

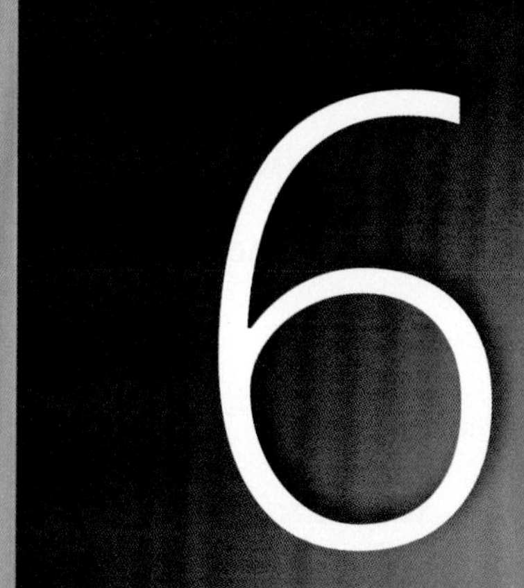

Pediatrics

EDITED BY

Jeffrey E. Martus, MD, MS, FAAOS

Associate Professor
Department of Orthopaedic Surgery
Monroe Carell Jr. Children's Hospital at Vanderbilt
Vanderbilt University Medical Center
Nashville, Tennessee

Wolters Kluwer

Philadelphia • Baltimore • New York • London
Buenos Aires • Hong Kong • Sydney • Tokyo

AAOS
American Academy of
Orthopaedic Surgeons

AAOS

AMERICAN ACADEMY OF ORTHOPAEDIC SURGEONS

Staff
American Academy of Orthopaedic Surgeons

Anna Salt Troise, MBA, *Chief Education Strategist*

Hans Koelsch, PhD, *Director, Publishing*

Lisa Claxton Moore, *Senior Manager, Editorial*

Steven Kellert, *Senior Editor*

Wolters Kluwer Health

Brian Brown, *Director, Medical Practice*

Stacey Sebring, *Senior Development Editor*

Emily Buccieri, *Senior Editorial Coordinator*

Ashley Pfeiffer, *Editorial Coordinator*

Erin Cantino, *Portfolio Marketing Manager*

David Saltzberg, *Production Project Manager*

Stephen Druding, *Design Coordinator*

Beth Welsh, *Senior Manufacturing Coordinator*

TNQ Technologies, *Prepress Vendor*

The material presented in the *Orthopaedic Knowledge Update®: Pediatrics, Sixth Edition* has been made available by the American Academy of Orthopaedic Surgeons (AAOS) for educational purposes only. This material is not intended to present the only, or necessarily best, methods or procedures for the medical situations discussed, but rather is intended to represent an approach, view, statement, or opinion of the author(s) or producer(s), which may be helpful to others who face similar situations. Medical providers should use their own, independent medical judgment, in addition to open discussion with patients, when developing patient care recommendations and treatment plans. Medical care should always be based on a medical provider's expertise that is individually tailored to a patient's circumstances, preferences and rights. Some drugs or medical devices demonstrated in AAOS courses or described in AAOS print or electronic publications have not been cleared by the Food and Drug Administration (FDA) or have been cleared for specific uses only. The FDA has stated that it is the responsibility of the physician to determine the FDA clearance status of each drug or device he or she wishes to use in clinical practice and to use the products with appropriate patient consent and in compliance with applicable law. Furthermore, any statements about commercial products are solely the opinion(s) of the author(s) and do not represent an Academy endorsement or evaluation of these products. These statements may not be used in advertising or for any commercial purpose.

ISBN 9781975152680

Library of Congress Control Number: Cataloging in Publication data available on request from publisher.

Printed in China

Published 2022 by the American Academy of Orthopaedic Surgeons
9400 West Higgins Road
Rosemont, Illinois 60018

CCS0121

Acknowledgments

Contributors

Joshua M. Abzug, MD
Associate Professor
Departments of Orthopedics and Pediatrics
University of Maryland School of Medicine
Director, University of Maryland Brachial Plexus Practice
Director of Pediatric Orthopedaics, University of Maryland Medical Center
Deputy Surgeon-in-Chief, University of Maryland Children's Hospital
Director and Founder, Camp Open Arms
Baltimore, Maryland

Benjamin A. Alman, MD, FAAOS
Chair of Orthopaedic Surgery
James R. Urbaniak, MD, Professor of Orthopaedic Surgery
Professor in Cell Biology
Professor in Pediatrics
Professor in the Department of Pathology
Duke University
Durham, North Carolina

Alexandre Arkader, MD
Pediatric Orthopedics and Orthopedic Oncology
The Children's Hospital of Philadelphia
Associate Professor of Orthopedic Surgery
Perelman School of Medicine at University of Pennsylvania
Philadelphia, Pennsylvania

Donald S. Bae, MD
Professor of Orthopedic Surgery
Department of Orthopedic Surgery
Boston Children's Hospital
Boston, Massachusetts

Pablo Marrero Barrera, MD
Pediatric Orthopedic Fellow
Arnold Palmer Hospital for Children
Orlando, Florida

Jennifer J. Beck, MD
Assistant Professor
Department of Orthopedic Surgery
Orthopaedic Institute for Children/UCLA
Los Angeles, California

James T. Beckmann, MD, MS, FAOA
Medical Director for the St. Luke's Athletic Training Residency Program
St. Luke's Hospital
Boise, Idaho

Craig Birch, MD
Instructor of Orthopedic Surgery
Harvard Medical School
Boston, Massachusetts

Richard E. Bowen, MD
Professor, Department of Orthopedic Surgery
Orthopaedic Institute for Children/UCLA
Los Angeles, California

Ravinder Brar, MD, MPH
Assistant Professor
Department of Orthopedic Surgery
University of California, San Francisco
San Francisco, California

Brian K. Brighton, MD, MPH
Associate Professor
Division Chief, Pediatric Orthopaedics
Atrium Musculoskeletal Institute
OrthoCarolina
Charlotte, North Carolina

Jessica D. Burns, MD, MPH
Clinical Assistant Professor
Department of Child Health
University of Arizona College of Medicine – Phoenix
Staff Orthopaedic Surgeon
Department of Orthopedic Surgery & Sports Medicine
Phoenix Children's Hospital
Phoenix, Arizona

Cordelia W. Carter, MD
Associate Professor of Pediatric Orthopedics and Sports Medicine
Department of Orthopedic Surgery
NYU Grossman School of Medicine
New York, New York

Johanna Chang, MD
Associate Professor of Clinical Health Sciences
University of California San Diego/Rady Children's Hospital
San Diego, California

Antonia F. Chen, MD, MBA
Associate Professor
Department of Orthopaedic Surgery
Brigham and Women's Hospital
Harvard Medical School
Boston, Massachusetts

Robert H. Cho, MD
Pediatric Orthopaedic Surgeon
Chief of Staff
Shriners for Children Medical Center
Pasadena, California

Ryan P. Coene, MS
Department of Orthopaedics
Boston Children's Hospital
Boston, Massachusetts

Lawson A. B. Copley, MD, MBA
Professor, Department of Orthopaedic Surgery and Pediatrics
University of Texas Southwestern
Texas Scottish Rite Hospital
Children's Medical Center of Dallas
Dallas, Texas

Patrick Curran, MD, MS
Clinical Fellow
Department of Orthopaedic Surgery
Boston Children's Hospital
Boston, Massachusetts

Jared William Daniel, MD
Pediatric Orthopedic Surgeon
Clinical Assistant Professor – Surgery
Sanford Health
University of South Dakota
Sanford School of Medicine
Sioux Falls, South Dakota

Matthew B. Dobbs, MD, FACS, FAOA
Director, Dobbs Clubfoot Center
Paley Orthopedic and Spine Institute
West Palm Beach, Florida

Kathryn S. Doughty, MD, MPH, MS
Pediatric Orthopaedic Surgeon
Director of Musculoskeletal Education
Department of Orthopaedic Surgery and Sports Medicine
Bassett Healthcare Network
Cooperstown, New York

Eric W. Edmonds, MD, FAOA
Professor, Department of Orthopaedic Surgery
University of California San Diego
Rady Children's Hospital–San Diego
San Diego, California

John B. Emans, MD
Professor, Department of Pediatric Orthopaedics
Boston Children's Hospital
Boston, Massachusetts

Corinna C. D. Franklin, MD
Associate Professor
Shriners Hospital for Children
Philadelphia, Pennsylvania

Brittany N. Garcia, MD
Adjunct Faculty Instructor
Department of Orthopaedic Surgery
University of Utah Hospital
Salt Lake City, Utah

Michael P. Glotzbecker, MD
Associate Professor
Department of Pediatric Orthopaedics
Rainbow Babies and Childrens Hospital
Cleveland, Ohio

Charles A. Goldfarb, MD, FAAOS
Professor and Executive Vice Chair
Department of Orthopaedic Surgery
Washington University School of Medicine
St. Louis, Missouri

Dorothy K. Grange, MD
Professor, Department of Pediatrics
Washington University School of Medicine
St. Louis, Missouri

John J. Grayhack, MD, MS
Professor, Department of Orthopaedic Surgery
Northwestern University Feinberg School of Medicine
Ann & Robert H. Lurie Children's Hospital of Chicago
Chicago, Illinois

Andrew J. M. Gregory, MD, FAAP, FACSM, FAMSSM
Associate Professor
Departments of Orthopedics, Pediatrics and Neurosurgery
Vanderbilt University Medical Center
Nashville, Tennessee

Christina A. Gurnett, MD, PhD
Professor, Department of Neurology
Washington University School of Medicine
St. Louis, Missouri

David H. Gutmann, MD, PhD
Professor, Department of Neurology
Washington University School of Medicine
St. Louis, Missouri

Matthew F. Halsey, MD
Associate Professor
Department of Orthopaedics and Rehabilitation
Oregon Health and Science University
Portland, Oregon

Jennifer Harrington, MBBS, PhD
Pediatric Endocrinologist, Assistant Professor
The Hospital for Sick Children
University of Toronto
Toronto, Ontario, Canada

Daniel J. Hedequist, MD
Associate Professor
Department of Pediatric Orthopaedics
Harvard Medical School
Boston, Massachusetts

Martin J. Herman, MD
Professor of Orthopedic Surgery and Pediatrics
Drexel University College of Medicine
St. Christopher's Hospital for Children
Philadelphia, Pennsylvania

José A. Herrera-Soto, MD
Director of Pediatric Orthopedic Fellowship
Arnold Palmer Hospital for Children
Orlando, Florida

Andrew W. Howard, MD, MSc, FRCSC
Pediatric Orthopaedic Surgeon
Department of Orthopaedic Surgery
Hospital for Sick Children
Toronto, Ontario, Canada

Elizabeth W. Hubbard, MD
Department of Orthopaedics
Duke University Hospital
Durham, North Carolina

Douglas T. Hutchinson, MD
Professor, Department of Orthopaedic Surgery
University of Utah Hospital
Salt Lake City, Utah

Christopher Iobst, MD
Clinical Associate Professor
Department of Orthopedic Surgery
Nationwide Children's Hospital
Columbus, Ohio

Megan E. Johnson, MD
Assistant Professor of Orthopedic Surgery
Texas Scottish Rite Hospital for Children
UT Southwestern Medical Center
Dallas, Texas

Scott P. Kaiser, MD
Attending Surgeon
Department of Orthopedic Surgery
Kaiser Permanente
Oakland, California

Simon P. Kelley, MBChB, PhD, FRCS (Tr and Orth)
Associate Professor
The Hospital for Sick Children
Department of Surgery
University of Toronto
Toronto, Ontario, Canada

Erik C. B. King, MD, MS
Associate Professor
Department of Orthopaedic Surgery
Northwestern University Feinberg School of Medicine
Ann & Robert H. Lurie Children's Hospital of Chicago
Chicago, Illinois

Mikhail A. Klimstra, MD
Department of Orthopedic Surgery
University of Minnesota
Minneapolis, Minnesota

Joel Kolmodin, MD
Pediatric Orthopaedic Surgeon
Essentia Health
Duluth, Minnesota

Pamela J. Lang, MD
Assistant Professor
Department of Orthopaedic Surgery
University of Wisconsin
Madison, Wisconsin

A. Noelle Larson, MD
Professor, Department of Orthopedic Surgery
Mayo Clinic
Rochester, Minnesota

David E. Lazarus, MD
Department of Orthopedic Surgery
Greenville Healthsystem
Greenville, South Carolina

Holly B. Leshikar, MD, MPH
Assistant Professor of Orthopedics
University of California at Davis
Shriners Hospital for Children, Northern California
Sacramento, California

Ying Li, MD
Associate Professor of Orthopaedic Surgery
C.S. Mott Children's Hospital
Michigan Medicine
Ann Arbor, Michigan

Kristin S. Livingston, MD
Assistant Professor
Department of Orthopedic Surgery
University of California, San Francisco
Benioff Children's Hospital
San Francisco, California

John F. Lovejoy III, MD
Associate Professor
Chair, Department of Orthopaedics and Sports Medicine
Nemours Children's Hospital
Orlando, Florida

Benjamin D. Martin, MD
Associate Professor, Orthopaedic Surgery and Pediatrics
The George Washington University School of Medicine and Health Sciences
Associate Chief, Division or Orthopaedic Surgery and Sports Medicine
Children's National Hospital
Washington, DC

David M. Matson, MD
Orthopedic Surgery Resident
Department of Orthopedic Surgery
University of Minnesota
Minneapolis, Minnesota

Douglas J. McDonald, MD, MS
Professor, Department of Orthopaedic Surgery
Washington University School of Medicine
St. Louis, Missouri

Amy L. McIntosh, MD
Professor of Orthopaedic Surgery
Texas Scottish Rite Hospital for Children
Dallas, Texas

Charles T. Mehlman, DO, MPH
Director, Musculoskeletal Outcomes Research
Co-Director, Brachial Plexus Center
Professor, Department of Surgery
University of Cincinnati
Cincinnati Children's Hospital
Cincinnati, Ohio

Matthew D. Milewski, MD
Assistant Professor
Division of Sports Medicine
Department of Orthopaedic Surgery
Boston Children's Hospital
Harvard Medical School
Boston, Massachusetts

Firoz Miyanji, MD, FRCSC
Clinical Professor
Department of Orthopedics
University of British Columbia
Vancouver, British Columbia, Canada

Stephanie N. Moore, BS
Department of Pharmacology
Vanderbilt University
Nashville, Tennessee

José A. Morcuende, MD, PhD
Professor, Department of Orthopedic Surgery and Rehabilitation, and Pediatrics
University of Iowa
Iowa City, Iowa

William Z. Morris, MD
Texas Scottish Rite Hospital
Assistant Professor
Department of Orthopaedic Surgery
University of Texas Southwestern
Dallas, Texas

Ryan D. Muchow, MD
Associate Professor
Department of Orthopaedic Surgery
University of Kentucky
Shriners Hospital for Children – Lexington
Lexington, Kentucky

Brian T. Muffly, MD
Resident Physician
Department of Orthopaedic Surgery
University of Kentucky
Lexington, Kentucky

Matthew E. Oetgen, MD, MBA
Chief, Division of Orthopaedic Surgery and Sports Medicine
Children's National Hospital
Associate Professor of Orthopaedic Surgery
George Washington University
Washington, DC

J. Lee Pace, MD
Director, Elite Sports Medicine
Assistant Professor
Connecticut Children's Medical Center
University of Connecticut School of Medicine
Hartford, Connecticut

Nirav K. Pandya, MD
Associate Professor
Chief, Pediatric Orthopedic Surgery
Department of Orthopedic Surgery
University of California, San Francisco
Benioff Children's Hospital
San Francisco, California

David A. Podeszwa, MD
Professor of Orthopedic Surgery
University of Texas Southwestern Medical Center
Scottish Rite for Children
Dallas, Texas

Robert H. Quinn, MD
Department Chair and Professor
Department of Orthopaedics
UT Health San Antonio
San Antonio, Texas

Suhas M. Radhakrishna, MD
Associate Professor
Department of Pediatrics
University of California, San Diego
San Diego, California

Deepak Ramanathan, MD
Chief Resident Physician
Orthopaedic & Rheumatologic Institute
Cleveland Clinic
Cleveland, Ohio

Karl C. Roberts, MD, FAOA
Program Director
Spectrum Health-Michigan State Orthopedic Surgery Residency
Clinical Assistant Professor
Department of Surgery
Michigan State College of Human Medicine
Grand Rapids, Michigan

Paul M. Saluan, MD
Director of Pediatric and Adolescent Sports Medicine
Orthopaedic and Rheumatologic Institute
Cleveland Clinic
Cleveland, Ohio

Anthony A. Scaduto, MD
Charles LeRoy Lowman Professor
Orthopaedic Institute for Children
University of California, Los Angeles
Department of Orthopaedic Surgery
Los Angeles, California

Brian P. Scannell, MD
Associate Professor of Orthopaedic Surgery
Carolinas Medical Center, Atrium Health
OrthoCarolina
Charlotte, North Carolina

Susan A. Scherl, MD
Professor, Department of Orthopaedics
The University of Nebraska
Omaha, Nebraska

Jonathan G. Schoenecker, MD, PhD
Associate Professor
Department of Orthopaedics
Vanderbilt University
Nashville, Tennessee

Mark Seeley, MD, FACS, FAOA
Associate Program Director
Geisinger Orthopaedic Surgery
Associate Professor
Geisinger Commonwealth School of Medicine
Danville, Pennsylvania

Apurva S. Shah, MD, MBA
Assistant Professor of Orthopaedic Surgery
Director of Clinical Research
Co-Director of the Brachial Plexus Program
Division of Orthopaedic Surgery
Children's Hospital of Philadelphia
University of Pennsylvania
Perelman School of Medicine
Philadelphia, Pennsylvania

Melinda S. Sharkey, MD
Associate Professor
Pediatric Orthopaedic Surgery
Department of Orthopaedic Surgery
Albert Einstein College of Medicine
New York, New York

Kevin G. Shea, MD
Chambers-Okamura Endowed Professor in Pediatric Orthopedics
Member of the Maternal & Child Health Research Institute (MCHRI)
Vice Chief of Pediatric Orthopedic Surgery for Research
Director of Pediatric Sports Medicine
Assistant Surgeon-in-Chief for Quality and Supply Chain Management
Department of Orthopaedic Surgery
Stanford University
Palo Alto, California

Robert M. Sheets, MD
Clinical Professor
Department of Pediatrics
University of California, San Diego
San Diego, California

Benjamin W. Sheffer, MD
Assistant Professor
Department of Orthopaedic Surgery
University of Tennessee Health Science Center
Campbell Clinic
Memphis, Tennessee

Eric D. Shirley, MD
Adjunct Associate Professor of Surgery
Department of Orthopaedic Surgery
Naval Medical Center Portsmouth
Portsmouth, Virginia

Mauricio Silva, MD
Clinical Professor
Department of Orthopaedic Surgery
David Geffen School of Medicine at UCLA
Medical Director
Orthopaedic Institute for Children
Los Angeles, California

Mark R. Sinclair, MD, FAAOS
Assistant Professor
Department of Orthopaedic Surgery
University of Missouri-Kansas City
Kansas City, Missouri

Brian D. Snyder, MD, PhD
Professor, Department of Orthopaedic Surgery
Harvard Medical School
Cerebral Palsy Center
Boston Children's Hospital
Boston, Massachusetts

David D. Spence, MD
Assistant Professor
Department of Orthopaedic Surgery
University of Tennessee Health Science Center
Campbell Clinic
Memphis, Tennessee

Christopher M. Stutz, MD
Pediatric Orthopaedic Surgeon
Assistant Professor
University of Texas Southwestern Medical Center
Dallas, Texas

Daniel J. Sucato, MD, MS
Texas Scottish Rite Hospital
Professor, Department of Orthopaedic Surgery
University of Texas Southwestern
Dallas, Texas

Michael D. Sussman, MD
Staff Surgeon
Former Chief of Staff
Shriners Hospital for Children
Portland, Oregon

Vineeta T. Swaroop, MD
Associate Professor
Department of Orthopaedic Surgery
Northwestern University Feinberg School of Medicine
Ann & Robert H Lurie Children's Hospital of Chicago
Chicago, Illinois

Mihir M. Thacker, MD
Attending Pediatric Orthopedic Surgeon
Orthopedic Oncologist
Director, Orthopedic Research Fellowship Program
Department of Orthopedic Surgery
Nemours/Alfred I. duPont Hospital for Children
Wilmington, Delaware
Orthopedic Oncologist
Helen F. Graham Cancer Center, Christiana Hospital
Newark, Delaware
Associate Professor of Orthopedic Surgery and Pediatrics
Sidney Kimmel Medical College at Thomas Jefferson University
Philadelphia, Pennsylvania

Rachel Mednick Thompson, MD
Assistant Professor-in-Residence of Orthopedic Surgery
David Geffen School of Medicine at UCLA
Orthopaedic Institute for Children
Los Angeles, California

Marc Tompkins, MD
Associate Professor
Division of Sports Medicine
Department of Orthopedic Surgery
University of Minnesota
Minneapolis, Minnesota

Caroline M. Tougas, MD
Clinical Assistant Professor
Department of Orthopedic Surgery
Children's Mercy Hospital and UMKC School of Medicine
Kansas City, Missouri

Natasha Trentacosta, MD
Department of Orthopaedic Surgery
Cedars-Sinai Kerlan-Jobe Institute
Los Angeles, California

Ann E. Van Heest, MD
Professor, Department of Orthopedic Surgery
Gillette Children's Hospital
Shriners Children's Twin Cities
University of Minnesota
Minneapolis, Minnesota

Anna D. Vergun, MD, FAAOS
Clinical Associate Professor
Division Chief of Pediatric Orthopedic Surgery
University of North Carolina, School of Medicine
Chapel Hill, North Carolina

Janet L. Walker, MD
Professor, Department of Orthopaedic Surgery and Sports Medicine
University of Kentucky
Shriners Hospital Medical Center – Lexington
Lexington, Kentucky

Lindley B. Wall, MD, MSc
Associate Professor
Department of Orthopaedic Surgery
Washington University School of Medicine
St. Louis, Missouri

Amanda T. Whitaker, MD
Clinical Associate Professor
Department of Orthopaedic Surgery
College of Medicine
The Ohio State University
Nationwide Children's Hospital
Columbus, Ohio

Klane K. White, MD, MSc
Director, Skeletal Health and Dysplasia Program
Professor, Orthopaedic Surgery and Sports Medicine
University of Washington
Seattle, Washington

Theresa O. Wyrick, MD
Associate Professor
Department of Orthopaedic Surgery
Arkansas Children's Hospital
University of Arkansas for Medical Sciences
Little Rock, Arkansas

Scott Yang, MD
Assistant Professor
Department of Orthopaedics and Rehabilitation
Oregon Health and Science University
Portland, Oregon

Preface

The sixth edition of *Orthopaedic Knowledge Update®: Pediatrics* is an extension of the previous editions of this series that focuses on musculoskeletal conditions in children and adolescents. This text is written for the experienced orthopaedic practitioner, not the superspecialist or the beginning student.

The goal of *OKU®: Pediatrics 6* is to describe the important developments in pediatric orthopaedics over the past 5 years, while providing core information for each topic. The editors and authors integrated new information with fundamental knowledge to provide an essential resource for the practicing general orthopaedic surgeon and pediatric subspecialist. The annotated reference list at the end of each chapter contains classic articles as well as updated references, with annotations provided for references published within the past 5 years.

Chapters new to the sixth edition include Developmental Biology, Metabolism, Cerebral Palsy: Upper Extremity, High-Energy Injury and Polytrauma, Elbow Trauma, Knee Trauma, and Disaster and Mass Casualty Preparedness.

The quality of this book is directly related to the efforts of the section editors: Brandon Ramo, Benjamin A. Alman, Henry G. Chambers, Charles A. Goldfarb, Vishwas R. Talwalkar, James O. Sanders, Mark R. Sinclair, and Jennifer M. Weiss. These individuals are leaders within the field of orthopaedics and worked hard to ensure that the content of this edition is complete, accurate, and of high quality. We are all indebted to the expert authors who volunteered their time and then spent many hours reviewing the literature and writing these excellent chapters.

The project would not have succeeded without the excellent work of the publications staff of the American Academy of Orthopaedic Surgeons and Wolters Kluwer. Special credit and thanks go to the entire team and in particular to Lisa Claxton Moore and Emily Buccieri. It has been a privilege to participate in this effort.

We hope that the readers find this book to be a useful resource in the treatment of children with musculoskeletal conditions. Suggestions to improve future editions would be appreciated.

Jeffrey E. Martus, MD, MS, FAAOS
Editor

Table of Contents

Section 1: General Topics

SECTION EDITOR:
Brandon A. Ramo, MD, FAAOS

Section 2: Basic Science

SECTION EDITOR:
Benjamin A. Alman, MD, FAAOS

Section 6: Spine

SECTION EDITOR:
James O. Sanders, MD, FAAOS

Section 7: Trauma

SECTION EDITOR:
Mark R. Sinclair, MD, FAAOS

Section 8: Sports-Related Topics

SECTION EDITOR:
Jennifer M. Weiss, MD, FAAOS

SECTION 1

General Topics

Section Editor:

Brandon A. Ramo, MD, FAAOS

CHAPTER 1

Quality, Safety, and Value

BRIAN K. BRIGHTON, MD, MPH • DONALD S. BAE, MD • APURVA S. SHAH, MD, MBA

ABSTRACT

The concepts of quality, safety, and value continue to receive attention in the rapidly changing healthcare landscape. An understanding of quality measures and quality improvement methodology, as well as using surgical simulation, implementing checklists, and creating a culture of safety, can improve the quality and safety of orthopaedic surgery. In turn, these efforts in quality and safety will improve patient outcomes and contain costs, thus improving value delivery in orthopaedic surgery.

Keywords: cost; quality; quality improvement; safety; value

INTRODUCTION

During the past decade, increased attention has been directed at improving the value of patient care through higher quality outcomes and improved patient safety. Two reports published by the Institute of Medicine at the beginning of the 21st century raised the collective awareness of patients, payers, hospitals, and providers regarding the importance of quality, safety, and value in the practice of medicine.[1,2] To further this effort, the Pediatric Orthopaedic Society of North America implemented a "Quality, Safety, and Value Initiative" in 2011 to involve society members in providing leadership, education, and direction to discussions on quality, safety, and value taking place both locally and nationally.[3-5] Each concept—quality, safety, and value—will be discussed, including specific applications to pediatric orthopaedic surgery.

Dr. Brighton or an immediate family member serves as a board member, owner, officer, or committee member of the American College of Surgeons and the Pediatric Orthopaedic Society of North America. Dr. Bae or an immediate family member serves as a paid consultant to or is an employee of OrthoPediatrics and serves as a board member, owner, officer, or committee member of the American Academy of Orthopaedic Surgeons, ASSH, and POSNA. Dr. Shah or an immediate family member serves as a board member, owner, officer, or committee member of the American Society for Surgery of the Hand and the Pediatric Orthopaedic Society of North America.

QUALITY

Physicians would universally agree that their top priority is to provide high-quality health care, but a challenging concept remains: What defines quality? The answer depends on who is answering the question and what is important to that individual. It also depends on who is defining quality and how the individual or organization is measuring it. Surgeons frequently refer to quality in the context of low infection, complication, and mortality rates, or adherence to process measures and practice guidelines. Patients and families may view quality from the perspective of rate of recovery and return to function. The Institute of Medicine defined quality as the "degree to which healthcare services for individuals and populations increase the likelihood of desired outcomes and are consistent with current professional knowledge."[1] In addition, the Institute of Medicine outlined six specific aims for improving health care that are focused on delivering care that is safe, effective, patient centered, timely, efficient, and equitable. In the equation, *value* = (*outcome* + *experience*)/*cost*,[6] quality is a composition of patient outcomes, safety, and patient experience. Improving the quality of care and patient outcomes provides an important opportunity to add value for a given cost.[7]

Quality Improvement

Quality improvement in health care is a systematic, data-guided activity designed to bring about immediate positive change in the delivery of health care in particular settings.[8] Quality improvement methodology is used to incorporate new knowledge into clinical practice and apply this information to fix existing problems in care delivery. The aim is to become more effective, safe, and efficient and continually improve processes of care. Such methodologies and principles originally were designed and implemented in the manufacturing industry and have been applied to health care to provide a framework for improving patient care. Commonly used methodologies include Lean, Six Sigma, and the Model for Improvement.

Lean is a quality improvement methodology that evolved from the Toyota Production System, which was a framework to map out and preserve the processes of value and eliminate waste and inefficiency.[9] One hallmark of the Lean process is the standardization of processes to ensure consistency. The Lean approach requires an understanding of the process, including how the process is intended to work and variations in the process that have evolved across time. This methodology has been used in several healthcare settings to improve the surgical care of patients.[10]

Six Sigma also has its origins in the manufacturing industry. This approach relies on precise and accurate measurements of process and outcomes using the improvement process known by the acronym DMAIC (define, measure, analyze, improve, and control). The problem within a process is defined, any defects are measured, the cause of the defects are analyzed, the process performance is improved by removing the causes of the defects, and the process is controlled to ensure that the defects do not recur. The Six Sigma goal is to identify and reduce error rates to the six sigma level (<3.4 defects per million opportunities).[11] Examples of Six Sigma methodology can be seen in reducing medication administration errors and improving operating room efficiency.[10,12]

Lean Six Sigma is a combination of Lean and Six Sigma principles that is often applied in health care. It aims to improve care by incorporating the Lean principles of eliminating waste and improving efficiency and the Six Sigma approach of pursuing accuracy and effectiveness.

The Model for Improvement is another example of a quality improvement methodology that provides a framework for improving a process or a system.[13] The model contains four essential components: an aim, measurement, change ideas, and tests of change. The first three components are examined by three key questions: (1) What are we trying to accomplish? (2) How will we know that a change is an improvement? and (3) What changes can we make that will result in an improvement? The final component involves using a technique for rapid testing and learning from change known as the plan-do-study-act cycle (**Figure 1**). Using a series of small plan-do-study-act cycles, changes on a larger scale can be made to improve and sustain improved patient care across time.

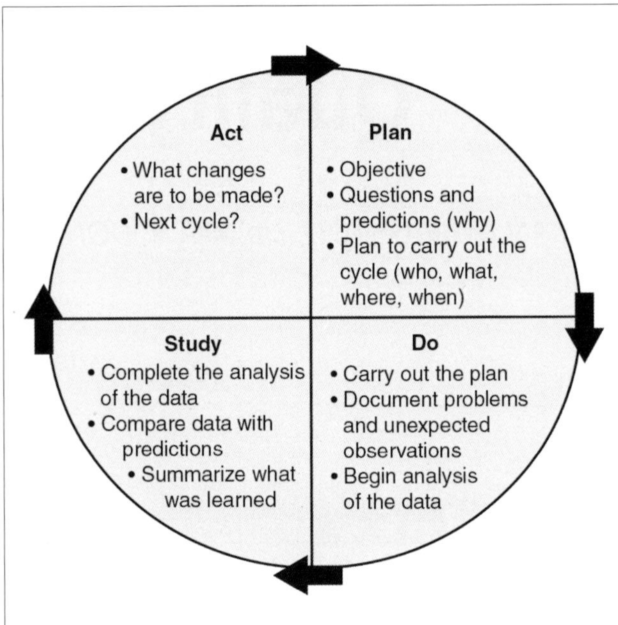

FIGURE 1 Illustration of the plan-do-study-act cycle for learning and improvement.

There are a number of examples of using quality improvement methodology in pediatric orthopaedic surgery. A 2017 article described an education and training program instituted at Boston Children's Hospital to reduce cast saw injuries.[14] Another example is the institutional investigation demonstrating that a dedicated orthopaedic trauma operating room in a pediatric trauma center was associated with fewer after-hours procedures, decreased wait time to the surgical procedure, reduced length of hospitalization, and lower cost.[15] The authors of a 2018 study, using the Model for Improvement quality improvement methodology, were able to implement evidence-based protocols for the treatment of pediatric supracondylar humerus fractures and distal radius buckle fractures to improve practice recommendations and reduce practice variation.[16] Some clinical examples of the application of quality improvement methodology [15,17-22] are listed in **Table 1**.

Quality Indicators and Measures

Quality indicators refer to a set of clear, measurable items that are ideally related to outcome. Numerous public and private agencies have already begun to define, measure, and report on healthcare quality.[23,24] In a systematic review of the pediatric orthopaedic surgery literature, researchers found mortality, postoperative complications, revision surgery, and readmission rates as the most commonly referenced quality indicators.[25]

Section 1: General Topics

TABLE 1

Examples of the Application of Quality Improvement Methodology to Patient Care

Methodology	Example
Improving efficiency of processes (streamlining)	Improving operating room efficiency, use of a dedicated orthopaedic trauma operating room in a pediatric trauma center
Eliminating waste associated with the process (logistics)	MRI use in musculoskeletal infection
Reducing errors and adverse events (safety)	Eliminating cast saw injuries
Decreasing variation in choosing and using processes (utilization and standardization)	Best-practice guidelines for high-risk spine surgery
Improving communication within the healthcare team (use of checklists)	Use of an intraoperative neuromonitoring checklist
Improving systematization of the process (care pathways)	Rapid recovery care pathways in adolescent idiopathic scoliosis
Maximizing health improvement (outcomes)	Patient-reported outcomes (PROMIS, PODCI)
Enhancing the patient's experience of care (satisfaction)	Patient satisfaction scores

PODCI = Pediatric Outcomes Data Collection Instrument, PROMIS = Patient-Reported Outcomes Measurement Information System

Adapted with permission from Jevsevar DS: Health system perspective: Variation, costs, and physician behavior. *J Pediatr Orthop* 2015;35(5 suppl 1):S14-S19.

Defining and measuring quality is essential to identify gaps in performance, make changes, and monitor and compare long-term performance. Process measures require defined criteria that can be determined by nationally derived evidence-based guidelines, institutional guidelines, or consensus guidelines. These often serve as surrogates to define the quality of care and may include compliance with clinical care pathways or adherence to evidence-based guidelines, with limited effect on value. Measures of patient expectations, satisfaction, function, and patient-reported outcomes all can be used to measure outcomes, yet no universal set of outcomes measures exist to clearly define the quality of care being delivered. The ideal measures should be clearly defined, easily obtainable, and risk adjusted to discriminate among levels of quality. The concept of standardization of outcomes measures remains on the near horizon.[26]

PATIENT SAFETY

Beginning with the Institute of Medicine report "To Err Is Human: Building a Safe Health System,"[2] recognizing the magnitude and scope of preventable errors and adverse events has led to the modern patient safety movement.[27] This movement has shifted focus away from individual errors because complications or adverse outcomes resulting from careless or technically incompetent providers are rare. Rather, current efforts aim to optimize care delivery systems, using principles such as standardization, simplification, reducing reliance on memory or experience, and crisis resource management.[27] Currently, patient safety is defined as the prevention and mitigation of harm caused by errors of omission or commission that are associated with health care, which involves the establishment of operational systems and processes that minimize the likelihood of errors and maximize the likelihood of intercepting them when they occur, before they reach the patient.

In pediatric orthopaedics, the first level of improving patient safety involves improving technical performance and minimizing technical error. Surgical simulation is an example of how performance may be improved through iterative, deliberate practice of surgery without patient risk.[28] Simulation training to improve technical performance has been used in several orthopaedic surgical disciplines, ranging from arthroscopy to complex spine surgery.[29-32] Although high-fidelity, virtual reality simulation trainers are available, effective training may be imparted with low-fidelity models focused on fundamental orthopaedic procedures. For example, recent publications highlight the use of a simple distal radius fracture cast model for improving both proficiency and safety in closed fracture treatment, cast application, and cast removal.[33,34] One simulation curriculum using this model was found to significantly decrease the rate of complications and, in doing so, yielded an 11:1 return on investment.[14] The authors of a 2019 study further reported that simulation training for distal radius fractures decreases the risk of loss of reduction and improves radiographic outcomes.[35]

In addition, the implementation of checklists has been an important measure to improve patient safety through error prevention. Most notably, the World Health Organization developed the Surgical Safety Checklist in 2008 as part of the Safe Surgery Saves Lives initiative. The checklist seeks to improve patient safety by promoting communication within surgical teams and minimizing the risk of preventable error. Therefore, the checklist provides a list of safety checks to be taken before inducing anesthesia (sign in), just before incision (time out), and at the conclusion of each procedure (sign out). Although compliance with the checklist is still variable, prior investigations have suggested that this simple measure may prevent adverse events and improve patient outcomes.[36,37] Various checklists have been similarly introduced in several orthopaedic subspecialties, including implant arthroplasty, anterior cruciate ligament reconstruction, spine surgery, and hand surgery; future work in pediatric orthopaedics is underway.[21,38-40]

The Safety Culture

Perhaps the most important, yet most challenging and elusive, step toward improving patient safety is to create a culture of safety.[27,41] Pediatric orthopaedic care is a complex and ever-changing field, yet safety cultures have been effectively nurtured in other equally complex industries, such as aviation and manufacturing. Effective individuals and organizations create a culture of safety by (1) acknowledging that errors occur; (2) participating in nonjudgmental mechanisms to identify, understand, and own the root sources of error; (3) recognizing expertise from stakeholders regardless of hierarchy; and (4) embracing changes in practice to minimize errors and potential complications.[42] Prior studies of practicing orthopaedic surgeons have identified that surgeons are concerned about the safety climate in their work environments and are enthusiastic about promoting improved communication and procedural standardization to improve patient safety.[43] These attitudes serve as an important foundation, given the traditional hierarchal structure of surgery and its reliance on autonomous individual providers.

It is critical that this process involve all providers involved in patient care, including the practicing surgeon. Improvement in individual behavior—and a decrease in disruptive behavior—may not only improve team dynamics but also decrease medical error and adverse patient outcomes.[44] Several initiatives have been developed to assist in provider education and training. Team Strategies and Tools to Enhance Performance and Patient Safety (TeamSTEPPS), for example, was developed by the Agency for Healthcare Research and Quality as a comprehensive, evidence-based teamwork system.[45] By providing means for site assessment, team training, implementation, and sustainment of change, TeamSTEPPS can improve team-based behavior and, ultimately, patient safety. Prior application of TeamSTEPPS programs improved perceptions of teamwork and communication and positively influenced clinical performance (eg, nosocomial infection rates and time to successful extracorporeal membrane oxygenation cannulation) in pediatric intensive care units.[46,47] Similar team training may improve patient outcomes and create a sustainable culture of patient safety within pediatric orthopaedics.[48]

Future Directions

Despite widespread efforts to improve patient safety, challenges remain. Some errors, such as wrong-site surgery, seem more refractory to time-outs and other systematic protocols. Systems initiatives that were proven effective in smaller pilot studies have not been appreciated with widespread implementation and generalization. Changing technology, rapidly advancing surgical techniques, organizational silos of healthcare systems, and persistent reliance on individual surgeons to manage patient care likely represent some of the reasons for these challenges. The current reimbursement system in the United States may further add challenges. Providers are typically incentivized and rewarded based on volume, not value. Work is underway to understand variations in compliance with checklists and other safety measures to improve adoption of and adherence to these helpful tools. In addition, continued cultural shifts away from individual autonomy and toward collaborative systems are needed to maximize patient care and safety.

VALUE

For decades, healthcare costs in the United States and other developed countries have steadily risen. In the United States, healthcare expenditures have increased at a greater rate than the economy as a whole for 31 of the past 40 years and now approach 18% of the gross domestic product.[49,50] This percentage is expected to reach 19.6% by 2024.[49] The Institute of Medicine has identified six domains of wasted expenditures including failure of care delivery, failure of care coordination, overtreatment or low-value care, pricing failure, fraud and abuse, and administrative complexity. When considering these six domains, the estimated cost of waste in the US healthcare system ranged from $760 to $935 billion, representing approximately 25% of total healthcare spending.[50]

Health economists have suggested that competition of the wrong type is responsible for this staggering level of waste in the US healthcare system.[51] In healthy competitive markets, motivation to improve efficiency and quality generally results in productive innovation, improved service, and decreased costs. However, in the current healthcare economy, competition occurs at the wrong level and has a poor focus.[51] In this market, costs continue to rise without concomitant improvements in quality. Leading health economists have suggested that competition within the US healthcare sector is a zero-sum game, where value is divided through cost shifting between patients, payers, and providers. Cost shifting increases administrative expenses without net cost reduction or value creation. Value-based competition is lacking in the United States.

How Do We Define and Measure Value?

Value is defined as "the health outcomes achieved per dollar spent" to achieve those outcomes.[6] Most thought leaders emphasize that the health outcomes of interest to patients include both the quality of health care plus patient and family satisfaction. The value of health care is represented by the equation: *value* = (*health outcomes* + *patient satisfaction*)/*cost*.

One of the most difficult challenges in creating value-based competition is measuring value. Outcomes can be measured by a wide variety of quality metrics (patient-related outcome measures, function, and safety), and satisfaction can be measured by a wide variety of service metrics (patient satisfaction, convenience, timeliness, and communication). Although less attention has historically been paid to measuring cost, costs have received increasing scrutiny given the apparent deficiency of financial sophistication in many healthcare provider organizations. Investigations in 2013 and 2018 demonstrated that only 10% to 45% of provider organizations could provide patients and families with cost estimates for common orthopaedic surgical procedures including total hip arthroplasty in adults and percutaneous pinning of distal radius fractures in children.[52,53]

How Do We Measure Patient Outcomes?

Patient-reported outcomes are important for assessing patient satisfaction and clinical outcomes. Some patient-reported outcome measures are generic and appropriate for use in a wide variety of conditions (eg, the Pediatric Quality of Life Inventory). Other patient-reported outcome measures are disease specific and focus on symptoms or side effects of a specific set of diseases, conditions, or treatments (eg, the Scoliosis Research Society Questionnaire). Disease-specific patient-reported outcome measures tend to be more sensitive to treatment-related changes and may help to precisely measure healthcare value.[54]

The advent of computer adaptive testing appears to offer major advantages in determining patient-centered outcomes. The National Institutes of Health has funded the development of the Patient-Reported Outcomes Measurement Information System (PROMIS), a well-used set of computer-adaptive patient-reported outcome measures. The use of PROMIS has increased in the measurement of musculoskeletal health outcomes. In 2014, researchers demonstrated that computerized adaptive testing using the PROMIS physical function item bank reduced testing burden and had a lower ceiling effect compared with a nonadaptive patient-reported outcome measure.[55] Several PROMIS physical function item banks have been validated for use in children.[56,57]

How Do We Measure Costs?

Most healthcare provider organizations measure costs using a cost-to-charge ratio or a relative value unit (RVU). In a cost-to-charge methodology, cost is estimated by multiplying charges set by the hospital charge master, which is a listing of every single procedure that a hospital can provide to its patients, by the cost-to-charge ratio. This type of methodology incorrectly assumes that each type of service consumes indirect costs in the same proportion; it tends to overallocate costs to some services and underallocate costs to others. As an example, a provider organization may falsely assume that procedures with high charges also have high costs. Because charges often reflect organizational pricing and negotiation strategies, the linkage of cost and charge may distort internal cost estimates.

An RVU methodology can theoretically generate refined cost estimates. RVUs are estimates of the relative time, complexity, and value of a service; they are used to more accurately allocate costs to individual procedures and activities. In theory, RVUs can accurately reflect real costs; however, in practice, the allocation methodologies tend to be imprecise. This lack of granularity often leads to unintended cost distortions. As an example, in an RVU methodology, the high cost of a robotic surgical system could be attributed to all surgical procedures rather than the small subset of procedures in urology and gynecology that require its use. It may be possible to improve cost estimates using RVUs with rigorous methodology.

These cost-measurement approaches have obscured value in health care and have led to cost reduction efforts that are incremental, ineffective, and occasionally counterproductive. Most healthcare organizations measure and accumulate costs according to departments, physician specialties, or discrete service lines—a reflection of internal organization and the financing of care. Costs, like outcomes, should instead be measured according to the patient and distributed across the entire care cycle. This type of cost accounting methodology could enable truly structural cost reduction by eliminating non–value-added services, improving capacity utilization, shortening cycle times, providing services in more efficient settings, and so forth.

In 2004, a new accounting technique, time-driven activity-based costing (TDABC), was introduced and has since gained popularity in leading healthcare organizations.[58,59] TDABC assigns costs based on the specific resource time each service or product requires and the unit cost of supplying capacity (labor, equipment, space): *resource cost* = *cost rate* × *time*. The total cost is the sum of each resource cost: ($cost\ rate_A \times time_A$) + ($cost\ rate_B \times time_B$) and so on. In this accounting technique, costs are carefully assigned based on actual labor and equipment utilization.

Data from a 2016 study suggest that TDABC may more accurately reflect costs in orthopaedic surgery than cost-to-charge or RVU methodologies.[60] An investigation published in 2016 suggests that traditional accounting systems that use cost-to-charge or RVU methodologies may overestimate costs associated with many surgical procedures. An investigation of carpal tunnel release in 2019 further demonstrated that TDABC appears to provide the granularity required to identify cost-reduction and value-improvement strategies.[59,61]

The measurement of value is the first step in improving value delivery in health care. Organizations that are able to precisely measure value, effectively eliminate practice pattern variations, and establish efficient clinical pathways will be best positioned to survive ongoing payment reform (eg, pay-for-performance, payment bundling, and accountable care organizations). The American Academy of Orthopaedic Surgeons has advocated the use of evidence-based clinical practice guidelines, which are systematically developed statements designed to support provider decision making in specific clinical scenarios. Such guidelines are based on available scientific evidence and attempt to reduce practice pattern variations and improve patient outcomes.

Standardized clinical assessment and management plans (SCAMPs) represent a promising adjunct to clinical practice guidelines.[62] A SCAMP is a flexible guideline that is designed to reduce practice variability while still permitting physicians the opportunity to exercise clinical judgment and offer treatment that is specific to a patient's clinical situation or personal preferences. SCAMP pathways are designed as decision trees that provide guidance based on the particular clinical scenario, such that management is individualized to the specific condition and patient. The first SCAMPs were developed and implemented at Boston Children's Hospital in 2009. Many features of SCAMPs are similar to the evidence-based care process models developed at the Intermountain Healthcare System in Utah.[63] In concept, either SCAMPS or evidence-based care process models could be seamlessly shared across provider organizations, resulting in rapid dissemination of actionable information. The transferability of these decision-support tools could permit provider organizations not initially involved in the design or implementation to rapidly reduce variation and create value.

SUMMARY

To improve value in pediatric orthopaedic surgery, there must be increased focus on improving outcomes and containing expenditures. Continuous quality measurement and rapid process change are critical aspects of any value improvement model. Although great challenges exist in outcome measurement, cost measurement, and the sharing of best practices across provider organizations, medical organizations, including the Pediatric Orthopaedic Society of North America, have taken a leadership role in uniting efforts across provider organizations.

KEY STUDY POINTS

- Quality in orthopaedic surgery often refers to process measures, patient-reported outcomes, patient experience, or patient safety measures.
- Quality improvement is a data-driven process using methods such as the Model for Improvement, Lean methodology, or Six Sigma to improve care in a particular setting.
- Patient safety is at the core of quality in health care, and activities such as the use of checklists, surgical simulation, and creating a safety culture are examples of methods to prevent harm and reduce errors.
- Value, although difficult to measure, is best thought of as a patient outcome or level of satisfaction achieved per unit of money spent to achieve said outcome.

ANNOTATED REFERENCES

1. Institute of Medicine (US) Committee on Quality of Health Care in America. *Crossing the Quality Chasm: A New Health System for the 21st Century*. Washington (DC), National Academies Press (US), 2001.
2. Kohn L: To err is human: An interview with the Institute of Medicine's Linda Kohn. *Jt Comm J Qual Improv* 2000;26(4):227-234.
3. Glotzbecker MP, Wang K, Waters PM, et al: Quality, safety, and value in pediatric orthopaedic surgery. *J Pediatr Orthop* 2016;36(6):549-557.

   The authors reflect on the POSNA Quality, Safety, and Value Initiative by defining quality, safety, and value; describing how they are measured; and discussing the principles of quality improvement. Level of evidence: V.
4. McCarthy JJ, Alessandrini EA, Schoettker PJ: POSNA quality, safety, value initiative 3 years old and growing strong. POSNA precourse 2014. *J Pediatr Orthop* 2015;35(5 suppl 1):S5-S8.
5. Waters PM, Flynn JM: POSNA Quality Safety Value Initiative: From vision to implementation to early results. *J Pediatr Orthop* 2015;35(5 suppl 1):S43-S44.
6. Porter ME: What is value in health care? *N Engl J Med* 2010;363(26):2477-2481.
7. Shore BJ, Murphy RF, Hogue GD: Quality, safety, value: From theory to practice management what should we measure? *J Pediatr Orthop* 2015;35(5 suppl 1):S61-S66.
8. Lynn J, Baily MA, Bottrell M, et al: The ethics of using quality improvement methods in health care. *Ann Intern Med* 2007;146(9):666-673.
9. Womack JP, Byrne AP, Fiume OJ, Kaplan GS, Toussaint J: *Going Lean in Health Care*. Cambridge, MA, Institute for Healthcare Improvement, 2005.
10. Mason SE, Nicolay CR, Darzi A: The use of Lean and Six Sigma methodologies in surgery: A systematic review. *Surgeon* 2015;13(2):91-100.

11. Liberatore MJ: Six Sigma in healthcare delivery. *Int J Health Care Qual Assur* 2013;26(7):601-626.
12. Cima RR, Brown MJ, Hebl JR, et al: Use of lean and six sigma methodology to improve operating room efficiency in a high-volume tertiary-care academic medical center. *J Am Coll Surg* 2011;213(1):83-92, discussion 93-94.
13. Langley GJ, Moen R, Nolan KM, et al: *The Improvement Guide: A Practical Approach to Enhancing Organizational Performance.* Hoboken, NJ, John Wiley & Sons, 2009.
14. Bae DS, Lynch H, Jamieson K, et al: Improved safety and cost savings from reductions in cast-saw burns after simulation-based education for orthopaedic surgery residents. *J Bone Joint Surg Am* 2017;99(17):e94.

    The authors created a novel tool that measured temperatures at the surface of a model used for casting practice. Through establishing the temperatures associated with pain, as well as burns, the model was used to teach residents how to remove casts without injuring the patient. Level of evidence: III.
15. Brusalis CM, Shah AS, Luan X, et al: A dedicated orthopaedic trauma operating room improves efficiency at a pediatric center. *J Bone Joint Surg Am* 2017;99(1):42-47.

    The use of a dedicated orthopaedic trauma room in a pediatric trauma center decreases the frequency of after-hours procedures, reduces wait time to surgery, reduces length of hospitalization, and lowers cost. Level of evidence: III.
16. Denning JR, Little KJ: Standardization of care of common pediatric fractures. *Orthop Clin North Am* 2018;49(4): 477-490.

    Using quality improvement methodology tools such as SMART aims, process mapping, failure mode effect analysis, and key driver diagrams, the authors show how to apply these techniques to help develop evidence-based protocols and reduce variation in the treatment of pediatric supracondylar humerus fractures and distal radius buckle fractures. Level of evidence: II.
17. Healey T, Peterson TC, Healey J, El-Othmani MM, Saleh KJ: Improving operating room efficiency, Part 1: General managerial and preoperative strategies. *JBJS Rev* 2015;3(10): 01874474-201510000-00002.
18. Healey T, Peterson TC, Healey J, El-Othmani MM, Saleh KJ: Improving operating room efficiency, Part 2: Intraoperative and postoperative strategies. *JBJS Rev* 2015;3(10):0187447 4-201510000-00003.
19. Mueller AJ, Kwon JK, Steiner JW, et al: Improved magnetic resonance imaging utilization for children with musculoskeletal infection. *J Bone Joint Surg Am* 2015;97(22): 1869-1876.
20. Shore BJ, Hutchinson S, Harris M, et al: Epidemiology and prevention of cast saw injuries: Results of a quality improvement program at a single institution. *J Bone Joint Surg Am* 2014;96(4):e31.
21. Vitale MG, Riedel MD, Glotzbecker MP, et al: Building consensus: Development of a best practice guideline (BPG) for surgical site infection (SSI) prevention in high-risk pediatric spine surgery. *J Pediatr Orthop* 2013;33(5):471-478.
22. Vitale MG, Skaggs DL, Pace GI, et al: Best practices in intraoperative neuromonitoring in spine deformity surgery: Development of an intraoperative checklist to optimize response. *Spine Deform* 2014;2(5):333-339.
23. Black KP, Armstrong AD, Hutzler L, Egol KA: Quality and safety in orthopaedics: Learning and teaching at the same time. AOA critical issues. *J Bone Joint Surg Am* 2015;97(21):1809-1815.
24. Bumpass DB, Samora JB, Butler CA, Jevsevar DS, Moffatt-Bruce SD, Bozic KJ: Orthopaedic quality reporting: A comprehensive review of the current landscape and a roadmap for progress. *JBJS Rev* 2014;2(8):01874474-201408000-00001.
25. Kennedy A, Bakir C, Brauer CA: Quality indicators in pediatric orthopaedic surgery: A systematic review. *Clin Orthop Relat Res* 2012;470(4):1124-1132.
26. Porter ME, Larsson S, Lee TH: Standardizing patient outcomes measurement. *N Engl J Med* 2016;374(6):504-506.

    This article presents the International Consortium for Health Outcomes Measurement working group approach to the standardization of outcomes measures.
27. Leape LL: Patient safety in the era of healthcare reform. *Clin Orthop Relat Res* 2015;473(5):1568-1573.
28. Bae DS: Simulation in pediatric orthopaedic surgery. *J Pediatr Orthop* 2015;35(5 suppl 1):S26-S29.
29. Butler A, Olson T, Koehler R, Nicandri G: Do the skills acquired by novice surgeons using anatomic dry models transfer effectively to the task of diagnostic knee arthroscopy performed on cadaveric specimens? *J Bone Joint Surg Am* 2013;95(3):e15.
30. Gottschalk MB, Yoon ST, Park DK, Rhee JM, Mitchell PM: Surgical training using three-dimensional simulation in placement of cervical lateral mass screws: A blinded randomized control trial. *Spine J* 2015;15(1):168-175.
31. Howells NR, Gill HS, Carr AJ, Price AJ, Rees JL: Transferring simulated arthroscopic skills to the operating theatre: A randomised blinded study. *J Bone Joint Surg Br* 2008;90(4):494-499.
32. Rambani R, Ward J, Viant W: Desktop-based computer-assisted orthopedic training system for spinal surgery. *J Surg Educ* 2014;71(6):805-809.
33. Brubacher JW, Karg J, Weinstock P, Bae DS: A novel cast removal training simulation to improve patient safety. *J Surg Educ* 2016;73(1):7-11.

    A novel simulation model is presented to assess competency and enhance performance in cast application and removal, with an emphasis on monitoring temperatures during cast saw use. Level of evidence: II.
34. Moktar J, Popkin CA, Howard A, Murnaghan ML: Development of a cast application simulator and evaluation of objective measures of performance. *J Bone Joint Surg Am* 2014;96(9):e76.
35. Jackson TJ, Shah AS, Buczek MJ, Lawrence JTR: Simulation training of orthopaedic residents for distal radius fracture reductions improves radiographic outcomes. *J Pediatr Orthop* 2020;40(1):e6-e13.

Simulation training of orthopaedic surgery residents for distal radius fracture reduction reduces the risk of loss of reduction and improves radiographic outcomes. Level of evidence: III.

36. Panesar SS, Noble DJ, Mirza SB, et al: Can the surgical checklist reduce the risk of wrong site surgery in orthopaedics? – Can the checklist help? Supporting evidence from analysis of a national patient incident reporting system. *J Orthop Surg Res* 2011;6:18.

37. Patel J, Ahmed K, Guru KA, et al: An overview of the use and implementation of checklists in surgical specialities – A systematic review. *Int J Surg* 2014;12(12):1317-1323.

38. Cobb TK: Wrong site surgery – Where are we and what is the next step? *Hand (NY)* 2012;7(2):229-232.

39. Rosenberg AD, Wambold D, Kraemer L, et al: Ensuring appropriate timing of antimicrobial prophylaxis. *J Bone Joint Surg Am* 2008;90(2):226-232.

40. van Eck CF, Gravare-Silbernagel K, Samuelsson K, et al: Evidence to support the interpretation and use of the anatomic anterior cruciate ligament reconstruction checklist. *J Bone Joint Surg Am* 2013;95(20):e153.

41. Morello RT, Lowthian JA, Barker AL, McGinnes R, Dunt D, Brand C: Strategies for improving patient safety culture in hospitals: A systematic review. *BMJ Qual Saf* 2013;22(1):11-18.

42. Sutcliffe W: *Managing the Unexpected: Assuring High Performance in an Age of Complexity*. New York, NY, John Wiley & Sons, 2006.

43. Janssen SJ, Teunis T, Guitton TG, Ring D, Herndon JH: Orthopaedic surgeons' view on strategies for improving patient safety. *J Bone Joint Surg Am* 2015;97(14):1173-1186.

44. Rosenstein AH, O'Daniel M: A survey of the impact of disruptive behaviors and communication defects on patient safety. *Jt Comm J Qual Patient Saf* 2008;34(8):464-471.

45. Agency for Healthcare Research and Quality: *TeamSTEPPS: Strategies and Tools to Enhance Performance and Patient Safety*. 2015. Available at: http://www.ahrq.gov/professionals/education/curriculum-tools/teamstepps/index.html. Accessed March 1, 2020.

46. Brodsky D, Gupta M, Quinn M, et al: Building collaborative teams in neonatal intensive care. *BMJ Qual Saf* 2013;22(5):374-382.

47. Mayer CM, Cluff L, Lin WT, et al: Evaluating efforts to optimize TeamSTEPPS implementation in surgical and pediatric intensive care units. *Jt Comm J Qual Patient Saf* 2011;37(8):365-374.

48. Weaver SJ, Dy SM, Rosen MA: Team-training in healthcare: A narrative synthesis of the literature. *BMJ Qual Saf* 2014;23(5):359-372.

49. Keehan SP, Cuckler GA, Sisko AM, et al: National health expenditure projections, 2014-24: Spending growth faster than recent trends. *Health Aff (Millwood)* 2015;34(8):1407-1417.

50. Shrank WH, Rogstad TL, Parekh N: Waste in the US health care system: Estimated costs and potential for savings. *J Am Med Assoc* 2019;322(15):1501-1509.

This study is a systematic review of the literature that characterizes the waste in the US healthcare system associated with six primary domains: failure of care delivery, failure of care coordination, overtreatment or low-value care, pricing failure, fraud and abuse, and administrative complexity. The annual estimate of waste is approximately $760 to $935 billion.

51. Porter ME, Teisberg EO: Redefining competition in health care. *Harv Bus Rev* 2004;82(6):64-76.

52. Rosenthal JA, Lu X, Cram P: Availability of consumer prices from US hospitals for a common surgical procedure. *JAMA Intern Med* 2013;173(6):427-432.

53. Racimo AR, Talathi NS, Zelenski NA, Wells L, Shah AS: How much will my child's operation cost? Availability of consumer prices from US hospitals for a common pediatric orthopaedic surgical procedure. *J Pediatr Orthop* 2018;38(7):e411-e416.

This study is a prospective investigation that used scripted telephone calls to demonstrate that price estimates for pediatric orthopaedic procedures are difficult to obtain. Level of evidence: II.

54. Wiebe S, Guyatt G, Weaver B, Matijevic S, Sidwell C: Comparative responsiveness of generic and specific quality-of-life instruments. *J Clin Epidemiol* 2003;56(1):52-60.

55. Hung M, Stuart AR, Higgins TF, Saltzman CL, Kubiak EN: Computerized adaptive testing using the PROMIS physical function item bank reduces test burden with less ceiling effects compared with the short musculoskeletal function assessment in orthopaedic trauma patients. *J Orthop Trauma* 2014;28(8):439-443.

56. Waljee JF, Carlozzi N, Franzblau LE, Zhong L, Chung KC: Applying the patient-reported outcomes measurement information system to assess upper extremity function among children with congenital hand differences. *Plast Reconstr Surg* 2015;136(2):200e-207e.

57. Wall LB, Vuillermin C, Miller PE, Bae DS, Goldfarb CA, CoULD Study Group: Convergent validity of PODCI and PROMIS domains in congenital upper limb anomalies. *J Hand Surg Am* 2019;45(1):33-40.

This study is a prospective evaluation of the perceived functional and psychosocial impact of upper limb congenital anomalies using the Pediatric Outcomes Data Collection Instrument (PODCI) and multiple PROMIS domains. Level of evidence: II.

58. Kaplan RS, Anderson SR: Time-driven activity-based costing. *Harv Bus Rev* 2004;82(11):131-138.

59. Kaplan RS, Witkowski M, Abbott M, et al: Using time-driven activity-based costing to identify value improvement opportunities in healthcare. *J Healthc Manag* 2014;59(6):399-412.

60. Akhavan S, Ward L, Bozic KJ: Time-driven activity-based costing more accurately reflects costs in arthroplasty surgery. *Clin Orthop Relat Res* 2016;474(1):8-15.

This article compares the accuracy of TDABC with that of traditional accounting techniques in total joint arthroplasty at a single institution. Level of evidence: III.

61. Koehler DM, Balakrishnan R, Lawler EA, Shah AS: Endoscopic versus open carpal tunnel release: A detailed analysis using time-driven activity-based costing at an academic medical center. *J Hand Surg Am* 2019;44(1):62 e1-62 e9.

This study is a matched cohort investigation of patients undergoing open versus endoscopic carpal tunnel release that defines the principle drivers of cost using time-driven activity-based costing. Level of evidence: II.

62. Shah AS, Waters PM, Bozic KJ: Orthopaedic healthcare worldwide: Standardized clinical assessment and management plans. An adjunct to clinical practice guidelines. *Clin Orthop Relat Res* 2015;473(6):1868-1872.

63. Byington CL, Reynolds CC, Korgenski K, et al: Costs and infant outcomes after implementation of a care process model for febrile infants. *Pediatrics* 2012;130(1):e16-e24.

CHAPTER 2

Evidence-Based Quality and Outcomes Assessment in Pediatric Orthopaedics

ANTONIA F. CHEN, MD, MBA • KARL C. ROBERTS, MD, FAOA
KEVIN G. SHEA, MD • CHARLES T. MEHLMAN, DO, MPH
ROBERT H. QUINN, MD • JAMES T. BECKMANN, MD, MS, FAOA

ABSTRACT

Evidence-based clinical practice guidelines, appropriate use criteria, outcome measures, and patient-reported outcome measures are critical tools to ensure the best clinical care for patients. These guidelines, criteria, and measures will be increasingly integrated into care pathways.

Keywords: appropriate use criteria (AUC); computerized adaptive testing; evidence-based clinical practice guidelines; outcome measures; Patient-Reported Outcomes Measurement Information System (PROMIS)

INTRODUCTION

Critical analysis of clinical care can lead to answers to a wide variety of clinical questions.[1-3] Pierre Charles Alexandre Louis, a French physician, applied the numerical method (early biostatistics) and helped end the practice of bloodletting.[4] The teachings and end result idea advocated by American surgeon Ernest Amory Codman influenced generations of outcomes researchers and inspired the American College of Surgeons and the Joint Commission for the Accreditation of Healthcare Organizations.[5] Randomized clinical trials and prospective study designs may produce the highest quality/lowest bias evidence; these types of studies, along with other forms of evidence, guide clinical care decisions.

Dr. Chen or an immediate family member serves as a paid consultant to or is an employee of 3M, ACI, American Medical Foundation, Avanos, bOne, Convatec, DePuy, a Johnson & Johnson Company, Heraeus, Irrimax, Recro, and Stryker; has stock or stock options held in Graftworx, Hyalex, Irrimax, Joint Purification Systems, and Sonoran; has received research or institutional support from Avanos; and serves as a board member, owner, officer, or committee member of the American Academy of Orthopaedic Surgeons, AJRR, the American Association of Hip and Knee Surgeons, the European Knee Association, the International Congress for Joint Reconstruction, and the Musculoskeletal Infection Society. Dr. Roberts or an immediate family member serves as a board member, owner, officer, or committee member of the American Academy of Orthopaedic Surgeons and MARCQI. Dr. Shea or an immediate family member serves as an unpaid consultant to Clinical Data Solutions and SourceTrust; has received research or institutional support from Vericel; and serves as a board member, owner, officer, or committee member of the American Academy of Orthopaedic Surgeons, the Pediatric Orthopaedic Society of North America, PRISM – the Pediatric Research in Sport Medicine, and ROCK – the Research for Osteochondritis Dissecans of the Knee. Dr. Mehlman or an immediate family member has received royalties from Oakstone Med Pub; serves as an unpaid consultant to Ortho Pediatrics; has stock or stock options held in Dyna Med Mobility; and serves as a board member, owner, officer, or committee member of the Denver Children's Hospital Visiting Professorship, the Michigan State University Visiting Professorship, the U.S. News and World Report Pediatric Orthopaedic Working Group, and the Vanderbilt University Visiting Professorship. Dr. Quinn or an immediate family member serves as a board member, owner, officer, or committee member of the American Academy of Orthopaedic Surgeons and the Wilderness Medical Society. Neither Dr. Beckmann nor any immediate family member has received anything of value from or has stock or stock options held in a commercial company or institution related directly or indirectly to the subject of this chapter.

It is important for orthopaedic surgeons to review the use of evidence for clinical care, with an emphasis on evidence-based clinical practice guidelines (CPGs), appropriate use criteria (AUC), and outcome measures, including those from the Patient-Reported Outcomes Measurement Information System (PROMIS) and computerized adaptive testing.

CLINICAL PRACTICE GUIDELINES AND SYSTEMATIC REVIEWS

The Institute of Medicine has called for the increased use of CPGs to reduce practice variation, improve quality of care, and decrease inefficiencies.[6-8] A CPG is a "systematically developed statement to assist practitioner and patient decisions about appropriate health care for one or more specific clinical circumstances."[7,8]

Historically, guidelines have been based on the consensus of expert groups, but consensus guidelines have several potential limitations: (1) Many guidelines do not consider all evidence. (2) Evidence integration and quality ranking may be flawed. (3) There may be a lack of transparency about conflicts of interest. (4) Results may not be reproducible by other groups. To address these limitations, the American Academy of Orthopaedic Surgeons (AAOS) guidelines are based on a systematic review of the literature and follow a rigorous, transparent, and reproducible methodology that meets all of the Institute of Medicine standards for developing trustworthy guidelines[9] (**Table 1**).

Clinical content experts develop systematically outlined research questions that define the patient, intervention, comparison, and outcome (PICO). Experts in the field of evidence analysis review the literature comprehensively, rank the quality of the study design and the risk of bias of the articles, and ensure that the evidence review is transparent, reproducible, reviewed by others, and updated.

TABLE 1

Institute of Medicine Standards for Evidence-Based Clinical Practice Guidelines

Transparency
Management of conflicts of interest
Composition of the guideline group
Standards for systematic reviews
Establishing evidence foundations for and rating strength of recommendations
Standard form for the articulation of the recommendations
External review
Updating

Overview: AAOS Guidelines and Systematic Review Process

For topics in which the published evidence contains a broad range of high-level/low-bias evidence, the CPG is an appropriate analysis. In cases in which the published evidence is not as robust to support a full CPG, a systematic review may be the best analysis. The AAOS addresses bias beginning with the selection of CPG and systematic review work group members, who function as the clinical content experts. Applicants with financial conflicts of interest related to the CPG or systematic review topic cannot participate if the conflict occurred within 1 year of the start date of the CPG or systematic review development, or if an immediate family member has a relevant financial conflict. In addition, all CPG or systematic review development group members sign an attestation form agreeing to remain free of relevant financial conflicts for 1 year following the publication of the CPG or the systematic review.

Physician and clinician groups (clinical experts) prepare CPGs and systematic reviews with the assistance of the AAOS Department of Clinical Quality and Value (expert evidence methodologists). These evidence methodologists include data analysts, health economics and outcomes research experts, and statisticians. As the physician experts, the CPG or systematic review work group defines the scope of the CPG or systematic review by creating PICO questions that direct the literature search. The medical librarian creates and executes the search or searches. The supporting group of expert methodologists reviews all abstracts, reviews pertinent full-text articles, and evaluates the quality of studies meeting the inclusion criteria. They also abstract, analyze, interpret, and summarize the relevant data for each PICO question and prepare the initial draft for the final work group meeting.

After completion of the systematic reviews, physician CPG work groups meet in person to participate in a 1-day meeting to develop the recommendations. To complete their charges, the physician experts and methodologists evaluate and integrate all material to develop the final recommendations. The final recommendations and rationales are edited, written, and voted on by the clinician work group. The CPG or systematic research work group may approve additional edits to the rationales via subsequent webinar meetings. The draft CPG or systematic review recommendations and rationales receive final review by the methodologists to ensure consistency with the data. The draft is then completed and subsequently undergoes a period of peer review.

After peer review and editing, the CPG or systematic review draft is distributed for public commentary. Thereafter, the AAOS Committee on Evidence-Based Quality and Value, AAOS Council on Research and Quality, and the AAOS Board of Directors sequentially approve the draft CPG or systematic review. All AAOS CPGs are reviewed and updated or retired approximately every 5 years. The process of AAOS CPG or systematic review development incorporates the benefits from clinical physician expertise and the statistical knowledge and interpretation of methodologists without conflict. The process also includes an extensive review process offering the opportunity for more than 200 clinical physician experts to provide input before publication. This process minimizes bias, enhances transparency, and ensures the highest level of accuracy for interpretation of the evidence.

The language used in the recommendations is based on the quality of the evidence, and a star system is used for ranking the strength of the recommendation based on the Grading of Recommendations Assessment, Development, and Evaluation (GRADE, more stars = greater strength; **Table 2**).

The AAOS has developed 20 evidence-based CPGs since 2007; 7 have clinical applicability to pediatric and adolescent care, and 3 are focused specifically on pediatric orthopaedics (**Table 3**). These guidelines can be accessed through the OrthoGuidelines website; a free mobile application is available (http://www.orthoguidelines.org/).

APPROPRIATE USE CRITERIA

The randomized clinical trial serves as the benchmark for clinical research, but these trials are complicated, expensive, and time-intensive and labor-intensive. Because they are performed under ideal circumstances, the results are not always generalizable. In many technical fields, including orthopaedic surgery, randomized clinical trials are complex (thereby limiting their construction and recruitment); may not have broad external applicability; or simply are not available. CPGs rely on higher-level evidence, but in many fields, higher-level evidence may be lacking. In areas in which the evidence base is less robust, AUC may be especially valuable. In 1986, a method was introduced for the detailed assessment of the appropriateness of medical

TABLE 2

American Academy of Orthopaedic Surgeons (AAOS) Clinical Practice Guideline Strength of Recommendation Descriptions

Strength of Recommendation	Overall Strength Of Evidence	Description of Evidence Quality	Strength Visual
Strong	**Strong or moderate**	Evidence from two or more high-quality studies with consistent findings for recommending for or against the intervention. Or Rec is upgraded from moderate using the EtD framework	★★★★
Moderate	**Strong. Moderate or limited**	Evidence from two or more moderate-quality studies with consistent findings, or evidence from a single high-quality study for recommending for or against the intervention. Or Rec is upgraded or downgraded from limited or strong using the EtD framework.	★★★☆
Limited	**Limited or moderate**	Evidence from one or more low-quality studies with consistent findings or evidence from a single moderate-quality study recommending for or against the intervention. Or Rec is downgraded from moderate using the EtD framework.	★★☆☆
Consensus	**No reliable evidence**	There is no supporting evidence, or higher quality evidence was downgraded due to major concerns addressed in the EtD framework. In the absence of reliable evidence, the guideline work group is making a recommendation based on their clinical opinion.	★☆☆☆

Reproduced from the American Academy of Orthopaedic Surgeons: *Appropriate Use Criteria Methodology.* Rosemont, IL, American Academy of Orthopaedic Surgeons, 2019. Available at: https://www.aaos.org/globalassets/quality-and-practice-resources/methodology/cpg-methodology.pdf. Accessed June 30, 2020.

TABLE 3

Published American Academy of Orthopaedic Surgeons (AAOS) Clinical Practice Guidelines

Acute Compartment Syndrome (2018) AUC
Anesthesia and Analgesia in TJA (2020) CPG Endorsement
Anterior Cruciate Ligament Injuries (2014) AUC
Carpal Tunnel Syndrome (2016) AUC
Distal Radius Fractures (2009) AUC
Glenohumeral Joint Osteoarthritis (2020)
Hip Fractures in the Elderly (2014) AUC
Limb Salvage or Early Amputation (2019) AUC
Osteoarthritis of the Hip (2017) AUC
Osteoarthritis of the Knee (Arthroplasty) (2015) AUC
Osteoarthritis of the Knee (Non-Arthroplasty) (2013) AUC
Osteochondritis Dissecans (2010) AUC
Pediatric Developmental Dysplasia of the Hip in Infants up to Six Months (2014) AUC
Pediatric Diaphyseal Femur Fractures (2015)
Pediatric Supracondylar Humerus Fractures (2011) AUC
Periprosthetic Joint Infections (2019)
Prevention of Orthopaedic Implant Infection in Patients Undergoing Dental Procedures (2012) AUC
Psychosocial Factors Influencing Trauma Recovery (2019)
Rotator Cuff Injuries (2019) AUC
Surgical Site Infections (2018) AUC
Tranexamic Acid in Total Joint Arthroplasty (2018) CPG Endorsement
Use of Imaging Prior to Referral to a Musculoskeletal Oncologist (2018) CPG Endorsement
Venous Thromboembolic Disease in Patients Undergoing Elective Hip and Knee Arthroplasty (2011)

Reproduced from the American Academy of Orthopaedic Surgeons: *OrthoGuidelines*. Rosemont, IL, American Academy of Orthopaedic Surgeons, 2020. Availabel at: http://www.orthoguidelines.org/guidelines. Accessed June 30, 2020.

technologies based on the concept that synthesizing expert medical opinion could simultaneously incorporate the knowledge gained from randomized clinical trials with that of clinical experience.[10] Expert panels were asked to rate the appropriateness of different interventions where "appropriate was defined to mean that the expected health benefit (ie, increased life expectancy, relief of pain, reduction in anxiety, improved functional capacity)...exceeded the expected negative consequences (ie, mortality, morbidity, anxiety of anticipating the procedure, pain produced by the procedure, time lost from work) by a sufficiently wide margin that the procedure was worth doing [exclusive of cost]." This early concept developed into the RAND/UCLA Appropriateness Method, which was developed by the RAND Corporation and clinicians at the University of California at Los Angeles (UCLA) as an instrument primarily designed to measure the overuse and underuse of medical and surgical procedures.[11,12]

Whereas a CPG indicates, based on best evidence, whether a given intervention is associated with a desirable outcome, the AUC indicates when (ie, in what specific clinical situation) the same intervention is best applied. The purpose of the AUC is to help determine the appropriateness of CPG recommendations for the heterogeneous patient populations routinely seen in practice. The best available scientific evidence is synthesized with collective expert opinion on topics where benchmark, randomized clinical trials are not available or are inadequately detailed for identifying distinct patient types. When there is evidence corroborated by consensus that expected benefits substantially outweigh potential risks, exclusive of cost, a procedure is determined to be appropriate. The AAOS uses the RAND/UCLA Appropriateness Method. The process includes the following steps: reviewing the results of the evidence analysis, compiling a list of clinical vignettes, and having an expert panel composed of representatives from multiple medical specialties determine the appropriateness of each of the clinical indications for treatment; classification is stratified as appropriate, may be appropriate, or is rarely appropriate.

In 2014, two AAOS AUC documents directly relevant to pediatric orthopaedic surgery were published: one addressing the management of pediatric supracondylar humerus fractures[13] and one on pediatric supracondylar fractures with vascular injury.[14] These follow the CPG on the treatment of pediatric supracondylar humerus fractures published by the AAOS in 2011.[15] There are also other AUCs that are applicable to the pediatric orthopaedic patient population, including anterior cruciate ligament injury prevention and treatment (two AUCs), osteochondritis dissecans, developmental dysplasia of the hip in infants up to 6 months of age for generalists and orthopaedic specialists (two AUCs), prevention of orthopaedic implant infection in patients undergoing dental procedures, and surgical site infections.

In developing an AAOS AUC document (and in keeping with the RAND/UCLA Appropriateness Method), a writing panel made up of orthopaedic specialists who have expertise in treating the specific condition is assembled. The panel follows the following guiding principles: Patient scenarios must include a broad spectrum of patients who may be eligible for treatment of pediatric supracondylar humerus fractures (comprehensive). Patient indications must classify patients into a unique

TABLE 4

Interpreting the Nine-Point Appropriateness Scale

Rating	Explanation
7-9	**Appropriate:** Appropriate for the indication provided, meaning treatment **is** generally acceptable and **is** a reasonable approach for the indication and **is** likely to improve the patient's health outcomes or survival.
4-6	**May Be Appropriate:** Uncertain for the indication provided, meaning treatment **may** be acceptable and **may** be a reasonable approach for the indication, but with uncertainty implying that more research and/or patient information is needed to further classify the indication.
1-3	**Rarely Appropriate:** Rarely an appropriate option for management of patients in this population due to the lack of a clear benefit/risk advantage; rarely an effective option for individual care plans; exceptions should have documentation of the clinical reasons for proceeding with this care option (i.e. procedure is not generally acceptable and is not generally reasonable for the indication).

Reproduced from the American Academy of Orthopaedic Surgeons: *Appropriate Use Criteria Methodology.* Rosemont, IL, American Academy of Orthopaedic Surgeons, 2019. Available at: https://www.aaos.org/globalassets/quality-and-practice-resources/methodology/auc-methodology_v1.1.pdf. Accessed June 30, 2020.

scenario (mutually exclusive). Patient indications must consistently classify similar patients into the same scenario (reliable, valid indicators).

The writing panel develops the scenarios by categorizing patients in terms of indications evident during the clinical decision-making process. These scenarios rely on definitions and general assumptions, mutually agreed on by the writing panel during the development of the scenarios. These definitions and assumptions are necessary to provide consistency in the interpretation of the clinical scenarios among experts voting on the scenarios and readers using the final criteria. The writing panel then organizes these indications into a matrix of clinical scenarios that address all combinations of the classifications.

When the work of the writing panel is completed, a separate independent voting panel is formed, composed of approximately 50% specialists and 50% nonspecialists (a specialist is defined as an orthopaedic surgeon who treats the condition addressed in the AUC that is under study). The panel uses a modified Delphi process to determine appropriateness ratings. The objective of this process is not to force consensus, but rather to determine whether discrepancies in the ratings are the result of actual clinical disagreement over the use of a procedure. The appropriateness of each scenario is rated as shown in **Table 4**. Following the final (second) round of voting, the final levels of appropriateness are determined as shown in **Tables 5** and **6**. Web-based AUC applications are available at the AAOS website. An example of the AUC application for pediatric supracondylar humerus fractures[16] is shown in **Figure 1**. The RAND/UCLA Appropriateness Method has now been used and studied in many procedural disciplines beyond orthopaedic surgery and found to be reliable.

TABLE 5

Defining Agreement and Disagreement for Appropriateness Ratings

Panel Size	Disagreement # of ratings between 1-3 or 7-9	Agreement # of ratings outside of appropriateness rating range
8, 9, 10	≥3	≤2
11, 12, 13	≥4	≤3
14, 15, 16	≥5	≤4

Reproduced from the American Academy of Orthopaedic Surgeons: *Appropriate Use Criteria Methodology.* Rosemont, IL, American Academy of Orthopaedic Surgeons, 2019. Available at: https://www.aaos.org/globalassets/quality-and-practice-resources/methodology/auc-methodology_v1.1.pdf. Accessed June 30, 2020.

TABLE 6

Interpreting Final Ratings of Criteria

Level of Appropriateness	Description
Appropriate	Median panel rating between 7 and 9 and no disagreement
May be appropriate	Median panel rating between 4 and 6 and no disagreement or median panel rating between 1 and 9 with disagreement
Rarely appropriate	Median panel rating between 1 and 3 and no disagreement

Adapted with permission of The Rand Corporation, from Fitch K, Bernstein SJ, Aguilar MD: *The Rand/UCLA Appropriateness Method User's Manual.* 2001.

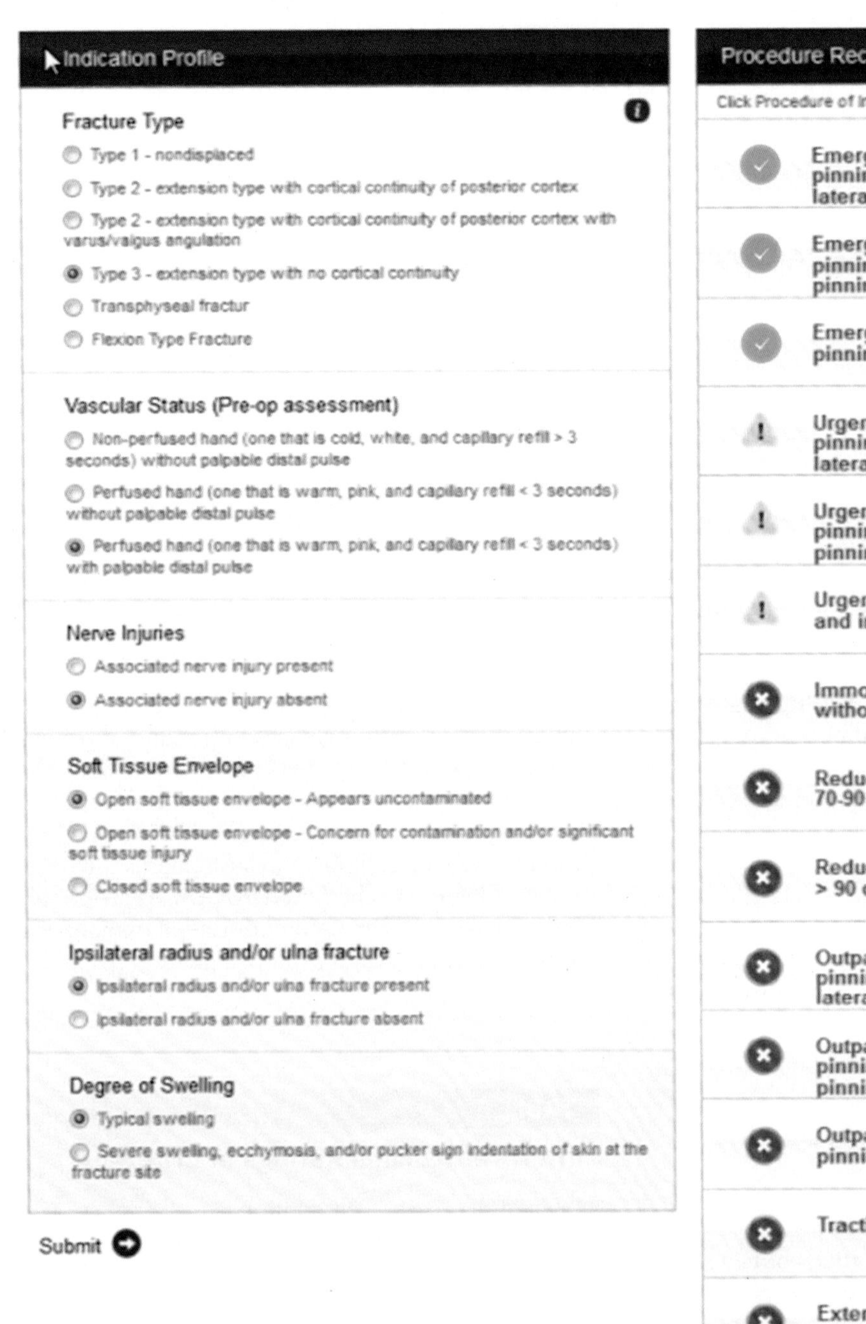

FIGURE 1 The given screenshot shows an example of the American Academy of Orthopaedic Surgeons (AAOS) Appropriate Use Criteria for pediatric supracondylar humerus fractures. (Reproduced from the American Academy of Orthopaedic Surgeons: *Appropriate Use Criteria on Pediatric Supracondylar Humerus Fractures: Treatment*. Rosemont, IL, American Academy of Orthopaedic Surgeons, 2014.)

OUTCOMES ASSESSMENT

Outcomes assessment is important.[17] Ernest Codman is often referred to as the father of outcomes research because of his common-sense notion that every hospital should follow every patient it treats long enough to determine whether the treatment has been successful. If treatment is unsuccessful, Codman advocated that the reason for the failure should be determined to preventing similar failures in the future.[18] Modern outcomes assessment in pediatric orthopaedics is dependent on the interrelated concepts of validity (measuring what is intended to be measured), reliability (measuring it in a reproducible fashion), responsiveness to change (detecting true improvement or worsening), and minimum clinically important difference (MCID; measuring differences that are important to patients and parents).[19] Collectively, these traits of outcome instruments are referred to as psychometrics or psychometric properties. These same principles apply to both traditional clinician-measured parameters (eg, radiographic angles, joint range of motion) and patient-generated measures (both general and disease-specific, health-related quality-of-life instruments).

Validity has several dimensions that must be considered.[20] The simplest is face validity, which amounts to passing the so-called sniff test or duck test. For example, using the Scoliosis Research Society Outcomes Questionnaire as the main outcome measure for a study of pediatric phalangeal neck fractures has no face validity.

Content validity relates to the fact that questions or measurements pertinent to the thing being assessed are appropriately included. The content validity of the Early Onset Scoliosis Questionnaire was established via a process that created questions based on recorded interviews focusing on factors that are important to parents.[21]

Construct validity refers to how consistent the new test or questionnaire seems to be when compared with existing tools that measure similar things. When the Muscular Dystrophy Spine Questionnaire was being developed, its construct validity was established by comparing it with two other established instruments (the Activity Scale for Kids and the Pediatric Outcomes Data Collection Questionnaire).[22]

Criterion validity relates specifically to how well the new measure correlates with an established benchmark (if one exists). In a 2013 study of a new shoulder instability scale, the authors tested its criterion validity by comparing it with the Rowe anterior shoulder instability scale.[23]

The types of reliability commonly assessed are interrater reliability (two or more raters) and intrarater reliability (the same rater on different occasions).[24] Moreover, these types of reliability may involve either continuous or categoric variables. The key aspect of statistical methods aimed at assessing reliability is that they control for chance agreement. The intraclass correlation coefficient is most commonly used for continuous variables, whereas the kappa coefficient (also known as the Cohen kappa) is usually used for categoric variables.[25] Interpretation of reliability data is similarly dictated by the type of data being analyzed (**Tables 7** and **8**).

The concept of responsiveness to change relates to whether the measuring instrument is appropriately able to detect improvement or worsening after a treatment intervention. Ceiling and floor effects play an important role in the responsiveness of a questionnaire. An example of the ceiling effect is when all students taking an examination get an "A" because the test was too easy. An example of the floor effect is when another group of students all get an "F" because the test was too hard. It may seem obvious to clinicians, but it also has been shown that retrospective methods of evaluating responsiveness to change are of little value because they consistently provide overestimates.[26] Responsiveness to change is directly related to effect size.[27]

Effect size refers to the inherent difference in statistically significant and clinically significant outcomes.[28,29] Estimates of the proportion of patients benefiting from a treatment based on effect size and so-called anchor-based approaches

TABLE 7

Fleiss Criteria (Typically Used for Continuous Variables)

ICC ≥ 0.75 = excellent

ICC ≥ 0.40 and <0.75 = fair to good

ICC <0.40 = poor

ICC = intraclass correlation coefficient

Data from Fleiss J, Levin B, Paik MC: *Statistical Methods for Rates and Proportions*, ed 2. New York, NY, John Wiley & Sons, 1981, pp 1-800.

TABLE 8

Criteria of Landis and Koch (Typically Used for Categoric Variables)

<0 = less than chance agreement

0.01-0.20 = slight agreement

0.21-0.40 = fair agreement

0.41-0.60 = moderate agreement

0.61-0.80 = substantial agreement

0.81-0.99 = almost perfect agreement

Adapted by permission of International Biometric Society from Landis JR, Koch GC: The measurement of observer agreement for categorical data. *Biometrics* 1977;33(1):159-174.

such as the MCID have been shown to perform equivalently.[30] The MCID (also known as a minimum important difference) is attractive because it reflects the importance of the patient.[31,32] When the MCID following scoliosis surgery (as measured by the Scoliosis Research Society Outcomes Questionnaire) was assessed, there was a large change in the appearance domain, but minimal change (within measurement error) was noted in the activity domain.[33] It is important to keep in mind that some trials may demonstrate a statistically significant difference in treatment outcome, but the difference may not be meaningful or perceptible to patients. Designing studies to assess MCID ensures outcomes are meaningful to patients.

A growing number of orthopaedic researchers are improving instrument development using Rasch analysis. These analytic methods have been applied in a wide variety of fields other than health care, including education, psychology, marketing, and economics.[34] Rasch analysis is a form of item response theory that mathematically models question difficulty and examiner aptitude. Recently, the Pediatric Outcomes Data Collection Instrument was subjected to Rasch analysis for cerebral palsy patients with Gross Motor Function Classification System levels 1 through 3. This process identified several redundant items as well as ceiling effect in all domains except the sports/physical function domain.[34]

PATIENT OUTCOMES: PROMIS, COMPUTERIZED ADAPTIVE TESTING

The National Institutes of Health has funded the development of PROMIS to address deficiencies associated with legacy instruments. The PROMIS marks a new paradigm for measuring patient-reported outcomes that is made possible through computerized adaptive testing. Instead of administering a fixed set of questions that are indivisibly validated (classic test theory),[35] computerized adaptive testing uses computer algorithms to dynamically administer only the most informative questions based on that individual's previous responses from a large question bank until a prespecified level of precision is met. This method paradoxically allows for maximal measurement precision through the fewest possible number of administered questions (typically only three to five per domain).[36,37] Pediatric-specific question banks are available for various domains, including global health, mental health, physical health, and social health[38] (**Table 9**).

TABLE 9

PROMIS Measures for Pediatric Patients (Ages 8 to 17 Years) and Parent Proxy Report (Ages 5 to 7 Years)

Domain	Subdomains
Global health	
Mental health	Cognitive function
	Emotional distress: anger
	Emotional distress: anxiety
	Emotional distress: depressive symptoms
	Life satisfaction
	Meaning and purpose
	Positive affect
	Psychologic stress experiences
Physical health	Fatigue
	Pain: behavior
	Pain: interference
	Pain quality (affective, sensory)
	Physical activity
	Physical activity: mobility
	Physical activity: upper extremity
	Physical stress experience
	Sleep-related disturbance
	Sleep-related impairment
	Strength impact
Social health	Peer relationships
	Family relationships

Reported benefits of computerized adaptive testing include reduced completion time that lowers the responder burden of the patient;[39,40] increases measurement precision with reduction of ceiling and floor effects;[41-43] and has the ability to add or subtract questions from the item bank without the need to re-create and validate an entirely new scale. The psychometric properties of computerized adaptive testing have outperformed legacy scales in adult orthopaedic patients.[39,41,42,44,45] Studies consistently show high correlation between the PROMIS and traditional instruments, but the PROMIS has increased reliability, decreased test length, and less unexplained variance in baseline studies. However, the responsiveness, or the ability of the PROMIS to detect change after treatment, has not been thoroughly evaluated in all orthopaedic patients, but has demonstrated limited improvement in cerebral palsy patients.[45]

The PROMIS has similarly been applied to pediatric orthopaedic patients to address the current limitations of existing instruments. The PROMIS can be used to assess multiple domains in pediatric patients, of which the most pertinent domains for pediatric orthopaedic patients include physical function, pain interference, anxiety, depression, and global health. The physical function domain may be scored singularly or broken into mobility (23-item question bank) and upper extremity (29-item question bank) domains that share approximately 35% common variance.[46] The PROMIS has shown good reliability in pediatric patients from 8 to 17 years of age, whether completed by the child or for the child by a parent.[47,48] When the parent completes the survey for the child, this is called parent-proxy. In addition, fewer children require parental assistance to complete the survey compared with legacy scales.[49,50] Finally, PROMIS for pediatric patients is available in multiple languages, depending on the domain being evaluated. For example, pain intensity is available in the following languages: Afrikaans, Arabic, Bosnian, Bulgarian, Chinese-Simplified, Chinese-Traditional, Croatian, Czech, Danish, Dutch, Finnish, French, Georgian, German, Greek, Gujarati, Hebrew, Hungarian, Italian, Kannada, Kazakh, Korean, Latvian, Lithuanian, Malay, Malayalam, Marathi, Norwegian, Orya, Polish, Portuguese, Punjabi, Romanian, Russian, Serbian, Slovak, Spanish, Swedish, Tamil, Telugu, Thai, Turkish, Ukrainian, Urdu, and Welsh.

The psychometric properties of computerized adaptive testing in pediatric orthopaedic patients have not been extensively researched, but have been compared with legacy scales in certain patient populations. PROMIS pediatric measures of general health have been shown to have excellent convergent and discriminant validity with the KIDSCREEN-10 and the Pediatric Quality of Life 15.[51] In pediatric patients with congenital hand deformities, the PROMIS was found to correlate with the Disabilities of the Arm, Shoulder and Hand score and the Pediatric Outcomes Data Collection Instrument, but was only mildly correlated with the Michigan Hand Questionnaire.[49] In children with cerebral palsy, the PROMIS physical function mobility portion showed good correlation with patient and parent assessments of mobility, but was less responsive to treatment than legacy scales (the Pediatric Outcomes Data Collection Instrument, the Functional Assessment Questionnaire, the Shriners Hospitals for Children with Cerebral Palsy Computer-Adapted Testing Battery) and did not distinguish between Gross Motor Function Measures as well as other instruments.[45,52] The investigators concluded that item-bank expansion may be needed before mobility computerized adaptive testing is applied to patients with cerebral palsy.

Pediatric orthopaedic surgeons should be aware of the PROMIS because it is likely that it will be used as a patient-reported outcome measure in the future. The number of scientific articles assessing or using PROMIS has increased exponentially in the past 10 years from 16 in 2005 to more than 150 in 2015. The measurement properties of the PROMIS appear favorable in adult orthopaedic patients across multiple specialties, but it is not known if they will translate into similar results in pediatric orthopaedic patients.

SUMMARY

Better outcomes for patients are based on evidence-based CPGs, AUC, outcome measures, and the PROMIS.

KEY STUDY POINTS

- Evidence-based CPGs inform patients and clinicians if a given intervention is associated with a desirable outcome.
- AUC documents indicate when (ie, in what specific clinical circumstance) the same intervention is best applied.
- Outcome measure assessments are dependent on the interrelated concepts of validity, reliability, responsiveness to change, and MCID.
- In addition to clinical measures that matter to clinicians, patient-reported outcome measures include variables that are important to patients. An increased emphasis on patient-reported outcome measures and computerized adaptive testing allows clinicians to better understand the effects of interventions on patients.

ANNOTATED REFERENCES

1. Farrokhyar F, Karanicolas PJ, Thoma A, et al: Randomized controlled trials of surgical interventions. *Ann Surg* 2010;251(3):409-416.
2. Ioannidis JP: Why most published research findings are false. *PLoS Med* 2005;2(8):e124.
3. Ioannidis JP: How to make more published research true. *PLoS Med* 2014;11(10):e1001747.
4. Morabia A: P.C.A. Louis and the birth of clinical epidemiology. *J Clin Epidemiol* 1996;49(12):1327-1333.
5. Mallon WJ: E. Amory Codman, surgeon of the 1990s. *J Shoulder Elbow Surg* 1998;7(5):529-536.
6. Institute of Medicine: *Crossing the Quality Chasm: A New Health System for the 21st Century.* Washington, DC, The National Academies Press, 2001, p 360.
7. National Institutes of Health: *Health Technology Assessment (HTA) 101: Glossary.* Available at: http://www.nlm.nih.gov/nichsr/hta101/ta101014.html. Accessed August 27, 2011.
8. Institute of Medicine: *Clinical Practice Guidelines: Directions for a New Program.* Washington, DC, The National Academies Press, 1990, p 168.
9. Institute of Medicine: *Clinical Practice Guidelines We Can Trust.* Washington, DC, The National Academies Press, 2011. Available at: http://www.nationalacademies.org/hmd/Reports/2011/Clinical-Practice-Guidelines-We-Can-Trust.aspx. Accessed April 5, 2016.
10. Brook RH, Chassin MR, Fink A, Solomon DH, Kosecoff J, Park RE: A method for the detailed assessment of the appropriateness of medical technologies. *Int J Technol Assess Health Care* 1986;2(1):53-63.
11. Fitch K, Bernstein SJ, Aguilar MD, et al: *The RAND/UCLA Appropriateness Method User's Manual.* Santa Monica, CA, RAND Corporation, 2001.

12. Lawson EH, Gibbons MM, Ko CY, Shekelle PG: The appropriateness method has acceptable reliability and validity for assessing overuse and underuse of surgical procedures. *J Clin Epidemiol* 2012;65(11):1133-1143.

13. American Academy of Orthopaedic Surgeons: *Appropriate Use Criteria for the Management of Pediatric Supracondylar Humerus Fractures.* Rosemont, IL, American Academy of Orthopaedic Surgeons, 2014. Available at: https://www.aaos.org/quality/quality-programs/pediatric-orthopaedic-programs/. Accessed November 20, 2020.

14. American Academy of Orthopaedic Surgeons: *Appropriate Use Criteria for the Management of Pediatric Supracondylar Humerus Fractures With Vascular Injury.* Rosemont, IL, American Academy of Orthopaedic Surgeons, 2015. Available at: https://www.aaos.org/quality/quality-programs/pediatric-orthopaedic-programs/. Accessed November 20, 2020.

15. American Academy of Orthopaedic Surgeons: *Clinical Practice Guideline on the Treatment of Supracondylar Humerus Fractures.* Rosemont, IL, American Academy of Orthopaedic Surgeons, 2011. Available at: https://www.aaos.org/quality/quality-programs/. Accessed November 20, 2020.

16. American Academy of Orthopaedic Surgeons: *Appropriate Use Criteria for the Management of Pediatric Supracondylar Humerus Fractures.* Rosemont, IL, American Academy of Orthopaedic Surgeons, 2014. Available at: https://www.aaos.org/quality/quality-programs/. Accessed November 20, 2020.

17. Poolman RW, Struijs PA, Krips R, et al: Reporting of outcomes in orthopaedic randomized trials: Does blinding of outcome assessors matter? *J Bone Joint Surg Am* 2007;89(3):550-558.

18. Brand RA: Ernest Amory Codman, MD, 1869-1940. *Clin Orthop Relat Res* 2009;467(11):2763-2765.

19. Mehlman CT: Clinical epidemiology, in Koval KJ, ed: *Orthopaedic Knowledge Update®*, ed 7. Rosemont, IL, American Academy of Orthopaedic Surgeons, 2002, pp 79-83.

20. Greenfield ML, Kuhn JE, Wojtys EM: A statistics primer: Validity and reliability. *Am J Sports Med* 1998;26(3):483-485.

21. Corona J, Matsumoto H, Roye DP, Vitale MG: Measuring quality of life in children with early onset scoliosis: Development and initial validation of the early onset scoliosis questionnaire. *J Pediatr Orthop* 2011;31(2):180-185.

22. Wright JG, Smith PL, Owen JL, Fehlings D: Assessing functional outcomes of children with muscular dystrophy and scoliosis: The Muscular Dystrophy Spine Questionnaire. *J Pediatr Orthop* 2008;28(8):840-845.

23. Weinstein SL, Dolan LA, Wright JG, Dobbs MB: Effects of bracing in adolescents with idiopathic scoliosis. *N Engl J Med* 2013;369(16):1512-1521.

24. Karanicolas PJ, Bhandari M, Kreder H, et al, Collaboration for Outcome Assessment in Surgical Trials (COAST) Musculoskeletal Group: Evaluating agreement: Conducting a reliability study. *J Bone Joint Surg Am* 2009;91(suppl 3):99-106.

25. Viera AJ, Garrett JM: Understanding interobserver agreement: The kappa statistic. *Fam Med* 2005;37(5):360-363.

26. Norman GR, Stratford P, Regehr G: Methodological problems in the retrospective computation of responsiveness to change: The lesson of Cronbach. *J Clin Epidemiol* 1997;50(8):869-879.

27. Norman GR, Wyrwich KW, Patrick DL: The mathematical relationship among different forms of responsiveness coefficients. *Qual Life Res* 2007;16(5):815-822.

28. Middel B, van Sonderen E: Statistical significant change versus relevant or important change in (quasi) experimental design: Some conceptual and methodological problems in estimating magnitude of intervention-related change in health services research. *Int J Integr Care* 2002;2:e15.

29. Streiner DL, Norman GR: Mine is bigger than yours: Measures of effect size in research. *Chest* 2012;141(3):595-598.

30. Norman GR, Sridhar FG, Guyatt GH, Walter SD: Relation of distribution- and anchor-based approaches in interpretation of changes in health-related quality of life. *Med Care* 2001;39(10):1039-1047.

31. Schünemann HJ, Guyatt GH: Commentary – Goodbye M(C)ID! Hello MID, where do you come from? *Health Serv Res* 2005;40(2):593-597.

32. Jevsevar DS, Sanders J, Bozic KJ, Brown GA: An introduction to clinical significance in orthopaedic outcomes research. *JBJS Rev* 2015;3(5):01874474-201503050-00002. Available at: http://reviews.jbjs.org/content/3/5/e2. Accessed April 5, 2016.

33. Carreon LY, Sanders JO, Diab M, Sucato DJ, Sturm PF, Glassman SD, Spinal Deformity Study Group: The minimum clinically important difference in Scoliosis Research Society-22 appearance, activity, and pain domains after surgical correction of adolescent idiopathic scoliosis. *Spine (Phila Pa 1976)* 2010;35(23):2079-2083.

34. Seok Park M, Youb Chung C, Min Lee K, et al: Rasch analysis of the pediatric outcomes data collection instrument in 720 patients with cerebral palsy. *J Pediatr Orthop* 2012;32(4):423-431.

35. Hudak PL, Amadio PC, Bombardier C, The Upper Extremity Collaborative Group (UECG): Development of an upper extremity outcome measure: The DASH (disabilities of the arm, shoulder and hand). *Am J Ind Med* 1996;29(6):602-608.

36. Chakravarty EF, Bjorner JB, Fries JF: Improving patient reported outcomes using item response theory and computerized adaptive testing. *J Rheumatol* 2007;34(6):1426-1431.

37. Hung M, Clegg DO, Greene T, Saltzman CL: Evaluation of the PROMIS physical function item bank in orthopaedic patients. *J Orthop Res* 2011;29(6):947-953.

38. Makhni EC, Meldau JE, Blanchett J, et al: Correlation of PROMIS physical function, pain interference, and depression in pediatric and adolescent patients in the ambulatory sports medicine clinic. *Orthop J Sports Med* 2019;7(6):2325967119851100.

    Administering PROMIS computer adaptive testing to pediatric and adolescent patients (aged 8 to 17 years) demonstrated similar correlations in physical function and upper extremity, depression, and pain interference as adults in a sports medicine clinic. Level of evidence: III.

39. Hung M, Stuart AR, Higgins TF, Saltzman CL, Kubiak EN: Computerized adaptive testing using the PROMIS physical function item bank reduces test burden with less ceiling effects compared with the Short Musculoskeletal Function Assessment in orthopaedic trauma patients. *J Orthop Trauma* 2014;28(8):439-443.
40. Hung M, Nickisch F, Beals TC, Greene T, Clegg DO, Saltzman CL: New paradigm for patient-reported outcomes assessment in foot & ankle research: Computerized adaptive testing. *Foot Ankle Int* 2012;33(8):621-626.
41. Beckmann JT, Hung M, Bounsanga J, Wylie JD, Granger EK, Tashjian RZ: Psychometric evaluation of the PROMIS physical function computerized adaptive test in comparison to the American Shoulder and Elbow Surgeons score and Simple Shoulder Test in patients with rotator cuff disease. *J Shoulder Elbow Surg* 2015;24(12):1961-1967.
42. Tyser AR, Beckmann J, Franklin JD, et al: Evaluation of the PROMIS physical function computer adaptive test in the upper extremity. *J Hand Surg Am* 2014;39(10):2047-2051.e4.
43. Hung M, Hon SD, Franklin JD, et al: Psychometric properties of the PROMIS physical function item bank in patients with spinal disorders. *Spine (Phila Pa 1976)* 2014;39(2):158-163.
44. Hung M, Baumhauer JF, Brodsky JW, et al, Orthopaedic Foot & Ankle Outcomes Research (OFAR) of the American Orthopaedic Foot & Ankle Society (AOFAS): Psychometric comparison of the PROMIS physical function CAT with the FAAM and FFI for measuring patient-reported outcomes. *Foot Ankle Int* 2014;35(6):592-599.
45. Mulcahey MJ, Haley SM, Slavin MD, et al: Ability of PROMIS pediatric measures to detect change in children with cerebral palsy undergoing musculoskeletal surgery. *J Pediatr Orthop* 2016;36(7):749-756.

    PROMIS was unable to detect changes after musculoskeletal surgery in patients with cerebral palsy, whereas other outcome measurements (Pediatric Quality of Life Cerebral Palsy, the Pediatrics Outcomes Data Collection Instrument, Gross Motor Functional Measure, and Timed Up and Go) had larger effect sizes and changes. Level of evidence: II.
46. Hays RD, Spritzer KL, Amtmann D, et al: Upper-extremity and mobility subdomains from the Patient-Reported Outcomes Measurement Information System (PROMIS) adult physical functioning item bank. *Arch Phys Med Rehabil* 2013;94(11):2291-2296.
47. Varni JW, Thissen D, Stucky BD, et al: Item-level informant discrepancies between children and their parents on the PROMIS pediatric scales. *Qual Life Res* 2015;24(8):1921-1937.
48. Irwin DE, Gross HE, Stucky BD, et al: Development of six PROMIS pediatrics proxy-report item banks. *Health Qual Life Outcomes* 2012;10:22.
49. Waljee JF, Carlozzi N, Franzblau LE, Zhong L, Chung KC: Applying the Patient-Reported Outcomes Measurement Information System to assess upper extremity function among children with congenital hand differences. *Plast Reconstr Surg* 2015;136(2):200e-207e.
50. Tucker CA, Bevans KB, Teneralli RE, Smith AW, Bowles HR, Forrest CB: Self-reported pediatric measures of physical activity, sedentary behavior, and strength impact for PROMIS: Item development. *Pediatr Phys Ther* 2014;26(4):385-392.
51. Forrest CB, Tucker CA, Ravens-Sieberer U, et al: Concurrent validity of the PROMIS pediatric global health measure. *Qual Life Res* 2016;25(3):739-751.

    The PROMIS pediatric global health measure summarizes a child's physical, mental, and social health into a single score. Level of evidence: II.
52. Kratz AL, Slavin MD, Mulcahey MJ, Jette AM, Tulsky DS, Haley SM: An examination of the PROMIS pediatric instruments to assess mobility in children with cerebral palsy. *Qual Life Res* 2013;22(10):2865-2876.

CHAPTER 3

Pediatric Anesthesia and Pain Management

ERIC D. SHIRLEY, MD • MARTIN J. HERMAN, MD

ABSTRACT

Appropriate planning for anesthesia and pain management is a critical component of orthopaedic surgery. For infants who require surgery, it is important to discuss the potential and uncertain risk of anesthetic neurotoxicity. Considerations during spine surgery include the preservation of neuromonitoring signals, fluid balance, and hemostasis. In the setting of forearm fracture reductions, both conscious sedation and intravenous regional anesthesia are safe and effective options. Perioperative and postoperative analgesia benefits from a multimodal strategy that addresses pain and muscle spasms while minimizing risks of developing opioid abuse.

Keywords: anesthetic neurotoxicity; antifibrinolytics; conscious sedation; multimodal anesthesia

Dr. Shirley or an immediate family member serves as a paid consultant to or is an employee of the U.S. Government; has stock or stock options held in Assertio Therapeutics and Lineage Medical; and serves as a board member, owner, officer, or committee member of the Pediatric Orthopaedic Society of North America. Dr. Herman or an immediate family member serves as a board member, owner, officer, or committee member of the American Academy of Orthopaedic Surgeons, the American Academy of Pediatrics: section on Orthopedics Executive Council member, and the Pediatric Orthopaedic Society of North America.

INTRODUCTION

Anesthesia and pain management options for the pediatric orthopaedic population include conscious sedation, regional and general anesthesia, and pharmacologic agents. These options must be used judiciously—alone or in combination—to optimize patient comfort. It is important to address recent research and intervention advancements in terms of potential neurotoxicity, spine surgery, fracture management, postoperative pain control, and opioid addiction.

ANESTHETIC NEUROTOXICITY AND THE DEVELOPING BRAIN

Selected pediatric orthopaedic conditions may require surgical treatment during infancy. The risk of general anesthetic neurotoxicity and subsequent learning deficits has been documented in mostly animal[1,2] and retrospective human[3,4] studies. However, these studies are limited by many factors, including the confounding effects of surgery and pathology. To coordinate additional research efforts regarding the risks of general anesthesia on the developing brain, the FDA, with assistance from the International Anesthesia Research Society, established SmartTots (Strategies for Mitigating Anesthesia-Related [Neuro]Toxicity in Tots) in 2011.

The General Anesthesia Compared to Spinal Anesthesia trial, which was facilitated by SmartTots in 2015, prospectively randomized 700 infants younger than 60 weeks to receive general or regional anesthesia for inguinal hernia repair.[5] The median duration of surgery in both groups was approximately 1 hour. At 2 years of age, evidence indicated that exposure to less than 1 hour of general

This chapter is adapted from Shirley ED, Bryskin RB: Pediatric anesthesia and pain management, in Martus JE, ed: *Orthopaedic Knowledge Update®: Pediatrics*, ed 5. Rosemont, IL, American Academy of Orthopaedic Surgeons, 2016, pp 25-33.

anesthesia in infancy did not increase the risk of adverse neurodevelopmental outcomes. Subsequent neurodevelopmental outcomes will be assessed when these children reach 5 years of age. The Pediatric Anesthesia and Neurodevelopmental Assessment prospective study, also facilitated by SmartTots, followed twin-sibling pairs, one of whom was exposed to anesthesia before the age of 3 years until the age of 8 to 15 years.[6] Analysis of neurocognitive performance and behavioral outcomes showed no significant difference between exposed and unexposed twins.[7] The lack of significant changes in cognitive performance in these two studies indicates that short-duration exposure to general anesthetics during infancy does not result in lasting cognitive deficiencies. This recommendation acknowledges the need for further long-term follow-up as well as further animal trials evaluating physiologic parameters delineating neurotoxic levels of anesthetics.

ANESTHETIC CONSIDERATIONS: SPINE SURGERY

Total intravenous anesthesia (TIVA) is the predominant method of anesthesia for pediatric patients undergoing spine surgery, especially when the evocation of motor potentials is involved.[8] The most commonly used agents are propofol, remifentanil, and midazolam[9-15] (**Table 1**). TIVA is now also preferred for pediatric patients over inhalational anesthesia because it has lower associated postoperative nausea and vomiting rates as well as fewer laryngeal complications.[16] Surgery for spinal deformities presents unique anesthetic challenges, such as the preservation of signals for neuromonitoring, fluid management, and bleeding. The complexity of these issues is greater in patients with neuromuscular conditions or those undergoing procedures requiring osteotomies. Recent research has evaluated the use of antifibrinolytics to reduce intraoperative blood loss and pharmacologic agents to assist in TIVA.

TABLE 1

Pharmacologic Agents and Dosing for Pediatric Spine surgery

Intraoperative

TIVA: propofol, remifentanil, and midazolam
Propofol: 100 μg/(kg × min) starting infusion rate
Remifentanil: 0.2 μg/kg/min induction rate, titration in increments of 0.05 μg/kg/min
Midazolam: 0.1 mg/(kg × hr) starting dose

Antifibrinolytics: EACA, TXA
TXA: >20 mg/kg loading dose and 10 mg/kg hr maintenance dose
EACA: 100 mg/(kg × hr) initiation dose and 10 mg/kg hr maintenance dose

Perioperative Pain Management

Ketorolac, gabapentin, morphine, hydromorphone
Ketorolac: 0.5 mg/kg every 6 hr for the first 72 hr
Gabapentin: 5 mg/kg every 3 times per day for 5 d
Morphine: 0.1 mg/(kg × hr) IV
Hydromorphone: 0.01 mg/(kg × hr)

EACA, epsilon-aminocaproic acid; TIVA, total intravenous anesthesia; TXA, tranexamic acid

Antifibrinolytics

Minimizing perioperative blood loss is a priority for avoiding transfusion risks, such as disease transmission, transfusion reaction, and increased risk of infection. Traditional methods of hemostasis include meticulous surgical technique, hypotensive anesthesia, muscle paralysis, acute hemodilution, and the use of cell salvage systems. According to the Pediatric Health Information Systems database for US children's hospitals, the median rates of transfusion for idiopathic and neuromuscular scoliosis are 24% and 43%, respectively.[17] Patients with neuromuscular scoliosis may have underlying coagulopathy from poor nutritional status, seizure medications, platelet abnormalities, and the depletion of clotting factors.[18] Fusion for neuromuscular scoliosis also has a higher risk of blood loss because it usually includes more fusion levels.

Antifibrinolytics, such as epsilon-aminocaproic acid (EACA) and tranexamic acid (TXA), have been used to minimize blood loss in adult patients during cardiac surgery, total joint arthroplasty, and spine surgery. Both EACA and TXA are synthetic derivatives that block lysine binding sites on plasminogen to impede blood clot degradation and have a low risk of adverse events.[19] A Cochrane systematic review concluded that these medications decrease blood loss in pediatric scoliosis surgery as well as the need for autologous and allogeneic blood transfusions.[20] A recent meta-analysis of both EACA and TXA also revealed significant reductions in blood loss during pediatric scoliosis surgery.[21]

The most pronounced effects of antifibrinolytics on blood loss are seen in spinal fusion for patients with neuromuscular scoliosis. Multiple studies on patients with neuromuscular scoliosis show that TXA treatment results in not only a reduction of blood loss but also a decrease in transfusion requirements compared with a placebo.[22,23] Current trends and evidence suggest similar results for adolescent idiopathic scoliosis and vertebral column resection procedures. Multiple studies using TXA perioperatively for these conditions have shown reductions in blood loss, necessary transfusion volumes, and transfusion rates when compared with control subjects.[24-28]

In direct comparisons, TXA tends to be favored over EACA. TXA is up to 10 times more potent in vitro than EACA,[29] has a longer half-life, and costs less. A prospective study in 2014 compared the two agents in patients with idiopathic or neuromuscular scoliosis.[30] TXA was associated with a lower overall transfusion requirement, less alteration in clotting studies, and a trend toward less blood loss. In patients with idiopathic scoliosis, TXA and EACA were found to be equally effective at reducing intraoperative blood loss, but TXA was more effective at reducing postoperative drainage and total blood loss.[27] In patients with cerebral palsy, TXA has been shown to be more effective than EACA in decreasing blood loss.[19]

The proper dosing of antifibrinolytics is under debate. So far research has shown that high-dose TXA (50 mg/kg loading dose with 5 mg/kg per hour maintenance dose) is more effective in reducing blood loss and transfusion requirements when compared with low-dose TXA (10 mg/kg loading dose and 1 mg/kg per hour maintenance dose).[24] TXA dosing of up to 100 mg/kg loading dose with 10 mg/kg per hour maintenance dose has been shown to be safe and effective.[31] A meta-analysis of TXA administration showed that TXA loading dosing >20 mg/kg is more effective than dosing <20 mg/kg in reducing perioperative blood loss in pediatric patients undergoing scoliosis surgery.[12] Specific EACA doses have not been shown to be clinically significant, but one dosing recommendation is a 100 mg/kg loading dose and 10 mg/kg per hour maintenance dose.[27]

Pharmacologic Agents

Pharmacologic agents given during spinal deformity surgery must not interfere with neuromonitoring. Dexmedetomidine, a selective alpha-2 adrenoceptor agonist with anesthetic and analgesic properties, has emerged as an effective adjuvant to total intravenous anesthesia for such cases. Its advantages include reduced intraoperative and postoperative analgesia requirements, shorter length of postoperative mechanical ventilation times, and a lower incidence of agitation and delirium.[32] When given during spine surgery, it provides hemodynamic stability, does not suppress evoked potentials, attenuates opioid-induced hyperalgesia, allows early neurologic assessment, and reduces analgesic needs postoperatively.[33-35] Ketorolac and gamma aminobutyric acid analogue have also been used as adjuvant pain medications resulting in shorter lengths of stay postoperatively as well as shortened periods of intravenous opioid use.[36]

Gabapentin, a common treatment for neuropathic pain, may also assist with postoperative analgesia by decreasing narcotic requirements, thus helping patients reach physical therapy goals more quickly. A 2014 retrospective chart review looked at 50 patients treated with perioperative gabapentin (in addition to normal opioids) compared with 51 control patients.[37] Patients in the gabapentin group received 5 mg/kg gabapentin before surgery, 5 mg/kg the evening of surgery, then 5 mg/kg three times a day for 2 days postoperatively. Patients in the gabapentin group were 5.3 times more likely than patients in the control group to complete the most challenging physical therapy goals in one day. A separate retrospective study analyzed the patient charts of 127 children who underwent posterior spinal fusion for adolescent idiopathic scoliosis.[38] Patients either received a patient-controlled analgesia (PCA) pump, a PCA pump with perioperative gabapentin (10 mg/kg up to 600 mg preoperatively and either 200 mg for >50 kg body weight or 100 mg for <50 kg body weight three times a day for 2 days postoperatively), or a PCA pump with gabapentin (same dosage as previously described) and clonidine (0.1 mg transdermal patch folded in half, placed for 7 days). Children who received gabapentin or gabapentin and clonidine in addition to their PCA pump had reduced opioid usage as well as shorter postoperative hospital stays. In another study, researchers found that a single preoperative dose of gabapentin (600 mg) before idiopathic scoliosis surgery was not associated with a substantial decrease in pain scores or total morphine consumption compared with placebo.[39] However, these authors suggested that their dose may have been too small to achieve a benefit.

ANESTHESIA AND SEDATION FOR FRACTURE MANIPULATION

Forearm and wrist fractures are common injuries in the pediatric population. Although open reduction and internal fixation is usually not required, displaced or angulated fractures often need closed reduction. Closed reduction may be performed either under general anesthesia or by means of conscious sedation using agents such as ketamine or nitrous oxide.

The optimal setting for forearm fracture reduction remains unclear. Closed reduction under general anesthesia in the operating room provides excellent sedation with muscle relaxation as needed and provides the opportunity to perform a percutaneous or open reduction and fixation when necessary. However, the potential disadvantages of treatment in the operating room include cost, efficiency, and access. Alternatively, conscious sedation in the emergency department often may be done immediately and at a lower cost but can negatively affect the efficiency of the emergency department. One study compared nonphyseal forearm fractures reduced in the emergency department under conscious sedation using nitrous oxide with those reduced in the operating room under general anesthesia.[40] Orthopaedic residents performed the reductions in both groups. Highly unstable fractures brought to the operating room for manipulation that underwent immediate internal fixation were excluded from the study. No substantial differences in the quality of reduction or the long arm plaster casts could be found, but the rate of repeat manipulation was substantially higher in fractures reduced in the emergency department compared with the operating room (32% versus 11%, respectively). The study authors proposed that the higher failure rate in the emergency department was the result of treating a larger number of unstable fracture patterns, which subsequently required immediate reduction in that setting.

Reductions in the emergency department also may be performed under intravenous regional anesthesia (Bier block). The block is performed by placing an intravenous line in the affected limb, inflating a brachial tourniquet, and then administering diluted lidocaine.[41] The use of intravenous regional anesthesia is associated with shorter lengths of stay and lower costs than conscious sedation.[41] Further study is needed to determine if intravenous regional anesthesia is contraindicated for certain fractures (such as those with significant shortening) or patient characteristics (age and/or weight).

PERIOPERATIVE AND POSTOPERATIVE PAIN MANAGEMENT

Pain management goals include relieving pain, decreasing the length of stay, allowing return to preoperative levels of activity, and minimizing adverse effects. Adequate postoperative pain control is essential to meet expectations and achieve an acceptable patient experience. Recent literature has focused on the complications of widespread opioid use and multimodal management strategies.

The Opioid Crisis

Opioids are the most powerful analgesics. They can be administered by injection or a PCA pump in patients aged 6 years and older with normal cognitive function and by proxy (eg, a nurse) in children younger than 6 years.[42] Oral opioids such as oxycodone and hydrocodone are used when the gastrointestinal tract is functioning properly. Adverse effects such as pruritus, drowsiness, respiratory depression, urinary retention, nausea, ileus, and constipation can be problematic. Codeine and tramadol are opioids metabolized via the cytochrome P450-metabolizing enzyme 2D6 phenotypes. Pediatric patients with overactive forms of these enzymes are at risk for oversedation, respiratory depression, and death. The FDA has contraindicated the use of codeine for pain or cough and tramadol for pain in children younger than 12 years.[43] The FDA has also placed a warning label on the use of both medications in children 12 to 18 years of age with obesity, sleep apnea, or severe pulmonary disease.[43]

The increase in opioid use, addiction, and overdose-related deaths is now an epidemic.[44] This problem is not limited to adults; prescription drug overdose is the most common cause of injury-related mortality in both children and adolescents.[45] Opioid poisoning is usually secondary to unintentional medicine cabinet access in children younger than 6 years, medication administration errors in children 6 to 12 years of age, and risk-taking behavior in adolescents.[46] A 2013 study found that this behavior among adolescents in not uncommon, with 13% of adolescents reporting nonmedical use of prescription opioids.[47]

Multimodal Approach to Pain Management

Multimodal strategies using NSAIDs, acetaminophen, and benzodiazepines were developed to minimize the use and complications of opioids.[48] Medications in each of these three classes can be administered intravenously in patients with abnormal gastrointestinal function. NSAIDs decrease prostaglandin production by inhibiting cyclooxygenase. Adverse effects include renal impairment, gastritis, and reversible platelet dysfunction. Although concerns about adverse effects on osseous healing have been raised in adult patients, they have not been substantiated in the pediatric setting following spinal fusion, fracture fixation, or osteotomies.[49-52] A 2017 randomized trial found that oral ibuprofen was as effective as oral morphine for pain control after minor outpatient orthopaedic surgery.[53] Combining NSAIDs with acetaminophen may provide superior analgesia than administering either medication alone.[54] Attention should be directed toward prescribing the appropriate dose of acetaminophen and NSAIDs because underdosage is common.[55] Finally, benzodiazepines can provide relief of postoperative muscle spasms in patients with fractures or neuromuscular conditions.

Additional research may result in the addition of other analgesics to multimodal protocols. Liposomal bupivacaine uses a multivesicular liposomal vehicle to provide increased extended drug release. This agent is currently FDA approved for surgical site injection in adult patients and as an interscalene brachial plexus nerve block. A 2018 study evaluating off-label injection just before skin closure during pediatric spine surgery did not find a decrease in pain medication requirements.[56] Further study is necessary to evaluate the safety and efficacy in pediatric patients.

Multimodal pain management extends far beyond the pharmaceutic agents.[57] The preoperative discussion includes screening for narcotic abuse, setting expectations for postoperative pain, and educating families about risk of narcotic addiction.[57] Published or institutional recommendations and state regulations should be used in determining the number of pills to describe, although exact guidelines for specific procedures are evolving.[44,58,59] It is also important to instruct patients and families to properly dispose of narcotics and avoid the opportunity for future nonmedical use.[44] After surgery, using pain scores alone or dosing to the numbers to determine analgesic requirements is not recommended because pain scores are subjective and medication requirements are multifactorial.[60] Follow-up phone calls are helpful to provide reassurance and further education regarding pain management.

Regional Anesthesia

Regional anesthesia for pediatric patients has seen substantial development in recent years, including further evaluation of potential complications from performing regional anesthesia under general anesthesia in children. The Pediatric Regional Anesthesia Network prospectively evaluated more than 53,000 cases of regional anesthesia performed between 2007 and 2012 in the United States.[61] The risk of neurologic complications was 8.3 per 1,000 in sedated patients, 3.4 per 1,000 in awake patients, 2.4 per 1,000 under general anesthesia with neuromuscular blockade, and 0.62 per 1,000 under general anesthesia without neuromuscular blockade.

Femoral nerve block is a common regional anesthetic for knee surgery. In 2015, a group of researchers evaluated strength and return to sports in pediatric patients receiving a femoral nerve block for anterior cruciate ligament (ACL) reconstruction.[62] The fast isokinetic extension strength deficit was significantly higher and meeting return to play criteria at 6 months was significantly lower in pediatric patients treated with a nerve block compared with patients who were not treated with a nerve block (17.6% versus 11.2% [$P = 0.01$] and 67.7% versus 90.2% [$P = 0.002$], respectively). Ultrasound-guided adductor canal block is a motor-sparing regional anesthesia technique that allows selective sensory nerve blockade, including the saphenous nerve, the medial femoral cutaneous nerve, the articular branches of the obturator nerve, and the nerve to the vastus medialis (sensory/motor) (**Figure 1**). In patients undergoing ACL reconstruction with patellar tendon autograft, the adductor canal block provided similar postoperative analgesia and narcotic consumption as a femoral nerve block.[63] Further study is needed to determine if adductor canal block is associated with any delays in return of strength similar to femoral nerve block.

Ideally, the use of regional anesthesia would decrease pain scores, complications, and postoperative opioid requirements. However, regional anesthesia has not resulted in a significant decrease in oral opioid use in pediatric patients after foot surgery or in adolescent and young adult patients after knee surgery.[58,64] This finding is likely explained by the duration of the postoperative pain exceeding the effect traditional regional anesthetics. Continuous peripheral nerve blocks are an option to extend the duration of postoperative analgesia and may have a larger effect on opioid use. The safety and

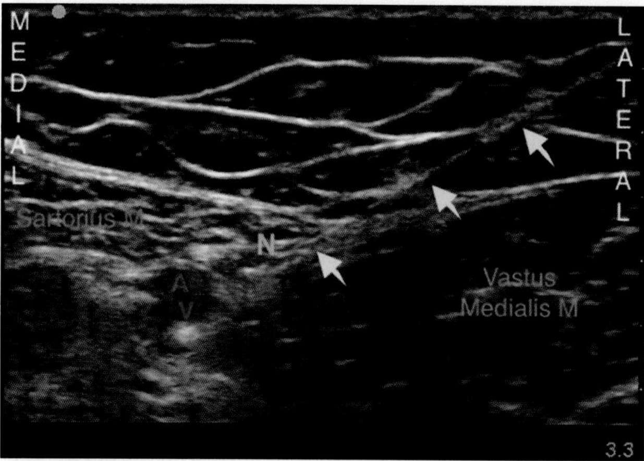

FIGURE 1 Ultrasound image demonstrating block needle placement in a 15-year-old during adductor canal block. A = superficial femoral artery, M = muscle, N = saphenous nerve, V = superficial femoral vein. Yellow arrows identify needle.

feasibility of continuous peripheral nerve blocks in pediatric hospitals under the careful supervision of a dedicated team performing placement and follow-up has been demonstrated.[65] Exact indications for the placement of continuous peripheral nerve blocks continue to evolve.

There are conflicting viewpoints on whether regional anesthesia delays the diagnosis of acute compartment syndrome (ACS). One survey found that 32% of orthopaedic surgeons had seen regional anesthesia mask the development of ACS.[66] This observation is supported by numerous case reports in the orthopaedic literature demonstrating delayed diagnosis of ACS in patients with regional anesthesia. Conversely, a 2017 review in the anesthesia literature suggested that there is no evidence that regional anesthesia delays the diagnosis in children.[67] However, anesthesiologists are not typically involved in the diagnosis of ACS and a motor or sensory blockade secondary to a regional anesthetic has the potential to compromise interpretation of physical examination findings. In addition, the presence of breakthrough pain after a nerve block is not diagnostic for compartment syndrome because some degree of pain and need for additional analgesia is not uncommon. A 2015 study of pediatric patients with cerebral palsy following hip osteotomies managed with an indwelling epidural catheter for 48 hours, a morphine PCA, scheduled valium, and scheduled ketorolac found that the mean total opioid use was 0.49 mg morphine/kg per day length of stay (range, 0.02 to 2.32).[68] None of the patients had compartment syndrome. Therefore, regional anesthesia is generally not advised following procedures or injuries at elevated risk for compartment syndrome.[48,69]

SUMMARY

Numerous advances have been made in pediatric anesthesia and pain management. It remains critical to further evaluate the risks of anesthetic neurotoxicity in infants. Future research also will help refine the dosing and indications for antifibrinolytics and regional anesthetic techniques in pediatric patients. Both conscious sedation and intravenous regional anesthesia have demonstrated safety and efficacy during closed reduction of fractures. Postoperative analgesia continues to consist of a multimodal strategy that addresses pain and muscle spasms while decreasing the risk of future opioid abuse. Further research may identify additional pharmacologic agents that are helpful in this setting.

KEY STUDY POINTS

- Antifibrinolytics decrease bleeding in pediatric spine deformity surgery, including patients with neuromuscular scoliosis, adolescent idiopathic scoliosis, and those undergoing vertebral column resection.
- Closed reduction of fractures in the emergency department under conscious sedation or Bier block represents a safe alternative to general anesthesia in the operating room.
- Multimodal pain management incorporates the use of acetaminophen, NSAIDs, regional anesthesia, and nonpharmacologic tactics to minimize the use of opioids and maximize pain control.

ANNOTATED REFERENCES

1. Brambrink AM, Evers AS, Avidan MS, et al: Isoflurane-induced neuroapoptosis in the neonatal rhesus macaque brain. *Anesthesiology* 2010;112(4):834-841.
2. Jevtovic-Todorovic V, Hartman RE, Izumi Y, et al: Early exposure to common anesthetic agents causes widespread neurodegeneration in the developing rat brain and persistent learning deficits. *J Neurosci* 2003;23(3):876-882.
3. Flick RP, Katusic SK, Colligan RC, et al: Cognitive and behavioral outcomes after early exposure to anesthesia and surgery. *Pediatrics* 2011;128(5):e1053-e1061.
4. Wilder RT, Flick RP, Sprung J, et al: Early exposure to anesthesia and learning disabilities in a population-based birth cohort. *Anesthesiology* 2009;110(4):796-804.
5. Davidson AJ, Disma N, de Graaff JC, et al, GAS Consortium: Neurodevelopmental outcome at 2 years of age after general anaesthesia and awake-regional anaesthesia in infancy (GAS): An international multicentre, randomized controlled trial. *Lancet* 2016;387(10015):239-250.

   A multicenter randomized trial of 700 infants examined the neurologic effects of anesthesia in children undergoing inguinal hernia repair under general anesthesia compared with awake regional anesthesia. No differences in neurodevelopmental outcomes were found at 2 years of age. Level of evidence: I.
6. Miller TL, Park R, Sun LS: Report of the fourth PANDA symposium on "Anesthesia and Neurodevelopment in Children". *J Neurosurg Anesthesiol* 2014;26(4):344-348.
7. Orser BA, Suresh S, Evers AS: SmartTots update regarding anesthetic neurotoxicity in the developing brain. *Anesth Analg* 2018;126(4):1393-1396.

   This statement incorporates previous studies to advise parents on the effect of short-term anesthesia on the developing brain of children. Level of evidence: V.
8. Lerman J: TIVA, TCI, and pediatrics: Where are we and where are we going? *Paediatr Anaesth* 2010;20(3):273-278.
9. Ngwenyama NE, Anderson J, Hoernschemeyer DG, Tobias JD: Effects of dexmedetomidine on propofol and remifentanil infusion rates during total intravenous anesthesia for spine surgery in adolescents. *Paediatr Anaesth* 2008;18(12):1190-1195.
10. Abu-Kishk I, Hod-Feins R, Anekstein Y, et al: Remifentanil use in pediatric scoliosis surgery-an effective alternative to morphine (a retrospective study). *Yonsei Med J* 2012;53(5):1014-1021.
11. Aydogan MS, Korkmaz MF, Ozgül U, et al: Pain, fentanyl consumption, and delirium in adolescents after scoliosis surgery: Dexmedetomidine vs midazolam. *Paediatr Anaesth* 2013;23(5):446-452.
12. Yuan QM, Zhao ZH, Xu BS: Efficacy and safety of tranexamic acid in reducing blood loss in scoliosis surgery: A systematic review and meta-analysis. *Eur Spine J* 2017;26(1):131-139.

    This systematic review and meta-analysis found that the use of TXA in pediatric scoliosis surgery reduced total blood loss. This review also found that high-dose TXA was more effective than low-dose TXA in reducing blood loss. Level of evidence: III.
13. Shrader MW, Nabar SJ, Jones JS, et al: Adjunctive pain control methods lower narcotic use and pain scores for patients with adolescent idiopathic scoliosis undergoing posterior spinal fusion. *Spine Deform* 2015;3(1):82-87.
14. Rusy LM, Hainsworth KR, Nelson TJ, et al: Gabapentin use in pediatric spinal fusion patients: A randomized, double-blind, controlled trial. *Anesth Analg* 2010;110(5):1393-1398.
15. Goodarzi M: Comparison of epidural morphine, hydromorphone and fentanyl for postoperative pain control in children undergoing orthopaedic surgery. *Paediatr Anaesth* 1999;9(5):419-422.
16. Lauder GR: Total intravenous anesthesia will supersede inhalational anesthesia in pediatric anesthetic practice. *Paediatr Anaesth* 2015;25(1):52-64.
17. McLeod LM, French B, Flynn JM, Dormans JP, Keren R: Antifibrinolytic use and blood transfusions in pediatric scoliosis surgeries performed at US children's hospitals. *J Spinal Disord Tech* 2015;28(8):E460-E466.

18. Brenn BR, Theroux MC, Dabney KW, Miller F: Clotting parameters and thromboelastography in children with neuromuscular and idiopathic scoliosis undergoing posterior spinal fusion. *Spine (Phila Pa 1976)* 2004;29(15):E310-E314.
19. Dhawale AA, Shah SA, Sponseller PD, et al: Are antifibrinolytics helpful in decreasing blood loss and transfusions during spinal fusion surgery in children with cerebral palsy scoliosis? *Spine (Phila Pa 1976)* 2012;37(9):E549-E555.
20. McNicol ED, Tzortzopoulou A, Schumann R, Carr DB, Kalra A: Antifibrinolytic agents for reducing blood loss in scoliosis surgery in children. *Cochrane Database Syst Rev* 2016;9(9):CD006883.

    This systematic review found that the use of antifibrinolytic agents reduced requirements for autologous and allogeneic blood transfusions in pediatric scoliosis surgery. Level of evidence: I.
21. Karimi S, Lu VM, Nambiar M, Phan K, Ambikaipalan A, Mobbs RJ: Antifibrinolytic agents for paediatric scoliosis surgery: A systematic review and meta-analysis. *Eur Spine J* 2019:28(5):1023-1034.

    This retrospective review found that the use of antifibrinolytics such as TXA and EACA resulted in significant reductions in blood loss and fresh-frozen plasma requirements. Level of evidence: III.
22. Sethna NF, Zurakowski D, Brustowicz RM, Bacsik J, Sullivan LJ, Shapiro F: Tranexamic acid reduces intraoperative blood loss in pediatric patients undergoing scoliosis surgery. *Anesthesiology* 2005;102(4):727-732.
23. Thompson GH, Florentino-Pineda I, Poe-Kochert C, Armstrong DG, Son-Hing J: Role of Amicar in surgery for neuromuscular scoliosis. *Spine (Phila Pa 1976)* 2008;33(24):2623-2629.
24. Johnson DJ, Johnson CC, Goobie SM, et al: High-dose versus low-dose tranexamic acid to reduce transfusion requirements in pediatric scoliosis surgery. *J Pediatr Orthop* 2017;37(8):e55 2-e557.

    This retrospective chart review found that high doses of TXA are better at limiting blood loss in adolescent idiopathic scoliosis surgery than low doses of TXA. Level of evidence: III.
25. Goobie SM, Zurakowski D, Glotzbecker MP, et al: Tranexamic acid is efficacious at decreasing the rate of blood loss in adolescent scoliosis surgery: A randomized placebo-controlled trial. *J Bone Joint Surg Am* 2018;100(23):2024-2032.

    A randomized trial of 111 patients undergoing surgery for adolescent idiopathic scoliosis found that the use of TXA significantly reduced blood loss when compared with placebo. Level of evidence: I.
26. Newton PO, Bastrom TP, Emans JB, et al: Antifibrinolytic agents reduce blood loss during pediatric vertebral column resection procedures. *Spine (Phila Pa 1976)* 2012;37(23):E14 59-E1463.
27. Verma K, Errico T, Diefenbach C, et al: The relative efficacy of antifibrinolytics in adolescent idiopathic scoliosis: A prospective randomized trial. *J Bone Joint Surg Am* 2014;96(10):e80.
28. Yagi M, Hasegawa J, Nagoshi N, et al: Does the intraoperative tranexamic acid decrease operative blood loss during posterior spinal fusion for treatment of adolescent idiopathic scoliosis? *Spine (Phila Pa 1976)* 2012;37(21):E1336-E1342.
29. Lecker I, Wang DS, Romaschin AD, Peterson M, Mazer CD, Orser BA: Tranexamic acid concentrations associated with human seizures inhibit glycine receptors. *J Clin Invest* 2012;122(12):4654-4666.
30. Halanski MA, Cassidy JA, Hetzel S, Reischmann D, Hassan N: The efficacy of Amicar versus tranexamic acid in pediatric spinal deformity surgery: A prospective, randomized, double-blinded pilot study. *Spine Deform* 2014;2:191-197.
31. Sui WY, Ye F, Yang JI: Efficacy of tranexamic acid in reducing allogeneic blood products in adolescent idiopathic scoliosis surgery. *BMC Musculoskeletal Disord* 2016;17(1):187.

    This retrospective review of 137 patients who underwent surgery for adolescent idiopathic scoliosis found that high doses of TXA reduced blood loss during surgery and the need for allogeneic blood transfusions. Level of evidence: II.
32. Pan W, Wang Y, Lin L, Zhou G, Hua X, Mo L: Outcomes of dexmedetomidine treatment in pediatric patients undergoing congenital heart disease surgery: A meta-analysis. *Paediatr Anaesth* 2016;26(3):239-248.

    This article is a systematic review of the perioperative use of dexmedetomidine in children undergoing congenital heart disease surgery. Level of evidence: V.
33. Rozet I, Metzner J, Brown M, et al: Dexmedetomidine does not affect evoked potentials during spine surgery. *Anesth Analg* 2015;121(2):492-501.
34. Bekker A, Haile M, Kline R, et al: The effect of intraoperative infusion of dexmedetomidine on the quality of recovery after major spinal surgery. *J Neurosurg Anesthesiol* 2013;25(1):16-24.
35. Hwang W, Lee J, Park J, Joo J: Dexmedetomidine versus remifentanil in postoperative pain control after spinal surgery: A randomized controlled study. *BMC Anesthesiol* 2015;15(1):21.
36. Rosenberg RE, Trzcinski S, Cohen M, Erickson M, Errico T, McLeod L: The association between adjuvant pain medication use and outcomes following pediatric spinal fusion. *Spine (Phila Pa 1976)* 2017;42(10):E602-E608.

    This retrospective review looked at the use of ketorolac and gamma aminobutyric acid analogue among 7,349 patients who underwent surgery for idiopathic scoliosis and found that the use of ketorolac and gamma aminobutyric acid analogue postoperatively were correlated with shorter IV opioid use durations. Level of evidence: III.
37. Thomas JJ, Levek C, Quick HD, Brinton JT, Garg S, Cohen MN: Utility of gabapentin in meeting physical therapy goals following posterior spinal fusion in adolescent patients with idiopathic scoliosis. *Paediatr Anaesth* 2018;28(6):558-563.

    This retrospective chart review found that the use of perioperative gabapentin was associated with significantly improved physical therapy outcomes in patients that have undergone surgery for adolescent idiopathic scoliosis. Level of evidence: III.

38. Choudhry DK, Brenn BR, Sacks K, Shah S: Evaluation of gabapentin and clonidine use in children following spinal fusion surgery for idiopathic scoliosis: A retrospective review. *J Pediatr Orthop* 2019;39(9):e687-e693.

This retrospective chart review found that the addition of gabapentin alone or the addition of gabapentin and clonidine to postoperative treatment reduced patient opioid use. Level of evidence: III.

39. Mayell A, Srinivasan I, Campbell F, Peliowski A: Analgesic effects of gabapentin after scoliosis surgery in children: A randomized controlled trial. *Paediatr Anaesth* 2014;24(12):1239-1244.

40. McKenna P, Leonard M, Connolly P, Boran S, McCormack D: A comparison of pediatric forearm fracture reduction between conscious sedation and general anesthesia. *J Orthop Trauma* 2012;26(9):550-555.

41. Aarons CE, Fernandez MD, Willsey M, Peterson B, Key C, Fabregas J: Bier block regional anesthesia and casting for forearm fractures: Safety in the pediatric emergency department setting. *J Pediatr Orthop* 2014;34(1):45-49.

42. Monitto CL, Greenberg RS, Kost-Byerly S, et al: The safety and efficacy of parent-/nurse-controlled analgesia in patients less than 6 years of age. *Anesth Analg* 2000;91(3):573-579.

43. US Food and Drug Administration: *FDA Restricts Use of Prescription Codeine Pain and Cough Medicines and Tramadol Pain Medicines in Children; Recommends Against Use in Breastfeeding Women: Drug Safety Communication.* 2017. Available at: https://www.fda.gov/drugs/drug-safety-and-availability/fda-drug-safety-communication-fda-restricts-use-prescription-codeine-pain-and-cough-medicines-and. Accessed October 7, 2019.

This safety announcement communicates the addition of contraindication and warning labels to use of codeine and tramadol in select pediatric patients. Level of evidence: V.

44. Raney EM, van Bosse HJ, Shea KG, Abzug JM, Schwend RM: Current state of the opioid epidemic as it pertains to pediatric orthopaedics from the Advocacy Committee of the Pediatric Orthopaedic Society of North America. *J Pediatr Orthop* 2018;38(5):e238-e244.

This article reviews the history, epidemiology, and treatment strategies to address the opioid crisis. Level of evidence: V.

45. Gaither JR, Leventhal JM, Ryan SA, Camenga DR: National trends in hospitalizations for opioid poisonings among children and adolescents, 1997 to 2012. *JAMA Pediatr* 2016;170:1195-1201.

This retrospective review found that pediatric hospitalizations for opioid poisoning doubled from 1997 to 2002. Level of evidence: III.

46. Allen JD, Casavant MJ, Spiller HA, Chounthirath T, Hodges NL, Smith GA: Prescription opioid exposures among children and adolescents in the United States: 2000-2015. *Pediatrics* 2017;139:e20163382.

This study analyzed data from the National Poison Data System to analyze to exposures in children younger than 20 years. Level of evidence: III.

47. McCabe SE, West BT, Boyd CJ: Motives for medical misuse of prescription opioids among adolescents: *J Pain* 2013;14:1208-1216.

48. Frizzell KH, Cavanaugh PK, Herman MJ: Pediatric perioperative pain management. *Orthop Clin North Am* 2017;48(4):467-480.

This article reviews the preoperative, intraoperative, and postoperative considerations including multimodal anesthesia in pediatric orthopaedic patients. Level of evidence: V.

49. Marquez-Lara A, Hutchinson ID, Nuñez F Jr, Smith TL, Miller AN: Nonsteroidal anti-inflammatory drugs and bone-healing: A systematic review of research quality. *JBJS Rev* 2016;4(3).

This systematic review did not find a clear consensus on the safety of NSAIDs in adult patients after orthopaedic surgery and suggested further studies with appropriate methodology. Level of evidence: III.

50. Sucato DJ, Lovejoy JF, Agrawal S, Elerson E, Nelson T, McClung A: Postoperative ketorolac does not predispose to pseudoarthrosis following posterior spinal fusion and instrumentation for adolescent idiopathic scoliosis. *Spine (Phila Pa 1976)* 2008;33(10):1119-1124.

51. Kay RM, Directo MP, Leathers M, Myung K, Skaggs DL: Complications of ketorolac use in children undergoing operative fracture care. *J Pediatr Orthop* 2010;30(7):655-658.

52. Kay RM, Leathers M, Directo MP, Myung K, Skaggs DL: Perioperative ketorolac use in children undergoing lower extremity osteotomies. *J Pediatr Orthop* 2011;31(7):783-786.

53. Poonai N, Datoo N, Ali S, et al: Oral morphine versus ibuprofen administered at home for postoperative orthopedic pain in children: A randomized controlled trial. *Can Med Assoc J* 2017;189(40):E1252-E1258.

This randomized trial found equivalent pain control efficacy of oral morphine (0.5 mg/kg, maximum 20 mg) and oral ibufprofen (10 mg/kg, maximum 600 mg) every 6 hours as needed for pain, for 48 hours after discharge following minor orthopaedic surgery. Level of evidence: II.

54. Ong CK, Seymour RA, Lirk P, Merry AF: Combining paracetamol (acetaminophen) with nonsteroidal antiinflammatory drugs: A qualitative systematic review of analgesic efficacy for acute postoperative pain. *Anesth Analg* 2010;110(4):1170-1179.

55. Milani GP, Benini F, Dell'Era L, et al: Acute pain management: Acetaminophen and ibuprofen are often under-dosed. *Eur J Pediatr* 2017;176(7):979-982.

This retrospective study of children presenting to the emergency room found that >60% were prescribed an underdose of acetaminophen (15 to 20 mg/kg, maximum 1,000 mg) and ibuprofen (10 mg/kg, maximum 400 mg). Level of evidence: III.

56. Cloyd C, Moffett BS, Bernhardt MB, Monico EM, Patel N, Hanson D: Efficacy of liposomal bupivacaine in pediatric patients undergoing spine surgery. *Paediatr Anaesth* 2018;28(11):982-986.

This retrospective matched study found that the injection of liposomal bupivacaine was not associated with a reductions in opioid use following pediatric spine surgery. Level of evidence: III.

57. Seymour RB1, Ring D, Higgins T, Hsu JR: Leading the way to solutions to the opioid epidemic: AOA critical issues. *J Bone Joint Surg Am* 2017;99(21):e113.

    This article reviews the pharmacologic options for the management of musculoskeletal pain and suggests solutions including system-wide interventions. Level of evidence: V.

58. Tepolt FA, Bido J, Burgess S, Micheli LJ, Kocher MS: Opioid overprescription after knee arthroscopy and related surgery in adolescents and young adults. *Arthroscopy* 2018;34(12):3236-3243.

    This retrospective case series of adolescent and young adult patients after knee arthroscopy found that patients were prescribed an average of 51 oxycodone pills and consumed an average of 17 pills. Level of evidence: III.

59. Reid DBC, Shah KN, Shapiro BH, Ruddell JH, Akelman E, Daniels AH: Mandatory prescription limits and opioid utilization following orthopaedic surgery. *J Bone Joint Surg Am* 2019;101(10):e43.

    This retrospective review found a decrease in the amount of opioid dispensed in the short and immediate term after orthopaedic surgery following the implementation of state prescription regulations. Level of evidence: III.

60. Pasero C, Quinlan-Colwell A, Rae D, Broglio K, Drew D: American society for pain management nursing position statement: Prescribing and administering opioid doses based solely on pain intensity. *Pain Manag Nurs* 2016;17(3):170-180.

    This position statement reviews how widespread use of pain intensity scales led to the problem of prescribing opioids solely based on pain intensity. Level of evidence: V.

61. Taenzer AH, Walker BJ, Bosenberg AT, et al: Asleep versus awake: Does it matter? Pediatric regional block complications by patient state. A report from the Pediatric Regional Anesthesia Network. *Reg Anesth Pain Med* 2014;39(4):279-283.

62. Luo TD, Ashraf A, Dahm DL, Stuart MJ, McIntosh AL: Femoral nerve block is associated with persistent strength deficits at 6 months after anterior cruciate ligament reconstruction in pediatric and adolescent patients. *Am J Sports Med* 2015;43(2):331-336.

63. Chisholm MF, Bang H, Maalouf DB, et al: Postoperative analgesia with saphenous block appears equivalent to femoral nerve block in ACL reconstruction. *HSS J* 2014;10(3):245-251.

64. Lloyd CH, Srinath AK, Muchow RD, et al: Efficacy of 2 regional pain control techniques in pediatric foot surgery. *J Pediatr Orthop* 2016;36(7):720-724.

    This retrospective review evaluated patients undergoing foot and ankle surgery managed with regional anesthesia (using ultrasound-guided or nerve stimulation) and general anesthesia. Patients with regional anesthesia received less morphine, but the amount of oxycodone use was similar. Level of evidence: III.

65. Gurnaney H, Kraemer FW, Maxwell L, Muhly WT, Schleelein L, Ganesh A: Ambulatory continuous peripheral nerve blocks in children and adolescents: A longitudinal 8-year single center study. *Anesth Analg* 2014;118(3):621-627.

66. Thonse R, Ashford RU, Williams TI, Harrington P: Differences in attitudes to analgesia in post-operative limb surgery put patients at risk of compartment syndrome. *Injury* 2004;35(3):290-295.

67. Lönnqvist PA, Ecoffey C, Bosenberg A, Suresh S, Ivani G: The European society of regional anesthesia and pain therapy and the American society of regional anesthesia and pain medicine joint committee practice advisory on controversial topics in pediatric regional anesthesia I and II: What do they tell us? *Curr Opin Anaesthesiol* 2017;30(5):613-620.

    This review article summarizes society guidelines regarding the use of regional anesthesia in children. Level of evidence: V.

68. Shrader MW, Jones J, Falk MN, White GR, Burk DR, Segal LS: Hip reconstruction is more painful than spine fusion in children with cerebral palsy. *J Child Orthop* 2015;9(3):221-225.

69. Noonan KJ, McCarthy JJ: Compartment syndromes in the pediatric patient. *J Pediatr Orthop* 2010:30(2):S96-S101.

CHAPTER 4

Musculoskeletal Infections

JOHN F. LOVEJOY III, MD • LAWSON A. B. COPLEY, MD, MBA

ABSTRACT

Diagnosing and managing pediatric musculoskeletal infections continues to be a challenge for pediatric orthopaedic surgery practitioners. Although the spectrum of disease has remained relatively consistent, the clinical presentation of these infections is highly variable, with a continuum of very mild to life-threatening disease. This wide range of severity coupled with acute, subacute, and chronic presentations that may involve one or more locations further complicates the evaluation process. Many centers now incorporate a team approach with involvement of specialists, such as emergency department physicians, hospitalists, pediatricians, infectious disease specialists, radiologists, and pathologists. Orthopaedic surgeons have an opportunity to play a leadership role in the establishment and guidance of multidisciplinary teams for pediatric musculoskeletal infection care. The expertise of the orthopaedic surgeon leads to less resource utilization and more timely interventions, whether in determining the correct study, constructing the differential diagnoses, or performing the definitive treatment. To improve outcomes for children with suspected bone, joint, and soft-tissue infections, orthopaedic surgeons must remain up to date with current trends in the diagnosis and management of these infections and play a decisive role in surgical care.

Dr. Lovejoy or an immediate family member serves as an unpaid consultant to OrthoPaediatrics and serves as a board member, owner, officer, or committee member of the Pediatric Orthopaedic Society of North America. Neither Dr. Copley nor any immediate family member has received anything of value from or has stock or stock options held in a commercial company or institution related directly or indirectly to the subject of this chapter.

Keywords: abscess; chronic recurrent multifocal osteomyelitis (CRMO); methicillin-resistant *Staphylococcus aureus* (MRSA); musculoskeletal infection; osteomyelitis; septic arthritis

INTRODUCTION

Pediatric musculoskeletal infections can present in an acute or chronic state with a wide range of severity. Infections can be superficial (septic bursitis, abscess, cellulitis, fasciitis, lymphangitis, and lymphadenitis) or deep (osteomyelitis, septic arthritis, and pyomyositis). Any soft tissue or bone is susceptible to infection. The initial presentation of children with a pediatric musculoskeletal infection is highly variable and necessitates a careful history and physical examination followed by appropriate imaging and laboratory studies. The data obtained should be analyzed to create a differential diagnosis and clarify the anatomic location and extent of disease. After a diagnosis is determined, a treatment algorithm should be used to facilitate rapid and timely resolution of the infection. Although most pediatric musculoskeletal infection occurs through hematogenous dissemination to deep tissues or microscopic penetrating inoculation for skin and soft-tissue infections, another form of infection includes surgical site infections. The challenge of treating infections is increased with the presence of implanted hardware.[1] The increasing trend toward establishing clinical practice guidelines indicates that there is a growing desire to reduce variation in care and improve short-term, intermediate-term, and long-term outcomes for these conditions.[1-3] In addition, efforts to reduce the costs of care while maintaining quality of care have yielded process and workflow improvements focusing on early transitions from intravenous to oral antibiotics and shortened lengths of hospital stay.[4-6] These treatment algorithms vary greatly as a function of the severity of illness, the child's response to therapy, and the need for surgical intervention.[7-9] Although progress has been made in the creation and utilization of treatment algorithms, variations in clinical evaluation and treatment of these conditions exist regionally and internationally and thus no universal algorithm has been accepted.[1,7,10-14]

It is important that the orthopaedic surgeon be mindful of the many conditions, such as neoplasms, inflammatory disorders, and trauma, which can mimic the clinical presentations of musculoskeletal infection. For example, early in the course of the child's disease, the orthopaedic surgeon must be mindful of conditions ranging from benign and self-limited processes, such as transient synovitis, to serious and life-threatening disorders, such as leukemia or Ewing sarcoma.[3] These workups often involve a multidisciplinary team. Orthopaedic surgeons should play an early, active leadership role within these teams as this often leads to less resource utilization (fewer laboratory and imaging studies) if the clinical scenario suggests a benign, self-limited problem (such as transient synovitis) or an orthopaedic problem (such as a fracture in a child with spina bifida) rather than an infectious problem.[3,15]

A CONTINUUM OF DISEASE

Musculoskeletal infections in children can occur in isolation, can be contiguous with other structures, can be multifocal, or can be part of a disseminated infection.[1,3,15-18] Because pediatric musculoskeletal infections can be complex and have life-threatening or limb-threatening complications, an early, accurate, and complete diagnosis is a priority.

Studies suggest that infections involving different tissue types behave differently according to the primary tissue of involvement, within a relative descending hierarchy from bone to joint to muscle to soft tissue.[1,18] Children with osteomyelitis in isolation or those who have osteomyelitis associated with septic arthritis have higher rates of bacteremia at presentation than do children with isolated septic arthritis.[18] Children with osteomyelitis require longer hospital stays and antibiotic treatment of longer durations than do children with isolated septic arthritis.[1,2,16,19] Children with osteomyelitis are susceptible to adverse outcomes from the infections, including physeal arrest, osteonecrosis, pathologic fracture, and deformity.[1,7,14,16] In contrast to children with osteomyelitis, children with skin and skin structure infections have a negligible rate of bacteremia and require the shortest duration of treatment.[18]

OSTEOMYELITIS

Evaluation

The clinical assessment of a child with osteomyelitis often reveals bone tenderness that is most pronounced over the epicenter of the disease. However, because increased pressure within the bone will be disseminated more widely, it is helpful to evaluate for tenderness of the bone away from the site of report. This helps to differentiate other causes of local tissue inflammation and swelling, such as cellulitis, bursitis, or even septic arthritis in which there appears to be local bone tenderness adjacent to the joint.

The workup for any possible musculoskeletal infection should include plain radiographs in at least two views, to assess for other potential causes of symptoms (eg, fracture or neoplasm) and for obvious radiographic changes that may occur in advanced disease (eg, lytic lesions, cortical erosions, sequestrum, or involucrum). These radiographic changes require time to develop and imply that the bone architecture has been substantially affected by the underlying process. Typically, a loss of approximately one-third of the local bone mineral density must occur before it is apparent on a plain radiograph. The most important initial plain radiographic finding in children with early presentation of acute hematogenous osteomyelitis is deep soft-tissue swelling.

MRI is an accurate and reliable imaging study to determine the anatomic and spatial extent of bone, joint, and soft-tissue infection (**Figure 1**). The use of MRI often provides a more complete understanding of the primary and contiguous tissues involved in the infection, as well as a determination of the presence and size of abscesses that may require surgical drainage.[3,9,18,19] Institutions are reporting an increased rate of MRI use to evaluate children with suspected musculoskeletal infection.[7] Challenges to obtaining MRIs include cost and the need for sedation or general anesthesia in younger children. In many busy pediatric centers, there are logistical challenges to obtaining MRI studies in a timely manner. Rapid image acquisition protocols can allow coronal screening MRI from the lumbar spine to the ankles with a minimal need for sedation. Evidence suggests

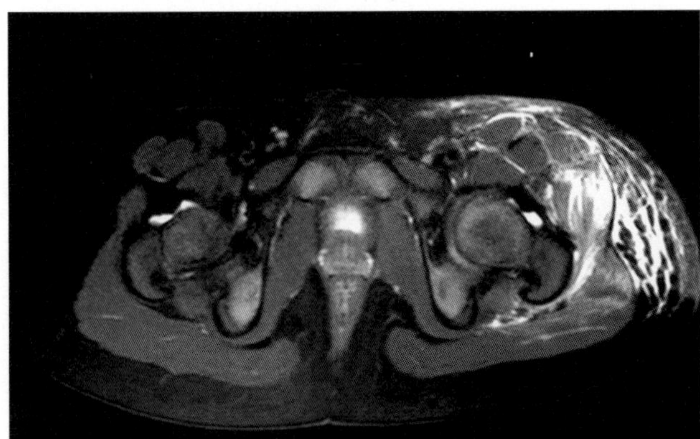

FIGURE 1 Magnetic resonance image from a patient with hip pyomyositis shows extensive edema within the musculature of the proximal left thigh.

Section 1: General Topics

that multispecialty care coordination of a child who has been sedated for MRI with continuation of anesthesia for immediate surgery can improve the efficiency of scanning and result in less scanning time, better coordination and timing of surgical intervention, and an overall shorter total length of hospitalization.[3] More recent literature suggests that scan duration, anesthesia duration, and contrast use may be significantly reduced when interdisciplinary communication and coordination are established between the key stakeholders of orthopaedic surgery, radiology, and anesthesia and when specific imaging processes and workflows are used.[4]

Clinical Practice Guidelines

Children with bone and joint infections have benefitted from the development and implementation of clinical guidelines or pathways to reduce variation in care.[1,2] The development of such guidelines for conditions, such as osteomyelitis, has led to improvements in the selection of antibiotics, greater consistency in the acquisition of culture material from the site of infection, a reduction in the time to obtain appropriate diagnostic imaging, and a trend toward reduction in the length of hospitalization[2] (**Figure 2**). The guidelines or pathways are best developed by an interdisciplinary group, including infectious disease and other pediatric specialties, using current literature and tailored to the specific needs of the institution and its available resources.

Severity of Illness

Determining the severity of illness for children with acute hematogenous osteomyelitis may help clinicians stratify children objectively based on the clinical and laboratory presentations.[15] Severity of illness determinations for children may also improve the study of disease cohorts that differ chronologically, geographically, or therapeutically, without being subjected to misleading assumptions about fundamental cohort differences caused by the relative severity of the underlying disease.[15] Comparative studies indicate that children with osteomyelitis caused by methicillin-resistant *Staphylococcus aureus* (MRSA) may be more ill than children with osteomyelitis caused by methicillin-sensitive *S aureus* (MSSA).[8,10-12,14-16] The awareness of the relative illness severity of children with osteomyelitis has implications for early identification of deep vein thrombosis and the risk of a hemodynamically significant pulmonary embolism.[17] One study demonstrated that children with osteomyelitis and deep vein thrombosis had a significantly higher severity of illness scores than children with osteomyelitis but without deep vein thrombosis (9.1 versus 2.7).[17] This study introduced the concept of pattern recognition that may be triggered in the presence of intensive care unit–admitted children with markedly elevated inflammatory markers, MRSA bacteremia, and the appearance of patchy infiltrates on chest radiograph suggestive of septic pulmonary emboli.[17] Another important implication of illness severity is the prognosis for long-term adverse clinical outcomes.[18] One center prospectively studied children with osteomyelitis for a minimum of 2 years (average 2.5 years, range 2 to 5 years) and found that children in the highest severity of illness group were significantly more likely to have osteochondrosis, chondrolysis, and deformity with 38.2% of children affected in comparison with only 1.3% of children with mild illness.[18] In an effort to anticipate which children will have confirmed MRSA infections before the culture results are available, a prediction algorithm has been created.[10] However, the use of such algorithms has not been confirmed in other communities, some of which have a higher incidence of MRSA osteomyelitis.[11]

Management

Antibiotic Therapy

A challenge in the management of musculoskeletal infection is the selection and timing of empiric antibiotic administration. In children who are hemodynamically stable, it is reasonable to withhold antibiotics until cultures are collected, thereby maximizing the sensitivity of the cultures obtained. In children showing signs of hemodynamic instability or signs of sepsis, early empiric antibiotic therapy should be administered early regardless of the timing of procurement of deep tissue cultures.[18] In all children, blood cultures should be obtained before antibiotic administration and may be drawn concurrent with other essential laboratory tests (including a complete blood count with differential, erythrocyte sedimentation rate [ESR], and C-reactive protein [CRP] level).[18]

Empiric antibiotic therapy should be chosen based on several considerations: the age of the child (eg, group B streptococcal osteomyelitis is common in young infants, but rare in older children; *Kingella kingae* is most common in children between the ages of 6 months and 4 years with a peak at 2 years of age), the presumed mode of infection (hematogenous spread or penetrating injury), underlying chronic diseases (eg, sickle cell anemia or primary immunodeficiency), and local epidemiology and antimicrobial susceptibilities of the most likely pathogens.[1,7,10,12,15] It is important to consider that the most likely pathogens may vary by region and change over time. In institutions that have an infectious disease department, an infectious disease consultation can be helpful in determining appropriate antibiotic selection, dosage, and efficacy of treatment. Infectious disease departments will generally be able to provide an up-to-date antibiogram and incidence of infection at the facility and within the region.

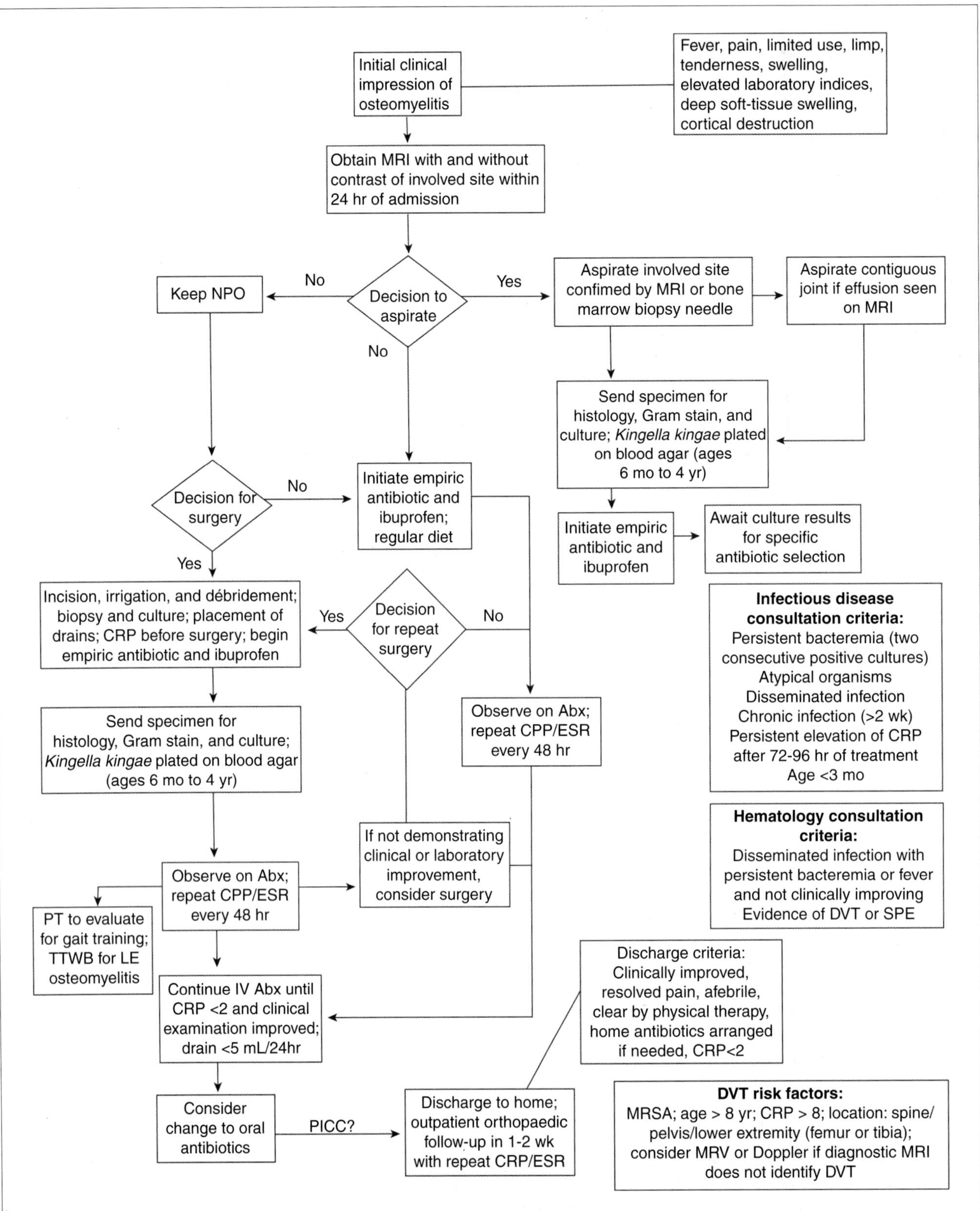

FIGURE 2 Flowchart of the Children's Medical Center of Dallas guideline for the evaluation and treatment of children with suspected osteomyelitis. Abx = antibiotics, CRP = C-reactive protein level, DVT = deep vein thrombosis, ESR = erythrocyte sedimentation rate, IV = intravenous, LE = lower extremity, MRSA = methicillin-resistant *Staphylococcus aureus*, MRV = magnetic resonance venography, NPO = nothing by mouth, PICC = peripherally inserted catheter, PT = physical therapist, SPE = septic pulmonary embolism, TTWB = toe-touch weight bearing. (Reproduced with permission from Copley LA, Kinsler MA, Gheen T, Shar A, Sun D, Browne R: The impact of evidence-based clinical practice guidelines applied by a multidisciplinary team for the care of children with osteomyelitis. *J Bone Joint Surg Am* 2013;95[8];686-693.)

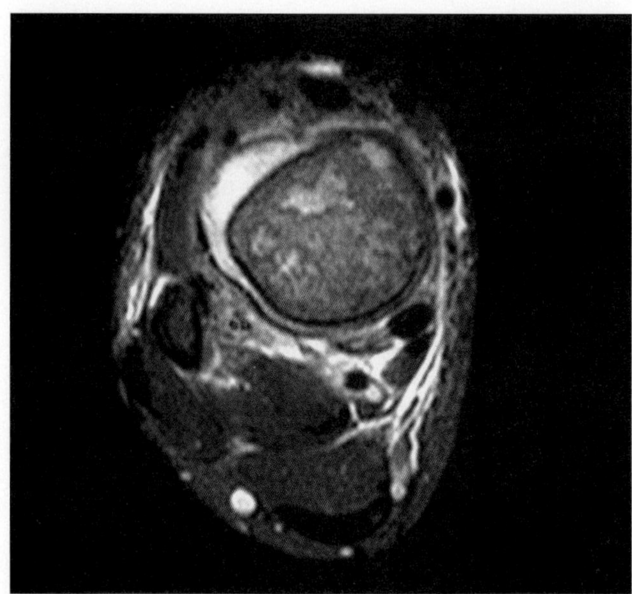

FIGURE 3 Magnetic resonance image shows tibial osteomyelitis with a subperiosteal abscess and extensive soft-tissue edema.

This is highlighted by the experience with MRSA. Over the past 2 decades, the predominance of community-acquired MRSA has been responsible for a high proportion of culture-positive bone, joint, and soft-tissue infections, leading to increased use of vancomycin and clindamycin instead of the cephalosporin drugs used when methicillin-sensitive staphylococcal infections predominated.[11,12,14,16] However, antimicrobial susceptibilities of bacterial pathogens, most notably *S aureus*, vary widely. It is important that clinicians monitor antibiotic resistance patterns within the communities because some communities are seeing an increase in methicillin-susceptible *S aureus* with up to one-third of these methicillin-susceptible strands being clindamycin resistant.[1,7,15,18,20]

Recommendations for the administration route and duration of antibiotic treatment of acute hematogenous osteomyelitis have changed substantially in recent years.[4,5,13] Historically, the standard practice was to administer intravenous antibiotics in the hospital for 4 to 6 weeks. With the advent of peripherally inserted central catheters, placement of the catheter and a short course of in-hospital–administered antibiotics followed by a course of parenteral antibiotics administered at home was shown to be safe and effective.[21]

Oral therapy after a course of intravenous antibiotics has now become an accepted practice. Many children are treated effectively with a limited course of intravenous antibiotics, followed by 3 to 4 weeks of oral therapy.[4,5,13,19] Oral antibiotics with good bioavailability to susceptible infecting organisms offer flexibility with respect to the route of administration. Sequential parenteral to oral antibiotic therapy is considered safe and effective and should be used whenever there are no contraindications (such as malabsorption or risk of noncompliance) or when antibiotic resistance of the causative organism necessitates the use of a parenteral antimicrobial agent.[19]

Antimicrobial therapy is finished when the prescribed course is completed, there are no physical examination findings suggesting inflammation, and inflammatory markers have normalized. Compliance can be challenging, particularly once the patient is no longer having active symptoms. To maximize outcomes, education of the parents and patient (when appropriate) regarding the importance of completing the full treatment course is essential.

If, at the completion of the planned antibiotic course of treatment, physical examination findings of inflammation persist, or if inflammatory indices remain elevated, antibiotic treatment should be continued with clinical and laboratory reassessment every 1 to 2 weeks until examination and laboratory findings normalize. If there is not a trend toward improvement, consideration should be given to evaluating the patient for a residual focus of infection (such as an abscess or sequestrum), which may be preventing resolution of the infection. Failure to improve or resolve the inflammatory indices is a sign of treatment failure, and the clinician should consider repeat MRI and possible repeat incision and débridement with new culture acquisition to ensure that the initially selected antibiotic remains the correct choice.[3]

Children receiving vancomycin for serious MRSA infections should have laboratory monitoring of vancomycin trough and serum creatinine levels assessed on a periodic basis. Some antibiotics, such as clindamycin, have excellent oral bioavailability and do not require routine serum concentration monitoring.[19]

Surgical Intervention

There is a dearth of evidence guiding the indications and methods for surgical intervention for children with osteomyelitis.[7,8] The clinician should consider whether surgery is indicated for children with osteomyelitis on the basis of clinical, laboratory, and imaging data. Although there is no clear guidance in the literature on this subject, surgery is generally indicated for children with osteomyelitis who demonstrate hemodynamic compromise consistent with septic shock or whose imaging studies have revealed findings consistent with a drainable abscess or abscesses (intraosseous, subperiosteal, or extraperiosteal) that will not likely resolve with antibiotic treatment alone[7,8] (**Figure 3**). Evidence suggests that, in children with osteomyelitis, the severity of illness at presentation is significantly associated with the occurrence of repeat surgery.[8,14] Children who have mild illness appear to do well without surgery, whereas children with severe illness (characterized by markedly elevated inflammatory markers; recurring febrile days on antibiotics; and evident disseminated disease, including deep vein thrombosis, septic pulmonary emboli, or pneumonia) appear to benefit from surgery and may even require more than one surgical procedure to resolve the infection.[8] In the era of MRSA, there appears to be a higher incidence of abscess formation, which may be responsible for a higher rate of surgical intervention for children with osteomyelitis.[10,14-16]

The literature also lacks evidence as to which surgical procedure or procedures to perform for osteomyelitis. Choices for the surgical treatment of osteomyelitis include drainage of subperiosteal abscesses; drilling of the bone; and incision of bone cortex, with irrigation and débridement of infected cancellous bone. Surgical decompression of infected bone has the potential benefit of reducing intraosseous pressure that may result in diminished perfusion and antibiotic delivery to the site of infection. In all drainage procedures, care should be taken to avoid injury to the epiphyseal plate and perichondrial ring. Surgical approach planning should incorporate a review of advanced imaging to account for all relevant foci of infection. Adjacent or contiguous abscess should be drained at the time of bone decompression. Involvement of adjacent joints in children with acute osteomyelitis may occur at a higher rate than initially anticipated.[1,17,19] Recent studies suggest methods to help anticipate contiguous disease.[17-19,22]

Repeat Surgery

If the child does not demonstrate satisfactory clinical or laboratory improvement within a few days of the initial surgical débridement, consideration should be given to repeat irrigation and débridement. Additional imaging is of limited use at this time unless a previously unaddressed focus of infection is suspected. Caution should be exercised in interpreting postoperative MRI scans, which will often appear to show a worsening condition as the infection progresses through its normal course.[3]

CHRONIC RECURRENT MULTIFOCAL OSTEOMYELITIS

Evaluation

Chronic recurrent multifocal osteomyelitis (CRMO) or chronic nonbacterial osteomyelitis is a self-limiting disease of variable course and location. Although poorly understood, a genetic predisposition is hypothesized.[23] CRMO presents primarily in late childhood and adolescence with a female to male ratio of 4:1. Initial presentation ranges from mild conditions to severe acute conditions with chronic pain and swelling of the involved area. CRMO may be associated with other inflammatory diseases.[24,25] The diagnosis of CRMO is based on the history and physical examination, radiographic, and laboratory findings. Compared with children with acute bacterial osteomyelitis, children with CRMO present with a more gradual onset, often with pain relieved by NSAIDs, and without a history of systemic infection or symptoms (such as fever). Although the ESR is often mildly elevated at presentation, both the ESR and the CRP levels are inconsistent and do not correlate with the initial clinical presentation or with the clinical course.[24,25] Children with CRMO typically have normal white blood cell (WBC) counts and, importantly, multiple bone lesions are typically seen on imaging studies. Management for some patients involves biopsy, débridement, obtaining cultures, and irrigation of the surgical field. Pathologic assessment of biopsy specimens typically shows chronic fibrotic and inflammatory changes, and cultures in patients with CRMO are generally sterile. Making a diagnosis of CRMO is challenging, and it is a diagnosis of exclusion.

Management

Management of CRMO is challenging. Because of the difficulty in distinguishing CRMO from acute osteomyelitis, most patients receive a trial of antibiotic therapy. Importantly, pain in patients with CRMO generally responds well to NSAIDs, activity modification, and immobilization. Management may require methotrexate or other biologic medications.

SEPTIC ARTHRITIS

Evaluation

Neonates are at high risk of musculoskeletal infection from community-acquired and hospital-acquired pathogens. *Streptococcus agalactiae* (group B streptococcus) and Enterobacteriaceae bacteria may be transmitted to the newborn in the peripartum period and lead to invasive infection in otherwise healthy neonates who typically go home with family, but in whom signs and symptoms of infection develop within weeks or months after birth. In comparison, premature infants in the neonatal intensive care unit are frequently exposed to invasive lines and catheters, which leads to a high risk for neonatal infections due to hospital-acquired pathogens, including MRSA; multidrug-resistant gram-negative rods; and *Candida* species, most often *Candida albicans* and *Candida parapsilosis*.

The immature immune system of neonates may result in an atypical presentation, such as lack of fever or normal inflammatory markers and less-than-expected pain. Neonates with musculoskeletal infections often present with pseudoparalysis as the only sign. After one site of musculoskeletal infection is found, a diligent search for other sites is indicated (perhaps including ultrasonography or other imaging given the difficulty of a physical examination) because up to 40% of neonates have multifocal musculoskeletal infections. However, with the rise of protocol-driven, evidence-based care in neonatal intensive care units, there has been a decline in occurrence of widely disseminated neonatal infections leading to devastating osteonecrosis. This may be due to the early administration of broad-spectrum antibiotics at the first sign of vital sign or feeding irregularity suggestive of evolving sepsis.

At all ages past early infancy, the most common cause of musculoskeletal infection is *S aureus*;[1,7,18] however, it should be noted that septic arthritis caused by *K kingae* is common in children 6 months to 4 years of age. Septic arthritis caused by *Streptococcus pneumoniae* or *Haemophilus influenzae* type b is still occasionally seen despite the widespread immunization efforts that had markedly minimized the occurrence. Most frequently these infections occur in unimmunized children, but these infections may also be caused by nonvaccine serotypes in fully immunized children due to the major genetic recombinations, which lead to serotype shifts among clinical isolates.[18,26-29]

A challenge in the assessment of children with suspected septic arthritis is recognition of the risk factors for and clinical features of osteomyelitis in the adjacent bones. The pathophysiology of concurrent infections of bone and joint are incompletely understood. It has been theorized that there are vascular channels that traverse the physis in neonates and remain open until approximately 18 months of age. Beyond that age group, it is surmised that bacteria enter the metaphyseal circulation and then leave the bloodstream in the area adjacent to the physis where the circulatory pattern makes a 180° turn. Because the blood vessels in that area are relatively more permeable and the blood flow is more sluggish, a permissive environment for bacterial seeding is created.

The role of minor trauma preceding the event of infection has been identified as a trend in some children, but most of these infections appear to evolve spontaneously.[30] Joints with intracapsular metaphysis, such as the proximal humerus and proximal femur, are most susceptible to the development of adjacent osteomyelitis. To evaluate young children with septic arthritis and possible adjacent osteomyelitis, advanced imaging should be considered.[17,31,32] However, in the specific case of septic arthritis of the hip, advanced imaging after ultrasonograpic assessment may be less valuable.[22]

To make a diagnosis of septic arthritis in children, clinicians often use supplemental laboratory tests, including nucleated cell count and differential of the joint fluid, peripheral WBC count, serum ESR, and serum CRP level.[33] Joint fluid samples from children with septic arthritis often have cell counts greater than 40,000 nucleated cells/mL, of which more than 75% are neutrophils. Children with infected joints typically have elevated peripheral WBC counts greater than 12,000 cells/mL, serum CRP levels greater than 2 mg/dL, and an initial ESR greater than 40 mm/hr. Improvements in these inflammatory markers after surgery and antibiotic administration support a diagnosis of acute septic arthritis.

Confirmation of the diagnosis of septic arthritis is also challenging because of the low rate of successful bacterial isolation from joint fluid. One recent study of children who had suspected septic arthritis based on clinical findings reported a positive culture rate of only 35%.[18] Because it is sufficiently difficult to grow bacteria from joint fluid, supplemental methods may be used.[26,31,34] An exciting, relatively new but increasingly available option is polymerase chain reaction (PCR) testing. PCR testing has increased sensitivity and specificity in identification of organisms infecting joints by amplifying bacterial DNA sequences in joint fluid being investigated. Because this method is currently experimental, PCR assessment of joint fluid is neither standardized nor widely available.[26,27]

Surgical Treatment

Septic arthritis may be treated surgically with either arthrotomy or arthroscopy, depending on the surgeon's level of comfort with these techniques.[29] Arthroscopic drainage has been found to be safe and effective in a wide variety of joints, including the hip, knee, ankle, shoulder, elbow, and wrist. Minimal soft-tissue disruption, a shorter hospital stay, and improved visualization of the joint space are reported as potential advantages of arthroscopy.[35]

Advanced imaging may be required if expected clinical and laboratory improvements are not demonstrated within the first 3 to 4 days after joint irrigation and drainage.[22] Particularly for presumed septic arthritis of the hip, pericapsular pyomyositis may mimic the classic clinical presentation of hip sepsis and should be suspected. In children in whom expected clinical and laboratory improvements are not seen, advanced imaging with MRI should be considered to identify any contiguous osteomyelitis or abscess.[32,36] Recognition of contiguous osteomyelitis in patients with septic arthritis is particularly important for patients with pyarthrosis, especially in joints where the metaphysis is predominantly intracapsular, such as the shoulder or the hip.

In children who are initially suspected to have septic arthritis, a few may have symptoms that evolve in a manner that suggests other disease processes, including inflammatory and reactive conditions, despite an initial impression that appeared to be that of infection. Children who are culture and/or PCR negative and lack substantial clinical or laboratory improvement despite appropriate surgical and antibiotic management may require additional evaluation and referral to rheumatology. Similarly, other noninfectious etiologies, such as leukemia, might be considered if anemia, thrombocytopenia, leukopenia, or leukocytosis with blasts is discovered with a complete blood count and differential.

Antibiotic Treatment

For most children with proven or suspected septic arthritis, therapy is initiated with appropriate empiric parenteral antibiotics. General coverage should include *S aureus* with consideration of extended coverage based on age-at-risk categories. For example, children in the *K kingae* age group should also be covered empirically with ceftriaxone, which is effective against the common pathogens identified in this age group. After culture results are obtained and there is a demonstrable decline in systemic inflammatory markers (eg, CRP level and ESR), patients may be transitioned to high-dose oral antibiotics.[37] If the patient evaluation suggests that the infection is isolated septic arthritis, antibiotics are typically given for 2 to 3 weeks. If there is concern for adjacent osteomyelitis, because of either the patient's young age or radiographic findings, a longer course of antibiotic therapy, often 4 to 8 weeks, is recommended.

LYME ARTHRITIS IN CHILDREN

Lyme arthritis may be difficult to differentiate from acute septic arthritis in children.[38-40] One study reported that there were no substantial differences in the synovial fluid WBC count, absolute neutrophil count, and percentage of segmented neutrophils in children with proven septic arthritis caused by pyogenic bacteria and children presenting with acute knee monoarthritis in Lyme-endemic areas.[38] It was also found that no child with a peripheral absolute neutrophil count of less than 10,000 cells/mL and an ESR of less than 40 mm/hr had septic arthritis.[39] In Lyme-endemic areas, the presentation of a child with an acutely swollen knee is more likely to be Lyme arthritis than bacterial septic arthritis.[40]

Lyme arthritis in children has an excellent prognosis after oral antibiotic treatment for approximately 4 weeks. Children with antibiotic-refractory disease respond well to NSAIDs, intra-articular steroid injection, or immunemodulatory drugs. Chronic arthritis, joint deformities, and recurrent infection usually do not develop in children with Lyme arthritis.

PYOMYOSITIS

Primary muscle infections are less common than infections of bones or joints. Children with suspected pyomyositis should be evaluated urgently for bacteremia (in children with pyomyositis, the rate of initial bacteremia is approximately 15%)[18] and for compartment syndrome. When an abscess develops within the muscle, surgical drainage is often needed for timely resolution. MRI is often helpful for the definitive diagnosis of pyomyositis and the assessment for surgical intervention. The identification of pyomyositis as a contiguous process related to adjacent osteomyelitis or septic arthritis is often challenging. Careful evaluation of MRI to look for substantial intramuscular inflammation is necessary and sufficient to make a diagnosis of pyomyositis.

SUMMARY

Children with musculoskeletal infections require careful evaluation to determine the specific diagnoses, relative severity of illness, and appropriate treatment. Although bone, joint, and muscle infections are common, it is important to consider other conditions that might mimic the diverse clinical and laboratory presentations of bone, joint, and deep soft-tissue infections. Evidence-based clinical pathways, improved communication between members of the healthcare team, and coordination of care can improve short-term and intermediate-term clinical outcomes and reduce the length of hospital stay. Such evidence-based clinical practice guidelines are now emerging and merit clinical and economic evaluation.

KEY STUDY POINTS

- Clinical and laboratory parameters appear to correlate with severity of illness and permit objective differentiation of children with acute hematogenous osteomyelitis who may be separated chronologically, geographically, or therapeutically.
- Clinical practice guidelines or pathways may be implemented in large pediatric medical centers and lead to better short-term and intermediate-term outcomes.
- Improved use of MRI with sedation through a careful pre-MRI evaluation and interdisciplinary communication results in shortened MRI duration, a reduced rate of preliminary scanning, and a shortened period of hospitalization.
- A team approach using the expertise, when available, of infectious disease and other medical services, with primary guidance by the pediatric orthopaedic surgeon, can better tailor treatments and improve outcomes.

ANNOTATED REFERENCES

1. Gafur OA, Copley LA, Hollmig ST, Browne RH, Thornton LA, Crawford SE: The impact of the current epidemiology of pediatric musculoskeletal infection on evaluation and treatment guidelines. *J Pediatr Orthop* 2008;28(7):777-785.
2. Copley LA, Kinsler MA, Gheen T, Shar A, Sun D, Browne R: The impact of evidence-based clinical practice guidelines applied by a multidisciplinary team for the care of children with osteomyelitis. *J Bone Joint Surg Am* 2013;95(8):686-693.
3. Mueller AJ, Kwon JK, Steiner JW, et al: Improved magnetic resonance imaging utilization for children with musculoskeletal infection. *J Bone Joint Surg Am* 2015;97(22):1869-1876.
4. Ojeaga PO, Hammer MR, Lindsay EA, Tareen NG, Jo CH, Copley LA: Quality improvement of magnetic resonance imaging for musculoskeletal infection in children results in decreased scan duration and decreased contrast use. *J Bone Joint Surg Am* 2019;101:1679-1688.

   The study illustrates the benefit of collaborative interdisciplinary communication and workflow redesign implemented through a continuous process improvement endeavor. The number of scan sequences, scan duration, anesthesia duration, and contrast use have been reduced progressively over a 6-year time frame. In the final 6 months of the study, average scan duration was 24.4 minutes and only 8.5% of children received contrast agents. Level of evidence: IV.
5. Jagodzinski NA, Kanwar R, Graham K, Bache CE: Prospective evaluation of a shortened regimen of treatment for acute osteomyelitis and septic arthritis in children. *J Pediatr Orthop* 2009;29(5):518-525.
6. Keren R, Shah SS, Srivastava R, et al, Pediatric Research in Inpatient Settings Network: Comparative effectiveness of intravenous vs oral antibiotics for post discharge treatment of acute osteomyelitis in children. *JAMA Pediatr* 2015;169(2):120-128.
7. Street M, Puna R, Huang M, Crawford H: Pediatric acute hematogenous osteomyelitis. *J Pediatr Orthop* 2015;35(6):634-639.
8. Tuason DA, Gheen T, Sun D, Huang R, Copley L: Clinical and laboratory parameters associated with multiple surgeries in children with acute hematogenous osteomyelitis. *J Pediatr Orthop* 2014;34(5):565-570.
9. Menge TJ, Cole HA, Mignemi ME, et al: Medial approach for drainage of the obturator musculature in children. *J Pediatr Orthop* 2014;34(3):307-315.
10. Ju KL, Zurakowski D, Kocher MS: Differentiating between methicillin-resistant and methicillin-sensitive Staphylococcus aureus osteomyelitis in children: An evidence-based clinical prediction algorithm. *J Bone Joint Surg Am* 2011;93(18):1693-1701.
11. Wade Shrader M, Nowlin M, Segal LS: Independent analysis of a clinical predictive algorithm to identify methicillin-resistant *Staphylococcus aureus* osteomyelitis in children. *J Pediatr Orthop* 2013;33(7):759-762.
12. Saavedra-Lozano J, Mejías A, Ahmad N, et al: Changing trends in acute osteomyelitis in children: Impact of methicillin-resistant Staphylococcus aureus infections. *J Pediatr Orthop* 2008;28(5):569-575.
13. Peltola H, Pääkkönen M, Kallio P, Kallio MJ, Osteomyelitis-Septic Arthritis Study Group: Short- versus long-term antimicrobial treatment for acute hematogenous osteomyelitis of childhood: Prospective, randomized trial on 131 culture-positive cases. *Pediatr Infect Dis J* 2010;29(12):1123-1128.
14. Sarkissian EJ, Gans I, Gunderson MA, Myers SH, Spiegel DA, Flynn JM: Community-acquired methicillin-resistant Staphylococcus aureus musculoskeletal infections: Emerging trends over the past decade. *J Pediatr Orthop* 2016;36(3):323-327.

    The authors report a threefold increase in community-acquired MRSA musculoskeletal infections. These infections were associated with a higher incidence of complications during inpatient management, with multiple surgical procedures, and longer inpatient hospitalization. Level of evidence: II.
15. Copley LA, Barton T, Garcia C, et al: A proposed scoring system for assessment of severity of illness in pediatric acute hematogenous osteomyelitis using objective clinical and laboratory findings. *Pediatr Infect Dis J* 2014;33(1):35-41.
16. Hawkshead JJ III, Patel NB, Steele RW, Heinrich SD: Comparative severity of pediatric osteomyelitis attributable to methicillin-resistant versus methicillin-sensitive *Staphylococcus aureus*. *J Pediatr Orthop* 2009;29(1):85-90.
17. Ligon JA, Journeycake JM, Josephs SC, Tareen NG, Lindsay EA, Copley LAB: Differentiation of deep venous thrombosis among children with or without osteomyelitis. *J Pediatr Orthop* 2018;38(10):e597-e603. doi:10.1097/BPO.0000000000001240.

    This study reports on 28 children with osteomyelitis and deep vein thrombosis and compares this cohort with children with deep vein thrombosis but without osteomyelitis and children with osteomyelitis but without deep vein thrombosis. The cohorts were significantly differentiated by severity of illness and comorbidities, which allow pattern recognition to expedite recognition of the cohort at risk. Level of evidence: II.
18. Vorhies JS, Lindsay EA, Tareen NG, Kellum RJ, Jo CH, Copley LA: Severity adjusted risk of long-term adverse sequelae among children with osteomyelitis. *Pediatr Infect Dis J* 2019;38:26-31.

    This study consecutively enrolled 195 children with osteomyelitis and followed up 139 (71.3%) for 2 to 5 years (average 2.5), finding that the initial severity of illness score significantly differentiated children at the greatest risk for long-term adverse outcomes. Children with high severity of illness scores (8 to 10) had a 32.0% rate of osteonecrosis, chondrolysis, deformity, or limb-length inequality. Level of evidence: II.
19. Erickson CM, Sue PK, Stewart K, et al: Sequential parenteral to oral clindamycin dosing in pediatric musculoskeletal infection. *Pediatr Infect Dis J* 2016;35:1092-1096.

This study illustrated that oral dosing of clindamycin at 30 mg/kg/ per day was effective for children with musculoskeletal infection in an MRSA-prevalent community. Level of evidence: III.

20. Schreckenberger PC, Llendo E, Ristow KL: Incidence of constitutive and inducible clindamycin resistance in *Staphylococcus aureus* and coagulase-negative staphylococci in a community and a tertiary care hospital. *J Clin Microbiol* 2004;42(6):2777-2779.
21. Zaoutis T, Localio AR, Leckerman K, Saddlemire S, Bertoch D, Keren R: Prolonged intravenous therapy versus early transition to oral antimicrobial therapy for acute osteomyelitis in children. *Pediatrics* 2009;123(2):636-642.
22. Laine JC, Denning JR, Riccio AI, Jo C, Joglar JM, Wimberly RL: The use of ultrasound in the management of septic arthritis of the hip. *J Pediatr Orthop B* 2015;24(2):95-98.
23. Golla A, Jansson A, Ramser J, et al: Chronic recurrent multifocal osteomyelitis (CRMO): Evidence for a susceptibility gene located on chromosome 18q21.3-18q22. *Eur J Hum Genet* 2002;10(3):217-221.
24. Huber AM, Lam PY, Duffy CM, et al: Chronic recurrent multifocal osteomyelitis: Clinical outcomes after more than five years of follow-up. *J Pediatr* 2002;141(2):198-203.
25. Kaiser D, Bolt I, Hofer M, et al: Chronic nonbacterial osteomyelitis in children: A retrospective multicenter study. *Pediatr Rheumatol Online J* 2015;13:25.
26. Carter K, Doern C, Jo CH, Copley LA: The clinical usefulness of polymerase chain reaction as a supplemental diagnostic tool in the evaluation and the treatment of children with septic arthritis. *J Pediatr Orthop* 2016;36(2):167-172.

    PCR was found to be a useful tool to supplement blood and joint fluid culture findings and improve the rate of positive identification of a causative bacterial organism among children with septic arthritis. Level of evidence: II.
27. Williams N, Cooper C, Cundy P: Kingella kingae septic arthritis in children: Recognizing an elusive pathogen. *J Child Orthop* 2014;8(1):91-95.
28. Basmaci R, Lorrot M, Bidet P, et al: Comparison of clinical and biologic features of *Kingella kingae* and *Staphylococcus aureus* arthritis at initial evaluation. *Pediatr Infect Dis J* 2011;30(10):902-904.
29. Ceroni D, Belaieff W, Cherkaoui A, et al: Primary epiphyseal or apophyseal subacute osteomyelitis in the pediatric population: A report of fourteen cases and a systematic review of the literature. *J Bone Joint Surg Am* 2014;96(18):1570-1575.
30. Morrissy RT, Haynes DW: Acute hematogenous osteomyelitis: A model with trauma as an etiology. *J Pediatr Orthop* 1989;9(4):447-456.
31. Montgomery CO, Siegel E, Blasier RD, Suva LJ: Concurrent septic arthritis and osteomyelitis in children. *J Pediatr Orthop* 2013;33(4):464-467.
32. Rosenfeld S, Bernstein DT, Daram S, Dawson J, Zhang W: Predicting the presence of adjacent infections in septic arthritis in children. *J Pediatr Orthop* 2016;36(1):70-74.

    Patient age, CRP level, duration of symptoms, platelet count, and absolute neutrophil count were found to provide guidance for determining the probability of contiguous disease. Patients with multiple risk factors should have a preoperative MRI. Level of evidence: III.
33. Caird MS, Flynn JM, Leung YL, Millman JE, D'Italia JG, Dormans JP: Factors distinguishing septic arthritis from transient synovitis of the hip in children. A prospective study. *J Bone Joint Surg Am* 2006;88(6):1251-1257.
34. Section J, Gibbons SD, Barton T, Greenberg DE, Jo CH, Copley LA: Microbiological culture methods for pediatric musculoskeletal infection: A guideline for optimal use. *J Bone Joint Surg Am* 2015;97(6):441-449.
35. Thompson RM, Gourineni P: Arthroscopic treatment of septic arthritis in very young children. *J Pediatr Orthop* 2017;37(1):e53-e57.

    A single portal inflow and outflow arthroscopic technique was shown to be safe and effective in a series of 24 children aged 3 weeks to 6 years. In addition, the technique allowed improved joint visualization and minimal soft-tissue dissection. Level of evidence: IV.
36. Monsalve J, Kan JH, Schallert EK, Bisset GS, Zhang W, Rosenfeld SB: Septic arthritis in children: Frequency of coexisting unsuspected osteomyelitis and implications on imaging work-up and management. *AJR Am J Roentgenol* 2015;204(6):1289-1295.
37. Chou AC, Mahadev A: The use of C-reactive protein as a guide for transitioning to oral antibiotics in pediatric osteoarticular infections. *J Pediatr Orthop* 2016;36(2):173-177.

    Conversion to oral antibiotic therapy and hospital discharge was guided by the combination of clinical improvement with a specific reduction in CRP level by 50% over 4 days. A persistently elevated CRP level was associated with adverse outcomes. Level of evidence: IV.
38. Deanehan JK, Nigrovic PA, Milewski MD, et al: Synovial fluid findings in children with knee monoarthritis in Lyme disease endemic areas. *Pediatr Emerg Care* 2014;30(1):16-19.
39. Deanehan JK, Kimia AA, Tan Tanny SP, et al: Distinguishing Lyme from septic knee monoarthritis in Lyme disease-endemic areas. *Pediatrics* 2013;131(3):e695-e701.
40. Tory HO, Zurakowski D, Sundel RP: Outcomes of children treated for Lyme arthritis: Results of a large pediatric cohort. *J Rheumatol* 2010;37(5):1049-1055.

CHAPTER 5

Benign and Malignant Musculoskeletal Neoplasms

MIHIR M. THACKER, MD • ALEXANDRE ARKADER, MD

ABSTRACT

Malignant bone and soft-tissue tumors in children are far less common than benign lesions. Most orthopaedic surgeons, as well as primary care practitioners, are frequently unfamiliar with these conditions. This can lead to inappropriate workup, delayed diagnoses, and, in some instances, improper initial treatment. It is helpful to be familiar with the principles of clinical and imaging evaluations of bone and soft-tissue lesions in children, along with the genetic syndromes that predispose children to tumor development. It is important to be knowledgeable about recent advances for imaging and treatment of the most common benign and malignant tumors in children.

Keywords: benign lesion; bone tumor; Ewing sarcoma; malignant tumor; osteosarcoma; rhabdomyosarcoma; sarcoma; soft-tissue tumor

INTRODUCTION

Cancer is the main cause of death from disease during childhood. Fortunately, most bone and soft-tissue tumors in children are benign. The correct and prompt diagnosis of these lesions can be challenging, leading to unnecessary stress and anxiety for families and patients. Understanding the steps in making a diagnosis and managing this broad group of conditions may allow early appropriate treatment, improving the child's prognosis and outcome.

The principles of approaching bone and soft-tissue lesions in children and the most common genetic syndromes that predispose children to the development of tumors are discussed. It is important to be knowledgeable about the recent advances in the management and prognosis for the most common benign and malignant lesions.

Dr. Arkader has received royalties from OrthoPediatrics; serves as a paid consultant to or is an employee of Clementia and OrthoPediatrics; and serves as a board member, owner, officer, or committee member of the Pediatric Orthopaedic Society of North America. Neither Dr. Thacker nor any immediate family member has received anything of value from or has stock or stock options held in a commercial company or institution related directly or indirectly to the subject of this article.

GENETIC SYNDROMES WITH AN INCREASED RISK FOR NEOPLASIA

Li-Fraumeni Syndrome

Li-Fraumeni syndrome is a rare autosomal dominant familial disorder that increases the risk for the development of several types of cancer, particularly in children and young adults. The hallmark of the syndrome is germline alterations of the *TP53* tumor suppressor gene; however, a smaller percentage of patients have inactivation of the *CHEK2* suppressor gene. Up to 10% of children with sporadic rhabdomyosarcoma or osteosarcoma carry germline *TP53* mutations; clinically, these patients tend to be younger and have poorer outcomes.[1]

The increased availability of next-generation sequencing and multigene panel testing has resulted in more frequent TP53 testing of families that do not meet classic clinical criteria. Patients with TP53+ by multigene panel testing do not tend to match the classic Li-Fraumeni criteria and are older at cancer presentation. These advances may lead to better understanding on the genetic basis of this syndrome.[2]

Beckwith-Wiedemann Syndrome

Beckwith-Wiedemann syndrome is a rare congenital overgrowth syndrome, with an incidence of 1 in 14,000 births. It occurs predominantly with a sporadic inheritance pattern; however, autosomal dominance with variable expression is possible. The responsible gene is located at 11p15.5, and the risk of recurrence in the same family is as high as 20%.

A diagnosis is usually made after birth based on the clinical features, including neonatal hypoglycemia and accelerated bone maturation, which is demonstrated by gigantism, metaphyseal flaring, and narrowing of the diaphysis. Patients may also present with craniofacial features, renal/endocrine involvement, abdominal wall defects, polycythemia, and cardiovascular anomalies. There is an increased risk of malignancy, particularly for embryonal tumors such as Wilms tumor, hepatoblastoma, rhabdomyosarcoma, and neuroblastoma.[3] The risk of malignancy may be associated to the specific genotype, and therefore recommendations regarding surveillance may need to be tailored on a patient-to-patient basis. Generally, surveillance is done with serial ultrasonography of the pelvis and abdomen at 3- to 4-month intervals for the first 5 years of life and alpha-fetoprotein measurements.[4]

McCune-Albright Syndrome

McCune-Albright syndrome is characterized by the classic triad of polyostotic fibrous dysplasia, café au lait spots, and endocrinopathies (precocious puberty being the most common).

The etiology of fibrous dysplasia has been linked to an activating mutation in the *GNAS* gene (located on 20q13.2-13.3) that encodes the Gsα protein. The result is failure of maturation from woven to lamellar bone, with a subsequent decrease in the mechanical strength of the affected bone; this leads to pain, fractures, and angular deformities.

The polyostotic form of this syndrome is less common but more severe, has the tendency to involve one side more severely, and causes deformities and limb-length discrepancies. Any bone may be involved, and craniofacial involvement occurs in 50% of patients.

The risk of malignant degeneration with monostotic fibrous dysplasia ranges from 0.5% to up to 6%, with higher incidence among children with polyostotic disease, McCune-Albright syndrome, or Mazabraud syndrome (fibrous dysplasia associated with intramuscular myxomas), most commonly to osteosarcoma, fibrosarcoma, chondrosarcoma, and malignant fibrous histiocytoma. Malignant degeneration should be suspected if there is an increase in pain and a radiographically detected interval growth of the lesion, especially with a new associated soft-tissue mass. The average age for malignant degeneration is in the fourth decade.[5]

Ollier Disease and Maffucci Syndrome

Both Ollier disease and Maffucci syndrome represent a spectrum of the same disease and are characterized by the presence of multiple enchondromas, typically in a unilateral pattern and associated with deformities. There is no evidence of a hereditary component, and the conditions affect both sexes and all races.

The risk of malignant degeneration with Ollier disease is approximately 5% to 30% by age 40 years (the risk of malignant degeneration of a solitary enchondroma is 1% or less). Increased growth of a lesion that is associated with pain is a cause for suspicion, especially in skeletally mature patients. Although no consensus exists on the best method to monitor these lesions, it is generally agreed that MRI is the first modality that should be used. Bone scans and positron emission tomography (PET) can be used to assess the level of activity within the lesion, but false positivity is an issue.[6]

The association of multiple enchondromas and multiple hemangiomas involving the soft tissues and other viscera characterizes Maffucci syndrome. This condition presents with a higher risk for malignant degeneration (approximately 50%; most commonly into chondrosarcoma or angiosarcoma), particularly among pelvic lesions.[6]

Multiple Hereditary Exostoses

Multiple hereditary exostosis is an autosomal dominant condition with a 96% penetrance rate. There are two main genes linked to the disease: *EXT1* located on 8q24.1 (responsible for approximately 50% of the cases) and *EXT2* located on 11p13 (seen in 30% of the patients). Both genes are suppressor genes that are responsible for regulating chondrocyte maturation and differentiation and are absent in this condition.

Clinical features include multiple osteochondromas, short stature, angular deformities, pain, and limited motion. The rate of secondary malignant degeneration has been reported ranging from 1% to 20% depending on the series (most recently 2.7%) and occurs after the third decade of life. Lesions in the axial skeleton more frequently become malignant.[7]

Screening for possible malignant degeneration should be performed on a case-by-case basis. Enlarged lesions seen after skeletal maturity should raise suspicion and should be screened with MRI. A cartilaginous cap larger than 2 cm in adults is highly suspicious for malignancy, and lesion excision is generally recommended.[8]

Hereditary Retinoblastoma

Retinoblastoma is a malignant tumor of the embryonic neural retina and is the most common intraocular malignancy in children with an annual incidence of 1 in 18,000 live births per year. The hereditary form (40% of all patients) is caused by heterozygous germline mutation in the *Rb1* suppressor gene and is usually bilaterally involved. In 10% of patients, there is a family history of retinoblastoma.

These children have high risk of second primary malignancy (up to 50%), including osteosarcoma and soft-tissue sarcomas, among others.[9,10]

PATIENT WORKUP

Imaging

After a thorough clinical evaluation has been completed, imaging modalities are critical for further workup of patients with bone and soft-tissue tumors. Plain radiographs are the best diagnostic imaging modality to establish a differential diagnosis for bone tumors and may be diagnostic in many instances (**Table 1**). The clinician should evaluate the anatomic location of the lesion (eg, which bone and which part of the bone), the zone of transition, the mineralization pattern, and the presence or absence of a soft-tissue extension. Radiographs of soft-tissue masses may reveal the presence of phleboliths (in a vascular malformation), extrinsic compression of the bone (in slow-growing lesions), or bone invasion (in aggressive lesions). Ultrasonography is extremely useful for differentiating between solid and cystic lesions, as well as for the evaluation of vascular lesions. Bone scans are essential for staging malignant bone lesions (such as osteosarcoma and Ewing sarcoma) and also for the evaluation of metastatic disease.

MRI has become standard for the diagnosis and evaluation of the local extent of most bone and soft-tissue lesions (with the notable exception of osteoid osteomas, which are better evaluated with a fine-cut CT scan). Full-body MRI is being increasingly used for screening in infantile myofibromatosis and Langerhans cell histiocytosis, and its use is being evaluated in soft-tissue sarcomas, although it is not as reliable as CT in detecting pulmonary metastases. Full-body MRI seems to be better for detecting lymph node and osseous involvement.

The role of PET continues to evolve. It has become standard in the staging of lymphomas and melanomas (in adults). PET scans are being used with increasing frequency to stage other tumors and predict the response to chemotherapy (potentially guiding the selection of proper margins of resection). PET is also being used to

TABLE 1

Differential Diagnoses of Bone Lesions

		Single Lesion		Multiple Lesions
Where is it?	Epiphysis	Chondroblastoma, GCT, clear cell CHSA, Brodie abscess, Trevor disease (DEH)	Osseous	Bone islands (osteopoikilosis), melorheostosis, multifocal osteosarcoma
	Metaphysis	Most tumors		
	Diaphysis	Fibrous dysplasia, Ewing sarcoma, osteofibrous dysplasia/adamantinoma, LCH, leukemia/lymphoma, osteoid osteoma		
What is it doing to the bone?	Sclerotic	—	Chondroid	Multiple osteochondromatosis, Trevor disease (DEH), Ollier disease, Maffucci syndrome
	Lucent			
What is the bone doing to it?	Zone of transition (margin)	Biologic behavior: narrow/geographic, less aggressive	Fibrous	Polyostotic fibrous dysplasia, multiple NOFs
	Periosteal reaction	Onion skin, sunburst, buttress type (solid)		
Is there any identifiable matrix mineralization pattern?	Cloudlike	Osseous	Miscellaneous	LCH, leukemia, lymphoma, brown tumors
	Rings, arcs, stipples	Chondroid		
	Ground glass	Fibro-osseous		

CHSA = chondrosarcoma, DEH = dysplasia epiphysealis hemimelica, GCT = giant cell tumor, LCH = Langerhans cell histiocytosis, NOF = nonossifying fibroma try to differentiate between plexiform neurofibromas and malignant peripheral nerve sheath tumors, although PET has higher sensitivity than specificity in this setting.

Imaging is nonspecific for soft-tissue tumors (except for lipomas, which can be reliably diagnosed on MRI), and biopsy becomes more critical in establishing a definitive diagnosis.

Biopsy Principles

Biopsy is an essential step in the diagnosis of many bone and soft-tissue lesions; however, there are risks associated with inappropriately performed biopsies. The Musculoskeletal Tumor Society has reported that biopsy has an 18% rate of diagnostic error and a 19% complication rate.[11] The definitive surgical procedure often needs to be modified as a result of an inappropriately performed biopsy, which can lead to a more complex resection and sometimes amputation (**Figure 1**). Biopsy-related complications are five times more common when the procedure is performed at a community or referring hospital compared with a tertiary care center.

Controversy still persists regarding the optimal biopsy modality. Core biopsy has a lower risk of contamination and cost compared with open incisional biopsy. The use of image guidance increases the accuracy of percutaneous biopsies, while reducing the risk of complications.[12]

For bone biopsy, planning should take into consideration the definitive surgery and the presence of a soft-tissue mass that may be more accessible than the bone. In general, for a soft-tissue biopsy, the most direct approach to the tumor is the preferred strategy.

Other strategies while planning a biopsy include reviewing the optimal location with the pathologist and radiologist because, in some instances, a second, more accessible lesion can be identified. For open biopsy, a longitudinal incision should be made without raising flaps. Meticulous homeostasis is essential to prevent the spread of tumor cells, thus limiting the size of the eventual resection to obtain clean margins. Obtaining an intraoperative frozen section is important to ensure adequate sampling, and specimens also should be sent for culture. Biopsy principles are outlined in **Table 2**. Routine use of immunohistochemistry has made it much easier to identify and classify tumors. The detection of specific mutations within tumor cells may determine the prognosis and even help target-specific treatments.

BENIGN BONE TUMORS

Benign bone tumors are very common and most frequently discovered incidentally. It is important for the evaluating physician to be familiar with the pathogenesis and prognosis for each skeletal lesion to guide the workup and treatment. The treatment of benign bone lesions depends on the natural history of the lesion, the risk of tumor progression, the risk of pathologic fracture, and

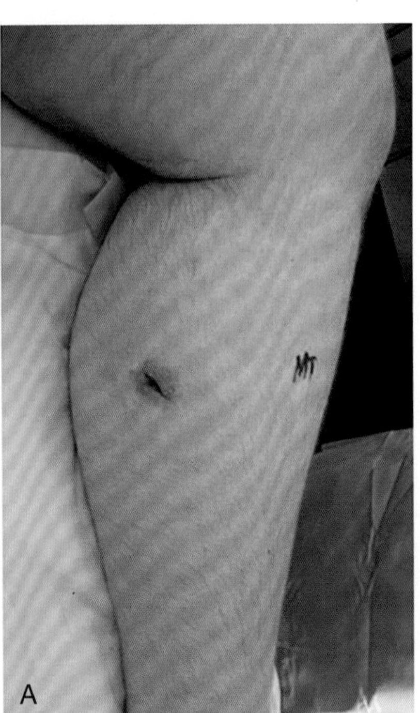

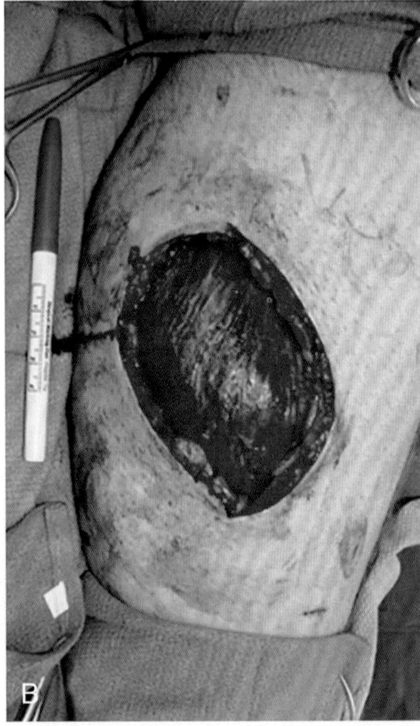

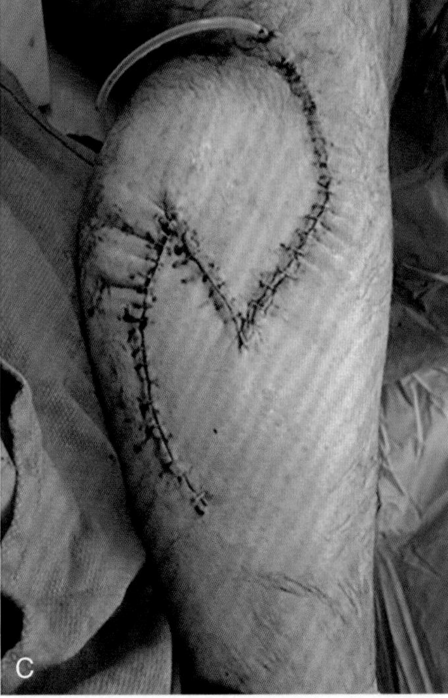

FIGURE 1 Clinical photographs showing an inappropriately performed biopsy. The incision is obliquely oriented on the calf (**A**), necessitating wide resection of the entire biopsy tract (**B**), and local flaps were used for coverage after definitive resection (**C**).

TABLE 2

Principles of Biopsy of Bone and Soft-tissue Tumors

The biopsy should be performed at the site of definitive treatment whenever possible.

Review clinical and radiographic findings with radiologist and pathologist before the biopsy.

Use a tourniquet but avoid expressive exsanguination (Esmarch bandage).

Use shortest possible incision, longitudinally placed, along the line of definitive resection.

Minimize soft-tissue dissection and contamination by dissecting through muscle, taking the most direct route feasible to the tumor.

Biopsy the advancing edge of the tumor, obtaining adequate lesional tissue (use of frozen section).

Obtain good hemostasis before closure, with use of a drain (brought out in line with the incision) as needed.

Sutures should be placed close to the skin edge to minimize amount of skin to be excised at definitive resection.

the current symptoms of the patient. Most benign active or aggressive bone lesions are treated surgically, although other modalities may be used in certain situations.

Osteoid Osteomas

Osteoid osteomas are characterized by night pain that is classically relieved by NSAIDs. In the past, these lesions were treated with surgical excision of the nidus (**Figure 2**). Radiofrequency ablation is now the standard treatment option for osteoid osteoma and also has achieved some success in the management of chondroblastoma. Other techniques such as cryoablation as well as microwave are also being used to manage these.[13]

Percutaneous image-guided laser photocoagulation has been used in spinal osteoid osteoma with good results. Special thermal protection techniques for the neural structures should be used if the nidus is within 1 to 2 cm of neural structures or in the absence of a protective cortex.[14]

Bone Cysts

Unicameral bone cysts are cystic lesions found in the metaphyses of long bones, most commonly in the proximal humerus (approximately 60%), proximal femur (approximately 30%), and the os calcis (typically under the angle of Gissane). These lesions cause thinning of the bone and may result in a pathologic fracture, often with the fallen leaf/fragment sign (**Figure 3**). Management of unicameral bone cysts remains controversial.[15] There is a prospective multicenter study currently underway (the Simple Bone Cysts in Kids clinical trial) that is evaluating the role of cyst perforation versus perforation and injection; recruitment is slow and results are not yet available.

Aneurysmal bone cysts may be primary (with characteristic USP6 rearrangements) or secondary to another underlying lesion. These lesions can be quite aggressive. Nodular enhancement of the cyst wall on postcontrast MRI as well as a lack of a peripheral rim of bone should raise suspicion for a possible telangiectatic

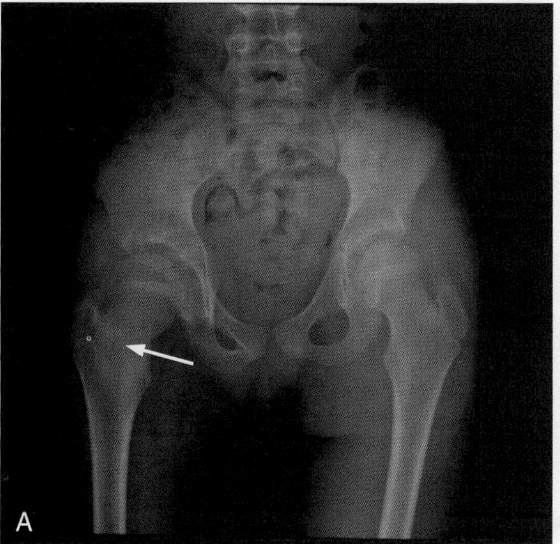

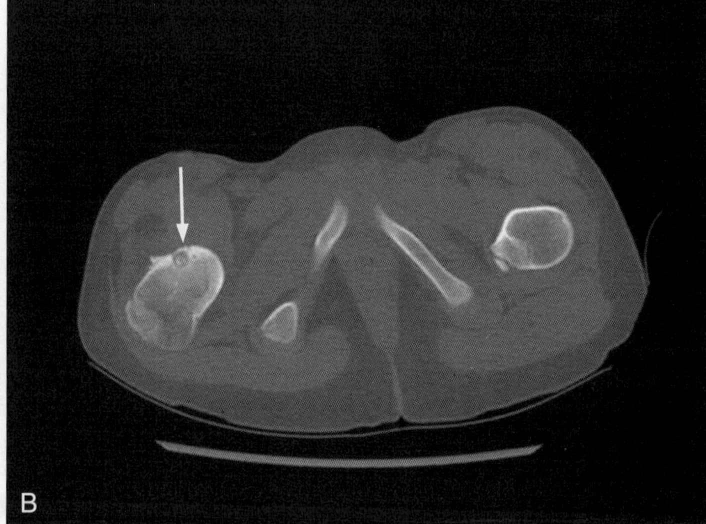

FIGURE 2 Imaging studies from a 10-yr-old girl who presented with right hip pain. **A**, AP radiograph demonstrates a lucent lesion in the intertrochanteric region with a sclerotic focus within it (arrow) and surrounding reactive new bone. **B**, CT scan demonstrates a cortically based nidus (arrow) that is suggestive of an osteoid osteoma.

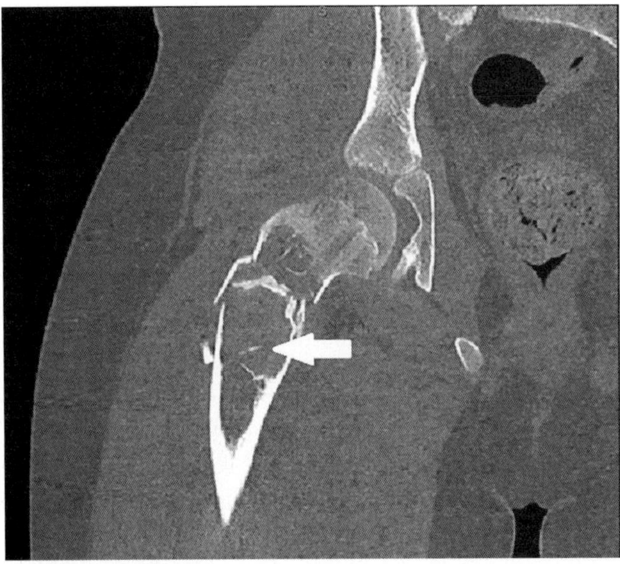

FIGURE 3 Coronal CT section shows a fracture through a proximal femoral unicameral bone cyst with a fallen leaf/ fragment sign (arrow).

osteosarcoma (**Figure 4**). The possibility of a secondary aneurysmal bone cyst must be considered, especially if it is in an epiphyseal location. The treatment of aneurysmal bone cysts is primarily surgical, with aggressive curettage (with or without the use adjuvant therapy). For aneurysmal bone cysts, especially those in surgically challenging locations, repeated embolization or injection of doxycycline foam has been used with moderate success.[16]

Chondroid Lesions

Osteochondromas are the most common chondroid lesions. These lesions may be single or multiple. Symptoms may be related to pressure or irritation of surrounding structures, fracture, limitation of motion, growth abnormality, or a rare malignant transformation (more likely in multiple osteochondromas). Mutations of the *EXT1* and *EXT2* genes result in disordered cartilage growth and account for most cases of multiple hereditary osteochondromatosis. These mutations are inherited in an autosomal dominant fashion. Given the increased appreciation of spinal osteochondromas, it is important to screen these patients for occipital headaches and neck and back pain and perform a thorough neurologic examination. Patients with multiple osteochondromas, especially those with shoulder and pelvic girdle involvement, should be counseled about potential for malignant transformation.

Chondroblastomas are the most common epiphyseal benign bone lesions in skeletally immature patients and typically cause pain. MRI will demonstrate characteristic perilesional edema around the lesion (**Figure 5**). Approximately one-third of these lesions will be associated with secondary aneurysmal bone cysts. Treatment

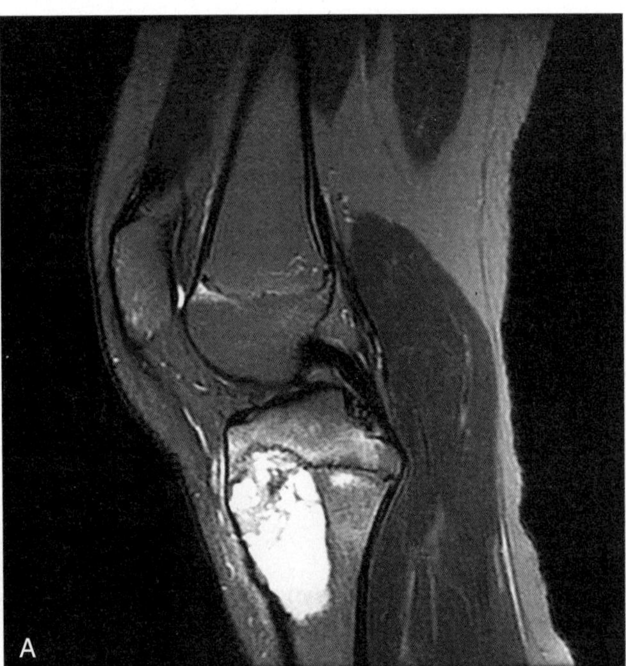

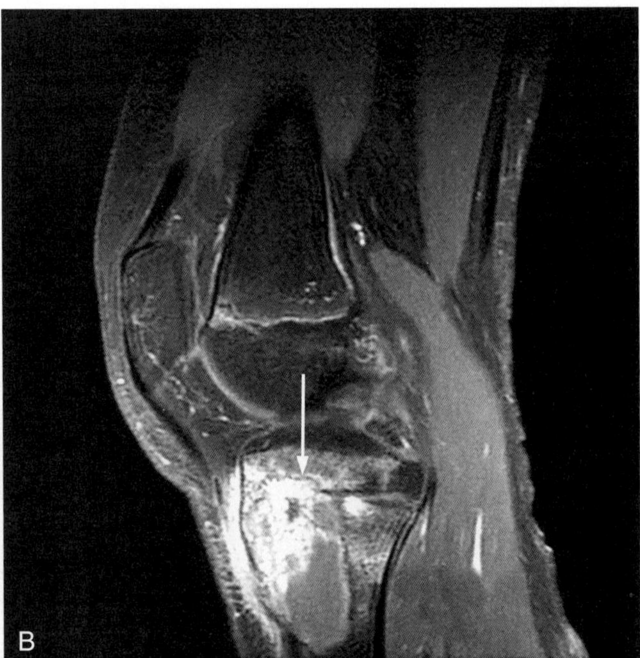

FIGURE 4 **A**, T2-weighted magnetic resonance image of a proximal tibial cystic lesion with multiple fluid levels is suggestive of an aneurysmal bone cyst. **B**, T1-weighted magnetic resonance image with nodular enhancement (arrow) with contrast raises suspicion of a telangiectatic osteosarcoma, which was the diagnosis in this case based on the biopsy.

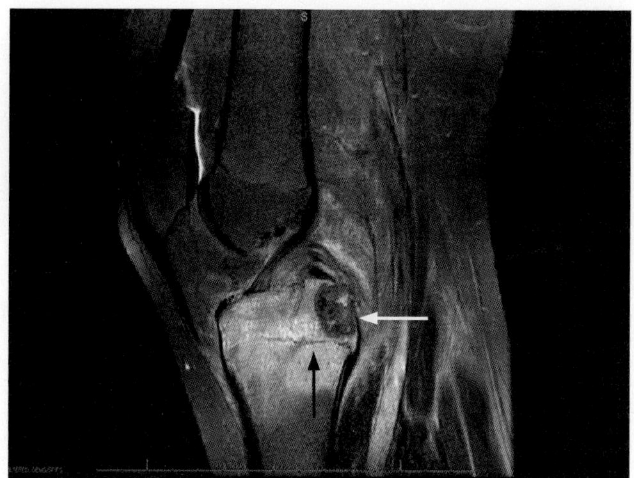

FIGURE 5 Proximal tibial epiphyseal lesion, with hypointense signal on a T2-weighted MRI sequence (white arrow) with characteristic perilesional edema (black arrow), is suggestive of a chondroblastoma.

is usually extended curettage and grafting, but there are recent reports of successful use of radiofrequency ablation for smaller lesions.[17]

Fibrous Dysplasia

Fibrous dysplasia results from a nonheritable missense mutation of the alpha subunit of the G-protein (*GNAS1* mutation). Approximately 80% of patients have monostotic involvement and 20% have polyostotic involvement. The combination of polyostotic fibrous dysplasia, café au lait spots with jagged or irregular (coast of Maine) borders, and endocrinopathy is referred to as McCune-Albright syndrome.[18] Indications for treatment in fibrous dysplasia include pain, fracture, and deformity (especially in the proximal femur-shepherd crook deformity; **Figure 6**). Because there is a high rate of bone graft resorption in fibrous dysplasia, the role of bone grafting has been questioned. Bulk allografts seem to offer the best resistance to resorption. Intramedullary fixation is preferred in patients with more extensive diaphyseal involvement.

The use of diphosphonates in polyostotic fibrous dysplasia remains controversial and is associated with reduction of biologic markers of bone turnover, improved bone mineral density, and improved radiographic appearance. Improvement in pain and function is not as clear.[19]

Langerhans Cell Histiocytosis

Langerhans cell histiocytosis is a disorder caused by clonal proliferation of CD1a+/CD207+ cells. Recent studies have identified MAPK pathway mutations in most patients with this lesion with *BRAF* V600E mutations in approximately 50% of patients and *MAP2K1* mutations in approximately 25% of the patients.[20] *BRAF* V600E mutations are associated with some increased risk of recurrence but do not affect overall survival. Spine involvement may result in vertebra plana deformity (**Figure 7**). Full-body MRI may be useful in determining other sites of involvement. Treatment is risk stratified. Single-site involvement is usually treated locally, but multiple-site involvement, especially with involvement of the liver, spleen, lung, or hematopoietic

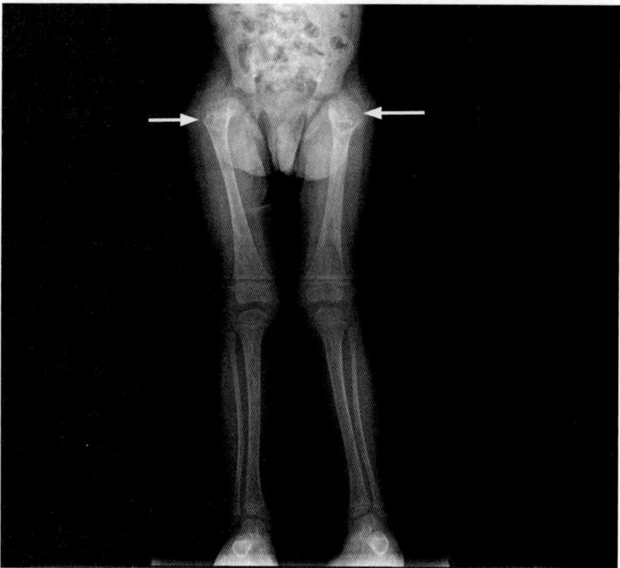

FIGURE 6 Radiograph from a child (age, 2 yr and 9 mo) with polyostotic fibrous dysplasia with bilateral coxa vara (arrows).

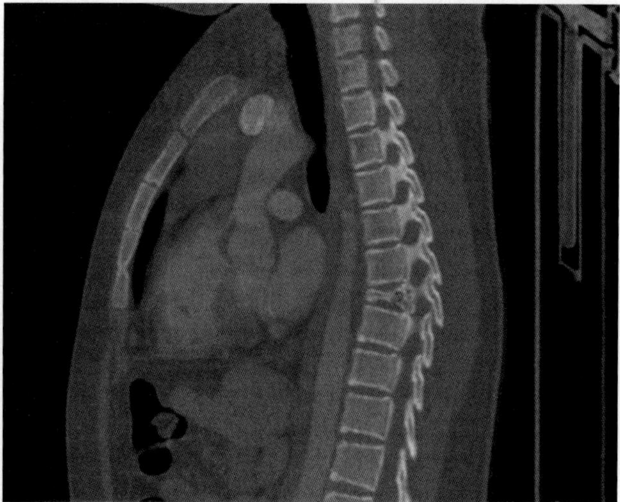

FIGURE 7 CT scan of the thoracic spine demonstrating a coin-shaped T7 vertebra (vertebra plana). The differential diagnosis includes Langerhans cell histiocytosis, leukemia, lymphoma, soft bone conditions such as osteogenesis imperfecta, trauma, and metastatic disease. (Figure courtesy Mihir Thacker, MD.)

Section 1: General Topics

system (high-risk organs), is treated more aggressively with chemotherapy. BRAF enzyme inhibitors (such as vemurafenib) have been used with some success.[21]

MALIGNANT BONE TUMORS

Osteosarcoma

Osteosarcoma is the most common primary bone sarcoma. It has two peak periods of incidence: during adolescence (>60% in the second decade of life) and during the sixth decade of life (often in Paget disease of bone). Although a genetic predisposition has been described, no constant genetic aberration has been identified.

Pain is the most common presenting symptom and is often associated with the presence of a firm, nonmobile mass. Pathologic fracture may occur in up to 10% of patients, and constitutional symptoms are usually a late sign. Most osteosarcomas occur around the knee (60%) or the shoulder.[22]

Radiographically, osteosarcoma is usually a destructive, poorly marginated blastic or mixed blastic-lytic lesion, arising in the metaphysis of long bones (**Figure 8**). Codman triangle and sunburst patterns of periosteal reaction are usually seen. MRI with and without contrast shows a heterogeneous-appearing mass with increased signal intensity on T2-weighted sequences and enhancement with gadolinium. There is typically a soft-tissue component to the bone tumor. Staging includes MRI of the entire affected bone (to look for skip lesions), a noncontrasted CT scan of the chest (most common site of metastasis), and screening for distant disease with a bone scan or PET scan (PET-CT or PET-MRI).

The treatment of osteosarcoma is multimodal, including neoadjuvant (presurgery) and adjuvant (postoperative) chemotherapy; most protocols use a combination of doxorubicin, ifosfamide, cisplatinum, and high-dose methotrexate. Local control is achieved with resection via limb salvage (90% of patients) or amputation. The overall survival rate for patients with localized disease is approximately 70% at 5 years, which has improved from the zero to 30% survival rates during the era before chemotherapy.[23]

A poor prognosis is associated with an axial location, a large tumor (>8 cm), the presence of metastases or skip lesions at presentation (approximately 20% of cases, with most of these lesions in the lungs), a less than 90% tumor necrosis rate after chemotherapy, and a highly elevated alkaline phosphatase level at diagnosis (greater than three times the normal level).

Ewing Sarcoma

Ewing sarcoma is in the family of primitive neuroectodermal tumors and is the second most common primary bone tumor in children. Although the cell of origin is unknown, it is characterized by a recurrent 11:22 translocation and the presence of the *EWS-FLI1* gene.

Similar to osteosarcoma, Ewing sarcoma often occurs around the knee and shoulder. However, it has a higher propensity to involve the axial skeleton. Ewing sarcoma is more common than osteosarcoma in the first decade of life, but in the second decade of life, osteosarcoma becomes approximately three times as common.

Clinically, Ewing sarcoma can present with constitutional symptoms in addition to the classic signs of pain and a palpable mass, and it thus may mimic infection. On imaging, Ewing sarcoma is often associated with a very large soft-tissue mass, and more often it arises from the diaphysis instead of the metaphysis. There is

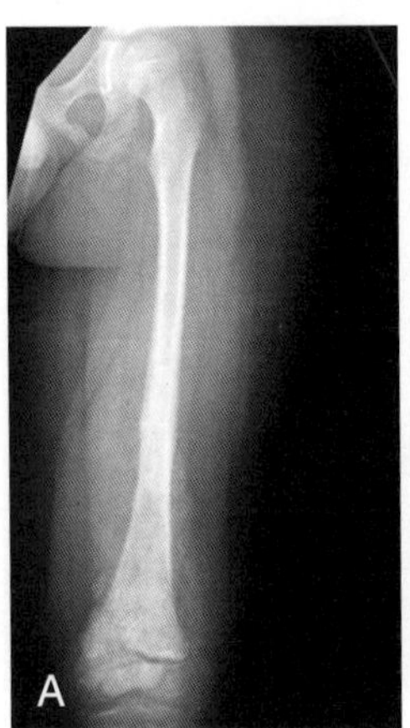

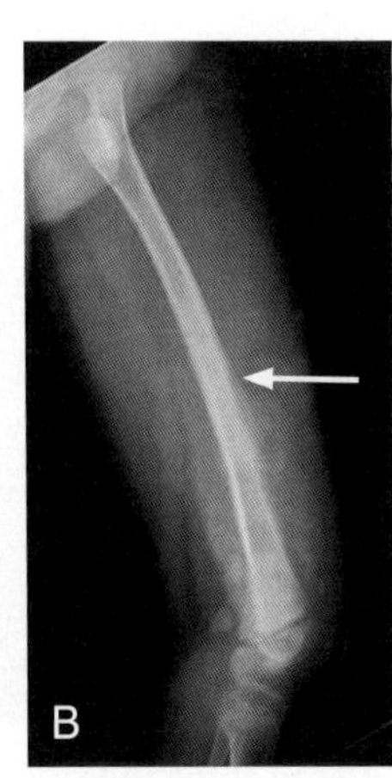

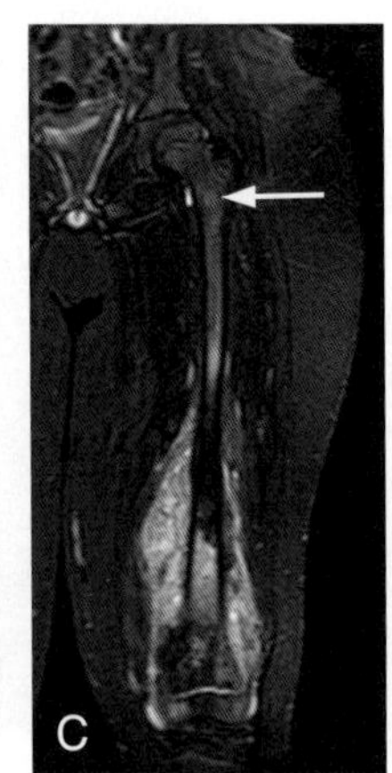

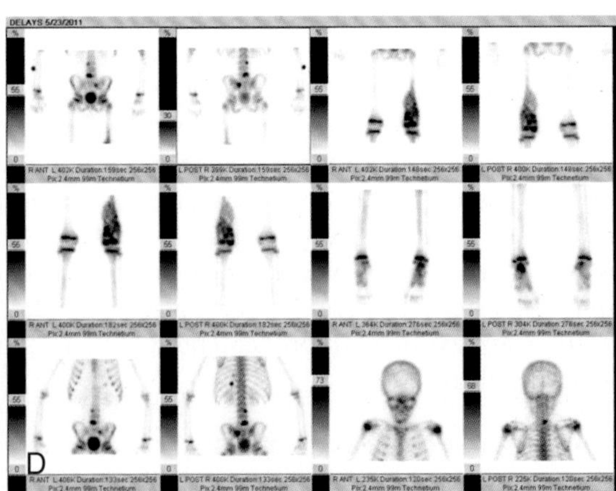

FIGURE 8 Images from a 9-yr-old child with thigh pain and a mass. **A**, Radiograph shows moth-eaten appearance of the distal femur, with a poorly defined sclerotic lesion in the metaphysis and distal diaphysis and mineralization in the soft-tissue. **B**, Radiograph shows a Codman triangle (arrow) created by the tumor, elevating the periosteum. **C**, Magnetic resonance image shows extensive involvement of the femur with a large soft-tissue mass as well as a skip lesion (arrow) in the proximal femoral metaphysis. **D**, A full-body bone scan shows multiple osseous metastatic lesions.

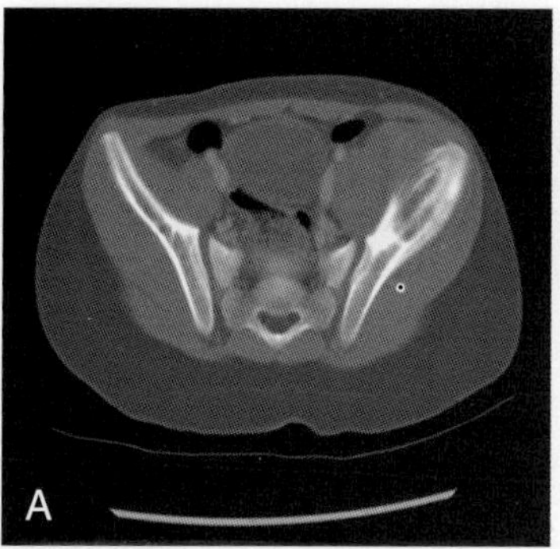

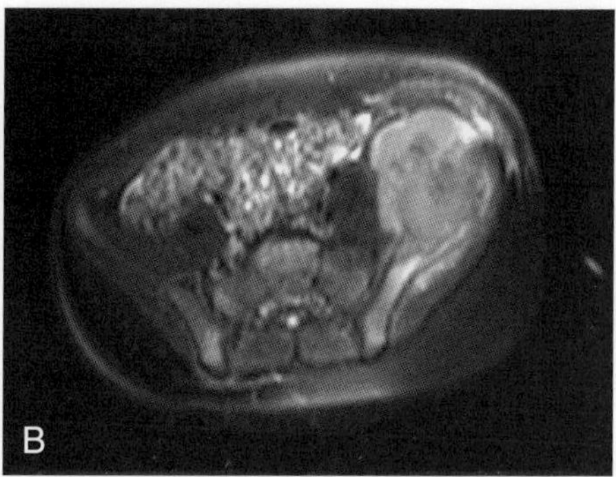

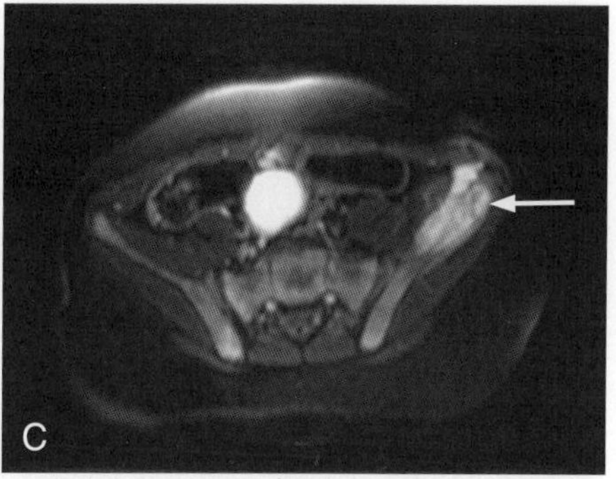

FIGURE 9 Images from a 6-yr-old child with a left-sided pelvic mass. **A**, Axial cut CT scan shows a soft-tissue mass on the inner table and a lytic lesion in the left ilium with a lamellated periosteal reaction (onion skin). T2-weighted magnetic resonance images before chemotherapy (**B**) and after chemotherapy (**C**) show substantial shrinkage of the soft-tissue component. This response is fairly typical in Ewing sarcoma.

no bone production. Onion skin (lamellated) periosteal reaction may be seen but is not diagnostic (**Figure 9**). Staging is similar to that performed for osteosarcoma, but additionally includes a bone marrow biopsy because around 20% of patients can have marrow involvement.

The management of Ewing sarcoma is also multimodal, with neoadjuvant and adjuvant chemotherapy. In contrast to osteosarcoma, radiation therapy is also an alternative to surgery for local control, but it has its own set of complications, especially in a growing child.[24] Some described complications include growth disturbance, neurologic compromise, contracture, pathologic fracture, and secondary sarcoma. Radiation therapy may also be used in patients with close or positive tumor margins. Current 5-year overall survival for patients with localized disease is around 75%. The presence of metastases leads to a 5-year overall survival <30%, and patients with recurrence have a dismal prognosis.[25]

RECONSTRUCTION OPTIONS AFTER MALIGNANT TUMOR RESECTION IN CHILDREN

Limb salvage is preferred over amputation, whenever feasible. Limitations in age/size-appropriate and growth-friendly reconstructive options make rotationplasty an attractive option in young children (especially younger than 5 to 8 years). Rotationplasties have been shown to be durable and have good functional outcomes. Biologic reconstructions (autogenous vascularized fibula, allograft, or combination of allograft with vascularized fibula using the Capanna technique) after tumor resection are preferred in the upper extremity. In the lower extremity, intercalary/joint-sparing reconstructions are best accomplished using biologic means (allograft ± autograft). Endoprosthetic reconstruction is often preferred around the knee in adolescents when the joint cannot be spared. There are limited endoprosthetic options for tumors distal to the elbow and leg/ankle. Expandable endoprostheses have been used in young children but have a high complication rate.[26]

BENIGN SOFT-TISSUE TUMORS

Lipoma and Lipoblastoma

Lipomas are the most common mesenchymal soft-tissue tumors. They are composed of mature white adipocytes, and most lipomas have a recurrent chromosomal aberration at 12q. These tumors have no malignant potential. Approximately 5% of lipomas are related to a familial predisposition. Most patients present with a painless mass and are adults past the fourth decade of life. MRI is diagnostic for lipomas with uniform fatty signal (hyperintense on both T1-weighted and T2-weighted MRIs) with uniform and complete suppression on fat-suppression sequences.

Lipoblastomas are characterized by nodules of adipose and myxoid tissue, which are demarcated by bands of fibrous tissue. Although they can be localized and clinically similar to lipomas, lipoblastomas also can present in a diffuse form that infiltrates surrounding muscles and soft tissues. These are exclusively tumors of infancy (most patients are younger than 3 years), with trunk and limb involvement occurring at similar incidences. The diffuse form is also known as lipoblastomatosis, and it has a 10% to 20% recurrence rate, with axial involvement being common.[27] The treatment of these lesions varies from observation alone to surgical resection.

Desmoid Tumors and Fibromatosis

Desmoid tumors and fibromatosis represent a benign fibroblastic proliferation with an infiltrative growth pattern. These lesions have a high recurrence rate and no metastatic potential. These lesions can be superficial (fibromatosis) or deep (aggressive fibromatosis or desmoid

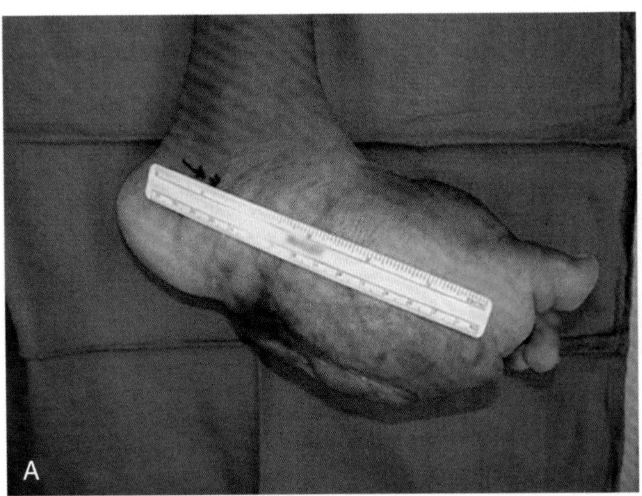

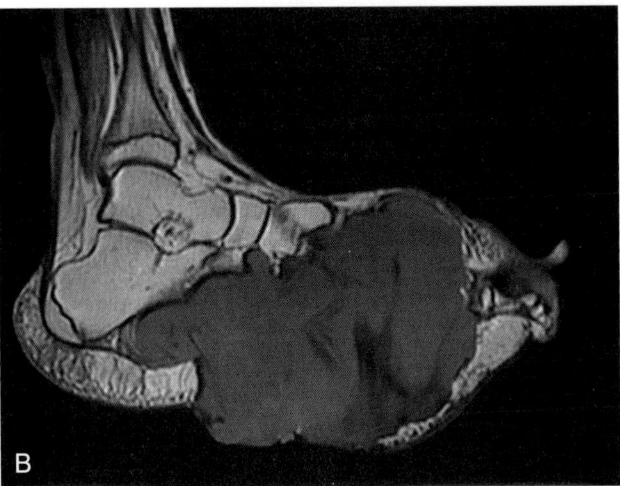

FIGURE 10 **A**, Clinical photograph of the foot of a 13-yr-old patient with aggressive fibromatosis. Magnetic resonance image shows that the lesion invades the soft tissues and extends from the dorsum to the plantar aspect of the foot and fungates through the bottom of the foot.

tumors). The superficial form is mostly limited to the fascia and includes Dupuytren (palmar), Ledderhose (plantar), and Peyronie disease (penile), or digital fibromatosis. Desmoid tumors can occur in a limb or in abdominal and retroperitoneal regions.

Although the etiology of these lesions is unknown, they have been associated with epilepsy, diabetes, and alcoholism in adults. A family history of the lesion may also exist.

Clinically, the disease starts as a painless firm mass (especially the superficial form). The rate of progression is variable, with some deep lesions being quite infiltrative. MRI demonstrates an irregular mass with poorly defined borders (unlike most other soft-tissue masses) and a variable degree of hypointense signal (depending on the degree of fibrosis; **Figure 10**). The degree of T2 signal may reflect the biologic behavior of the lesion, with larger extent of high T2 signal associated with more aggressive disease. WNT/beta catenin (*CTNNB1*) mutations have been identified in these tumors. The *S45F* mutation has been associated with very rapid recurrence, and identification of this mutation may suggest use of nonsurgical modalities.[28]

The wait-and-see strategy has become standard for the nonsymptomatic or minimally symptomatic patients. For failure of this approach or more symptomatic patients, surgical resection is the mainstay of treatment, with adjuvant radiation treatment for those with positive margins. In situations where morbidity is unacceptable, various nonsurgical treatments with NSAIDs, tamoxifen, methotrexate, vinblastine, and sorafenib have been described. The two main concerns with this condition are the high recurrence rate and the potential for infiltration of surrounding tissues.[29] With improvement in the understanding of the pathogenesis of desmoid tumors and fibromatosis (involvement of the WNT/beta catenin pathway and Notch signaling), targeted medical treatments are being explored.[30]

Peripheral Nerve Tumors

The most common peripheral nerve tumors are neuromas, schwannomas, and neurofibromas. Neuromas are a result of a trauma and are a nonneoplastic proliferation. These tumors are most commonly seen after amputation.

Schwannomas are encapsulated nerve sheath tumors. Although they are more common between the ages of 20 and 50 years, they may occur in children. The most common locations are the head, the neck, and flexor surfaces. Schwannomas are usually solitary and sporadic lesions and are rarely associated with neurofibromatosis type 2. The risk of malignant degeneration is minimal. Histology reveals characteristic Antoni A and Antoni B areas with nuclear palisading (Verocay bodies).

Neurofibromas can be isolated or associated with neurofibromatosis type 1. Neurofibromas are usually painless, superficial, slow-growing lesions generally involving small nerves. These are more difficult to separate from the parent nerve at surgery compared with schwannomas. The diffuse/plexiform form is associated with neurofibromatosis type 1. Atypical neurofibromas or globular areas within plexiform neurofibromas degenerate into malignant peripheral nerve sheath tumor and warrant monitoring.[31,32]

Giant Cell Tendon Sheath Tumors and Pigmented Villonodular Synovitis

Giant cell tendon sheath tumors and pigmented villonodular synovitis (PVS) are tumors of the synovium and can be localized or diffuse. Increased levels of colony-stimulating factor-1 have been demonstrated in these tumors. This attracts macrophages that have a receptor for colony-stimulating factor-1 and induce inflammation and consequent joint damage. Giant cell tendon sheath tumors often involve the limbs and present as a painless growing mass, whereas PVS can be intra-articular, with the knee as the most common location, or extra-articular. PVS is often diffuse, and patients have recurrent joint swelling and pain.

These lesions characteristically present as low signal on both T1-weighted and T2-weighted MRIs. Gradient-recalled echo imaging highlights the presence of hemosiderin, which results in the typical blooming artifact.

The mainstay of treatment is surgical resection, although there are studies researching the use of chemotherapy (such as tyrosine kinase inhibitor).[33] The local recurrence risk (approximately 20%) in patients with diffuse PVS is much higher than in patients with localized disease in whom surgery is often curative and has a very low recurrence rate.[34]

MALIGNANT SOFT-TISSUE TUMORS

Pediatric soft-tissue sarcomas account for 7% of all childhood tumors. The clinical presentation of soft-tissue sarcomas may be somewhat misleading because they often present as painless soft-tissue masses with a variable growth rate. Some tumors, such as infantile fibrosarcoma, may be present at birth and can be mistaken for vascular lesions. A careful clinical evaluation (including transillumination) can often help differentiate solid from cystic lesions. Many soft-tissue sarcomas are associated with characteristic cytogenetic abnormalities (**Table 3**).

TABLE 3

Cytogenetic Abnormalities in Some Common Tumors

Tumor	Cytogenetic Abnormality
Embryonal rhabdomyosarcoma	Loss of heterozygosity at 11p15
Alveolar rhabdomyosarcoma	t(2;13) (q35;q14) or t(1;13) (q36;q14) or 25%-40% of cases without either
Synovial sarcoma	t(X;18) (p11;q11)
Infantile fibrosarcoma	t(12;15) (9p13;q25)
Epithelioid sarcoma-proximal	22q11.2 alterations
Alveolar soft-part sarcoma	(der17) (x;17) (p11.2;q25)
Myxoid liposarcoma	t(12;16) (q13;11) and t(2;22) (q13;q12)
Extraskeletal myxoid chondrosarcoma	t(9;22) (q22;q12) or t(9;17) (q22;q12) or t(9;15) (q22;q21)
Extraskeletal Ewing sarcoma	t(11;22) (q24;q12) and other less common variants

Rhabdomyosarcoma

Rhabdomyosarcoma accounts for 50% of the soft-tissue sarcomas in children from birth to 14 years of age. The prevalence of rhabdomyosarcoma is approximately 4.5 per 1 million individuals.[35] Approximately 20% of rhabdomyosarcomas affect the limbs. Embryonal and alveolar are the two main types of rhabdomyosarcoma. Alveolar rhabdomyosarcoma is more common in the limbs and is usually seen in older children (5 to 15 years of age). Lymph node involvement is also more common in patients with alveolar rhabdomyosarcoma. Translocations (*PAX3-FOXO1*, *PAX7-FOXO1*) are seen in most patients with alveolar rhabdomyosarcoma. The prognosis of patients with embryonal rhabdomyosarcoma, nontranslocation-associated alveolar rhabdomyosarcoma, and alveolar rhabdomyosarcoma with *PAX7-FOXO1* translocation is better than for those with *PAX3-FOXO1* translocation. Staging includes MRI of the local area (including lymph nodes), bone marrow biopsies, and CT of the chest.

The role of PET-CT combination imaging or a full-body MRI for staging and estimating the response to chemotherapy is being investigated. Treatment is risk stratified and usually is a combination of multiagent chemotherapy, with surgery with or without radiation therapy for local control.

Nonrhabdomyosarcoma Soft-tissue Sarcomas

Nonrhabdomyosarcoma soft-tissue sarcomas are less common and comprise a heterogeneous group of malignancies. Synovial sarcoma, malignant peripheral nerve sheath tumors, and fibrosarcomas are among the more common nonrhabdomyosarcoma soft-tissue sarcomas in the pediatric population.

Synovial Sarcoma

Synovial sarcoma is the second most common soft-tissue sarcoma in children and young adults. The name is misleading because the cell of origin is not a synovial cell, and a joint is involved in only 0.5% to 5% of patients; however, it frequently occurs close to joints. The lower extremity is the most common location (especially the knee and the ankle; **Figure 11**). Histologically, the tumor may be monophasic with spindle cells (fibrous) or epithelial variants, or biphasic with epithelial and spindled areas. These lesions often have the characteristic X:18 translocation with fusion of the *SYT* gene on chromosome

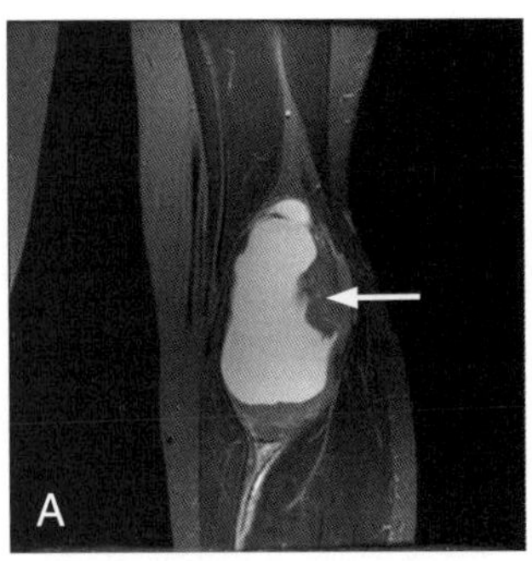

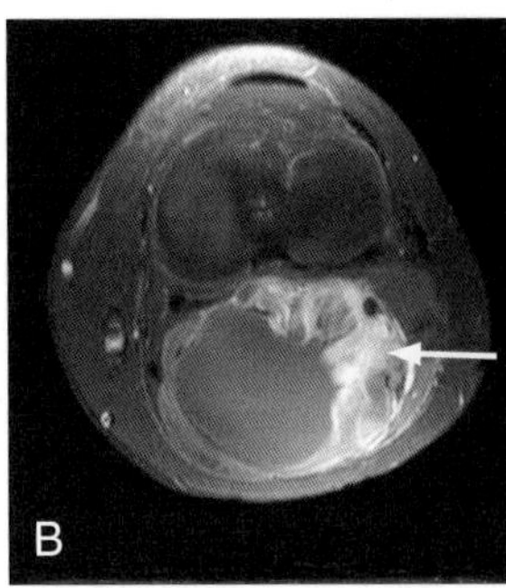

FIGURE 11 Images from a 17-yr-old patient with synovial sarcoma in the popliteus fossa that presented with deep vein thrombosis secondary to mass effect and invasion of the popliteus vein. The lesion is complex with cystic as well as solid components (arrows) on both coronal (**A**) and axial (**B**) MRI.

18 to the *SSX* genes on the X chromosome. Surgery is the mainstay of treatment, with radiation also useful in decreasing local recurrence. The role of chemotherapy is still unclear.

Malignant Peripheral Nerve Sheath Tumors

The diagnosis of 10% to 20% of malignant peripheral nerve sheath tumors is made in the first 2 decades of life. The lifetime risk of these tumors in patients with neurofibromatosis type 1 is 2% to 10% higher in patients younger than 30 years. In contrast to adults, fewer than 50% of malignant peripheral nerve sheath tumors in children arise in the setting of neurofibromatosis type 1. Radiation is also a risk factor for the development of malignant peripheral nerve sheath tumors. The clinical presentation is a progressively enlarging soft-tissue mass, with pain or neurologic symptoms frequently absent. Treatment is primarily wide surgical excision, because chemotherapy and radiation have limited efficacy. The prognosis is poor, with a 5-year survival rate of 38% to 51%.

SUMMARY

Appropriate workup of pediatric bone and soft-tissue tumors includes a thorough clinical evaluation, judicious use of imaging studies, and a well-planned and executed biopsy (when needed). Making the correct diagnosis and knowing the natural history of a particular tumor helps the physician to devise the most appropriate treatment plan. With improved understanding of the mechanisms involved in tumorigenesis, new therapeutic targets are being identified. Improved imaging with better interpretation of the response to neoadjuvant treatment may help determine the best surgical margins. Newer surgical techniques such as intraoperative navigation will help improve the ability of surgeons to obtain appropriate margins. Improvements in metallurgy and tailoring implants to the resection with improved efficacy using computerized planning should help improve reconstruction outcomes. Future innovations should improve the care of children with bone and soft-tissue tumors.

KEY STUDY POINTS

- The differential diagnosis of a tumor or lesion is driven primarily by the age of the patient and the location of the tumor.
- Radiographs are extremely useful in the evaluation of osseous lesions and often may be diagnostic by themselves.
- Soft-tissue sarcomas may not have substantial pain associated with them (at least in the initial stages), grow centrifugally, and push rather than invade the surrounding tissues (hence, are well circumscribed), leading to diagnostic confusion with benign lesions.
- Imaging is less often diagnostic in soft-tissue tumors compared with osseous tumors, and biopsy is needed much more frequently in the evaluation of soft-tissue tumors.
- Osteosarcoma and rhabdomyosarcoma are the most common bone and soft-tissue sarcomas, respectively, in children (alveolar rhabdomyosarcoma is more common than embryonal rhabdomyosarcoma in the extremities).

ANNOTATED REFERENCES

1. Mirabello L, Yeager M, Mai PL, et al: Germline TP53 variants and susceptibility to osteosarcoma. *J Natl Cancer Inst* 2015;107(7):djv101.

2. Rana HQ, Gelman R, LaDuca H, et al: Differences in TP53 mutation carrier phenotypes emerge from panel-based testing. *J Natl Cancer Inst* 2018;110(8):863-870.

   The authors found that TP53+ individuals ascertained by single gene mutation testing were more likely than those determined by multiple gene testing panels to have earlier onset cancer and be more likely to meet dianostic criteria for Li-Fraumeni syndrome. Level of evidence: IV.

3. DeBaun MR, Tucker MA: Risk of cancer during the first four years of life in children from the Beckwith-Wiedemann Syndrome Registry. *J Pediatr* 1998;132(3 pt 1):398-400.

4. Maas SM, Vansenne F, Kadouch DJ, et al: Phenotype, cancer risk, and surveillance in Beckwith-Wiedemann syndrome depending on molecular genetic subgroups. *Am J Med Genet A* 2016;170(9):2248-2260.

   The group attempted to define molecular risk factors in 1941 patients with Beckwith-Wiedemann syndrome. Tumor risks were highest in the IC1 (H19/IGF2:IG-DMR) hypermethylation subgroup (28%) and pUPD subgroup (16%). Level of evidence: II.

5. Qu N, Yao W, Cui X, Zhang H: Malignant transformation in monostotic fibrous dysplasia: Clinical features, imaging features, outcomes in 10 patients, and review. *Medicine (Baltimore)* 2015;94(3):e369.
6. Verdegaal SH, Bovee JV, Pansuriya TC, et al: Incidence, predictive factors, and prognosis of chondrosarcoma in patients with Ollier disease and Maffucci syndrome: An international multicenter study of 161 patients. *Oncologist* 2011;16(12):1771-1779.
7. Czajka CM, DiCaprio MR: What is the proportion of patients with multiple hereditary exostoses who undergo malignant degeneration? *Clin Orthop Relat Res* 2015;473(7):2355-2361.
8. Bernard SA, Murphey MD, Flemming DJ, Kransdorf MJ: Improved differentiation of benign osteochondromas from secondary chondrosarcomas with standardized measurement of cartilage cap at CT and MR imaging. *Radiology* 2010;255(3):857-865.
9. Ren W, Gu G: Prognostic implications of RB1 tumour suppressor gene alterations in the clinical outcome of human osteosarcoma: A meta-analysis. *Eur J Cancer Care (Engl)* 2017;26(1):e12401.

   A meta-analysis of 491 patients demonstrated that loss of *RB1* gene function results in increased metastatic and mortality rates for patients with osteosarcoma and a substantial reduction in the histologic response of osteosarcoma to chemotherapy. Level of evidence: I.
10. Dommering CJ, Marees T, van der Hout AH, et al: RB1 mutations and second primary malignancies after hereditary retinoblastoma. *Fam Cancer* 2012;11(2):225-233.
11. Mankin HJ, Mankin CJ, Simon MA: The hazards of the biopsy, revisited. Members of the Musculoskeletal Tumor Society. *J Bone Joint Surg Am* 1996;78(5):656-663.
12. Skrzynski MC, Biermann JS, Montag A, Simon MA: Diagnostic accuracy and charge-savings of outpatient core needle biopsy compared with open biopsy of musculoskeletal tumors. *J Bone Joint Surg Am* 1996;78(5):644-649.
13. Rinzler ES, Shivaram GM, Shaw DW, Monroe EJ, Koo KSH: Microwave ablation of osteoid osteoma: Initial experience and efficacy. *Pediatr Radiol* 2019;49(4):566-570.

    The authors report their initial experience with use of microwave ablation for osteoid osteomas, with clinical success in all 24 patients treated and only minor complications in 4/24 or 17% patients. Level of evidence: IV.
14. Tsoumakidou G, Thenint MA, Garnon J, Buy X, Steib JP, Gangi A: Percutaneous image-guided laser photocoagulation of spinal osteoid osteoma: A single-institution series. *Radiology* 2016;278(3):936-943.

    The authors report on 58 patients with spinal osteoid osteomas treated at a single institution. Recurrences (5.3% of the patients) were successfully treated with laser photocoagulation. In osteoid osteomas with less than 8 to 10 mm of surrounding cortical bone, thermal protection techniques were recommended. Level of evidence: I.
15. Kadhim M, Thacker M, Kadhim A, Holmes L Jr: Treatment of unicameral bone cyst: Systematic review and meta analysis. *J Child Orthop* 2014;8(2):171-191.
16. Shiels WE II, Beebe AC, Mayerson JL: Percutaneous doxycycline treatment of juxtaphyseal aneurysmal bone cysts. *J Pediatr Orthop* 2016;36(2):205-212.

    This study of 16 patients with juxtaphyseal aneurysmal bone cysts treated with doxycycline foam demonstrated a recurrence rate of 6%. All patients needed multiple injections (2 to 14 injections) for their treatment. Level of evidence: IV.
17. Xie C, Jeys L, James SL: Radiofrequency ablation of chondroblastoma: Long-term clinical and imaging outcomes. *Eur Radiol* 2015;25(4):1127-1134.
18. Javaid MK, Boyce A, Appelman-Dijkstra N, et al: Best practice management guidelines for fibrous dysplasia/McCune-Albright syndrome: A consensus statement from the FD/MAS international consortium. *Orphanet J Rare Dis* 2019;14(1):139.

    This was a consensus statement by a group of experts regarding the clinical guidelines for best clinical practice for the definition, diagnosis, staging, treatment, and monitoring for fibrous dysplasia/McCune Albright syndrome. Level of evidence: V.
19. Boyce AM, Kelly MH, Brillante BA, et al: A randomized, double blind, placebo-controlled trial of alendronate treatment for fibrous dysplasia of bone. *J Clin Endocrinol Metab* 2014;99(11):4133-4140.
20. Berres ML, Lim KP, Peters T, et al: BRAF-V600E expression in precursor versus differentiated dendritic cells defines clinically distinct LCH risk groups. *J Exp Med* 2015;212(2):281.
21. Haroche J, Cohen-Aubart F, Emile JF, et al: Dramatic efficacy of vemurafenib in both multisystemic and refractory Erdheim-Chester disease and Langerhans cell histiocytosis harboring the BRAF V600E mutation. *Blood* 2013;121(9):1495-1500.
22. Cates JM: Pathologic fracture a poor prognostic factor in osteosarcoma: Misleading conclusions from meta-analyses? *Eur J Surg Oncol* 2016;42(6):883-888.

    The authors of this multivariable survival analysis of 131 patients with high-grade osteosarcoma of the extremity long bones concluded that pathologic fracture was not an important prognostic factor for osteosarcoma of the limbs.
23. Luetke A, Meyers PA, Lewis I, Juergens H: Osteosarcoma treatment – Where do we stand? A state of the art review. *Cancer Treat Rev* 2014;40(4):523-532.
24. Biswas B, Rastogi S, Khan SA, et al: Outcomes and prognostic factors for Ewing-family tumors of the extremities. *J Bone Joint Surg Am* 2014;96(10):841-849.
25. Gaspar N, Hawkins DS, Dirksen U, et al: Ewing sarcoma: Current management and future approaches through collaboration. *J Clin Oncol* 2015;33(27):3036-3046.
26. Groundland JS, Ambler SB, Houskamp LD, Orriola JJ, Binitie OT, Letson GD: Surgical and functional outcomes after limb-preservation surgery for tumor in pediatric patients: A systematic review. *JBJS Rev* 2016;4(2):01874474-201602000-00002.

    This was a systematic review of studies describing limb salvage after pediatric extremity tumor resection and found most studies are level IV and had significant limiations. However, they concluded that despite all the study limitations children had satisfactory initial surgical and functional outcomes. Level of evidence: IV.

27. Coffin CM, Lowichik A, Putnam A: Lipoblastoma (LPB): A clinicopathologic and immunohistochemical analysis of 59 cases. *Am J Surg Pathol* 2009;33(11):1705-1712.

28. Colombo C, Miceli R, Lazar AJ, et al: CTNNB1 45F mutation is a molecular prognosticator of increased postoperative primary desmoid tumor recurrence: An independent, multicenter validation study. *Cancer* 2013;119(20):3696-3702.

29. Garbay D, Le Cesne A, Penel N, et al: Chemotherapy in patients with desmoid tumors: A study from the French Sarcoma Group (FSG). *Ann Oncol* 2012;23(1):182-186.

30. Shang H, Braggio D, Lee YJ, et al: Targeting the Notch pathway: A potential therapeutic approach for desmoid tumors. *Cancer* 2015;121(22):4088-4096.

31. Varan A, Sen H, Aydin B, Yalcin B, Kutluk T, Akyuz C: Neurofibromatosis type 1 and malignancy in childhood. *Clin Genet* 2016;89(3):341-345.

    In this study, nonneurofibroma neoplasms developed in 26 of 473 patients (5%) with neurofibromatosis type 1. These included 12 soft-tissue tumors (6 malignant peripheral nerve sheath tumors, 5 rhabdomyosarcomas, and 1 malignant fibrous histiocytoma), 11 brain tumors (6 low-grade gliomas, 3 high-grade gliomas, and 2 medulloblastomas), 2 neuroblastomas, and 1 non-Hodgkin lymphoma. Level of evidence: IV.

32. Miettinen MM, Antonescu CR, Fletcher CDM, et al: Histopathologic evaluation of atypical neurofibromatous tumors and their transformation into malignant peripheral nerve sheath tumor in patients with neurofibromatosis 1-a consensus overview. *Hum Pathol* 2017;67:1-10.

    This is a consensus overview by a group of experts defining the diagnostic criteria of nerve sheath tumors and describing the spectrum of nerve sheath tumors in neurofibromatosis 1. Level of evidence: V.

33. Cassier PA, Gelderblom H, Stacchiotti S, et al: Efficacy of imatinib mesylate for the treatment of locally advanced and/or metastatic tenosynovial giant cell tumor/pigmented villonodular synovitis. *Cancer* 2012;118(6):1649-1655.

34. Mollon B, Lee A, Busse JW, et al: The effect of surgical synovectomy and radiotherapy on the rate of recurrence of pigmented villonodular synovitis of the knee: An individual patient meta-analysis. *Bone Joint J* 2015;97-B(4):550-557.

35. Ognjanovic S, Linabery AM, Charbonneau B, Ross JA: Trends in childhood rhabdomyosarcoma incidence and survival in the United States, 1975-2005. *Cancer* 2009;115(18):4218-4226.

CHAPTER 6

Growth of the Musculoskeletal System

CHRISTOPHER IOBST, MD • BRIAN P. SCANNELL, MD

ABSTRACT

Growth is unique in pediatric patients compared with adult patients. Growth is a complex and well-synchronized phenomenon. It is important that orthopaedic surgeons who care for children have a good understanding of normal growth to better address deviations from normal that can result in progressive deformity, impaired function, or future pain.

Keywords: bone age; growth; peak height velocity; skeletal maturity

INTRODUCTION

Growth is unique in pediatric care compared with adult care. Because growth is a complex and well-synchronized phenomenon,[1] orthopaedic surgeons who care for children should understand what normal growth is to better address deviations from normal that can result in progressive deformity, impaired function, or pain.

Growth is divided into two areas: microgrowth and macrogrowth.[2] Microgrowth occurs at the cellular level in the epiphyseal plate. Macrogrowth is the total effect of microgrowth and allows for changes in height, weight, and body proportion. From birth through adulthood, height increases 350% and weight increases 20-fold.[3]

Dr. Iobst or an immediate family member is a member of a speakers' bureau or has made paid presentations on behalf of Smith & Nephew and serves as a paid consultant to or is an employee of Orthofix Inc. and Nuvasive. Neither Dr. Scannell nor any immediate family member has received anything of value from or has stock or stock options held in a commercial company or institution related directly or indirectly to the subject of this chapter.

NORMAL GROWTH

Height

It is important to document the standing height of children at regular physician visits. Standing height is the composition of sitting height (trunk) and subischial height (lower limbs).[3] Each component grows at different rates and times. A child's overall standing height increases rapidly from birth to age 5 years. It then slows down until beginning another rapid increase during puberty.[3] At age 2 years, a child's standing height is approximately 50% of his or her adult height; at puberty, a child's standing height is approximately 86% of adult height.

In the same manner as standing height, sitting height can be measured supine in young children. Sitting height has been used to anticipate the onset of puberty. In an average population, puberty starts when the sitting height is approximately 75 cm in girls and 78 cm in boys. At 84 cm of sitting height, 80% of girls have reached menarche.[2]

Subischial height is determined by subtracting the sitting height from the standing height.[2] Over time, the subischial height contributes a far greater growth percentage in height than does the sitting height.[2] In a newborn, the proportion of sitting height to subischial height is 65:35. At skeletal maturity, this ratio is 52:48. Thus, as children age, a much higher percentage of growth occurs in the lower limbs compared with growth in the trunk.[3]

Weight

Similar to height, weight gain is not constant. The average male weighs 10 kg at age 1 year, 20 kg at age 5 years, 30 kg at age 10 years, and 60 kg at age 17 years.[2,4] Weight nearly doubles from ages 10 to 17 years during puberty.[3] These estimates are from studies several decades ago, but newer studies suggest that children and adolescents are heavier than previously thought.[5] The National Center for Health Statistics in 2015 documented an obesity rate of 17.5% in children aged 3 to 19 years in the United States.[6]

Body Mass Index

The body mass index (BMI) is an estimate of body fat based on weight and height. It is calculated by taking a person's weight and dividing it by the person's height squared (kg/m^2). Because the body composition of children is different from that of adults, the BMI is calculated based on both age and sex. Normal or healthy weight is the 5th percentile to less than the 85th percentile for children of the same age and sex. Overweight is defined as being in the 85th percentile to less than the 95th percentile for children of the same age and sex. Obesity is defined as greater than the 95th percentile.

With increasing obesity rates in children, it is important to understand the basic effects of obesity on the growing skeleton.[7] The increasing BMI seen in children may lead to increased mechanical load encouraging bone strength; however, endocrine-related changes including insulin resistance, increased inflammatory cytokine production, altered leptin production, and vitamin D deficiency will lead to lower ratio of bone mass compared with overall patient weight.[7-10] The result of the obesity and the effects on the skeleton can lead to future issues with effects on pattern of injury, nonorthopaedic complications (deep vein thrombosis, ulcers, wound infections), and the development of orthopaedic disease (Blount disease).[7]

Chronologic Growth

Within the first year of life, growth in both sitting height and subischial limb length substantially accelerates. This higher rate of growth commonly continues until approximately age 5 years.[3] During the first 5 years of life, the proportions of growth change as the cephalic end becomes relatively smaller compared with increases seen in subischial limb length.

From 5 years to the onset of puberty, the growth rate markedly decelerates. On average, standing height increases 5.5 cm/yr.[3] Approximately two-thirds of growth occur in the lower limbs, and one-third occurs in the sitting height. The trunk grows at a slower rate than the lower limbs, thus altering the body's proportions.[4]

Acceleration of growth velocity characterizes the beginning of puberty, which occurs at approximately age 10 years in girls and 12 years in boys. During puberty, standing height increases approximately 1 cm/mo, with more growth occurring in the trunk compared with the subischial limbs. The four main characteristics of puberty are as follows: (1) dramatic increase in stature; (2) changing proportions of the upper and lower body; (3) change in overall morphology, including fat distribution, shoulder width, and pelvic diameter; and (4) the development of secondary sexual characteristics (testicular growth, breast buds).[3]

Puberty and Peak Height Velocity

The exact onset of puberty and a determination of future growth can be difficult. It requires assessing the following: bone age, the Tanner classification of secondary sexual characteristics, height changes, the onset of menstruation, and the Risser sign. The issue with using menstruation onset and the Risser sign in isolation is that they typically occur later in puberty.[2] More recently the Sanders classification has been used to assess skeletal maturity and its relationship to peak height velocity (PHV).

Growth has two primary phases during puberty (**Figure 1**). The first phase is the ascending phase of the growth velocity curve. This phase lasts approximately 2 years; during this phase, the PHV, or the maximum growth rate, occurs. PHV occurs between 13 and 15 years of bone age (according to a 1959 study[11]) in boys and 11 to 13 years of bone age in girls.[3] Determining whether children are in the ascending phase of the growth velocity curve can be difficult, but it can be accomplished with serial height measurements. Height commonly increases at least 8 cm/yr during PHV. As seen on radiographs, the triradiate cartilage commonly closes about halfway through the ascending phase. The Risser sign is not very useful in determining PHV because most patients have a Risser grade of 0 during this phase (**Figure 1**). In girls with idiopathic scoliosis, the PHV was correlated with a Risser grade of 0 and open triradiate cartilage.[12] Peak height velocity has also been shown to correspond to 90% final height, and stages of growth correlate better to hand radiographic morphology according to the Sanders classification.[13,14]

The second phase is the descending phase of the growth velocity curve (**Figure 1**). During this phase, the growth rate slows, children are becoming more skeletally mature (elbow physis closure and Risser progression), and

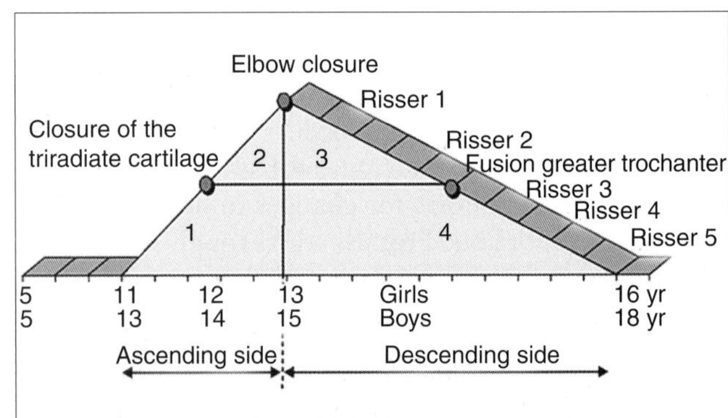

FIGURE 1 Illustration of a pubertal growth diagram that shows ascending and descending growth phases with corresponding radiographic findings. (Reproduced with permission from Diméglio A: Growth in pediatric orthopaedics, in Morrissey RT, Weinstein SL, eds: *Lovell and Winter's Pediatric Orthopaedics*, ed 6. Philadelphia, PA, Lippincott Williams and Wilkins, 2006, p 52.)

girls commonly begin menarche. Using the Sauvegrain method, the olecranon apophysis typically closes near the beginning of the descending phase.[4] Menarche occurs after closure of this apophysis in girls, but this can be variable.[3] Girls experience menarche variably according to the Risser grades: 42% before Risser grade 1, 31% at Risser grade 1, 13% at Risser grade 2, 8% at Risser grade 3, and 5% at Risser grade 4.[15]

SPINE GROWTH

Growth of the Spinal Column

The overall development of the spine includes both longitudinal (vertical) and axial growth. The spine is approximately 60% of sitting height. The overall height of the spine nearly triples between birth and adulthood, with peak growth rates in the first 5 years of life and again during puberty.[3,4]

Growth of the spinal canal occurs at each vertebral level through essentially three primary ossification centers: the posterior spinous process synchondrosis and two neurocentral synchondroses at the junction of each pedicle and vertebral body. The diameter of the canal reaches adult size sometime between ages 6 and 8 years.[16-18] In addition, spinal growth occurs at each vertebral level at the ring apophysis (two per vertebral body) to contribute to longitudinal growth. The posterior elements also contribute to longitudinal growth.[19]

The cervical spine will grow approximately 9 cm from birth to adulthood, reaching an adult length of 12 to 13 cm, and is approximately 15% of sitting height.[3] Two-thirds of this growth occur by age 5 years, and the remaining growth occurs during puberty. All vertebral body growth occurs as previously discussed, with the exception of C1 (atlas) and C2 (axis). C1 is unique because the primary anterior ossification center is present in less than 20% of neonates.[20] The anterior ossification center typically develops between 9 and 12 months, and two neurocentral synchondroses are formed with the posterior ossification centers.[19] C2 is unique because it involves the dens. The dens is more similar to a long bone, with a cartilaginous epiphysis at each end.

The thoracic spine will grow approximately 18 cm from birth to adulthood, reaching an adult length of approximately 28 cm in men and 26 cm in women.[4] It comprises approximately 30% of sitting height. Similar to the cervical spine, a growth spurt occurs from birth to age 5 years and again during puberty. The posterior components of the spine grow at a faster rate than the anterior counterparts.[3] By knowing and understanding the growth of the thoracic spine, it is possible to calculate the effect of a thoracic fusion on final height.[3,4]

The lumbar spine will grow approximately 9 cm from birth to adulthood, reaching an adult length of 16 cm in men and 15.5 cm in women. It comprises approximately 18% of sitting height.[3,4] Growth of the vertebral elements occurs in reverse from the thoracic spine; the anterior elements grow at a faster rate than the posterior elements.[3]

Scoliosis and Spine Growth

A close relationship has been demonstrated to exist between increased height and scoliosis progression.[21] Curve progression markedly increases at the time of adolescent growth spurts for idiopathic and neuromuscular curves. In addition, curve progression slows or ceases when skeletal maturity is achieved.

Studies have attempted to look at the natural history of curve progression during puberty. In the ascending phase of the growth diagram, any spinal curvature increasing by 1° per month or 12° per year is likely to be progressive and require treatment. Any curve increase of less than 0.5° per month is mild and less likely to need treatment.[4] Female patients with a curve of less than 30° at the time of PHV were demonstrated to have only a 4% chance of progression to a surgical range.[22] However, female patients with a curve greater than 30° at the time of PHV had an 84% chance of requiring surgical intervention. This risk of progression appears similarly in males, with nearly a 100% chance of progression to surgical range with curves greater than 30° at PHV.[23]

Even in the descending phase of the growth diagram, the risk for scoliosis progression is present. The Risser grades are not the best indicators of risk progression; however, based on previous literature,[24-27] they can be used to predict progression (**Table 1**). Some authors recommend using radiographs of the hand to determine skeletal age. One group of researchers found that curve acceleration most closely correlated with the Tanner-Whitehouse III scoring system for hand radiographs.[28] This scoring system provides better maturity and prognosis determination during adolescence.

A more recent simplified classification for skeletal maturity has been developed. Authors of a 2008 study developed a simpler classification based on the Tanner-Whitehouse III score and Digital Skeletal Age score.[14]

TABLE 1

Risk of Curve Progression (5° or More)

	20° Curve	30° Curve
Risser grade 0	30%	100%
Risser grade 1	10%	60%
Risser grade 2	2%	30%

They demonstrated that this eight-stage scoring system is reliable and correlates with scoliosis curve progression more strongly than the Risser sign or Greulich and Pyle skeletal age. A further study validated the Sanders Skeletal Maturity Staging System or what is now simply the Sanders classification.[29] This study demonstrated a strong predictive correlation between the Sanders stage and initial Cobb angle in regard to the probability of idiopathic scoliosis progression. With the development of the Sanders classification and its high reliability and accuracy, this method for assessing skeletal maturity is preferred given the limited sensitivity of the Risser sign.[29]

Arthrodesis for scoliosis often is required before skeletal maturity. For some patients undergoing surgery, the risk for a crankshaft phenomenon secondary to remaining growth of the spine is present. The crankshaft phenomenon was first described in 1989 and occurs when a solid posterior arthrodesis is performed while growth remaining anteriorly produces rotation of the spine or trunk with progression of the spinal curvature.[30] Patients at Tanner stage 1 with open triradiate cartilage have the greatest risk for the crankshaft phenomenon. Another group of researchers observed crankshaft deformities in 10 of 23 patients who had open triradiate cartilage but only 1 of 20 patients with closed triradiate cartilage.[31] The strongest predictor of the crankshaft phenomenon appears to be when arthrodesis is performed in the setting of open triradiate cartilage before or during PHV.[32] Ultimately, understanding the growth of the spine can help determine treatment and the timing of treatment of patients with scoliosis.

GROWTH REMAINING

In discussing growth, it is important to not only ascertain how much total growth a child will accrue but also determine how much growth is remaining for a child at a particular point in time. This information often is necessary when determining treatment strategies for patients who are skeletally immature and have limb-length discrepancy (LLD) or an angular deformity. Traditionally, the three most widely used methods of determining the amount of growth remaining were the arithmetic method, the Anderson-Green-Messner growth-remaining charts, and the Moseley straight-line method. The arithmetic method states that girls cease growing at age 14 years and boys at age 16 years.[33] This method also assumes a yearly growth rate of 0.375 inches from the distal femoral physis and 0.25 inches from the proximal tibial physis. Growth remaining at each physis can be calculated by multiplying the number of years of growth remaining by the amount of growth expected from each physis. This simplistic approach is a quick method that can be used in the clinic and does not require graphs or complex computations.

In 1969, growth-remaining graphs were published to determine the amount of growth remaining in the femur and the tibia until skeletal maturity was reached.[34] Using these growth data, a straight-line graph method was created in 1977 to predict LLD in a lower extremity and the amount of growth remaining.[35] Both methods require a child's skeletal age and a determination of the growth percentile of the patient. In addition, the straight-line method requires a special graph and a minimum of three measurements. One important concern with both the growth-remaining charts and the straight-line method is that they are based on a population of children living under conditions different than those experienced by the current population of children. Because growth data can be affected by regional, racial, ethnic, and generational differences, it may not be possible to extrapolate these methods to the current population of children and expect accurate predictions.

The multiplier method is an alternative method for assessing the amount of growth remaining.[36-41] Lower limb growth is thought to follow a biologic constant based on age and sex. Children of all generations and ethnic backgrounds grow the same percentage of their limb length at the same age. The multiplier method characterizes the pattern of normal human growth by using an age-specific and sex-specific coefficient. The multiplier for each age and sex is a measure of the percentage of growth remaining. The multiplier method is, therefore, viewed as a universal method for predicting lower limb length because it is independent of percentile, regional, racial, ethnic, and generational differences in growth data. The multiplier values for boys and girls differ from each other only because growth in boys continues for approximately 2.25 years longer than growth in girls. The patterns of the multipliers are otherwise the same.

To predict limb or bone length, the current limb or bone length is multiplied by the current age multiplier to obtain the predicted limb or bone length at maturity. Lower limb length, upper limb length, total height, foot length, and foot height have each been characterized by the multiplier method.[36-41] Predictions are based on a single radiograph obtained at any age for congenital conditions and two radiographs obtained at any age for developmental conditions. The multiplier method provides a simple, rapid method of predicting remaining growth. It is especially valuable when attempting to evaluate the growth pattern of a patient without previous radiographs or a very young patient with few previous radiographs. In these situations, the multiplier method provides a concise way of providing information and guidance to families who want to know the predicted LLD at skeletal maturity to allow for long-term treatment planning.

Relying on chronologic age to estimate the amount of growth remaining may lead to errors. Chronologic age has been found to correspond to skeletal age within a 6-month range in only 49% of boys and 51% of girls.[2] Chronologic age is superior to skeletal age for predicting ultimate limb length before the adolescent growth spurt but is inferior once the growth spurt begins.[42] Therefore, skeletal age is preferable for making predictions in adolescents. With the multiplier method, the multiplier corresponding to skeletal age can be used rather than the multiplier corresponding to chronologic age.

Knowing when an adolescent child is about to enter his/her growth spurt is an important marker of growth remaining. The authors of a 2017 study[13] found that in healthy children, the adolescent growth spurt is standardized at 90% of final height, with similar patterns for children of both sexes beginning at the initiation of the growth spurt. Once children enter the growth spurt, their growth pattern is consistent between children, with peak growth at 90% of final height and skeletal maturity closely reflecting growth remaining. The corresponding Greulich and Pyle[11] skeletal ages were 11.0 years for average girls and just younger than 13.5 years for boys.

Even though various mathematical formulas have been designed to capture the complexity of growth, it is unwise to rely solely on these equations. When attempting to understand the growth dynamics of a patient, the ideal approach should use multiple methods that complement each other. For example, checking the Anderson-Green-Messner growth-remaining chart in addition to the arithmetic method or the multiplier method is better than using only one method. If the different methods agree with each other, then the probability exists that the calculations are reliable. If, however, the calculations produce widely disparate results, then further investigation may be necessary. Combining these methods with an evaluation of a child's Tanner stages and annual growth velocity can further refine the accuracy of prediction. In the best-case scenario, the clinician should accumulate multiple, meticulous, lower limb measurements while continuously monitoring the onset of puberty (acceleration of the annual lower limb growth velocity, the onset of Tanner stages, double ossification of the olecranon, and ossification of the sesamoid of the thumb).[43] The beginning of puberty corresponds to 11 years of skeletal age in girls and 13 years of skeletal age in boys.[44]

Skeletal Maturity

Similar to the growth-remaining predictions, the bone age assessment in children is influenced by sex, race, nutritional status, living environment, and social resources.[39] Different methods for determining skeletal age have been described, using hand, elbow, foot, knee, or pelvic radiographs.[45] Accurate measurements of skeletal maturity should yield better growth-remaining predictions, but the optimal method or a combination of methods for assessing skeletal maturity remains controversial. The *Radiographic Atlas of the Hand and Wrist* is the most common tool for evaluating bone age, and many practitioners consider it the preferred method.[11] However, this method has known weaknesses that limit its effectiveness. It relies on the subjective analysis of subtle morphologic changes described within the atlas and has long intervals between reference standards, especially during the critical pubertal growth period. The standards for 11.5 and 12.5 years of skeletal age in girls and 14.5 years of skeletal age in boys are absent. Furthermore, training in the technique is required to become proficient, and access to the atlas in hard copy form is necessary for its use.

The shorthand bone age assessment is an abridged method of bone age assessment based on the basic principles of the Greulich and Pyle method (also known as the atlas method).[45] It allows the assessment of skeletal maturity in males aged 12.5 to 16 years and females aged 10 to 14 years (**Table 2**). The relatively simple set of radiographic criteria for interpreting skeletal age can be easily referenced in tabular form or committed to memory. The shorthand assessment method has been shown to have high intraobserver and interobserver reliability and can be quickly mastered by practitioners at all levels of training. Because it is derived from the Greulich and Pyle method, the shorthand bone age has some limitations. For example, skeletal half-age determinations such as 12.5 and 15.5 years in females and 14.5 years in both males and females are not included in the shorthand bone age. In addition, similar to the Greulich and Pyle method, the shorthand bone age depends on the patient having a normal left-hand radiograph, which may not be applicable for patients with skeletal dysplasias affecting the left hand or other hand abnormalities. In such cases, a method of skeletal age determination using radiographs of other body parts should be used.

To address these limitations, other methods of bone age estimation have been proposed as alternatives to the Greulich and Pyle method or the shorthand bone age. The Sauvegrain method uses changes in the radiographic appearance of the ossification centers of the elbow to determine skeletal age.[46] The elbow undergoes regular morphologic changes at the epiphysis ossification centers that are clearly identifiable before and during puberty. For this reason, elbow radiographs are helpful to study skeletal age near and during the adolescent growth spurt. Elbow radiographs should be obtained between 10 and 13 years of skeletal age in girls and between 12 and 15 years of skeletal age in boys. In younger children, elbow radiographs cannot be used to assess skeletal age because

TABLE 2

Description of Radiographic Criteria Used to Determine Skeletal Age in Males Aged 12.5 to 16 Years and Females Aged 10 to 14 Years, According to the Shorthand Bone Age Assessment Method

Criterion	Males (Years)	Females (Years)
Appearance of the hook of hamate ossific nucleus	12.5	10
Appearance of the thumb sesamoid ossific nucleus	13	11
Proximal aspect of the distal radius epiphysis has extended to meet the maximum width of the distal width of the distal aspect of distal radius metaphysis but has not yet begun to cap	13.5	—
Capping of the distal radius epiphysis	14	12
Closure of the thumb distal phalanx physis	15	13
Closure of the index finger distal phalanx physis	15.5	13.5
Closure of the index finger proximal phalanx physis	16	14

the elbow is still mainly cartilaginous, and the ossification centers do not yet show any remarkable morphologic characteristics.

The Sauvegrain method is based on a 27-point scoring system of four anatomic landmarks: the lateral condyle/epicondyle, the trochlea, the olecranon apophysis, and the proximal radial epiphysis. Skeletal age is determined by summing the individual scores of each landmark to arrive at a total score. The score is then plotted on a graph (separate graphs for girls and boys), which gives the corresponding skeletal age. A score of 26 or higher indicates that a child has passed PHV.

In 2005, a group of researchers simplified the original Sauvegrain method by condensing the method from evaluating four different ossification centers in the elbow to one ossification center.[47] These researchers demonstrated that the morphology of the olecranon apophysis on lateral radiographs goes through five distinct and characteristic appearances (**Table 3**). It allows skeletal age to be determined in regular 6-month intervals in girls aged 11 to 13 years and boys aged 13 to 15 years. Furthermore, the learning curve of this simplified method is short. Studies have shown that this modified Sauvegrain method is reliable and accurate.[47-49] Clinically, the maturation of the olecranon is relevant because it occurs during the pubertal growth spurt, when the Risser grade is still 0. During this phase of accelerated growth, the information obtained from the olecranon apophyseal lines complements the assessment of the triradiate cartilage, and it helps identify patients who are skeletally immature. Closure of the epiphyses at the elbow indicates the end of the accelerated growth spurt, when the adolescent is entering the decelerating phase of pubertal growth.

As another alternative to the Greulich and Pyle method, a group of researchers presented a method of digital (phalangeal) skeletal age assessment derived from the Tanner-Whitehouse III method.[14] This technique is based on a radiologic analysis of the metacarpals and fingers on AP hand radiographs. The simplified digital method is useful from the prepubertal growth period to skeletal maturity. It divides this period into eight stages and includes several markers before Risser grade 1. The

TABLE 3

Modified Sauvegrain Method for Skeletal Age

	Males (Years)	Females (Years)
Two ossification centers at the level of the olecranon apophysis	13	11
Half-moon shape of the olecranon apophysis	13.5	11.5
Rectangular shape of the olecranon apophysis	14	12
Beginning of fusion of the olecranon apophysis	14.5	12.5
Complete fusion of the olecranon apophysis	15	13

eight stages are as follows: stages 1 and 2 correspond to the prepubertal period, stages 3 and 4 correspond to the pubertal growth spurt (Risser grade 0), and stages 5 to 8 cover the period from Risser grade 1 to 5, when full skeletal maturity has occurred. Although this technique is less detailed than the modified Sauvegrain method during the 2-year phase of accelerated growth, the digital method can be combined with the Sauvegrain method to cover every Risser grade until skeletal maturity.

Two recent publications highlight more practical methods to calculate skeletal age without having to obtain additional specialized radiographs. The authors of a 2017 study developed a formula for determining skeletal age using cervical vertebrae (C3 and C4).[50] This technique can be used in patients with scoliosis who are already undergoing regular spine radiographic examinations. Similarly, estimating skeletal maturity using the distal femoral central physeal peak value has also been described.[51,52] Because this measurement can be made comparably on isolated AP knee or standing hip-to-ankle leg-length radiographs, the central physeal peak value provides a quick, quantitative and easily reproducible method that avoids exposing patients with LLD to additional radiation exposure.

Each method has its own strengths and weaknesses. The proper strategy should be to take advantage of each method's strengths and apply it at the proper time. For example, a lateral elbow radiograph may be more effective than a hand radiograph when assessing skeletal maturity during puberty. A hand radiograph is preferable before puberty and from Risser grade 1 to skeletal maturity. A combination of both methods adequately covers the gap between elbow fusion and Risser grade 1 because one complements the other.

Because many of the commonly used methods of skeletal age assessment are associated with some intraobserver and interobserver variability, there may be a future role for automated bone age assessment.[53] Evidence shows that using computer software to evaluate radiographs for skeletal age may be faster and more accurate than subjective readings by radiologists.[38] The software also may allow an evaluation that is applicable across different racial and ethnic groups. At this time, however, automated techniques require further testing before they can be considered as a valid alternative to current methods.

Angular Correction

Gradual correction of angular deformity by asymmetric physeal suppression is an attractive option in growing children. Creating a tether on the convex side of the physis allows subsequent growth from the opposite side of the physis to correct the angular deformity. However, when using this method, the chosen physis must retain enough viable growth potential to successfully respond to growth guidance. Percutaneous hemiepiphyseal drilling, hemiepiphyseal stapling, hemitransphyseal screws, and tension-band plating are the most commonly used techniques. With the exception of percutaneous hemiepiphyseal drilling, these methods are potentially reversible and minimally invasive in nature. After angular correction has been achieved, the tethering device (staple, screw, plate) may be removed, and normal linear growth should resume. However, the response of the physis can be unpredictable after the removal of a tethering device. Recurrence of deformity as a rebound effect (accelerated growth on the side of the physis that was temporarily restrained) is known to occur in some patients.[54]

Determining the appropriate timing of hemiepiphysiodesis is one of the most difficult aspects of using guided growth to correct angular deformity. Incorrect timing can lead to either overcorrection or undercorrection. When planning to use any of these techniques, the surgeon should consider the magnitude of the deformity and the amount of remaining growth available. In general, the speed of angular correction is a function of two variables: the growth rate of the physis and the distance from the tether to the far edge of the epiphyseal plate (the narrower the width of the physis, the faster the rate of correction will be).[55] The rate of correction, however, also is known to be influenced by the age and sex of the patient, the surgical method used (staples, transphyseal screws, or flexible plate), etiology, and the location of the physis being treated.

In 1985, a technique for determining the timing of hemiepiphysiodesis was published.[55] Data were incorporated from the Anderson-Green-Messer growth-remaining chart, skeletal age, and physeal width for development of a chart guiding angular deformity versus growth remaining for coronal plane deformities about the knee. Based on these data, correction was estimated at 7° per year following distal femoral hemiepiphysiodesis and 5° per year in the proximal tibia. This chart is helpful when applied to a patient with a normally functioning physis. However, when considering patients with abnormal physes, such as in skeletal dysplasias and Blount disease, the chart is less reliable.

The multiplier method can also be used to predict the timing of angular correction. The authors of a 2019 study[56] found that the multiplier method underpredicted the time needed for angular correction in 69% of the cases. They suggest that hemiepiphysiodesis before skeletal maturity should be started 2 to 4 months earlier than predicted by the multiplier method.

Further studies on guided growth, however, have provided additional guidelines.[54,57-61] For example, the rate of improvement in mechanical axis alignment that is derived from the tibial segment is slower than that from the femoral segment. The correction rates of coronal angular deformity at the distal femur range from 0.56° to 1.0° per month and range from 0.36° to 0.82° per month at the proximal tibia.[54,57-61] The fastest rates of correction are achieved in two instances: (1) when the distal femoral and proximal tibial physes are treated concurrently and (2) when the technique is used in children younger than 10 years. One study reported that the overall rates of correction for children younger than 10 years was 1.4° and 0.6° per month for children older than 10 years.[60] A 2012 study of valgus deformity found that in boys 14 years or younger and girls 12 years or younger, the rates of correction at the distal femur, the proximal tibia, and the distal tibia were 0.71° per month (8.5° per year), 0.40° per month (4.8° per year), and 0.48° per month (5.8° per year), respectively.[61] In older children, the rates of correction at the distal femur, the proximal tibia, and the distal tibia were 0.39° per month (4.7° per year), 0.29° per month (3.5° per year), and 0.48° per month (5.8° per year), respectively.[61] Measuring the rates of correction per month allows the surgeon to estimate the overall treatment time. Visual appreciation of the effect of gradual correction usually does not occur until near the end of the treatment period. Consequently, providing the patient and parents with counseling about the expected time needed for correction will help diffuse any anxiety over what may initially appear to be a lack of improvement.

Smartphone Applications

Two free smartphone apps (Multiplier, Paley Growth) have been developed to help the clinician make growth assessments quickly and conveniently. The equations for limb-length inequality can be complicated and are prone to arithmetic errors when computed manually. With smartphone apps, the user simply enters the patient's sex and age and the direct measurements from the limb-length study. All calculations and predictions are then processed by the app. Such apps allow faster and more accurate determination of the timing of epiphysiodesis compared with traditional methods.[62] For example, the Multiplier has multiple platforms that allow a comprehensive evaluation of growth. The formulas and tables available in the Multiplier include calculating LLD at maturity (congenital and developmental), growth remaining (femur, tibia, and entire leg), and bone length at maturity for both the upper and lower limbs. Functions also are available for calculating the timing of both epiphysiodesis and angular correction. In addition, the Multiplier contains helpful supplemental information, such as the standard deformity measurements of the lower limbs and the foot, the Sauvegrain bone age method, the shorthand bone age assessment method, height and growth charts from the Centers for Disease Control and Prevention, oblique plane deformity calculation, and multiplier tables and formulas. Having a comprehensive wealth of information at the click of a button allows the clinician to provide practical information to the patient and his or her family in a quick and accurate manner.

Reversible Growth Arrest

With the advent of tension-band plating to achieve guided growth of angular deformities in patients who are skeletally immature, some surgeons have attempted to apply this technique to reversible epiphysiodesis.[63-69] By implanting tension-band plates on both the medial and lateral sides of the physis, it is theoretically possible to slow longitudinal physeal growth without damaging the physis. Physeal growth would then resume after the plates are removed. The need for accurate prediction would be less critical because the plates could be removed after equality in leg length has been obtained. This technique would allow surgeons to treat LLDs at a younger age, not necessarily according to the age of maturity. The correction also could potentially be performed more than once during a child's growth period.

Although reversible epiphysiodesis in an animal model was successful by using tension-band plating, the duration that a physis may be tethered with the expectation of growth after implant removal remains unknown.[63] The resumption of growth after the removal of medial and lateral tension-band plates has not yet been clinically demonstrated in the literature. Other concerns with the technique include creating an angulation by asymmetric growth retardation if the screws do not reach maximum splay at the same time. In addition, the eight-Plate (Orthofix) seems to allow for central physeal growth.[64] The authors of a 2018 study[67] found the eight-plate epiphysiodesis caused a change in the bony morphology of the tibial plateau. The current recommendation is that surgeons use the 2-year rule, which states that it is safe to leave tethering over a physis for up to 2 years in a growing child before permanent epiphysiodesis takes place.[63]

The use of tension-band plates for definitive epiphysiodesis has also been investigated. The authors of a 2019 study[68] do not recommend the use of tension-band plates for LLD correction because of inferior correction rates with higher complication and revision rates than traditional percutaneous epiphysiodesis. Similarly, the authors of a 2016 study[69] found poor efficiency of tension-band plates in the management of LLD when compared with percutaneous epiphysiodesis using transphyseal screws.

SUMMARY

It is important to understand the pattern of normal growth. Management decisions for pediatric orthopaedic conditions can be guided by knowing the expected growth rate of a child. Estimating growth remaining and skeletal maturity, however, is still not an exact science. Using multiple complementary methods to calculate these parameters will help to decrease the chance of error.

KEY STUDY POINTS

- A basic understanding of growth in children is necessary to better assess deviations from the normal.
- Knowledge of PHV can be used to guide decision making in children with scoliosis.
- The multiplier method is independent of percentile, regional, racial, ethnic, and generational differences in growth data.
- When assessing bone age, a hand radiograph is preferable before puberty and from Risser grade 1 to skeletal maturity. A lateral elbow radiograph should be obtained during puberty.

ANNOTATED REFERENCES

1. Buckwalter JA, Ehrlich MG, Sandell LJ, Trippel SB, eds: *Skeletal Growth and Development: Clinical Issues and Basic Science Advances*. Rosemont, IL, American Academy of Orthopaedic Surgeons, 1997, p 577.
2. Diméglio A: Growth in pediatric orthopaedics. *J Pediatr Orthop* 2001;21(4):549-555.
3. Diméglio A: Growth in pediatric orthopaedics, in Morrissey RT, Weinstein SL, eds: *Lovell and Winter's Pediatric Orthopaedics*, ed 6. Philadelphia, PA, Lippincott Williams and Wilkins, 2006, pp 35-63.
4. Diméglio A: *La croissance en orthopedie*. Montpellier, France, Sauramps Medical, 1987.
5. Adair LS: Child and adolescent obesity: Epidemiology and developmental perspectives. *Physiol Behav* 2008;94(1): 8-16.
6. Carroll MD, Navaneelan T, Bryan S, Ogden C: *Prevalence of Obesity Among Children and Adolescents in the United States and Canada*. National Center for Health Statistics Data Brief, 211. Available at: http://www.cdc.gov/nchs/data/databriefs/db211.htm. Accessed March 11, 2016.

   This online article discusses the prevalence of obesity in children in the United States and Canada. Both countries have seen a substantial increase in obesity in the past 30 years.
7. Nowicki P, Kemppainen J, Maskill L, Cassidy J: The role of obesity in pediatric orthopedics. *J Am Acad Orthop Surg Glob Res Rev* 2019;3(5):e036.

   This review article concerning the mounting evidence demonstrated that obesity itself increases the risk of complications related to fracture and surgical management along with physiologic changes to the growing skeleton compared with healthy weight patients. Level of evidence: III.
8. da Silva VN, Fiorelli LNM, da Silva CC, Kurokawa CS, Goldberg TBL: Do metabolic syndrome and its components have an impact on bone mineral density in adolescents? *Nutr Metab (Lond)* 2017;14:1.

   This review performs a critical analysis of articles that specifically focus on the adolescent age group, evaluating the influence of metabolic syndrome and its components on bone mineral density in adolescents. Level of evidence: III.
9. Pollock NK: Childhood obesity, bone development, and cardiometabolic risk factors. *Mol Cell Endocrinol* 2015;410:52-63.
10. Turner CB, Lin H, Flores G: Prevalence of vitamin D deficiency among overweight and obese US children. *Pediatrics* 2013;131:e152-e161.
11. Greulich WW, Pyle SI: *Radiographic Atlas of Skeletal Development of the Hand and Wrist*, ed 2. Stanford, CA, Stanford University Press, 1959.
12. Sanders JO, Browne RH, Cooney TE, Finegold DN, McConnell SJ, Margraf SA: Correlates of the peak height velocity in girls with idiopathic scoliosis. *Spine (Phila Pa 1976)* 2006;31(20):2289-2295.
13. Sanders JO, Qiu X, Lu X, et al: The uniform pattern of growth and skeletal maturation during the human adolescent growth spurt. *Sci Rep* 2017;7:16705.

    The ability to use 90% of final height as easily identified important maturity standard with its close relationship to skeletal maturity represents a significant advance allowing accurate prediction of future growth for individual children and accurate maturity comparisons for future studies of children's growth. Level of evidence: III.
14. Sanders JO, Khoury JG, Kishan S, et al: Predicting scoliosis progression from skeletal maturity: A simplified classification during adolescence. *J Bone Joint Surg Am* 2008;90(3):540-553.
15. Needlman RD: Growth and development, in Behrman RE, ed: *Nelson Textbook of Pediatrics*, ed 16. Philadelphia, PA, WB Saunders, 2000, pp 23-65.
16. Ford DM, McFadden KD, Bagnall KM: Sequence of ossification in human vertebral neural arch centers. *Anat Rec* 1982;203(1):175-178.
17. Hinck VC, Hopkins CE, Clark WM: Sagittal diameter of the lumbar spinal canal in children and adults. *Radiology* 1965;85(5):929-937.
18. Yousefzadeh DK, El-Khoury GY, Smith WL: Normal sagittal diameter and variation in the pediatric cervical spine. *Radiology* 1982;144(2):319-325.
19. Labrom RD: Growth and maturation of the spine from birth to adolescence. *J Bone Joint Surg Am* 2007;89(suppl 1):3-7.
20. Ogden JA: Radiology of postnatal skeletal development: XI. The first cervical vertebra. *Skeletal Radiol* 1984;12(1): 12-20.
21. Duval-Beaupere G: Pathogenic relationship between scoliosis and growth, in Zorab PA, ed: *Scoliosis and Growth*. Edinburgh, Scotland, Churchill Livingstone, 1971, pp 58-64.

22. Little DG, Song KM, Katz D, Herring JA: Relationship of peak height velocity to other maturity indicators in idiopathic scoliosis in girls. *J Bone Joint Surg Am* 2000;82(5):685-693.

23. Song KM, Little DG: Peak height velocity as a maturity indicator for males with idiopathic scoliosis. *J Pediatr Orthop* 2000;20(3):286-288.

24. Bunch WH, Dvonch VM: Pitfalls in the assessment of skeletal immaturity: An anthropologic case study. *J Pediatr Orthop* 1983;3(2):220-222.

25. Bunnell WP: The natural history of idiopathic scoliosis before skeletal maturity. *Spine (Phila Pa 1976)* 1986;11(8):773-776.

26. Lonstein JE, Carlson JM: The prediction of curve progression in untreated idiopathic scoliosis during growth. *J Bone Joint Surg Am* 1984;66(7):1061-1071.

27. Perdriolle R, Vidal J: Thoracic idiopathic scoliosis curve evolution and prognosis. *Spine (Phila Pa 1976)* 1985;10(9):785-791.

28. Sanders JO, Browne RH, McConnell SJ, Margraf SA, Cooney TE, Finegold DN: Maturity assessment and curve progression in girls with idiopathic scoliosis. *J Bone Joint Surg Am* 2007;89(1):64-73.

29. Sitoula P, Verma K, Homles L, et al: Prediction of curve progression in idiopathic scoliosis: Validation of the Sanders Skeletal Maturity Staging System. *Spine* 2015;40(13):1006-1013.

30. Dubousset J, Herring JA, Shufflebarger H: The crankshaft phenomenon. *J Pediatr Orthop* 1989;9(5):541-550.

31. Sanders JO, Herring JA, Browne RH: Posterior arthrodesis and instrumentation in the immature (Risser-grade-0) spine in idiopathic scoliosis. *J Bone Joint Surg Am* 1995;77(1):39-45.

32. Sanders JO, Little DG, Richards BS: Prediction of the crankshaft phenomenon by peak height velocity. *Spine (Phila Pa 1976)* 1997;22(12):1352-1356, discussion 1356-1357.

33. Menelaus MB: Correction of leg length discrepancy by epiphysial arrest. *J Bone Joint Surg Br* 1966;48(2):336-339.

34. Anderson M, Green WT, Messner MB: Growth and predictions of growth in the lower extremities. *J Bone Joint Surg Am* 1963;45:1-14.

35. Moseley CF: A straight-line graph for leg-length discrepancies. *J Bone Joint Surg Am* 1977;59(2):174-179.

36. Paley D, Bhave A, Herzenberg JE, Bowen JR: Multiplier method for predicting limb-length discrepancy. *J Bone Joint Surg Am* 2000;82(10):1432-1446.

37. Paley J, Talor J, Levin A, Bhave A, Paley D, Herzenberg JE: The multiplier method for prediction of adult height. *J Pediatr Orthop* 2004;24(6):732-737.

38. Aguilar JA, Paley D, Paley J, et al: Clinical validation of the multiplier method for predicting limb length at maturity, part I. *J Pediatr Orthop* 2005;25(2):186-191.

39. Aguilar JA, Paley D, Paley J, et al: Clinical validation of the multiplier method for predicting limb length discrepancy and outcome of epiphysiodesis, part II. *J Pediatr Orthop* 2005;25(2):192-196.

40. Lamm BM, Paley D, Kurland DB, Matz AL, Herzenberg JE: Multiplier method for predicting adult foot length. *J Pediatr Orthop* 2006;26(4):444-448.

41. Paley D, Gelman A, Shualy MB, Herzenberg JE: Multiplier method for limb-length prediction in the upper extremity. *J Hand Surg Am* 2008;33(3):385-391.

42. Sanders JO, Howell J, Qiu X: Comparison of the Paley method using chronological age with use of skeletal maturity for predicting mature limb length in children. *J Bone Joint Surg Am* 2011;93(11):1051-1056.

43. Kelly PM, Diméglio A: Lower-limb growth: How predictable are predictions? *J Child Orthop* 2008;2(6):407-415.

44. Canavese F, Charles YP, Dimeglio A, et al: A comparison of the simplified olecranon and digital methods of assessment of skeletal maturity during the pubertal growth spurt. *Bone Joint J* 2014;96-B(11):1556-1560.

45. Heyworth BE, Osei DA, Fabricant PD, et al: The shorthand bone age assessment: A simpler alternative to current methods. *J Pediatr Orthop* 2013;33(5):569-574.

46. Sauvegrain J, Nahum H, Bronstein H: Study of bone maturation of the elbow [French]. *Ann Radiol (Paris)* 1962;5:542-550.

47. Diméglio A, Charles YP, Daures JP, de Rosa V, Kaboré B: Accuracy of the Sauvegrain method in determining skeletal age during puberty. *J Bone Joint Surg Am* 2005;87(8):1689-1696.

48. Charles YP, Diméglio A, Canavese F, Daures JP: Skeletal age assessment from the olecranon for idiopathic scoliosis at Risser grade 0. *J Bone Joint Surg Am* 2007;89(12):2737-2744.

49. Hans SD, Sanders JO, Cooperman DR: Using the Sauvegrain method to predict peak height velocity in boys and girls. *J Pediatr Orthop* 2008;28(8):836-839.

50. Turkoz C, Kaygisiz E, Ulusoy C, Ates C: A practical formula for determining growth. *Diagn Interv Radiol* 2017;23:194-198.

    This study develops a formula derived for evaluating skeletal age in cephalometric radiographs that is reliable and can be applied to both girl and boy subjects for legal requirements or therapeutic needs of age estimation. Level of evidence: III.

51. Knapik DM, Sanders JO, Gilmore A, Weber DR, Cooperman DR, Liu RW: A quantitative method for the radiological assessment of skeletal maturity using the distal femur. *Bone Joint J* 2018;100-B:1106-1111.

    This article demonstrates that chronological age + gender + central peak value provides more accurate prediction of 90% of final height compared with chronological age + gender and Greulich and Pyle bone age + gender. Level of evidence: III.

52. Knapik DM, Duong MM, Liu RW: Evaluation of skeletal maturity using the distal femoral physeal central peak is not significantly affected by radiographic projection. *J Pediatr Orthop* 2019;39(10):e782-e786.

    This study describes the central peak value, which is a quick, quantitative method for estimating skeletal maturity from standard AP radiographs of the knee. Level of evidence: III.

53. De Sanctis V, Soliman AT, Di Maio S, Bedair S: Are the new automated methods for bone age estimation advantageous over the manual approaches? *Pediatr Endocrinol Rev* 2014;12(2):200-205.
54. Lykissas MG, Jain VV, Manickam V, Nathan S, Eismann EA, McCarthy JJ: Guided growth for the treatment of limb length discrepancy: A comparative study of the three most commonly used surgical techniques. *J Pediatr Orthop B* 2013;22(4):311-317.
55. Bowen JR, Leahey JL, Zhang ZH, MacEwen GD: Partial epiphysiodesis at the knee to correct angular deformity. *Clin Orthop Relat Res* 1985;198:184-190.
56. Eltayeby HH, Gwam CU, Frederick MM, Herzenberg JE: How accurate is the multiplier method in predicting the timing of angular correction after hemiepiphysiodesis? *J Pediatr Orthop* 2019;39:e91-e94.

    This article found that the multiplier method has a tendency to underpredict angular correction. Therefore, doing a guided growth right before skeletal maturity should be started 2 to 4 months earlier than suggested by the multiplier method. Level of evidence: IV.
57. Castañeda P, Urquhart B, Sullivan E, Haynes RJ: Hemiepiphysiodesis for the correction of angular deformity about the knee. *J Pediatr Orthop* 2008;28(2):188-191.
58. Wiemann JM IV, Tryon C, Szalay EA: Physeal stapling versus 8-plate hemiepiphysiodesis for guided correction of angular deformity about the knee. *J Pediatr Orthop* 2009;29(5):481-485.
59. Shin SJ, Cho TJ, Park MS, et al: Angular deformity correction by asymmetrical physeal suppression in growing children: Stapling versus percutaneous transphyseal screw. *J Pediatr Orthop* 2010;30(6):588-593.
60. Ballal MS, Bruce CE, Nayagam S: Correcting genu varum and genu valgum in children by guided growth: Temporary hemiepiphysiodesis using tension band plates. *J Bone Joint Surg Br* 2010;92(2):273-276.
61. Sung KH, Ahn S, Chung CY, et al: Rate of correction after asymmetrical physeal suppression in valgus deformity: Analysis using a linear mixed model application. *J Pediatr Orthop* 2012;32(8):805-814.
62. Wagner P, Standard SC, Herzenberg JE: *Abstract: Evaluation of a Mobile Application for Multiplier Method Growth and Epiphysiodesis Predictions. ILLRS Congress, Miami 2015.* Montreal, Canada, Limb Lengthening and Reconstruction Society of North America, 2015, p 141.
63. Gottliebsen M, Møller-Madsen B, Stødkilde-Jørgensen H, Rahbek O: Controlled longitudinal bone growth by temporary tension band plating: An experimental study. *Bone Joint J* 2013;95-B(6):855-860.
64. Lauge-Pedersen H, Hägglund G: Eight plate should not be used for treating leg length discrepancy. *J Child Orthop* 2013;7(4):285-288.
65. Stewart D, Cheema A, Szalay EA: Dual 8-plate technique is not as effective as ablation for epiphysiodesis about the knee. *J Pediatr Orthop* 2013;33(8):843-846.
66. Siedhoff M, Ridderbusch K, Breyer S, Stucker R, Rupprecht M: Temporary epiphysiodesis for limb-length discrepancy: 8- to 15-year follow-up of 34 children. *Acta Orthop* 2014;85:626-632.
67. Sinha R, Weigl D, Mercado E, Becker T, Kedem P, Bar-On E: Eight-plate epiphysiodesis: Are we creating an intra-articular deformity? *Bone Joint J* 2018;100-B:1112-1116.

    The article found the use of eight-plates in the proximal tibia for deformity correction, and limb-length equalization causes a change in the bony morphology of the tibial plateau in a significant number of patients and the effect is more pronounced in the correction of limb-length discrepancy. Level of evidence: IV.
68. Borbas P, Agten CA, Rosskopf AB, Hingsammer A, Eid K, Ramseier LE: Guided growth with tension band plate or definitive epiphysiodesis for treatment of limb length discrepancy? *J Orthop Surg Res* 2019;14:99.

    This article does not recommend the use of tension band plates for limb-length discrepancy correction due to inferior correction with higher complication and revision rate. Level of evidence: III.
69. Gaumetou E, Mallet C, Souchet P, Mazda K, Ilharreborde B: Poor efficiency of eight-plates in the treatment of lower limb discrepancy. *J Pediatr Orthop* 2016;36:715-719.

    This article concluded that eight-plate procedures cannot be considered as an efficient epiphysiodesis technique in comparison with standard technique. Level of evidence: IV.

SECTION 2

Basic Science

Section Editor:

Benjamin A. Alman, MD, FAAOS

CHAPTER 7

Genetics and Personalized Medicine

CHRISTINA A. GURNETT, MD, PhD • DOROTHY K. GRANGE, MD
DAVID H. GUTMANN, MD, PhD • DOUGLAS J. MCDONALD, MD, MS
MATTHEW B. DOBBS, MD, FACS, FAOA

ABSTRACT

Physicians are striving to develop treatment and prevention strategies that can be targeted to meet a patient's unique genetic and environmental milieu. Genetic advances that facilitate comprehensive and inexpensive genome-wide testing are largely driving personalized medicine. Rich opportunities exist for developing personalized treatment approaches for pediatric orthopaedic disorders. It is helpful to be aware of the latest advances in genetic technology and pharmacogenetics, the new discoveries of somatic mutations in bone cancers and segmental overgrowth syndromes, and the new insights into the etiology of clubfoot and adolescent idiopathic scoliosis.

Dr. Gurnett or an immediate family member has received royalties from D-Bar Enterprises; serves as a paid consultant to or is an employee of D-Bar Enterprises; and serves as a board member, owner, officer, or committee member of the Association of Bone and Joint Surgeons. Dr. Grange or an immediate family member has received research or institutional support from Biomarin Pharmceuticals Inc. and Shire. Dr. Dobbs or an immediate family member has received royalties from D-Bar Enterprises; serves as a paid consultant to or is an employee of C-Pro Direct, D-Bar Enterprises, MD Orthopaedics, and Orthopediatrics; and serves as a board member, owner, officer, or committee member of the Association of Bone and Joint Surgeons, the Orthopaedic Research and Education Foundation, SICOT, and WOC. None of the following authors or any immediate family member has received anything of value from or has stock or stock options held in a commercial company or institution related directly or indirectly to the subject of this chapter: Dr. Gutmann and Dr. McDonald.

Keywords: personalized medicine; pharmacogenetics; segmental overgrowth; somatic mutation

INTRODUCTION

In January 2015, President Barack Obama launched a new $215-million initiative to advance the research and implementation of precision medicine.[1] Personalized medicine promises to (1) deliver pharmaceutical agents with minimal toxicity and optimal efficacy and (2) guide treatment and preventive interventions informed by a patient's unique biology. Abandoning a one-size-fits-all approach to health care will require more research into the genetic and environmental factors that influence disease presentations and surgical outcomes for pediatric orthopaedic conditions. Recent advances in genetic technology and new insights into rare and common pediatric orthopaedic disorders that will pave the way for personalized medicine in the next decade are highlighted.

COMPREHENSIVE GENETIC PROFILING

The first wave of genetic and genomic discoveries followed the development of microarray technology, which facilitated the simultaneous ascertainment of an extremely large number (often >1 million) of known single-nucleotide polymorphic genotypes (**Table 1**). Microarray technology also allows the identification of genomic abnormalities, including microdeletions and microduplications of small chromosomal regions that are too small to be viewed microscopically, on a routine karyotype.[2] Single-nucleotide polymorphisms (SNPs) are informative for some disorders because a plethora of genome-wide association studies (GWASs), mostly for common and complex diseases, have yielded SNPs or groups of SNPs that increase the risk for complex human diseases.[3] Genetic risk factors for common diseases identified through GWASs are mostly associated with a small

TABLE 1

Common Genetic Terms

Term	Definition and Characteristic
Complex genetic disease	A disorder caused by multiple genetic variations in a single individual.
De novo	Arising newly in the genome in either somatic cells or the germline, germline de novo mutations can be identified by sequencing unaffected parents and the affected child, whereas somatic de novo mutations can be detected by paired sequencing of normal and abnormal tissues.
DNA variant	Differences in DNA between individuals.
Genetic association	DNA sequence variants that are more common in a group of patients compared with a control group.
Germline mutation	A mutation that occurs in the ova or the sperm before fertilization.
Mendelian genetic disorder	A genetic disorder that is caused by a single genetic variation and is highly heritable.
Microdeletion/microduplication	A small deletion or duplication of DNA that is undetectable under the microscope but detectable with other methods.
Mosaic	Differences in genetic composition between different cells in an organism result from a somatic mutation.
Pharmacogenetic variant	A genetic variant that influences a drug response, by altering drug absorption, distribution, metabolism, or the drug target.
Segmental overgrowth syndrome	One of many syndromes that results from abnormal growth of a region of the body.
Single-nucleotide polymorphism (SNP)	A variant that consists of a change of one nucleotide between individuals. The term is often used to indicate a common SNP that is present in more than 1% and up to 5% of the population.
Somatic mutation	A mutation during cell division that occurs at any time after fertilization. Depending on the temporal and spatial patterns of the mutational event, these mutations may cause cancer or congenital malformations.
Ultrarapid metabolizer	An individual who has a genetic variant that results in better metabolism of a prodrug into the active drug.

to modest increase in risk, increasing the odds ratio from 1.0 to approximately 1.1 to 1.4. These SNPs are typically variants that are present in approximately 5% to 40% of the population, and the variants may be either protective or risk alleles. Although most of these genetic risk factors are not highly predictive of disease within a single individual, collectively they provide an understanding of the pathways involved and the overall landscape of a single disease in terms of how much disease risk is predicted by common versus rare genetic variants.

The investigation of de novo variants, defined as mutations that are present in an affected child but not the unaffected parents, has made possible extensive new genetic discoveries for patients with rare genetic diseases. De novo variants may arise in two places: (1) the germline (the ova or the sperm), where they would then be incorporated into all cells in the developing fetus, or (2) in somatic cells during cell division, where they would be present only in a subset of cells depending on the location and timing of the mutational event. De novo germline mutations play an important role in the causality of diseases and are associated with reduced life expectancy and/or diminished reproductive fitness, which often occurs in children with severe autism or developmental disabilities.[4] Whole-genome sequencing studies of healthy trios (a healthy child and both healthy parents) estimate that the germline mutation rate is approximately 1.0×10^{-8}, which results in 10 to 20 de novo coding sequence variants per child.[5] Although all human genomes harbor de novo variants, most do not negatively affect the coding genes. Congenital disorders occur when de novo mutations deleteriously affect genes that are important for development. Because more germ cell divisions occur in males than in females, most de novo missense mutations arise on paternally derived chromosomes. The male germline accumulates mutations during normal aging, such that approximately twice as many de novo mutations are present in the child of a 40-year-old father compared with the child of a 20-year-old father. As a consequence of recent de novo gene discovery for children with presumed genetic disease, exome sequencing of trios is rapidly becoming a first-line test for children with severe cognitive and developmental disabilities and results in a diagnosis in nearly 50% of all patients. This approach is useful to study severe, sporadic disorders that arise without any family history of the disorder.

In addition to revealing the cause of a disease for which clinical diagnostic exome sequencing is performed, comprehensive gene sequencing often reveals mutations in disease genes that are found incidentally because all genes are sequenced in this test. In 2013, the American College of Medical Genetics compiled a list of 56 disease genes that are clinically actionable because treatments are available and routinely used to prevent or reduce the severity of a disorder.[6] Information on mutations in clinically actionable genes are typically provided to the patient, even when they are found incidentally; however, during the genetic testing consent process, some patients may opt not to learn about possible mutations. Clinically actionable disease genes include the breast cancer genes *BRCA1* and *BRCA2*, along with several genes responsible for disorders frequently encountered in orthopaedic clinics, including Marfan syndrome and Loeys-Dietz syndrome, because the cardiac manifestations of these syndromes can be prevented with early diagnosis. As comprehensive genetic testing becomes routine, it is likely that patients with clinically actionable disease gene mutations will receive an earlier diagnosis, which will provide additional opportunities for improvements in care.

High-coverage next-generation sequencing is revealing a major role for somatic mutations in the pathogenesis of both developmental disorders and cancer.[7] The mutation rate in somatic cells is estimated to be 4 to 25 times higher than in the germline cells; therefore, dividing cells accumulate a high burden of mutations during the course of a lifetime, which contributes to the development of cancer.[5] Likewise, somatic mutations occurring during development contribute to the pathogenesis of congenital malformations and overgrowth syndromes. Somatic mutations contribute to a mosaic phenotype in which only a fraction of all cells contain the disease mutation, resulting in differentially affected tissues and organs. In these heterogeneous and mosaic disorders, the resultant phenotype is highly dependent on the spatial and temporal course of mutagenesis.

PHARMACOGENETIC VARIABILITY IN CODEINE METABOLISM

Pharmacogenetic testing to reduce the frequency of adverse drug events is moving quickly to the clinic. Such testing includes evaluating the metabolism of cancer drugs, carbamazepine, and warfarin.[8] Of particular interest to orthopaedic surgeons are data regarding codeine, a commonly prescribed opioid. Codeine and other opioids, such as tramadol, hydrocodone, and oxycodone, are metabolized to morphine in the liver by means of the cytochrome P450 CYP2D6 enzyme. Individuals who are ultrarapid metabolizers make up 1% to 2% of the general population and are at higher risk for toxicity.[9] In 2006, the death of a breast-fed infant by a mother taking codeine, who was an ultrarapid metabolizer, was attributed to opioid toxicity secondary to morphine secretion into breast milk.[10] Even at normal codeine dosages, deaths in children undergoing a tonsillectomy or an adenoidectomy have been attributed to CYP2D6 polymorphisms leading to ultrarapid metabolism,[9] resulting in an FDA warning against codeine use for postoperative pain for tonsillectomies or adenoidectomies.[11] Although the FDA did not comment on the use of codeine for pain control in other situations, some pediatric hospitals have completely removed codeine from their pharmacopeia. Individuals who are ultrarapid metabolizers are at high risk for life-threatening respiratory depression or signs of overdose, including sleepiness, confusion, and shallow breathing, even at approved doses, particularly combined with airway swelling from surgery or infection. Because these CYP2D6 variants have lesser roles in the metabolism of other opioids, the primary concerns have been with codeine. Carrier frequency of ultrarapid metabolizer variants varies by ethnicity and, for example, is approximately 4% in Caucasians in North America, 10% in Greece and Portugal, 20% in Saudi Arabia, and 30% in Ethiopia. Some CYP2D6 polymorphisms can also reduce the conversion to morphine and result in poor analgesic response. Poor metabolizer polymorphisms are present in 6% to 10% of Caucasian Americans, 3% to 6% of Mexican Americans, 2% to 5% of African Americans, and 1% of Asian Americans. Genetic testing for CYP2D6 polymorphisms to identify individuals who are ultrarapid or poor metabolizers is available but typically takes days to weeks to obtain; therefore, testing needs to be performed well in advance of codeine administration. Some healthcare systems are now generating and storing pharmacogenetic data on patients within the electronic medical record system, so that it is accessible at the point of care.[12] Genetic testing has not yet been advocated for other types of opioid anesthetics.

SOMATIC MUTATIONS IN EWING SARCOMA AND OSTEOSARCOMA

Germline and somatic mutations play a role in cancer pathogenesis, but the relative contributions of each and the specific genes involved differ substantially among tumor types.[13] Recent data suggest that approximately 8% of pediatric cancers are associated with a germline mutation in a known inherited cancer predisposition gene.[14] Although relatively rare cancers (representing 6% to 8% of all primary

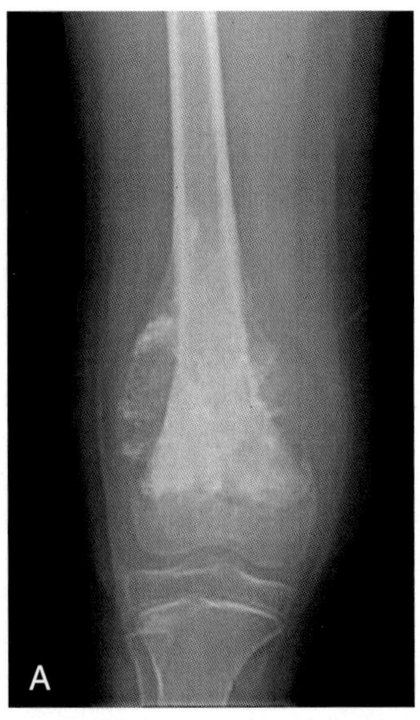

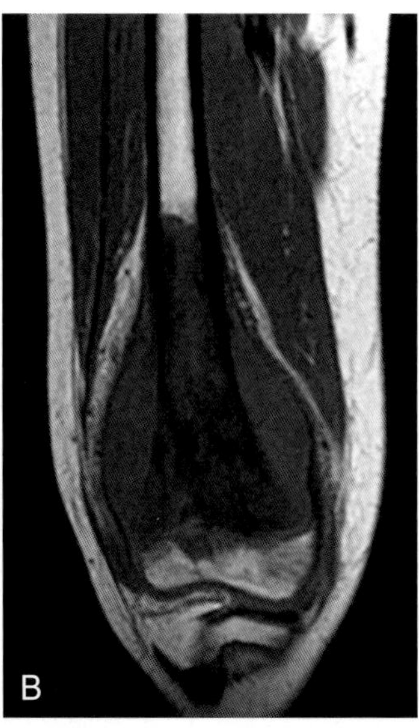

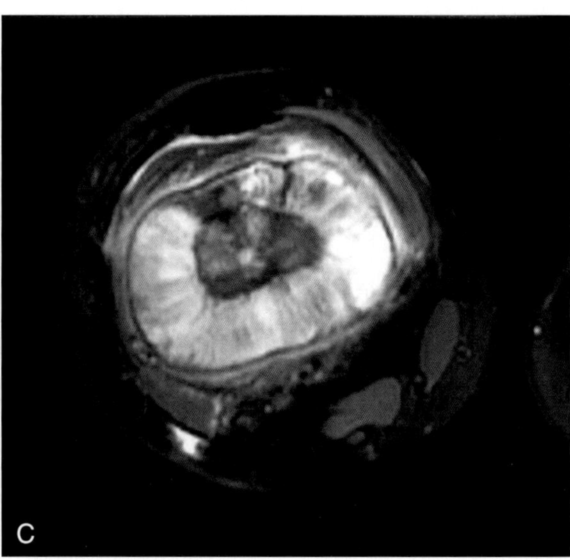

FIGURE 1 Images of osteosarcoma in a 9-year-old girl. **A**, AP radiograph of the distal right femur shows an obvious mixed lytic and blastic lesion in the metaphysis with a classic sunburst pattern of periosteal new bone formation in the soft tissue. **B**, T1-weighted coronal magnetic resonance image shows the intraosseous and soft-tissue implant. **C**, T2-weighted fat-suppressed axial magnetic resonance image delineates the extensive soft-tissue involvement surrounding the distal femoral metaphysis.

malignant bone tumors), Ewing sarcoma and osteosarcoma are the two most frequently encountered tumors in pediatric orthopaedics. Importantly, the genetic etiologies and landscapes of these tumors are very different.[15]

Osteosarcoma is the most common primary bone tumor that affects both children and young adults, with an incidence of 5 to 10 new cases per 1 million individuals each year (**Figure 1**). The overall survival rate of patients with this cancer is approximately 60%. In contrast to Ewing sarcoma, osteosarcoma tumors are genomically unstable and exhibit high rates of somatic mutations and rearrangements.[16] As such, the median somatic nonsilent mutational frequency has been estimated at 1.2 mutations per megabase.[13,16] Genes commonly mutated in osteosarcoma include the *TP53* gene as well as genes converging on the phosphatidylinositol 3-kinase/mammalian target of rapamycin (*PI3K/mTOR*) gene pathway.[16] Germline mutations in *TP53* are common in Li-Fraumeni syndrome,[17] a cancer predisposition condition in which multiple tumor types, including osteosarcoma, develop in affected individuals.[18] Unfortunately, despite substantial research, *TP53* has not been amenable to pharmacologic intervention.[19] Because the *PI3K/mTOR* gene pathway is amenable to pharmacologic intervention, future therapies might use drugs already in clinical use for other cancers.[20]

Ewing sarcoma is an aggressive primary bone (neuroectodermal) tumor that affects male children slightly more often than female children during adolescence or young adulthood, with an incidence of three new cases per 1 million individuals annually (**Figure 2**). Severe pain with or without an associated mass is the most common clinical symptom. In many patients, current therapy can be curative, although the prognosis for those with disseminated disease remains dismal. It has been known for more than 20 years that Ewing sarcoma is nearly always caused by a chimeric fusion between the EWS (Ewing sarcoma) and the ETS (E26 transformation-specific) family transcription factors,[21] with a paucity of additional somatic mutations detected in most tumors. However, somatic loss of the *STAG2*, *INK4A*, or *TP53* tumor suppressor genes is present in approximately 10% to 20% of tumors, where these molecular alterations have been associated with metastatic disease and a poor prognosis.[22,23]

Inherited genetic risk factors play a more important role than had previously been appreciated in Ewing sarcoma and may explain the low somatic mutational burden. A GWAS of 401 patients showed an association of Ewing sarcoma with high-risk common variants near the *TARDBP* and *EGR2* genes.[24] EGR2 is a zinc-finger transcription factor that promotes proliferation, differentiation, and survival. Relevant to Ewing sarcoma pathogenesis, the chimeric EWS-ETS fusion protein differentially binds and regulates its expression, depending on the presence or absence of the risk allele within its enhancer.[25] *EGR2* also is overexpressed in Ewing sarcoma, suggesting that pharmaceutical interventions aimed at reducing its expression may be a logical therapeutic option. Interestingly, the lower prevalence of this genetic risk variant in African American populations is likely responsible for the ninefold lower incidence of Ewing sarcoma in African Americans than in Caucasian Americans.[26] Overall, targeted therapies to correct these molecular defects, including cytosine arabinoside to suppress EWS-ETS expression, may yield new treatment strategies.

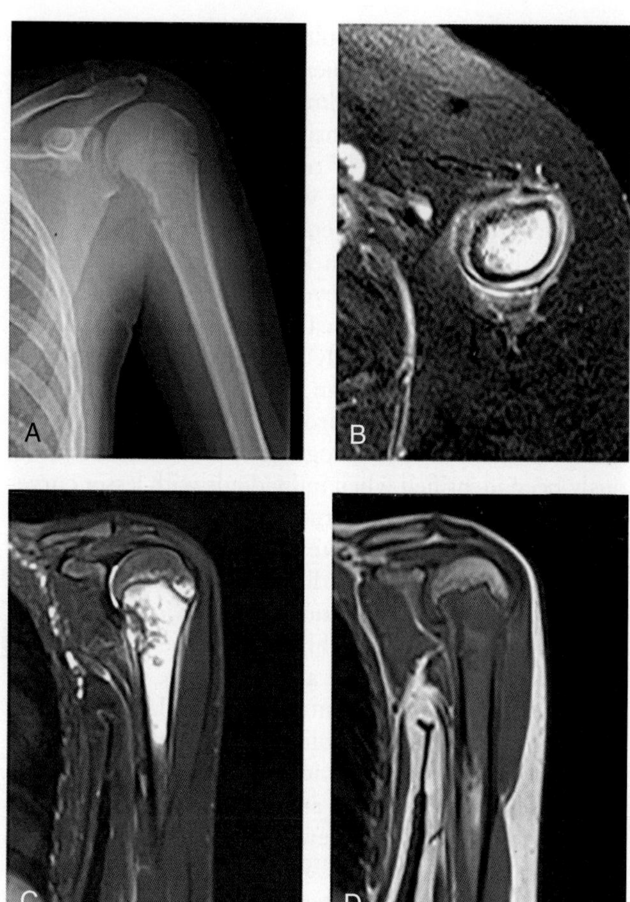

FIGURE 2 Images of Ewing sarcoma in an 11-year-old girl. **A**, AP radiograph of the left proximal humerus demonstrates medial lytic cortical destruction with a subtle permeative pattern of bone destruction throughout the metaphysis along with a lateral periosteal reaction. **B**, T2-weighted fat-suppressed axial magnetic resonance image shows minimal soft-tissue mass but the clear onion-skin pattern of a circumferential periosteal reaction. **C**, T1-weighted coronal magnetic resonance image reveals distal intraosseous involvement of the shaft with proximal extension up to the physis. **D**, T2-weighted fat-suppressed coronal magnetic resonance image shows the intraosseous involvement and periosteal reaction.

SOMATIC MUTATIONS IN SEGMENTAL OVERGROWTH SYNDROMES

A major shift in the understanding of sporadic overgrowth syndromes resulted from the discovery of a recurrent activating somatic mutation in Proteus syndrome.[27] The characteristic features of Proteus syndrome include overgrowth of skin, connective, fat, brain, and other tissues. Sequencing of paired samples taken from affected and unaffected tissues revealed somatic activating (gain-of-function) mutations in the growth-promoting serine/threonine kinase gene *AKT1*, which was only present in highly enriched affected tissue.[27] Interestingly, these *AKT1* mutations all occurred at the same nucleotide and resulted in a constitutively activated AKT1 kinase. In addition to *AKT1*, somatic mutations in the *PIK3CA* gene, now collectively referred to as *PIK3CA*-related overgrowth syndrome,[28] cause a wide spectrum of congenital abnormalities depending on the cell type containing the somatic mutations. Manifestations of these mutations include macrodactyly;[29] fibroadipose overgrowth;[30] muscle hemihypertrophy; congenital lipomatous overgrowth with vascular, epidermal, and skeletal anomalies syndrome;[31] isolated brain malformations;[32] and other fibroadipose vascular anomalies[33] (**Figure 3**). Further genetic studies have revealed that additional mutations in genes that regulate the *PI3K/AKT/mTOR* gene pathway, including *PIK3R2*, *AKT3*, and *TOR*, are responsible for a wide spectrum of human segmental overgrowth syndromes.[34]

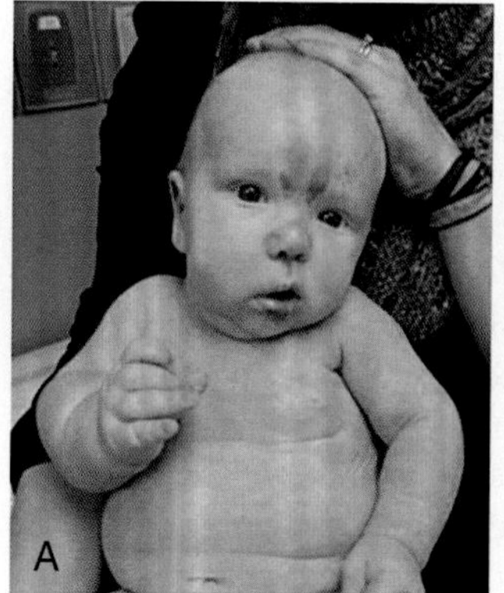

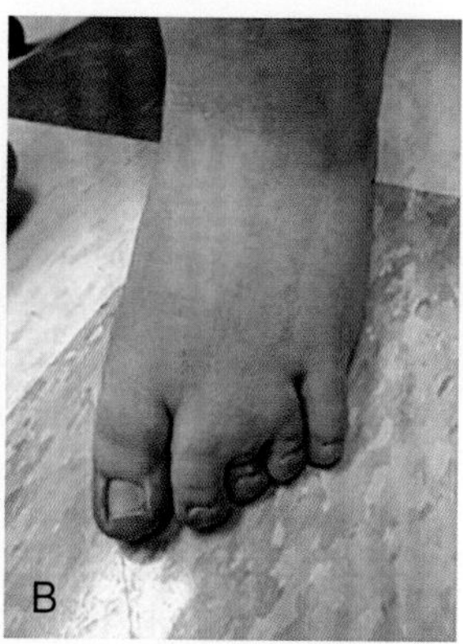

FIGURE 3 Clinical photographs of phenotypic manifestations of *PIK3CA*-related overgrowth syndrome. **A**, A male infant with facial asymmetry, midline facial capillary malformation, and hemimegalencephaly who has *PIK3CA* somatic mutation. **B**, A child with *PIK3CA* mutation showing two-three-four toe syndactyly.

Genetic testing of genes that operate within the *PI3K/AKT/mTOR* gene pathway is warranted in clinically suspicious cases to guide tumor surveillance as well as personalize treatments using pharmacologic agents to inhibit these hyperactivated growth pathways. In many biopsy specimens, the percentage of cells harboring these somatic mutations may be quite small, arguing for the use of diagnostic testing with high-density sequence coverage. Although many of the genes implicated in overgrowth have also been demonstrated in sporadic cancers, the risk of true malignancy in affected tissues appears to be quite low.

GENETIC PREDICTION OF COMORBIDITIES AND OUTCOME IN CLUBFOOT

Although the genetic basis for clubfoot in most patients remains unknown, evidence supports an important role for genes regulating early leg development. Disruption of genes in the *PITX1/TBX4/HOXC* gene pathway, by either point mutations or through microdeletions or microduplications,[35-38] is present in some families with autosomal dominant inherited clubfoot. Although clubfoot is the most common orthopaedic condition in these disorders, vertical talus is more common in families with *HOXC* gene cluster microdeletions.[39] Limb patterning defects, with small peroneus muscles and arteries supplying the lateral lower limb, appear to be present in patients with mutations in the *PITX1/TBX4/HOXC* gene pathway, possibly contributing to the greater incidence of treatment resistance. Additional orthopaedic abnormalities, including hip dysplasia, polydactyly, and tibial hemimelia, are more common in these conditions. Although genetic testing is not yet recommended for all children with clubfoot because the yield of testing remains low, chromosomal microarray testing to identify microdeletions or microduplications may be helpful in familial cases or for children in whom additional congenital anomalies are present. Chromosomal microarray testing has the additional benefit of detecting large-scale chromosomal abnormalities, including trisomy and Klinefelter syndrome, which are both associated with an increased incidence of congenital foot contractures.[19,37]

ADVANCES IN THE GENETIC BASIS OF ADOLESCENT IDIOPATHIC SCOLIOSIS

In addition to addressing the basic mechanisms of the pathogenesis of adolescent idiopathic scoliosis (AIS), genetic studies are now identifying the factors responsible for female sex bias and scoliotic curve progression. Although common genetic variants likely play only a minor role in overall AIS pathogenesis,[40] multiple large-scale GWASs have strongly confirmed the importance of SNPs near *LBX1* (ladybird homeobox 1), a gene that is involved in muscle cell migration and cardiac and neural tube development.[41-43] AIS also is associated with a SNP near *GPR126* (G protein–coupled receptor 126) that is essential for cardiac, neural, and ear development.[44] Interestingly, *GPR126* also regulates human height and binds to collagen, suggesting a possible role in mediating extracellular matrix stability.

In the first study to reveal an explanation for female sex bias in AIS, researchers reported an association of AIS with a SNP located in an enhancer near *PAX1* (paired box 1) that is present only in females.[45] *PAX1* is a transcription factor involved in spine development that has been implicated in congenital scoliosis in mice. Early-onset alopecia in males was previously associated with these risk alleles, suggesting the possibility that hormonal modulation of these regulatory sites contributes to both sexually dimorphic phenotypes. The paucity of males with scoliosis highlights the extent of the problem but also may hinder the identification of sex-specific risk factors because large numbers of male cases may be needed to definitively exclude an association. Notably, several GWASs used only females as cases, and therefore, some of the previously reported loci may apply only to females.

The identification of genetic factors responsible for scoliotic curve progression is of major clinical importance because these markers could be used to prospectively design personalized treatment methods. Previous studies reported SNPs near calmodulin, estrogen receptors, tryptophan hydroxylase, insulinlike growth factor, neurotrophin-3, interleukin 17 receptor, melatonin receptor, and a group of SNPs that were predictive of scoliotic curve progression. However, a systematic review and a meta-analysis concluded a limited predictive value of these studies and a low level of evidence; none could be recommended for clinical use as a diagnostic criterion.[46] An association study using female patients with scoliotic curves greater than 40° demonstrated an association of AIS with SNPs around SOX9, a transcription factor involved in chondrogenesis, that had not previously been identified when individuals with lesser curves were included.[47] Genetic studies also suggest that there may be overlap between the genetic factors responsible for AIS and intervertebral disk degeneration with adult spinal deformity.[48] Rare genetic variants in the extracellular matrix genes *FBN1* (fibrillin 1), the gene responsible for Marfan syndrome, are also predictive of AIS curve progression.[49] *FBN1* variants present in the genomes of patients with congenital scoliosis also highlight the overlap between structural and idiopathic scoliosis.[50]

Mendelian forms of AIS are rare. Although large families have been described, few causative genes have been identified. Variants in *POC5*, a centriolar protein gene, and *CHD7*, a gene associated with CHARGE syndrome (coloboma of the eye, heart defects, atresia choanae, retarded growth and development, genital abnormalities, and ear abnormalities), may play a role in AIS pathogenesis in some families.[51,52] Because the genetic inheritance of AIS is complex, it is more likely that a polygenic burden of rare variants will contribute to disease susceptibility, which was recently shown for extracellular matrix genes as a whole.[53] Much larger studies are needed to confirm the genetic associations that have already been published and identify new disease and gene associations, particularly with rare variants that only recently have begun to be investigated in AIS. Eventually, if algorithms that take into account the role of both common and rare genetic variants can be applied, it is possible that better predictions of scoliotic risk and curve progression can be developed.

SUMMARY

Technology is driving new disease gene discovery and genetic associations for pediatric orthopaedic disorders. These technologies have resulted in the identification of somatic mutations that may lead to cancer or segmental overgrowth syndromes. In the future, new pharmacogenetic data will be implemented in clinical practice to optimize efficacy and reduce the risk of adverse effects in selected populations.

KEY STUDY POINTS

- Pharmacogenetic variants can identify individuals who are ultrarapid metabolizers of codeine and are at risk for adverse respiratory suppression and death.
- The genetic landscapes of Ewing sarcoma and osteosarcoma are very different; insights about these differences may lead to new therapeutic strategies.
- Segmental overgrowth syndromes are associated with somatic mutations that may increase cancer risk. Treatment with pharmacotherapeutic interventions may be possible.
- Rare genetic factors are predictive of comorbidities and treatment outcomes in some families with clubfoot.
- The genetic inheritance of AIS is complex, but factors responsible for female sex bias and scoliotic curve progression have recently been revealed.

ANNOTATED REFERENCES

1. Collins FS, Varmus H: A new initiative on precision medicine. *N Engl J Med* 2015;372(9):793-795.
2. Alkan C, Coe BP, Eichler EE: Genome structural variation discovery and genotyping. *Nat Rev Genet* 2011;12(5):363-376.
3. Manolio TA: Genomewide association studies and assessment of the risk of disease. *N Engl J Med* 2010;363(2):166-176.
4. Ronemus M, Iossifov I, Levy D, Wigler M: The role of de novo mutations in the genetics of autism spectrum disorders. *Nat Rev Genet* 2014;15(2):133-141.
5. Shendure J, Akey JM: The origins, determinants, and consequences of human mutations. *Science* 2015;349(6255):1478-1483.
6. Green RC, Berg JS, Grody WW, et al, American College of Medical Genetics and Genomics: ACMG recommendations for reporting of incidental findings in clinical exome and genome sequencing. *Genet Med* 2013;15(7):565-574.
7. Biesecker LG, Spinner NB: A genomic view of mosaicism and human disease. *Nat Rev Genet* 2013;14(5):307-320.
8. Lee JW, Aminkeng F, Bhavsar AP, et al: The emerging era of pharmacogenomics: Current successes, future potential, and challenges. *Clin Genet* 2014;86(1):21-28.
9. Madadi P, Amstutz U, Rieder M, et al, CPNDS Clinical Recommendations Group: Clinical practice guideline: CYP2D6 genotyping for safe and efficacious codeine therapy. *J Popul Ther Clin Pharmacol* 2013;20(3):e369-e396.
10. Koren G, Cairns J, Chitayat D, Gaedigk A, Leeder SJ: Pharmacogenetics of morphine poisoning in a breastfed neonate of a codeine-prescribed mother. *Lancet* 2006;368(9536):704.
11. US Food and Drug Administration: *Codeine Product Labeling Changes*. Available at: http://www.fda.gov/Safety/MedWatch/SafetyInformation/ucm356221.htm. Accessed May 26, 2016.

    The FDA issued a policy statement after deaths were reported in patients taking appropriately prescribed codeine dosages.
12. Gammal RS, Crews KR, Haidar CE, et al: Pharmacogenetics for safe codeine us in sickle cell disease. *Am Acad Pediatr* 2016;138(1)e20153479.

    Using genetics to tailor analgesic prescribing retained an important therapeutic option by limiting codeine use to patients who could safely receive and benefit from it.
13. Lawrence MS, Stojanov P, Polak P, et al: Mutational heterogeneity in cancer and the search for new cancer-associated genes. *Nature* 2013;499(7457):214-218.
14. Zhang J, Walsh MF, Wu G, et al: Germline mutations in predisposition genes in pediatric cancer. *N Engl J Med* 2015;373(24):2336-2346.
15. HaDuong JH, Martin AA, Skapek SX, Mascarenhas L: Sarcomas. *Pediatr Clin North Am* 2015;62(1):179-200.
16. Perry JA, Kiezun A, Tonzi P, et al: Complementary genomic approaches highlight the PI3K/mTOR pathway as a common vulnerability in osteosarcoma. *Proc Natl Acad Sci USA* 2014;111(51):E5564-E5573.
17. Srivastava S, Zou ZQ, Pirollo K, Blattner W, Chang EH: Germline transmission of a mutated p53 gene in a cancer-prone family with Li-Fraumeni syndrome. *Nature* 1990;348(6303):747-749.
18. Gorlick R: Current concepts on the molecular biology of osteosarcoma. *Cancer Treat Res* 2009;152:467-478.
19. Vogelstein B, Papadopoulos N, Velculescu VE, Zhou S, Diaz LA Jr, Kinzler KW: Cancer genome landscapes. *Science* 2013;339(6127):1546-1558.
20. Yap TA, Bjerke L, Clarke PA, Workman P: Drugging PI3K in cancer: Refining targets and therapeutic strategies. *Curr Opin Pharmacol* 2015;23:98-107.
21. Delattre O, Zucman J, Plougastel B, et al: Gene fusion with an ETS DNA-binding domain caused by chromosome translocation in human tumours. *Nature* 1992;359(6391):162-165.
22. Crompton BD, Stewart C, Taylor-Weiner A, et al: The genomic landscape of pediatric Ewing sarcoma. *Cancer Discov* 2014;4(11):1326-1341.
23. Tirode F, Surdez D, Ma X, et al, St. Jude Children's Research Hospital–Washington University Pediatric Cancer Genome Project and the International Cancer Genome Consortium: Genomic landscape of Ewing sarcoma defines an aggressive subtype with co-association of STAG2 and TP53 mutations. *Cancer Discov* 2014;4(11):1342-1353.
24. Postel-Vinay S, Véron AS, Tirode F, et al: Common variants near TARDBP and EGR2 are associated with susceptibility to Ewing sarcoma. *Nat Genet* 2012;44(3):323-327.
25. Grünewald TG, Bernard V, Gilardi-Hebenstreit P, et al: Chimeric EWSR1-FLI1 regulates the Ewing sarcoma susceptibility gene EGR2 via a GGAA microsatellite. *Nat Genet* 2015;47(9):1073-1078.
26. Jawad MU, Cheung MC, Min ES, Schneiderbauer MM, Koniaris LG, Scully SP: Ewing sarcoma demonstrates racial disparities in incidence-related and sex-related differences in outcome: An analysis of 1631 cases from the SEER database, 1973-2005. *Cancer* 2009;115(15):3526-3536.

27. Lindhurst MJ, Sapp JC, Teer JK, et al: A mosaic activating mutation in AKT1 associated with the Proteus syndrome. *N Engl J Med* 2011;365(7):611-619.

28. Keppler-Noreuil KM, Sapp JC, Lindhurst MJ, et al: Clinical delineation and natural history of the PIK3CA-related overgrowth spectrum. *Am J Med Genet A* 2014;164A(7):1713-1733.

29. Rios JJ, Paria N, Burns DK, et al: Somatic gain-of-function mutations in PIK3CA in patients with macrodactyly. *Hum Mol Genet* 2013;22(3):444-451.

30. Lindhurst MJ, Parker VE, Payne F, et al: Mosaic overgrowth with fibroadipose hyperplasia is caused by somatic activating mutations in PIK3CA. *Nat Genet* 2012;44(8):928-933.

31. Kurek KC, Luks VL, Ayturk UM, et al: Somatic mosaic activating mutations in PIK3CA cause CLOVES syndrome. *Am J Hum Genet* 2012;90(6):1108-1115.

32. Poduri A, Evrony GD, Cai X, et al: Somatic activation of AKT3 causes hemispheric developmental brain malformations. *Neuron* 2012;74(1):41-48.

33. Alomari AI, Spencer SA, Arnold RW, et al: Fibro-adipose vascular anomaly: Clinical-radiologic-pathologic features of a newly delineated disorder of the extremity. *J Pediatr Orthop* 2014;34(1):109-117.

34. Lee JH, Huynh M, Silhavy JL, et al: De novo somatic mutations in components of the PI3K-AKT3-mTOR pathway cause hemimegalencephaly. *Nat Genet* 2012;44(8):941-945.

35. Alvarado DM, Aferol H, McCall K, et al: Familial isolated clubfoot is associated with recurrent chromosome 17q23.1q23.2 microduplications containing TBX4. *Am J Hum Genet* 2010;87(1):154-160.

36. Alvarado DM, McCall K, Aferol H, et al: Pitx1 haploinsufficiency causes clubfoot in humans and a clubfoot-like phenotype in mice. *Hum Mol Genet* 2011;20(20):3943-3952.

37. Alvarado DM, Buchan JG, Frick SL, Herzenberg JE, Dobbs MB, Gurnett CA: Copy number analysis of 413 isolated talipes equinovarus patients suggests role for transcriptional regulators of early limb development. *Eur J Hum Genet* 2013;21(4):373-380.

38. Gurnett CA, Alaee F, Kruse LM, et al: Asymmetric lower-limb malformations in individuals with homeobox *PITX1* gene mutation. *Am J Hum Genet* 2008;83(5):616-622.

39. Alvarado DM, McCall K, Hecht JT, Dobbs MB, Gurnett CA: Deletions of 5' HOXC genes are associated with lower extremity malformations, including clubfoot and vertical talus. *J Med Genet* 2016;53(4):250-255.

Small microdeletions of the *HOXC* gene cluster were identified in three families with clubfoot or vertical talus, and point mutations in *HOXC12* segregate with familial clubfoot.

40. Kou I, Otomo N, Takeda K, et al: Genome-wide association study identifies 14 previously reported susceptibility loci for adolescent idiopathic scoliosis in Japanese. *Nat Commun* 2019;10(1):3685.

The authors identify 20 loci significantly associated with AIS, including 14 previously not reported loci. These loci explain 4.6% of the phenotypic variance of AIS.

41. Takahashi Y, Kou I, Takahashi A, et al: A genome-wide association study identifies common variants near LBX1 associated with adolescent idiopathic scoliosis. *Nat Genet* 2011;43(12):1237-1240.

42. Zhu Z, Tang NL, Xu L, et al: Genome-wide association study identifies new susceptibility loci for adolescent idiopathic scoliosis in Chinese girls. *Nat Commun* 2015;6:8355.

43. Londono D, Kou I, Johnson TA, et al, TSRHC is Clinical Group, International Consortium for Scoliosis Genetics, Japanese Scoliosis Clinical Research Group: A meta-analysis identifies adolescent idiopathic scoliosis association with LBX1 locus in multiple ethnic groups. *J Med Genet* 2014;51(6):401-406.

44. Kou I, Takahashi Y, Johnson TA, et al: Genetic variants in GPR126 are associated with adolescent idiopathic scoliosis. *Nat Genet* 2013;45(6):676-679.

45. Sharma S, Londono D, Eckalbar WL, et al, TSRHC Scoliosis Clinical Group, Japan Scoliosis Clinical Research Group: A PAX1 enhancer locus is associated with susceptibility to idiopathic scoliosis in females. *Nat Commun* 2015;6:6452.

46. Noshchenko A, Hoffecker L, Lindley EM, et al: Predictors of spine deformity progression in adolescent idiopathic scoliosis: A systematic review with meta-analysis. *World J Orthop* 2015;6(7):537-558.

47. Miyake A, Kou I, Takahashi Y, et al: Identification of a susceptibility locus for severe adolescent idiopathic scoliosis on chromosome 17q24.3. *PLoS One* 2013;8(9):e72802.

48. Takeda K, Kou I, Hosogane N, et al: Association of susceptibility genes for adolescent idiopathic scoliosis and intervertebral disc degeneration with adult spinal deformity. *Spine (Phila Pa 1976)* 2019;44(23):1623-1629.

49. Buchan JG, Alvarado DM, Haller GE, et al: Rare variants in FBN1 and FBN2 are associated with severe adolescent idiopathic scoliosis. *Hum Mol Genet* 2014;23(19):5271-5282.

50. Lin M, Zhao S, Liu G, et al: Identification of novel FBN1 variations implicated in congenital scoliosis. *J Hum Genet* 2020;65(3):221-230.

One missense variant, c.2613A>C (p.Leu871Phe) was recurrent in two unrelated CS subjects, and in vitro functional experiments for the variant suggest that FBN1 may contribute to CS by upregulating the transforming growth factor beta (TGF-β) signaling.

51. Patten SA, Margaritte-Jeannin P, Bernard JC, et al: Functional variants of POC5 identified in patients with idiopathic scoliosis. *J Clin Invest* 2015;125(3):1124-1128.

52. Gao X, Gordon D, Zhang D, et al: CHD7 gene polymorphisms are associated with susceptibility to idiopathic scoliosis. *Am J Hum Genet* 2007;80(5):957-965.

53. Haller G, Alvarado D, Mccall K, et al: A polygenic burden of rare variants across extracellular matrix genes among individuals with adolescent idiopathic scoliosis. *Hum Mol Genet* 2016;25(1):202-209.

An exome sequencing study revealed excess extracellular matrix gene variation in patients with AIS compared with control subjects. Although rare variants across multiple collagen genes were associated with AIS, the association was strongest with *COL11A2*.

CHAPTER 8

Skeletal Dysplasias

JOSÉ A. MORCUENDE, MD, PhD

ABSTRACT

Skeletal dysplasias are a group of more than 450 heterogeneous genetic disorders characterized by abnormal differentiation, development, growth, and maintenance of bone and cartilage. Albeit individually rare, collectively, the incidence of these disorders is estimated to be approximately 1 per 5,000 live births, representing 5% of children born with a birth defect. An accurate diagnosis based on clinical and radiographic features is important to predict final height, allow specific genetic counseling, and permit the selection of the best treatment approaches to avoid potential complications. A multidisciplinary approach is highly recommended for the treatment of patients with skeletal dysplasia. It is helpful to be familiar with background information related to genetics, classifications, and key clinical characteristics, including the natural history and treatment options for some of the most common skeletal dysplasias seen in orthopaedics.

Keywords: classification; genetics; skeletal dysplasia

INTRODUCTION

The vertebrate skeleton is a fascinating and complex organ system, composed of 206 bones with many different shapes and sizes. Like every other organ system, the skeleton has specific developmental and functional characteristics that define its identity in biologic and pathologic terms. For normal skeletogenesis to take place, the coordination of temporal and spatial gene expression patterns is a crucial prerequisite. Any disturbances in these processes will lead to abnormalities of the skeleton.

It is important for those interested in the musculoskeletal system to be aware of not only the clinical characteristics of these disorders but also the genetic causes to make appropriate referrals for genetic counseling and to refine the prognosis and natural history in each individual patient. Given the large number of inherited musculoskeletal abnormalities and the power and speed of current genetic and developmental biology information, a few selected disorders will be discussed. Fundamental general concepts on the genetic basis of musculoskeletal disorders and current classifications are addressed; key clinical characteristics including natural history and treatment options are focused; and the most recent developments in the understanding of the pathogenesis are reflected.

THE GENETIC BASIS OF MUSCULOSKELETAL DISORDERS

Broadly defined, birth defects or congenital abnormalities occur in 6% of all live births, with 20% of infant deaths due to congenital anomalies. Currently, the cause of approximately 50% of birth defects is unknown, with chromosomal abnormalities accounting for 6% to 7%, specific gene mutations causing 7% to 8%, and environmental teratogens responsible for 7% to 10% of defects. Combined genetic predisposition with environmental factors causes the remaining 20% to 25% of congenital abnormalities.

Genetic disorders of the skeleton comprise a large group of clinically distinct and genetically heterogeneous conditions now comprising 456 forms. Of these conditions, 316 are associated with one or more of 226

Dr. Morcuende or an immediate family member serves as an unpaid consultant to Clubfoot Solutions and serves as a board member, owner, officer, or committee member of Ponseti International Association.

different genes. This reflects the continued delineation of unique phenotypes that in aggregate represents about 5% of children with birth defects. Therefore, although individually rare, the different forms add to produce a significant number of affected individuals, with significant mortality and morbidity.

Their clinical diversity makes these disorders often difficult to diagnose, and many attempts have been made to delineate single entities or groups of diseases to facilitate the diagnosis. The criteria used for their distinction have been based on a combination of clinical, morphologic, radiographic, and, in some instances, biochemical and molecular characteristics.[1,2] The Nosology and Classification of Genetic Skeletal Disorders has been commonly used since its first publication in 1970 (with its latest revision in 2010).[3] However, it is now becoming increasingly clear that several distinctive classifications that reflect, on the one hand, the clinical signs and symptoms and, on the other hand, the molecular pathology are needed. Several reviews of the rapidly changing molecular basis of the skeletal dysplasias have been published, focusing either on a molecular-pathogenetic classification, on more specific aspects such as transcriptional deregulation, or on a combination of molecular pathology and developmental biology of the musculoskeletal system. These new concepts directly link the clinical phenotype to key cellular processes of skeletal biology and should assist in providing a framework accessible to clinicians as well as basic scientists for future understanding of these disorders.[4-7] It is likely that future insights will lead to reclassification.

Conceptually, it is useful to classify musculoskeletal disorders caused by gene mutations into groups broadly categorized by the function of the causative gene. Mutations in early patterning genes cause disorders called dysostoses: these affect only specific skeletal elements, leaving the rest of the skeleton largely unaffected. In contrast, mutations in genes that are involved primarily in cell differentiation cause disorders called osteochondrodysplasias, which affect the development and growth of most skeletal elements in a generalized fashion (by affecting endochondral bone formation).

These skeletal disorders can be broadly classified into those caused by mutation in genes encoding one of the following types of proteins: structural proteins; proteins that regulate developmentally important signaling pathways; proteins that play a role in metabolic macromolecular processing; proteins implicated in neoplasia; and proteins that play a role in nerve or muscle function. In addition, many genes have important functions in both of these processes, so that some inherited disorders can display features of both dysostoses and osteochondrodysplasias. Finally, genes used during skeletal development may also be important in other organs so that when mutated, the resulting skeletal defects are part of a syndrome.

Finally, there are numerous online services that allow access to public information and services relevant to the genetics of musculoskeletal disorders. One database that contains a wealth of clinical and genetic data is the Online Mendelian Inheritance in Man. It provides free text overviews of genetic disorders and gene loci, with the correspondent mouse correlate. In addition, it is linked to a wealth of other genetic databases, allowing the users to obtain information on gene structure, map location, function, phenotype, literature references, etc. It is found at http://ww.ncbi.nlm.nih.gov/omim/.

CLINICAL EVALUATION

With the increased availability of ultrasonographic prenatal screening, more patients with skeletal dysplasias are being diagnosed before birth.[8] When there is suspicion of a skeletal dysplasia on ultrasonography, the femoral length is the best biometric parameter. Further testing may be performed, if indicated, by chorionic villous sampling and karyotype/genetic mutation analysis.

Most skeletal dysplasias result in short stature, defined as height more than two standard deviations below the mean for the population at a given age. The resultant growth disproportion is commonly referred to as short trunk or short limb. The short-limb types are further subdivided into categories based on the segment of the limb that is affected. Rhizomelic refers to shortening of the proximal part of the limb (humerus and femur); mesomelic refers to the middle segment (radius, ulna, tibia, and fibula); and acromelic refers to the distal segment (hands and feet).

In evaluating a patient with short stature or abnormal bone development, several aspects of the medical history and the physical examination should be investigated. The accurate history regarding time of onset of short stature is essential before physical examination. Among the 456 skeletal dysplasias, 100 or so have prenatal onset, whereas others may only present either as newborns or beyond 2 to 3 years of age. Individuals with disproportionate short stature are likely to be affected by a skeletal dysplasia. Therefore, whenever an individual presents with short stature, it is essential to measure body proportions.

A history of heart disease, respiratory difficulty, immune deficiency, precocious puberty, and malabsorption should also be sought because they are associated with some of these disorders. Birth length, head circumference, and weight should be recorded, and pertinent family history of short stature or dimorphism should be sought. The height and weight percentile should be determined using standard charts. The physical examination should include careful characterization of the facial features of the patients and presence of cleft palate, abnormal teeth, position of the ears, and extremity malformations. A thorough neurologic evaluation is needed because of the frequent incidence of spinal compromise in many of these syndromes.

Following the history and physical examination, radiographs are used to identify the area of bone involvement.[9] The so-called skeletal survey may vary from institution to institution, but it should include the following views: skull (AP and lateral), thoracolumbar spine (AP and lateral), chest, pelvis, one upper limb, one lower limb, and left hand. Flexion-extension views of the cervical spine should be ordered if instability is suspected. In some instances, imaging of other family members suspected of having the same condition may be helpful.

Laboratory tests may include calcium, phosphate, alkaline phosphatase, serum thyroxin, and protein to rule out metabolic disorders. Urine should be checked for storage products if a progressive disorder is found. Referral to a pediatric geneticist is often very helpful in reaching a diagnosis in complex cases, in providing genetic counseling to the family, and to manage the many medical problems associated with these disorders.

DISORDERS CAUSED BY DEFECTS IN STRUCTURAL PROTEINS

A variety of proteins play important roles in the connective tissues, including the bones, articular cartilage, ligaments, and skin. Mutations in such genes disrupt the structural integrity of the connective tissues in which they are expressed. In most cases, the phenotype is absent or there are only minor manifestations present at birth; the phenotype evolves with time because the abnormal structural components slowly fail or wear out as the individual grows. Deformity often recurs after surgery because the structural components are abnormal and will wear out again. In cases where the structural abnormality involves cartilage, there may be growth abnormality caused by physeal mechanical failure or early degenerative disease of the joints caused by articular cartilage failure. When a protein that is important for ligament or tendon strength is affected, joints are often subluxated. There can be substantial heterogeneity in the severity of the phenotype, depending on the exact way in which the mutation alters the protein function. In patients with mild disease, life expectancy is normal; however, in patients with more severe disease, life expectancy may be shortened because of secondary effects of the structural defects on vital organs. These disorders tend to be inherited in an autosomal dominant manner.

Multiple Epiphyseal Dysplasia

Multiple epiphyseal dysplasia (MED) is one of the most widely known and commonly occurring skeletal dysplasias. It is most commonly inherited in an autosomal dominant fashion, although autosomal recessive forms have been described as well. Its prevalence is estimated at 1 in 10,000 individuals. The predominant feature of MED is the delayed and irregular ossification of numerous epiphyses. In most cases, there is pain and stiffness in the joints, with hips and knees being most commonly affected. In general, affected patients have mild short stature and early-onset osteoarthritis.

Historically, it was described as occurring in two separate forms: Ribbing dysplasia, having mild involvement, and Fairbank dysplasia, a more severe type. However, with the current genetic understanding, MED is now considered to represent a continuous spectrum from mild to severe, and these eponyms have been abandoned.

MED shows considerable genetic heterogeneity. To date, mutations have been reported in 40 patients or families with MED, and 15 of these are allelic with pseudoachondroplasia and result from mutations in the gene encoding cartilage oligomeric matrix protein (COMP). MED can also result from mutations in the genes encoding the α1, α2, and α3 chains of type IX collagen, COL9A1, COL9A2, COL9A3, respectively. Furthermore, mutations in the gene encoding matrilin-3, a member of the matrilin family of extracellular oligomeric proteins, can cause a distinctive mild form of MED. Finally, it has been demonstrated that a form of recessively inherited MED, with a distinctive clinical presentation including clubfoot and bilateral double-layered patellae, can result from mutations in the solute carrier family 26, member 2 gene (SLC26A2). Therefore, MED is one of the more genetically heterogeneous conditions of the bone dysplasias.[10]

Patients typically present in early adolescence because of joint stiffness and contractures, lower extremity pain, angular deformities of the knees, gait disturbance, or short stature.[11] Depending on the severity of the epiphyseal dysplasia, symptoms may develop as early as 4 or 5 years. It is not uncommon, however, for patients with milder forms to go unrecognized until young adult life. Most patients have minimal short stature and are above the third percentile for standing height, so true dwarfism is not present. The face and spine are normal. There are no associated neurologic findings. Intelligence is not affected. The epiphyses of the upper extremities can be involved, but patients rarely complain of any significant symptoms in this area. Mild limitation of motion in the elbow, wrist, and shoulder is occasionally found.

The principal finding on radiographs is a delay in the appearance of the ossification centers. When the epiphyses do appear, they are fragmented, mottled, and flattened. The more fragmentation there is in the capital femoral epiphysis, the earlier the onset of osteoarthritis. The proximal femur is most often affected, and its appearance may be easily confused with those of bilateral Legg-Calvé-Perthes disease. Several radiographic clues may be helpful in differentiating the two. In Legg-Calvé-Perthes disease, usually one hip is involved before the other, so that each hip is in a different stage of the disease. This is not the case in MED. In addition, acetabular changes are primary in MED and are more pronounced. Metaphyseal cysts are seen in Legg-Calvé-Perthes disease but not in MED. Radiographs of the knees, ankles, shoulders, and wrists should be obtained in any child when the diagnosis of Legg-Calvé-Perthes disease is being entertained to rule out MED.[12]

Coxa vara occurs in some patients. Radiographs of the knees often demonstrate flattening of the femoral condyles as well as genu valgum deformity. Osteochondritis dissecans may be superimposed. Lateral radiographs of the knees demonstrate a double-layered patella in some patients. When this is present, it is characteristic for MED. The ankles in MED are also in valgus due to deformity in the talus predominantly. Upper extremity involvement is less severe. The metacarpals and phalanges usually are short with irregular epiphyses. MED is distinguished from spondyloepiphyseal dysplasia by the absence of severe vertebral changes. Mild end plate irregularities may be present.

Hip pain or subluxation is a common reason patients with MED seek orthopaedic care in adolescence. Containment surgery can be considered for those hips that show progressive subluxation. Although the principle of coverage is the same as that used in Legg-Calvé-Perthes disease, there is often preexisting coxa vara in hips with MED, which contraindicates the use of a proximal femoral varus osteotomy. In those cases, a shelf acetabular augmentation can improve coverage of the misshapen femoral head. If hinged abduction is present on arthrography, a valgus proximal femoral osteotomy may improve congruency and therefore relieve pain. Osteotomies may be helpful in realigning angular deformities at the knees. For optimal surgical correction, the site of the deformity must be ascertained preoperatively as the distal femur, proximal tibia, or both. Degenerative joint disease is the biggest problem, and it usually occurs in the second or third decade. If the femoral head is well formed at maturity, the onset of arthritis is delayed. The hip is the most common location of arthritis in this patient group and often leads to total joint arthroplasty.[13]

Pseudoachondroplasia

Pseudoachondroplasia is a form of short-limbed dwarfism that has a prevalence of approximately four per million, making it one of the more common skeletal dysplasias. It is characterized by involvement of both the epiphyses and metaphyses with affected individuals having significantly short stature and a predisposition to premature osteoarthritis. The spine is also involved with this disorder.

Pseudoachondroplasia is usually transmitted as an autosomal dominant trait. The molecular genetics of pseudoachondroplasia has been extensively studied, and it now appears that this disease results almost exclusively from mutations in the gene encoding COMP. The *COMP* gene consists of 19 exons, and most mutations to date (95%) are clustered within exons 8 to 14, which encode the type III repeats. The fact that most of these mutations are in the conformationally sensitive type III repeats indicates that this region is critical for protein function. The remaining 5% of mutations are in exons 16 and 18, which encode specific segments of the C-terminal globule.[10]

The cell-matrix pathology of pseudoachondroplasia resulting from *COMP* mutations has been well documented. Abnormal COMP is retained within the rough endoplasmic reticulum of cartilage, tendon, and ligament cells. This results in the secondary retention of type IX collagen, chondroitin sulfate proteoglycan 1 (aggrecan), and link protein. This retention of proteins leads to a reduction in the amount of these molecules available for interactions within the extracellular matrix of cartilage, resulting in cell death and the phenotypic picture of pseudoachondroplasia.[14-16] Additional studies are needed to delineate the mechanism leading to excessive retention of proteins to develop treatment modalities.

Pseudoachondroplasia is a relatively straightforward disease to provide molecular diagnosis because it results almost exclusively from mutations along a very compact region in the *COMP* gene. Molecular diagnosis for pseudoachondroplasia is currently provided on a commercial basis (www.genetests.com) and also as part of the service provision of the European Skeletal Dysplasia Network for research and diagnosis (www.ESDN.man.ac.uk).

Children with pseudoachondroplasia have no apparent abnormality at birth and the condition is usually diagnosed at 2 years of age after the onset of a waddling gait and at the time rhizomelic shortening becomes noticeable. Adult height ranges from 106 to 130 cm. Growth curve charts specific to pseudoachondroplasia are available. The clinical features are limited to the skeleton. The skull and facial features in pseudoachondroplasia are normal, and this is helpful in differentiating it from achondroplasia, in which frontal bossing and midface hypoplasia are present. Abnormalities of the lower extremities are common and include genu valgum and varum deformities. In some patients windswept deformity of the knees develops in which genu valgum is present on one side and genu varum on the other side. The joints are extremely lax, especially in childhood and adolescence, and there is a predisposition to early osteoarthropathy. The large weight-bearing joints (hips and knees) are the ones most often affected, and approximately one-third of patients need total hip arthroplasty by their mid thirties. Scoliosis may occur in adolescence but is generally not severe. Cervical spine instability is seen in 10% to 20% of individuals. Development milestones and intelligence are normal, and premature mortality is not a reported problem.[17]

Typical radiographic changes include small, irregular epiphyses and metaphyseal changes. Hand radiographs reveal delayed epiphyseal ossification resulting in delayed bone age. In the long bones, these changes are seen as epiphyseal ossification delay. When the epiphyses do ossify, they appear irregular and fragmented. The hip and knee are most severely affected. In the pelvis, there is delay in ossification of the capital femoral epiphysis, and when ossified, they are small and flattened. The femoral heads may resemble what is seen in other spondyloepiphyseal dysplasias or bilateral Legg-Calvé-Perthes disease. Sclerosis and irregularity of the acetabular roof are commonly observed.[12] Subluxation of the hips often occurs, and degenerative arthritis develops in response to the incongruity. The vertebral changes in pseudoachondroplasia are characteristic and consist of anterior beaking in childhood that resolves in adolescence. The interpedicular distance in the lumbar spine is normal in pseudoachondroplasia, unlike achondroplasia. Odontoid hypoplasia may be present, resulting in atlantoaxial instability.

Patients with pseudoachondroplasia often have significant angular deformities of the lower extremities that require corrective osteotomies. Careful preoperative assessment is necessary to properly realign the mechanical axis through the hip, knee, and ankle. For instance, in genu varum associated with achondroplasia, the deformity is present solely in the tibia; however, in pseudoachondroplasia, the deformity is often present in both the femur and the tibia, requiring osteotomies in both the distal femur and the proximal tibia. Care must also be taken in assessing the contribution of ligamentous laxity to the bowing deformity. After corrective osteotomy, recurrence of the deformity with growth is not uncommon.

Premature osteoarthritis of the hip in early adulthood is a frequent problem in pseudoachondroplasia. Patients with symptomatic subluxation or incongruity may benefit from a realignment osteotomy of the proximal femur. Varus osteotomy of the proximal femur usually creates more incongruity. If hinged abduction is present, demonstrated by the femoral head levering out of the joint with abduction of the hip, a proximal femoral valgus osteotomy may improve joint congruity and improve abductor function. Before performing a proximal femoral valgus osteotomy, preoperative arthrography should be performed to demonstrate improved congruity with 15° to 20° of flexion and adduction of the femur. Abduction of the hip should demonstrate hinged abduction of the femoral head. Reconstructive pelvic osteotomies, such as the Salter osteotomy or the triple innominate osteotomy of Steel, are contraindicated in pseudoachondroplasia because a concentric reduction is not present preoperatively, which is a prerequisite for these osteotomies. Salvage procedures such as the shelf augmentation or the Chiari osteotomy can be done in select cases. As many as 50% of adult patients have undergone total hip arthroplasty.

Type II Collagenopathies

This group includes the lethal forms of achondrogenesis II and hypochondrogenesis (not discussed) and the congenital forms of spondyloepiphyseal dysplasia, Kniest syndrome, and Stickler syndrome.

Spondyloepiphyseal Dysplasia

This skeletal dysplasia mainly affects the spine, but also involves the epiphysis of long bones. The congenital type is diagnosed at birth, and its mode of inheritance is autosomal dominant, whereas the late onset is X-linked or autosomal recessive. Most cases of congenital type are attributable to new mutations on type II collagen (COL2A1), and the late onset is thought to involve the *SEDL* gene.[18,19]

Patients with the congenital form have a pronounced coxa vara and short stature at birth. Hip flexion contracture and hyperlordosis of the lumbar spine are also present, with a characteristic barrel chest. Radiographically, the femoral neck shows a reminiscent of pseudarthrosis and the greater trochanter is displaced upward, whereas the femoral heads are normally centered. Platyspondyly and delayed epiphyseal ossification are present in both types. The cervical spine demonstrates a dysplastic dens with risk for atlantoaxial instability. Kyphosis and scoliosis frequently develop. Possible associated abnormalities include cleft palate, hearing loss, myopia, cataracts, retinal detachment, and clubfeet. Early referral to ophthalmology and ear, nose, and throat (ENT) specialists is important, with orthopaedic treatment directed to early correction of the lower extremity and spine deformities, especially coxa vara and atlantoaxial instability.[20,21]

Kniest Syndrome

This is a rare, autosomal dominant, skeletal dysplasia, resulting from deletion of several amino acids in type II collagen (COL2A1). It is characterized by normal trunk at birth with shortened extremities. Both the epiphysis and metaphysis of the long bones are affected. However, there is usually development of scoliosis and kyphosis. The face is unusually flat with hypertelorism. There are joint contractures of the knees and hips, dumbbell-shaped femurs, cleft palate, retinal detachment, otitis/hearing loss, and early osteoarthritis. Early referral to ophthalmology and ENT specialists is important, with orthopaedic treatment directed to correction of progressive lower extremity and spine deformities.

Stickler Syndrome

This syndrome, also known as arthro-ophthalmopathy, is genetically and phenotypically heterogeneous, with variations in both the signs and symptoms and the age of onset. Most striking are the ocular problems (myopia, retinal detachment, glaucoma, and blindness). In addition, patients suffer from micrognathia, cleft palate, and hearing loss. Patients are of normal height, and they even show a marfanoid habitus with mitral valve prolapse often present. Joint involvement demonstrates some stiffness and pain with radiographic flat epiphysis with remodeling defects and fairly narrow diaphysis. Signs of early osteoarthritis are common as young adults. As in Kniest syndrome, early referral to ophthalmology, ENT specialists, and pediatric cardiology is important, with orthopaedic treatment directed to correction of progressive lower extremity and spine deformities.

DISORDERS CAUSED BY DEFECTS IN DEVELOPMENTALLY IMPORTANT SIGNALING PATHWAYS

Achondroplasia and Related Disorders

Achondroplasia is by far the most common osteochondrodysplasia in humans, occurring in about 1 in 30,000 live births. It is inherited as an autosomal dominant trait, although it results from sporadic mutations in at least 80% of the patients (with increased risk associated with paternal age). The mutation is always in the same location of the gene (a G-to-A change at nucleotide 1,138 most commonly and that the remaining patients had a G-to-C change at the same nucleotide) and results in uncontrolled activation of the FGFR3 receptor that leads to an impaired growth in the proliferative zone of the physis. Intramembranous and periosteal ossification processes are normal. It has been demonstrated that, as previously expected, *FGFR3* mutations in sporadic cases of achondroplasia occur exclusively on the parentally derived allele.

Because the FGFR3 mutation in achondroplasia was recognized, similar observations regarding the conserved nature of *FGFR3* mutations and resulting phenotype have been made regarding hypochondroplasia, the lethal thanatophoric dysplasia, severe achondroplasia with developmental delay and acanthosis nigricans, and recently two craniosynostosis disorders: Muenke coronal craniosynostosis and Crouzon syndrome with acanthosis nigricans. More importantly, the relationship between mutations in the *FGFR3* gene and other *FGFR* genes and the phenotypes that result from these mutations have improved the understanding of these disorders, and it has been observed that there is a highly conserved relationship between mutations at a particular amino acid and the resulting phenotype.[22-25]

The skeletal manifestations of achondroplasia are related to a defect in endochondral bone formation.[26,27] The resulting growth disturbances are variable, affecting proximal segments to a greater extent than the distal segments of the limbs (rhizomelia), and with relatively minor involvement of the growth of the spine. Achondroplasia is recognized at birth, and the appearance of a person with achondroplasia has numerous features that are uniform and predictable. Intelligence is normal, and life expectancy is not significantly diminished. The predicted adult height is 132 cm for men and 122 cm for women. Obesity is more common than in the general population. Developmental milestones are met later in children with achondroplasia than the average-stature children.

There is enlargement of the cranium with frontal bossing, midface hypoplasia, flattening of the nasal bridge, and prominent mandible. The foramen magnum is frequently narrowed, and it is associated with neurologic complications from compression of the brain stem (quadriparesis, spasticity, sleep apnea and respiratory insufficiency, and sudden death). The spine length is in the lower range of normal, whereas the extremities are much shorter than normal, with the proximal segments—the humeri and femora—the most foreshortened (rhizomelic). There is kyphosis of the thoracolumbar junction during infancy, and it usually improves with increasing age. Scoliosis is rare. Hyperlordosis of the lumbar spine increases with age, and there is a high incidence of symptomatic spinal stenosis (narrowing of the interpedicular distances with shortening of the pedicles). Clinically, patients will present with low back and leg pain, paresthesias, dysesthesias, weakness, or bowel and bladder incontinence.

There is limitation of extension of the elbows, and some patients may have asymptomatic radial head dislocations. Patients had a classic trident hand characterized by a persistent space between the long and ring fingers. The main functional limitations of the upper extremities are related to shortening of the humeri, which lead to difficulties in personal hygiene and dressing. Radiographically, the pelvis is broad with a diminished vertical height. The iliac crest has a square appearance, and the superior acetabular roof is horizontal. There is flaring of the distal femoral metaphysis. Genu varum is very common, with ligamentous laxity, and the fibula overgrows the tibia. Internal tibial torsion is common with varus of the ankle.

Children with achondroplasia should be closely monitored in the first 2 years of life for signs of foramen magnum stenosis.[28] If the diagnosis is made and symptoms are persistent, decompression of the brain stem is indicated.[29] In some patients, there may be associated hydrocephalus that will require shunting. ENT problems are frequently secondary to the facial abnormalities. Recurrent otitis media may result in hearing loss, thus early hearing screening should be performed. Maxillary hypoplasia leads to dental crowding and malocclusion, which may require orthodontic treatment. Sleep apnea treatment, if necessary, begins with adenotonsillectomy and may progress to include more complex procedures.

The main orthopaedic problems include thoracolumbar kyphosis, spinal stenosis, shortening of the extremities, and angular deformities of the knees. Kyphosis is noncongenital, and it is centered in the thoracolumbar junction. Treatment may be indicated to prevent further development of the deformity and to assist in those that do not correct with time (bracing treatment) and, in adulthood, to correct surgically those cases in which kyphosis contributes to symptomatic spinal stenosis. Spinal stenosis is the most serious problem and usually develops in the third decade of life. Spinal decompression is indicated as soon as the diagnosis is made. Limb lengthening remains controversial but is gradually gaining greater acceptance. If the lower extremities are lengthened, the humeri should also be lengthened to facilitate personal care. Treatment of the genu varum usually requires surgery because bracing treatment is not effective. Fibular head epiphysiodesis, fibular shortening, and tibial osteotomies can be performed to correct the deformity usually not until age 4 years at the earliest. Interestingly, severe degenerative arthritis is not common in adults with achondroplasia.

Hypochondroplasia manifestations are similar but milder than those of achondroplasia. The gene mutation is in different locations than achondroplasia; thus, there is more variability in the phenotype.[30] Clinically, the stunted growth first become apparent around 2 to 3 years of age or in some cases not until the 5 or 6 years of age. The children otherwise have a normal appearance apart from the disproportionately small stature, which is attributable solely to the shortening of the extremities with small hands. Genu varum and flexion contractures of knees and elbows develop over time, as well as lumbar hyperlordosis and mild stenosis. Radiographically, the long bones are broad and short, with the acetabular roof often more horizontal than normal and the sciatic notch slightly smaller. At the lumber level, there is some reduction in the interpedicular distance. Patients with hypochondroplasia attain a height of 130 to 140 cm and have normal life expectancy. Orthopaedic treatment may be required for corrective osteotomies and management of symptomatic spinal stenosis.

Thanatophoric dysplasia is very severe and almost always fatal before the patient reaches 2 years of age. It is characterized by severe disproportionate small stature with rhizomelic shortening, platyspondyly, protuberant abdomen, and small, narrow thoracic cavity that results in cardiorespiratory insufficiency, from which the children usually die immediately after birth. Given its early lethality, pediatric orthopaedic surgeons are rarely confronted with this condition.

Campomelic Dysplasia

The term campomelic refers to bowing of the long bones, primarily the tibiae and femora, that appears to be due to an abnormality in the formation of the cartilage anlage during fetal development. Endochondral ossification is normal, but diaphyseal cylinderization is markedly abnormal. The first transcription factor discovered to cause a skeletal dysplasia was SOX9 in campomelic dysplasia. The transcriptional targets of this gene include several cartilage matrix proteins such as types II and XI collagen and aggrecan. Hence, the skeletal manifestations are in part caused by decreased expression of these molecules and explain some of the phenotypic overlap with some of the severe type II collagenopathies.

This dominantly inherited condition is a severe and rare form of short-limbed skeletal dysplasia that is sometimes fatal. It is characterized by congenital bowing and angulation of long bones (campomelia), primarily involving the tibiae and femora, and disproportionate short-limb stature. There is relative macrocephaly, distinctive face (flattened face with a high forehead), low nasal bridge, and a specific pattern of defective mineralization, including areas of the spine with progressive scoliosis that further compromises pulmonary function leading to death if untreated. Hydromyelia and diastematomyelia have been reported, and neurologic complications and pseudarthrosis after spinal treatment are very common.[31,32] There is also defective cartilage in the tracheal rings and lower respiratory tract that may cause respiratory failure. Other clinical features include flattened head, cleft palate, micrognathia, defects of the heart and kidneys, and sex reversal (female with XY karyotype).

Treatment is symptomatic and directed to the deformities. However, there is a high degree of complications such as pseudarthrosis and neurologic complications.

Cleidocranial Dysplasia

Although the name may suggest that only two bones are affected, this is a true dysplasia because there are numerous abnormalities in all parts of the skeleton, primarily those bones of membranous origin (primarily clavicles, cranium, and pelvis). It is transmitted as an autosomal dominant condition, and the defect is in the *CBFA1* gene that encodes for an osteoblast-specific transcription factor required for osteoblast differentiation.[33-35] Approximately two-thirds are familial, and the rest are new mutations.

Typically, the disorder is identified within the first 2 years of life. Classic features include a widening of the cranium and dysplasia of the clavicles and pelvis. The patients have mild to moderate short stature. There is bossing in the frontal parietal and occipital regions. There is maxillary micrognathism and common high palate and dental abnormalities. The clavicles are partially or completely absent (10% of the time). This defect causes the shoulders to look droopy, the chest to be narrow, and the neck longer. The defect may be palpable. When it is bilateral, the classic diagnostic feature is that the child can touch the shoulders together, an ability that helped one college wrestler to escape holds. Brachial plexus irritation occurs in rare occasions. Pectus excavatum and sternal abnormalities are also common. Scoliosis and syringomyelia have been described, and it is recommended to obtain an MRI in patients with progressive scoliosis. The iliac wings appear small and coxa vara may occur, causing limitation of abduction and Trendelenburg gait. Widening of the symphysis pubis and coxa vara with short femoral necks are common, and 24% of patients have lumbar spondylolysis.[36]

There is no need for treatment for the clavicles. If there is brachial plexus irritation with pain and numbness, excision of the clavicular fragments can be performed to decompress. Coxa vara is managed by corrective femoral osteotomies. Scoliosis should be managed as idiopathic scoliosis.[37]

Nail-Patella Syndrome

The gene mutation in this syndrome is *LMX1B*, a transcription factor involved in patterning of the dorsoventral axis of the limbs and early morphogenesis of the glomerular basement membrane. It is inherited as an autosomal dominant trait, but there is marked intrafamilial and interfamilial variation in clinical features.[38,39] Characteristically, there is dystrophy of the nails, absent or hypoplastic patella, and iliac horns. Femoral condyle dysplasia and genu valgum are common. There is also varying degrees of cubitus valgus (hypoplasia lateral side humerus) with radial head posterior subluxation or dislocation. Other associated abnormalities include abnormal pigmentation of the iris in 50% of patients with glaucoma and nephropathy, leading to renal failure developing in the third or fourth decade.

Cornelia de Lange Syndrome

Heterozygous mutations in the gene *NIPBL* have been documented in 47% of unrelated individuals, with autosomal dominant inheritance in familial cases. This gene codes for a protein (delangin) important for chromosomal function and DNA repair.[40] Orthopaedic manifestations show a wide variability in the severity from short thumbs, clinodactyly of the fifth finger, flexion contractures of the elbow with radial head dislocations, and radial hemimelia with ray deficiencies. In the lower extremities, hip dysplasia, syndactyly of the second and third toes, and hallux valgus have been described. Patients also have short stature, microcephaly, mental retardation, cleft palate, and distinctive facial features (bushy eyebrows, small nose, and full eyelashes). Congenital heart malformations are present in about 30% of patients.[41]

DISORDERS CAUSED BY DEFECTS IN METABOLIC MACROMOLECULAR PROCESSING

Enzymes modify molecules or other proteins. They often modify substances for degradation and cause cell dysfunction when mutated because of the accumulation of these substances. Mutations in genes that encode for enzymes can have a wide variety of effects on cells, resulting in a broad range of abnormalities in cell function and a wide range of clinical findings. Many of these disorders result in the excess accumulation of proteins in cells. In these cases, the cells become larger than normal. This results in increased pressure in bones, causing osteonecrosis, and in increased extradural material in the spine, potentially causing paralysis. Multiple systems are almost always involved in these disorders. Medical treatments to replace the defective enzyme have been developed for many of these disorders, and such treatments will often arrest, but not reverse, the skeletal manifestations of the disorder. Early diagnosis and appropriate medical treatment are slowly decreasing the number of these individuals who present to orthopaedic surgeons with musculoskeletal problems. Most enzyme disorders are inherited in an autosomal recessive manner.

Mucopolysaccharidoses

This group of genetic disorders is characterized by mucopolysaccharide excretion in the urine, and they have been among the first skeletal dysplasias to be described and also among the first to be understood at the biochemical level.[42,43] There are at least 13 types, and each type produces a particular sugar in the urine because of a specific enzyme defect (**Table 1**). The incidence is about 1 in 20,000 live births.

All the mucopolysaccharidoses (MPSs) are autosomal recessive except for MPS type II (Hunter syndrome), which is X-linked. The most common MPSs are type I (Hurler syndrome) and type IV (Morquio syndrome). The MPS can be diagnosed by urine screening, using a toluidine blue spot test. If the initial results are positive, specific blood testing is done for the associated sugar abnormality.

Each MPS has a deficiency of a specific lysosomal enzyme that degrades the sulfated glycosaminoglycans: heparan sulfate, dermatan sulfate, keratan sulfate, and chondroitin sulfate. The incomplete degradation product accumulates in the lysozymes themselves. The incomplete product accumulates in the tissues such as the brain, the viscera, and the joints. This accumulation is responsible for the development of osteonecrosis, presumably because of too much material in the intramedullary space, and also contributes to spinal cord compressive symptoms, because of accumulation of material in the spinal canal.

TABLE 1

Mucopolysaccharidoses

Designation	Name	Enzyme Defect	Stored Substance	Inheritance Pattern
MPS I	Hurler/Scheie	α-L-Iduronidase	HS + DS	Autosomal recessive
MPS II	Hunter	Iduronidase-2-sulfatase	HS + DS	X-linked recessive
MPS IIIA	Sanfilippo A	Heparan sulfatase (sulfamidase)	HS	Autosomal recessive
MPS IIIB	Sanfilippo B	α-*N*-Acetylglucosaminidase	HS	Autosomal recessive
MPS IIIC	Sanfilippo C	Acetyl-CoA: α-glucosaminide *N*-acetyltransferase	HS	Autosomal recessive
MPS IIID	Sanfilippo D	Glucosamine-6-sulfatase	HS	Autosomal recessive
MPS IVA	Morquio A	*N*-Acetylgalactosamine-6-sulfate sulfatase	KS, CS	Autosomal recessive
MPS IVB	Morquio B	β-D-Galactosidase	KS	Autosomal recessive
MPS IVC	Morquio C	Unknown	KS	Autosomal recessive
MPS V	Formerly Scheie disease, no longer used	—	—	—
MPS VI	Maroteaux-Lamy	Arylsulfatase B, *N*-acetylgalactosamine-4-sulfatase	DS, CS	Autosomal recessive
MPS VII	Sly	β-D-Glucuronidase	CS, HS, DS	Autosomal recessive
MPS VIII	—	Glucosamine-6-sulfatase	CS, HS	Autosomal recessive

CS = chondroitin sulfate, DS = dermatan sulfate, HS = heparan sulfate, KS = keratan sulfate, MPSs = mucopolysaccharidoses

This unremitting process leads to the clinical progression of the disorders. The child has no apparent abnormality at birth, with the disorder being biochemically detectable by 6 to 12 months of age, and clinically symptomatic by 2 years of age. All these disorders lead to abnormally short stature. In some cases, there is severe mental retardation (Hurler, Hunter, and Sanfilippo syndromes). There are also abnormalities of the skull (enlarged, with thick calvarium) and facial features (coarse, gargoyle) and deafness. In some cases, there is hepatosplenomegaly and cardiovascular abnormalities. Radiographically, the clavicles are broad, and the scapulae are short and stubby. The vertebral bodies are ovoid, and scoliosis and kyphosis are frequent. There is acetabular dysplasia and coxa valga, and the iliac wings are flared.

The clinical course is variable, but most patients die in the first 2 decades of life if untreated. Treatment is evolving, and some of these patients have been treated successfully with bone marrow transplantation. The preferred donor is an HLA-identical sibling. Following successful transplantation, accumulation of the mucopolysaccharide stops, and there is improvement in the coarse facial features, hepatosplenomegaly, and partial improvement in hearing.[44-47] Research is currently underway in the field of gene therapy for some of these syndromes.

Orthopaedic treatment is directed to correct the functionally impairing musculoskeletal deformities. Hip flexion contractures and dysplasia often require surgical reconstruction, including reduction, femoral, and pelvis osteotomies. Cervical instability may be present and C1-C2 fusion, and halo immobilization may be necessary. Kyphosis requires orthotic treatment or even surgical spine fusion. Genu valgus may be managed with corrective osteotomies.

MPS Type I

MPS type I is characterized by a deficiency of L-iduronidase, the enzyme that degrades dermatan sulfate and heparan sulfate. The Hurler and Scheie forms represent the severe and mild ends of the clinical spectrum in MPS I. Children with the Hurler form have progressive mental retardation, severe, multiple skeletal deformities, and considerable organ and soft-tissue deformities and die before the age of 10 years.[48] The Scheie form is characterized by stiffness of the joints and corneal clouding, but no mental retardation; the diagnosis is usually made during the teenage years and affected patients have a normal life expectancy. Marrow transplantation is used in the management of the more severe forms. However, the results on the bones are variable, with the typical skeletal phenotypic features developing in most children despite undergoing successful bone marrow transplant. Some long-term studies cast doubt on the long-term effectiveness of marrow transplantation, but marrow transplant still provides short-term improvement, especially in the nonosseous manifestations. Musculoskeletal deformities that persist after marrow transplant still require treatment.[49]

Malalignment of the limbs can occur, and guided growth techniques or osteotomies may be necessary for management of genu valgum. Osteotomies may be associated with recurrence, and as such, guided growth approaches are an attractive alternative; however, comparative series are lacking in the literature. Approximately one-fourth of the patients have an abnormality of the upper cervical spine. The accumulation of degradation products in closed anatomic spaces, such as the carpal tunnel, causes triggering of the fingers and carpal tunnel syndrome.

MPS Type II and III

Hunter syndrome (MPS type II) and Sanfilippo syndrome (MPS type III) usually demonstrate milder skeletal manifestations.[50,51] Carpal tunnel syndrome is almost universal in Hunter syndrome, with ankle equinus contractures present in both types. Hip dysplasia is usually mild in these disorders and typically does not require surgical treatment. All patients with Sanfilippo syndrome sustain persistent neurocognitive decline, which is more variable in patients with Hunter syndrome.

MPS Type IV

There are three types of Morquio syndrome, which are classified as subtypes of MPS IV. All are caused by enzyme defects involved in the degradation of keratan sulfate. All the patients have no apparent abnormality at birth. For patients with the severe type IVA, the diagnosis is made between 1 and 3 years of age; those with the mild type IVC are diagnosed as teens; and those with the intermediate form (type IVB) are diagnosed somewhere in the middle of this age range. Intelligence is normal in patients of all of the MPS IV types, and only rarely are the facial features coarsened. All are short-trunked dwarfs with ligamentous laxity. The degree of genu valgus is significant, aggravated by the lax ligaments. Management of the knee proves difficult because of the osseous malalignment and the lax ligaments. Realignment osteotomies can restore plumb alignment, but recurrence may occur, and osteotomies may not control the instability during ambulation. The prophylactic use of braces to prevent initial valgus or recurrent deformity after surgery has not been effective. Guided growth is an attractive alternative to osteotomies, avoiding issues of recurrence, but comparative studies are lacking. Early arthritis develops in the hips and knees. The hips show a progressive acetabular dysplasia. Radiographs may show a small femoral ossific nucleus, but MRI or arthrogram will show a much larger cartilaginous femoral head. The femoral capital epiphyses are initially advanced for the patient's age, but between 4 and 9 years of age, the femoral heads grow smaller and then disappear altogether. The pathophysiology of the progressive hip disease is not completely understood, and to date, there is no pharmacologic or surgical approach to improve the prognosis. Patients may require total joint replacement surgery.

Odontoid hypoplasia or aplasia is common, with resultant C1-C2 instability. There is a soft-tissue mass in the spinal canal, contributing to cord compression. The upper and lower extremity findings are often of flaccidity rather than spasticity. Sudden deaths of patients with Morquio disease have been reported, and they are typically attributed to the C1-C2 subluxation. C1-C2 fusion before the onset of symptoms is controversial, but promoted by some, whereas others recommend surgical intervention for symptomatic patients. There are no comparative studies evaluating the outcomes of each of the different management approaches. Elsewhere in the spine, the vertebrae show a progressive platyspondyly with a thoracic kyphosis. Progressive deformity should be surgically stabilized. Despite these problems, many patients with Morquio disease live for decades. Cardiorespiratory disease is common, but the problems at the upper cervical spine account for most disabilities.

Diastrophic Dysplasia

This condition is an autosomal recessive disorder characterized by rhizomelic dwarfism associated with multiple severe spinal deformities that can be life threatening at times.[52] It is the result of a sulfate transport protein defect (SLC26A2) that affects proteoglycan sulfation in cartilage. Interestingly, it is present in 1 in 70 Finnish citizens. The disorder is apparent at birth, and patients can have cleft palate and develop cauliflower ears from cystic swelling in the ear cartilage. The hands are short, and there is characteristic hitchhiker thumbs. Joint contractures are common in the hips (which can be often dislocated in both sides) and knees, with genu valgus and dislocated patellae. Severe clubfeet are very often present.

Cervical kyphosis occurs in up to 40% of the cases but resolves spontaneously in most children by 6 years of age. Severe thoracic kyphosis (>60°) is usually associated with hypoplastic vertebrae and has a tendency to progress. In addition, there is a high incidence (75%) of spina bifida occulta, and surgeons must be aware when planning surgical stabilization.[53-56]

Compressive wrapping is used with good results for the cystic ear swelling. Progressive lower extremity deformities are difficult to manage and have a great tendency to recur. Hip dislocations are very difficult to reduce, and their reduction should be carefully discussed with the parents because the prognosis is poor even when they are centered. Treatment is indicated for progressive spinal deformity or cord compromise. However, severe complications can be expected with multiple reports of quadriplegia and cardiopulmonary failure.

DISORDERS CAUSED BY DEFECTS IN TUMOR SUPPRESSOR GENES

There are a variety of cellular proteins that are important in regulating cell reproduction or proliferation. A mutation that results in dysregulation of such pathways can cause overgrowth of a cell type or organ, and these pathways are frequently dysregulated in neoplasia. In many of these conditions, when a single copy (one of the two alleles) of a gene is mutated in the germ line, the result is an overgrowth phenotype, but when the second copy (the other allele) becomes mutated in a somatic manner (in a certain cell type), the result is the development of a tumor. Because many of these disorders are usually caused by one copy of a defective gene, they are inherited in an autosomal dominant manner.

Hereditary Multiple Exostoses

Hereditary multiple exostoses (HME), or diaphyseal aclasis, is a highly penetrant, autosomal dominant trait characterized by slightly stunted growth of long bones and multiple osteochondromas. Osteochondromas are cartilage-capped excrescences of bone that develop at the epiphyseal plate level during growth. These osteochondromas are indistinguishable morphologically from the solitary cases. HME has an incidence of about 1 in 50,000 live births.[57] The median age at the time of diagnosis in affected individuals is approximately 3 years. By the second decade of life, almost all affected individuals will have exostoses because the penetrance of the disorder has been found to be 96% to 100%. Many patients with HME require resection of the lesions because of a mass effect or neurovascular impingement symptoms. Importantly, up to 3% of patients with HME will eventually develop a malignant chondrosarcoma.

Over the past decade, advances in molecular biology and genetics have permitted a better understanding into the molecular players underlying these lesions. Linkage analysis has located three etiologic genes for HME: *EXT1*, *EXT2*, and *EXT3*. Interestingly, mutations in any of these genes demonstrate very similar clinical manifestations.[58,59] These EXT loci have defined a new class of putative tumor suppressor genes, to which three related genes—*EXTL1*, *EXTL2*, and *EXTL3*—have been recently added.

Because both HME and sporadic osteochondromas have been associated with loss of heterozygosity at one or more of the EXT loci, a neoplastic model of pathogenesis has been suggested. The Knudson two-hit theory of carcinogenesis derived from familial retinoblastoma has been applied to HME. Both copies of the *EXT1* gene have been observed to be deleted, and gene losses and mutations have been observed in chondrosarcomas arising from osteochondromas. However, it is still unclear how *EXT1* and *EXT2* can function as tumor suppressors.

Patients will present with several hard, knobby lumps near the joints. Numerous sites can be involved, and typically five or six exostoses can be found in the upper and lower extremities.[60-65] The most common locations are distal femur (70%), proximal tibia (70%), humerus (50%), and proximal fibula (30%). Over time, there will be some shortening of the extremities in relation to the trunk, and there may be leg length inequality. As the lesions enlarge, they may cause discomfort secondary to mechanical pressure to adjacent soft tissues and muscles. They rarely cause neurologic dysfunction. Often, patients complain of an undesirable cosmetic appearance. Valgus deformity of the knee and ankle is not uncommon, and osteochondromas of the proximal femur may lead to dysplasia of the hip, which may require corrective osteotomies. In adults, sarcomatous transformation will present as a painful and enlarging mass in an area of previous deformity.

Treatment for multiple hereditary exostoses is surgical excision. However, not all the exostoses should be removed. Established indications for surgery include growth disturbances leading to angular deformities or hip dysplasia; functional limitation of joint range of motion; spinal cord compression with neurologic compromise; painful mass and obvious cosmetic deformity; and rapid increase in the size of the lesion. Deformities in the forearm should be managed early to prevent further progression and to reduce disability. Knee osteotomies are associated with a high incidence of peroneal nerve palsy.

Russell-Silver Syndrome

Patients with Russell-Silver syndrome have a low birth weight with average head circumference, but a triangular shape to the face. Hemihypertrophy is present in 80% of affected individuals. Managing leg length equality can be difficult because individual growth curves may vary, not following normal predictive charts. Growth hormone has been administered in an attempt to improve stature, and although the use of growth hormone will increase growth velocity, it is not yet known whether the ultimate height is increased. There is a case report of Wilms tumor developing in an affected patient, leading some to recommend screening for Wilms tumor in these patients as would be done in other causes of hemihypertrophy.[66,67]

Proteus Syndrome

Proteus syndrome includes hemihypertrophy, macrodactyly, and partial gigantism of the hands or feet, or both, with a characteristic appearance to the plantar surface of the feet, often described as similar to the surface of the brain.[68] There is worsening of existing symptoms and the appearance of new ones over time. Unlike in other overgrowth syndromes, an increased incidence of malignancy has not been reported in Proteus syndrome. There is an array of cutaneous manifestations including hemangiomas and pigmented nevi of various intensities and subcutaneous lipomas. Varicosities are present, although true arteriovenous malformations are rare.

Skeletal deformities include focal and regional gigantism, scoliosis, and kyphosis. Rather large vertebral bodies, known as megaspondylodysplasia, are present. Angular malformations of the lower extremities, especially genu valgus, are common. Recurrences after surgical interventions are very common. This is probably due to an underlying growth advantage in affected tissues that cannot be corrected surgically. Thus, musculoskeletal deformities caused by Proteus syndrome can be very difficult to manage. Osteotomies can correct angular malformations, but the decision to undertake surgical correction must take into account the possibility of a rapid recurrence of the deformity after corrective surgery. The use of growth modulation (eg, 8-plate) to manage limb angular deformity is a rather promising approach, but publications on the results of this approach are lacking. Nerve compression can be managed using decompression, but spinal cord compression is difficult, if not impossible, to successfully manage surgically because of the overgrowth of the vertebrae. Scoliosis seems to be caused by overgrowth of one side of the spine. Functional ability depends on the severity of the limb deformity and the presence of intracranial abnormalities.

SUMMARY

Skeletal dysplasias are a group of heterogenous genetic disorders characterized by abnormal differentiation, development, growth, and maintenance of bone and cartilage. Diagnosis of these conditions is sometimes difficult. An individualized multidisciplinary treatment approach is recommended for affected patients.

KEY STUDY POINTS

- The clinical diversity of skeletal dysplasias makes these disorders often difficult to diagnose, and the criteria used for their distinction have been based on a combination of clinical, morphologic, radiographic, and, in some instances, biochemical and molecular characteristics.
- It is important to be aware of not only the clinical characteristics of these disorders but also the genetic causes to make appropriate referrals for genetic counseling and to refine the prognosis and natural history in each individual patient.
- Conceptually, it is useful to classify musculoskeletal disorders caused by gene mutations into groups broadly categorized by the function of the causative gene. Mutations in early patterning genes cause disorders called dysostoses. In contrast, mutations in genes that are involved primarily in cell differentiation cause disorders called osteochondrodysplasias.

ANNOTATED REFERENCES

1. Carey JC, Viskochil DH: Status of the human malformations map: 2002. *Am J Med Genet* 2002;115:205-220.
2. Krakow D, Rimoin DL: The skeletal dysplasias. *Genet Med* 2010;12:327-341.
3. Warman ML, Cormier-Daire V, Hall C, et al: Nosology and classification of genetic skeletal disorders: 2010 revision. *Am J Med Genet* 2011;155:943-968.
4. Kornak U, Mundlos S: Genetic disorders of the skeleton: A developmental approach. *Am J Hum Genet* 2003;73:447.
5. Hermanns P, Lee B: Transcriptional dysregulation in skeletal malformations syndromes. *Am J Hum Genet* 2001; 106:258.
6. Unger S: A genetic approach to the diagnosis of skeletal dysplasia. *Clin Orthop Relat Res* 2002;401:32-38.
7. Mortier GR: The diagnosis of skeletal dysplasias: A multidisciplinary approach. *Eur J Radiol* 2001;40:161-167.
8. Parilla B, Leeth E, Kambich M, Chilis P, MacGregor S: Antenatal detection of skeletal dysplasias. *J Ultrasound Med* 2003;22:255-258.
9. Alanay Y, Lachman RS: A review of the principles of radiological assessment of skeletal dysplasias. *J Clin Res Pediatr Endocrinol* 2011;3:163-178.
10. Briggs MD, Chapman KL: Pseudoachondroplasia and multiple epiphyseal dysplasia: Mutation review, molecular interactions, and genotype to phenotype correlations. *Hum Mutat* 2002;19:465.
11. Ingram RR: Early diagnosis of multiple epiphyseal dysplasia. *J Pediatr Orthop* 1992;12:241-244.

12. Crossan JF, Wynne-Davies R, Fulford GE: Bilateral failure of the capital femoral epiphysis: Bilateral Perthes disease, multiple epiphyseal dysplasia, pseudoachondroplasia, and spondyloepiphyseal dysplasia congenita and tarda. *J Pediatr Orthop* 1983;3(3):297-301.
13. Treble NJ, Jensen FO, Bankier A, Rogers JG, Cole WG: Development of the hip in multiple epiphyseal dysplasia. Natural history and susceptibility to premature osteoarthritis. *J Bone Joint Surg Br* 1990;72:1061-1064.
14. Acharya C, Yik JH, Kishore A, Van Dinh V, Di Cesare PE, Haudenschild DR: Cartilage oligomeric matrix protein and its binding partners in the cartilage extracellular matrix: Interaction, regulation and role in chondrogenesis. *Matrix Biol* 2014;37:102-111.

    The interactions of COMP with other proteins in the cartilage extracellular matrix were compiled and their importance in maintaining the structural integrity of cartilage and regulating cellular functions was discussed.
15. Posey KL, Alcron JL, Hecht JT: Pseudoachondroplasia/COMP—Translating from the bench to the bedside. *Matrix Biol* 2014;37:167-173.

    Pseudoachondroplasia is a skeletal dysplasia caused by muations in the *COMP* gene. Information learned from mutant *COMP* mouse model systems and how it may translate to clinical therapies is discussed.
16. Cooper RR, Ponseti IV, Maynard JA: Pseudoachondroplastic dwarfism: A rough-surfaced endoplasmic reticulum storage disorder. *J Bone Joint Surg Am* 1973;55:475-484.
17. McKeand J, Rotta J, Hecht JT: Natural history study of pseudoachondroplasia. *Am J Med Genet* 1996;63:406.
18. Reardon W, Hall CM, Shaw DG, Kendall B, Hayward R, Winter RM: New autosomal dominant form of spondyloepiphyseal dysplasia presenting with atlanto-axial instability. *Am J Med Genet* 1994;52:432-437.
19. Zabel B, Hilbert K, Stoss H, Superti-Furga A, Spranger J, Winterpacht A: A specific collagen type II gene (COL2A 1) mutation presenting as spondyloperipheral dysplasia. *Am J Med Genet* 1996;63:123-128.
20. Miyoshi K, Nakamura K, Haga N, Mikami Y: Surgical treatment for atlantoaxial subluxation with myelopathy in spondyloepiphyseal dysplasia congenita. *Spine (Phila Pa 1976)* 2004;29(21):E488-E491.
21. Svensson O, Aaro S: Cervical instability in skeletal dysplasia: Report of 6 surgically fused cases. *Acta Orthop Scand* 1988;59(1):66-70.
22. Shiang R, Thompson LM, Zhu YZ, et al: Mutations in the transmembrane domain of FGFR3 cause the most common genetic form of dwarfism, achondroplasia. *Cell* 1994; 78:335.
23. Horton WA: Fibroblast growth factor receptor 3 and the human chondrodysplasias. *Curr Opin Pediatr* 1997;9:437.
24. Yamanaka Y, Ueda K, Seino Y, et al: Molecular basis for the treatment of achondroplasia. *Horm Res* 2003;60(suppl 3):60-64.
25. Maynard JA, Ippolito EG, Ponseti IV, Mickelson MR: Histochemistry and ultrastructure of the growth plate in achondroplasia. *J Bone Joint Surg Am* 1981;63: 969-979.
26. Ponseti IV: Skeletal growth in achondroplasia. *J Bone Joint Surg Am* 1970;52:701-716.
27. Hall JG: The natural history of achondroplasia. *Basic Life Sci* 1988;48:3-9.
28. Lutter LD, Lonstein JE, Winter RB, Langer LO: Anatomy of the achondroplastic lumbar canal. *Clin Orthop Relat Res* 1977;126:139-142.
29. Baca KE, Abdullah MA, Ting BL, et al: Surgical decompression for lumbar stenosis in pediatric achondroplasia. *J Pediatr Orthop* 2010;30(5):449-454.
30. Rousseau F, Bonaventure J, Legeai-Mallet L, et al: Clinical and genetic heterogeneity of hypochondroplasia. *J Med Genet* 1996;33:749.
31. Coscia MF, Bassett GS, Bowen JR, Ogilvie JW, Winter RB, Simonton SC: Spinal deformities in camptomelic dysplasia. *J Pediatr Orthop* 1989;9:6.
32. Thomas S, Winter RB, Lonstein JE: The treatment of progressive kyphoscoliosis in camptomelic dysplasia. *Spine (Phila Pa 1976)* 1997;22(12):1330-1337.
33. Lee B, Thirunavukkarasu K, Zhou L, et al: Missense mutations abolishing DNA binding of the osteoblast-specific transcription factor OSF2/CBFA1 in cleidocranial dysplasia. *Nat Genet* 1997;16:307.
34. Mundlos S: Cleidocranial dysplasia: Clinical and molecular genetics. *J Med Genet* 1999;36:177.
35. Otto F, Kanegame H, Mundlos S: Mutations in the RUNX2 gene in patients with cleidocranial dysplasia. *Hum Mutat* 2002;19:209.
36. Cooper SC, Flaitz CM, Johnston DA, Lee B, Hecht JT: A natural history of cleidocranial dysplasia. *Am J Med Genet* 2001;104:1-6.
37. Richie NF, Johnston CE: Management of developmental coxa vara in cleidocranial dysplasia. *Orthopedics* 1989;12:1001-1004.
38. Bongers EM, Gubler MC, Knoers NV: Nail-patella syndrome: Overview on clinical and molecular findings. *Pediatr Nephrol* 2002;17:703.
39. Beguiristain JL, de Rada PD, Barriga A: Nail-patella syndrome: Long term evolution. *J Pediatr Orthop B* 2003;12:13-16.
40. Gillis LA, McCallum J, Kaur M, et al: NIPBL mutational analysis of 120 individuals with Cornelia de Lange syndrome and evaluation of genotype-phenotype correlations. *Am J Hum Genet* 2004;75:610.
41. Joubin J, Pettrone CF, Pettrone FA: Cornelia de Lange's syndrome: A review article (with emphasis on orthopedic significance). *Clin Orthop Relat Res* 1982;171:180.
42. Muenzer J: The mucopolysaccharidoses: A heterogenous group of disorders with variable pediatric presentations. *J Pediatr* 2004;144:S27-S34.

43. Kircher S, Bajbouj M, Beck M: *Mucopolysaccharidoses: A Guide for Physicians and Parents*. Bremen, Germany, Uni-Med Verlag AG, 2007.

44. Sauer M, Grewal S, Peters C: Hematopoietic stem cell transplantation for mucopolysaccharidoses and leukodystrophies. *Klin Padiatr* 2004;216:163.

45. Wraith JE, Clarke LA, Beck M, et al: Enzyme replacement therapy for mucopolysaccharidosis I: A randomized, double-blind, placebo-controlled, multinational study of recombinant human α-L-iduronidase (laronidase). *J Pediatr* 2004;144:561.

46. Muenzer J, Fisher A: Advances in the treatment of mucopolysaccharidosis type I. *N Engl J Med* 2004;350:1932-1934.

47. Giugliani R, Federhen A, Rojas MY, et al: Mucopolysaccharidosis I, II, and VI: Brief review and guidelines for treatment. *Genet Mol Biol* 2010;33(4):589-604.

48. Taylor C, Brady P, O'Meara A, Moore D, Dowling F, Fogarty E: Mobility in Hurler syndrome. *J Pediatr Orthop* 2008;28:163-168.

49. Malm G, Gustafsson B, Berglund G, et al: Outcome in six children with mucopolysaccharidosis type IH, Hurler syndrome, after haematopoietic stem cell transplantation (HSCT). *Acta Paediatr* 2008;97:1108-1112.

50. White KK, Hale S, Goldberg MJ: Musculoskeletal health in Hunter disease (MPS II): ERT improves functional outcomes. *J Pediatr Rehabil Med* 2010;3(2):101-107.

51. White KK, Karol LA, White DR, Hale S: Musculoskeletal manifestations of Sanfilippo Syndrome (mucopolysaccharidosis type III). *J Pediatr Orthop* 2011;31(5):594-598.

52. Carten M, Gagne V: Diastrophic dysplasia. Available at: http://www.pixelscapes.com/ddhelp/DD-booklet/. Accessed December 2, 2020.

53. Bethem D, Winter RB, Lutter L: Disorders of the spine in diastrophic dwarfism. *Bone Joint Surg Am* 1980;62(4): 529-536.

54. Poussa M, Merikanto J, Ryoppy S, Marttinen E, Kaitila I: The spine in diastrophic dysplasia. *Spine (Phila Pa 1976)* 1991;16(8):881-887.

55. Remes V, Marttinen E, Poussa M, Kaitila I, Peltonen J: Cervical kyphosis in diastrophic dysplasia. *Spine (Phila Pa 1976)* 1999;24(19):1990-1995.

56. Ryoppy S, Poussa M, Merikanto J, Marttinen E, Kaitila I: Foot deformities in diastrophic dysplasia. An analysis of 102 patients. *J Bone Joint Surg Am* 1992;74:441-444.

57. Black B, Dooley J, Pyper A, Reed M: Multiple hereditary exostoses. An epidemiologic study of an isolated community in Manitoba. *Clin Orthop Relat Res* 1993;287:212-217.

58. Hall CR, Cole WG, Haynes R, Hecht JT: Reevaluation of a genetic model for the development of exostoses in hereditary multiple exostoses. *Am J Med Genet* 2002;112:1-5.

59. Zak BM, Crawford BE, Esko JD: Hereditary multiple exostoses and heparin sulfate polymerization. *Biochem Biophys Acta* 2002;1573:346.

60. Peterson HA: Deformities and problems of the forearm in children with multiple hereditary osteochondromata. *J Pediatr Orthop* 1994;14:92-100.

61. Ballantyne JA, Simpson AH, Porter DE, Fraser M: Wrist and forearm dysfunction in hereditary multiple exostoses. *J Hand Surg* 2003;28(suppl 1):26.

62. Porter DE, Benson MK, Hosney GA: The hip in hereditary multiple exostoses. *J Bone Joint Surg Br* 2001;83:988-995.

63. Nawata K, Teshima R, Minamizaki T, Yamamoto K: Knee deformities in multiple hereditary exostoses. A longitudinal radiographic study. *Clin Orthop Relat Res* 1995;313:194-199.

64. Noonan KJ, Feinberg JR, Levenda A, Snead J, Wurtz LD: Natural history of multiple osteochondromatosis of the lower extremity and ankle. *J Pediatr Orthop* 2002;22:120.

65. Schmale GA, Conrad EU III, Raskind WH: The natural history of hereditary multiple exostoses. *J Bone Joint Surg Am* 1994;76:986-992.

66. Siklar Z, Berberoglu M: Syndromic disorders with short stature. *J Clin Res Pediatr Endocrinol* 2014;6:1-8.

    Syndromes associated with short stature are discussed. These disorders are associated with endocrinopathies as well as developmental, systemic, and behavioral issues.

67. Azzi S, Abi Habib W, Netchine I: Beckwith-Wiedemann and Russell-Silver syndromes: From new molecular insights to the comprehension of imprinting regulation. *Curr Opin Endocrinol Diabetes Obes* 2014;21:30-38.

    A discussion of molecular abnormalities at 11p15.5 involved in Silver-Russell and Beckwith-Wiedemann syndromes is presented.

68. Cohen MM Jr: Proteus syndrome review: Molecular, clinical, and pathologic features. *Clin Genet* 2014;85:111-119.

    An overview of Proteus syndrome is provided, along with a discussion of diagnostic criteria, natural history, management, psychological issues, and differential diagnosis.

CHAPTER 9

Orthopaedic-Related Syndromes

KLANE K. WHITE, MD, MSc • CRAIG BIRCH, MD • BENJAMIN A. ALMAN, MD, FAAOS

ABSTRACT

Syndromes are characterized by a constellation of phenotypic findings that run together. Many syndromes are caused by genetic mutation; others may be caused by fetal environmental factors that alter cell behavior, often in a manner that mimics genetic mutation. Each class of syndromes commonly shares similar clinical findings and responses to treatment. Advances in the understanding of the sequelae of the various genetic mutations also have identified novel possible treatment methods for some syndromes. Such therapies are being adopted in select patients. During the next decades, it is predicted that many such therapies will alter the orthopaedic manifestations of these conditions.

Dr. White or an immediate family member is a member of a speakers' bureau or has made paid presentations on behalf of Biomarin and Genzyme; serves as a paid consultant to or is an employee of Biomarin; has received research or institutional support from Biomarin and Ultragenyx; has received nonincome support (such as equipment or services), commercially derived honoraria, or other non–research-related funding (such as paid travel) from Genzyme; and serves as a board member, owner, officer, or committee member of the Pediatric Orthopaedic Society of North America. Dr. Alman or an immediate family member serves as an unpaid consultant to SpringWorks Therapeutics; has stock or stock options held in ScarX; and serves as a board member, owner, officer, or committee member of the Foundation for Advancing Pediatric Orthopedics and the Shrine research advisory board. Neither Dr. Birch nor any immediate family member has received anything of value from or has stock or stock options held in a commercial company or institution related directly or indirectly to the subject of this chapter.

Keywords: development; dysplasia; overgrowth; syndrome

INTRODUCTION

Numerous syndromes affect the musculoskeletal system. As such, it is useful to group them into classes. As more is learned about the underlying genetic causes of syndromes, they can be categorized according to the function of the causative gene. Syndromes within each broad group share similarities in the mode of inheritance and clinical behavior.

DISORDERS CAUSED BY STRUCTURAL GENES

Marfan Syndrome

Marfan syndrome results from mutations in the gene encoding for the fibrillin protein. Fibrillin is an extracellular glycoprotein essential in the formation of the elastic fibers found in connective tissues and has an important role in resistance to cyclic stresses of the cardiovascular, ocular, and skeletal systems.[1,2] Increased recognition of transforming growth factor beta (TGF-β) and the bone morphogenetic proteins to SMAD cell receptors promote skeletal growth, leading to the typical phenotype of tall stature and long, thin fingers and toes.[3]

Scoliosis in Marfan syndrome is treated in a manner similar to idiopathic scoliosis, although bracing treatment appears to be less effective, with a reported success rate of only 17% for a group of patients with mild to moderate curves.[4] Dural ectasia is common in these patients, and CT and MRI are recommended for all patients before surgical intervention. Small pedicles in the lumbar spine, particularly on the concave side, make pedicle screw fixation more challenging.[5] Infection, implant failure, pseudarthrosis, or coronal and sagittal curve decompensation are reported to occur in 10% to 20% of patients. Infection often is associated with a dural tear, and perioperative death from valvular insufficiency has been reported.

Osteopenia is commonly found in patients with Marfan syndrome; however, this is not associated with an increased risk of fractures. Protrusio acetabula may be treated with prophylactic fusion of the triradiate cartilage. Correction of this deformity is not predictable, and therefore this procedure is not advocated for in most patients.

Loeys-Dietz syndrome is a disorder genetically related (TGF-β family) to Marfan syndrome, with similar skeletal manifestations of skeletal overgrowth, including pectus excavatum or pectus carinatum, scoliosis, joint laxity, arachnodactyly, clubfeet, cervical spine malformations and/or instability.[6] Heterozygous variants in *SMAD2*, *SMAD3*, *TGFB2*, *TGFB3*, *TGFBR1*, or *TGFBR2* are associated with Loeys-Dietz syndrome. Progressive spondylolisthesis and severe pes planus are seen in older patients. Spinal manifestations often require surgical interventions, whereas foot deformities can typically be managed nonsurgically.

Ehlers-Danlos Syndrome

Ehlers-Danlos syndrome (EDS) is a group of clinically and genetically heterogeneous, connective tissue disorders characterized by joint hypermobility, skin hyperextensibility, and tissue fragility. The most recent nosology recognizes 13 subtypes, with variations in which tissue types are involved, including skin, ligament, joints, eyes, intestines, and cardiovascular structures[7] (**Table 1**). 90%

TABLE 1

Nosology of Ehlers-Danlos Syndrome (EDS)

Clinical EDS Subtype	Abbreviation	IP	Genetic Basis	Protein
1. Classical EDS	cEDS	AD	Major: COL5A1, COL5A2 Rare: COL1A1 c.934C>T, p.(Arg312Cys)	Type V collagen Type I collagen
2. Classical-like EDS	clEDS	AR	TNXB	Tenascin XB
3. Cardiac-valvular	cvDS	AR	COL1A2 (biallelic mutations that lead to COL1A2 NMD and absence of pro α2(1) collagen chains)	Type III collagen
4. Vascular EDS	vEDS	AD	Major: COL3A1 Rare: COL1A1 c.934C>T, p.(Arg312Cys) c.1720>T, p.(Arg574Cys) c.3227>T, p.(Arg1093Cys)	Type I collagen
5. Hypermobile EDS	hEDS	AD	Unknown	Unknown
6. Arthrochalasia EDS	aEDS	AD	COL1A1, COL1A2	Type I collagen
7. Dermatosparaxis EDS	dEDS	AR	ADAMTS2	ADAMTS-2
8. Kyphoscoliotic EDS	kEDS	AR	PLOD1 FKBP14	LH1 FKBP22
9. Brittle cornea syndrome	BCS	AR	ZNF469 PRDM5	ZNH469 PRDM5
10. Spondylodysplastic EDS	spEDS	AR	B4GALT7 B3GALT6 SLC39A13	β4GalT7 β3GalT6 ZIP13
11. Musculocontractural EDS	mcEDS	AR	CHST14 DSE	D4ST1 DSE
12. Myopathic EDS	mEDS	AD or AR	COL12A1	Type XII collagen
13. Periodontal EDS	pEDS	AD	C1R C1S	C1r C1s

AD = autosomal dominant, AR = autosomal recessive, IP = inheritance patterns, MDN = nonsense-mediated mRNA decay.

Adapted from Malfait F, Francomano C, Byers P, et al: The 2017 international classification of the Ehlers-Danlos syndromes. *Am J Med Genet C Semin Med Genet* 2017;175(1):8-26. © 2017 Wiley Periodicals, Inc.

of EDS is represented by two of these subtypes: classical EDS and hypermobile EDS. Classical EDS is an autosomal dominant disorder, with >90% associated with mutations in COL5A1 or COL5A2. Classical EDS can also be associated with COL1A1 and COL1A2 mutations when clinical criteria are met. Hypermobile EDS also appears to be transmitted in an autosomal dominant fashion, but no certain genetic underpinning has been identified.

Chronic musculoskeletal pain, recurrent joint dislocations, or frank instability in the absence of trauma are seen in hypermobile EDS.[8] There are no pathognomonic radiographic findings associated with EDS. Physical therapy focused on core muscle strength or stabilization of specific joints may be successful. Recognition that patients with EDS have loose joints and tight muscles is requisite to the rehabilitation success, but exercise programs that emphasize range of motion or repetitive, forceful actions may make symptoms worse.

Higher complication rates after surgery are commonly associated with EDS.[9] Avoidance of surgical complications depends on observation of appropriate and strict indications. Surgery is an option for a select number of specific conditions in EDS, including the spine, shoulders, elbows, and hands as well as hips and lower extremities. The rate of failure of surgical intervention is higher in EDS, particularly for conditions where ligaments are repaired. Wound healing is generally good, but may result in widened scars.

Osteogenesis Imperfecta

Osteogenesis imperfecta results from a mutation in the genes that code for type I collagen (*COL1A1* and *COL1A2*) or the genes that encode for processing of these strands.[10] The Sillence classification includes the original four types of osteogenesis imperfecta and has been subsequently modified to include, at present, 11 forms based on clinical, radiographic, biochemical, and genetic information[11] (**Table 2**). Despite an increase in the frequency of fractures in patients with osteogenesis imperfecta during childhood, bone healing occurs at a normal rate, but with abnormal bone.

Pharmacologic treatment with diphosphonates is commonly used in the care for children with osteogenesis imperfecta sustaining two or more long-bone fractures per year.[12] Cyclic treatment with intravenous pamidronate results in improved bone mineral density, reduction in fracture incidence, reduction in pain, and improved remodeling of vertebral body compression fractures. Animal models suggest that impaired bone healing may occur in the presence of diphosphonate therapy. Infusions can be given any time before osteotomy but should then be delayed for approximately 3 months afterward. Several protocols exist for pamidronate use and typically intravenous infusions every 3 months, 4 hours a day, for 3 days are administered. Smaller, more frequent dosing is often used in children younger than 3 years to avoid hypocalcemia.[13] Maintenance dosing (one 3-hour infusion every 6 months) is recommended after 2 years of therapy until growth is completed. Treatment beyond 5 years in skeletally mature patients may paradoxically result in increased fracture risk because of overmineralization. Zoledronic acid allows for shorter less frequent infusion times and is likely equally effective.[14]

Nonsurgical management of fractures consists of a short course of splinting to minimize the effects of disuse osteoporosis and cyclic fracturing. Realignment osteotomy with intramedullary fixation is the standard treatment in children with bone deformities that interfere with function. Age at realignment is dictated by the size of the patient, frequency of fractures, and severity of deformity and can be performed as early as 18 months of age, but in smaller individuals may have to wait until 4 to 5 years of age.

Fassier-Duval telescoping rods are the mainstay for orthopaedic management of lower extremity deformities in osteogenesis imperfecta. Fassier-Duval rods can be placed using relatively minimally invasive techniques. Short-term and medium-term (4 to 5 years) outcomes are good, with regard to reducing fracture recurrence and improving mobility. Complications include refracture, pseudarthrosis, rod migration, and failure to deploy. Revision surgery rates for lower extremities are approximately 50% by 4 years, and about 35% at 3 years for upper extremities.

Craniocervical junction abnormalities are seen in 37% of patients with osteogenesis imperfecta, including basilar invagination (13%), basilar impression (15%), and platybasia (29%).[15] The presence of skull base abnormalities is clearly correlated with the severity of disease and older age.[16]

Management of basilar invagination may be by odontoid resection, foramen magnum decompression, or both and may require occipitocervical fusion.[17] Brace treatment has not been found to be effective and is difficult to use because of the fragility of the rib cage.[18] Recommendations for surgical intervention for scoliosis in osteogenesis imperfecta are variable; treatment delay to 50° is unlikely to significantly compromise pulmonary function or increase difficulty in treatment.[19]

DISORDERS CAUSED BY TUMOR-RELATED GENES

Neurofibromatosis

Neurofibromatosis is the most common single-gene disorder in humans, and neurofibromatosis type 1 (NF-1) is the type most frequently encountered by orthopaedic

TABLE 2

Sillence Classification for COL1A1/2-related Osteogenesis Imperfecta (OI)

Type	MOI	Severity	Fractures	Bone Deformity	Stature	DI	Sclerae	Hearing Loss
I. Classic nondeforming OI w/blue sclerae	AD	Mild	Few to 100	Uncommon	Normal or slightly short for a family	Rare	Blue	Present in ~50%
II. Perinatally lethal OI	AD	Perinatal lethal	Multiple fracture of the ribs, minimal calvarial mineralization, platyspondyly, marked compression of long bones	Severe	Severely short stature	+	Dark blue	—
III. Progressively deforming OI	AD	Severe	Thin ribs, platyspondyly, thin gracile bones w/ many fractures, popcorn epiphyses	Moderate to severe	Very short	+	Blue	Frequent
IV. Common variable OI w/normal sclerae	AD	Moderate to mild	Multiple	Mild to moderate	Variably short stature	—	—	—

AD = autosomal dominant, DI = dentinogenesis imperfecta, MOI = mode of inheritance.

Adapted from Steiner RD, Basel D: COL1A1/2 osteogenesis imperfecta, in *Gene Reviews*. Available at: https://www.ncbi.nlm.nih.gov/books/NBK1295/. © 1993-2020 University of Washington.

surgeons. Two of following cardinal clinical findings are required to make the diagnosis: six café au lait spots larger than 5 mm in diameter in children, and larger than 15 mm in diameter in adults; two neurofibromas or a single plexiform neurofibroma; freckling in the axillae or inguinal region; an optic glioma; at least two Lisch nodules (hamartoma of the iris); a distinctive osseous lesion such as vertebral scalloping or cortical thinning; and a first-degree relative with NF-1.[20]

Neurofibromatosis is caused by a mutation in the *NF1* gene. Its protein product, neurofibromin, acts as a tumor suppressor. The mutation stimulates the conversion of Ras-GTP (guanosine-5′-triphosphate) to Ras-GDP (guanine diphosphate), activating Ras signaling, which is involved in the control of cell growth.[21] Farnesyl transferase and statin inhibitors have been investigated as agents to treat NF-1, but results have been mixed.[22-25] Two approaches to treat the bone-specific phenotype target pyrophosphate, which accumulates at high levels in bone.[26,27] Another approach is to target β-catenin signaling, which is hyperactive in osteogenesis in neurofibromatosis, preventing bone formation. Inhibiting its activity improves bone repair.[27]

Scoliosis is common, with curves classified as dystrophic or nondystrophic. Dystrophic scoliosis is associated with a short, sharp, single curve involving six or fewer vertebrae, deformity of the ribs and vertebrae, and dural ectasia and rib penetration of the spinal canal. The onset is early in childhood; and it is relentlessly progressive. The most important risk factors for progression are early age of onset; a high Cobb angle; an apical vertebra that is severely rotated; and scalloped bone (concave loss of bone) in the middle to lower thoracic area.[28] Dystrophic curves are refractive to brace treatment. Other spinal deformities such as kyphosis also can occur. In severe cases, the scoliosis has so much rotation that curve progression is more obvious on lateral rather than AP radiographs.[28] In those with severe angular kyphosis, a high risk of paraplegia is present.

Pseudarthrosis of bone can occur and most frequently affects the tibia. Tibial dysplasia with a characteristic anterolateral bow, which in infancy can progress to pseudarthrosis, is associated with NF-1. The characteristic anterolateral bow is apparent in infancy and may progress to fracture, with spontaneous union being rare.[29] Hamartoma of undifferentiated mesenchymal cells occurs at the pseudarthrosis site, which sometimes is associated with loss of the normal allele of the *NF1* gene.[30,31] Direct installation of bone morphogenetic protein to the pseudarthrosis site may help to achieve union, but variable results have been reported, and it is not known if the use of bone morphogenetic protein in patients with an inherited premalignant condition has long-term consequences.[32]

The incidence of malignancy in neurofibromatosis is reported to range from less than 1% to more than 20%. The most common tumor location is in the central nervous system. Malignant degeneration of a peripheral neurofibroma to a neurofibrosarcoma is a risk, and it can be difficult to distinguish a malignant lesion from a benign lesion. CT scans show areas of low-enhancing density in neurofibrosarcomas.[33] Similar patterns also can be visualized using MRI. Routine surveillance for sarcomatous change is difficult because of the large number of neurofibromas. In children with a neurofibroma, the propensity also exists for the development of other malignancies such as Wilms tumors or rhabdomyosarcomas.

Hereditary Multiple Osteochondroma

Hereditary multiple osteochondroma (HMO), also known as multiple hereditary exostoses, is an autosomal dominant disorder characterized by multiple osteochondromas and associated skeletal deformities.[34] Two genes have been identified to be associated with HMO, *EXT1* and *EXT2*, which account for 50% and 33% of cases respectively.[35]

The most common skeletal deformities associated with HMO are short stature, limb-length discrepancies, and valgus deformity of the knee or ankle. Upper extremity deformities are classically ulnar shortening leading to limited forearm rotation, and subluxation of the radial head.[36] The spine has been reported to be involved in 7% of patients with multiple hereditary exostoses and may result in spinal cord compression, with MRI screening recommended by some authors.[37]

General treatment approach is observation and surveillance unless the lesions become painful. Treatment consists of surgical excision. Recurrence may occur if a portion of the stalk or cartilage cap remains. Angular deformities are treated with osteotomy or guided growth. Malignant transformation of osteochondromas in patients with HMO is around 5% by current estimation.[38,39] A lesion that enlarges after the age of 30 years warrants further imaging and excision. In adults, a cartilage cap larger than 2 cm is generally accepted to indicate malignant transformation; however, in the pediatric population, the normal cartilage cap may be 2 to 3 cm thick.[40] Secondary malignancy in the pediatric age group is extremely rare, but patients should be counseled regarding their lifetime risk.

Enchondromatosis Syndromes

There are two well-established syndromes of enchondromatosis: Ollier disease and Maffucci disease. The distinguishing factor for Maffucci is the presence of hemangiomata. Most cases of enchondromatosis are due to sporadic mutations.[41-43] Patients typically present with bilateral involvement with a mosaic pattern. Both longitudinal and angular deformities of the extremities can exist. Epiphysiodesis, lengthening, and acute or gradual correction are all effective in these disorders. Ollier disease has a reported malignant degeneration rate of up to 25%, specifically with transition to chondrosarcoma.[44,45] This rate exceeds 40% in patients with lesions of the axial skeleton, specifically the pelvis.[46] For Maffucci syndrome, the malignant degeneration rate of an enchondroma to chondrosarcoma is estimated to be 18%, whereas the overall risk of malignancy, skeletal or nonskeletal, is nearly 100%, necessitating long-term oncology surveillance.[45,47]

Polyostotic Fibrous Dysplasia

Polyostotic fibrous dysplasia may involve several small regions or up to 75% of the skeleton, with most cases identified before age 10 years.[48,49] There appears to be a postzygotic somatic activating pathogenic variant in *GNAS* (encoding the cAMP pathway-associated G-protein, $G_s\alpha$) in both mono and polyostotic fibrous dysplasia. This somatic rather than germ line mutation leads to focal proliferation of mesenchymal osteoblastic progenitor cells.[50-52] Polyostotic fibrous dysplasia is a part of McCune-Albright syndrome (fibrous dysplasia, café au lait spots, and endocrinopathy) and Mazabraud syndrome (fibrous dysplasia and soft-tissue myxomas). Various endocrinopathies including hyperparathyroidism, hypophosphatemia, acromegaly, hyperprolactinemia, and Cushing disease have all been associated with polyostotic fibrous dysplasia.[48,53,54]

The most frequently involved sites are femur, tibia, pelvis, and foot at 91%, 81%, 78%, and 73% respectively.[55] Asymptomatic lesions should be followed up for progression or development of deformity during skeletal immaturity. Symptoms tend to diminish with age, possibly because of a failure of mutant stem cells to self-renew, leaving their progeny to be consumed by apoptosis, allowing residual normal stem cells to survive and self-renew, enabling the formation of a normal structure. Surgery is undertaken for larger lesions associated with progressive deformity, pain, or pathologic fracture. Standard treatment of the lesion is curettage, bone grafting, and internal fixation. Graft may be rapidly incorporated and recurrence rates remain high.[56,57] Associated angular deformities should be addressed concurrently with the lesion itself, specifically the common proximal femoral varus deformity. Valgus-producing osteotomy may be required for progressive deformity, using cephalomedullary fixation.[57] Medical management of polyostotic fibrous dysplasia with diphosphonates has been associated with improved cortical thickness, improved function, reduced pain, and a lower rate of pathologic fracture.[58,59]

Proteus Syndrome

A characteristic appearance on the plantar surface of the feet, which is similar to the surface of the brain, occurs in Proteus syndrome. Both hemihypertrophy and macrodactyly are present. A mosaic distribution of lesions, a progressive course, and sporadic occurrence are characteristics required to make the diagnosis. An increased incidence of malignancy has not been associated with this disorder. Hemangiomas, pigmented nevi, and subcutaneous lipomas are present in the skin. A somatic mosaic mutation (mutant only in involved cells) activating *AKT1* is associated with Proteus syndrome.[60]

Spinal deformity, including scoliosis, kyphosis, and large vertebral bodies, known as megaspondylodysplasia, can be present.[61] Angular malformations of the lower extremities, especially genu valgum, are common, along with regional gigantism. Recurrence after surgical intervention is very common.[61] Osteotomies can correct angular malformations, but the decision to undertake surgical correction must consider the possibility of rapid recurrence of the deformity after corrective surgery. The use of guided growth to manage limb angular deformity is a promising approach,[45] but published results are lacking. Nerve compression can be managed with decompression, but spinal cord compression is difficult, if not impossible, to successfully treat surgically because of vertebrae overgrowth.[45]

Around 20% of patients with Proteus syndrome have premature death, with deep vein thrombosis or pulmonary embolism being the most common cause.[62] Chemoprophylaxis following orthopaedic procedures is warranted.[63] Pulmonary evaluation to determine presence of underlying pulmonary varicosities or bullous lung disease should also be undertaken before surgical intervention.[64]

DISORDERS CAUSED BY MULTIPLE GENES AND CHROMOSOME ABNORMALITIES

Down Syndrome (Trisomy 21)

Down syndrome is the most common trisomy, and its incidence increases with maternal age. Most patients have three copies of chromosome 21; 4% have a translocation involving this chromosome; and 1% are mosaic (with some normal cells). Many features attributable to Down syndrome are found in a specific chromosomal region (D21S55), including hypotonia and joint hyperlaxity, with abnormalities in the upper cervical spine (atlantoaxial and occipitoatlantal). Patients have relatively short stature, a flat face, and varying degrees of mental retardation. Acetabular dysplasia or hip dislocations occur in 5% of patients aged 2 to 10 years, and slipped capital femoral epiphysis and osteonecrosis often are present.[65] Wide variability in acetabular version occurs, which must be taken into account to effectively reconstruct the hip.[66] Other common characteristics include short, broad hands; patellofemoral instability; flatfoot and hallux valgus; congenital heart defects; and thyroid dysfunction.

A broad variety of radiographic abnormities of the cervical spine are present, but radiographic findings often do not correlate with the symptoms. In addition, a high complication rate associated with cervical spine fusion occurs in Down syndrome. Modern instrumentation techniques can decrease but not eliminate the associated complication rate. For children who want to participate in the Special Olympics and are asymptomatic but have radiographic findings, the most prudent approach is to have these children avoid tumbling activities.[67,68]

Turner Syndrome

Turner syndrome is caused by complete or partial absence of one of the X chromosomes in females; a lack of this chromosome in males is incompatible with life. Clinical features include short stature, webbed neck, low-set ears and hairline, cubitus and genu valgum, Madelung deformity, scoliosis, and a broad, flat chest shaped like a shield. Patients usually experience gonadal dysfunction, which results in absent or incomplete development at puberty, infertility, diabetes, increased weight, and osteoporosis. Life expectancy is normal.[69]

Madelung deformity of the wrist is common in Turner syndrome. Asymptomatic Madelung deformity may be observed.[70] If symptoms develop, initial treatment is rest, bracing treatment, and activity modification. Persistence or progression in skeletally immature patients may warrant epiphyseolysis and interposition fat graft of the region of growth disturbance at the volar-ulnar aspect of the distal radius physis, with or without release of Vicker ligament. There is risk of further injury to the physis and possible greater growth disturbance.[71] As one approaches skeletal maturity, dome osteotomy to correct the multiplanar deformity with or without an ulnar shortening osteotomy is recommended for symptomatic deformities.[72] Wrist arthrodesis is recommended as a salvage procedure for severe pain in the skeletally mature.

Prader-Willi Syndrome

Prader-Willi syndrome (PWS) is caused by a partial deletion of the 15th chromosome involving a group of methylated (imprinted) genes inherited from the father. PWS is characterized by hypotonia, short stature, a failure to thrive in the early years (later followed by an extreme and insatiable appetite often resulting in morbid obesity), hypogonadism, and mild mental retardation. Patients with PWS have complications from surgery secondary to an abnormal physiologic response to hypercapnia and hypoxia, obstructive sleep apnea, thick pulmonary secretions, obesity, prolonged exaggerated response to sedatives, and increased risk for aspiration. Growth hormone therapy is used in this disorder, which improves weight and behavior.[73] The effect of growth hormone therapy on skeletal deformity is unclear, but the results of a 2009 randomized controlled trial suggest that it does not negatively affect the sequelae of spinal deformity.[74]

Scoliosis is most frequently juvenile-onset, affecting anywhere from 40% to 80% of individuals.[75,76] Coronal and sagittal plane deformities are seen in PWS, with an increased incidence of kyphosis associated with obesity.[77,78] Early intervention with serial casting or growing constructs has been attempted in PWS with variable success.[76] The complication rate of growth friendly surgery was higher than in non-PWS cases with a rate of 85% compared with the normal group of 58% to 67%.[79,80] Hip dysplasia has recently been reported to have a higher incidence in PWS (upward of 30%).[81,82] There is also an increased rate of limb malalignment including genu valgum, genu varum, and limb-length difference.[83,84] The extremity manifestations of PWS have not been observed to have a significant impact on activity level and rarely require intervention. There exists an increased risk of fracture secondary to reduced bone density.[85]

CONTRACTURE SYNDROMES

Arthrogryposis Multiplex Congenita

Arthrogryposis multiplex congenita (AMC or amyoplasia) is the most affected syndrome of the arthrogryposis family.[86] AMC is not genetically mediated, but is thought to be related to decreased fetal movement during development.[87,88] All four extremities are involved in 50% to 60% of cases: lower limbs, in 30% to 40%, and upper limbs, in 10% to 15%.

Outcomes appear to be improved if surgery is performed at ages younger than 4 to 6 years, before secondary intra-articular deformity occurs. Up to 25% of affected patients are nonambulatory, and many others are household ambulators. Hip dislocation is common, and treatment is controversial, particularly for bilateral dislocations.[89] Medial approach, open reduction has yielded excellent results, and at least one early attempt at surgical reduction of bilaterally dislocated hips may be worthwhile.[90] Hip flexion contractures exceeding 30° impair ambulation, and soft-tissue releases should be considered for this group.[91] External rotation deformities tend to resolve, but abduction contractures do not, and may benefit from proximal femoral osteotomies, which adduct (varus) and internally rotate the femurs to promote sitting.

Flexion and extension deformities of the knee are common in AMC. During infancy, serial casting may improve knee position. In the hyperextended knee, surgical lengthening (percutaneous or open) of the extensor apparatus may be helpful.[92] For true knee dislocations recalcitrant to nonsurgical interventions, open reduction with quadriceps V-Y plasty and supracondylar extension osteotomies of the femur can be helpful to correct residual deformity. Anterior growth modulation of the distal femur, using plates or transphyseal screws, may be used to correct milder, residual flexion deformities of the knee.[93]

Foot deformities, clubfoot or congenital vertical talus, occur in 80% to 90% of children with AMC.[94] Ponseti casting has demonstrated good results in several studies and should be considered as the first line of treatment.[95] A prolonged course of casting should be expected. Limited posterior ankle release or continued serial casting may be required to achieve dorsiflexion above neutral. Congenital vertical talus generally responds to accepted treatments including reverse-Ponseti casting with limited release and pinning.[96]

Splinting and casting are first-line treatment for hand and wrist deformities, but the recurrence rate is high.[97] Deepening of the first web with thenar release and thumb stabilization may be required for contractures that involve both the thumb-index webspace and the flexor aspect of the thumb.[98] For elbows with extension contractures, 90° of elbow flexion is desired.[99] Distal humeral external rotation osteotomy has been proposed to treat the internal rotation deformity of the humerus.[100] One treatment algorithm for upper extremity deformities is to address elbow contractures with a posterior release and triceps lengthening at approximately 1 year of age, followed by dorsal closing wedge osteotomy of the wrist and thenar release with first web space deepening as needed. Tendon transfers for flexion and distal humerus rotational osteotomies are performed later, at about 6 years of age. Bilateral distal humeral osteotomies should be staged by 3 months to allow for healing and to regain motion.

Complex and rigid spinal deformities develop in approximately one-third of patients with AMC.[101] Bracing treatment and casting may be useful in slowing the progression of moderate deformities (20° to 40°), but cure should not be expected.[102] For severe deformities, a course of gravity halo traction may be considered, and for younger patients, growth friendly constructs are encouraged.[103]

Distal Arthrogryposis/Freeman-Sheldon Syndrome

Distal arthrogryposis is a group of syndromes (**Table 3**) with primarily distal joint contractures (ie, the hands and feet). The three most common forms are DA1 with distal joint involvement and no facial or other organ system involvement; DA2A (Freeman-Sheldon syndrome) with distal joint involvement, but varying proximal joint and facial contractures, small whistling mouth, short stature, scoliosis; and DA2B (Sheldon-Hall syndrome) an intermediate form between DA1 and DA2A. Distal arthrogryposis syndromes are often hereditary. Distal arthrogryposis was originally defined as arthrogryposis with congenital hand and foot involvement.[86] Ten different forms are now identified.[104,105]

TABLE 3

Distal Arthrogryposis (DA) Conditions and Genetics

Type of DA	Condition Name	Associated Gene Mutations
DA1	Classic DA	*TNNI2*, TPM2, MYBPC1, MYH3
DA2A	Freeman-Sheldon syndrome	MYH3
DA2B	Sheldon-Hall syndrome	TNNAS, TNNT2, TPM2, MYH3
DA3	Gordon syndrome (short stature, cleft palate, and ptosis)	PIEZO2
DA4	DA with severe scoliosis	—
DA5	DA with ophthalmoplegia, ptosis, and retinal involvement	*PIEZO2, ECEL1* (for DA5 without ophthalmoplegia)
DA6	DA with sensorineural hearing loss and microcephaly	—
DA7	Trismus-pseudocamptodactyly syndrome	*MYH8*
DA8	Autosomal dominant multiple pterygium syndrome	*MYH3*
DA9	Congenital contractural arachnodactyly/Beals syndrome	*FBN2*
DA10	DA with congential plantar flexion contractures	—

ECEL = neuronal endopeptidase, FBN2 = fibrillin 2, MYBPC1 = myosin binding protein C1, *MYH3* = embryonic myosin heavy chain 3, MYH8 = fetal myosin chain 8, PIEZO2 = piezo-type mechanosensitive ion channel component 2, *TNNI2* = troponin I subunit, *TNNT3* = troponin T subunit, TPM2 = tropomypsin or β-troponin myosin.

Adapted from Hall JG, Kimber E, van Bosse HJP: Genetics and classifications. *J Pediatr Orthop* 2017;37(5):S4-S8.

Associated gene mutations have been identified in genes encoding for sarcomeric muscle proteins, b tropomyosin (*TPM2*), fast troponin I (*TNNI2*), fast troponin T (*TNNT3*), embryonic myosin heavy chain (*MYH3*), and fetal myosin heavy chain (*MYH8*).[87] Management of foot/ankle and hand/wrist deformities follows the same principles outlined for AMC. Clubfeet tend to be highly recalcitrant to casting, but may still achieve partial correction, thus reducing the extent of surgical correction ultimately required. Splinting for hand and wrist deformities is first line of therapy, with surgical intervention required on an *a la carte* basis.

SUMMARY

Orthopaedic-related syndromes are caused by genetic mutations or fetal environmental factors that alter cell behavior, often in a manner that mimics genetic mutation. An understanding of genetic etiology allows the classification of syndromes based on the function of the causative gene product. Each class of syndromes shares common clinical findings, surveillance and medical care requirements, and responses to treatment.

KEY STUDY POINTS

- Knowledge about the genetic cause of a syndrome can explain the phenotype and predict treatment outcomes.
- Syndromes caused by mutations in genes encoding proteins that regulate cell growth can predispose individuals to cancers.
- Syndromes caused by large chromosomal abnormalities such as a trisomy are not inherited.
- Overgrowth conditions can be caused by mosaic (or somatic) mutations.
- Contracture syndromes may be environmental or genetic in disorder, but follow common treatment strategies.

ANNOTATED REFERENCES

1. Pyeritz RE, McKusick VA: The Marfan syndrome: Diagnosis and management. *N Engl J Med* 1979;300(14):772-777.
2. Doman I, Kover F, Illes T, Doczi T: Subluxation of a lumbar vertebra in a patient with Marfan syndrome. Case report. *J Neurosurg* 2001;94(1):154-157.
3. Pearson GD, Devereux R, Loeys B, et al: Report of the National Heart, Lung, and Blood Institute and National Marfan Foundation Working Group on research in Marfan syndrome and related disorders. *Circulation* 2008;118(7):785-791.
4. Sponseller PD, Bhimani M, Solacoff D, Dormans JP: Results of brace treatment of scoliosis in Marfan syndrome. *Spine (Phila Pa 1976)* 2000;25(18):2350-2354.
5. Qiao J, Zhu F, Xu L, et al: Accuracy of pedicle screw placement in patients with Marfan syndrome. *BMC Musculoskelet Disord* 2017;18(1):123.

   CT scanning was performed to analyze accuracy of pedicle screw placement in patients with Marfan syndrome. A total of 976 pedicle screws were evaluated: 924 (94.7%) screws were considered as acceptable, and 52 (5.3%) as unacceptable. Placement of pedicle screws in Marfan syndrome was deemed accurate and safe. Special attention should be paid when screws were placed at the lumbar spine and the concave side of spine deformity to avoid a higher rate of complications. Level of evidence: IV.
6. MacCarrick G, Black JH III, Bowdin S, et al: Loeys-Dietz syndrome: A primer for diagnosis and management. *Genet Med* 2014;16(8):576-587.
7. Malfait F, Francomano C, Byers P, et al: The 2017 international classification of the Ehlers-Danlos syndromes. *Am J Med Genet C Semin Med Genet* 2017;175(1):8-26.

   The International EDS Consortium proposed a revised EDS classification, which recognized 13 subtypes. For each subtypes, they proposed a set of clinical criteria that are suggestive for the diagnosis. Definitive diagnosis of all EDS subtypes, except for the hypermobile type, relies on molecular confirmation with identification of a causative genetic variant or variants. They also revised the clinical criteria for hypermobile EDS to allow for a better distinction from other joint hypermobility disorders. Level of evidence: V.
8. Ericson WBJ, Wolman R: Orthopaedic management of the Ehlers-Danlos syndromes. *Am J Med Genet C Semin Med Genet* 2017;175(1):188-194.

   This is an expert review for orthopaedic management of EDS. Both surgical and nonsurgical recommendations for hypermobile and painful joints are made. Level of evidence: V.
9. Freeman RK, Swegle J, Sise MJ: The surgical complications of Ehlers-Danlos syndrome. *Am Surg* 1996;62(10):869-873.
10. Sillence DO, Senn A, Danks DM: Genetic heterogeneity in osteogenesis imperfecta. *J Med Genet* 1979;16(2):101-116.
11. Van Dijk FS, Pals G, Van Rijn RR, Nikkels PG, Cobben JM: Classification of osteogenesis imperfecta revisited. *Eur J Med Genet* 2010;53(1):1-5.
12. Glorieux FH, Ward LM, Rauch F, Lalic L, Roughley PJ, Travers R: Osteogenesis imperfecta type VI: A form of brittle bone disease with a mineralization defect. *J Bone Miner Res* 2002;17(1):30-38.
13. Plotkin H, Rauch F, Bishop NJ, et al: Pamidronate treatment of severe osteogenesis imperfecta in children under 3 years of age. *J Clin Endocrinol Metab* 2000;85(5):1846-1850.
14. Lv F, Liu Y, Xu X, et al: Zoledronic acid versus alendronate in the treatment of children with osteogenesis imperfecta: A 2-year clinical study. *Endocr Pract* 2018;24(2):179-188.

   A total of 161 patients with osteogenesis imperfecta ranging from 2 to 16 years old were randomized to receive either weekly oral alendronate or a once-yearly infusion of zoledronic acid for 2 years. The primary endpoints were percentage change from baseline in lumbar spine bone mineral density (BMD) and change in Z-scores of lumbar spine BMD.

Once-yearly infusion of zoledronic acid and weekly oral alendronate had similar effects in increasing BMD and reducing bone resorption in children and adolescents with osteogenesis imperfecta. Zoledronic acid was superior to alendronate in reducing the clinical fracture rate. Level of evidence: II.

15. Arponen H, Makitie O, Haukka J, et al: Prevalence and natural course of craniocervical junction anomalies during growth in patients with osteogenesis imperfecta. *J Bone Miner Res* 2012;27(5):1142-1149.
16. Cheung MS, Arponen H, Roughley P, et al: Cranial base abnormalities in osteogenesis imperfecta: Phenotypic and genotypic determinants. *J Bone Miner Res* 2011;26(2):405-413.
17. Klekamp J: Treatment of basilar invagination. *Eur Spine J* 2014;23(8):1656-1665.
18. Benson DR, Donaldson DH, Millar EA: The spine in osteogenesis imperfecta. *J Bone Joint Surg Am* 1978;60(7):925-929.
19. Kocher MS, Shapiro F: Osteogenesis imperfecta. *J Am Acad Orthop Surg* 1998;6(4):225-236.
20. Ferner RE, Gutmann DH: Neurofibromatosis type 1 (NF1): Diagnosis and management. *Handb Clin Neurol* 2013;115:939-955.
21. Abramowicz A, Gos M: Neurofibromin in neurofibromatosis type 1 – Mutations in NF1 gene as a cause of disease. *Dev Period Med* 2014;18(3):297-306.
22. Widemann BC, Salzer WL, Arceci RJ, et al: Phase I trial and pharmacokinetic study of the farnesyltransferase inhibitor tipifarnib in children with refractory solid tumors or neurofibromatosis type I and plexiform neurofibromas. *J Clin Oncol* 2006;24(3):507-516.
23. Widemann BC, Babovic-Vuksanovic D, Dombi E, et al: Phase II trial of pirfenidone in children and young adults with neurofibromatosis type 1 and progressive plexiform neurofibromas. *Pediatr Blood Cancer* 2014;61(9):1598-1602.
24. Korf BR: Statins, bone, and neurofibromatosis type 1. *BMC Med* 2008;6:22.
25. Kolanczyk M, Kühnisch J, Kossler N, et al: Modelling neurofibromatosis type 1 tibial dysplasia and its treatment with lovastatin. *BMC Med* 2008;6:21.
26. de la Croix Ndong J, Makowski AJ, Uppuganti S, et al: Asfotase-α improves bone growth, mineralization and strength in mouse models of neurofibromatosis type-1. *Nat Med* 2014;20(8):904-910.
27. Ghadakzadeh S, Kannu P, Whetstone H, Howard A, Alman BA: β-Catenin modulation in neurofibromatosis type 1 bone repair: Therapeutic implications. *FASEB J* 2016;30(9):3227-3237.

    Using a surgically induced tibial fracture model in conditional knockout Nfl mice, for those treated with a Cre-expressing adenovirus, there was a localized knockdown of Nf1 in the healing fracture, and a subsequent development of a fibrous pseudarthrosis. Consistent with human data, elevated β-catenin levels were found in the murine fracture sites. The murine pseudarthrosis phenotype was also rescued by conditional β-catenin gene inactivation. An upregulation of β-catenin in NF1 causes a shift away from osteoblastic differentiation resulting in a pseudarthrosis in vivo. Level of evidence: I.

28. Feldman DS, Jordan C, Fonseca L: Orthopaedic manifestations of neurofibromatosis type 1. *J Am Acad Orthop Surg* 2010;18(6):346-357.
29. Turra S, Santini S, Cagnoni G, Jacopetti T: Gigantism of the foot: Our experience in seven cases. *J Pediatr Orthop* 1998;18(3):337-345.
30. Cho TJ, Seo JB, Lee HR, Yoo WJ, Chung CY, Choi IH: Biologic characteristics of fibrous hamartoma from congenital pseudarthrosis of the tibia associated with neurofibromatosis type 1. *J Bone Joint Surg Am* 2008;90(12):2735-2744.
31. Stevenson DA, Zhou H, Ashrafi S, et al: Double inactivation of NF1 in tibial pseudarthrosis. *Am J Hum Genet* 2006;79(1):143-148.
32. Senta H, Park H, Bergeron E, et al: Cell responses to bone morphogenetic proteins and peptides derived from them: Biomedical applications and limitations. *Cytokine Growth Factor Rev* 2009;20(3):213-222.
33. Filippi G: The de Lange syndrome. Report of 15 cases. *Clin Genet* 1989;35(5):343-363.
34. Stieber JR, Dormans JP: Manifestations of hereditary multiple exostoses. *J Am Acad Orthop Surg* 2005;13(2):110-120.
35. Philippe C, Porter DE, Emerton ME, Wells DE, Simpson AH, Monaco AP: Mutation screening of the EXT1 and EXT2 genes in patients with hereditary multiple exostoses. *Am J Hum Genet* 1997;61(3):520-528.
36. Shapiro F, Simon S, Glimcher MJ: Hereditary multiple exostoses. Anthropometric, roentgenographic, and clinical aspects. *J Bone Joint Surg Am* 1979;61(6A):815-824.
37. Mermer MJ, Gupta MC, Salamon PB, Benson DR: Thoracic vertebral body exostosis as a cause of myelopathy in a patient with hereditary multiple exostoses. *J Spinal Disord Tech* 2002;15(2):144-148.
38. Voutsinas S, Wynne-Davies R: The infrequency of malignant disease in diaphyseal aclasis and neurofibromatosis. *J Med Genet* 1983;20(5):345-349.
39. Noonan KJ, Feinberg JR, Levenda A, Snead J, Wurtz LD: Natural history of multiple hereditary osteochondromatosis of the lower extremity and ankle. *J Pediatr Orthop* 2002;22(1):120-124.
40. Unni KK: Chondrosarcoma (primary, secondary, dedifferentiated, and clear-cell), in Unni KK, Dahlin DC, eds: *Dahlin's Bone Tumors: General Aspects and Data on 11,087 Cases*, ed 5. Philadelphia, PA, Lippincott-Raven, 1996, pp 11-23.
41. Muramatsu K, Kawakami Y, Tani Y, Taguchi T: Malignant transformation of multiple enchondromas in the hand: Case report. *J Hand Surg Am* 2011;36(2):304-307.
42. Schwartz HS, Zimmerman NB, Simon MA, Wroble RR, Millar EA, Bonfiglio M: The malignant potential of enchondromatosis. *J Bone Joint Surg Am* 1987;69(2):269-274.
43. Sun TC, Swee RG, Shives TC, Unni KK: Chondrosarcoma in Maffucci's syndrome. *J Bone Joint Surg Am* 1985;67(8):1214-1219.

44. Stevens PM, Klatt JB: Guided growth for pathological physes: Radiographic improvement during realignment. *J Pediatr Orthop* 2008;28(6):632-639.

45. Choi ML, Wey PD, Borah GL: Pediatric peripheral neuropathy in Proteus syndrome. *Ann Plast Surg* 1998;40(5):528-532.

46. Verdegaal SH, Bovée JV, Pansuriya TC, et al: Incidence, predictive factors, and prognosis of chondrosarcoma in patients with Ollier disease and Maffucci syndrome: An international multicenter study of 161 patients. *Oncologist* 2011;16(12):1771-1779.

47. Yamashita A, Morioka M, Kishi H, et al: Statin treatment rescues FGFR3 skeletal dysplasia phenotypes. *Nature* 2014;513(7519):507-511.

48. Danon M, Robboy SJ, Kim S, Scully R, Crawford JD: Cushing syndrome, sexual precocity, and polyostotic fibrous dysplasia (Albright syndrome) in infancy. *J Pediatr* 1975;87(6 pt 1):917-921.

49. Dorfman HD: Fibroosseous lesions, in Dorfman HD, Czerniak B, eds: *Bone Tumors*. St. Louis, MO, Mosby, 1998, pp 441-491.

50. Gaiddon C, Boutillier AL, Monnier D, Mercken L, Loeffler JP: Genomic effects of the putative oncogene G α s. Chronic transcriptional activation of the c-fos proto-oncogene in endocrine cells. *J Biol Chem* 1994;269(36):22663-22671.

51. Candeliere GA, Glorieux FH, Prud'homme J, St-Arnaud R: Increased expression of the c-fos proto-oncogene in bone from patients with fibrous dysplasia. *N Engl J Med* 1995;332(23):1546-1551.

52. Weisstein JS, Majeska RJ, Klein MJ, Einhorn TA: Detection of c-fos expression in benign and malignant musculoskeletal lesions. *J Orthop Res* 2001;19(3):339-345.

53. Mirra JM, Gold RH, Picci P: Osseous tumors of intramedullary origin, in Mirra JM, Picci P, Gold RH, eds: *Bone Tumors: Clinical, Radiologic, and Pathologic Correlations*. Philadelphia, PA, Lea & Febiger, 1989, pp 143-438.

54. Lee PA, Van Dop C, Migeon CJ: McCune-Albright syndrome. Long-term follow-up. *J Am Med Assoc* 1986;256(21):2980-2984.

55. Kumar R, Madewell JE, Lindell MM, Swischuk LE: Fibrous lesions of bones. *Radiographics* 1990;10(2):237-256.

56. Enneking WF, Gearen PF: Fibrous dysplasia of the femoral neck. Treatment by cortical bone-grafting. *J Bone Joint Surg Am* 1986;68(9):1415-1422.

57. Parekh SG, Donthineni-Rao R, Ricchetti E, Lackman RD: Fibrous dysplasia. *J Am Acad Orthop Surg* 2004;12(5):305-313.

58. Lane JM, Khan SN, O'Connor WJ, et al: Bisphosphonate therapy in fibrous dysplasia. *Clin Orthop Relat Res* 2001;382:6-12.

59. Weinstein RS: Long-term aminobisphosphonate treatment of fibrous dysplasia: Spectacular increase in bone density. *J Bone Miner Res* 1997;12(8):1314-1315.

60. Lindhurst MJ, Sapp JC, Teer JK, et al: A mosaic activating mutation in AKT1 associated with the Proteus syndrome. *N Engl J Med* 2011;365(7):611-619.

61. Azouz EM, Costa T, Fitch N: Radiologic findings in the Proteus syndrome. *Pediatr Radiol* 1987;17(6):481-485.

62. Slavotinek AM, Vacha SJ, Peters KF, Biesecker LG: Sudden death caused by pulmonary thromboembolism in Proteus syndrome. *Clin Genet* 2000;58(5):386-389.

63. Biesecker LG, Happle R, Mulliken JB, et al: Proteus syndrome: Diagnostic criteria, differential diagnosis, and patient evaluation. *Am J Med Genet* 1999;84(5):389-395.

64. Lim GY, Kim OH, Kim HW, et al: Pulmonary manifestations in Proteus syndrome: Pulmonary varicosities and bullous lung disease. *Am J Med Genet A* 2011;155(4): 865-869.

65. Talmac MA, Kadhim M, Rogers KJ, Holmes L Jr, Miller F: Legg-Calvé-Perthes disease in children with Down syndrome. *Acta Orthop Traumatol Turc* 2013;47(5):334-338.

66. Abousamra O, Bayhan IA, Rogers KJ, Miller F: Hip instability in Down syndrome: A focus on acetabular retroversion. *J Pediatr Orthop* 2016;36(5):499-504.

    Pelvic CT or MRI scans were evaluated in 10 patients with 13 unstable hips and 13 patients with 26 stable hips in children with Down syndrome. Acetabular anteversion was compared between groups. Extrusion index, Tonnis, Sharp, lateral center edge, and neck shaft angles were measured. Presence of Shenton line disruption, crossover, and posterior wall signs were recorded. A wide range of acetabular anteversion measurements were identified. With proper preoperative imaging, good results with a low complication rate can be expected over the intermediate term after hip reconstruction. Level of evidence: III.

67. Caird MS, Wills BP, Dormans JP: Down syndrome in children: The role of the orthopaedic surgeon. *J Am Acad Orthop Surg* 2006;14(11):610-619.

68. McKay SD, Al-Omari A, Tomlinson LA, Dormans JP: Review of cervical spine anomalies in genetic syndromes. *Spine (Phila Pa 1976)* 2012;37(5):E269-E277.

69. Levitsky LL, Luria AH, Hayes FJ, Lin AE: Turner syndrome: Update on biology and management across the life span. *Curr Opin Endocrinol Diabetes Obes* 2015;22(1):65-72.

70. Tauber M, Lounis N, Coulet J, Baunin C, Cahuzac JP, Rochiccioli P: Wrist anomalies in Turner syndrome compared with Leri-Weill dyschondrosteosis: A new feature in Turner syndrome. *Eur J Pediatr* 2004;163(8):475-481.

71. Vickers D, Nielsen G: Madelung deformity: Surgical prophylaxis (physiolysis) during the late growth period by resection of the dyschondrosteosis lesion. *J Hand Surg Br* 1992;17(4):401-407.

72. Harley BJ, Brown C, Cummings K, Carter PR, Ezaki M: Volar ligament release and distal radius dome osteotomy for correction of Madelung's deformity. *J Hand Surg Am* 2006;31(9):1499-1506.

73. Festen DA, de Lind van Wijngaarden R, van Eekelen M, et al: Randomized controlled GH trial: Effects on anthropometry, body composition and body proportions in a large group of children with Prader-Willi syndrome. *Clin Endocrinol (Oxf)* 2008;69(3):443-451.

74. de Lind van Wijngaarden RF, de Klerk LW, Festen DA, Duivenvoorden HJ, Otten BJ, Hokken-Koelega AC: Randomized controlled trial to investigate the effects of growth hormone treatment on scoliosis in children with Prader-Willi syndrome. *J Clin Endocrinol Metab* 2009;94(4):1274-1280.

75. Gurd AR, Thompson TR: Scoliosis in Prader-Willi syndrome. *J Pediatr Orthop* 1981;1(3):317-320.

76. Nakamura Y, Murakami N, Iida T, et al: The characteristics of scoliosis in Prader-Willi syndrome (PWS): Analysis of 58 scoliosis patients with PWS. *J Orthop Sci* 2015;20(1):17-22.

77. Weiss HR, Goodall D: Scoliosis in patients with Prader Willi syndrome – Comparisons of conservative and surgical treatment. *Scoliosis* 2009;4:10.

78. Odent T, Accadbled F, Koureas G, et al: Scoliosis in patients with Prader-Willi syndrome. *Pediatrics* 2008;122(2):e499-e503.

79. Bess S, Akbarnia BA, Thompson GH, et al: Complications of growing-rod treatment for early-onset scoliosis: Analysis of one hundred and forty patients. *J Bone Joint Surg Am* 2010;92(15):2533-2543.

80. Lucas G, Bollini G, Jouve JL, et al: Complications in pediatric spine surgery using the vertical expandable prosthetic titanium rib: The French experience. *Spine (Phila Pa 1976)* 2013;38(25):E1589-E1599.

81. Trizno AA, Jones AS, Carry PM, Georgopoulos G: The prevalence and treatment of hip dysplasia in Prader-Willi syndrome (PWS). *J Pediatr Orthop* 2018;38(3):e151-e156.

    This is a retrospective review of 90 patients with PWS. Hip dysplasia was identified in 30%. A higher prevalence of hip dysplasia was seen in patients with PWS than previously documented. The age at which hip dysplasia develops was not determined; therefore ultrasound screening for all infants with PWS and subsequent radiographic studies at 1, 2, 5, 10, and 15 years of age are recommended. Level of evidence: IV.

82. West LA, Ballock RT: High incidence of hip dysplasia but not slipped capital femoral epiphysis in patients with Prader-Willi syndrome. *J Pediatr Orthop* 2004;24(5):565-567.

83. Torrado M, Foncuberta ME, Perez MF, et al: Change in prevalence of congenital defects in children with Prader-Willi syndrome. *Pediatrics* 2013;131(2):e544-e549.

84. Kroonen LT, Herman M, Pizzutillo PD, Macewen GD: Prader-Willi syndrome: Clinical concerns for the orthopaedic surgeon. *J Pediatr Orthop* 2006;26(5):673-679.

85. Goldstone AP: Prader-Willi syndrome: Advances in genetics, pathophysiology and treatment. *Trends Endocrinol Metab* 2004;15(1):12-20.

86. Hall JG: Arthrogryposis multiplex congenita: Etiology, genetics, classification, diagnostic approach, and general aspects. *J Pediatr Orthop B* 1997;6(3):159-166.

87. Bamshad M, Van Heest AE, Pleasure D: Arthrogryposis: A review and update. *J Bone Joint Surg Am* 2009;91(suppl 4):40-46.

88. Kalampokas E, Kalampokas T, Sofoudis C, Deligeoroglou E, Botsis D: Diagnosing arthrogryposis multiplex congenita: A review. *ISRN Obstet Gynecol* 2012;2012:264918.

89. Bradish C: The hip in arthrogryposis. *J Child Orthop* 2015;9(6):459-463.

90. Staheli LT, Chew DE, Elliott JS, Mosca VS: Management of hip dislocations in children with arthrogryposis. *J Pediatr Orthop* 1987;7(6):681-685.

91. Hoffer MM, Swank S, Eastman F, Clark D, Teitge R: Ambulation in severe arthrogryposis. *J Pediatr Orthop* 1983;3(3):293-296.

92. Roy DR, Crawford AH: Percutaneous quadriceps recession: A technique for management of congenital hyperextension deformities of the knee in the neonate. *J Pediatr Orthop* 1989;9(6):717-719.

93. Bouchard M: Guided growth: Novel applications in the hip, knee, and ankle. *J Pediatr Orthop* 2017;37(suppl 2):S32-S36.

    This article reviews applications of screw hemiepiphysiodesis for coronal and sagittal plane deformities in the lower extremity. Indications, technical pearls, and pitfalls are discussed. Level of evidence: V.

94. van Bosse HJP, Pontén E, Wada A, et al: Treatment of the lower extremity contracture/deformities. *J Pediatr Orthop* 2017;37(suppl 1):S16-S23.

    This is a review article the discusses treatment strategies for lower extremity deformity in arthrogryposis, presented in September 2014 in Saint Petersburg, Russia at the second international symposium on arthrogryposis. Level of evidence: V.

95. Kowalczyk B, Lejman T: Short-term experience with Ponseti casting and the Achilles tenotomy method for clubfeet treatment in arthrogryposis multiplex congenita. *J Child Orthop* 2008;2(5):365-371.

96. Dobbs MB, Purcell DB, Nunley R, Morcuende JA: Early results of a new method of treatment for idiopathic congenital vertical talus. Surgical technique. *J Bone Joint Surg Am* 2007;89(suppl 2, pt 1):111-121.

97. Smith DW, Drennan JC: Arthrogryposis wrist deformities: Results of infantile serial casting. *J Pediatr Orthop* 2002;22(1):44-47.

98. Ezaki M, Oishi SN: Index rotation flap for palmar thumb release in arthrogryposis. *Tech Hand Up Extrem Surg* 2010;14(1):38-40.

99. Gogola GR, Ezaki M, Oishi SN, Gharbaoui I, Bennett JB: Long head of the triceps muscle transfer for active elbow flexion in arthrogryposis. *Tech Hand Up Extrem Surg* 2010;14(2):121-124.

100. Wall LB, Calhoun V, Roberts S, Goldfarb CA: Distal humerus external rotation osteotomy for hand position in arthrogryposis. *J Hand Surg Am* 2017;42(6):473.e1-473.e7.

    Nine patients with amyoplasia were treated with distal humeral external rotation osteotomy (DHO). All patients had an improved resting posture of the upper extremity after DHO surgery. DHO was an effective procedure for correcting the internal rotation position of the upper extremity in arthrogryposis, and the surgery improved hand opposition with minimal complications. There were perceived improved function by families and high postoperative Pediatric Outcomes Data Collection Instrument Happiness scores. Level of evidence: IV.

101. Fassier A, Wicart P, Dubousset J, Seringe R: Arthrogryposis multiplex congenita. Long-term follow-up from birth until skeletal maturity. *J Child Orthop* 2009;3(5):383-390.

102. Komolkin I, Ulrich EV, Agranovich OE, van Bosse HJP: Treatment of scoliosis associated with arthrogryposis multiplex congenita. *J Pediatr Orthop* 2017;37(suppl 1):S24-S26.

This article reviews treatment of scoliosis in children with arthrogryposis, including casting, bracing, expandable implant surgery, and spinal fusion. Level of evidence: V.

103. Astur N, Flynn JM, Flynn JM, et al: The efficacy of rib-based distraction with VEPTR in the treatment of early-onset scoliosis in patients with arthrogryposis. *J Pediatr Orthop* 2014;34(1):8-13.

104. Bamshad M, Jorde LB, Carey JC: A revised and extended classification of the distal arthrogryposes. *Am J Med Genet* 1996;65(4):277-281.

105. Stevenson DA, Swoboda KJ, Sanders RK, Bamshad M: A new distal arthrogryposis syndrome characterized by plantar flexion contractures. *Am J Med Genet A* 2006;140(24):2797-2801.

CHAPTER 10

Medical Therapy in Pediatric Orthopaedics

ANDREW W. HOWARD, MD, MSc, FRCSC • STEPHANIE N. MOORE, BS
JONATHAN G. SCHOENECKER, MD, PhD

ABSTRACT

The need for medical therapy in children with orthopaedic conditions is limited typically to analgesia, antibiotics, and medications that are designed to optimize bone integrity. It is helpful to have a broad overview of these therapies, including specific pathologic conditions in which these therapies are used, the mechanisms of action, and adverse effects.

Keywords: analgesics; antibiotic; antibiotic resistance; diphosphonate; pain relief

INTRODUCTION

Pediatric orthopaedic surgeons manage a variety of conditions, including traumatic injuries, developmental and genetic skeletal manifestations, and musculoskeletal infections. Four overarching categories of therapeutics are commonly prescribed for this wide range of conditions: antibiotics targeting infection, analgesics targeting traumatic and postoperative pain, therapeutics targeting degenerative phenotypes, and therapies aimed at enhancing tissue regeneration. Although the management of traumatic injuries and musculoskeletal infections is common in orthopaedics as a whole, the pediatric orthopaedic specialty also regularly manages premature skeletal degeneration from pathologic causes (such as osteogenesis imperfecta, cerebral palsy, or Duchenne muscular dystrophy) and environmental causes (such as diet, obesity, and vitamin D deficiency). Numerous pharmacologic therapies are available for limiting skeletal degeneration, but no therapies have been approved by the FDA to improve musculoskeletal regeneration. As such, substantial activity is ongoing in both the development of novel therapeutics and the off-label use of currently approved therapeutics, although the latter must be prescribed with great caution. A broad overview of the common therapeutics used in pediatric orthopaedics to treat trauma-induced or postoperative pain, musculoskeletal degeneration, and infections is provided.

ANALGESIA

Principles of Acute Pain Relief

For the management of acute pain, the ladder concept espoused by the World Health Organization in 1986 (that was initially related to cancer pain) still applies.[1] This approach says that if pharmacologic agents are needed to manage pain, it is appropriate to start with simple analgesics (acetaminophen or ibuprofen) and progress to an opioid if pain is severe. The role of opioid use in chronic pain is being increasingly questioned because of its limited clinical effectiveness and the severe secondary problems for both patients and society associated with chronic opioid use.[2] The recent evidence regarding the pharmacologic management of acute pain in children's orthopaedics is discussed. Typically, acute pain includes pain from fractures and postoperative pain.

Dr. Schoenecker or an immediate family member has received research or institutional support from Ionis pharmaceuticals. Neither of the following authors nor any immediate family member has received anything of value from or has stock or stock options held in a commercial company or institution related directly or indirectly to the subject of this chapter: Dr. Howard and Ms. Moore.

This chapter is reprinted from Howard AW, Moore, SN, Schoenecker JG: Medical therapy in pediatric orthopaedics, in Martus JE, ed: Orthopaedic Knowledge Update®: Pediatrics, ed 5. Rosemont, IL, American Academy of Orthopaedic Surgeons, 2016, pp 107-119.

Pain Relief for Fractures

Multiple recent randomized controlled trials (RCTs) are available to guide the selection of analgesics to treat fracture pain in the emergency department. For nondisplaced fractures, all recent randomized trials indicate that ibuprofen is the preferred agent rather than morphine, codeine, acetaminophen, or codeine plus acetaminophen.[3-5] Ibuprofen provided equal or better analgesia compared with the other agents and had a better adverse event profile and better patient and parent satisfaction.

In displaced fractures requiring emergency department reduction, equal effectiveness was reported for fentanyl administered intranasally compared with intravenous morphine.[6,7] A Cochrane review confirmed this finding for nonfracture pain as well.[8]

Postoperative Pain Relief

The American Society of Anesthesiologists produces and updates practice guidelines that combine high-level scientific evidence with opinions from the society or experts when high-level evidence is lacking.[9] For pediatric postoperative pain, the guidelines emphasize multimodal approaches, a reduction of anxiety and emotional distress, and proactive and aggressive pain management based on the concern that pediatric postoperative pain has traditionally been undertreated.[9]

Combinations of nonopioid analgesics are the rational starting point for postoperative pain management. A meta-analysis of three RCTs involving 1,647 adult patients with wisdom tooth extraction (a common model for moderate pain) showed that a combination of ibuprofen and paracetamol was superior to either agent used alone.[10]

Postoperative pain that is more severe often is treated with an opioid in addition to simple analgesics. As with many common practices in medicine, the level of evidence supporting this practice is low. A 2014 Cochrane systematic review examined 10 RCTs that evaluated nalbuphine (an opioid) for postoperative pain management in children. Interestingly, five trials compared nalbuphine with a placebo, but nalbuphine was not superior to placebo or other comparator opioid medications based on the trials available.[11] The absence of evidence of effectiveness, however, should not be mistaken as evidence of no effectiveness. It would be difficult to design a proper placebo-controlled trial of opioid use for severe pain.

Patient-controlled analgesia is a means of administering a postoperative intravenous opioid with an automatic pump that responds to patient demand but limits total dosing. A 2015 Cochrane review of RCTs found that in adults, pain scores were better, opioid use was a little higher, and patient satisfaction was higher with patient-controlled analgesia compared with the conventional administration of opioid medications.[12] In pediatric patients, it is common to use a background infusion in addition to the on-demand analgesia; a recent systematic review found such infusions to be equally safe and effective.[13]

Adjunctive medications given intraoperatively can reduce postoperative pain and postoperative opioid requirements. In a systematic review of 11 RCTs involving 742 children, clonidine, an α-agonist, was found to be beneficial in reducing postoperative pain.[14] More recently, in a review of 14 RCTs involving 1,463 children, dexmedetomidine was shown to be effective in reducing postanesthesia care unit (PACU) pain scores and opioid use.[15] A second systematic review of 20 RCTs linked reduced PACU pain to a reduction in emergence agitation when dexmedetomidine was used as an adjunct to pediatric anesthesia.[16] Dexmedetomidine is a highly selective agonist of α-2 receptors that has a favorable profile in children regarding anxiolysis, analgesia, sympatholysis, and anesthetic-sparing effect with minimal respiratory depression.[17] Ketamine also can be used as an adjunct to general anesthesia; a systematic review of 35 pediatric RCTs showed that ketamine produced a reduction in PACU pain scores but did not have an opioid-sparing effect.[18]

Epidural, caudal, or regional anesthetics are commonly used to improve postoperative pain management and reduce opioid requirements in children's orthopaedics. According to a meta-analysis of four RCTs, epidural anesthesia was superior to patient-controlled morphine for pain relief after scoliosis surgery.[19] Evidence is less conclusive for other types of surgery. A comprehensive systematic review of regional blocks in pediatrics found six trials for an upper extremity, one trial for a hip, and five trials for a lower extremity and concluded that the literature supported the use of blocks, but the studies had low methodologic quality.[20]

Epidural, caudal, and regional blocks can be potentiated by adding agents to the local anesthetic. One meta-analysis compared neostigmine with clonidine and tramadol as adjuncts to a single-shot caudal anesthetic and found that neostigmine provided the greatest increase (8 hours) in the duration of effective analgesia.[21] A similar 8-hour increase in the duration of analgesia was noted in a 2014 meta-analysis of six pediatric RCTs that evaluated dexmedetomidine as an adjunct to caudal anesthetic.[22]

A delay in the diagnosis of compartment syndrome is an ongoing concern with epidural or regional anesthesia. A 2009 review article evaluated all published cases (pediatric and adult) of compartment syndrome in the presence of regional anesthesia and concluded that the classic signs of compartment syndrome were present in 32 of 35 patients.[23] Although the authors determined that no conclusive evidence linked regional anesthesia to diagnostic delay, the important message is that a high index of clinical suspicion and ongoing assessment must apply. This observation is particularly true for children because invasive compartment pressure monitoring may not be indicated and may be less reliable.

Opioid Dependence and Withdrawal

Children can manifest withdrawal symptoms from the abrupt cessation of an opioid after as few as 5 to 7 days. Withdrawal symptoms can include anxiety, agitation, insomnia, and tremors and often are missed or misinterpreted in pediatric patients. Patients who have been in intensive care units for prolonged periods are most at risk because of both pain and procedural sedation. Current guidelines suggest that after 14 days or more of opioid use, children should be weaned with a gradually decreasing dose, and those who have been given an opioid for 7 to 14 days should be considered for weaning and monitored for withdrawal symptoms. Abrupt discontinuation of opioid use is generally well tolerated by children who have received such medication for less than 7 days.[24]

OSTEOPOROSIS

Calcium and Phosphate

Calcium and phosphorus, in the form of phosphate, are essential elements in many biologic processes. They are not only required for proper cellular function and signaling but also combine to make biologic crystals, most notably, hydroxyapatite, which is found in bone (**Figure 1**). Because of their essential nature, their anatomic distribution is tightly regulated, with 10,000 times more calcium and phosphate circulating in the extracellular space compared with the intracellular microenvironment. This ideal biologic gradient provides excess calcium and phosphate for cellular function; however, calcium and phosphate are at their saturation points when circulating in plasma (**Figure 2**). Although this is ideal for maintaining bone integrity, calcium and phosphate can aggregate in soft tissues, such as muscle, skin, and blood vessels. The fact that most soft tissues are free of calcium phosphate aggregates indicates that specialized biologic mechanisms are in place to prevent aberrant aggregation. Pyrophosphate directly inhibits calcium and phosphate aggregation, thus preventing in vivo mineralization. Circulating levels of pyrophosphate are maintained by pyrophosphate pumps, which, in turn, provide the frontline defense against soft-tissue calcification[25] (**Figure 2**). Thus, calcium, phosphate, and pyrophosphate homeostasis is critical for maintaining bone integrity and cellular function while also preventing soft-tissue calcification.

It follows that genetic mutations to elements of the pyrophosphate pump are considered the potential underlying cause of soft-tissue calcification disorders, such as pseudoxanthoma elasticum and generalized arterial calcification of infancy.[26] More commonly, pediatric orthopaedic surgeons are tasked with addressing deficiencies or disorders of calcium and/or phosphate that result in osteoporosis. Childhood osteoporosis is divided into primary and secondary causes. Osteogenesis imperfecta represents the prototypical primary osteoporosis of childhood. Secondary pediatric osteoporosis, incited by underlying diseases and/or their treatment, can be placed into two broad categories: glucocorticoid-treated diseases and disorders that compromise normal weight bearing and mobility.

First-line measures to optimize pediatric osteoporosis can be placed into three main categories: improve nutrition, increase physical activity, and treat the underlying condition and associated comorbidities.[27] The most well-described nutritional factors for pediatric bone health are vitamin D and calcium (**Figure 1**). However, several other nutrients also play a role in bone metabolism, including protein; potassium; magnesium; copper; iron; fluoride; zinc; and vitamin A, C, and K supplementation. Diphosphonates are synthetic analogues of pyrophosphate and are the most extensively published agents for treating childhood osteoporosis in the United States,[28] although their use remains off-label in many other countries.

Vitamin D

Vitamin D, a fat-soluble hormone that is synthesized and metabolized by all mammals, is a critical component of calcium homeostasis and, as a result, has a substantial effect on bone quality and mineralization (**Figure 1**). Vitamin D is first synthesized in the skin as a provitamin, 7-dehydrocholesterol, where subsequent exposure to sunlight converts 7-dehydrocholesterol to vitamin D_3 (cholecalciferol). Vitamin D also can be obtained from dietary supplementation, where it is absorbed from the small intestine and circulated into the blood. Whether from endogenous or dietary sources, all circulating vitamin D requires two successive modifications within the liver and kidneys to become the biologically active form, calcitriol [1,25$(OH)_2$D]. Although the primary function of vitamin D is regulation of calcium homeostasis, it is now well understood that vitamin D also plays important roles in multiple components of the musculoskeletal system. Specifically, vitamin D stimulates the intestinal absorption of calcium, which, in turn, indirectly promotes bone mineralization. Conversely, vitamin D also has been demonstrated to directly regulate the mobilization of calcium from bone back into circulation. In addition to effects on the skeletal system, vitamin D affects the function of skeletal muscle.[27,29,30]

Severe vitamin D deficiency causes rickets and/or hypocalcemia in infants and children. The clinical

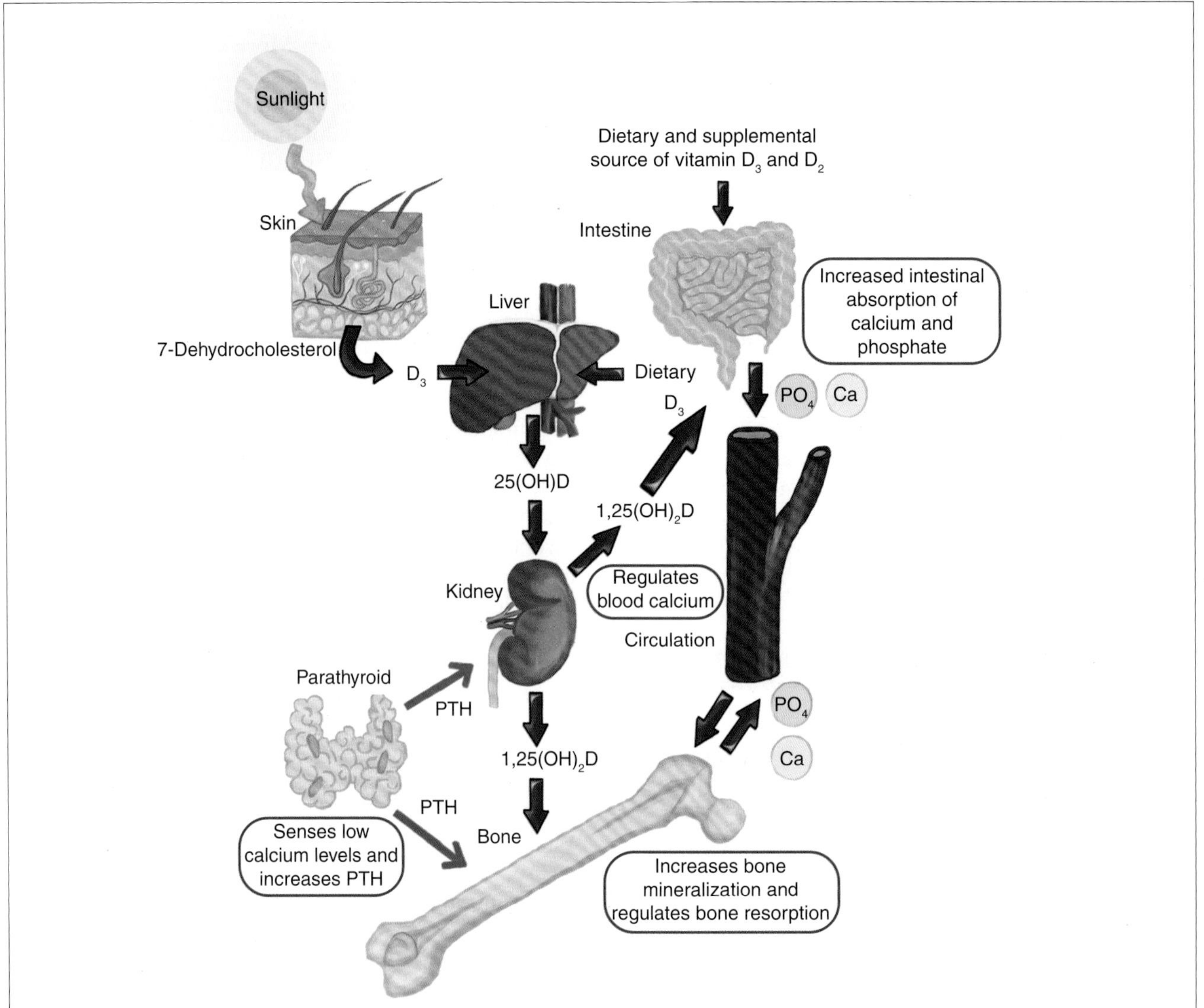

FIGURE 1 Illustration of calcium, phosphate, and vitamin D homeostasis. The classic pathway begins with either endogenous, dietary, or supplemental sources of vitamin D_3. Following metabolism by the liver to produce 25-hydroxyvitamin D [25(OH) D], the renal system converts 25(OH)D to the active form of vitamin D, calcitriol [$1,25(OH)_2D$], which circulates throughout the body in the picomolar range. $1,25(OH)_2D$ acts both on bone and the intestinal system to regulate circulating levels of calcium and phosphate. Because bone contains the body's primary reserve of calcium (Ca) and phosphate (PO_4), in the form of hydroxyapatite, resorption of bone via $1,25(OH)_2D$ signaling through osteoblasts and osteoclasts serves as a critical regulatory mechanism for circulating calcium and phosphate levels. In addition, $1,25(OH)_2D$ acts on the intestinal system to increase dietary absorption of calcium and phosphate by regulating both passive and active ion transport through the intestinal epithelium. Together, this system tightly regulates circulating calcium and phosphate levels, thereby allowing for proper intracellular signaling, muscle cell contraction, nerve cell activity, and bone and teeth health. D_2 = vitamin D_2 (ergocalciferol), D_3 = vitamin D_3 (cholecalciferol), PTH = pituitary hormone

consequences of mild vitamin D deficiency are less well established. However, chronically low vitamin D levels are associated with the development of low bone mineral density and other measures of reduced bone health, even in the absence of rickets. Vitamin D deficiency is common in infants who are dark skinned and exclusively breastfed beyond ages 3 to 6 months.[27] More commonly, the pediatric orthopaedic surgeon should be aware of vitamin D deficiency when managing fracture repair, osteotomies, or fusion. These populations include children with chronic illnesses, on vegetarian or unusual diets, who are dark skinned, who use anticonvulsant or antiretroviral medications, or with malabsorptive conditions. Additional risk factors include residence at higher latitudes, the winter season, and other causes of low sun exposure.[27] Vitamin D deficiency in children in

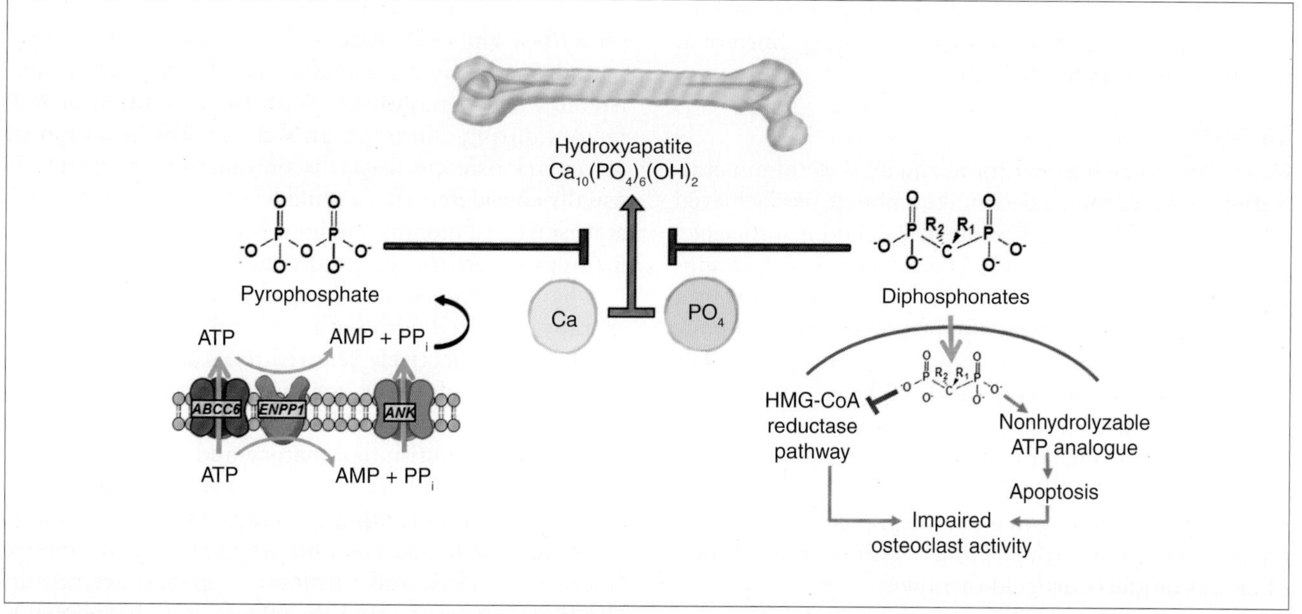

FIGURE 2 Illustration of pyrophosphate (PP_i) and diphosphonate mechanisms of regulating mineralization. Pyrophosphate is a well-described antimineralization molecule that, as early as the 1930s, was shown to inhibit calcium (Ca) crystal buildup when used in small amounts as a water softener. Since that time, substantial research has been conducted to identify the biologic source and roles of pyrophosphate, such that pyrophosphate prevents calcification in soft tissues such as the skin, kidney, and smooth muscles while regulating bone mineralization. Pyrophosphate is regulated in circulation by a group of proteins found primarily within the liver and referred to as the pyrophosphate pump. ATP-binding cassette C subfamily, member 6 (ABCC6) exports ATP from inside the cell to the extracellular space where the enzyme ENPPI cleaves ATP to produce pyrophosphate and AMP (adenosine monophosphate). In addition to extracellular conversion, pyrophosphate also can be produced from ATP intracellularly and exported to the extracellular space by the transporter ANK (ANKH inorganic pyrophosphate transport regulator). Together, this system and enzymes that hydrolyze pyrophosphate to inorganic phosphate tightly regulate circulating pyrophosphate levels, which are critical for proper bone and teeth mineralization. Diphosphonates are nonhydrolyzable analogues of pyrophosphate. As such, they possess the same antimineralization properties as pyrophosphate but cannot be removed from circulation by using hydrolyzing enzymes. Therefore, the half-lives of diphosphonates are long, at times being present in the body for years after their initial administration. In addition to their antimineralization properties, diphosphonates also impair osteoclast activity by inhibiting the HMG-CoA reductase pathway and/or becoming intercalated into DNA as an ATP analogue, thereby inducing cellular apoptosis. Because of their effects on osteoclast activity, the predominant clinical application of diphosphonates has been concentrated on their antibone resorptive properties.

the United States and several other developed nations has been reported with increasing frequency since the mid 1980s.[29] According to large population-based studies, the overall prevalence of vitamin D deficiency or insufficiency in children in the United States is approximately 15%.[31]

Because of improved analytic methods for measuring vitamin D and more comprehensive data collection, low circulating levels of vitamin D and the reemergence of vitamin D–dependent rickets are common clinical findings. The level of calcifediol, also known as 25-hydroxyvitamin D [25(OH)D], is the best indicator of vitamin D status and stores because it is the main circulating form of vitamin D and has a half-life of 2 to 3 weeks. In contrast, $1,25(OH)_2D$ has a much shorter half-life (4 hours), circulates in much lower concentrations than 25(OH)D, and is susceptible to fluctuations induced by the pituitary hormone in response to subtle changes in calcium levels. The optimal serum 25(OH) D level remains controversial, and no clinical consensus exists for optimal vitamin D intake levels for children and infants. However, a minimum 25(OH)D level of 50 nmol/L (20 ng/mL) is recommended in youth through diet and/or supplementation. As such, the American Academy of Pediatrics recently recommended a vitamin D dietary allowance of 400 IU or 10 µg daily from the time of infancy through adolescence.[30] The initial basis for selecting this dose was from a well-established source of vitamin D supplementation, cod liver oil, in which 10 µg represents the amount of vitamin D found in 1 teaspoon, which had long been considered safe and effective at preventing rickets.[29] Beyond the time of adolescence and skeletal development, the recommendations for optimal vitamin D levels are less precise, resulting in reports that recommend daily vitamin D intake ranging from 200 to 4,000 IU/d. Therapeutic adverse effects and adverse consequences of vitamin D are rare and include toxicity associated with increased intestinal calcium and phosphate absorption; hypercalcemia and/or hyperphosphatemia; and suppression of the pituitary hormone, which results in renal pathology.

Calcium

Calcium is a key nutrient for adequate skeletal mineralization, with recommended intake amounts best achieved through a healthy diet. Pathologic calcium insufficiency is less common than vitamin D deficiency. Calcium supplementation in childhood was recently investigated by a meta-analysis, but it showed only a small effect on bone mineral density that is unlikely to alter fracture risk.[30] The Institute of Medicine recommends 700 mg/d for children aged 1 to 3 years, 1,000 mg/d for children aged 4 to 8 years, and 1,300 mg/d for children and adolescents aged 9 to 18 years.[30] Higher daily supplementation may be required for children with malabsorption or those taking medications that impair calcium retention or absorption (diuretics or glucocorticoid therapy).

Diphosphonates

Diphosphonates are a powerful family of pharmaceuticals that have been used by clinicians for more than 40 years to prevent osteoporosis.[28] These stable forms of pyrophosphate freely pass into cells and act as effective inhibitors of the HMG-CoA (3-hydroxy-3-methyl-glutaryl-coenzyme A) reductase pathway (**Figure 2**). In addition, diphosphonates induce osteoclast apoptosis when they are metabolized into nonhydrolyzable adenosine triphosphate (ATP) analogues, which, following incorporation into replicating DNA, accumulate in cells and induce apoptosis (**Figure 2**). Diphosphonates have pleiotropic effects on cellular function,[31] most notably attenuating osteoclast activity and reducing the ability to resorb bone. However, the industrial use of diphosphonates to protect against aberrant mineralization predates their use to preserve bone by at least a century. Diphosphonates were first used to soften public water supplies in the 1800s, thereby preventing the calcification of pipes. In addition, the first clinical studies regarding diphosphonates and their uses in vivo in the 1960s also focused on their ability to prevent calcium and phosphate aggregation. Despite the well-documented antimineralization properties of diphosphonates, their predominant clinical application has instead been concentrated on their antibone resorptive properties.

Most studies that describe the effects of diphosphonate therapy in children are observational preadministration and postadministration reports; relatively few controlled studies of diphosphonate therapy in children exist, and even fewer studies have been sufficiently powered to assess fracture outcomes. Diphosphonate therapy is typically reserved for children with a history of low-trauma fractures; it also has limited potential for spontaneous (medication-unassisted) recovery caused by permanent or persistent osteoporosis risk factors. The most frequently prescribed diphosphonate regimen is cyclic intravenous pamidronate (divided equally over 3 days and administered every 4 months).[28] With the resolution of risk factors during children's growth (eg, the cessation of secondary osteoporosis), discontinuation of therapy is usually considered after a child has been fracture free for at least 6 to 12 months and bone mineral density z-scores are appropriate for the child's height.

The most frequent adverse effects of diphosphonate therapy, reported with both oral and intravenous treatment,[28] are collectively referred to as acute-phase reactions and include fever, malaise, back and bone pain, nausea, and vomiting. These reactions are effectively managed with anti-inflammatory and antiemetic medications. The more serious acute adverse effects associated with diphosphonate therapy in adults (such as osteonecrosis of the jaw and atypical subtrochanteric fractures, uveitis, and thrombocytopenia) are rare in children. Concerns about the effects of diphosphonates on linear growth have ultimately been quelled by studies that confirm expected growth rates in children with diphosphonate-treated osteogenesis imperfecta and osteoporosis; some studies have reported improved growth with long-term diphosphonate therapy, which is likely attributable to the positive effect on vertebral height.[32]

Antibiotics

Antibiotic use is common in pediatric orthopaedic practice for two reasons: (1) spontaneous bone and joint infections are prevalent among children, and (2) infection is a potentially severe and potentially preventable complication of elective orthopaedic surgery. The broad mechanisms of action are depicted in **Figure 3**.

The antibiotics in current use have actually changed the nature of the infections being treated. For example, methicillin-resistant *Staphylococcus aureus* (MRSA) is rapidly increasing in prevalence as a community-acquired pediatric musculoskeletal infection in many jurisdictions in the United States. MRSA infections can be more severe and difficult to treat than infections caused by methicillin-sensitive *S aureus* (MSSA). Careful, conscientious, and evidence-informed stewardship of antibiotic management is required of both individual clinicians and the medical community if orthopaedic surgeons are to maintain their ability to easily and effectively treat musculoskeletal infections.

ACUTE HEMATOGENOUS OSTEOMYELITIS AND SEPTIC ARTHRITIS

Local signs of inflammation and systemic signs of infection characterize hematogenous osteomyelitis; antibiotic treatment alone often is curative.[33] With septic arthritis,

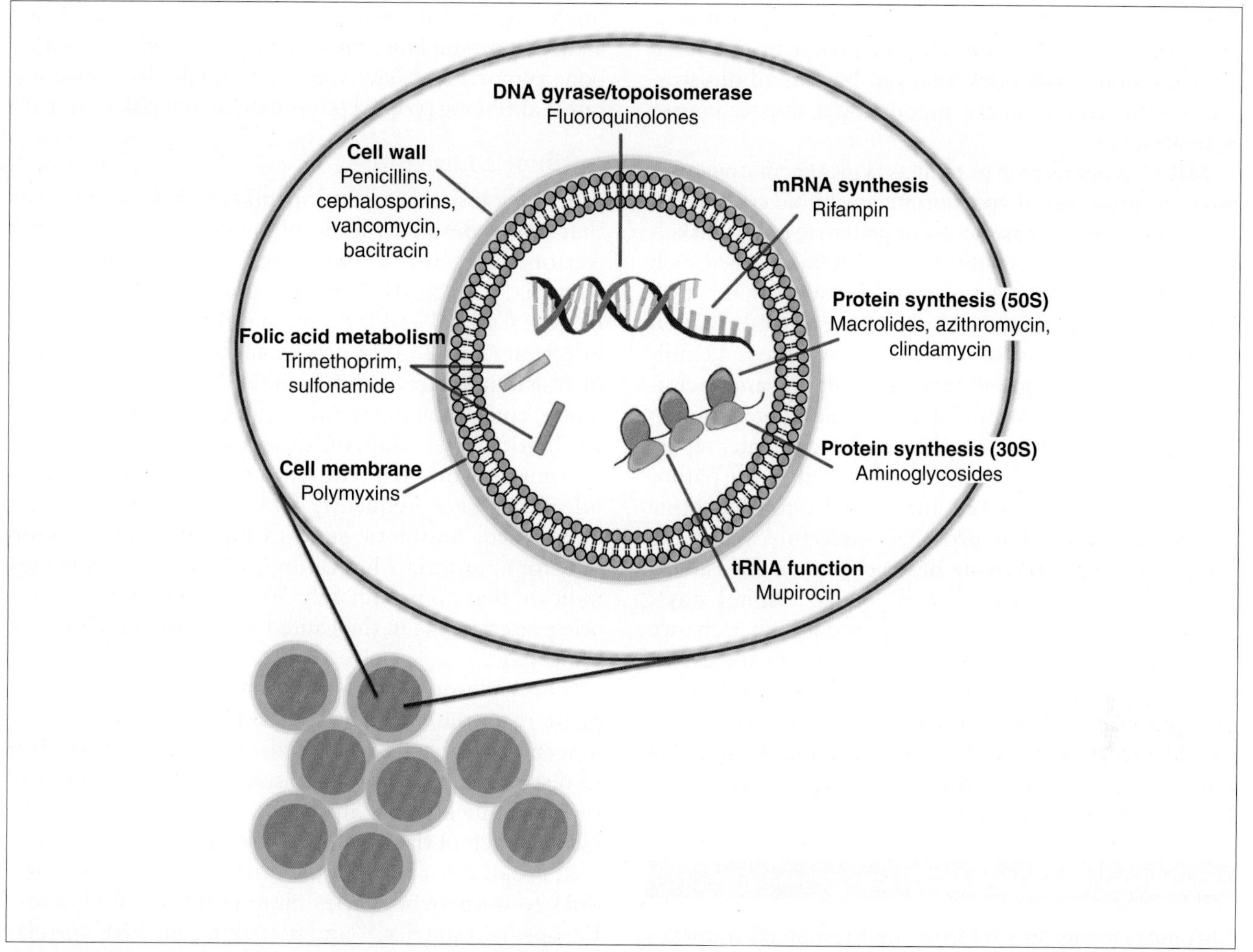

FIGURE 3 Illustration of the mechanism of action for common classes of antibiotics. Commonly prescribed antibiotics and their target(s) within the pathogen are depicted. Antibiotics are naturally occurring or chemically synthesized compounds that inhibit a wide range of critical bacterial functions. Specifically, antibiotics can impair cell wall and cell membrane structure, function, and synthesis; DNA replication and messenger RNA (mRNA) synthesis; protein production and folding; and cellular metabolism and folic acid synthesis of the pathogen. tRNA = transfer RNA

initial surgical drainage and irrigation of the joint are the mainstays of treatment, but antibiotic therapy is an important adjunct. In either case, the initial choice of antibiotic therapy is made based on the anatomic location (bone versus joint); the community prevalence of infectious agents; and the age, immunization status, and comorbidities of the patient.

For most children in most locations, *S aureus* is the most common cause of both osteomyelitis and septic arthritis.[33] The ongoing emergence of community-acquired MRSA is likely the most important determinant of the choice of empiric antibiotic coverage. Current recommendations are for a first-generation cephalosporin or antistaphylococcal penicillin if the community prevalence of MSSA is 90% or greater and for clindamycin or vancomycin if the community prevalence of MRSA is 10% or greater. The current prevalence of MRSA is higher than 10% in most states in the United States according to data from the Centers for Disease Control and Prevention.[34]

Recent trends are for a shorter course of intravenous therapy and a shorter total course of treatment of uncomplicated acute osteomyelitis treated within 4 days of symptom onset. A systematic review comparing intravenous dosing regimens of less than 1 week and more than 1 week showed no differences in response rates or complications, a result that has been shown in RCTs and multihospital cohort studies and is the subject of a current systematic review.[35-38] Recommendations for prolonged (6 weeks) intravenous treatment of patients with acute hematogenous osteomyelitis date back to a time when the condition had an appreciable mortality and long-term morbidity, but this is no longer the case in the United States and Europe.[33] Trends in the treatment of septic arthritis are similar—toward a brief course of intravenous antibiotics followed by oral administration—with RCT evidence supporting a shorter course of treatment.[36]

MRSA is not as easy to treat as typical hematogenous osteomyelitis, even if appropriate antibiotic coverage is selected. An initial case series of pediatric musculoskeletal MRSA infections published in 2009 described such infections as a game changer and reported that, of 27 children with MRSA musculoskeletal sepsis, 12 children required care in an intensive care unit. Of those 12 children, 5 children required inotrope support, and 4 children required extracorporeal membrane oxygenation in the presence of multisystem organ failure.[39] A later report contrasted MRSA with MSSA and described the pathogenic mechanisms involved, including Panton-Valentine leukocidin genes that produce powerful cytotoxins leading to increased tissue destruction and invasion.[40] MRSA remains associated with longer hospital stays, a higher chance of repeat surgery, and a higher chance of intensive care admission, although not to the extent described in the 2009 report. For patients with MRSA, the appropriate timing for changing from intravenous to oral antibiotic therapy is unknown, and the decision should be based on the clinical course in consultation with infectious disease specialists.

CHRONIC OSTEOMYELITIS

Chronic osteomyelitis is rare in well-resourced countries but remains very common in less-resourced settings. An established sequestrum (devitalized bone separated from circulation) and an evolving involucrum (new periosteal bone created by a healing process) create an environment where surgical intervention is necessary to remove dead bone, and antibiotics may not be important to achieve healing—at least according to authors with experience in managing chronic osteomyelitis in less-resourced settings.[41] However, patients who are systemically ill with invasive infection should be treated with antibiotics, guided by the particular clinical presentation and the results of a blood culture.[41]

Surgical Prophylaxis

Strong evidence shows that prophylactic antibiotics are important in preventing surgical site infections,[42] although much of this evidence has been derived from adult populations undergoing total joint arthroplasty or spinal instrumentation procedures. A systematic review and meta-analysis found no benefit of additional antibiotics beyond a single preincision dose in closed fracture surgery.[43] Large, single-center retrospective studies have evaluated low-risk orthopaedic procedures in children (including percutaneous pinning of fractures, knee arthroscopy, implant removal, and the excision of benign bone tumors) and have found an equally low infection rate if antibiotic prophylaxis is used in low-risk settings.[44]

Antibiotic Resistance

Antibiotic resistance is an emerging public health crisis that has prompted the development of the National Action Plan for Combating Antibiotic-Resistant Bacteria.[45] According to this plan, the Centers for Disease Control and Prevention estimate that 2 million infections and 23,000 deaths annually occur because of resistant bacteria in the United States; more importantly, epidemiologic trends suggest that without good antibiotic stewardship, the drug resistance problem will continue to worsen. A return to a preantibiotic era where infections were frequently fatal is foreseen and must be avoided. Antibiotic stewardship means prescribing only for appropriate indications, whereas best estimates indicate that approximately 30% of outpatient antibiotic prescriptions in the United States are not clinically indicated.[46]

The widespread use of antibiotics creates selective pressure for the emergence of resistant organisms, a phenomenon predicted by Alexander Fleming in 1946 when he discovered penicillin.[47] Substantial evidence indicates that the clinical use of antibiotics in humans is responsible for much of the development of antibiotic resistance seen today. For example, the rate of prescribing antibiotics to outpatients varies more than threefold across European countries,[48] and a striking positive correlation exists between the volume of antibiotics consumed and the presence of antibiotic resistance across multiple classes of pathogenic bacteria.[48]

More than 15 classes of antibiotics are in current use, and bacterial resistance mechanisms exist for all these classes.[49] Antibiotics are naturally occurring compounds that inhibit a range of critical bacterial functions, including cell wall structure, function, and synthesis; protein production and folding; DNA synthesis and replication; RNA synthesis; and folic acid synthesis[49] (**Figure 3**). Bacteria acquire resistance either gradually by a stepwise process of mutation in relevant chromosomes or more rapidly through the sharing of genetic material by means of bacteriophages, plasmids, naked DNA, or transposons. Drug resistance can be transferred from one bacterium to another across taxonomic groups.[49] Membrane proteins that pump drugs from the bacterial cell can provide resistance to multiple classes of antibiotics simultaneously.[47]

Strategies to prevent and manage drug resistance include tracking the resistance frequency, reducing the prescription of antibiotics, isolating hospital patients with resistant infections, and developing new antibiotic agents.[49] Mathematical modeling supports the empiric observation that resistant organisms appear relatively quickly, but take a much longer time to disappear even if antibiotic use is restricted. However, empiric work from Finland has shown that a national program to restrict the outpatient use of macrolide antibiotics was successful in decreasing the frequency of erythromycin resistance among streptococcal infections.[50]

The development of new antibiotics has always been and will remain an important strategy in combatting resistance. A valid concern is that the pace of discovery and marketing of new antibiotic agents has slowed down.[51] Drug companies are said to have little incentive for the development of new antibiotics because a new antibiotic likely will be prescribed for only brief periods, for chronic use, and it eventually will become worthless when resistance develops. Regulatory agencies often restrict the use of new drugs, even if they are effective, to slow the development of resistance. In addition, the traditional source of antibiotic agents (soil organisms that can be cultured in the laboratory) has perhaps already yielded most of the useful agents possible.[51] Some of these marketplace and regulatory realities need to be considered and addressed by the medical community as part of its social responsibility and extended role in antibiotic stewardship.

A relatively new approach—culturing in soil—has opened up the possibility of discovering natural antibiotics among an estimated remaining 99% of soil organisms that cannot be cultured under traditional laboratory conditions.[52] The first of these new antibiotics, teixobactin, targets a bacterial cell wall lipid and shows high antibacterial activity and low toxicity to mammalian cells. Furthermore, its mechanism of action suggests that it evolved to minimize the development of antibiotic resistance. Other such natural compounds with similarly low susceptibility to resistance are likely present in nature. Thus, the development of new antibiotics and good stewardship of the use of current antibiotics should allow physicians to stay ahead in the antimicrobial arms race.

SUMMARY

The overall treatment and care of pediatric orthopaedic patients is diverse. As such, a variety of pharmaceutical agents is used throughout treatment, including interventional, preoperative, and postoperative care. Common pharmacologic agents include analgesics, vitamin D supplementation, calcium supplementation, diphosphonates, and antibiotics. Understanding their mechanisms of action, potential adverse effects, and the pathologic conditions where the therapies are used will aid in providing the best care to pediatric patients.

KEY STUDY POINTS

- A multimodal therapeutic approach to analgesic use in pediatric patients is paramount.
- Dependency and withdrawal after analgesic administration can occur rapidly in pediatric patients. Physicians should recognize and act on the signs of analgesic dependency and withdrawal.
- The regulation of vitamin D and calcium levels is critical to maintain pediatric bone health.
- Given limited controlled studies, diphosphonates should be prescribed with caution.
- No FDA-approved therapies currently exist to improve bone regeneration. Off-label uses of therapies must be used with caution.
- Therapeutics and recommendations for the treatment of infection are consistently changing. Pediatric orthopaedic surgeons must stay up-to-date to provide the most informed care. Strategies for minimizing antibiotic resistance are critical in pediatric orthopaedics.

ANNOTATED REFERENCES

1. McGrath PA: Development of the World Health Organization guidelines on cancer pain relief and palliative care in children. *J Pain Symptom Manage* 1996;12(2):87-92.
2. Ballantyne JC, Kalso E, Stannard C: WHO analgesic ladder: A good concept gone astray. *Br Med J* 2016;352:i20.

   This editorial addresses the World Health Organization's analgesic ladder for use in chronic pain. The authors state that although the ladder approach is a valuable tool for guiding the treatment of excruciating and short-lived pain, such an approach is not appropriate for highly complex chronic pain. Level of evidence: V.
3. Drendel AL, Gorelick MH, Weisman SJ, Lyon R, Brousseau DC, Kim MK: A randomized clinical trial of ibuprofen versus acetaminophen with codeine for acute pediatric arm fracture pain. *Ann Emerg Med* 2009;54(4):553-560.
4. Poonai N, Bhullar G, Lin K, et al: Oral administration of morphine versus ibuprofen to manage postfracture pain in children: A randomized trial. *Can Med Assoc J* 2014;186(18):1358-1363.
5. Ali S, Klassen TP: Ibuprofen was more effective than codeine or acetaminophen for musculoskeletal pain in children. *Evid Based Med* 2007;12(5):144.
6. Borland M, Jacobs I, King B, O'Brien D: A randomized controlled trial comparing intranasal fentanyl to intravenous morphine for managing acute pain in children in the emergency department. *Ann Emerg Med* 2007;49(3):335-340.
7. Ali S, Klassen TP: Intranasal fentanyl and intravenous morphine did not differ for pain relief in children with closed long-bone fractures. *Evid Based Med* 2007;12(6):176.

8. Murphy A, O'Sullivan R, Wakai A, et al: Intranasal fentanyl for the management of acute pain in children. *Cochrane Database Syst Rev* 2014;10(10):CD009942.
9. American Society of Anesthesiologists Task Force on Acute Pain Management: Practice guidelines for acute pain management in the perioperative setting: An updated report by the American Society of Anesthesiologists Task Force on Acute Pain Management. *Anesthesiology* 2012;116(2):248-273.
10. Moore RA, Derry S, Aldington D, Wiffen PJ: Single dose oral analgesics for acute postoperative pain in adults: An overview of Cochrane reviews. *Cochrane Database Syst Rev* 2015;9:CD008659.
11. Schnabel A, Reichl SU, Zahn PK, Pogatzki-Zahn E: Nalbuphine for postoperative pain treatment in children. *Cochrane Database Syst Rev* 2014;7:CD009583.
12. McNicol ED, Ferguson MC, Hudcova J: Patient controlled opioid analgesia versus non-patient controlled opioid analgesia for postoperative pain. *Cochrane Database Syst Rev* 2015;6:CD003348.
13. Hayes J, Dowling JJ, Peliowski A, Crawford MW, Johnston B: Patient-controlled analgesia plus background opioid infusion for postoperative pain in children: A systematic review and meta-analysis of randomized trials. *Anesth Analg* 2016;123(4):991-1003.

    No substantial differences were found in patient pain scores 12 and 24 hours after surgery with the addition of an opioid background infusion to patient-controlled analgesia bolus doses of opioid. Further high-quality studies are required. Level of evidence: II.
14. Lambert P, Cyna AM, Knight N, Middleton P: Clonidine premedication for postoperative analgesia in children. *Cochrane Database Syst Rev* 2014;1:CD009633.
15. Bellon M, Le Bot A, Michelet D, et al: Efficacy of intraoperative dexmedetomidine compared with placebo for postoperative pain management: A meta-analysis of published studies. *Pain Ther* 2016;5(1):63-80.

    A meta-analysis demonstrated that the intraoperative administration of a dexmedetomidine bolus (>0.5 μg/kg) in children reduces postoperative opioid consumption and pain in the PACU. Level of evidence: II.
16. Zhu M, Wang H, Zhu A, Niu K, Wang G: Meta-analysis of dexmedetomidine on emergence agitation and recovery profiles in children after sevoflurane anesthesia: Different administration and different dosage. *PLoS One* 2015;10(4):e0123728.
17. Mahmoud M, Mason KP: Dexmedetomidine: Review, update, and future considerations of paediatric perioperative and periprocedural applications and limitations. *Br J Anaesth* 2015;115(2):171-182.
18. Dahmani S, Michelet D, Abback PS, et al: Ketamine for perioperative pain management in children: A meta-analysis of published studies. *Paediatr Anaesth* 2011;21(6):636-652.
19. Taenzer AH, Clark C: Efficacy of postoperative epidural analgesia in adolescent scoliosis surgery: A meta-analysis. *Paediatr Anaesth* 2010;20(2):135-143.
20. Suresh S, Schaldenbrand K, Wallis B, De Oliveira GS Jr: Regional anaesthesia to improve pain outcomes in paediatric surgical patients: A qualitative systematic review of randomized controlled trials. *Br J Anaesth* 2014;113(3):375-390.
21. Engelman E, Marsala C: Bayesian enhanced meta-analysis of post-operative analgesic efficacy of additives for caudal analgesia in children. *Acta Anaesthesiol Scand* 2012;56(7):817-832.
22. Tong Y, Ren H, Ding X, Jin S, Chen Z, Li Q: Analgesic effect and adverse events of dexmedetomidine as additive for pediatric caudal anesthesia: A meta-analysis. *Paediatr Anaesth* 2014;24(12):1224-1230.
23. Mar GJ, Barrington MJ, McGuirk BR: Acute compartment syndrome of the lower limb and the effect of postoperative analgesia on diagnosis. *Br J Anaesth* 2009;102(1):3-11.
24. Galinkin J, Koh JL, Committee on Drugs, Section on Anesthesiology and Pain Medicine, American Academy of Pediatrics: Recognition and management of iatrogenically induced opioid dependence and withdrawal in children. *Pediatrics* 2014;133(1):152-155.
25. Dabisch-Ruthe M, Kuzaj P, Götting C, Knabbe C, Hendig D: Pyrophosphates as a major inhibitor of matrix calcification in pseudoxanthoma elasticum. *J Dermatol Sci* 2014;75(2):109-120.
26. Uitto J, Jiang Q, Váradi A, Bercovitch LG, Terry SF: Pseudoxanthoma elasticum: Diagnostic features, classification, and treatment options. *Expert Opin Orphan Drugs* 2014;2(6):567-577.
27. Misra M, Pacaud D, Petryk A, Collett-Solberg PF, Kappy M, Drug and Therapeutics Committee of the Lawson Wilkins Pediatric Endocrine Society: Vitamin D deficiency in children and its management: Review of current knowledge and recommendations. *Pediatrics* 2008;122(2):398-417.
28. Russell RG: Bisphosphonates: The first 40 years. *Bone* 2011;49(1):2-19.
29. Weisberg P, Scanlon KS, Li R, Cogswell ME: Nutritional rickets among children in the United States: Review of cases reported between 1986 and 2003. *Am J Clin Nutr* 2004;80(6 suppl):1697S-1705S.
30. Wagner CL, Greer FR, American Academy of Pediatrics Section on Breastfeeding, American Academy of Pediatrics Committee on Nutrition: Prevention of rickets and vitamin D deficiency in infants, children, and adolescents. *Pediatrics* 2008;122(5):1142-1152.
31. Ohba T, Cates JM, Cole HA, et al: Pleiotropic effects of bisphosphonates on osteosarcoma. *Bone* 2014;63:110-120.
32. Thomas IH, DiMeglio LA: Advances in the classification and treatment of osteogenesis imperfecta. *Curr Osteoporos Rep* 2016;14(1):1-9.

    Osteogenesis imperfecta, a rare collagen disorder characterized by an increased susceptibility to bony fractures, is now routinely treated with diphosphonates. New therapies, such as anabolic agents, transforming growth factor-β antibodies, and other antiresorptive drugs, are currently under development. Level of evidence: III.

33. Peltola H, Pääkkönen M: Acute osteomyelitis in children. *N Engl J Med* 2014;370(4):352-360.

34. *Methicillin-Resistant: Staphylococcus aureus (MRSA). MRSA Tracking.* Centers for Disease Control and Prevention. Available at: http://www.cdc.gov/mrsa/tracking/. Accessed June 27, 2016.

The number and kind of MRSA infections throughout the United States are tracked using the National Healthcare Safety Network and the Emerging Infections Program.

35. Le Saux N, Howard A, Barrowman NJ, Gaboury I, Sampson M, Moher D: Shorter courses of parenteral antibiotic therapy do not appear to influence response rates for children with acute hematogenous osteomyelitis: A systematic review. *BMC Infect Dis* 2002;2:16.

36. Peltola H, Pääkkönen M, Kallio P, Kallio MJ, Osteomyelitis-Septic Arthritis (OM-SA) Study Group: Prospective, randomized trial of 10 days versus 30 days of antimicrobial treatment, including a short-term course of parenteral therapy, for childhood septic arthritis. *Clin Infect Dis* 2009;48(9):1201-1210.

37. Zaoutis T, Localio AR, Leckerman K, Saddlemire S, Bertoch D, Keren R: Prolonged intravenous therapy versus early transition to oral antimicrobial therapy for acute osteomyelitis in children. *Pediatrics* 2009;123(2):636-642.

38. Grimbly C, Odenbach J, Vandermeer B, Forgie S, Curtis S: Parenteral and oral antibiotic duration for treatment of pediatric osteomyelitis: A systematic review protocol. *Syst Rev* 2013;2:92.

39. Vander Have KL, Karmazyn B, Verma M, et al: Community-associated methicillin-resistant Staphylococcus aureus in acute musculoskeletal infection in children: A game changer. *J Pediatr Orthop* 2009;29(8):927-931.

40. Sarkissian EJ, Gans I, Gunderson MA, Myers SH, Spiegel DA, Flynn JM: Community-acquired methicillin-resistant Staphylococcus aureus musculoskeletal infections: Emerging trends over the past decade. *J Pediatr Orthop* 2016;36(3):323-327.

At the Children's Hospital of Philadelphia, community-acquired pediatric MRSA musculoskeletal infections increased threefold, and the risk for complications during inpatient management was elevated. Regional epidemiologic trends will help facilitate timely and accurate clinical diagnosis and treatment. Level of evidence: II.

41. Jones HW, Beckles VL, Akinola B, Stevenson AJ, Harrison WJ: Chronic haematogenous osteomyelitis in children: An unsolved problem. *J Bone Joint Surg Br* 2011;93(8):1005-1010.

42. Tsai DM, Caterson EJ: Current preventive measures for health-care associated surgical site infections: A review. *Patient Saf Surg* 2014;8(1):42.

43. Slobogean GP, Kennedy SA, Davidson D, O'Brien PJ: Single-versus multiple-dose antibiotic prophylaxis in the surgical treatment of closed fractures: A meta-analysis. *J Orthop Trauma* 2008;22(4):264-269.

44. Formaini N, Jacob P, Willis L, Kean JR: Evaluating the use of preoperative antibiotics in pediatric orthopaedic surgery. *J Pediatr Orthop* 2012;32(7):737-740.

45. White House: *National Action Plan for Combatting Antibiotic-Resistant Bacteria.* 2015. Available at: https://www.whitehouse.gov/sites/default/files/docs/national_action_plan_for_combating_antibotic-resistant_bacteria.pdf. Accessed June 20, 2016.

46. Fleming-Dutra KE, Hersh AL, Shapiro DJ, et al: Prevalence of inappropriate antibiotic prescriptions among US ambulatory care visits, 2010-2011. *J Am Med Assoc* 2016;315(17):1864-1873.

Researchers estimated the total number of antibiotic prescriptions written in the US by sampling national ambulatory care databases. They applied national guidelines and regional variation to estimate the appropriate prescriptions. They found that each year 506 antibiotic prescriptions are written per 1000 population of which 353 were likely appropriate, and 153 likely inappropriate. They advocate for establishing goals for outpatient antibiotic stewardship. Level of evidence: II.

47. Alekshun MN, Levy SB: Molecular mechanisms of antibacterial multidrug resistance. *Cell* 2007;128(6):1037-1050.

48. Goossens H, Ferech M, Vander Stichele R, Elseviers M, ESAC Project Group: Outpatient antibiotic use in Europe and association with resistance: A cross-national database study. *Lancet* 2005;365(9459):579-587.

49. Levy SB, Marshall B: Antibacterial resistance worldwide: Causes, challenges and responses. *Nat Med* 2004;10(12 suppl):S122-S129.

50. Seppälä H, Klaukka T, Vuopio-Varkila J, et al, Finnish Study Group for Antimicrobial Resistance: The effect of changes in the consumption of macrolide antibiotics on erythromycin resistance in group A streptococci in Finland. *N Engl J Med* 1997;337(7):441-446.

51. Wright G: Antibiotics: An irresistible newcomer. *Nature* 2015;517(7535):442-444.

52. Ling LL, Schneider T, Peoples AJ, et al: A new antibiotic kills pathogens without detectable resistance. *Nature* 2015;517(7535):455-459.

Developmental Biology

SIMON P. KELLEY, *MBChB, PhD, FRCS (TR AND ORTH)*

ABSTRACT

The bones of the human skeleton develop via two distinct processes: intramembranous and endochondral ossification. Intramembranous ossification is a process where osteochondroprogenitor cells differentiate directly to osteoblasts, which form bone directly. Endochondral bone formation is a more complex process, whereby cartilage is formed as an intermediate step and acts as a template, which is subsequently replaced by bone. Endochondral ossification is responsible for most skeletal bone growth including all of the appendicular bones, vertebral column, ribs, and bones of the face.

Keywords: chondrocyte; endochondral ossification; epiphyseal plate; intramembranous ossification; osteoblast

INTRODUCTION

Despite the varied size, shape, and function, all 206 bones of the adult human skeleton develop in a remarkably tightly controlled fashion, via two distinct processes: intramembranous and endochondral ossification. Intramembranous ossification is a process where osteochondroprogenitor cells differentiate directly to osteoblasts, which form bone directly.[1] This type of ossification is responsible for development of the bones of the dermatocranium and the medial ends of the clavicles.[2] Endochondral bone formation is a more complex process, whereby cartilage is formed as an intermediate step and acts as a template, which is subsequently replaced by bone.[3] Endochondral ossification is responsible for most skeletal bone growth, including all of the appendicular bones, vertebral column, ribs, and bones of the face.

Although it is conventional to categorize bones as to whether they form by intramembranous or endochondral ossification, bones that form primarily by endochondral ossification also incorporate elements of intramembranous ossification, for the purpose of forming a central bone collar for structural integrity and developmental morphology.[4] When a fractured bone heals, both endochondral and intramembranous ossification occur in varying degrees based on the anatomic location in the fracture and the overall mechanical environment.[5] Distraction osteogenesis is a bone regenerative process, which is distinct from development and fracture repair, and is commonly seen during bone lengthening surgeries. Distraction osteogenesis is primarily achieved by intramembranous ossification aided by elements of endochondral ossification in the earliest phases.[6] There is emerging evidence that a third type of ossification may also occur, which sits somewhere between intramembranous and endochondral ossification, where mature chondrocytes actually transdifferentiate into osteoblasts that lay down bone in specific developmental processes, such as the formation of an ossific nucleus at the growing ends of the long bone.[7-9]

What was long considered to be two quite distinct methods of bone formation may actually be just two ends of a spectrum that are more intrinsically linked than was originally supposed. Whether a bone forms for development, fracture repair, or distraction osteogenesis, the same fundamental cells, signaling pathways, and niches are present, and understanding the nuances of each processes, the cellular interactions, variations in signaling, and the importance of niche is essential for the advancement of

Dr. Kelley or an immediate family member is a member of a speakers' bureau or has made paid presentations on behalf of Smith & Nephew; serves as a paid consultant to or is an employee of Smith & Nephew; and serves as a board member, owner, officer, or committee member of the International Hip Dysplasia Institute.

fundamental knowledge, development of novel therapies for the management of genetic bone diseases, enhancement of fracture repair, and tissue regeneration.

MESENCHYMAL CONDENSATION

The first step in the development of a bone is the migration and condensation of mesenchymal progenitors. The mesenchymal progenitors that form the cranium, mandible, and medial clavicles (intramembranous bones) are derived from the neural crest. The mesenchymal progenitors that form the endochondral facial bones, vertebrae, and limbs are derived from the neural crest, the paraxial mesoderm, and the lateral plate mesoderm, respectively. Mesenchymal condensation reflects the aggregation of mesenchymal cells and is mediated by cell-cell interactions, including the transient expression of neural cell adhesion molecule and N-cadherin.[10]

ENDOCHONDRAL OSSIFICATION

The next step in the development of a long bone occurs when the central cells of the mesenchymal condensation differentiate into chondrocytes. Not all the cells of the condensation will differentiate to chondrocytes, however, as there is second subpopulation of mesenchymal cells, which differentiate directly into osteoblasts and are positioned peripherally, which demarcates the bone from the surrounding mesenchymal tissue. The differentiation of chondrocytes expands out from the central portion of the condensation both longitudinally and transversely patterning the shape of the bone in the process. The initiation of chondrogenesis is accompanied by the expression of a number of important molecules. SOX9 is the earliest identified molecule associated with chondrogenesis in the limb bud, and it is considered the master regulator of chondrogenesis, which acts on the newly differentiated chondrocytes to generate the extracellular matrix proteins collagen type II, collagen type IX, and collagen type XI in addition to aggrecan and cartilage oligomeric matrix protein.[11]

Soon after the undifferentiated mesenchymal cells have become chondrocytes, the centrally located chondrocytes stop proliferating, start to exit the cell cycle, and undergo terminal differentiation to become hypertrophic chondrocytes. Hypertrophic chondrocytes drive bone formation and are characterized by the production of collagen type X. They also secrete matrix metalloproteinase 13 and vascular endothelial growth factor.[11] Vascular endothelial growth factor and matrix metalloproteinase 13 stimulate the ingrowth of blood vessels and cleavage of extracellular matrix proteins, respectively, to facilitate further vascular ingrowth to the central area of chondrocyte hypertrophy, which delivers both osteoclasts and osteoblasts. The hypertrophic chondrocytes undergo apoptosis, leaving gaps within the extracellular matrix. Osteoclasts further remove the deposited chondrocytic matrix to allow more space for osteoblasts and blood vessels to invade. Osteoblasts then lay down bone matrix composed primarily of collagen type I and then mineralize this matrix to form the primary spongiosa in the center of the developing bone.

This spreading wave of chondrocyte terminal differentiation moves longitudinally away from the center of the anlage toward both ends of the growing bone. Simultaneously the chondrocytes at the ends of the growing bone continue to proliferate, thus increasing the length of bones. The wave of cellular hypertrophic differentiation never actually reaches the end of the bone. Instead, the cells slow their rate of proliferation and differentiation and organize themselves into a disklike structure called the epiphyseal plate, which is bordered by the primary spongiosa on one side and the epiphysis, made of proliferative chondrocytes, in the juxtarticular region. The epiphyses are largely cartilaginous in most bones in the early postnatal period, but during growth, a secondary ossification center forms. This occurs when the central epiphyseal chondrocytes undergo terminal differentiation to hypertrophic chondrocytes and, via the same mechanisms outlined previously, encourage vascular invasion and the formation of an ossific nucleus, which expands to replace the cartilaginous epiphysis, leaving just a layer of highly specialized articular cartilage surrounding the end of the bone forming the joint surface. This bony epiphysis is separated from the metaphysis of the bone by the epiphyseal plate.[1,3,12,13]

The epiphyseal plate structurally consists of a layer of round resting chondrocytes that lie oriented parallel to the joint, which form a ready supply of cells to enter a proliferative state during skeletal growth. Beneath the layer of resting cells are neatly organized columns of disk-shaped proliferative cells. The proliferative layer then transitions into a prehypertrophic layer and subsequently a hypertrophic layer of chondrocytes that undergo apoptosis and direct bone formation as previously described. The rate of proliferation and differentiation in the epiphyseal plate determines how rapidly a bone gains length. According to a 2018 study, there is emerging evidence that the epiphyseal plate actually contains a unique class of skeletal stem cell within its resting zone. These stem cells exist as a subset of unipotent parathyroid hormone–related peptide ($PTHrP^+$) chondrocytes that become columnar cells of the physis in the proliferative zone but then develop multipotent capacity to differentiate into osteoblasts and stromal cells controlled by the balance of signaling from nearby Indian hedgehog (IHH) signaling and PTHrP signaling chondrocytes.[14] In adolescence, the epiphyseal plate disappears and is replaced by bone, thus ending the phase of skeletal growth[13,15] (**Figure 1**).

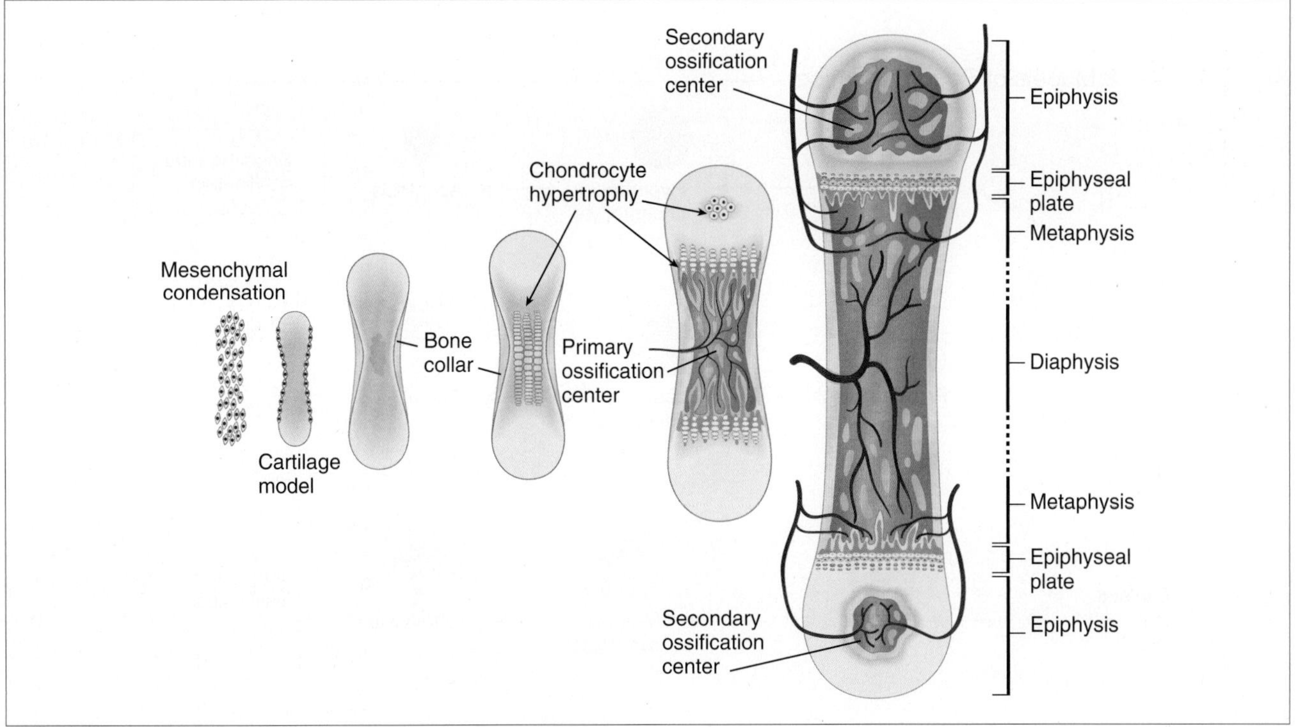

FIGURE 1 Illustration of the stages of bone development.

ORIGIN OF OSTEOBLASTS IN ENDOCHONDRAL OSSIFICATION

An emerging concept in bone development is that rather than the linear model, whereby osteochondroprogenitors become specified to differentiate to either an osteoblast or chondrocyte lineage, chondrocytes may actually be able to transdifferentiate to osteoblasts. This line of investigation came about because of differences in opinion about the fate of hypertrophic chondrocytes.[16] It has long been known that chondrocytes undergo apoptosis or autophagy as their terminal event and as a key step in driving local osteogenesis,[17] but in vitro observations suggested that hypertrophic chondrocytes might be able to transdifferentiate to osteoblasts.[18] In addition, it is known that hypertrophic chondrocytes express many of the same markers as osteoblasts, such as RUNX2, Osterix (OSX), alkaline phosphatase, bone sialoprotein, osteopontin, and osteocalcin.[19] It was not until very recently that a number of publications gave more weight to the hypothesis that transdifferentiation or dedifferentiation of hypertrophic chondrocytes actually occurs, with convincing in vivo demonstrations of this phenomenon. Through lineage tracing experiments using conditionally labeled cells, it has been shown that some hypertrophic chondrocytes are able to dedifferentiate to an immature osteoblast type cell, which further differentiate to mature osteoblasts, or alternatively, hypertrophic chondrocytes may transdifferentiate directly to mature osteoblasts (**Figure 2**). These processes are seen in the region of the lower hypertrophic zone at the mineralization front of the epiphyseal plate. The mature osteoblasts derived from these hypertrophic chondrocytes can be seen in the primary spongiosa of the bone marrow alongside osteoblasts derived from the perichondrium.[7-9,20] Not only does it appear that hypertrophic chondrocytes can form up to 60% of osteoblasts in endochondral bone both prenatally and postnatally (in 1-month-old mice), the same process also occurs in fracture healing with the direct transdifferentiation of hypertrophic chondrocytes to osteoblasts in the healing callus, adding to the pool of osteoblasts differentiated from dedicated progenitors in the periosteum.[9]

TRANSCRIPTIONAL CONTROL OF EPIPHYSEAL PLATE FUNCTION

Following the initial differentiation of mesenchymal cells to chondrocytes, which requires SOX9 expression, the subsequent terminal differentiation of chondrocytes to hypertrophic chondrocytes is then accompanied by a reduction in SOX9 expression.[21] An increase in RUNX2 expression is also seen at this time, which positively regulates terminal chondrocyte

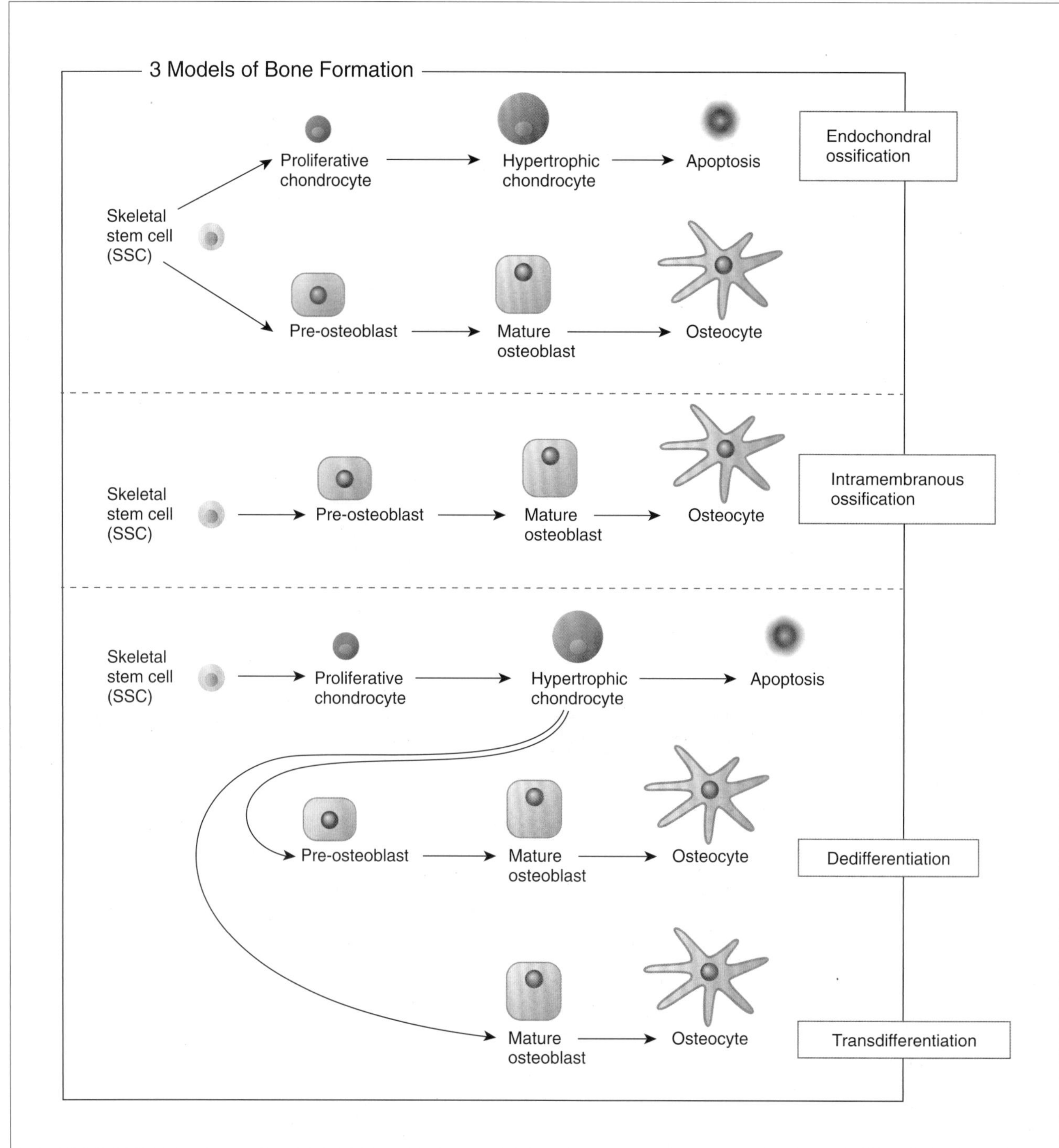

FIGURE 2 Illustration of models of bone formation.

differentiation (and osteoblast differentiation).[22,23] Because RUNX2 is also a major transcriptional regulator of osteoblast differentiation, the expression of OSX is more specific for differentiation of the osteoblast lineage.[24]

IHH/PTHrP SIGNALING LOOP

The IHH/PTHrP signaling loop is critical for controlling the balance of chondrocyte proliferation and differentiation in the epiphyseal plate of the developing bone.[3]

PTHrP is expressed at the end of the developing bone in perichondrial cells and in the epiphyseal plate by proliferating chondrocytes. The action of PTHrP positively regulates chondrocyte proliferation by acting on its own receptors on proliferating chondrocytes to maintain a proliferative state and prevent differentiation.[25,26] Proliferating chondrocytes receive less signal from PTHrP as they move distally away from their resting progenitors through the epiphyseal plate, which would tend to cause them to stop proliferating and undergo differentiation; however, they become increasingly signaled by IHH,[27] which acts to prevent further chondrocyte differentiation.[28] In addition, IHH also acts by signaling back to the proliferative chondrocytes at the ends of the bone to secrete PTHrP, thus further maintaining the proliferating pool and closing the feedback loop.[27,29,30] Developmental control of the epiphyseal plate is therefore modulated by the gradient of IHH and PTHrP, which exists because of the spatial organization of the physeal zones and the fact that these signaling molecules are expressed by cells at either end of the epiphyseal plate (**Figure 3**).

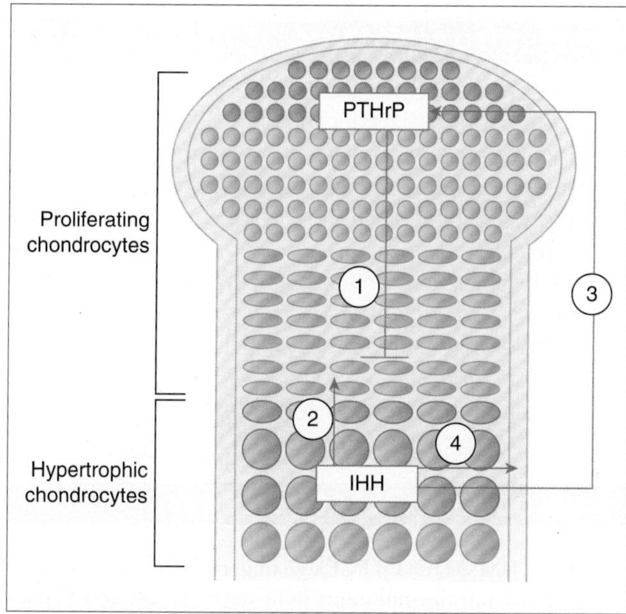

FIGURE 3 Illustration of Indian hedgehog (IHH)/parathyroid hormone–related peptide (PTHrP) negative-feedback loop. PTHrP is secreted from perichondrial and chondrocytes at the ends of long bones (1). PTHrP acts on receptors on proliferating chondrocytes to keep the chondrocytes proliferating and, thereby, to delay the production of IHH. When the source of PTHrP production is sufficiently distant, then IHH is produced. The IHH acts on its receptors on chondrocytes to increase the rate of proliferation (2) and, through a poorly understood mechanism, stimulates the production of PTHrP at the ends of bones (3). IHH also acts on perichondrial cells to convert these cells into osteoblasts of the bone collar (4). (Reprinted with permission from Kronenberg HM: Developmental regulation of the growth plate. *Nature* 2003;423:332-336.)

Through this intricately controlled feedback loop the developing bone is able to grow in length, by controlling and maintaining the pool of proliferating chondrocytes and determining the rate and extent of osteoblast differentiation. This controls the rate of terminal differentiation, which adds structure and integrity to the bone by controlling the rate of terminal differentiation of chondrocytes to hypertrophic chondrocytes which, as discussed previously, stimulates osteogenesis following apoptosis or autophagy, or transdifferentiate directly into osteoblasts.

The first elements of osteogenesis that occur in the developing bone are during the formation of the bone collar, as previously discussed. The perichondrial cells that secrete PTHrP and differentiate directly to bone to form the bone collar are also stimulated by IHH, secreted by the nearby differentiating chondrocytes, which occurs in the center of the cartilage anlage.[28]

BONE MORPHOGENETIC PROTEIN SIGNALING IN THE EPIPHYSEAL PLATE

Bone morphogenetic proteins (BMPs) are members of the transforming growth factor beta superfamily of growth and differentiation factors.[3] BMPs are known to be potent drivers of endochondral ossification, readily forming ectopic endochondral bone when injected subcutaneously in rats.[31] BMP signaling is critical in the formation of mesenchymal condensations, to the extent that when BMP signaling is repressed by noggin (a BMP inhibitor) in chick limbs, then the mesenchymal condensations fail to form.[32] In addition, it has been found that BMPs are essential for early cartilage development in three main areas—proliferation, cell survival, and differentiation—and act through SOX9, SOX5, and SOX6.[33,34] Signaling to the epiphyseal plate from the perichondrium are numerous BMP ligands: BMP2, BMP3, BMP4, BMP5, and BMP7. Hypertrophic chondrocytes express BMP2 and BMP6, whereas proliferating chondrocytes express BMP7.[3] BMP increases the expression of IHH from prehypertrophic chondrocytes, which in addition to its own direct mechanisms allows BMP ligands to increase chondrocyte proliferation through the IHH/PTHrP signaling pathway.[35]

INTRAMEMBRANOUS OSSIFICATION

During the development of endochondral bone, and despite the name, there is a role for direct intramembranous bone formation. An increase in fibroblast growth factor receptor 1 expression corresponds to the development of the zone of intramembranous ossification called the bone collar, which is formed by the differentiation of cells within the perichondrium to osteoblasts, which then lay down bone.[4]

There are, however, bones that form completely by intramembranous bone formation, where no cartilage template is seen, and mesenchymal cells differentiate directly to bone. Examples of intramembranous bones (and their origins) include the bones of the dermatocranium (mesoderm and neural crest), the mandible (neural crest), and the medial ends of the clavicles (neural crest and mesoderm).[2] The embryologic origins of the cells that make up the intramembranous bones are not actually defined by the mode of ossification but rather by the attachment of muscles and have varied through evolution.[2,36]

The intramembranous bones, as with endochondral bones, form from an initial condensation of mesenchymal cells, which can be of neural crest or mesodermal origin, often sharing cells of these two sources.[2] Ossification occurs directly from osteoblasts that have differentiated from these mesenchymal condensations. The bones of the cranial vault expand during development but do not fuse because of the presence of sutures, which are specialized fibrous joints separating the bony plates.[37] Osteoblastic differentiation of osteoprogenitor cells occurs mainly at the margins of the condensation at the suture line. The osteoblasts lay down matrix composed mostly of collagen type I. Other extracellular matrix proteins expressed by osteoblasts include osteopontin, bone sialoprotein, and osteocalcin. Osteocalcin is the most specific marker of a terminally differentiated osteoblast. Following matrix deposition, osteoblasts then mineralize the extracellular matrix to form bone.[38]

TRANSCRIPTIONAL REGULATION OF INTRAMEMBRANOUS OSSIFICATION

Intramembranous bone formation is transcriptionally controlled at different stages by different factors. The four most important are from (upstream to downstream) RUNX2, OSX, ATF4, and MSX2.[24] RUNX2 is expressed in early mesenchymal condensations and is important for both osteoblast and chondrocyte differentiation and thus defines a common progenitor.[39] Mice deficient in RUNX2 fail to undergo development of cartilage or bony elements to their skeleton and die shortly after birth.[22] SOX9 downregulates RUNX2 expression, which allows specification of the chondrocyte lineage, whereas unchecked RUNX2 along with the expression of OSX steers the osteochondroprogenitor down the osteoblast lineage. OSX is therefore considered the master regulator of osteoblast differentiation.[40] In OSX-null mice, cartilaginous components of the skeleton develop but fail to ossify; furthermore, RUNX2 is still expressed in the cartilaginous tissues of OSX-null mice, confirming that OSX is downstream of RUNX2.[40] ATF4 is downstream of OSX and is involved in expressing genes such as osteocalcin that are critical for terminal differentiation of osteoblasts. ATF4 is partly dispensable in osteoblast differentiation because in the absence of ATF4, bone can still form, albeit at a reduced rate and volume.[41] MSX2 is also an important transcriptional regulator for the commitment of mesenchymal cells into osteoblasts, particularly in the setting of craniofacial bone formation, which is induced by BMPs.[42] Deficiencies in MSX2 cause defects in calvarial ossification in both mice and humans, and mice overexpressing MSX2 show enhanced growth of calvariae and increased number of osteoprogenitor cells.[43]

SUMMARY

Human skeletal development is controlled by a complex series of tightly coordinated biologic processes. There are known methods of bone formation, endochondral and intramembranous ossification. These two distinct processes are involved in bone development but also in repair and regeneration. By intimately understanding the processes underpinning bone development this can potentially provide the keys to being able to manipulate bone repair and regeneration such that new therapies can be sought for fractures that are slow to heal, to reconstruct bone defects, or to equalize limb differences in individuals with congenital deficiencies.

KEY STUDY POINTS

- Bones form by either intramembranous ossification or endochondral ossification.
- Fracture repair and distraction osteogenesis recapitulate processes of bone development.
- Epiphyseal plates contain a unique class of skeletal stem cell.
- The origin of osteoblasts is an area of controversy and intense current research.
- Complex signaling pathways, including IHH, PTHrP, BMP, and fibroblast growth factor, tightly control the coordination of bone development.

ANNOTATED REFERENCES

1. Ornitz DM, Marie PJ: FGF signaling pathways in endochondral and intramembranous bone development and human genetic disease. *Genes Dev* 2002;16(12):1446-1465.
2. Matsuoka T, Ahlberg PE, Kessaris N, et al: Neural crest origins of the neck and shoulder. *Nature* 2005;436(7049):347-355.
3. Kronenberg HM: Developmental regulation of the growth plate. *Nature* 2003;423(6937):332-336.
4. Syftestad GT, Weitzhandler M, Caplan AI: Isolation and characterization of osteogenic cells derived from first bone of the embryonic tibia. *Dev Biol* 1985;110(2):275-283.
5. Perren SM, Fernandez A, Regazzoni P: Understanding fracture healing biomechanics based on the "strain" concept and its clinical applications. *Acta Chir Orthop Traumatol Cech* 2015;82(4):253-260.

6. Bouletreau PJ, Warren SM, Longaker MT: The molecular biology of distraction osteogenesis. *J Craniomaxillofac Surg* 2002;30(1):1-11.
7. Park J, Gebhardt M, Golovchenko S, et al: Dual pathways to endochondral osteoblasts: A novel chondrocyte-derived osteoprogenitor cell identified in hypertrophic cartilage. *Biol Open* 2015;4(5):608-621.
8. Yang L, Tsang KY, Tang HC, Chan D, Cheah KSE: Hypertrophic chondrocytes can become osteoblasts and osteocytes in endochondral bone formation. *Proc Natl Acad Sci U S A* 2014;111(33):12097-12102.
9. Zhou X, von der Mark K, Henry S, Norton W, Adams H, de Crombrugghe B: Chondrocytes transdifferentiate into osteoblasts in endochondral bone during development, postnatal growth and fracture healing in mice. *PLoS Genet* 2014;10(12):e1004820.
10. Oberlender S, Tuan RS: Expression and functional involvement of N-cadherin in embryonic limb chondrogenesis. *Development* 1994;120(1):177-187.
11. Degnin CR, Laederich MB, Horton WA: FGFs in endochondral skeletal development. *J Cell Biochem* 2010;110(5): 1046-1057.
12. Berendsen AD, Olsen BR: Bone development. *Bone* 2015;80:14-18.
13. Long F, Ornitz DM: Development of the endochondral skeleton. *Cold Spring Harb Perspect Biol* 2013;5(1):a008334.
14. Mizuhashi K, Ono W, Matsushita Y, et al: Resting zone of the growth plate houses a unique class of skeletal stem cells. *Nature* 2018;563(7730):254-258.

    Using a mouse model, the authors show that skeletal stem cells are formed among PTHrP-positive chondrocytes within the resting zone of the postnatal growth plate.
15. Kronenberg HM: The role of the perichondrium in fetal bone development. *Ann N Y Acad Sci* 2007;1116:59-64.
16. Shapiro IM, Adams CS, Freeman T, Srinivas V: Fate of the hypertrophic chondrocyte: Microenvironmental perspectives on apoptosis and survival in the epiphyseal growth plate. *Birth Defects Res C Embryo Today* 2005;75(4):330-339.
17. Aizawa T, Kokubun S, Tanaka Y: Apoptosis and proliferation of growth plate chondrocytes in rabbits. *J Bone Joint Surg Br* 1997;79(3):483-486.
18. Descalzi Cancedda F, Gentili C, Manduca P, Cancedda R: Hypertrophic chondrocytes undergo further differentiation in culture. *J Cell Biol* 1992;117(2):427-435.
19. Lefebvre V, Smits P: Transcriptional control of chondrocyte fate and differentiation. *Birth Defects Res C Embryo Today* 2005;75(3):200-212.
20. Yang G, Zhu L, Hou N, et al: Osteogenic fate of hypertrophic chondrocytes. *Cell Res* 2014;24(10):1266-1269.
21. Haruhiko A, Marie-Christine C, Martin JF, Schedl A, de Crombrugghe B: The transcription factor Sox9 has essential roles in successive steps of the chondrocyte differentiation pathway and is required for expression of Sox5 and Sox6. *Genes Dev* 2002;16(21):2813-2828.
22. Komori T, Yagi H, Nomura S, et al: Targeted disruption of Cbfa1 results in a complete lack of bone formation owing to maturational arrest of osteoblasts. *Cell* 1997;89(5): 755-764.
23. Otto F, Thornell AP, Crompton T, et al: Cbfa1, a candidate gene for cleidocranial dysplasia syndrome, is essential for osteoblast differentiation and bone development. *Cell* 1997;89(5):765-771.
24. Franceschi RT, Ge C, Xiao G, Roca H, Jiang D: Transcriptional regulation of osteoblasts. *Cells Tissues Organs* 2009;189(1-4):144-152.
25. Lee K, Lanske B, Karaplis AC, et al: Parathyroid hormone-related peptide delays terminal differentiation of chondrocytes during endochondral bone development. *Endocrinology* 1996;137(11):5109-5118.
26. Weir EC, Philbrick WM, Amling M, Neff LA, Baron R, Broadus AE: Targeted overexpression of parathyroid hormone-related peptide in chondrocytes causes chondrodysplasia and delayed endochondral bone formation. *Proc Natl Acad Sci U S A* 1996;93(19):10240-10245.
27. Vortkamp A, Lee K, Lanske B, Segre GV, Kronenberg HM, Tabin CJ: Regulation of rate of cartilage differentiation by Indian hedgehog and PTH-related protein. *Science* 1996;273(5275):613-622.
28. St-Jacques B, Hammerschmidt M, McMahon AP: Indian hedgehog signaling regulates proliferation and differentiation of chondrocytes and is essential for bone formation. *Genes Dev* 1999;13(16):2072-2086.
29. Karp SJ, Schipani E, St-Jacques B, Hunzelman J, Kronenberg H, McMahon AP: Indian hedgehog coordinates endochondral bone growth and morphogenesis via parathyroid hormone related-protein-dependent and -independent pathways. *Development* 2000;127(3):543-548.
30. Kronenberg HM, Chung U: The parathyroid hormone-related protein and Indian hedgehog feedback loop in the growth plate. *Novartis Found Symp* 2001;232:144-152.
31. Wozney JM, Rosen V, Celeste AJ, et al: Novel regulators of bone formation: Molecular clones and activities. *Science* 1988;242(4885):1528-1534.
32. Pizette S, Niswander L: BMPs are required at two steps of limb chondrogenesis: Formation of prechondrogenic condensations and their differentiation into chondrocytes. *Dev Biol* 2000;219(2):237-249.
33. Yoon BS, Ovchinnikov DA, Yoshii I, Mishina Y, Behringer RR, Lyons KM: Bmpr1a and Bmpr1b have overlapping functions and are essential for chondrogenesis in vivo. *Proc Natl Acad Sci U S A* 2005;102(14):5062-5067.
34. Zou H, Wieser R, Massagué J, Niswander L: Distinct roles of type I bone morphogenetic protein receptors in the formation and differentiation of cartilage. *Genes Dev* 1997;11(17):2191-2203.
35. Minina E, Kreschel C, Naski MC, Ornitz DM, Vortkamp A: Interaction of FGF, Ihh/Pthlh, and BMP signaling integrates chondrocyte proliferation and hypertrophic differentiation. *Dev Cell* 2002;3(3):439-449.

36. Graham A: Vertebrate evolution: Turning heads. *Curr Biol* 2005;15(18):R764-R766.

37. Hall BK, Miyake T: All for one and one for all: Condensations and the initiation of skeletal development. *BioEssays* 2000;22(2):138-147.

38. Aubin JE: Advances in the osteoblast lineage. *Biochem Cell Biol* 1998;76(6):899-910.

39. Ducy P, Zhang R, Geoffroy V, Ridall AL, Karsenty G: Osf2/Cbfa1: A transcriptional activator of osteoblast differentiation. *Cell* 1997;89(5):747-754.

40. Nakashima K, Zhou X, Kunkel G, et al: The novel zinc finger-containing transcription factor Osterix is required for osteoblast differentiation and bone formation. *Cell* 2002;108(1):17-29.

41. Yang X, Karsenty G: ATF4, the osteoblast accumulation of which is determined post-translationally, can induce osteoblast-specific gene expression in non-osteoblastic cells. *J Biol Chem* 2004;279(45):47109-47114.

42. Ichida F, Nishimura R, Hata K, et al: Reciprocal roles of MSX2 in regulation of osteoblast and adipocyte differentiation. *J Biol Chem* 2004;279(32):34015-34022.

43. Jabs EW, Müller U, Li X, et al: A mutation in the homeodomain of the human MSX2 gene in a family affected with autosomal dominant craniosynostosis. *Cell* 1993;75(3):443-450.

CHAPTER 12

Metabolism

ELIZABETH W. HUBBARD, MD

ABSTRACT

The skeletal system is involved in complex interactions with multiple organ systems, including the renal, gastrointestinal, and endocrine systems. The main determinant of bone mineralization and turnover is the need to maintain calcium homeostasis. However, phosphate and vitamin D metabolism, nutritional status, hormonal status, and physical activity also play key roles in bone metabolism and bone turnover.

Keywords: bone metabolism; bone mineralization; calcium; hyperparathyroidism; phosphate; rickets; vitamin D

INTRODUCTION

The skeletal system can be perceived as a stagnant structure that serves as both a scaffold for soft tissue and a protective structure for internal organs. However, the bone is a complex organism that is in a constant state of remodeling. This process requires a complex interaction between osteoblasts, osteocytes, and osteoclasts.

Osteoblasts release type 1 collagen as well as noncollagenous proteins, which combine to form osteoid, the unmineralized matrix that is the basis for new bone.[1] Deposition of calcium and phosphate converts osteoid into the mature mineralized matrix of bone. Once an osteoblast is surrounded by mineralized matrix, the cells change and become osteocytes.

Changing from an osteoblast to osteocyte requires a transition from the initial cuboid shape to a smaller central cell body with long tentacles that extend through the mineralized matrix. The dendritic processes create a network that spans the entire bone and can also extend into bone marrow and vascular channels.[1,2] This creates a network that allows osteocytes to communicate with one another as well as a potential route that osteocytes can secrete hormones that alter remote organ systems. Osteocytes are involved in sensing the mechanical loads applied to the bone as well as play a role in bone remodeling and calcium and phosphate homeostasis.[3,4]

Osteoclasts are the cells that break down the extracellular matrix of the bone. Osteoclasts are not always present and activated. Instead, osteoblasts, osteocytes, and other stromal cells release receptor activator of nuclear factor-κ B ligand (RANKL), which stimulates the precursor hematopoietic cells to both travel toward a specific region of the bone and combine with one another to form the multinucleated cell, which is the mature osteoclast.[1] This multinucleated cell then attaches to the edge of the bone and secretes protons and proteolytic enzyme that break down the matrix and release calcium and phosphate. Although RANKL stimulates osteoclast formation and ultimately bone matrix degradation, osteoblasts also produce osteoprotegerin. Osteoprotegerin binds available RANKL and inhibits it from stimulating osteoclasts and pre-osteoclasts, thereby inhibiting bone resorption.[5] Varying the concentrations of RANKL and osteoprotegerin is a determinate of osteoclast activity and rate of bone resorption.

Bone mass is determined by the balance between bone formation and bone degradation. The musculoskeletal system plays an integral role in calcium-phosphate homeostasis, and as a result, calcium homeostasis is the primary determinate in the balance of bone formation and degradation.[6] Hormones, such as estrogen, play a secondary role in determining bone mass. Physical force also plays a role, but the body's response to mechanical loads is a less potent determinant of bone mass compared with calcium homeostasis and hormonal effects.[7]

Dr. Hubbard or an immediate family member serves as an unpaid consultant to Orthofix, Inc.

CALCIUM HOMEOSTASIS

The skeletal system acts as a reservoir for 99% of the body's calcium. It is complexed with phosphate to form hydroxyapatite [$Ca_5(PO_4)_6(OH)_2$].[6,8] About 40% of the extracellular calcium is complexed with plasma proteins, particularly albumin, whereas the remainder is either complexed with anions or exists as free ionized calcium.[9] The free ionized calcium (Ca^{2+}) is the only biologically active form of calcium in the body. It is typically maintained at a concentration of 5 mg/dL, whereas the total calcium level in the blood is about 10 mg/dL. Changes in the free ionized calcium concentration can have profound complications. For this reason, the free ionized calcium concentration is carefully controlled by the interaction of multiple signaling pathways.

Calcium plays a critical role in neurologic and muscular signaling pathways. Hypocalcemia causes increased excitability of nerves and muscle resulting in tingling, paresthesia, muscle cramping, and hyperreflexia. In contrast, hypercalcemia can cause hyporeflexia, lethargy, and potentially death.[9] Changes in calcium concentration can be due to changes in available extracellular protein concentration, such as hypoalbuminemia in the setting of malnutrition, alterations of acid-base balance, or disruption of the hormonal pathways involved in calcium homeostasis. The skeletal system is used as a source for calcium when the calcium concentration starts to decline as well as a repository for calcium when the concentration begins to rise.[8] Absorption and deposition in the skeletal system also need to balance calcium absorption from the gastrointestinal tract and excretion via the renal system to effectively maintain homeostasis. Alterations in any of these pathways can affect how the calcium is being stored within the skeletal system.

Vitamin D also has a major role in maintaining calcium homeostasis. The precursors of vitamin D are created within the skin in response to ultraviolet light or absorbed from the gut, as calciferol (D2) or cholecalciferol (D3).[6] The liver then converts D2 and D3 to 25-hydroxyvitamin D. This is then converted to either 24,25-dihydroxyvitamin D or 1,25-dihydroxyvitamin D in the kidney.[9] The 1,25-dihydroxyvitamin D is the most potent form and acts both independently and in conjunction with parathyroid hormone (PTH) to help increase calcium bioavailability, but the ratio of 1,25-dihydroxyvitamin D to 24,25-dihydroxyvitamin D is directly related to serum calcium concentration. Low serum calcium combined with elevated PTH levels stimulates increased production of 1,25-dihydroxyvitamin D, which in turn helps increase calcium absorption in the gut and reabsorption in the renal tubules.[6] Elevated serum calcium and phosphate levels combined with low PTH result in greater production of the 24,25-dihydroxyvitamin D, resulting in diminished calcium absorption and reabsorption.[9]

PTH is the primary hormone involved in calcium homeostasis. The chief cells of the parathyroid gland release PTH in response to hypocalcemia.[10,11] In the gut and kidney, PTH acts with 1,25-dihydroxyvitamin D to stimulate calcium absorption from the gastrointestinal tract and reabsorption in the renal tubules to help increase calcium levels.[12] Simultaneously, PTH directly activates osteoblasts to directly degrade surrounding osteoid to release calcium. PTH also drives osteoblasts to increase production of RANKL, which ultimately stimulates both production and activity of osteoclasts, leading to further bone matrix degradation and calcium release.[12] PTH also prevents phosphate reabsorption in the renal tubules, which decreases the overall availability of phosphate.[9] This prevents formation of hydroxyapatite, resulting in increased calcium concentration.

Conditions that alter the available PTH concentration can have significant effects on bone mass. Under normal conditions, the release of PTH is tightly regulated and correlated with the serum calcium concentration. Hypocalcemia triggers the release of intracellular stores of PTH and also triggers an increase in production of PTH mRNA, which allows the parathyroid glands to both respond to hypocalcemia quickly and have the ability to sustain the release of PTH over time if needed.[10-13] In contrast, hypercalcemia leads to degradation of intracellular PTH stores and leads to reduced PTH mRNA production.[13] Most patients with primary hyperparathyroidism have an adenoma, which secretes PTH. The cells within the adenoma do not respond to the feedback loops that normally regulate PTH secretion, so PTH secretion is sustained, despite hypercalcemia. This results in persistent release of RANKL from osteoblasts, resulting in excessive osteoclast recruitment and activation and sustained bone resorption.[6] This condition is known as osteitis fibrosa cystica, and these patients develop generalized bone weakness, which can result in abnormal bowing and fragility fractures.[14-17]

Secondary hyperparathyroidism is typically triggered by chronic renal insufficiency. Renal insufficiency results in a decreased production of 1,25-dihydroxyvitamin D.[18,19] This results in diminished calcium absorption from the gastrointestinal tract as well as increased phosphate retention in the kidneys. Both the hypocalcemia and hyperphosphatemia trigger an increased production and release of PTH.[12] In addition, the impaired production of 1,25-dihydroxyvitamin D compounds the PTH release, as 1,25-dihydroxyvitamin D normally acts to suppress PTH.[20,21] Unlike primary hyperparathyroidism, the resulting sustained bone resorption is the body's way of

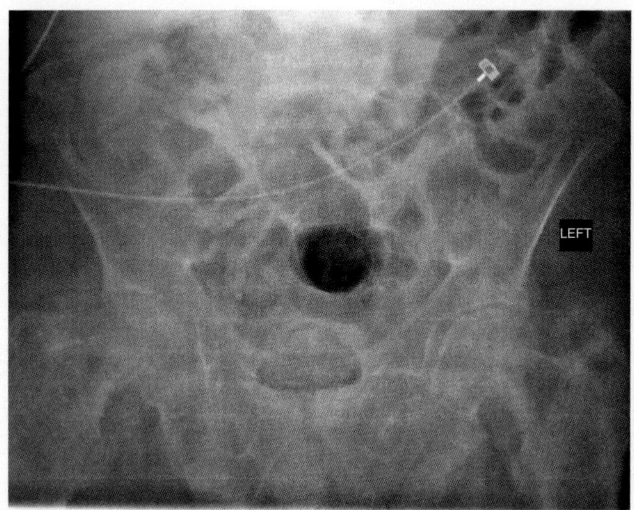

FIGURE 1 AP pelvis radiograph from a patient with chronic renal failure and severe osteoporosis due to secondary hyperparathyroidism. This patient presented with 2 weeks of progressive bilateral groin pain with no history of trauma and diagnosed with bilateral nondisplaced femoral neck fractures.

compensating for the hypocalcemia caused by the renal insufficiency. Severe forms of this result in renal osteodystrophy which, like osteitis fibrosis cystica, can result in abnormal bowing deformities and fragility fractures[19] (**Figure 1**).

Parathyroid hormone–related peptide (PTHrP) is similar but structurally larger and more complex than PTH.[12] It was originally described as a source of hypercalcemia of malignancy.[22-24] As with primary hyperparathyroidism, the neoplastic cells that secrete PTHrP do not respond to the standard negative feedback loops, resulting in sustained hypercalcemia and bone resorption. However, unlike primary hyperparathyroidism, patients have low PTH levels because the parathyroid glands respond appropriately to the hypercalcemia. More recently, additional roles of PTHrP have been identified, although they are less well understood. PTHrP has been shown to be important in maintaining fetal calcium levels and is critical during fetal skeletal development.[25,26]

PHOSPHATE HOMEOSTASIS

Similar to calcium, the skeletal system is the primary repository for most of the phosphate in the body, with about 80% to 90% of phosphate stored as hydroxyapatite within mineralized bone matrix.[27] The remaining is found within soft tissue and in the extracellular fluid. Phosphate is absorbed in the gastrointestinal tract and enters the extracellular fluid. Incorporation into the skeletal system is a passive process as phosphate gets incorporated into hydroxyapatite crystals.[28] Release of phosphate from the hydroxyapatite is driven by mechanisms designed to release calcium from bone rather than an active process to alter serum phosphate levels. However, the degree to which phosphate is reabsorbed from the renal tubules is actively regulated and affected by the concentration of PTH, which inhibits phosphate reabsorption, thereby increasing its excretion in the urine.[27]

RICKETS

Rickets is a disorder of formation of the immature skeletal system. It is caused by impaired endochondral ossification at the physes of long bones.[7] Radiographically, this results in widening and cupping deformities of the physes (**Figure 2**). It also leads to impaired longitudinal growth of long bones with resulting osteomalacia, bone softening due to impaired mineralization of the osteoid matrix.[29] Consequentially, in addition to the changes seen at the physes, patients with rickets develop long bones that are preternaturally short and often bowed. Internationally, the leading cause of rickets is vitamin D deficiency in the setting of malnutrition.[30] The vitamin D concentration within breast milk is low, so infants rely on both maternal intake of vitamin D and sunlight exposure to maintain their vitamin D levels.[31] Milk product supplementation with vitamin D has played a major role in reducing the incidence of vitamin D deficiency rickets in developed nations. Internationally, poverty and malnutrition can be compounded by a range of factors that limit ultraviolet light exposure and vitamin D production, including geographic location and distance from the equator, overcrowding of urban communities, and cultural factors that affect clothing choices.[32] The American Academy of Pediatrics recommends the infants of age 0 to 12 months receive 400 IU of vitamin D daily and children older than 12 months receive 600 IU daily to prevent vitamin D–deficient rickets.[33] Poor calcium intake and resultant hypocalcemia can compound the effects of hypovitaminosis D, and the current recommendations for calcium intake are 1,300 mg/d in preadolescents and adolescents.[33]

Impaired vitamin D metabolism and abnormalities in the signaling pathway of vitamin D can also result in rickets, even in the presence of appropriate vitamin D intake and ultraviolet light exposure. The enzyme 1-alpha-hydroxylase converts 25-hydroxyvitamin D to the active form 1,25-dihydroxyvitamin D. Patients with 1-alpha-hydroxylase deficiency present very early in life because of severe hypocalcemia.[34] These infants can demonstrate muscle weakness, gross motor delay, general growth retardation, and seizures. Laboratory studies demonstrate severe hypocalcemia, very low 1,25-dihydroxyvitamin D, high PTH, and high alkaline phosphatase but normal levels of 25-hydroxyvitamin D.[35]

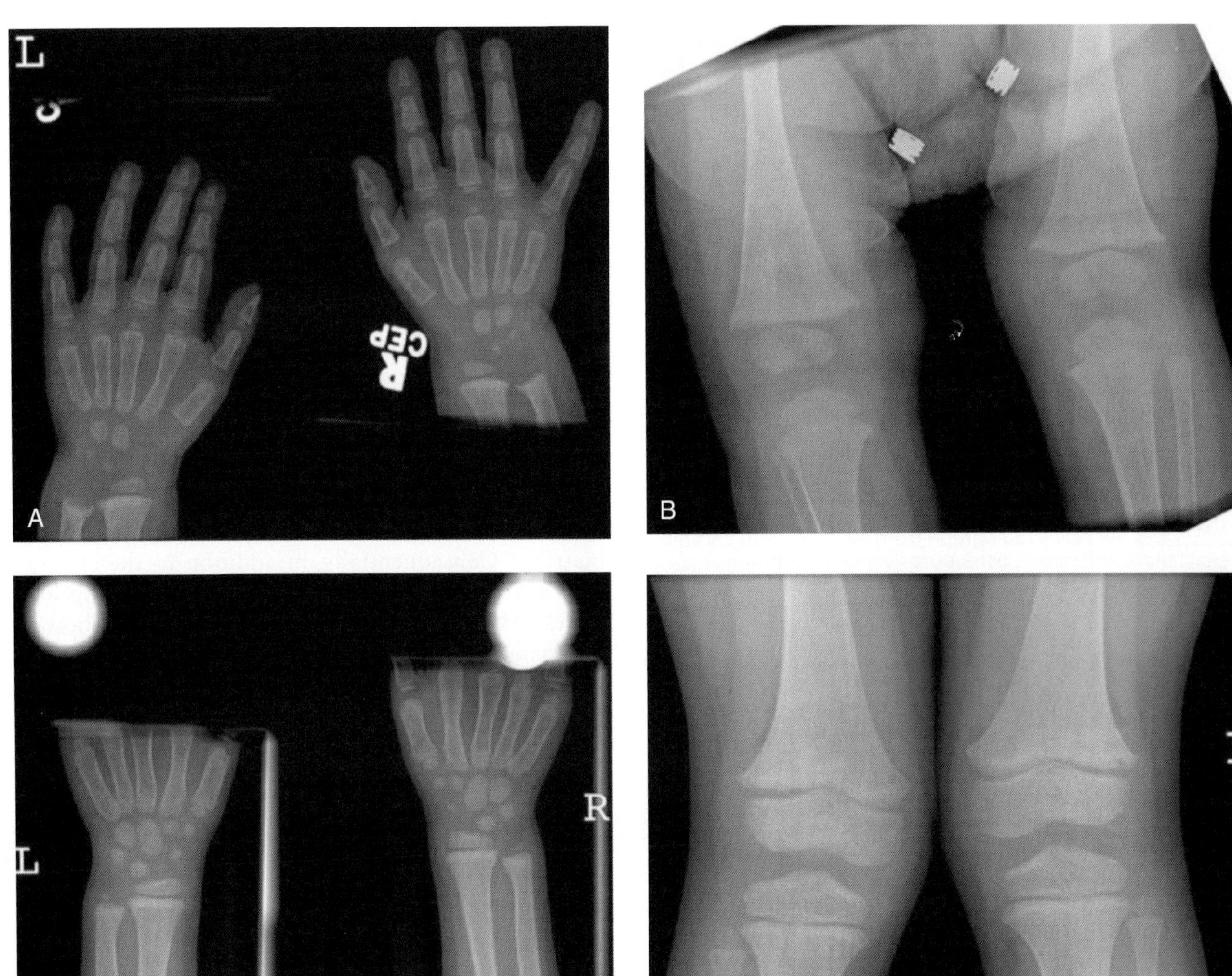

FIGURE 2 Radiographic changes associated with vitamin D–deficient rickets. **A** and **B**, Radiographs demonstrate physeal widening and cupping seen in a 1-year-old child diagnosed with hypophosphatemic rickets. **C** and **D**, Radiographs demonstrate resolution of the radiographic features after medical management. (Reprinted with permission from Howard AW, Alman BA: Metabolic and endocrine abnormalities, in Weinstein SL, Flynn JM: *Lovell & Winter's Pediatric Orthopaedics*, ed 7. Wolters Kluwer, 2014.)

These patients are treated with oral supplementation of the activated form of vitamin D_3, which circumvents the impaired enzyme.

In contrast, patients with vitamin D–resistant rickets have normal 1-alpha-hydroxylase function, and therefore normal production of 1,25-dihydroxyvitamin D, but a mutation in the vitamin D receptor leads to end-organ insensitivity to vitamin D.[36] These patients also have clinical and radiographic manifestations of rickets but can have significantly elevated levels of 1,25-dihydroxyvitamin D. In addition, most of these patients have very limited body hair or complete alopecia, which can be an early clinical finding and is unique to this form of rickets.[37] Some patients can have clinical improvement with administration of high levels of vitamin D_3. Successful clinical improvement has also been seen when patients are treated with high levels of intravenous elemental calcium, but this requires sustained supplementation for several years and also has significant health risks relating to the effects of hypercalcemia.[34]

In the United States, the most common form of rickets is X-linked hypophosphatemic rickets.[38] This form of rickets is related to impaired renal absorption of phosphate. This is an X-linked dominant condition in which there is a mutation in the production of the PHEX enzyme, which regulates the bioavailability of fibroblast growth factor-23 (FGF-23).[39,40] In the absence of PHEX enzymatic activity, FGF-23 levels rise, resulting in downregulation of the sodium-phosphate transporters that allow for reabsorption of phosphate in the renal tubules. In addition, FGF-23 suppresses 1-alpha-hydroxylase function, resulting in decreased levels of 1,25-dihydroxyvitamin D in patients with X-linked hypophosphatemic rickets.[39] These patients are treated with calcitriol but can still develop mild short stature as well as long bone angular deformities, which may require surgical intervention[41,42] (**Figure 3**). Autosomal dominant and autosomal recessive forms of hypophosphatemic rickets have also been identified, but these are less common and involve other alterations in the metabolic pathways that affect renal reabsorption of phosphate. In addition, mutations that affect FGF-23 levels independent of PHEX enzyme activity have also been identified and can result in a similar clinical picture to X-linked hypophosphatemic rickets.[40]

Alkaline phosphatase is an enzyme involved in normal bone mineralization and phosphate metabolism. It plays a critical role in the synthesis of inorganic phosphate necessary for osteoid production and mineralization. Elevated levels of alkaline phosphatase are a sign of active bone formation and remodeling. Hypophosphatasia is a rare disorder that results in alkaline phosphatase deficiency and creates a clinical picture similar to rickets.[43] Multiple genetic mutations resulting in hypophosphatasia have been identified. The most severe form is lethal in the perinatal period, but infants with other forms of hypophosphatasia can develop failure to thrive, increased intracranial pressure, and craniosynostosis.[44] These patients also have abnormal dentition and early tooth loss.

HORMONAL EFFECTS ON BONE MASS

Hormones can have a significant effect on bone mass. Estrogen seems to have the strongest effect, with increased estrogen levels being linked to improved bone mass.[45,46] Although the mechanism is not well understood, this relationship was the basis for hormonal supplementation for postmenopausal women as a means to prevent osteoporosis. However, this treatment is no longer widely recommended given the demonstrated increased risk of heart disease–related morbidity and mortality among women receiving hormonal supplementation.[47] Similarly, children who are born with an impaired ability to produce estrogen, such as Turner syndrome, can have significant morbidity related to low bone density.[48] Androgen levels also affect bone mass, with low levels being tied to diminished mass. However, these pathways are not well understood.[7,49]

Corticosteroids can also significantly alter bone density. The adrenal glands produce glucocorticoids that have widespread effects on metabolism, the

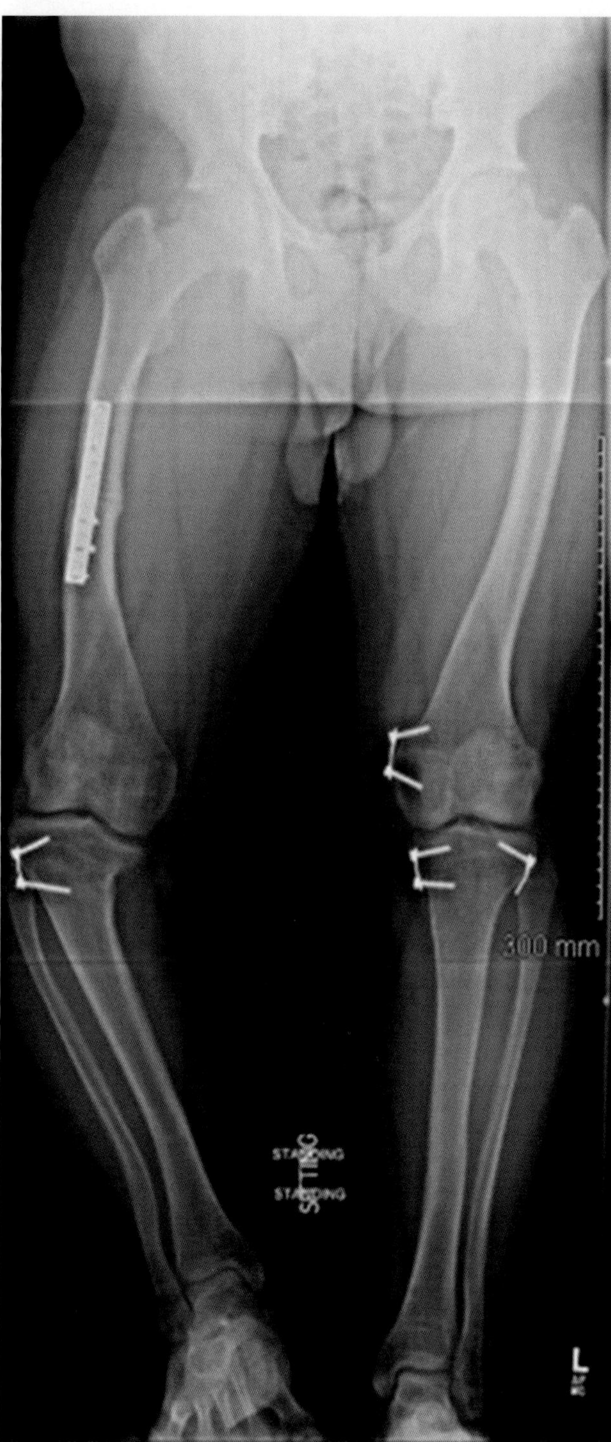

FIGURE 3 Long-standing radiograph from a 15-year-old boy with hypophosphatemic rickets and right knee pain. The patient presented with persistent right genu varum despite prior attempted surgical management with corrective osteotomies and growth modulation on the femoral and tibial sides.

immune system, the skeletal system, and the gastrointestinal tract. Excessive exposure to cortisol and other glucocorticoids can result in decreased type 1 collagen production, decreased production of osteoid

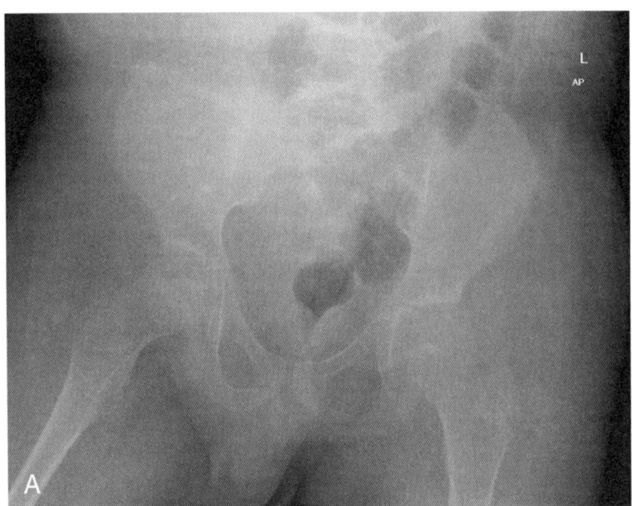

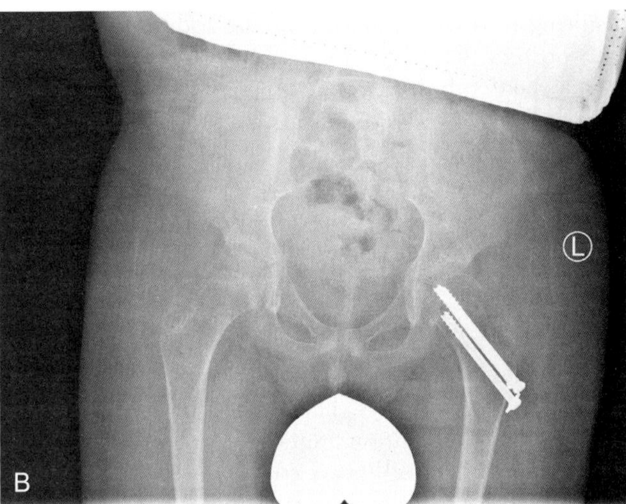

FIGURE 4 Radiographs from a 12-year-old boy with Duchenne muscular dystrophy and a left femoral neck fracture. The patient sustained a mild displaced left femoral neck fracture when attempting to transfer from a wheelchair to a regular chair at school (**A**). The patient underwent closed reduction and percutaneous screw fixation with three cannulated screws, and radiographs demonstrated fracture healing at his 6-week postoperative visit (**B**).

by osteoblasts, and reduced calcium absorption from the gastrointestinal tract, resulting in osteomalacia.[6] In the pediatric orthopaedic patient, this is well demonstrated in patients with Duchenne muscular dystrophy. Because of absent or limited dystrophin production, these patients have accelerated degeneration of the extracellular matrix of smooth and skeletal muscle. Historically, patients with Duchenne muscular dystrophy demonstrated early onset weakness with progressive loss of gross motor skills, decreased ability to ambulate independently, and then ultimately early mortality relating to pulmonary and cardiac failure.[50] However, sustained treatment with corticosteroids such as prednisone or fluticasone slows the rate of disease progression.[51-53] These patients remain ambulatory longer and are significantly less likely to develop scoliosis.[51,54,55] However, there are significant drawbacks to sustained corticosteroid therapy relating to the widespread effects on multiple organ systems. Despite being more mobile, the altered glucose metabolism contributes to excessive weight gain.[56] Because of the effects on osteoblast function and decreased collagen production, patients develop osteomalacia and are predisposed to fragility fractures[57,58] (**Figure 4**). The steroids can also interfere with wound and bone healing in patients who undergo surgery to address fractures. Because of the known complications of corticosteroid therapy, the decision to use fluticasone or prednisone can be a difficult choice for patients and families. New advances in gene therapy for patients with Duchenne muscular dystrophy offer a promising alternative to steroid treatment, but early clinical trials are still ongoing, and this is not widely available.[59]

PHYSICAL ACTIVITY

Osteocytes can detect and signal information regarding the mechanical loads applied to the skeletal system to other osteocytes.[1] Physical activity, including running and weight lifting, has been shown to have beneficial effects for building bone mass in younger adults and preserving bone mass in older adults.[60-62] Compared with the need to maintain calcium homeostasis and the effects of hormones, physical activity has the least overall effect on bone density.[7] However, in the pediatric population, nonambulatory or minimally ambulatory patients are at risk for significant osteopenia and fragility fractures. This has been a particular problem in patients with cerebral palsy, who are minimally ambulatory or nonambulatory.[63] For these patients, supplemental calcium and vitamin D are recommended to try to help prevent progressive osteopenia, and in specific instances, initiating osteoporosis treatment with medications such as diphosphonates can be beneficial to prevent serial fractures.[64,65]

SUMMARY

Bones are constantly undergoing a process of breakdown and remodeling, both as a response to complex signaling pathways designed to minimize fluctuations in our systemic calcium and phosphate levels and in response to physical stress. This requires interactions between the renal, gastrointestinal, and endocrine systems as well as local signalizing between osteoblasts, osteocytes, and osteoclasts within bone. A disruption of these interactions can have a profound effect on the integrity of the skeletal system as well as affect a patient's overall health.

KEY STUDY POINTS

- The skeletal system is the body's main repository for calcium and plays a critical role in maintaining calcium homeostasis.
- Skeletal remodeling is the result of a complex interaction of endocrine and paracrine signaling, resulting in changes to the activity of osteoblasts, osteoclasts, and osteocytes.
- Genetic and acquired disorders of the renal, endocrine, and gastrointestinal systems can result in altered phosphate, vitamin D, and calcium metabolism, resulting in significant changes in bone formation and skeletal remodeling.
- Physical activity and weight bearing affect bone turnover and bone density. Patients who are nonambulatory due to chronic underlying conditions, such as cerebral palsy, can be at significant risk for osteoporosis and fragility fractures.

ANNOTATED REFERENCES

1. Jahn K, Bonewald LF: Bone cell biology: Osteoclasts, osteoblasts, osteocytes, in Glorieux FH, Pettifor JM, Jüppner H, eds: *Pediatric Bone*. Amsterdam, the Netherlands, Academic Press, 2012, pp 1-7.
2. Kerschnitzki M, Kollmannsberger P, Burghammer M, et al: Architecture of the osteocyte network correlates with bone material quality. *J Bone Miner Res* 2013;28:1837-1845.
3. Raggatt LJ, Partridge NC: Cellular and molecular mechanisms of bone remodeling. *J Biol Chem* 2010;285:25103-25108.
4. Schaffler MB, Cheung WY, Majeska R, Kennedy O: Osteocytes: Master orchestrators of bone. *Calcif Tissue Int* 2014;94:5-24.
5. Bradley EW, Oursler MJ: Osteoclast culture and resorption assays. *Methods Mol Biol* 2008;455:19-35.
6. Costanzo LS: Endocrine physiology, in Costanzo LS, ed: *Physiology*, ed 6. Philadelphia, PA, Elsevier, 2018, pp 395-460.

   The author details the pathways of normal physiology for the human body. Her embryology chapter details the way calcium homeostasis is maintained as well as the effects of failure to maintain calcium homeostasis.
7. Howard AW, Alman BA: Metabolic and endocrine abnormalities, in Lovell WW, Weinstein SL, Flynn JM, eds: *Lovell and Winter's Pediatric Orthopaedics*, ed 7. Philadelphia, PA, Wolters Kluwer Health, 2014, vol 1, pp 140-176.
8. Maes C, Kronenberg HM: Bone development and remodeling, in Jameson JL, ed: *Endocrinology: Adult & Pediatric*, ed 7. Philadelphia, PA, Elsevier Saunders, 2016, pp 1038-1062.

   This a two-volume text detailing the function and regulation of the endocrine system in pediatric and adult patients. The authors described the mechanisms of bone development as well as principles of remodeling and regulation of bone mass.
9. Costanzo LS: Renal physiology, in Costanzo LS, ed: *Physiology*, ed 6. Philadelphia, PA, Elsevier, 2018, pp 245-310.

   The author details the pathways of normal physiology for the human body. The renal chapter details the specific pathways by which calcium and phosphate are managed in the kidneys as well as the role the renal system plays in vitamin D metabolism.
10. Brown EM: Extracellular Ca^{2+} sensing, regulation of parathyroid cell function, and role of Ca^{2+} and other ions as extracellular (first) messengers. *Physiol Rev* 1991;71:371-411.
11. Hanley DA, Takatsuki K, Sultan JM, Schneider AB, Sherwood LM: Direct release of parathyroid hormone fragments from functioning bovine parathyroid glands in vitro. *J Clin Invest* 1978;62:1247-1254.
12. Potts JT, Gardella TJ: Parathyroid hormone and calcium homeostasis, in Glorieux FH, Pettifor JM, Jüppner H, eds: *Pediatric Bone*. Amsterdam, the Netherlands, Academic Press, 2012, pp 109-140.
13. Habener JF, Kemper B, Potts JT Jr: Calcium-dependent intracellular degradation of parathyroid hormone: A possible mechanism for the regulation of hormone stores. *Endocrinology* 1975;97:431-441.
14. Silverberg SJ, Bilezikian JP: Primary hyperparathyroidism, in Jameson JL, ed: *Endocrinology: Adult & Pediatric*, ed 7. Philadelphia, PA, Elsevier Saunders, 2016, pp 1105-1124.

    This a two-volume text detailing the function and regulation of the endocrine system in pediatric and adult patients. The authors detail the pathology, clinical presentation, and multiorgan effects of primary hyperparathyroidism.
15. Walker MD, Silverberg SJ: Primary hyperparathyroidism. *Nat Rev Endocrinol* 2018;14:115-125.

    This is a review of etiology and management of primary hyperparathyroidism, with a discussion on both surgical and medical treatment options for patients. Level of evidence: IV.
16. Silverberg SJ, Shane E, de la Cruz L, et al: Skeletal disease in primary hyperparathyroidism. *J Bone Miner Res* 1989;4:283-291.
17. Khan AA, Hanley DA, Rizzoli R, et al: Primary hyperparathyroidism: Review and recommendations on evaluation, diagnosis, and management. A Canadian and international consensus. *Osteoporos Int* 2017;28:1-19.

    This is a review of the management of primary hyperparathyroidism and recommendations for patient evaluation, diagnosis, and treatment. Level of evidence: II.
18. Portillo MR, Rodriguez-Ortiz ME: Secondary hyperparthyroidism: Pathogenesis, diagnosis, preventive and therapeutic strategies. *Rev Endocr Metab Disord* 2017;18:79-95.

    This study reviewed the effects of chronic renal failure on phosphate, vitamin D, and calcium, resulting in secondary hyperthyroidism. Authors also reviewed the latest evidence on treatment options. Level of evidence: II.

19. Jamal SA, Miller PD: Secondary and tertiary hyperparathyroidism. *J Clin Densitom* 2013;16:64-68.
20. Komaba H, Kakuta T, Fukagawa M: Management of secondary hyperparathyroidism: How and why? *Clin Exp Nephrol* 2017;21:37-45.

    This is a review of current treatment options available for patients with secondary hyperparathyroidism. Authors also discuss that associated abnormalities in levels of PTH and FGF-23 these patients may have detrimental systemic effects that extend beyond the muscular skeletal system. Level of evidence: II.
21. Cocchiara G, Fazzotta S, Palumbo VD, et al: The medical and surgical treatment in secondary and tertiary hyperparathyroidism [Review]. *Clin Ter* 2017;168:e158-e167.

    This is a review of causes and potential treatment options for patients with secondary and tertiary hyperparathyroidism. Level of evidence: II.
22. Albright F: Case records of the Massachusetts General Hospital; Case 27461. *N Engl J Med* 1941;225:789-791.
23. Stewart AF, Horst R, Deftos LJ, Cadman EC, Lang R, Broadus AE: Biochemical evaluation of patients with cancer-associated hypercalcemia: Evidence for humoral and nonhumoral groups. *N Engl J Med* 1980;303:1377-1383.
24. Goldner W: Cancer-related hypercalcemia. *J Oncol Pract* 2016;12:426-432.

    This is a review of the most common causes of hypercalcemia related to malignancy as well as diagnosis and treatment strategies for each. Level of evidence: II.
25. Kronenberg HM: PTHrP and skeletal development. *Ann N Y Acad Sci* 2006;1068:1-13.
26. Kovacs CS: Calcium, phosphorus, and bone metabolism in the fetus and newborn. *Early Hum Dev* 2015;91:623-628.
27. Bergwitz C, Jüppner H: Phosphate homeostasis regulatory mechanisms, in Glorieux FH, Pettifor JM, Jüppner H, eds: *Pediatric Bone: Biology & Diseases*, ed 2. Amsterdam, the Netherlands, Academic Press, 2012, pp 141-161.
28. Manghat P, Sodi R, Swaminathan R: Phosphate homeostasis and disorders. *Ann Clin Biochem* 2014;51:631-656.
29. Pettifor JM: Nutritional rickets, in Glorieux FH, Pettifor JM, Jüppner H, eds: *Pediatric Bone: Biology & Diseases*, ed 2. Amsterdam, the Netherlands, Academic Press, 2012, pp 625-654.
30. Creo AL, Thacher TD, Pettifor JM, Strand MA, Fischer PR: Nutritional rickets around the world: An update. *Paediatr Int Child Health* 2017;37:84-98.

    In this systematic review of causes of nutritional rickets, authors discussed the economic and cultural factors that contribute to the prevalence, causes, and potential preventative measures and treatment options for rickets in different geographic regions. Level of evidence: II.
31. Taylor SN, Wagner CL, Hollis BW: Vitamin D supplementation during lactation to support infant and mother. *J Am Coll Nutr* 2008;27:690-701.
32. Munns CF, Shaw N, Kiely M, et al: Global consensus recommendations on prevention and management of nutritional rickets. *J Clin Endocrinol Metab* 2016;101:394-415.

    In this consensus statement that defines nutritional rickets and reviews the diagnosis and clinical management of rickets and osteomalacia, authors reviewed the multifactorial risk factors for nutritional rickets and offer prevention recommendations including food fortification and supplementation. Level of evidence: IV.
33. Golden NH, Abrams SA, Committee on Nutrition: Optimizing bone health in children and adolescents. *Pediatrics* 2014;134:e1229-e1243.
34. Portale AA, Perwad F, Miller WL: Rickets due to hereditary abnormalities of vitamin D. Synthesis or action, in Glorieux FH, Pettifor JM, Jüppner H, eds: *Pediatric Bone: Biology & Diseases*, ed 2. Amsterdam, the Netherlands, Academic Press, 2012, pp 679-698.
35. Miller WL, Portale AA: Vitamin D biosynthesis and vitamin D 1α-hydroxylase deficiency. *Endocr Dev* 2003;6:156-174.
36. Marx SJ, Spiegel AM, Brown EM, et al: A familial syndrome of decrease in sensitivity to 1,25-dihydroxyvitamin D. *J Clin Endocrinol Metab* 1978;47:1303-1310.
37. Rosen JF, Fleischman AR, Finberg L, Hamstra A, DeLuca HF: Rickets with alopecia: An inborn error of vitamin D metabolism. *J Pediatr* 1979;94:729-735.
38. Bitzan M, Goodyer PR: Hypophosphatemic rickets. *Pediatr Clin North Am* 2019;66:179-207.

    This is a review of the cause, diagnosis, and treatment of hypophosphatemic rickets with a discussion on new therapeutic options available and potential pharmacologic treatment approaches being studied. Level of evidence: II.
39. Goldsweig BK, Carpenter TO: Hypophosphatemic rickets: Lessons from disrupted FGF23 control of phosphorus homeostasis. *Curr Osteoporos Rep* 2015;13:88-97.
40. Holm IA, Econs MJ, Carpenter TO: Familial hypophosphatemia and related disorders, in Glorieux FH, Pettifor JM, Jüppner H, eds: *Pediatric Bone: Biology & Diseases*, ed 2. Amsterdam, the Netherlands, Academic Press, 2012, pp 699-726.
41. Pavone V, Testa G, Gioitta Iachino S, Evola FR, Avondo S, Sessa G: Hypophosphatemic rickets: Etiology, clinical features and treatment. *Eur J Orthop Surg Traumatol* 2015;25:221-226.
42. Acar S, Demir K, Shi Y: Genetic causes of rickets. *J Clin Res Pediatr Endocrinol* 2017;9:88-105.

    This study reviewed the etiologies of various forms of rickets. The authors discussed vitamin D–related etiologies as well as syndromes involving phosphate metabolism. Clinical, laboratory, and genetic characteristics of various types of hereditary rickets as well as differential diagnosis and treatment approaches are covered. Level of evidence: II.
43. Whyte MP: Hypophosphatasia, in Glorieux FH, Pettifor JM, Jüppner H, eds: *Pediatric Bone: Biology & Diseases*, ed 2. Amsterdam, the Netherlands, Academic Press, 2012, pp 771-794.

44. Osteochondrodysplasias: Hypophosphatasia, in Jones KL, Jones MC, del Campo M, eds: *Smith's Recognizable Patterns of Human Malformation*, ed 7. Philadelphia, PA, Elsevier Saunders, 2013, p 506.

45. Vaananen HK, Harkonen PL: Estrogen and bone metabolism. *Maturitas* 1996;23(suppl):S65-S69.

46. Okano H: Calcium and bone metabolism across women's life stages. The effects of oral contraceptives/low dose estrogen-progestin on bone metabolism, bone mass and geometry in adolescent and young adult women [Japanese]. *Clin Calcium* 2017;27:661-671.

Estrogens have a biphasic action on pubertal and/or adolescent skeletal growth. Low levels of estrogen may increase the periosteal expansion through the increase in the sensitivity of bone for mechanical stimuli and the secretion of insulinlike growth factor-1. However, high estrogen concentrations may inhibit periosteal bone formation. Use of oral contraceptive/low-dose estrogen-progestin during adolescence, with exposure to high levels of estrogen, may prevent the acquisition of physiologic peak of bone mass. Level of evidence: III.

47. Cintron D, Rodriguez-Gutierrez R, Serrano V, Latortue-Albino P, Erwin PJ, Murad MH: Effect of estrogen replacement therapy on bone and cardiovascular outcomes in women with Turner syndrome: A systematic review and meta-analysis. *Endocrine* 2017;55:366-375.

In this meta-analysis of the effects of chronic estrogen replacement therapy in patients diagnosed with Turner syndrome, patients who received estrogen replacement, regardless of the route of administration, demonstrated improved bone mineral density. Authors were unable to conclude whether the improved density measured correlated with a clinical reduction in either osteoporosis or fragility fractures in this population based on the available evidence. Studies also showed increased low-density lipoprotein levels in patients receiving hormonal therapy, but there was insufficient evidence regarding whether increased low-density lipoprotein correlated with an increased cardiovascular risk in these patients. Level of evidence: II.

48. Nadeem M, Roche EF: Bone mineral density in Turner's syndrome and the influence of pubertal development. *Acta Paediatr* 2014;103:e38-e42.

49. Mohamad NV, Soelaiman IN, Chin KY: A concise review of testosterone and bone health. *Clin Interv Aging* 2016;11:1317-1324.

Although studies have shown that estrogen plays an important role in maintaining bone density, androgens play a critical role in osteoblast differentiation and development and ultimately in bone formation. Authors also reviewed available evidence on the effects androgens have on bone development. Level of evidence: II.

50. Yiu EM, Kornberg AJ: Duchenne muscular dystrophy. *J Paediatr Child Health* 2015;51:759-764.

51. McAdam LC, Mayo AL, Alman BA, Biggar WD: The Canadian experience with long-term deflazacort treatment in Duchenne muscular dystrophy. *Acta Myol* 2012;31:16-20.

52. Biggar WD, Politano L, Harris VA, et al: Deflazacort in Duchenne muscular dystrophy: A comparison of two different protocols. *Neuromuscul Disord* 2004;14:476-482.

53. Alman BA: Duchenne muscular dystrophy and steroids: Pharmacologic treatment in the absence of effective gene therapy. *J Pediatr Orthop* 2005;25:554-556.

54. Lebel DE, Corston JA, McAdam LC, Biggar WD, Alman BA: Glucocorticoid treatment for the prevention of scoliosis in children with Duchenne muscular dystrophy: Long-term follow-up. *J Bone Joint Surg Am* 2013;95:1057-1061.

55. Alman BA, Raza SN, Biggar WD: Steroid treatment and the development of scoliosis in males with Duchenne muscular dystrophy. *J Bone Joint Surg Am* 2004;86:519-524.

56. Salera S, Menni F, Moggio M, Guez S, Sciacco M, Esposito S: Nutritional challenges in Duchenne muscular dystrophy. *Nutrients* 2017;9(6):594.

In this study, the authors reviewed components of a multidisciplinary approach to nutrition in pediatric and adult patients with Duchenne muscular dystrophy. This study reviewed the literature on the prevalence and risks associated with overnutrition and undernutrition; gastrointestinal complications; infectious diseases; dysphagia; and reduced bone mass in this population. Level of evidence: III.

57. Bell JM, Shields MD, Watters J, et al: Interventions to prevent and treat corticosteroid-induced osteoporosis and prevent osteoporotic fractures in Duchenne muscular dystrophy. *Cochrane Database Syst Rev* 2017;1:CD010899.

In this meta-analysis of studies examining treatment of patients with Duchenne muscular dystrophy who have corticosteroid-induced osteoporosis, only two studies that met inclusion criteria for the review were identified, and these did not provide sufficient evidence to guide treatment for these patients. Level of evidence: II.

58. Ward LM, Hadjiyannakis S, McMillan HJ, Noritz G, Weber DR: Bone health and osteoporosis management of the patient with Duchenne muscular dystrophy. *Pediatrics* 2018;142:S34-S42.

This is an approach to the detection and management of poor bone health in patients with Duchenne muscular dystrophy. Authors discussed the importance of early detection of compromised bone health as well as therapeutic treatments for symptomatic patients and medical management of osteoporosis. The article offers detailed recommendations of pharmacologic strategies available, including specific drugs, dosing, length of therapy, contraindications, and monitoring of treatment efficacy and safety. Level of evidence: III.

59. Duchene B, Iyombe-Engembe JP, Rousseau J, Tremblay JP, Ouellet DL: From gRNA identification to the restoration of dystrophin expression: A dystrophin gene correction strategy for Duchenne muscular dystrophy mutations using the CRISPR-induced deletion method. *Methods Mol Biol* 2018;1687:267-283.

This is a protocol of how CRISPR technology can be used to restore the dystrophin gene in patients with Duchenne muscular dystrophy. Level of evidence: II.

60. Scofield KL, Hecht S: Bone health in endurance athletes: Runners, cyclists, and swimmers. *Curr Sports Med Rep* 2012;11:328-334.

61. Ravnholt T, Tybirk J, Jorgensen NR, Bangsbo J: High-intensity intermittent "5-10-15" running reduces body fat, and increases lean body mass, bone mineral density, and performance in untrained subjects. *Eur J Appl Physiol* 2018;118:1221-1230.

In this study, untrained subjects initiated running regimens three times per week over a 7-week period. At the completion of training, subjects showed improvements in endurance and a reduction of body fat mass as well as lean body mass. Subjects also demonstrated both a significant increase in bone mineral density of 0.9% ($P < 0.01$) and significant increase in bone turnover markers as well as markers of collagen cross-linking. Level of evidence: II.

62. Watson SL, Weeks BK, Weis LJ, Harding AT, Horan SA, Beck BR: High-intensity resistance and impact training improves bone mineral density and physical function in postmenopausal women with osteopenia and osteoporosis: The LIFTMOR randomized controlled trial. *J Bone Miner Res* 2018;33:211-220.

In this study of 101 postmenopausal women randomized to initiate either a home-based weight training program or a high-intensity formal resistance and impact training program (HiRIT) over an 8-month period, subjects underwent dual-energy x-ray absorptiometry testing before and after the intervention. Compared with the home-based resistance training, subjects who underwent HiRIT showed improved bone density measures both in the proximal femur and lumbar spine with no significant difference in injury or complications relating to the training. Level of evidence: II.

63. Shin YK, Yoon YK, Chung KB, Rhee Y, Cho SR: Patients with non-ambulatory cerebral palsy have higher sclerostin levels and lower bone mineral density than patients with ambulatory cerebral palsy. *Bone* 2017;103:302-307.

This study provided a comparison of ambulatory status, bone mineral density, and sclerostin levels in patients with cerebral palsy. Compared with ambulatory patients, nonambulatory patients have both significantly lower bone density measures and elevated plasma sclerostin levels. Authors highlighted that sclerostin levels may be an important serum marker for fragility fracture risk in this population as well as a potential pharmacologic target for future treatment options. Level of evidence: III.

64. Houlihan CM: Bone health in cerebral palsy: Who's at risk and what to do about it? *J Pediatr Rehabil Med* 2014;7:143-153.

65. Trinh A, Fahey MC, Brown J, Fuller PJ, Milat F: Optimizing bone health in cerebral palsy across the lifespan. *Dev Med Child Neurol* 2017;59:232-233.

This is a summary of the osteoporosis care pathway published by the American Academy of Cerebral Palsy and Developmental Medicine. Authors reviewed the current literature and recommended the importance of diagnosis and treatment of hypogonadism in this population as well as the utility of alternative dual-energy x-ray absorptiometry (DXA) scanning sites and whole-body DXA scanning in this population. Level of evidence: II.

SECTION 3

Neuromuscular, Metabolic, and Inflammatory Disorders

Section Editor:

Henry G. Chambers, MD, FAAOS

CHAPTER 13

Cerebral Palsy

NIRAV K. PANDYA, MD • SCOTT P. KAISER, MD • RAVINDER BRAR, MD, MPH

ABSTRACT

Cerebral palsy is a static encephalopathy that affects movement, tone, and posture. This upper motor neuron syndrome is caused by injury to the immature brain in the prenatal, perinatal, or postnatal periods. The clinical manifestations of this disorder vary widely based on the location and degree of injury to the motor cortex. In addition, other areas of the brain may be affected, which leads to cognitive, speech, and sensory difficulties. Although it is considered a nonprogressive disorder, its effects on the skeleton can be progressive and children need to be routinely surveilled. Multiple advances have been made in the treatment of this disorder over the past several years.

Keywords: cerebral palsy; motor function; neuromuscular; spasticity; treatment

INTRODUCTION

Cerebral palsy (CP) is a static encephalopathy that affects movement, tone, and posture. It is caused by injury to the immature brain in the prenatal, perinatal, or postnatal periods. The clinical manifestations of this disorder vary widely based on the location and degree of injury to the motor cortex. In addition, other areas of the brain may be affected, which leads to cognitive, speech, and sensory difficulties. Although it is considered a nonprogressive disorder, its effects on the skeleton can be progressive and children need to be routinely surveilled. Multiple advances have been made in the treatment of this disorder over the past several years.

EPIDEMIOLOGY

CP is the most common motor disability in children and currently has a prevalence ranging from 1.5 to 4 individuals per 1,000 live births.[1] Approximately 1 in 323 children is identified with cerebral palsy.[2] In particular, low birth weight (less than 1,500 g) drastically increases the risk of this condition.[3] Additional risk factors include premature birth (before 31 weeks) and multiple births (ie, twins or triplets).[4,5] With improved neonatal care, there is an increased incidence.

In addition to motor disease, nearly 50% of patients have concurrent epilepsy.[2] Other manifestations include cognitive impairment, sensory deficits, strabismus, gastrointestinal dysfunction, impaired oral motor function, decreased bone mass, spasticity, contractures, urinary incontinence, and emotional and behavioral problems. Functionally, approximately 60% of patients with CP are able to walk independently, approximately 10% use a mobility device, and approximately 30% have limited or no walking ability.[2]

ETIOLOGY

The etiology of CP in most patients is unknown. Although prematurity combined with very low birth weight is a risk factor, full-term birth is more common than premature birth in patients with CP. Prenatal, perinatal, and postnatal causes also should be considered. In the prenatal period, congenital brain defects, intrauterine infections, placental complications, Rh/ABO hemolytic disease, fetal anoxia, coagulopathies, and maternal disease (ie, seizure,

Dr. Pandya or an immediate family member serves as a paid consultant to or is an employee of OrthoPediatrics and serves as a board member, owner, officer, or committee member of the Pediatric Orthopaedic Society of North America. Neither of the following authors nor any immediate family member has received anything of value from or has stock or stock options held in a commercial company or institution related directly or indirectly to the subject of this chapter: Dr. Kaiser and Dr. Brar.

hyperthyroidism, and chorioamnionitis) should be considered. Ischemic stroke is a major cause of CP in the perinatal period. Intracranial hemorrhage, hypoglycemia, trauma, hypoxic ischemic encephalopathy, infection, and hypothyroidism also are possible causes. A very small number of cases are caused by obstetric trauma. Possible postnatal causes of CP also include hypoxia, acidosis, bacterial meningitis, viral encephalitis, hyperbilirubinemia, traumatic brain injury, and toxin exposure. The common link, regardless of the specific etiology, is an insult to the developing motor system of the brain. This can include the motor cortex, but also includes the periventricular regions of the brain and, in those with associated dystonia, the basal ganglia.

DIAGNOSIS

Before the initiation of treatment, an appropriate diagnosis should be made. Because of the varied manifestations of the disorder, making a diagnosis of CP can be challenging for the clinician. From a global standpoint, a patient with a developmental delay and/or persistence of primitive reflexes may have CP. Many patients do not achieve gross motor milestones such as head control by the age of 2 months, the ability to sit by the age of 6 months, or the ability to walk by the age of 14 months. On physical examination, patients may exhibit preferential use of limbs and abnormal tone. The differential diagnosis should include other metabolic or neurodegenerative disorders, particularly if the neurologic manifestations are progressive or there is a loss of previously acquired motor milestones.[6] Laboratory studies can be used to investigate genetic, metabolic, and endocrine disorders. Although MRI findings have been shown to be abnormal in 86% of patients with CP (patients with ataxia are more likely to have normal MRI findings), there is substantial heterogeneity in the clinical meaning of these imaging findings.[7] As a result, CP is usually diagnosed using clinical methods.

CLASSIFICATION

Accurate classification of CP also can be challenging because of its heterogeneous presentations. Geographic, physiologic, and functional classifications have been developed. The pattern of limb involvement is described by the geographic classification and reflects the location of the insult to the motor cortex. Monoplegia (the involvement of one limb), hemiplegia (the involvement of both limbs on the same side), diplegia (greater involvement of both lower limbs than both upper limbs), and quadriplegia (all four/three limbs equally involved) are common geographic terms used to describe CP. Poor reliability has been reported with this classification system.[8]

Even in instances in which the geographic classification accurately describes the pattern of limb involvement, the manner in which the involvement manifests can vary. The physiologic classification attempts to describe the nature of the involvement. In the most common form, spastic, patients exhibit an increase in muscle tone with rapid passive stretching. Joint contractures are frequently present in patients with spasticity.[2,9] Spasticity is a stretch reflex disorder that involves the pyramidal area of the brain. It is both velocity dependent (worse when the stretch is faster) and length dependent (worse when the muscle is shorter).

When CP involves the extrapyramidal areas of the brain, patients exhibit dyskinesia, which manifests as involuntary motor movements. Athetosis (purposeless movements with rare joint contractures), choreiform (continual purposeless movements), and dystonia (increased tone without spasticity, clonus, or hyperreflexia) may be present. Rigidity may be present in patients with severe involvement, but this manifestation is rare in children with CP. If the cerebellum is involved, patients may exhibit ataxia. This condition is less common and involves difficulty with coordinated movements and balance, particularly walking. In addition, some patients may be hypotonic and exhibit low muscle tone in the context of normal reflexes.

Not all patients can receive an accurate diagnosis using these specific physiologic definitions, because some patients may have a mixture of disease manifestations resulting from injury to multiple overlapping areas of the brain.[9]

From an orthopaedic standpoint, interventions are chosen to optimize function. Although terms such as household ambulator and community ambulator attempt to capture the functional ability of patients with CP, they do not recognize the unique functional needs of this patient population. The Gross Motor Function Classification System (GMFCS) describes the functional abilities of patients with developmental differences[10] (**Figure 1**). Different age-based criteria have been developed.[11] The GMFCS focuses on functional limitations for certain motor tasks such as walking and sitting as well as the need for assistive devices. This system has been shown to be reliable for classifying patients and helping to determine proper interventions.[11-13]

GOAL SETTING

The orthopaedic surgeon is one member of a multidisciplinary team of healthcare providers that should be involved in the management of patients with CP. The clinicians should be able to make a correct diagnosis; determine the etiology of the disease (if possible); identify the type, extent, and severity of the neuromuscular deficit;

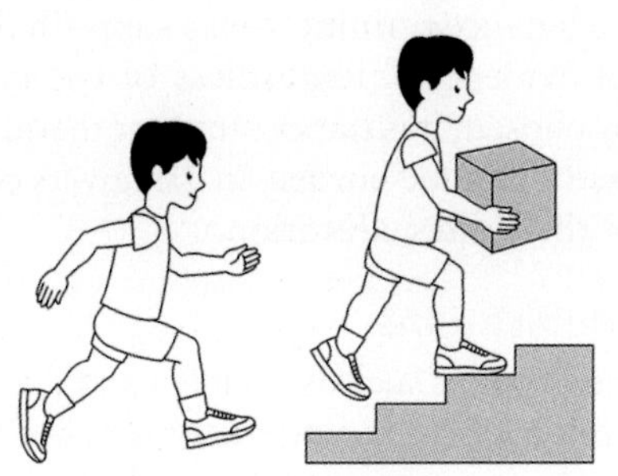

GMFCS Level I
Children walk at home, school, outdoors, and in the community. They can climb stairs without the use of a railing. Children perform gross motor skills such as running and jumping, but speed, balance, and coordination are limited.

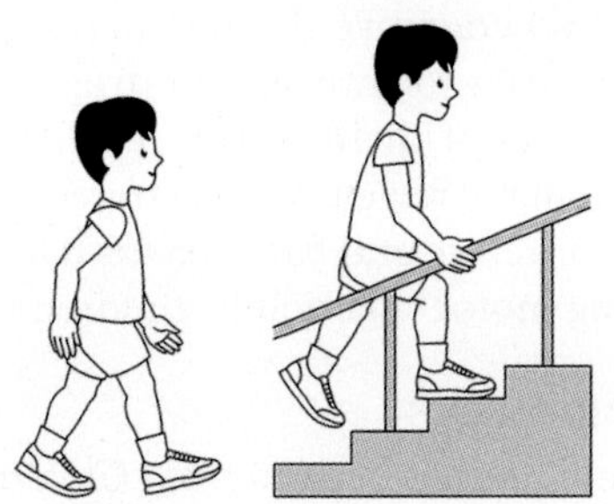

GMFCS Level II
Children walk in most settings and climb stairs holding onto a railing. They may experience difficulty walking long distances and balancing on uneven terrain, inclines, in crowded areas or confined spaces. Children may walk with physical assistance, a hand-held mobility device, or use wheeled mobility over long distances. Children have only minimal ability to perform gross motor skills such as running and jumping.

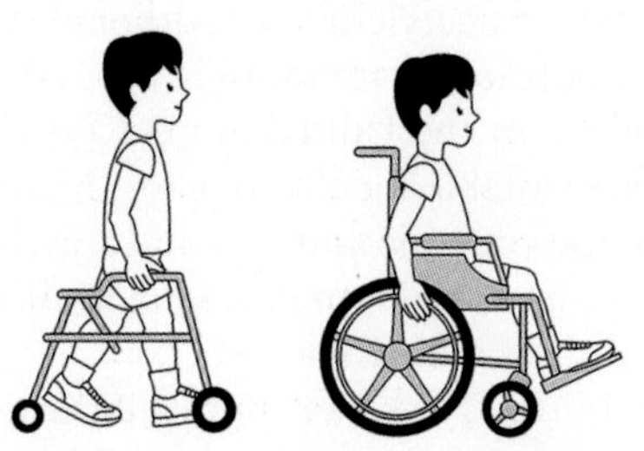

GMFCS Level III
Children walk using a hand-held mobility device in most indoor settings. They may climb stairs holding onto a railing with supervision or assistance. Children use wheeled mobility when traveling long distances and may self-propel for shorter distances.

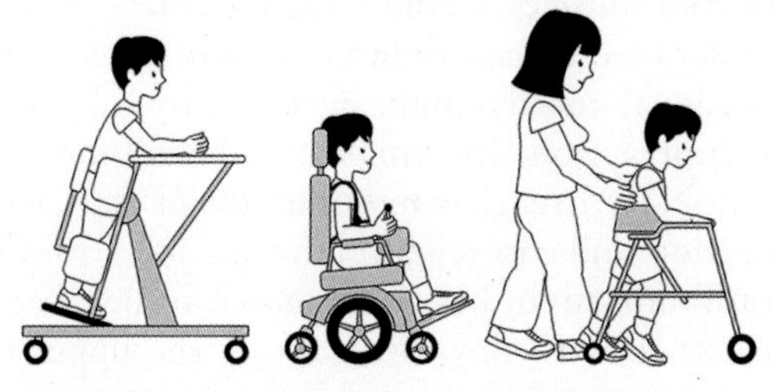

GMFCS Level IV
Children use methods of mobility that require physical assistance or powered mobility in most settings. They may walk for short distances at home with physical assistance or use powered mobility or a body support walker when positioned. At school, outdoors, and in the community, children are transported in a manual wheelchair or use powered mobility.

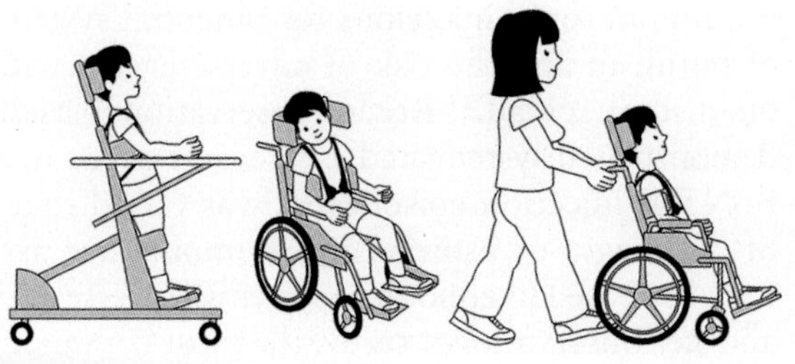

GMFCS Level V
Children are transported in a manual wheelchair in all settings. Children are limited in their ability to maintain antigravity head and trunk postures and control leg and arm movements.

FIGURE 1 Illustration of the expanded and revised Gross Motor Function Classification System (GMFCS) for children between the ages of 6 and 12 years. (Copyright Kerr Graham, Bill Reid, and Adrienne Harvey, The Royal Children's Hospital, Melbourne, Australia.)

and address any associated conditions. Multiple aspects of the patient's condition should be addressed, including the interplay between pathophysiology, organ dysfunction, task performance, roles (responsibilities in society), and the various influences of each of these factors.[14] In combination with the family and other healthcare providers, goals need to be established that address independence, working, communication, activities of daily living, mobility, and walking. It is important for clinicians to balance the perceived benefits of any intervention with the risks of disruption to education, social relationships, future employment, and independence. The clinicians and family should discuss treatments intended to correct the secondary issues resulting from the brain insult, not methods to reverse the brain injury.

Because goal setting for many caregivers focuses on the patient's ability to walk, clinicians should set realistic goals and discourage unrealistic expectations. Prognostic factors for poor ambulatory ability include the persistence of two or more primitive reflexes after the age of 1 year and the inability to sit independently by the age of 2 years.[15,16] It is critical to balance the patient's desire to walk with other desires such as the abilities to communicate and be mobile (not necessarily to achieve ambulation).

NONORTHOPAEDIC TREATMENT

Multiple nonsurgical and surgical treatment modalities are at the disposal of the clinician. A 2013 systematic review found the following interventions effective in the treatment of patients with CP: botulinum toxin, diazepam/baclofen, and selective dorsal rhizotomy (SDR) for reducing muscle spasticity; casting for improving and maintaining ankle range of motion; hip surveillance for maintaining hip joint integrity; various physical and occupational therapy programs for improving motor activity, self-care, and fitness; diphosphonates for treating low bone mineral density; pressure care for preventing ulcers; and anticonvulsant administration for managing seizures.[17]

Physical Therapy

Physical therapy is critical in the treatment of patients with CP, particularly before the age of 3 years and in postoperative periods. A 2013 study demonstrated a positive effect in older children with CP, but the largest effect was seen in younger patients and those with level II GMFCS.[18] However, the efficacy of physical therapy on the long-term function of patients with CP remains controversial. In a 2015 study that evaluated the effect of exercise on postural control in children with CP, the effectiveness of five interventions—gross motor task training, hippotherapy (horseback riding), treadmill training with no body-weight supported, trunk-targeted training, and reactive balance training—was supported by a moderate level of evidence.[19] Regardless of the type of physical therapy chosen, it is important that therapy programs do not place an undue burden on caregivers or unnecessarily disrupt the child's education.

Oral Medications

Oral medications such as baclofen and diazepam (gamma-aminobutyric acid receptor agonists) both act on spasticity by reducing muscle tone but also can cause sedation, balance and cognitive dysfunction, increased drooling, increased drug tolerance, and drug withdrawal symptoms because of their central mechanism of action. A 2016 systematic review demonstrated insufficient data to promote or refute oral baclofen for reducing spasticity or improving motor function in children with spastic CP.[20]

Botulinum Toxin

Botulinum toxin is derived from *Clostridium botulinum* and works at the neuromuscular junction by preventing the release of acetylcholine. Although there are several forms of botulinum toxin, only types A and B are available for use in the United States. Type A toxin, which has been available for the longest amount of time, lacks many of the systemic and regional anticholinergic effects of type B toxin, and more data are available regarding its use in patients with CP.

In 2015, the FDA has approved the use of botulinum toxin injections in treatment of children with upper and lower limb spasticity. Injections are performed in the affected muscles in the location where there is a preponderance of neuromuscular junctions. It is used to treat local and dynamic spasticity by suppressing muscle contraction. Intramuscular botulinum toxin type A (BoNT-A) reaches maximal effect by 4 weeks post-injection and can remain effective for 3 to 6 months.[21] Botulinum toxin has been shown to be effective when combined with physiotherapy in the upper limbs and improves ease of care and comfort for nonambulatory children.[22,23] The FDA issued a black box warning on botulinum toxin injections for potential systemic signs of botulism and the risk of adverse events with possible distant spread.[24] Recent observational studies have demonstrated systemic adverse events occur in 3.6% of BoNT-A injection episodes. It was found that history of dysphagia or aspiration pneumonia are associated with increased likelihood of systemic adverse events.[25] In another observational study, the most common adverse events were found to be mild and self-limiting. Still, the study noted that the GMFCS IV and V pediatric cohort had increased rates of systemic adverse events.[26]

Botulinum toxin injections have reliably improved joint range of motion and focal spasticity in the short term; however, there have been no long-term proven clinical benefits.[27] Botulinum toxin is also widely used in attempts to delay surgery. A randomized controlled trial comparing the effect of intramuscular BoNT-A adductor injections combined with hip abduction bracing treatment demonstrated no benefit in the prevention of progressive hip displacement.[28]

There has been increasing controversy and debate over the number of injection episodes patients should undergo before progression to surgical muscle-tendon lengthening. Muscle morphology in children with CP is known to be weaker secondary to loss of muscle mass, reduced contractile material, increased amounts of connective tissue and fat, and overstretched sarcomeres.[29] Historical animal studies demonstrated recovery of skeletal muscle after BoNT-A injection and reversible effects. The animal studies in 2009 demonstrate partial, incomplete recovery and acute muscle atrophy from the chemodenervation after BoNT-A injections.[30] Animal studies have also demonstrated deleterious osteopenic effects with incomplete recovery of bone density on the bone adjacent to the muscle injected.[29] There is renewed focus to find interventions to strengthen the muscles of children with CP and not deplete their skeletal muscle reserves with repeated injections. The transient therapeutic benefits of BoNT-A must be weighed against the long-term sarcopenic effects and potential loss of further muscle function.[29] Other therapies such as collagenase injections are being investigated.[31]

Intrathecal Baclofen

Because of its local administration, intrathecal baclofen (ITB) has a much lower risk of systemic adverse effects compared with oral baclofen. It is administered via a pump, which is implanted in the submuscular tissue of the anterior abdomen. The pump can be controlled by a clinician, who may vary the dosage based on the patient's clinical presentation. These pumps are generally used in nonambulatory patients with severe spasticity. A 2015 systematic review demonstrated a short-term benefit in the treatment of spasticity, with limited long-term data suggesting continued efficacy.[32] Complications with this treatment modality include infection, catheter problems, and pump malfunction. Because of limited battery life, these pumps should be reimplanted every 6 to 7 years. In addition, there is some concern that the incidence or progression of scoliosis is increased after pump insertion.

Selective Dorsal Rhizotomy

Selective dorsal rhizotomy (SDR) is a surgical, permanent procedure that decreases lower limb spasticity and tone by selectively cutting the dorsal afferent nerve fibers from L1 to S1. The major goal of SDR is to improve quality of gait by selectively decreasing tone. The ideal patient for this procedure is generally ambulatory, has spastic diplegia, and is aged 3 to 8 years. A preoperative evaluation is needed to assess the patient's ambulatory ability and strength (which should be good, particularly in the trunk) as well as his or her motivation and cognitive ability to engage in intensive physical therapy. A multidisciplinary healthcare team is necessary to assess a patient's suitability for the procedure and ensure a good postoperative outcome. Although reported results have been mixed, a retrospective review demonstrated that the benefits of SDR lasted throughout adolescence and early adulthood, particularly in patients with spastic diplegia at levels I through III GMFCS.[33] The benefits include decreased muscle tone, improved activities of daily living performance, and a decreased need for soft-tissue orthopaedic procedures and botulinum toxin injections. Some studies have demonstrated improvement in GMFCS level post-SDR.[34,35]

SDR addresses tone management, but does not change the bony abnormalities, dysplasia, or lever arm dysfunction of children with CP. Therefore, it does not decrease the need for bony surgeries, even though it may reduce the need for soft-tissue surgeries. When considering timing of orthopaedic interventions and SDR, orthopaedic surgery is usually delayed until at least one year post-SDR so as not affect the rehabilitation protocol after SDR. The few exceptions are progressive hip subluxation that may need to be addressed before SDR and equinus contracture that may impede plantigrade ambulation after SDR.[36] Classically, SDR is indicated for ambulatory children. However, there is a trend toward performing SDRs in GMFCS level IV and V children instead of ITB implantation. Compared with ITB, SDR can be overall less expensive, less invasive (avoiding replacements, refills, pump complications, infections), and more effective in reducing spasticity and improving ease of care.[37]

ORTHOPAEDIC TREATMENT

Orthopaedic surgical treatment of children with cerebral palsy can reduce or eliminate joint contractures, stabilize or relocate joints, correct bony deformity, and improve lever arm function and biomechanics of gait. As previously discussed, orthopaedic surgery can not decrease underlying neurologic causes of these deformities such as hypertonicity, spasticity, and dystonia. Surgical decision making should be made with the goals of pain reduction or prevention, or improvement of gait function. The primary goal is improvement of quality of life. Although newer validated patient-reported outcome measures such as the Child Health Index of Life with Disabilities (CPCHILD) enable measurements of quality of life, there remains a paucity of data to guide the surgeon when deciding whether a surgery will benefit a patient.[38] Surgical decision making is best shared with the families and with input from the child's pediatrician, physiatrist, and physical therapist. Social factors must be considered to ensure the family is supported and equipped to manage postoperative recovery and rehabilitation.

Upper Extremity

The goal of surgery in upper extremity cerebral palsy should be to address impairment to improve activity and participation.[39] Splinting and botulinum toxin injections can be used to prevent progressive and fixed contractures, including adduction at the shoulder, flexion at the elbow, pronation of the forearm, flexion of the wrist, adduction of the thumb into the palm, or flexion of the fingers. Surgery to achieve better cosmesis, such as repositioning the wrist, may alleviate anxiety about the social stigma of CP and may be considered for the cognitively aware patient.

The most common upper extremity contracture in CP results from spasticity and leads to imbalance in the forearm musculature. The deformity is a combination of forearm pronation, wrist flexion and adduction, with opposition of the thumb into the palm. Forearm pronation can be addressed with tenotomy or transfer of the pronator teres.[40] Wrist flexion can be addressed with transfer of the flexor carpi ulnaris to the extensor carpi radialis brevis or common digital extensors, or a wrist fusion in the setting of fixed contracture. Thumb-in-palm deformity can be addressed with adductor pollicis slide and extensor pollicis longus transfer from the third extensor compartment to the first extensor compartment. A prospective multicenter study at the Shriner's Hospital for Children network examined forearm surgery (including transfer of the flexor carpi ulnaris to the extensor carpi radialis brevis, pronator teres release, and extensor pollicis longus rerouting with adductor pollicis release) in children with CP and adequate selective control.[41] The authors reported that surgery achieved substantial sustained improvements compared with botulinum toxin injections and continued physical therapy.

A thorough patient assessment can help evaluate potential functional gains from surgery. When assessing the need for surgical intervention, specifically at the wrist, activity measurement tools can be helpful. Physical examination measurements such as range of motion have been shown to have poor correlation with measurements of activity. The Assisting Hand Assessment and the Shriners Hospital Upper Extremity Evaluation Dynamic Positional Analyses have been validated as activity limitation measurement tools.[42] Gripping ability may be improved by repositioning the wrist; however, adequate selective control of finger extension and flexion should exist. The grasp and release test can be performed to assess whether the patient can position his or her fingers with the wrist extended. Patients are given six objects to grasp, lift, and release to test their level of functioning, including lateral pinch and palmar grasp. Without adequate selective control, functional gains will not occur with surgical correction. When selective control is present, fusion of the wrist in the neutral position may enable grip, even in a child who could not grip before surgery. Recent data support that careful patient selection based on the level of impairment, goals of the patient and family, presence of selective control in the fingers, and level of involuntary movement in the hand can result in clinically relevant improvement with surgical treatment of upper extremity cerebral palsy.[43] In patients without selective control or potential use of the hand, surgical release may be necessary to facilitate proper hygiene when nonsurgical management is unsuccessful.

Shoulder adduction and elbow contractures are often associated with more severe CP. Shoulder adduction can be improved with intramuscular lengthening of the pectoralis major.[44] Elbow contractures can be improved with release of the lacertus fibrosus, lengthening of the biceps and brachialis tendons, and anterior capsule release. Postoperative extension casting with long-term intermittent splinting is needed to maintain the gains in range of motion made possible by these surgical procedures.

Spine

Orthopaedic surgeons are questioning the role of arthrodesis in nonambulatory patients with cerebral palsy in light of a lack of evidence that arthrodesis results in any quality of life benefits.[45-47] The risk-to-benefit ratio should be evaluated for each patient, especially those with level V GMFCS.[48] Neuromuscular scoliosis may be progressive after skeletal maturity. Bracing treatment will not alter the course of the scoliosis but can potentially influence sitting balance. Spinal fusion is indicated when a curve is progressive and sitting balance is compromised. The goals of fusion are to establish a balanced spine and a level pelvis. A straightened spine may improve intestinal motility and absorption and result in improved nutritional status.[49]

Complications are higher during and after spinal arthrodesis in the neuromuscular population compared with the idiopathic population. Medical comorbidities increase surgical risk. Specifically, low preoperative albumin, chronic respiratory insufficiency, bladder dysfunction, and epilepsy have been associated with increased perioperative complications, increased length of stay, and increased readmission rates.[50,51] Lower gross motor functional level and greater magnitude curves are predictors of higher complication rates. Patients with CP have an increased risk of infection after posterior spinal fusion compared with other patient populations. The presence of gastrostomy and gastrojejunostomy tubes, a higher preoperative serum white blood cell count, and longer surgical time are risk factors for infection.[52]

Neuromuscular scoliosis and neuromuscular hip dislocation are very common in children with CP, and both conditions increase in frequency and severity with increased GMFCS levels. Dislocation of a reduced hip is common after spinal fusion. If the dislocated hip is the down hip, it is more likely to become painful after dislocation.[53] Therefore, assessment of the hips before and after spinal fusion is crucial.

Hip

Hip pain prevalence in patients with cerebral palsy increases with age, lower gross motor function, and higher degree of hip displacement.[54] Treatment for neuromuscular hip subluxation can be divided into proactive and reactive strategies. Proactive strategies aim to slow the progression of subluxation and prevent dislocation. The goals are to prevent pain and progressive limitations in perineal care. A prevention strategy coupling radiographic surveillance with proactive surgical treatment can nearly eliminate hip dislocations in patients with CP. This was demonstrated by a prevention program undertaken in Sweden that eliminated hip dislocations in the CP population.[55] The recently published 5-year follow-up from this surveillance program demonstrated continued success, but a high rate of recurrence requiring additional operations.[56] Beginning at the age of 2 years, the hips of children with CP should be monitored with annual pelvic radiography up to the age of 5 years in ambulatory patients (levels I through III GMFCS) and up to skeletal maturity in nonambulatory patients (levels IV and V GMFCS). Monitoring may be discontinued at these end points if the hip is normal. If subluxation is present, the Reimer migration index is used to measure the progression of subluxation (**Figure 2**). When the Reimer migration index exceeds the 50% threshold, hip reconstruction is recommended.[57] Recent data have supported the long-held belief that severe hip displacement or dislocation decreases quality of life in children with cerebral palsy.[58] A 2017 survey of Pediatric Orthopedic Society of North America (POSNA) members found 90% agreement that a dislocated hip could become painful and 93% agreement to follow a surveillance strategy.[59]

A persistence of immature hip morphology, characterized by coxa valga and greater anteversion, contribute to neuromuscular hip dysplasia. A delay in walking prevents the normal pressure relationship between the femoral head and the acetabulum. Without early weight bearing, and in the setting of muscle spasticity (especially spasticity of the adductor and flexor muscles) and weakness of the hip extensor and abductor muscles, the neck-shaft angle and anteversion of the femur remain increased, and the triradiate cartilage is not stimulated to cover the femoral head with a deep acetabulum.

In the femur, coxa valga and excess anteversion can be treated with proximal varus derotation osteotomy

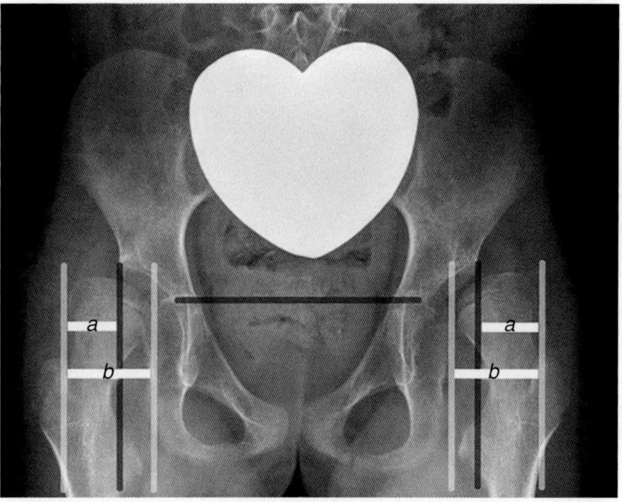

FIGURE 2 Pelvic radiograph shows parameters for measuring the Reimer migration index. The index equals *a* divided by *b* and is measured by drawing lines perpendicular to the axis of the triradiate cartilage at the lateral acetabular margins (black lines). Parallel lines are drawn at the lateral and medial margins of the proximal femoral physis (white lines). The Reimer migration index is the ratio of the width of the femoral head lateral to the acetabulum *a* divided by the total width of the femoral head *b*.

(**Figure 3**). The goal is to maximize coverage of the femoral head at the time of surgery. The amount of varus depends on the child's preoperative ambulatory status and the potential for future ambulation. Hip coverage can be improved by increasing the degree of varus correction, but varus greater than 110° to 115° increases the risks of excessive shortening of the abductors and impairment of postoperative gait.

Acetabular dysplasia in CP is characterized by superior and posterior insufficiency. Therefore, incomplete osteotomies (eg, Pemberton, Dega, San Diego, and incomplete periacetabular osteotomies) are recommended over a complete innominate osteotomy (as described by Salter). The Pemberton and Dega osteotomies provide more anterior coverage and are not recommended for patients with levels IV and V GMFCS who have posterior acetabular insufficiency.

Maximizing coverage of the femoral head during hip reconstruction is important because the muscle imbalance that preceded the reconstruction will persist after the reconstruction. Unlike in developmental dysplasia of the hip, redirecting the femoral head toward the triradiate cartilage in neuromuscular hip subluxation does not reliably stimulate acetabular remodeling around the femoral head with continued growth. The risk of recurrent hip dislocation is proportional to potential growth remaining and disease severity. Recurrence of dysplasia and dislocation after hip reconstruction is very rare in levels II and III GMFCS hips but does occur in levels IV and V GMFCS hips.[60]

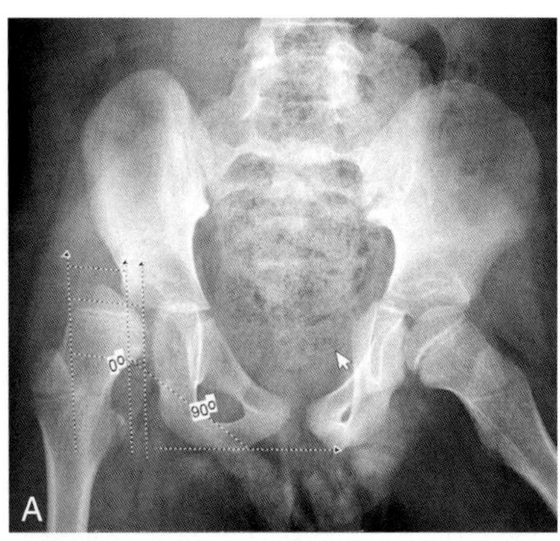

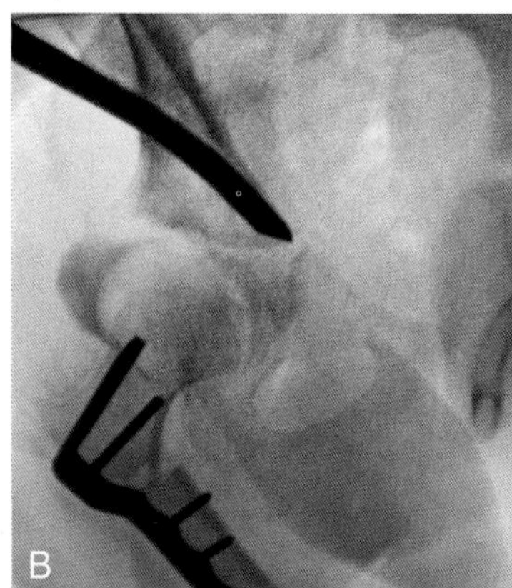

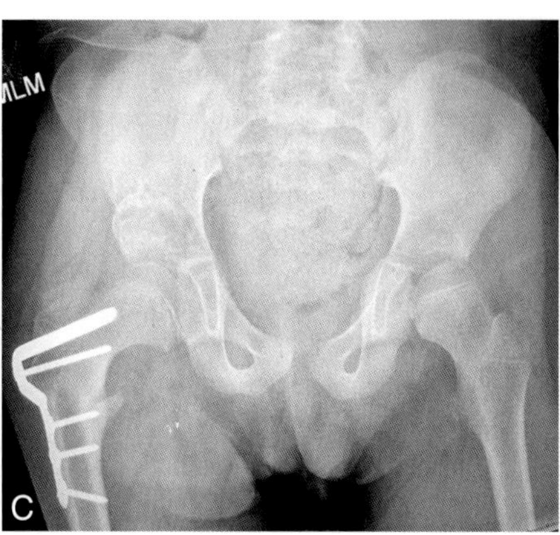

FIGURE 3 **A,** AP pelvis radiograph shows Reimer migration percentage > 50% in this preteen girl with cerebral palsy and neuromuscular hip dysplasia. **B,** Intraoperative fluoroscopy with arthrogram shows correction achieved after varus derotation osteotomy with fixation with a blade plate construct, and with curved osteotome inserted to the triradiate cartilage to affect an acetabuloplasty. **C,** One-year postoperative AP pelvis radiograph shows coverage and deep seating of the femoral head in the acetabulum with healing at both osteotomy sites.

If a hip dislocates, the decision for hip reconstruction or salvage should take into consideration the patient's ambulatory status and level of pain, as well as the radiographic characteristics of the hip. A hip that remains subluxated will have progressive wear from the capsule and spastic abductor muscles. Because obvious wear can generate pain, reducing an arthritic femoral head into the acetabulum may be ill advised. In this case, salvage surgery is an option (**Figure 4**). Techniques include proximal femoral resection (Castle procedure) or proximal femoral valgus osteotomy with or without resection of the femoral head or neck.

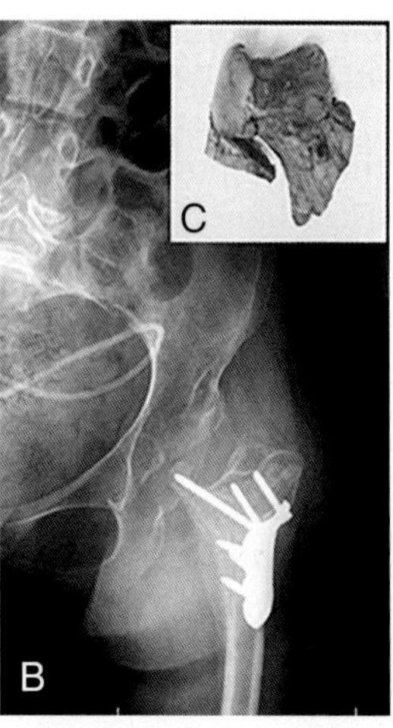

FIGURE 4 Radiographic images from a patient with cerebral palsy and level IV Gross Motor Function Classification System (GMFCS) who had severe groin pain in the left hip. **A**, AP pelvic radiograph shows a dislocated left hip, with extensive wear of the lateral femoral head. **B**, The patient was treated with salvage hip reconstruction. **C**, At the time of surgery, the resected femoral head showed severe wear laterally with destruction of the articular surface and exposed epiphyseal bone. After surgery, there was immediate improvement in pain; however, spasms continued for 8 months after surgery.

The Castle procedure was originally described with a required period of 3 months of postoperative traction. A 2014 study reported improved success rates without postoperative traction.[61] Systematic review of salvage surgeries for painful dislocated hips in patients with CP found that each technique had approximately a 70% success rate. Complications included persistent pain, heterotopic ossification, and skin ulceration.[62] Arthrodesis of the painful neuromuscular hip has a lower success rate and higher complication rate when compared with other techniques of salvage surgery.[63] There is a limited role for total hip arthroplasty in a select group of patients with cerebral palsy. Increased tone, lack of muscular control, and muscular imbalance would increase the risk of recurrent dislocations in the spastic population.

LOWER EXTREMITY SURGERY IN AMBULATORY CHILDREN

The surgical treatment of gait abnormalities in children with CP involves release of contractures that prevent joint range of motion at various levels (the hip, knee, and ankle), correction of rotation of the long bones, and realignment of tendons and osseous structures to better lever arm function. These procedures are done to improve kinetics and gait efficiency.

The decision for or against surgical treatment depends on the nature of the patient's disability and the potential for successful rehabilitation. Children with CP may have neurologic manifestations such as dystonia, ataxia, or choreoathetosis that limit gait and will not be improved by surgery. There may be an underlying weakness that prevents ambulation or behavioral or cognitive limitations that prevent participation in preoperative and/or postoperative therapy. These limitations can result in failed improvement in joint contractures or in malrotation. Inappropriate or excessive lengthening of tendons can decrease the patient's motor strength, and the surgeon should always consider the risk of an ambulatory child becoming nonambulatory after a major orthopaedic intervention.

Quantitative three-dimensional gait analysis provides substantial research benefits and serves as a clinical tool to analyze the relationship among forces (center of mass, ground reaction force, kinetics), joint motion (video-based kinematics), and muscle activity (electromyography) during each moment of the gait cycle. Quantitative data can be combined with observational and video-based gait analyses and physical examination findings to accurately diagnose gait pathology and develop a surgical plan. Because spasticity is eliminated by anesthesia, examination under anesthesia is the most useful method for determining the true mechanical limitations in range of motion. The limitations are caused by fixed contractures of muscle tendon units or capsular contractures at the joint. The decision for or against surgery should not be made until the examination under anesthesia has been completed so that the final decision can be made based on all available data. For example, a knee flexion contracture, perceived to be due solely to hamstring contractures, may have an underlying fixed contracture that becomes clear under anesthesia. In this case, to enable full extension of the knee, the fixed contracture must be addressed with a posterior capsular release or accommodated through a distal femoral extension osteotomy. Understanding the effects of each procedure is key: A distal femoral extension osteotomy will lengthen the hamstrings further and shorten the extensor mechanism, and a patellar shortening or advancement surgery is subsequently required to maintain the lever arm of the extensor mechanism[64,65] (**Figure 5**).

The five priorities of gait have been described as follows: stability in stance phase, clearance in swing phase, appropriate prepositioning before heel strike, adequate stride length, and conservation of energy.[66] Each priority builds on the preceding priorities. The goal of surgery in ambulatory patients with CP is to eliminate joint contractures and rotational abnormalities that affect gait biomechanics and impair function. Focusing on the priorities of gait allows the surgeon to define the impairment and

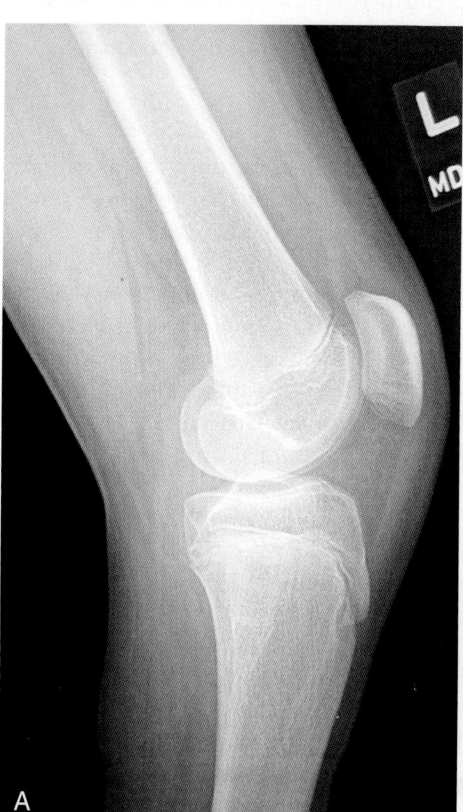

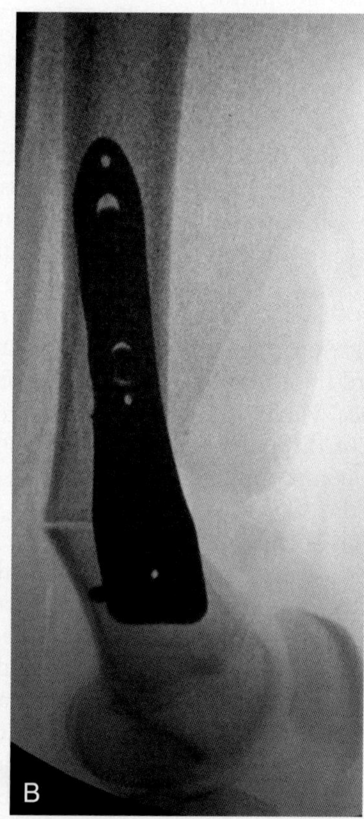

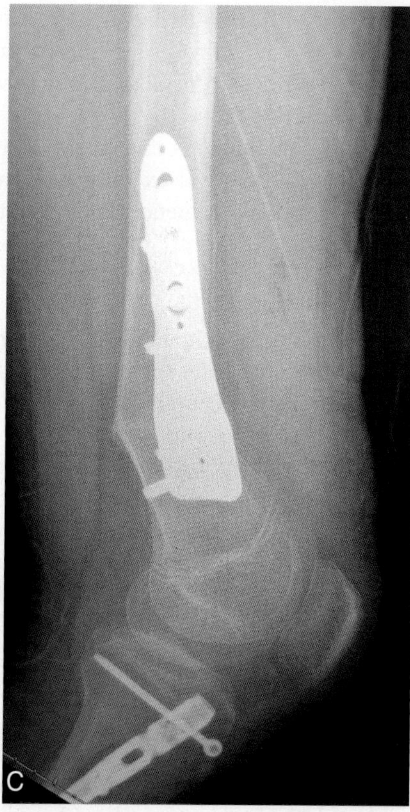

FIGURE 5 **A** and **B,** AP and lateral fluoroscopy of the knee showing intraoperative results of a distal femoral extension osteotomy using a closing wedge osteotomy and distal femoral locking plate, coupled with a patellar shortening procedure. **C,** A follow-up radiograph at 18 months postoperatively demonstrates maintained correction despite interval growth.

determine the potential benefit of surgery. For example, the first priority of gait—stability in stance—is vital to gait. Without stability on the stance limb, gait is not possible. Ataxia will manifest as instability in the stance phase, and, subsequently, all other priorities of gait will be affected. Because orthopaedic surgery cannot change ataxia, surgery will fail to improve gait. However, if stability in stance is limited because of a fixed equinus contracture manifesting as a small base of contact, then stability may be improved with lengthening of the gastrocnemius-soleus complex. An equinus contracture also results in poor clearance, with the toe catching at the midswing phase, poor prepositioning caused by limited dorsiflexion at terminal swing, decreased stride length caused by the inability to advance the center of mass over the talus during the stance phase, and poor conservation of energy caused by loss of the foot rockers. Orthopaedic surgery can reduce contractures (specifically, contractures at the hip, knee, and ankle) to increase stride length during the swing phase, decrease energy expenditure during the stance phase, and improve weight transition over the ankle during second rocker phase. Bony realignment, patellar tendon shortening, and tendon transfers can improve the biomechanics of gait to prevent collision of the knees during gait (scissoring) and improve the efficiency of existing strength to maximize ambulatory capacity. Although expectations should not include a jump in GMFCS level, single event multi level surgery has been shown in a meta-analysis to improve gait in children with CP.[67]

Fixed contractures can occur around any or all of the joints in the lower extremity. A patient's gait can be classified by the influence of contractures at each level (**Figure 6**).

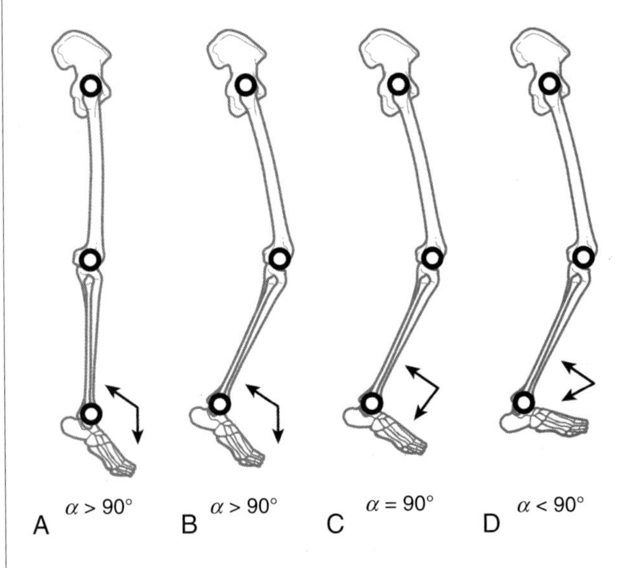

FIGURE 6 Illustrations of gait patterns seen in patients with spastic diplegia. Arrows show the alpha (α) angle. **A**, Group 1: true equinus is driven by a gastrocnemius contracture without flexion contracture at the knee or hip. **B**, Group 2: jump gait is characterized by an equinus contracture with compensatory knee and/or hip flexion contracture. **C**, Group 3: apparent equinus is similar to jump gait in appearance, but the toe walking is driven by a flexion contracture at the knee and/or hip, and there is no associated contracture of the gastrocnemius-soleus complex. **D**, Group 4: crouched gait is characterized by excessive ankle dorsiflexion and contractures at the knee and/or hip.

True Equinus Gait

In true equinus gait, inadequate dorsiflexion through the ankle joint shifts first contact toward the forefoot. To maintain the center of mass, the knee, which does not have a fixed contracture, is kept bent through the midstance phase. When there is a fixed contracture of the gastrocnemius and/or soleus muscle, the patient will benefit from lengthening the gastrocnemius-soleus complex.[68] This may be done through various gastrocnemius lengthening techniques such as the Vulpius, Strayer, and Baker techniques or Z-lengthening. A risk of overlengthening the gastrocnemius-soleus complex exists with any of these techniques and can lead to excessive dorsiflexion, weakness in plantar flexion, and iatrogenic progression into the crouched gait. A gastrocnemius recession procedure decreases the risk of overcorrection, compared with Achilles tendon lengthening, and does not weaken the gastrocnemius-soleus complex as much as Achilles tendon lengthening. Lengthening only the gastrocnemius fascia is preferable, if possible, to prevent weakness and maintain the plantar flexion–knee extension couple. Ankle dorsiflexors are weak in the setting of equinus. Lengthening of the gastrocnemius-soleus complex has the secondary benefit of improving active ankle dorsiflexion, because it enables increased function of antagonist muscles and active ankle dorsiflexion during the swing phase, thereby improving clearance.[55] This benefit has been shown to be maintained at least 1 year after surgery.[69]

Jump Gait

When a fixed equinus at the ankle is coupled with a fixed flexion contracture at the knee and/or hip, the patient has jump gait. The ankle equinus and contractures at the knee and hip should be concurrently addressed. At the hip, psoas muscle lengthening should be performed at the pelvic brim as a fractional lengthening. If the psoas muscle is released from the lesser trochanter, the result will be weakened hip flexion, and ambulatory capacity will be affected. Gait analysis coupled with physical examination is important to accurately identify contractures, because overlengthening can degrade gait. Recently proposed criteria for decision-making in proximal fractional psoas muscle lengthening highlight these risks. The criteria involve a complex decision algorithm that combines variables, including age, mass, speed, stride time, dimensionless stride time, the pelvis-hip deviation index, minimum swing phase pelvic rotation, and swing phase knee flexion range of motion. In children who met the criteria, 82% had good outcomes, and in those who did not meet the criteria, only 27% had good outcomes.[70]

Crouched Gait

Crouched gait is defined as increased hip and knee flexion with increased dorsiflexion of the ankle. Overlengthening the gastrocnemius-soleus complex is the most common cause of this gait deviation, but it also is seen in patients who are overweight or have severe pes valgus, which can mimic the effect of increased dorsiflexion of the ankle. Solid ankle-foot orthoses can be used to support the ankle and foot and attempt to prevent collapse of the foot into planovalgus; however, this is often unsuccessful. Ground reaction (or floor reaction) ankle-foot orthoses can be used to place an extension moment on the knee during the stance phase. Chronic knee flexion leads to traction injury of the knee extensor mechanism. This manifests as progressive elongation of the patellar tendon, and it often results in fragmentation of the distal patella. The quadriceps become inefficient and weak, and anterior knee pain ensues. Any single-event multilevel surgery in this setting should address the extensor mechanism with a patellar tendon shortening or advancement.[71]

Rotational Abnormalities

Rotational abnormalities can manifest at the femur or tibia. This so-called lever arm syndrome is secondary to persistent femoral anteversion and internal tibial torsion, but external tibial torsion may develop in response to the increased femoral anteversion. Excessive femoral anteversion mimics the scissoring seen with true adduction contractures. There is also an apparent valgus leading to the knees colliding during gait. Children with excessive femoral anteversion coupled with excessive hip internal rotation benefit from proximal or distal femoral derotation osteotomy. However, femoral derotation osteotomy to correct excessive femoral anteversion in children with mild increases of hip internal rotation on examination can lead to overcorrection with an externally rotated foot-progression angle.[72] Long-standing proximal internal rotation may couple with secondary deformities in the lower limb segment such as tibial external rotation, distal tibial valgus, and foot planovalgus. The downstream effects of proximal derotation should be considered in surgical planning for each patient.

Foot and Ankle

The goal of foot and ankle surgery in an ambulatory patient with CP is restoration of a plantigrade, well-positioned foot to maximize gait efficiency. In a nonambulatory patient, the goal is to preserve adequate positioning of the foot to prevent or heal chronic skin breakdown and prevent osteomyelitis. Equinus usually is present and is a major factor in foot deformities in CP. It can be present in isolation or in conjunction with other deformities caused by muscle imbalance.

Contracture of the Achilles tendon combined with contractures of the anterior and/or posterior tibial tendons result in equinocavovarus foot deformity. Contracture of the Achilles tendon combined with collapse of the midfoot and/or contractures of the peroneal tendons lead to equinoplanovalgus foot deformity. Secondary deformities encountered include hallux valgus, toe flexion contractures, and distal tibial valgus. Successful surgical treatment requires identifying the contributing deforming forces and defining each as dynamic or fixed. Dynamic contractures can be corrected with manipulation and spasticity management such as botulinum toxin injections. They can be addressed with tendon lengthening, tendon transfer, and/or capsular release. Fixed contractures are not reducible, even in the absence of spasticity, and require bony realignment or fusion. It is often impossible to determine the true nature of the foot deformity until all spasticity is relieved with the patient under anesthesia. Foot reconstructions may be staged rather than included in single-event multilevel surgeries, because the combination may increase the risks of long-term pain and complex regional pain syndrome.[73]

The loss of the medial arch and external rotation of the foot in equinoplanovalgus reduces the lever arm and results in weakness. Dorsiflexion through the midfoot can result in a crouched gait. Correcting the foot and restoring the lever arm can improve gait and increase extension at the knee.[74] Options for equinoplanovalgus deformity correction include lateral column lengthening (the modified Evans procedure) and calcaneo-cuboid-cuneiform osteotomies (medial slide calcaneal osteotomy, open wedge cuboid osteotomy, and closing wedge cuneiform osteotomy). In severe equinoplanovalgus deformity, lateral column lengthening may fail, which can lead to subluxation of the calcaneocuboid joint, unless it is augmented medially with a tibialis posterior reefing or talonavicular arthrodesis.[75]

In equinocavovarus deformity, differentiation of the deforming force between the tibialis anterior and tibialis posterior should guide the plan for correction. If the hindfoot is correctable into valgus, then isolated soft-tissue surgeries can be used to correct the deformity. A split transfer of the tibialis anterior tendon to the lateral cuneiform can maintain active dorsiflexion while reorienting the force vector out of varus. This tendon transfer is often coupled with lengthening of the tibialis posterior tendon and, occasionally, posteromedial capsular release. If the tibialis anterior tendon is weak, then a split tibialis posterior tendon transfer to the peroneus brevis should be used. If the hindfoot is not correctable into valgus, tendon transfer should be coupled with a calcaneal lateral closing wedge osteotomy or a slide osteotomy. The contribution of cavus and equinus to restriction of dorsiflexion also should be assessed. Cavus can be addressed with a plantar fascia release through either a plantar or a medial incision. Equinus can be addressed through Achilles tendon lengthening. If both are present, their correction should be staged because the surgeon cannot control the contributions of each procedure if done concurrently.

When deformities are too severe to correct through reconstruction, or when reconstruction fails, triple arthrodesis is an option. To address severe deformity, the addition of a lateral column lengthening to the triple arthrodesis has been described.[76] Although this results in good correction, it also results in a stiff foot that is at higher risk for skin breakdown. Reconstruction is preferred when possible.

SUMMARY

CP is a nonprogressive disorder of movement, tone, and posture caused by an injury to the brain during early development that has progressive effects on the growing skeleton. Because CP manifests with great variability, the GMFCS classification helps to describe the functional ability of patients as they age. A multidisciplinary approach is necessary to optimize the patient's function. Nonsurgical treatment modalities such as botulinum toxin can aid in spasticity control and are a useful adjunct to physical and occupational therapy. Surgery can aid in improving function; however, before the decision for surgical intervention is made, it is important to identify the ambulatory potential and ability of a child and whether his or her contractures are dynamic (necessitating tendon transfer and/or lengthening) versus static or fixed (requiring bony surgery). Hip surveillance is important for all patients, and the high complication rate with spinal fusion should be noted. In the ambulatory patient, careful preoperative planning is necessary to identify gait abnormalities so that function can be improved and weakness prevented.

KEY STUDY POINTS

- CP is a nonprogressive disorder of movement, tone, and posture caused by injury to the immature brain, which can occur in the prenatal, perinatal, or postnatal period. It has progressive effects on the growing skeleton.
- Orthopaedic surgery can address issues of anatomy (contractures, torsional abnormalities, dysplasia, lever arm dysfunction, and malalignment). Limitations caused by spasticity might be addressed with nonsurgical treatment or SDR. Functional limitation and need for self-care should be addressed.
- Dynamic contractures for which nonsurgical treatments have been unsuccessful can be addressed with tendon transfer and/or lengthening. Fixed contractures require joint release or bony surgery.
- Surgery to address lever arm dysfunction such as increased femoral anteversion, excessive internal or external tibial torsion, and pes valgus should be considered in ambulatory patients.
- Spinal fusion in children with CP has a high complication rate, and the risks of surgery may outweigh the benefits in some patients.
- Screening with pelvic radiography should be performed for all children with CP and neuromuscular hip subluxation until at least 5 years of age. A Reimer migration index greater than 50% is an indication for hip reconstruction surgery.

ANNOTATED REFERENCES

1. Centers for Disease Control and Prevention: *Data and Statistics for Cerebral Palsy.* Available at: http://www.cdc.gov/ncbddd/cp/data.html. Updated May 2, 2016. Accessed June 1, 2020.

   This report provides an overview of the prevalence, characteristics, and risk factors for CP. Level of evidence: IV.

2. Christensen D, Van Naarden Braun K, Doernberg NS, et al: Prevalence of cerebral palsy, co-occurring autism spectrum disorders, and motor functioning: Autism and Developmental Disabilities Monitoring Network, USA, 2008. *Dev Med Child Neurol* 2014;56(1):59-65.
3. Winter S, Autry A, Boyle C, Yeargin-Allsopp M: Trends in the prevalence of cerebral palsy in a population-based study. *Pediatrics* 2002;110(6):1220-1225.
4. Pakula AT, Van Naarden Braun K, Yeargin-Allsopp M: Cerebral palsy: Classification and epidemiology, in Michaud LJ, ed: *Cerebral Palsy*. Philadelphia, PA, WB Saunders, 2009, pp 425-452.
5. Bonellie SR, Currie D, Chalmers J: Comparison of risk factors for cerebral palsy in twins and singletons. *Dev Med Child Neurol* 2005;47(9):587-591.
6. Zarrinkalam R, Russo RN, Gibson CS, van Essen P, Peek AK, Haan EA: CP or not CP? A review of diagnoses in a cerebral palsy register. *Pediatr Neurol* 2010;42(3):177-180.

7. Reid SM, Dagia CD, Ditchfield MR, Carlin JB, Reddihough DS: Population-based studies of brain imaging patterns in cerebral palsy. *Dev Med Child Neurol* 2014;56(3):222-232.
8. Blair E, Stanley F: Interobserver agreement in the classification of cerebral palsy. *Dev Med Child Neurol* 1985;27(5):615-622.
9. Reid SM, Carlin JB, Reddihough DS: Distribution of motor types in cerebral palsy: How do registry data compare? *Dev Med Child Neurol* 2011;53(3):233-238.
10. Palisano R, Rosenbaum P, Walter S, Russell D, Wood E, Galuppi B: Development and reliability of a system to classify gross motor function in children with cerebral palsy. *Dev Med Child Neurol* 1997;39(4):214-223.
11. Palisano RJ, Rosenbaum P, Bartlett D, Livingston MH: Content validity of the expanded and revised gross motor function classification system. *Dev Med Child Neurol* 2008;50(10):744-750.
12. Shi W, Yang H, Li CY, et al: Expanded and revised gross motor function classification system: Study for Chinese school children with cerebral palsy. *Disabil Rehabil* 2014;36(5):403-408.
13. Godwin EM, Spero CR, Nof L, Rosenthal RR, Echternach JL: The gross motor function classification system for cerebral palsy and single-event multilevel surgery: Is there a relationship between level of function and intervention over time? *J Pediatr Orthop* 2009;29(8):910-915.
14. US Department of Health and Human Services, National Institutes of Health, National Institute of Child Health and Human Development: *National Center for Medical Rehabilitation Research: Report to the NACHHD Council.* Washington, DC, US Department of Health and Human Services, 2006. Available at: https://www.nichd.nih.gov/publications/pubs/documents/ncmrr_report_online_2006_historical.pdf. Accessed December 14, 2015.
15. Sala DA, Grant AD: Prognosis for ambulation in cerebral palsy. *Dev Med Child Neurol* 1995;37(11):1020-1026.
16. Wu YW, Day SM, Strauss DJ, Shavelle RM: Prognosis for ambulation in cerebral palsy: A population-based study. *Pediatrics* 2004;114(5):1264-1271.
17. Novak I, McIntyre S, Morgan C, et al: A systematic review of interventions for children with cerebral palsy: State of the evidence. *Dev Med Child Neurol* 2013;55(10):885-910.
18. Chen YN, Liao SF, Su LF, Huang HY, Lin CC, Wei TS: The effect of long-term conventional physical therapy and independent predictive factors analysis in children with cerebral palsy. *Dev Neurorehabil* 2013;16(5):357-362.
19. Dewar R, Love S, Johnston LM: Exercise interventions improve postural control in children with cerebral palsy: A systematic review. *Dev Med Child Neurol* 2015;57(6):504-520.
20. Navarrete-Opazo AA, Gonzalez W, Nahuelhual P: Effectiveness of oral baclofen in the treatment of spasticity in children and adolescents with cerebral palsy. *Arch Phys Med Rehabil* 2016;97(4):604-618.

    This systematic review identified six randomized controlled trials examining the use of oral baclofen in the treatment of spasticity in children with CP. The authors found conflicting evidence regarding reduction of muscle tone and improvements in motor function and level of activity. Level of evidence: III.
21. Tilton AH: Evidence-based review of safety and efficacy in cerebral palsy. *Toxicon* 2015;107:105-108.
22. Ferrari A, Maoret AR, Muzzini S, et al: A randomized trial of upper limb botulinum toxin versus placebo injection, combined with physiotherapy, in children with hemiplegia. *Res Dev Disabil* 2014;35(10):2505-2513.
23. Copeland L, Edwards P, Thorley M, et al: Botulinum toxin A for nonambulatory children with cerebral palsy: A double blind randomized controlled trial. *J Pediatr* 2014;165(1):140-146.e4.
24. *Botox. Prescribing Information, Food and Drug Administration.* Available at: https://www.accessdata.fda.gov/drugsatfda_docs/label/2011/103000s5232lbl.pdf. Accessed September 26, 2019.
25. Paget SP, Swinney CM, Burton KLO, Bau K, O'Flaherty SJ: Systemic adverse events after botulinum neurotoxin A injections in children with cerebral palsy. *Dev Med Child Neurol* 2018;60(11):1172-1177.

    This prospective observational study of 591 children with 2,219 injections demonstrated a 3.6% rate of adverse events; particularly in patients who were GMFCS level IV and V and those with a history of dysphagia, gastrostomy, aspiration pneumonia, and increased BoNT-A dose. Level of evidence: V.
26. Swinney CM, Bau K, Burton KLO, O'Flaherty SJ, Bear NL, Paget SP: Severity of cerebral palsy and likelihood of adverse events after botulinum toxin A injections. *Dev Med Child Neurol* 2018;60(5):498-504.

    This observational study of 591 children who underwent BoNT-A treatment reported a 22% systemic adverse event rate particularly in GMFCS level IV and V patients. Of note, these severely involved patients reported less local weakness and pain. Level of evidence: III.
27. Bradley LJ, Huntley JS: Question 2: Is there any long-term benefit from injecting botulinum toxin-A into children with cerebral palsy? *Arch Dis Child* 2014;99(4):392-394.
28. Graham HK, Boyd R, Carlin JB, et al: Does botulinum toxin A combined with bracing prevent hip displacement in children with cerebral palsy and "hips at risk"? A randomized, controlled trial. *J Bone Joint Surg Am* 2008;90(1):23-33.
29. Multani I, Manji J, Tang MJ, Herzog W, Howard JJ, Graham HK: Sarcopenia, cerebral palsy, and botulinum toxin type A. *JBJS Rev* 2019;7(8):e4.

    This review paper discusses the risk of sarcopenia from the injection of botulinum toxin type A into the muscles of patients with cerebral palsy. Level of evidence: V.
30. Schroeder AS, Ertl-Wagner B, Britsch S, et al: Muscle biopsy substantiates long-term MRI alterations one year after a single dose of botulinum toxin injected into the lateral gastrocnemius muscle of healthy volunteers. *Mov Disord* 2009;24(10):1494-1503.
31. Howard JJ, Huntley JS, Graham HK, Herzog WL: Intramuscular injection of collagenase clostridium histolyticum may decrease spastic muscle contracture for children with cerebral palsy. *Med Hypotheses* 2019;122:126-128.

    The authors examine the use of collagenase to treat muscle spasticity rather than tone-reducing agents. Level of evidence: V.

32. Hasnat MJ, Rice JE: Intrathecal baclofen for treating spasticity in children with cerebral palsy. *Cochrane Database Syst Rev* 2015;13(11):CD004552.

33. Dudley RW, Parolin M, Gagnon B, et al: Long-term functional benefits of selective dorsal rhizotomy for spastic cerebral palsy. *J Neurosurg Pediatr* 2013;12(2):142-150.

34. Munger ME, Aldahondo N, Krach LE, Novacheck TF, Schwartz MH: Long-term outcomes after selective dorsal rhizotomy: A retrospective matched cohort study. *Dev Med Child Neurol* 2017;59(11):1196-1203.

    This study examined long-term (10- to 17-year) outcomes after SDR and without SDR in 24 patients. SDR and non-SDR groups had significant improvement in gait pathology. The non-SDR group had more gait improvement. Energy cost, pain, and quality of life were similar between groups although non-SDR participants underwent significantly more orthopaedic surgery and antispasticity injections. Level of evidence: III.

35. Josenby AL, Wagner P, Jarnlo GB, Westbom L, Nordmark E: Motor function after selective dorsal rhizotomy: A 10-year practice-based follow-up study. *Dev Med Child Neurol* 2012;54(5):429-435.

36. Wang KK, Munger ME, Chen BP, Novacheck TF: Selective dorsal rhizotomy in ambulant children with cerebral palsy. *J Child Orthop* 2018;12(5):413-427.

    This review paper discusses the indications, techniques, and outcomes of selective dorsal rhizotomy; highlighting controversies in utilization. Level of evidence: V.

37. Ingale H, Ughratdar I, Muquit S, Moussa AA, Vloeberghs MH: Selective dorsal rhizotomy as an alternative to intrathecal baclofen pump replacement in GMFCS grades 4 and 5 children. *Childs Nerv Syst* 2016;32(2):321-325.

    This was a prospective review of 10 children with severe spasticity who required ITB replacement. Rather than undergoing replacement, patients underwent SDR. SDR was found to be cheaper, less intrusive, easier for nursing care, and reduced spasticity more than ITB replacement. Level of evidence: IV.

38. Narayanan UG, Fehlings D, Weir S, Knights S, Kiran S, Campbell K: Initial development and validation of the Caregiver Priorities and Child Health Index of Life with Disabilities (CPCHILD). *Dev Med Child Neurol* 2006;48(10):804-812.

39. James MA, Bagley A, Vogler JB, Davids JR, Van Heest AE: Correlation between standard upper extremity impairment measures and activity-based function testing in upper extremity cerebral palsy. *J Pediatr Orthop* 2017;37(2):102-106.

    A cohort study comparing measurements of impairment (active and passive range of motion) and measurements of activity (Assisting Hand Assessment, Box and Blocks test, and the Shriners Hospitals Upper Extremity Evaluation Dynamic Positional Analyses), and participation. Impairment measures showed inconsistent correlation with activity measures. Level of evidence: II.

40. Strecker WB, Emanuel JP, Dailey L, Manske PR: Comparison of pronator tenotomy and pronator rerouting in children with spastic cerebral palsy. *J Hand Surg* 1988;13(4):540-543.

41. Van Heest AE, Bagley A, Molitor F, James MA: Tendon transfer surgery in upper-extremity cerebral palsy is more effective than botulinum toxin injections or regular, ongoing therapy. *J Bone Joint Surg Am* 2015;97(7):529-536.

42. James MA, Bagley A, Vogler JB IV, Davids JR, Van Heest AE: Correlation between standard upper extremity impairment measures and activity-based function testing in upper extremity cerebral palsy. *J Pediatr Orthop* 2015;37:102-106.

43. Louwers A, Warnink-Kavelaars J, Obdeijn M, Kreulen M, Nollet F, Beelen A: Effects of upper-extremity surgery on manual performance of children and adolescents with cerebral palsy: A multidisciplinary approach using shared decision-making. *J Bone Joint Surg Am* 2018;100(16):1416-1422.

    This case series of patients with cerebral palsy demonstrated that eligibility could be determined in a multi-disciplinary fashion with shared decision making resulting in clinical relevant improvement. Level of evidence: IV.

44. Domzalski M, Inan M, Littleton AG, Miller F: Pectoralis major release to improve shoulder abduction in children with cerebral palsy. *J Pediatr Orthop* 2007;27(4):457-461.

45. Miller DJ, Flynn JJ, Pasha S, et al: Improving health-related quality of life for patients with nonambulatory cerebral palsy: Who stands to gain from scoliosis surgery? *J Pediatr Orthop* 2020;40(3):e186-e192.

    Prospective multicenter registry study that evaluated patients with nonambulatory CP (GMFCS level IV and V) with over 2 years follow-up after posterior spinal fusion. 36.3% of patients demonstrated an increase in health-related quality of life as measured with the CPCHILD tool. Level of evidence: II.

46. Jain A, Sullivan BT, Shah SA, et al: Caregiver perceptions and health-related quality-of-life changes in cerebral palsy patients after spinal arthrodesis. *Spine (Phila Pa 1976)* 2018;43(15):1052-1056.

    Health-related quality of life data reported from a multicenter prospective database of GMFCS level IV or V patients with cerebral palsy ($n = 212$) demonstrated significant improvement in five CPCHILD domains, including the general quality of life domain. Level of evidence: II.

47. Jain A, Sponseller PD, Shah SA, et al: Subclassification of GMFCS level-5 cerebral palsy as a predictor of complications and health-related quality of life after spinal arthrodesis. *J Bone Joint Surg Am* 2016;98(21):1821-1828.

    Data reported from a multicenter prospective database were used to subclassify GMFCS level-V patients with cerebral palsy. GMFCS level-V was subdivided according to central neuromotor impairments in feeding and/or swallowing, respiratory function, speech, and cortical stability (seizures). Major complication rates were significantly greater for patients with more central neuromotor impairments. Level of evidence: III.

48. Whitaker AT, Sharkey M, Diab M: Spinal fusion for scoliosis in patients with globally involved cerebral palsy: An ethical assessment. *J Bone Joint Surg Am* 2015;97(9):782-787.

49. DeFrancesco CJ, Miller DJ, Spiegel D, Flynn J, Baldwin KD: Does spinal fusion in children with cerebral palsy and neuromuscular scoliosis result in weight gain and improvement of nutritional status? *Pediatrics* 2018;142(1):319.

    This abstract presented at the 2018 American of Pediatrics Annual Meeting was a retrospective cohort study showing that weight percentiles increased reliably in the first year after posterior spinal fusion. These initial data raise the question as to whether spinal deformity may impact nutritional status and, if so, might decreased abdominal pressure because straightening of the spinal deformity enables better nutritional management in children with cerebral palsy and scoliosis. Level of evidence: IV.

50. Berry JG, Glotzbecker M, Rodean J, Leahy I, Hall M, Ferrari L: Comorbidities and complications of spinal fusion for scoliosis. *Pediatrics* 2017;139(3):e20162574.

 This is a retrospective multicenter analysis of 7,252 children younger than 5 years with an underlying complex medical condition undergoing spinal fusion. Chronic respiratory insufficiency, bladder dysfunction, and epilepsy had significant associations with hospital resource use for CMC undergoing spinal fusion. Level of evidence: IV.

51. Jackson T, Yaszay B, Sponseller PD, et al, Harms Study Group: Factors associated with surgical approach and outcomes in cerebral palsy scoliosis. *Eur Spine J* 2019;28(3):567-580.

 Retrospective study of prospective data on 222 patients from the Harms Study Group database found that staged and circumferential approaches tend to be used for greater deformity, but were not associated with superior deformity correction, and were associated with longer surgical time, hospital stays, intensive care unit stays, and days intubated. Level of evidence: III.

52. Sponseller PD, Jain A, Shah SA, et al: Deep wound infections after spinal fusion in children with cerebral palsy: A prospective cohort study. *Spine (Phila Pa 1976)* 2013;38(23):2023-2027.

53. Crawford L, Herrera-Soto J, Ruder JA, Phillips J, Knapp R: The fate of the neuromuscular hip after spinal fusion. *J Pediatr Orthop* 2015;37(6):403-408.

54. Marcström A, Hägglund G, Alriksson-Schmidt AI: Hip pain in children with cerebral palsy: A population-based registry study of risk factors. *BMC Musculoskelet Disord* 2019;20(1):62.

 A cross-sectional retrospective study on the 20-year results of a population-based hip surveillance prevention program in Sweden demonstrated a significantly lower incidence of hip dislocation in CP patients. This follow-up study reports a 7% prevalence of hip pain overall in cerebral palsy, with risk factors of of migration percentage and decreased ROM identified in multivariate analysis. Level of evidence: IV.

55. Hägglund G, Alriksson-Schmidt A, Lauge-Pedersen H, Rodby-Bousquet E, Wagner P, Westbom L: Prevention of dislocation of the hip in children with cerebral palsy: 20-year results of a population-based prevention programme. *Bone Joint J* 2014;96-B(11):1546-1552.

56. Kiapekos N, Broström E, Hägglund G, Åstrand P: Primary surgery to prevent hip dislocation in children with cerebral palsy in Sweden: A minimum 5-year follow-up by the national surveillance program (CPUP). *Acta Orthop* 2019;90(5):495-500.

 This cross-sectional retrospective study of prospectively collected data in the Swedish CPUP demonstrates high rates of recurrent surgery in neuromuscular hip dysplasia. Rates of revision surgery were similar in soft-tissue surgery (adductor and iliopsoas lengthening) at 43% recurrent surgery, and osseous reconstruction (femoral osteotomy with or without acetabuloplasty) at 39%. Level of evidence: III.

57. Shore B, Spence D, Graham H: The role for hip surveillance in children with cerebral palsy. *Curr Rev Musculoskelet Med* 2012;5(2):126-134.

58. Ramstad K, Jahnsen RB, Terjesen T: Severe hip displacement reduces health-related quality of life in children with cerebral palsy: A population-based study of 67 children. *Acta Orthop* 2017;88(2):205-210.

 A cross-sectional study from the Norwegian CP register compared quality of life outcomes between patients with and without hip displacement (migration percentage > 40%). Hip displacement was significantly associated with lower scores on the CPCHILD domains 3 (Comfort and Emotions) and 5 (Health), but not with domains 1 (Activities of Daily Living/Personal Care), 2 (Positioning, Transfer, and Mobility), and 6 (Overall Quality of Life). GMFCS level V was a significant predictor of low scores in all the domains. Level of evidence: III.

59. Shore BJ, Shrader MW, Narayanan U, Miller F, Graham HK, Mulpuri K: Hip surveillance for children with cerebral palsy: A survey of the POSNA membership. *J Pediatr Orthop* 2017;37(7):e409-e414.

 In a survey of POSNA membership, with a response rate of 27%, 90% of respondents agree that a dislocated hip could be painful and 93% would follow a national surveillance program if available. Level of evidence: V.

60. Bayusentono S, Choi Y, Chung CY, Kwon SS, Lee KM, Park MS: Recurrence of hip instability after reconstructive surgery in patients with cerebral palsy. *J Bone Joint Surg Am* 2014;96(18):1527-1534.

61. Dartnell J, Gough M, Paterson JM, Norman-Taylor F: Proximal femoral resection without post-operative traction for the painful dislocated hip in young patients with cerebral palsy: A review of 79 cases. *Bone Joint J* 2014;96-B(5):701-706.

62. Boldingh EJ, Bouwhuis CB, van der Heijden-Maessen HC, Bos CF, Lankhorst GJ: Palliative hip surgery in severe cerebral palsy: A systematic review. *J Pediatr Orthop B* 2014;23(1):86-92.

63. Kolman SE, Ruzbarsky JJ, Spiegel DA, Baldwin KD: Salvage options in the cerebral palsy hip: A systematic review. *J Pediatr Orthop* 2016;36(6):645-650.

 A systematic review of the available literature found similar success rates for pain relief in painful dislocated hips in nonambulatory cerebral palsy, nearly 90% for femoral head resection, valgus osteotomy, and total hip arthroplasty, but a far lower rate of pain relief (56.3%) for arthrodesis. Complication rates for arthrodesis were greater than 100%. Level of evidence: IV.

64. Bittmann MF, Lenhart RL, Schwartz MH, Novacheck TF, Hetzel S, Thelen DG: How does patellar tendon advancement alter the knee extensor mechanism in children treated for crouch gait? *Gait Posture* 2018;64:248-254.

Using retrospective data and computational modelling, the effect of distal femoral extension osteotomy on hamstring and extensor mechanism lengths were calculated. Preoperatively 80% of knees demonstrated patella alta; postoperatively 86% of the knees demonstrated patella baja. Distal femoral extension osteotomy coupled with patellar tendon advancement resulted in a 13% increase in the patellar moment arm in extended knee postures. This study provides biomechanical supporting evidence that patellar tendon advancement enhances the lever arm of the knee extensor mechanism, and this factor may be important in resolving crouch gait. Level of evidence: IV.

65. Klotz M, Krautwurst BK, Hirsch K, et al: Does additional patella tendon shortening influence the effects of multilevel surgery to correct flexed knee gait in cerebral palsy: A randomized controlled trial. *Gait Posture* 2018;60:217-224.

    A randomized controlled study of 22 patients who underwent single-event multilevel surgery with and without the addition of patellar tendon shortening found that the addition of patellar tendon shortening lead to superior stance phase knee extension, but carries the risk of a stiff knee gain and increased anterior pelvic tilt. Level of evidence: I.

66. Gage JR, DeLuca PA, Renshaw TS: Gait analysis: Principle and applications with emphasis on its use in cerebral palsy. *Instr Course Lect* 1996;45:491-507.

67. Amirmudin NA, Lavelle G, Theologis T, Thompson N, Ryan JM: Multilevel surgery for children with cerebral palsy: A meta-analysis. *Pediatrics* 2019;143(4):e20183390.

    A meta-analysis of 74 studies (3,551 participants) found that GMFCS level was not influenced by multilevel surgery, but that gait was improved after multilevel surgery. Level of evidence: III.

68. Davids JR, Rogozinski BM, Hardin JW, Davis RB: Ankle dorsiflexor function after plantar flexor surgery in children with cerebral palsy. *J Bone Joint Surg Am* 2011;93(23): e1381-e1387.

69. Dreher T, Buccoliero T, Wolf SI, et al: Long-term results after gastrocnemius-soleus intramuscular aponeurotic recession as a part of multilevel surgery in spastic diplegic cerebral palsy. *J Bone Joint Surg Am* 2012;94(7):627-637.

70. Schwartz MH, Rozumalski A, Truong W, Novacheck TF: Predicting the outcome of intramuscular psoas lengthening in children with cerebral palsy using preoperative gait data and the random forest algorithm. *Gait Posture* 2013;37(4):473-479.

71. Novacheck TF, Stout JL, Gage JR, Schwartz MH: Distal femoral extension osteotomy and patellar tendon advancement to treat persistent crouch gait in cerebral palsy: Surgical technique. *J Bone Joint Surg Am* 2009;91(suppl 2):271-286.

72. Schwartz MH, Rozumalski A, Novacheck TF: Femoral derotational osteotomy: Surgical indications and outcomes in children with cerebral palsy. *Gait Posture* 2014;39(2):778-783.

73. Høiness PR, Capjon H, Lofterød B: Pain and rehabilitation problems after single-event multilevel surgery including bony foot surgery in cerebral palsy: A series of 7 children. *Acta Orthop* 2014;85(6):646-651.

74. Kadhim M, Miller F: Crouch gait changes after planovalgus foot deformity correction in ambulatory children with cerebral palsy. *Gait Posture* 2014;39(2):793-798.

75. Sung KH, Chung CY, Lee KM, Lee SY, Park MS: Calcaneal lengthening for planovalgus foot deformity in patients with cerebral palsy. *Clin Orthop Relat Res* 2013;471(5):1682-1690.

76. Frost NL, Grassbaugh JA, Baird G, Caskey P: Triple arthrodesis with lateral column lengthening for the treatment of planovalgus deformity. *J Pediatr Orthop* 2011;31(7):773-782.

CHAPTER 14

Cerebral Palsy: Upper Extremity

BRITTANY N. GARCIA, MD • DOUGLAS T. HUTCHINSON, MD

ABSTRACT

Cerebral palsy affects approximately 3 per 1,000 births in the United States and is the most common motor disability afflicting children.[1,2] Brain injury in cerebral palsy results in nonprogressive, irreversible neurologic deficits in motor, sensory, and cognitive areas.[1,2] Patients with cerebral palsy often depend on sufficient upper extremity function for hand-operated mobility devices, hygiene, and activities of daily living, and the management of upper extremity manifestations should focus on such functional goals. Furthermore, treatment demands a careful history and physical examination, expectation management, and a thorough evaluation of family goals and support.

Keywords: cerebral palsy; thumb-in-palm deformity; upper extremity cerebral palsy; wrist spasticity

INTRODUCTION

Patients with upper extremity cerebral palsy (UECP) can be challenging to evaluate given the number of subtypes, impairment heterogeneity, and variations in cognitive disability.[3] The upper extremity is rarely affected in isolation in patients with cerebral palsy. It is typically treated with manifestations elsewhere in the body as seen in hemiplegia, diplegia, or quadriplegia. Although evaluation of the entire patient is imperative, the focus will be on the treatment algorithm for the upper extremity. Spastic cerebral palsy is the most common subtype seen in the upper extremity, although patients may present with mixed movement disorders as well.[1,4] Patients with UECP exhibit predictable patterns of joint contractures and deformities, which result in both functional disability and skin and soft-tissue issues.[4,5] Treatment of these patients should involve a multidisciplinary approach, including pediatricians, neurologists, surgeons, rehabilitation physicians, and therapy and social services. The primary focus of management should emphasize improving function and hygiene; however, aesthetics and self-esteem concerns can be particularly important to families as well. Surgical goals should focus on muscle balance, correcting deformities, stabilizing joints, and improvement in object grasp and release.[2,3,5,6]

Neither of the following authors nor any immediate family member has received anything of value from or has stock or stock options held in a commercial company or institution related directly or indirectly to the subject of this chapter: Dr. Garcia and Dr. Hutchinson.

PATIENT EVALUATION

Activity Level and Use

Evaluation of a patient with UECP should begin with a thorough history and physical examination, including birth history, achievement of developmental milestones, medical history, and current upper extremity use. Patients should be evaluated over multiple clinic visits to fully appreciate the extent of their disability. Patients affected by UECP will typically demonstrate findings within the first year of life, such as difficulty with crawling, oppositional pinch, and object grasp. Patients also demonstrate maintenance of primitive reflexes and early handedness.[2,3]

Several assessment tools have been developed to evaluate the functional status of patients with UECP and assist with treatment decision making. Frequently used assessment tools include the Shriners Hospital for Children Upper Extremity Evaluation; the Assisting Hand Assessment; and the House, Zancolli, and Manual Ability Classification Systems.[2,7-11] Together these assessments help to categorize activity level, motor functions such as grasp and object stabilization, independence in activities of daily living (ADLs), and severity of spasticity.[5,8,12]

Classification of Movement Disorders

Spastic cerebral palsy is caused by a lesion of the medullary pyramid and is manifested by velocity-dependent, increased tone, with brisk externally applied resistance to a joint. Upper motor neuron signs, such as hyperreflexia, clonus, and myostatic contractures, are present in spastic UECP. Patients who have spastic hemiplegic cerebral palsy often yield the greatest benefit from surgical intervention. Dyskinetic cerebral palsy, in contrast, is a result of extrapyramidal lesions, manifested by recurrent involuntary motor movements, and therefore is inherently difficult to balance surgically, yielding a poorer prognosis.[1,3,5]

Joint Contractures and Range of Motion

A thorough evaluation of shoulder, elbow, wrist, finger, and thumb contractures should be assessed and documented. Both passive and active range of motion of each joint of the upper extremity should be noted. In patients with spasticity, it is important to get the patient to relax to accurately evaluate motion and the presence or absence of contractures. Classic upper extremity spastic joint contractures include shoulder adduction and internal rotation; elbow, wrist, and finger flexion; and thumb-in-palm deformity[5-7] (**Figure 1**).

Sensory and Motor Function

To evaluate motor and sensory function, the examiner should ask the patient to perform simple active movements, such as clapping their hands together or alternating hand positions from one point to another. Asking the patient to toss an object to the examiner can allow for evaluation of grasp and release function. Patients may be prompted to grasp and hold small objects, such as a coin or pen, to evaluate stereognosis.[2] Ability to grasp, stabilize, and manage objects should be noted and documented. Inability to perform thumb opposition may be helpful for diagnosis in infants.[2,3,5,8] Strength should be evaluated by serial physical examinations, and muscles should be assessed for function, tone, bulk, and ability to be transferred. Sensory function may be difficult to evaluate in patients with cerebral palsy but is integral to treatment decisions. Videography and electromyography can also be useful adjunct tools for functional assessment.[3,5,6]

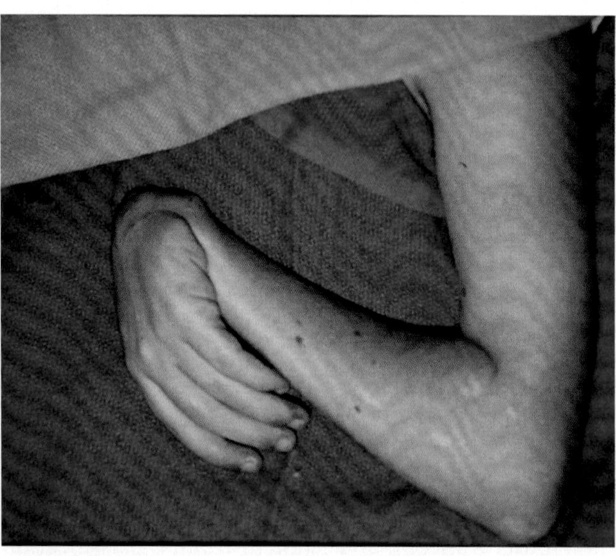

FIGURE 1 Clinical photograph showing classic deformity of the upper extremity in spastic cerebral palsy: shoulder adduction and internal rotation, forearm pronation, and elbow, wrist, and finger flexion. Patients also present with a thumb-in-palm deformity that is not pictured here.

Imaging

Radiography and CT can sometimes be helpful to assess joint congruity and bone quality; however, advanced imaging is rarely needed.

MANAGEMENT

Treatment Considerations

Goals of treatment should be discussed with the patient and family early in management and reevaluated often. Surgery has historically been indicated in less than 20% of patients with UECP.[2,6,13] Major goals of intervention should include improving hygiene, providing independence in ADLs, managing spasticity and deformity, and providing comfort.[2,5] To achieve successful outcomes, patient and family expectations should be realistic and discussed preoperatively and should emphasize that surgical intervention is aimed at the aforementioned goals rather than restoration of a normal limb.

Nonsurgical Therapies

Nonsurgical treatment modalities for UECP have traditionally focused on therapy, splinting, assisted devices, and neuromuscular agents.[9] These treatment options are aimed at preserving joint motion, improving function, and preventing contractures and deformities.[6] Static and dynamic splinting, bracing treatment, casting, and passive and active range-of-motion exercises are important for preventing the progression to permanent deformity. Care should be taken with bracing treatment and splinting, however, to prevent skin complications in limbs with altered sensibility.[2,5,9,14]

Pharmacologic Therapies

Pharmacologic agents such as spasmolytic and neuromuscular blocking agents are helpful in symptom management and may be administered orally, intramuscularly, or intrathecally. Common agents used include botulinum toxin, benzodiazepines, seizure medications (eg, gabapentin), and baclofen. Intramuscular administration of botulinum toxin A has become popularized, is typically used for spasticity, and can be helpful in times of growth, to assist with aggressive therapy, and/or to be used as a diagnostic tool for preoperative planning.[5,9,13,15-17]

Surgical Interventions

A limited number of patients with UECP are candidates for surgical intervention, and patients with poor voluntary control, significant dystonia, and severely limited sensibility are less likely to improve from surgery.[2,13] Surgical goals should focus on optimizing function in the affected upper extremity to assist with ADLs and hygiene, although improved aesthetics is frequently important to patients and families as well. Mainstays of surgical treatment in UECP include tendon lengthening and transfers, neurectomies, contracture releases, and joint stabilization procedures[2,3,5,6,9,18,25] (**Table 1**).

Timing

The earliest timing for surgical intervention in patients with UECP is thought to be between 5 and 7 years of age. Patients with appropriate cognition can typically participate in examination and postoperative therapies by this age.[13] In addition, there are correlations between increasing age and worsening joint contractures, with children older than 12 years having a 5.5 times greater likelihood of contracture, indicating the need for intervention, where appropriate, before this age.[9] Projected growth potential is also an important consideration. Bones typically grow faster than muscles, and therefore spastic muscles may cause increased contracture during periods of growth and alter surgical outcomes. Frequently, multiple procedures can and should be performed in a reliable manner during one surgery (elbow, wrist, hand, fingers).[2,18]

Several basic principles must be adhered to during surgery for UECP.[5,13] **Table 2** demonstrates these principles.[2,3,5]

SHOULDER

The most common deformity of the shoulder in UECP is glenohumeral adduction and internal rotation contractures. It is often associated with more severe forms of cerebral palsy, and treatment is aimed at assisting with repositioning the limb in space (increasing external rotation) and providing joint stability.[6,13]

TABLE 1

Summary of Surgical Procedures Used to Treat Deformity in Upper Extremity Cerebral Palsy

Joint	Deformity	Procedures
Shoulder	Glenohumeral internal rotation contracture	Pectoralis major and/or subscapularis tendon lengthening or releases; latissimus or teres major tendon transfer; severe—humeral derotational osteotomy
Elbow	Flexion contracture	Elbow flexor tendon lengthening or myotomies; musculocutaneous neurectomy (rare); severe—flexor-pronator mass release; capsulotomy
Forearm	Pronation contractures	PT insertion release or rerouting/transfer to dorsal radial shaft
Wrist	Flexion contractures, extension weakness	Wrist flexor tendon lengthenings; *augment w/ tendon transfers:* FDS to FDP tendon (STP) transfer; FCU → ECRB (Green transfer); severe—wrist arthrodesis
Fingers	Flexion contractures, extension weakness	Finger flexor tendon lengthenings; *augment w/ tendon transfers:* ECU or PT → ECRB; FCU → EDC
Thumb	Thumb-in-palm—adduction/flexion contracture, MCP joint instability, extensor mechanism laxity	First DI release; FPL lengthening; EPL rerouting; MCP joint capsulodesis, arthrodesis, or tenodesis; *tendon transfers*: BR → EPB or APL

APL = abductor pollicis longus, BR = brachioradialis, DI = dorsal interossei, ECRB = extensor carpi radialis brevis, ECU = extensor carpi ulnaris, EDC = extensor digitorum communis, EPB = extensor pollicis brevis, EPL = extensor pollicis longus, FCU = flexor carpi ulnaris, FDP = flexor digitorum profundus, FDS = flexor digitorum superficialis, FPL = flexor pollicis longus, MCP = metacarpophalangeal, PT = pronator teres, STP = superficialis-to-profundus

Data from Kozin SH, Lightdale-Miric N: Spasticity: Cerebral palsy and traumatic brain injury, in Wolfe SW, Hotchkiss RN, Pederson WC, Kozin SH, Cohen MS, eds: *Green's Operative Hand Surgery.* Philadelphia, PA, Elsevier, 2017, pp. 1081-1121; Skoff H, Woodbury DF: Management of the upper extremity in cerebral palsy. *J Bone Joint Surg Am* 1985;67(3):500-503; Lomita C, Ezaki M, Oishi S: Upper extremity surgery in children with cerebral palsy. *J Am Acad Orthop Surg* 2010;18(3):160-168; Koman LA, Sarlikiotis T, Smith BP: Surgery of the upper extremity in cerebral palsy. *Orthop Clin North Am* 2010;41(4):519-529; Leafblad ND, Van Heest AE: Management of the spastic wrist and hand in cerebral palsy. *J Hand Surg Am* 2015;40(5):1035-1040, quiz 1041; Oishi S, Butler L: Technique of pronator teres rerouting in pediatric patients with spastic hemiparesis. *J Hand Surg Am* 2016;41(10):e389-e392; Van Heest AE: Surgical technique for thumb-in-palm deformity in cerebral palsy. *J Hand Surg Am* 2011;36(9):1526-1531.

TABLE 2

Basic Surgical Principles in Upper Extremity Cerebral Palsy Management

1. When feasible, the elbow, wrist, and fingers should be addressed in the same surgical procedure.
2. A preoperative plan, including the order of each surgical component, use of tourniquet time, and total surgical and anesthetic time, should be considered.
   a. A plan should address the entire limb and determine how procedures on one area of the extremity will affect the rest of the extremity.
3. Basic principles of tendon transfer should be followed and tendon transfers should not be used for rigid bony deformities/contractures.
4. Soft-tissue deficits created by deformity correction should be anticipated and incorporated into the preoperative plan.

Data from Kozin SH, Lightdale-Miric N: Spasticity: Cerebral palsy and traumatic brain injury, in Wolfe SW, Hotchkiss RN, Pederson WC, Kozin SH, Cohen MS, eds: *Green's Operative Hand Surgery*. Philadelphia, PA, Elsevier, 2017, pp. 1081-1121; Skoff H, Woodbury DF: Management of the upper extremity in cerebral palsy. *J Bone Joint Surg Am* 1985;67(3):500-503; Lomita C, Ezaki M, Oishi S: Upper extremity surgery in children with cerebral palsy. *J Am Acad Orthop Surg* 2010;18(3):160-168.

Surgical Technique

The most common procedures used for glenohumeral internal rotation deformities are humeral derotational osteotomies and/or tendon releases or lengthenings. Dynamic internal rotation contractures can be addressed with pectoralis major and subscapularis tendon releases or lengthenings. This may be coupled with a latissimus dorsi and teres major transfer to the posterolateral humerus to assist with external rotation. For patients with fixed shoulder contractures or significant shoulder instability, tendon releases are less effective and can result in instability. In these patients, humeral derotational osteotomies are more appropriate.[2,6,13,16] Rarely, shoulder arthrodesis may be used for fixed deformities or advanced arthritis.[6,16]

ELBOW

Flexion contractures are the most common deformity of the elbow in UECP. In spastic cerebral palsy, elbow flexion contractures can be exacerbated with use, such as running or playing.[19] Elbow flexion deformity is the result of contracted biceps, brachialis, and brachioradialis tendons. In severe, long-standing flexion deformities, the elbow capsular tissue can also be significantly contracted. Deformities of greater than 40° to 60° can be functionally limiting, cause skin breakdown and infections, and necessitate surgery. Goals of surgery are aimed at elbow joint stabilization and improving extension; however, simply decreasing high flexion tone encountered while running/playing can be very satisfactory from an appearance standpoint to both the patient and caregivers.[2,6,20] Parents should be counseled that patients will typically gain a maximum of approximately 40° of additional extension following the procedures listed.[5,19]

Surgical Technique

There are three major techniques that can be used to improve elbow extension in UECP.[2,19,21]

1. **Elbow flexor tendon fractional lengthening and/or myotomies:** In dynamic spasticity, the biceps tendon, brachioradialis tendon/muscle, brachialis tendon/muscle, and lacertus fibrosus can be lengthened at the elbow to provide elbow extension.
2. **Flexor–pronator mass release:** For more advanced or fixed contractures, a flexor–pronator mass release and elbow joint capsulotomy, in addition to lengthenings, may also be helpful for gaining extension.[6]
3. **Musculocutaneous neurectomy:** This is a rarely used procedure because it requires full passive range of motion and results in significant elbow weakness. Selective branch neurectomies may be more useful instead.

The antecubital fossa is typically approached with either a curvilinear (S-shaped) incision or Z-plasty to prevent further skin contractures. Vertical incisions should not be used.[5,19]

Following the aforementioned procedures, patients should be immobilized in some extension for approximately 4 weeks, and therapy and splinting should ensue thereafter.

Risks and Considerations

One of the most common consequences of the procedures noted previously is postoperative elbow flexion weakness. It is imperative that patients have strong elbow flexion preoperatively to proceed with flexor tendon lengthenings. In addition, in long-standing, severe contractures, tendon releases can cause soft-tissue deficits. The surgical team should be prepared for such occurrences preoperatively and have a plan for soft-tissue and/or flap coverage if needed. Several major neurovascular structures are at risk during the aforementioned surgical procedures, including the radial nerve, median nerve, and brachial artery. These structures may limit the degree of extension gained in severe cases and should be identified and protected throughout the procedure. Tethering of the lateral antebrachial cutaneous nerve may occur with brachioradialis release or lengthening, and this nerve may be released if needed.[6]

FOREARM

Pronation is the most common deformity and contracture of the forearm in UECP. The deformity is caused by increased tone in the pronator teres and pronator quadratus musculature. The primary surgical interventions for forearm contractures include pronator teres release or pronator teres rerouting procedures. The decision regarding which procedure to perform is based on the patient's preoperative active and passive supination of the forearm and surgeon preference.[5,6,18,22] From a timing perspective as mentioned previously, this should typically be performed before age 12 years because the limb is more supple in younger children.[1,9]

Surgical Technique

Pronator teres release is routinely performed through a longitudinal 3-cm incision in the midforearm. Dissection is carried down between the brachioradialis and extensor carpi radialis longus to identify and completely release its insertion off the radius. If the pronation contracture is more severe and rerouting is chosen, the insertion is lengthened by taking a 1-cm strip of periosteum distally off the bone with the tendon. The tendon is then rerouted through the interosseous membrane and reinserted at the same level dorsally on the radius to provide a supination moment. The authors perform this procedure very infrequently, however, to avoid the risk of a debilitating supination contracture.[5,18]

Following the aforementioned procedures, patients may wear a cast with the arm in supination for 3 to 4 weeks and then begin a formalized hand therapy protocol.[5,18]

Risks and Considerations

Pronator teres release or especially rerouting in an inappropriately indicated patient can lead to a fixed supination deformity of the limb and greater disability.[18] Pronator teres and pronator quadratus should not be released in the same surgery because this would prevent active pronation necessary for normal ADLs.[2] Care should be taken when combining flexor carpi ulnaris (FCU) to extensor carpi radialis brevis (ECRB) transfers (to assist with wrist extension, discussed later) in the setting of pronator teres rerouting procedures because this can also cause fixed forearm supination. Several neurovascular structures are at risk during dissection of the pronator teres. The radial sensory nerve and lateral antebrachial cutaneous nerve should be identified and protected during pronator teres release and rerouting procedures.[5] In patients with fixed pronation and elbow flexion deformities, it is important to obtain elbow radiographs to ensure anatomic position of the radiocapitellar joint and no radial head subluxation.[13,23] In fixed deformities/contractures, tendon transfers in isolation are contraindicated, and interosseous membrane release or radial shaft osteotomy may be necessary.

WRIST

Flexion contracture is the most common deformity of the wrist in UECP. Patients may present with a flexed, ulnarly deviated wrist due to tightness of wrist flexors and the FCU and/or extensor carpi ulnaris (ECU). Wrist extensors are frequently weak, whereas wrist flexors are spastic. The most common goal of wrist surgery is to improve wrist extension.

Surgical Technique

Flexion contractures of the wrist are commonly addressed by fractional tendon lengthening and tenotomies. The most common tendons to be lengthened include the FCU, flexor carpi radialis, and palmaris longus. **Figure 2** demonstrates a flexor tendon lengthening in a patient with a wrist flexion contracture. To augment fractional lengthenings of the flexor tendons, various tendon transfers may be used to improve wrist extension. This typically entails transfers to ECRB given its central location in the dorsal wrist. Transfer options include extensor carpi ulnaris or pronator teres to ECRB or a Green transfer, which entails the transfer of the FCU tendon to the ECRB tendon. A Green transfer is indicated in patients with dynamic flexion deformities and maintained wrist flexibility in the setting of weak wrist extension. It is performed by making multiple smaller transverse or one single ulnar-based incision or incisions over the FCU tendon. The tendon is then mobilized, freed of any intervening septum, and tunneled subcutaneously and ulnarly to the dorsal wrist

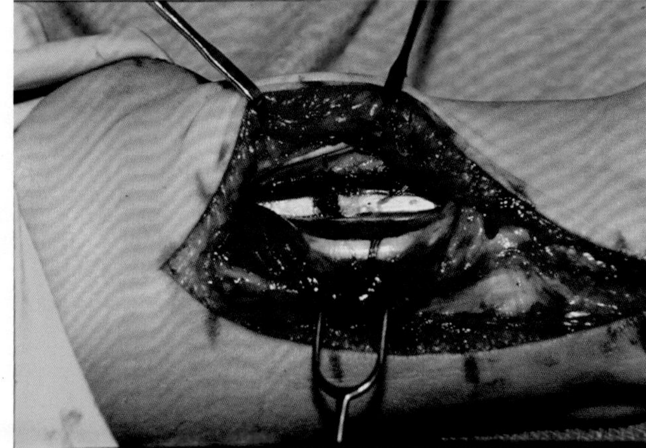

FIGURE 2 Intraoperative photograph demonstrates fractional tendon lengthening of the forearm flexor tendons for wrist flexion contractures.

above the extensor tendons. Here, it is incorporated into the ECRB tendon via a Pulvertaft weave at the level of the dorsal wrist.[2,5] In patients with severe, fixed flexion contractures with hygiene or functional concerns, a proximal row carpectomy with wrist arthrodesis can be performed. Patients with athetoid or other dyskinetic-type movement disorders may do better with a wrist fusion (typically reserved for skeletal maturity), as opposed to tendon transfers.[2,5,6,17,24]

Following the aforementioned procedures, the wrist should be immobilized in relative extension with forearm supination for 3 to 4 weeks before hand therapy and additional splinting commence.

Risks and Considerations

It is important for flexor carpi radialis to have volitional function to perform a Green transfer to prevent a loss of active wrist flexion post transfer. In addition, the ulnar neurovascular bundle should be identified and protected during this transfer given the proximity to FCU tendon.

FINGERS

Finger deformity in UECP should be addressed concurrently while addressing wrist contractures or spasticity. Flexion contractures are also the most common deformity of the fingers in UECP. The goal of surgery for addressing these contractures is to provide improved finger extension while allowing for grasp and release of objects. Tendon transfers and lengthenings are most commonly performed to address finger flexion deformities in patients with cerebral palsy.

Surgical Technique

If finger flexors are tight after correcting wrist deformity, flexor tendon lengthening procedures, such as fractional tendon lengthenings or Z lengthenings, can be performed. If the finger contractures are severe and the fingers cannot be extended without substantial wrist flexion, pronator origin release or flexor digitorum superficialis to flexor digitorum profundus tendon transfer (also known as superficialis-to-profundus tendon transfer) can be considered[6] (**Figure 3**). Tendon transfers can also be used to augment tendon lengthenings and the most frequently used procedure entails transfer of the FCU tendon to the EDC tendon. To perform tendon transfers, the patient must possess good passive extension of the digits.[2,5,6,17]

Risks and Considerations

If a patient's fingers cannot be passively extended with the wrist in flexion, a fractional tendon lengthening alone will likely not produce desirable results. During an FCU to extensor digitorum communis tendon transfer, the surgeon should ensure the patient has a functioning flexor carpi radialis to prevent loss of active wrist flexion after transfer.

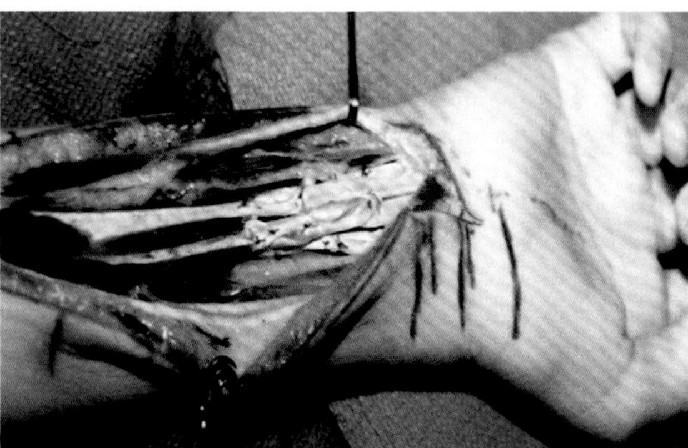

FIGURE 3 Intraoperative photograph shows flexor digitorum superficialis to flexor digitorum profundus tendon transfer for severe finger flexion contractures.

THUMB

The most common deformity of the thumb in UECP is thumb-in-palm deformity. This prevents patients from being able to efficiently grasp objects or form pinching motions. The deformity is a result of varying levels of contracture and spasticity of the flexor pollicis longus (FPL), flexor pollicis brevis, first dorsal interosseous, and adductor pollicis muscles. The metacarpophalangeal (MCP) joint is frequently unstable, and the thumb abductors and extensors may be overstretched and weak in this deformity as well. Goals of surgery are aimed at repositioning the thumb in space (ie, greater abduction and extension), resulting in improved pinch and grasp.[2,6,25]

Surgical Technique

Surgery should include correction of the adduction deformity, reinforcement of thumb abduction and extension, and MCP joint stabilization. These deformities can be corrected by coupling several different procedures, but treatment depends on thumb extensor and abductor tendon function—particularly volitional extensor pollicis longus tendon function, degree of first web space contracture, extensor mechanism laxity, and intrinsic versus extrinsic muscles involved in the adduction and flexion contractures. The following procedures can be considered for specific deformity corrections:[2,5-7,13,26]

1. For adduction contractures, the first dorsal interosseous and adductor pollicis can be released from their origin, whereas fixed flexion deformities of the interphalangeal joint can be addressed with an FPL tendon or muscle lengthening.

2. In the setting of laxity of the extensor and abductor mechanisms, several tendon procedures can be performed, such as brachioradialis → extensor pollicis brevis or abductor pollicis longus tendon transfers or rerouting of the extensor pollicis longus tendon through the first dorsal compartment to the thumb extensor mechanism.[27]
3. An unstable MCP joint can be treated by a capsulodesis, arthrodesis, or extensor tendon reinforcement–type procedures (eg, extensor pollicis brevis tenodesis).
4. Finally, the goals of surgery must be adjusted for the particular deformity. The Tonkin and Lawson Modification of the House Classification system can be used as a guide. This classification groups thumb deformities into type 1, intrinsic deformity (spasticity of abductor pollicis longus, flexor pollicis brevis, and first dorsal interosseous); type 2, extrinsic deformity (predominant tightness of FPL, comparatively weak extensor pollicis longus, and less significant adduction); and type 3, combined (spasticity of FPL + intrinsics).[5,26] Types 1 and 2 deformities typically require release of the thenar musculature at their origin. Types 2 and 3 typically require FPL lengthening.[26] The additional deformities, including adduction deformity, abduction and extensor weakness, and MCP instability, may come in combination with the aforementioned types and should be managed based on manifestation.

Following the aforementioned procedures, the thumb should be immobilized for 4 to 5 weeks before hand therapy and additional splinting commence.

Risks and Considerations

Kirschner wire fixation should be used for MCP fusion in the setting of open growth plates (chondrodesis). First web space contractures may be addressed with a Z-plasty type soft-tissue and skin procedure.[25]

SUMMARY

Patients with cerebral palsy frequently have spastic upper extremity manifestations, including joint contractures and deformities, which may make performing hygiene tasks, ADLs, and use of assistive devices challenging. The treatment of patients with UECP includes a diverse team of caretakers from family and social support to therapists, surgeons, and neurologists. Many patients can be treated nonsurgically; however, where appropriate, tenotomies, tendon transfers, and selective arthrodesis can be very useful in attaining improved function.

KEY STUDY POINTS

- Most common joint deformities in UECP include shoulder adduction and internal rotation, elbow flexion, forearm pronation, wrist and finger flexion, and thumb-in-palm contractures.
- Management of UECP should include a multidisciplinary approach with a thorough family/caregiver discussion regarding functional needs and surgical outcome expectations.
- Goals of surgical intervention include improving hygiene, function of the affected extremity, and aesthetics as appropriate.
- Nonsurgical treatment is the first-line treatment and includes a combination of hand therapy, splinting, casting, bracing treatment, and neuromuscular medications.
- Surgical treatment options involve a combination of tendon lengthenings, transfers, and/or releases and joint arthrodesis, and care must be taken to fully evaluate each area of the upper extremity to correctly indicate patients.

ANNOTATED REFERENCES

1. Pakula AT, Van Naarden Braun K, Yeargin-Allsopp M: Cerebral palsy: Classification and epidemiology. *Phys Med Rehabil Clin N Am* 2009;20(3):425-452.
2. Kozin SH, Lightdale-Miric N: Spasticity: Cerebral palsy and traumatic brain injury, in Wolfe SW, Hotchkiss RN, Pederson WC, Kozin SH, Cohen MS, eds: *Green's Operative Hand Surgery*. Philadelphia, PA, Elsevier, 2017, pp. 1081-1121.

   A detailed description of the spastic upper extremity and surgical approaches to deformities of the shoulder, elbow, wrist, and digits is presented.
3. Skoff H, Woodbury DF: Management of the upper extremity in cerebral palsy. *J Bone Joint Surg Am* 1985;67(3):500-503.
4. James MA, Bagley A, Vogler JB, Davids JR, Van Heest AE: Correlation between standard upper extremity impairment measures and activity-based function testing in upper extremity cerebral palsy. *J Pediatr Orthop* 2017;37(2):102-106.

   The correlation between activity and impairment measures is evaluated using validated measures of activity in children with UECP. Level of evidence: II.
5. Lomita C, Ezaki M, Oishi S: Upper extremity surgery in children with cerebral palsy. *J Am Acad Orthop Surg* 2010;18(3):160-168.
6. Koman LA, Sarlikiotis T, Smith BP: Surgery of the upper extremity in cerebral palsy. *Orthop Clin North Am* 2010;41(4):519-529.
7. House JH, Gwathmey FW, Fidler MO: A dynamic approach to the thumb-in palm deformity in cerebral palsy. *J Bone Joint Surg Am* 1981;63(2):216-225.

8. Eliasson AC, Krumlinde-Sundholm L, Rosblad B, et al: The Manual Ability Classification System (MACS) for children with cerebral palsy: Scale development and evidence of validity and reliability. *Dev Med Child Neurol* 2006;48(7):549-554.
9. Leafblad ND, Van Heest AE: Management of the spastic wrist and hand in cerebral palsy. *J Hand Surg Am* 2015;40(5):1035-1040, quiz 1041.
10. Eliasson AC, Ekholm C, Carlstedt T: Hand function in children with cerebral palsy after upper-limb tendon transfer and muscle release. *Dev Med Child Neurol* 1998;40(9):612-621.
11. Davids JR, Peace LC, Wagner LV, Gidewall MA, Blackhurst DW, Roberson WM: Validation of the Shriners Hospital for Children Upper Extremity Evaluation (SHUEE) for children with hemiplegic cerebral palsy. *J Bone Joint Surg Am* 2006;88(2):326-333.
12. Gong HS, Chung CY, Park MS, Shin HI, Baek GH: Functional outcomes after upper extremity surgery for cerebral palsy: Comparison of high and low Manual Ability Classification System levels. *J Hand Surg Am* 2010;35(2):277-283.e1-e3.
13. Koman LA, Gelberman RH, Toby EB, Poehling GG: Cerebral palsy. Management of the upper extremity. *Clin Orthop Relat Res* 1990;253:62-74.
14. Ozer K, Chesher SP, Scheker LR: Neuromuscular electrical stimulation and dynamic bracing for the management of upper-extremity spasticity in children with cerebral palsy. *Dev Med Child Neurol* 2006;48(7):559-563.
15. Koman LA, Paterson Smith B, Balkrishnan R: Spasticity associated with cerebral palsy in children: Guidelines for the use of botulinum A toxin. *Paediatr Drugs* 2003;5(1):11-23.
16. Koman LA, Smith BP, Williams R, et al: Upper extremity spasticity in children with cerebral palsy: A randomized, double-blind, placebo-controlled study of the short-term outcomes of treatment with botulinum A toxin. *J Hand Surg Am* 2013;38(3):435-446.e1.
17. Van Heest AE, Bagley A, Molitor F, James MA: Tendon transfer surgery in upper-extremity cerebral palsy is more effective than botulinum toxin injections or regular, ongoing therapy. *J Bone Joint Surg Am* 2015;97(7):529-536.
18. Oishi S, Butler L: Technique of pronator teres rerouting in pediatric patients with spastic hemiparesis. *J Hand Surg Am* 2016;41(10):e389-e392.

    This is a technique article describing treatment for forearm pronation deformities in children with spasticity of the upper extremity. This includes a detailed description of the technique of rerouting the pronator teres to provide active supination and improved function in the spastic pediatric upper extremity.
19. Manske PR, Langewisch KR, Strecker WB, Albrecht MM: Anterior elbow release of spastic elbow flexion deformity in children with cerebral palsy. *J Pediatr Orthop* 2001;21(6):772-777.
20. Mital MA, Sakellarides HT: Surgery of the upper extremity in the retarded individual with spastic cerebral palsy. *Orthop Clin North Am* 1981;12(1):127-141.
21. Maarrawi J, Mertens P, Luaute J, et al: Long-term functional results of selective peripheral neurotomy for the treatment of spastic upper limb: Prospective study in 31 patients. *J Neurosurg* 2006;104(2):215-225.
22. Gschwind C, Tonkin M: Classification and surgical treatment of pronation deformity in cerebral palsy [German]. *Handchir Mikrochir Plast Chir* 1993;25(3):155-159.
23. Pletcher DF, Hoffer MM, Koffman DM: Non-traumatic dislocation of the radial head in cerebral palsy. *J Bone Joint Surg Am* 1976;58(1):104-105.
24. Alexander RD, Davids JR, Peace LC, Gidewall MA: Wrist arthrodesis in children with cerebral palsy. *J Pediatr Orthop* 2000;20(4):490-495.
25. Van Heest AE: Surgical technique for thumb-in-palm deformity in cerebral palsy. *J Hand Surg Am* 2011;36(9):1526-1531.
26. Lawson RD, Tonkin MA: Surgical management of the thumb in cerebral palsy. *Hand Clin* 2003;19(4):667-677.
27. Manske PR: Redirection of extensor pollicis longus in the treatment of spastic thumb-in-palm deformity. *J Hand Surg Am* 1985;10(4):553-560.

CHAPTER 15

Myelomeningocele

VINEETA T. SWAROOP, MD

ABSTRACT

The orthopaedic care of patients with myelomeningocele has continued to evolve over the past 5 years. It is helpful to review the early outcomes of fetal surgery and issues affecting the function of patients with myelomeningocele.

Keywords: fetal surgery; myelomeningocele; neural tube defect; spina bifida

INTRODUCTION

Neural tube defects result from failure of the neural tube to close during embryogenesis. Although the incidence of these defects has declined in recent decades, it remains at 1 per 2,000 births in the United States.[1] Myelomeningocele, the most common neural tube defect, is a myelodysplasia of the neural elements that manifests in the vertebrae as a defect in the posterior elements. Dysplasia of the spinal cord and nerve roots leads to bowel, bladder, motor, and sensory paralysis below the level of the lesion. Patients may have concomitant lesions of the spinal cord, such as diastematomyelia or hydromyelia, or structural abnormalities of the brain, such as hydrocephalus or Arnold-Chiari malformation, which also can compromise neurologic function.

With advances in the management of several important complications, the survival rate into early adulthood for patients born with an open myelomeningocele has improved from 10% in the 1950s to 75% in the early 2000s.[2] Comprehensive treatment is necessary to prevent, monitor, and treat a variety of potential complications that can affect function, quality of life, and survival. Treatment is best accomplished using a multidisciplinary team approach, including orthopaedic surgeons, neurosurgeons, urologists, rehabilitation specialists, physical and occupational therapists, and orthotists. Access to nutritionists, social workers, wound specialists, and psychologists also is helpful.

Both congenital and acquired orthopaedic deformities occur in patients with myelomeningocele. Congenital deformities include kyphosis, teratologic hip dislocation, clubfoot, and vertical talus. Acquired deformities, such as external tibial torsion and cavovarus foot, are related to the level of involvement and are caused by muscle imbalance, paralysis, and decreased sensation in the lower extremities.[3]

Since the advent of computerized gait analysis (CGA) in the late 1980s, the orthopaedic care of myelomeningocele has changed substantially. The most important change has been a shift from the goal of radiographic improvement to a focus on functional improvement. The use of gait analysis as a preoperative diagnostic tool has provided a major step in establishing these changes. The main goal of orthopaedic care is to correct deformities that may prevent the patient from using an orthosis for ambulation. The negative effects of spasticity, poor balance, and tethered cord syndrome on ambulatory function are now better appreciated than in the past.[4] Functional outcome assessments, including gait analysis, oxygen consumption, and patient-based outcomes, provide better feedback for surgeons and families regarding which patients may achieve the most benefit from surgery.

ETIOLOGY

Myelomeningocele results from failure of fusion of the neural folds during the fourth week of embryogenesis. In contrast, conditions such as meningocele, lipomeningocele,

Neither Dr. Swaroop nor any immediate family member has received anything of value from or has stock or stock options held in a commercial company or institution related directly or indirectly to the subject of this chapter.

and diastematomyelia arise from abnormalities during the canalization phase and are referred to as postneurulation defects.[5] The cause of these embryonic failures is suspected to be multifactorial in origin and includes genetic and environmental contributors. Folate deficiency is an important factor in the cause of neural tube defects, as evidenced by the 20% decline of anencephaly and 34% decline of myelomeningocele since folic acid fortification was added to the US food supply.[1] Other environmental factors examined for a potential role in neural tube defects include temperature; drug exposure; substance abuse; maternal infection; and other nutritional factors, including vitamin B_{12} and zinc deficiency.[6]

Genetic factors also play a role in the development of myelomeningocele. Some studies suggest a higher incidence of neural tube defects in siblings of affected children compared with the general population, with a positive family history reported in 6% to 14% of cases.[7,8] Association with single gene defects, increased recurrence risk among siblings, and higher frequency in twins also seem to indicate a genetic factor; however, the low frequency of families with a substantial number of neural tube defects makes research into genetic causation challenging. Animal studies have shown as many as 100 mutant genes that affect neurulation, and almost all have homologs in humans.[6] These candidate genes include those that are important in folic acid metabolism, glucose metabolism, retinoid metabolism, apoptosis, and the planar cell polarity pathway.[9,10] Future research directions such as genome-wide association studies and whole genome sequencing may help to identify genes affecting the risk for human neural tube defects.

OUTCOMES OF FETAL SURGERY

Prenatal diagnosis of myelomeningocele has increased considerably since second-trimester ultrasound evaluation has become routine. The current standard of neurosurgical care is closure of the defect within 48 to 72 hours of birth to prevent further deterioration. Prenatal surgery to perform intrauterine closure of the defect arose as an attempt to improve neurologic function based on the two-hit hypothesis. Under this hypothesis, the first hit is failure of neurulation in the embryonic period causing myelodysplasia, and the second hit is persistent exposure of neural tissue to the intrauterine environment, which leads to tissue damage and irreversible loss of neurologic function.[11]

The goal of fetal surgery for myelomeningocele is to prevent progressive neural tissue destruction and improve neurologic outcome at birth. In addition, in utero repair may stop leakage of cerebrospinal fluid, thus reducing hindbrain herniation and hydrocephalus. An endoscopic technique was first used to perform intrauterine repair in the mid 1990s but was abandoned because of poor outcomes. The first open intrauterine surgeries were performed in the late 1990s, with encouraging outcomes of a decreased need for ventriculoperitoneal shunt (VPS) placement and reversion of brainstem herniation compared with postnatal surgery.[12] However, many complications were reported, including preterm labor, premature rupture of membranes, premature delivery, uterine dehiscence, and perinatal death. As a result of controversy over the benefits versus risks of intrauterine repair, a randomized controlled trial, Management of Myelomeningocele Study (MOMS), was conducted between 2003 and 2008 at three US medical centers. Although the intent of the study was to randomize 200 pregnant women to either intrauterine repair or postnatal surgery, the trial was stopped after 183 patients were treated because of the benefits of intrauterine surgery.

A report on the initial results of 158 of those patients showed rates of VPS placement of 40% in the group who received prenatal surgery compared with 82% in the group receiving postnatal surgery.[13] Prenatal surgery led to an improved composite score for mental development and motor function at 30 months, improved outcomes of hindbrain herniation by 12 months, and improved ambulation by 30 months. However, prenatal surgery was associated with an increased risk of preterm delivery and uterine dehiscence. After the trial, the participating medical centers published their post-MOMS experiences, reporting better outcomes mainly in the rates of uterine dehiscence and premature rupture of membranes.[14]

In terms of lower extremity function, the primary outcome most studies to date have focused on is whether prenatal surgery can improve the functional level of involvement compared with the neurologic level of involvement. The functional level of involvement is established from a manual muscle test (MMT) and predicted from the lowest functional muscle group, defined as strength ≥ 3 out of 5. In comparison, the neurologic level of involvement is based on the anatomic location of the spinal defect. Although there is some correlation between the functional and neurologic level, many other factors influence the actual functional level achieved including tethered cord, VPS revision, balance disturbances, spasticity, and obesity. Multiple studies without a control group have reported motor function and walking ability better than what would be predicted from the neurologic level.[14-16] The early data from the MOMS trial showed patients with prenatal repair were significantly more likely to function two or more levels better than predicted from anatomic level, less likely to function two or more levels worse than predicted, and more likely to be able to ambulate without orthotic devices compared with patients who have undergone postnatal repair.[13] In 2018, 30-month outcomes for the entire cohort of 183 MOMS patients were published, confirming these findings, despite a higher lesion level and increased preterm delivery in the prenatal surgery group.[17]

CLASSIFICATION

Functional Classification

The classification of myelomeningocele is based on the neurologic level of the lesion. Four main groups were identified based on the lesion level and associated functional capabilities (**Table 1**).

Functional Mobility Scale

The Functional Mobility Scale (FMS) was initially intended to describe functional mobility in children with cerebral palsy. Application of the FMS in the classification of populations with myelomeningocele reflects the increased focus on functional outcomes. The unique value of the FMS is that it allows quick, practical scoring of mobility over three distinct distances representing home (5 m), school (50 m), and community (500 m) (**Figure 1**). A score is assigned for each distance based on the assistive devices used, including crutches, a walker, or a wheelchair. The FMS provides an accurate clinical picture of a patient's functional status at a distinct point in time. A major advantage of the FMS is its ability to account separately for distances representing the home, the school, and the community, hence addressing the complexities of functional mobility in the real world.[5]

Prognosis for Ambulation

Among the many factors affecting the ambulatory potential of a patient with myelomeningocele, the most important is

TABLE 1

Functional Classification of Myelomeningocele

Group	Neurologic Level of Lesion	Prevalence (%)	Functional Capacity	Ambulatory Capability	Functional Mobility Scale[a]
Thoracic/high lumbar	L1 or above	30	No functional quadriceps (≤ grade 2)	During childhood, require bracing to level of pelvis for ambulation (RGO, HKAFO)	1,1,1
Low lumbar	L3-L5	30	Quadriceps, medial hamstring (≥ grade 3) No functional activity (≤ grade 2) of gluteus medius and maximus, gastrocnemius-soleus complex	Require AFOs for ambulation 80%-95% of patients maintain community ambulation in adulthood	3,3,1
High sacral	S1-S3	30	Quadriceps, gluteus medius (≥ grade 3) No functional activity (≤ grade 2) of gastrocnemius-soleus complex	Require AFOs for ambulation 94%-100% of patients maintain community ambulation in adulthood	6,6,6
Low sacral	S3-S5	5-10	Quadriceps, gluteus medius, gastrocnemius-soleus complex (≥ grade 3)	Ambulate without braces or support 94%-100% of patients maintain community ambulation in adulthood	6,6,6

AFO = ankle-foot orthosis, HKAFO = hip-knee-ankle-foot orthosis, RGO = reciprocating gait orthosis

[a]The three numbers represent ratings for the level of function achieved at three separate distances, representing home, school, and community environments.

Adapted with permission from Kay RM, Swaroop VT: Other neuromuscular disorders, in Weinstein SL, Flynn JM, Crawford H, eds: *Lovell and Winter's Pediatric Orthopaedics*, ed 8. Philadelphia, PA, Wolters Kluwer, 2020, pp 591-658.

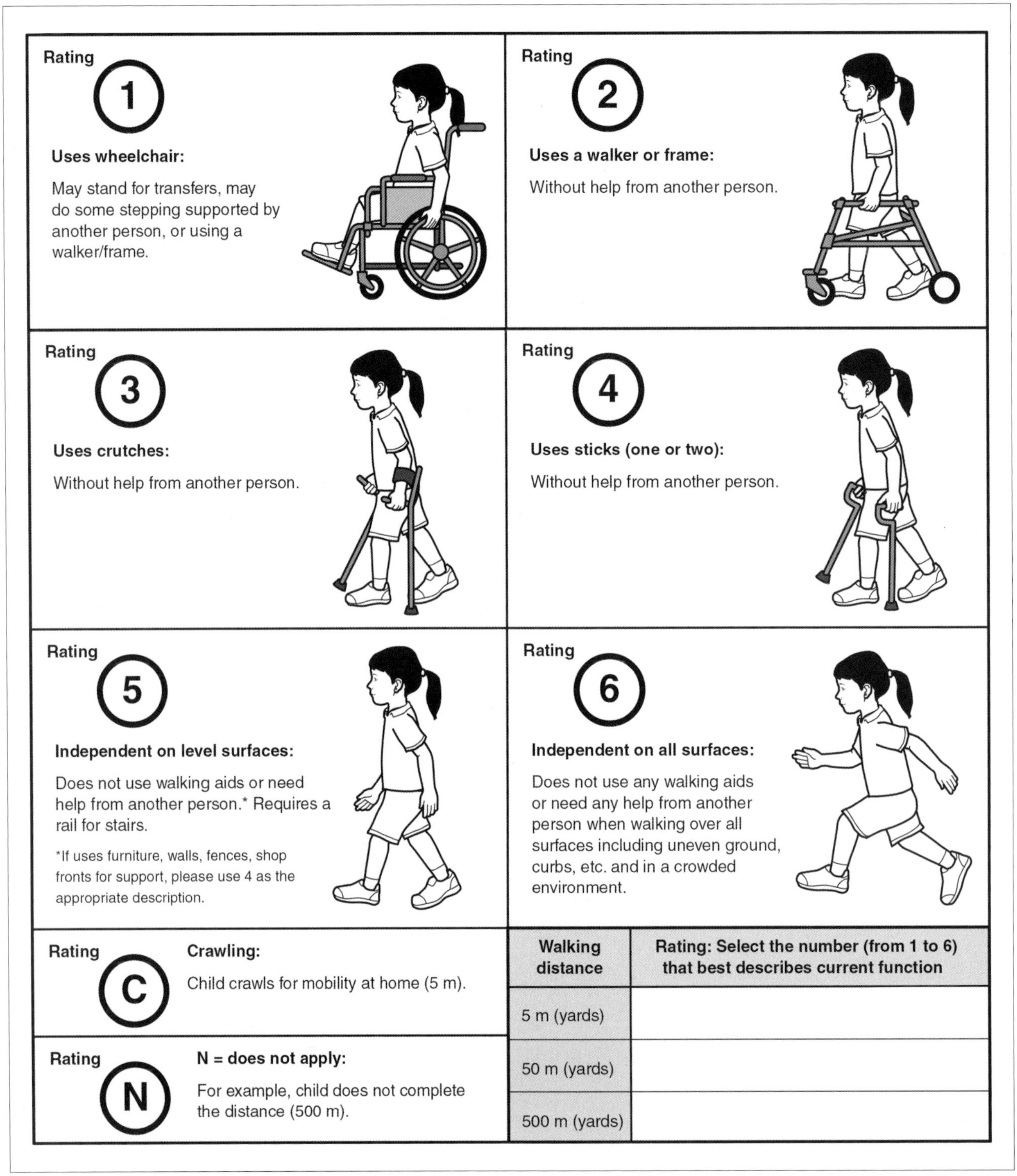

Rating **1**

Uses wheelchair:

May stand for transfers, may do some stepping supported by another person, or using a walker/frame.

Rating **2**

Uses a walker or frame:

Without help from another person.

Rating **3**

Uses crutches:

Without help from another person.

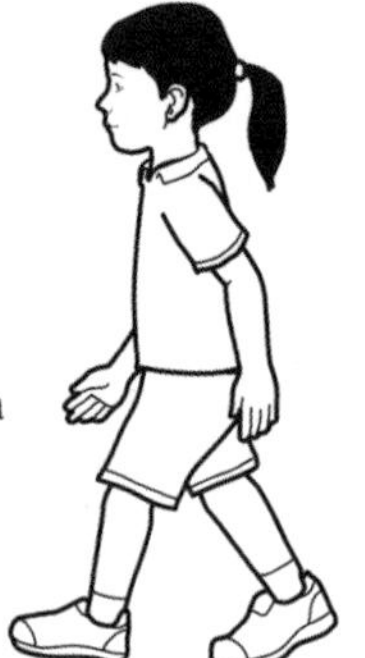

Rating **4**

Uses sticks (one or two):

Without help from another person.

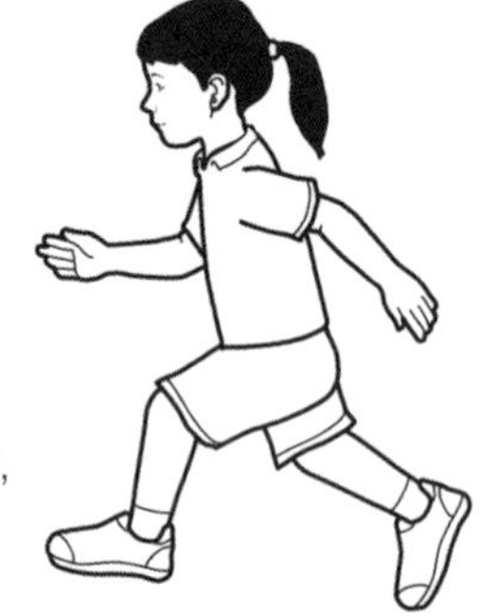

Rating **5**

Independent on level surfaces:

Does not use walking aids or need help from another person.* Requires a rail for stairs.

*If uses furniture, walls, fences, shop fronts for support, please use 4 as the appropriate description.

Rating **6**

Independent on all surfaces:

Does not use any walking aids or need any help from another person when walking over all surfaces including uneven ground, curbs, etc. and in a crowded environment.

Rating **C**

Crawling:

Child crawls for mobility at home (5 m).

Rating **N**

N = does not apply:

For example, child does not complete the distance (500 m).

Walking distance	Rating: Select the number (from 1 to 6) that best describes current function
5 m (yards)	
50 m (yards)	
500 m (yards)	

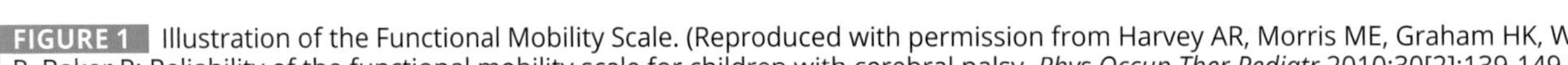

FIGURE 1 Illustration of the Functional Mobility Scale. (Reproduced with permission from Harvey AR, Morris ME, Graham HK, Wolfe R, Baker R: Reliability of the functional mobility scale for children with cerebral palsy. *Phys Occup Ther Pediatr* 2010;30[2]:139-149.)

the neurologic level of involvement. Multiple studies have shown the critical role that neurologic level and resulting muscle group strength plays in achieving and maintaining ambulation. In particular, functional iliopsoas and quadriceps strength (grade 4 or 5) have shown a strong correlation with ambulatory ability.[18,19] Many other factors affect ambulation and, when present, can prevent a patient from reaching his or her expected potential based on muscle strength. These factors include poor balance; spasticity; the number of VPS revisions; tethered cord syndrome; age; obesity; and musculoskeletal conditions, including hip contractures, scoliosis, and foot and ankle deformity.

The MMT, which is performed by a physical therapist, helps to assign a functional level to patients with myelomeningocele (**Figure 2**). The results allow providers to counsel families from an early age regarding the expected potential for ambulation with or without assistive devices and orthoses. In general, patients with thoracic or high lumbar levels (L1 or above) of neurologic involvement require a walker and a hip-spanning orthosis, such as a reciprocating gait orthosis or a hip-knee-ankle-foot orthosis (**Figure 3**), for short-distance ambulation during childhood. For these patients, achievement of independent sitting balance (a proxy for function of the central nervous system) is another predictor of potential for ambulation with orthoses. Most patients with high-level lesions require a wheelchair for mobility in adulthood because of the high energy cost of ambulation and the high incidence of scoliosis and hip and knee flexion contractures, which are prone to recurrence in adulthood despite aggressive treatment during childhood. Some controversy exists regarding whether patients in this group should be assisted to attain early ambulation. It was found that patients with high-level lesions who participated in a walking program early in life were more independent and better able to accomplish transfers later in life compared with those who did not achieve early walking.[20]

Patients with low lumbar lesions lack functional hip abductor strength and require crutches and ankle-foot orthoses (AFOs) for ambulation. Most patients in this group retain the ability for community ambulation in adulthood. Because of the muscle imbalance, patients in this group are at high risk for orthopaedic deformities, including hip contractures, rotational malignment of the tibia, and foot and ankle deformities. Aggressive surgical treatment is warranted to preserve ambulatory capability. Patients with high sacral lesions have functional activity of the quadriceps and gluteus medius but lack functional activity of the gastrocnemius-soleus complex; they usually can ambulate at the community level with AFOs and no assistive devices. The relatively rare patient with neurologic involvement at the low sacral level retains gastrocnemius-soleus complex function and can ambulate into adulthood without orthoses or assistive devices.

ISSUES AFFECTING FUNCTION

Bone Density and Fractures

Long bone fractures occur in up to 40% of patients with myelomeningocele.[21,22] The increased risk for fracture is related to a variety of factors, including disuse osteoporosis, joint contractures, and postoperative immobilization, especially spica casting. A lesion at a higher level also has been shown to correspond to a higher incidence of fracture, with the risk of fracture six times greater with neurologic involvement at the thoracic level compared with the sacral level.[23] The correlation with the lesion level is thought to be caused by osteopenia related to mobility, and *z*-scores have been shown to vary substantially based on neurologic level, with lower scores in patients who have a lesion at a higher level. Fractures may occur with minor trauma; hence, caregivers must have a high index of suspicion. In this population with impaired sensation, a presentation of a warm, erythematous, swollen extremity is a fracture until proven otherwise, and radiographs should always be obtained. If caregivers are not aware of this characteristic presentation for fracture, a mistaken diagnosis of cellulitis may be made and delay proper treatment. Bone health should be monitored closely from an early age to identify patients who would benefit from a directed bone health program.

Hydrocephalus

Some degree of hydrocephalus will develop in many infants after closure of a spinal defect. The use of newer protocols may help to avoid VPS placement and its inherent long-term complications. Currently, approximately 50% of infants with postnatal closure of myelomeningocele require a VPS.[24] Patients who do not require a VPS may have improved functional outcomes in terms of upper extremity function, trunk balance, and independent ambulation.[25] In addition, studies in adults have found a relationship between lifetime VPS revisions and increased mortality, achievement, IQ, memory, and quality of life.[24]

Obesity

Childhood and adolescent obesity is common in patients with myelomeningocele, affecting 40% of patients and likely resulting from a complex interaction of factors, including energy intake and the degree of motor impairment.[26] Studies have shown that many patients with myelomeningocele have a higher percentage of body fat compared with age-matched children with normal development.[27] Both neurologic level and ambulatory ability are associated with the percentage of body fat in a patient. In addition, a correlation has been shown between body fat and hydrocephalus, which suggests that the metabolic and nutritional maladaptation may be caused not only by inactivity but also by the underlying condition itself.[28] Nutritional counseling and mobility programs should be initiated from a very early age to prevent the development of obesity.

Myelomeningocele MMT/ROM
PATIENT: **DATE:**
DIAGNOSIS: Myelomeningocele **DOB:** **PHYSICIAN:**

RANGE OF MOTION °

HIP	RIGHT	LEFT
Flexion		
Abduction (hip extended)		
Adductor stretch reflex		
Abduction (hip flexed)		
Adduction		
Internal/external rotation		
Hip flexion contracture		
Ober test		

KNEE	RIGHT	LEFT
Flexion (prone)		
Flexion (supine)		
Extension		
Straight leg raise		
Popliteal angle (bilateral)		

ANKLE	RIGHT	LEFT
Dorsiflexion (knee flexed)		
Dorsiflexion (knee extended)		
Plantar flexor stretch (R1) (knee flexed/knee extended)		
Clonus (knee flexed/knee extended)		
Plantar flexion		
Thigh-foot angle		
Thigh foot angle range (ext/int)		
Forefoot abd/add		

Ligamentous Laxity	RIGHT	LEFT
Medial coll. (Knee Flexed)		
Medial coll. (knee extended)		
Lateral coll. (Knee Flexed)		
Lateral coll.(Knee extended)		

WEIGHT BEARING	RIGHT	LEFT
hindfoot valgus		
hindfoot varus		
correctable		
equinus		
correctable		
hallux valgus/varus		
rocker bottom midfoot		

MEASUREMENTS*	RIGHT	LEFT
leg length		
calf circumference		

*in centimeters

STRENGTH

		RIGHT		LEFT	
	COMMENTS:	CC	IP	CC	IP
Iliopsoas					
Sartorius					
Gluteus maximus					
Gluteus medius					
Tensor					
Adductors					
Medial hamstrings					
Lateral hamstrings					
Quadriceps					
Anterior tibialis					
Posterior tibialis					
Gastroc (hand test)					
Gastroc (standing)					
Soleus					
Peroneus longus					
Brevis					
Toe ext. longus					
Brevis					
Toe flex. Longus					
Brevis					
EHL					
EHB					
FHL					
FHB					
Lumbricales					

CC = cerebral control / IP = in pattern

		DEFINITION
X	Present	**Unable to be graded, but working**
5	Normal	**Complete range of motion against gravity with full resistance**
4	Good	**Complete range of motion against gravity with moderate resistance**
4-	Good Minus	**Complete range of motion against gravity with some resistance**
3+	Fair	**Complete range of motion against gravity with slight resistance**
3	Fair	**Complete range of motion against gravity**
3-	Fair Minus	**Incomplete (greater than 1/2 way) range of motion against gravity**
2+	Poor Plus	**Less than 1/2 way against gravity or full ROM with gravity eliminated plus slight resistance**
2	Poor	**Complete range of motion with gravity eliminated**
2-	Poor Minus	**Incomplete range of motion with gravity eliminated**
1	Trace	**Contraction is felt but there is no visible joint movement**
0	Zero	**No contraction is felt in the muscle**

rev. 2/03

FIGURE 2 A sample of a manual muscle test form. (Adapted with permission from Tasos Karakostas, MPT, PhD BEng. Motion Analysis laboratory, Shirley Ryan AbilityLab, Chicago, IL.)

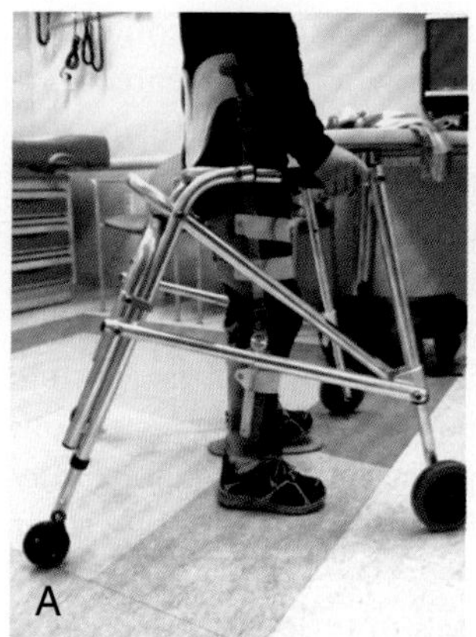

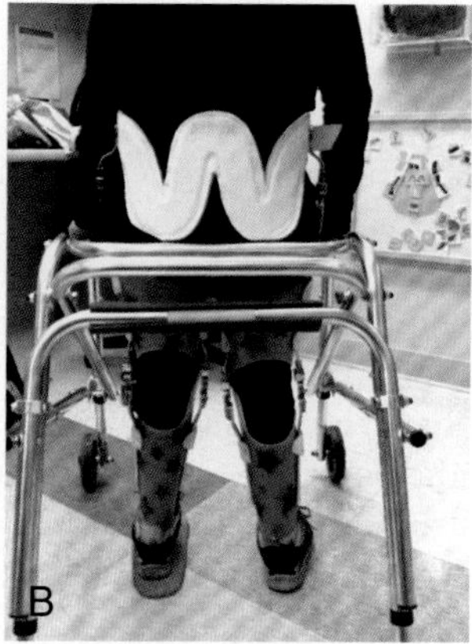

FIGURE 3 Photographs showing lateral (**A**) and PA (**B**) views of a patient with a hip-knee-ankle-foot orthosis.

Tethered Cord

Tethered cord syndrome occurs in 10% to 30% of patients with myelomeningocele. The most common clinical symptom is progressive scoliosis; other common symptoms are gait changes, loss of muscle strength, spasticity, back and leg pain, and bladder changes. If tethered cord is suspected, a VPS malfunction should be ruled out first. When the diagnosis of tethered cord is made, surgical untethering is indicated to prevent further deterioration. Improvements may be seen in pain, strength, gait, spasticity, bladder function, and other symptoms after surgical untethering.

OVERVIEW OF ORTHOPAEDIC TREATMENT

The goal of orthopaedic care of patients with myelomeningocele is to prevent or correct deformities to maximize mobility, function, and independence. The role of the orthopaedic surgeon is to assist the patient and family in developing realistic individualized goals based on the patient's functional neurosegmental level and provide the necessary care to meet established goals. To promote increased independence, care providers should emphasize intellectual and personality development through wheelchair mobility, wheelchair sports programs beginning in preschool, and educational mainstreaming.

At the time of the newborn examination of a patient with myelomeningocele, any associated conditions such as clubfoot or hip or knee contractures should be recognized and treated appropriately. A MMT performed by a skilled physical therapist is done to evaluate the neurologic level of function for each limb. This should occur before closure of the spinal defect and should be repeated 10 to 14 days after closure. Based on the clinical examination and the results of the MMT, the orthopaedic surgeon can provide families with a reasonable expectation for short-term and long-term mobility outcomes and ambulatory potential and anticipated orthoses or assistive devices necessary to achieve those outcomes.

Orthopaedic follow-up examinations should occur every 3 to 4 months during the first year of life, every 6 months until 12 years of age, and annually thereafter. Each visit should include assessment and monitoring of motor and sensory function, gait, spinal alignment, skin integrity, and orthotic devices. Range of motion and alignment of the lower extremities should be tracked over time, and any changes that limit function should be addressed. In addition, the orthopaedic surgeon should remain vigilant for tethered cord syndrome and must monitor spinal balance and deformity and assist in monitoring the neurologic status of each patient. For this reason, a MMT should be obtained at least annually. Any major change in muscle strength on the MMT may signal a tethered cord.

COMPUTERIZED GAIT ANALYSIS

In patients with myelomeningocele, accurate identification of gait pathologies and their underlying causes is crucial to achieve the goal of maintaining ambulatory capacity and functional ability. CGA provides important quantitative information about movement patterns and has been used in the evaluation of patients with myelomeningocele since the late 1980s. For patients with neurologic involvement at the low lumbar or sacral level, CGA has played a role in the identification of deformities affecting function such as hip and knee contractures, rotational deformities of the femur and tibia, and foot deformities. The authors of a 2019 study found that the addition of gait analysis data, compared with clinical examination and video analysis alone, led to a change in pathology identification for common gait problems in patients with myelomeningocele including crouch (28% of cases), tibial rotation (35%), pes valgus (18%), excessive hip flexion (70%), and abnormal femur rotation (75%).[29]

CGA also has a major influence on the selection of functional surgical procedures. In the same study referenced previously, the authors also found that the consideration of gait analysis data altered surgical recommendations for 44% of patients.[29] Furthermore, CGA has helped to identify the importance of hip abductor strength and its effect on gait. Knowing that hip abductor weakness causes excessive pelvic obliquity and rotation has led to the understanding that any surgery that affects pelvic motion will make gait more difficult. In addition, CGA has helped to identify negative effects on gait caused by surgical procedures that decrease the strength of the power-generation muscles, iliopsoas, gluteus, and hamstrings. CGA also has been used to evaluate the relationship between energy consumption and gait, using oxygen cost to compare various orthoses and gait patterns.

SPINAL DEFORMITY

Spinal deformity in patients with myelomeningocele may occur as a congenital deformity resulting from a malformation such as hemivertebrae or unsegmented bar or may occur as an acquired developmental deformity related to the level of neurologic involvement.[5] The incidence of spinal deformity correlates with the neurologic level of involvement. The development of scoliosis in patients with involvement at the low lumbar or sacral levels should alert the care provider to the possibility of a tethered spinal cord because patients with neurologic involvement at these levels have a low incidence of scoliosis.

Scoliosis

Scoliosis is present in 60% to 90% of patients with myelomeningocele. Many factors, including functional level of involvement, ambulatory status, level of last intact laminar arch, hip displacement, and lower extremity spasticity, correlate with the development and progression of scoliosis. The goals for scoliosis treatment in patients with myelomeningocele are to prevent deformity progression, achieve solid fusion, maximize functional independence, increase sitting tolerance, and achieve a level pelvis with a balanced spine.[4]

Patients with a curve magnitude of less than 20° should be observed using serial radiographs. For patients with a curve magnitude greater than 20°, brace treatment may be considered; however, the general consensus is that brace treatment does not halt curve progression in this population. Rather, a brace may be used for postural support of the trunk in a functional position and to control the curve during growth in an attempt to delay surgical treatment. If a brace is prescribed, proper fitting and daily skin assessments are essential to avoid skin complications.

Surgical treatment is generally indicated for progressive curves greater than 50° that interfere with sitting balance. For each patient, the benefits of surgical treatment must be weighed against the increased risk of complications associated with scoliosis surgery in the myelomeningocele population. Complications include hardware problems in approximately 30% of the patients. These problems often lead to a loss of correction and pseudarthrosis in up to 75% of the patients, depending on the surgical technique (the highest rates are associated with isolated posterior fusion). Other common complications include infection and postoperative lower limb fractures. Neurologic complications occur infrequently but can be permanent.

Consideration should be given to the functional consequences of surgical treatment. Multiple studies have shown no substantial difference in the ability to perform activities of daily living after surgical intervention.[30,31] Comparisons of the long-term outcomes of scoliosis in patients with myelomeningocele who were treated surgically or nonsurgically showed that spinal fusion for scoliosis is effective in halting curve progression but has no clear effect on walking capability, motor level, sitting balance, or health-related quality of life (HR-QOL).[32] Multiple authors have reported that ambulation may be more difficult after surgery.[30,31] However, it is possible that evolving surgical techniques, newer instrumentation, and improvements in postoperative management may eventually lead to improved functional outcomes for surgically treated patients.

For most patients, combined anterior and posterior instrumented arthrodesis is the treatment of choice to achieve fusion and provide the best long-term correction. The benefits of the combined approach include increased strength of the fusion mass from anterior interbody fusion and diskectomy to improve curve flexibility. The posterior-only approach has been associated with higher failure rates, hardware complications, and loss of correction. Regardless of the approach, achieving rigid fixation proximally and distally is crucial to successful treatment. Controversy exists as to whether it is necessary to extend posterior fusion to the pelvis to address associated pelvic obliquity. In general, the fusion should include all curves and should extend to the sacrum for nonambulators. Because preservation of pelvic motion is essential for function in ambulatory patients, lumbosacral arthrodesis should be avoided whenever possible.

Pedicle screw instrumentation in patients with myelomeningocele allows for posterior segmental fixation in the spine, which is difficult to achieve with other forms of fixation that require intact laminae such as multihook systems or sublaminar wires. Pedicle screws allow for preservation of lumbar lordosis and motion in ambulatory patients. The limitations of this technique arise from the abnormal pedicles in patients with myelomeningocele, which are often small, dysplastic, and rotated or are small, tightly packed vertebrae in lordotic segments.[5] Pelvic fixation has evolved to more rigid, segmental fixation, and improved results have been shown with the use of sacral-alar-iliac screw fixation, including in the neuromuscular population.[33] In addition to reliable fixation, sacral-alar-iliac screws are less prominent, which is a benefit in patients with myelomeningocele with poor soft-tissue envelope and impaired sensation.

For skeletally immature patients, growing spine instrumentation may be needed to allow for correction and stabilization of spinal deformity while maintaining adequate respiratory function until sufficient growth of the thorax has occurred to perform definitive fusion. This instrumentation consists of proximal and distal anchors with the central portion unfused to allow for lengthenings every 4 to 6 months. Multiple options exist, including spine or rib-anchored spine instrumentation, vertical expandable prosthetic titanium rib, or more recently, magnetic lengthening rods.

Kyphosis

Rigid kyphotic deformities of the lumbar or thoracolumbar spine, which occur in 8% to 21% of patients with myelomeningocele, can lead to difficulty with sitting or lying supine and are prone to skin breakdown and the resulting risk of infection. Patients may have a large, rigid curve at birth; curve progression is related to the level of the neurologic lesion. Nonsurgical treatment with orthoses or modified seating systems has been largely ineffective. Surgical treatment is indicated to correct sitting posture, prevent skin breakdown, and prevent deformity progression.

Various surgical treatment options exist; however, surgery for rigid kyphosis is technically demanding and carries a high risk of associated complications, including skin issues, infection, and pseudarthrosis. Multiple studies have shown a high rate of revision surgery and lengthy hospital stays.[34,35] The standard surgical treatment is kyphectomy with osteotomy and resection of the vertebral bodies combined with cordotomy and segmental spinal instrumentation and fusion down to the pelvis (**Figure 4**). Despite the high complication rate, surgical treatment has been shown to achieve lasting correction, with improved seating balance and resolution of skin problems in most patients.

Growth-friendly techniques recently have been applied as an alternative to fusion after kyphectomy in patients with myelomeningocele to prevent further compromise of trunk height. Growth-friendly options include growing rods and the Luque trolley with Galveston instrumentation. Medium-term results suggest both options are reasonable alternatives to fusion to allow extra growth; however, the use of these techniques must be balanced against the risk of an increased number of surgeries.[36]

Hip Instability

Paralytic hip dislocation is a common and difficult problem in patients with myelomeningocele, and its management represents an example of a radical change in treatment strategy in recent years that has resulted from the increased emphasis on functional outcomes. CGA assessment of patients with neurologic involvement at a low lumbar level and a unilateral hip dislocation has shown that gait symmetry corresponds to the absence of hip contractures and is not related to hip dislocation.[37] An examination of functional results after surgical hip reduction showed no improvement in hip range of motion, ambulatory ability, decreased pain, or a decreased need for bracing. A review of the literature confirmed that current treatment goals should focus on maintaining hip range of motion, with contracture release as necessary. No role was identified for hip reduction in patients with low lumbar or higher functional levels of involvement.[38] In a 2019 study, the authors assessed functional outcomes in adulthood across three cohorts of patients with myelomeningocele and found no statistically significant difference in any of the outcomes measures between groups.[39]

Optimal treatment remains controversial for the relatively rare patient who has sacral-level involvement, a dislocated hip, and the ability to walk without support. Without treatment, these patients may experience a decline in gait function caused by limb-length discrepancy and increased lurch caused by the loss of a fulcrum resulting from the dislocated hip. These patients may benefit from surgical reduction to preserve independent gait function; however, surgical outcomes in this subgroup of patients are unknown and merit further study.[3]

KNEE DEFORMITY AND PAIN

Knee Flexion Contracture

Knee flexion contracture, which is common in patients with myelomeningocele, causes a crouch gait with high energy cost in ambulatory patients. Studies have shown that a fixed knee flexion contracture greater than 10° may lead to anterior knee pain, decreased endurance, difficulty fitting an orthotic device, and a progressive crouch gait.[40,41] CGA is useful to quantify the amount of knee flexion during gait, which can be substantially greater than that seen during a static clinical examination. To preserve ambulatory potential, surgical treatment is indicated for knee flexion contracture greater than 20°.[42] Surgical options include anterior distal femoral epiphysiodesis, radical knee flexor release of the hamstrings and posterior capsule, or, for severe cases, distal femur supracondylar extension osteotomy. Epiphysiodesis has been shown to be safe and effective for knee flexion contracture in patients with myelomeningocele, with a rate of correction of approximately 1° per month. CGA has documented improvements in clinical knee flexion contracture, dynamic sagittal kinematics, and walking velocity after radical posterior knee capsulectomy.[42]

Knee Valgus Stress

Valgus knee deformity occurs frequently in patients with neurologic involvement at the low lumbar and sacral levels and can lead to instability, pain, and arthritis in adulthood. Knee pain plays an important role in a patient's decision not to walk. CGA has facilitated a better understanding of the multiple factors that can contribute to abnormal valgus stress. During the stance phase, the knee is subjected to forces of the upper body and ground reaction forces coming through the foot,

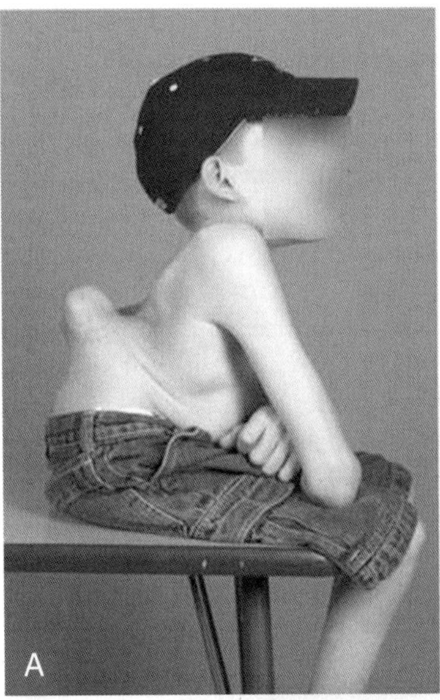

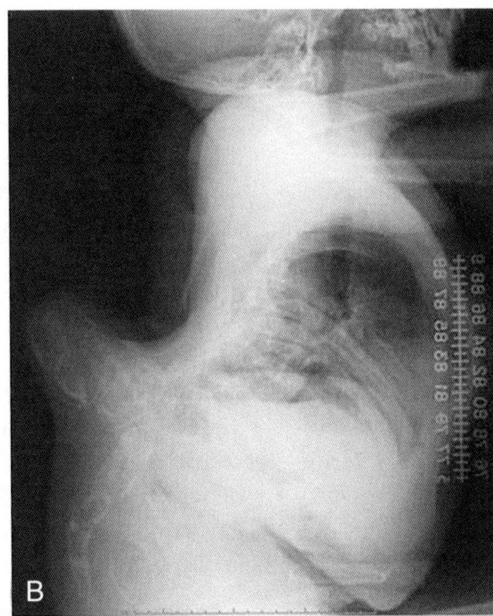

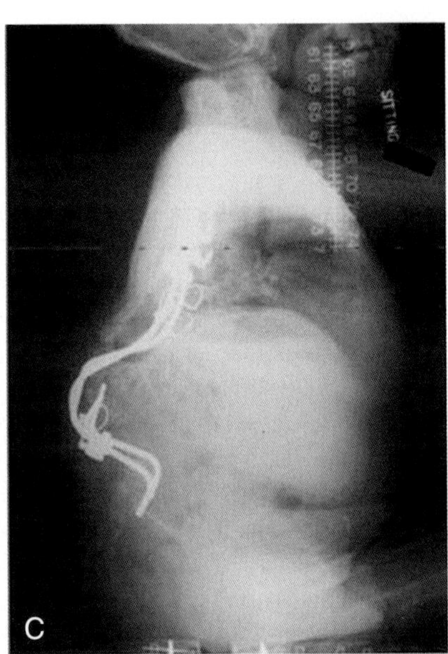

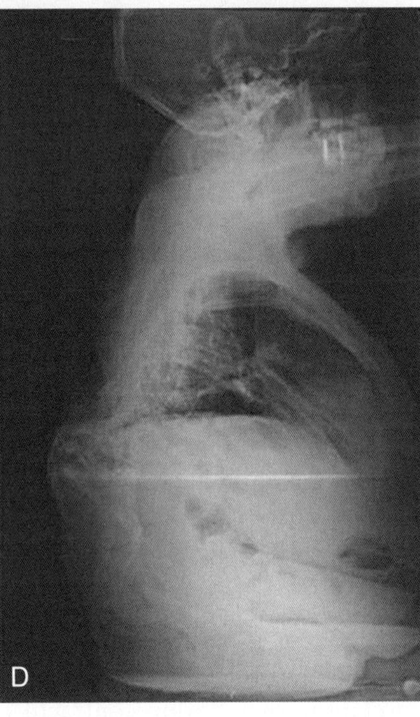

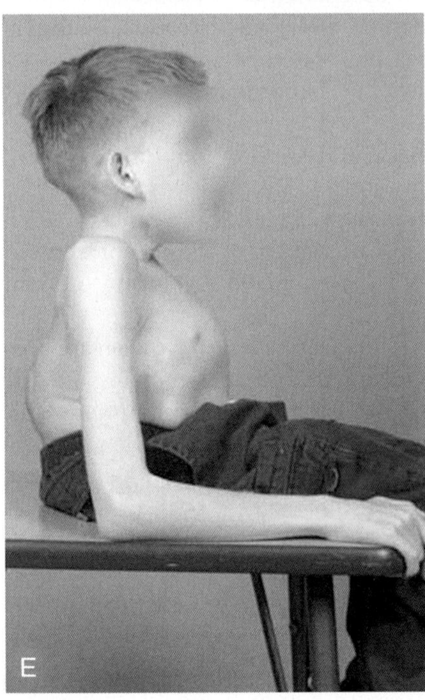

FIGURE 4 Images from a patient with thoracic-level myelomeningocele and a severe rigid kyphotic deformity. Preoperative lateral photograph (**A**) and lateral radiograph (**B**). **C**, Postoperative lateral radiograph after kyphectomy with segmental proximal fixation and distal sacral fixation. A deep infection developed and was treated with anterior fusion; a posterior infection was suppressed. Infection recurred after suppression therapy was discontinued, and implant removal was required. **D**, Final lateral radiograph shows solid anterior fusion. **E**, Photograph shows the final clinical appearance of the patient. (Reproduced with permission from Garg S, Oetgen M, Rathjen K, et al: Kyphectomy improves sitting and skin problems in patients with myelomeningocele. *Clin Orthop Relat Res* 2011;469[5]:1279-1285.)

which can lead to valgus positioning.[4] Contributing factors to knee valgus stress include rotational malalignment of the femur, femoral anteversion in association with excessive external tibial torsion, excessive trunk and pelvic motion, knee flexion contractures, and valgus foot deformities.

Although surgical correction of excessive rotational abnormalities leads to improvement in knee stress, it may not completely normalize the knee moment because of the many involved factors. Tibial derotation osteotomy can lead to improvement in knee pain and may prevent the onset of late degenerative changes,[43] but crutches still may be recommended to compensate for weak hip abductor muscles and protect the knees from excessive lateral sway. AFOs also should be used to increase stance-phase stability. If knee flexion contracture or hindfoot valgus is present, these conditions should be corrected surgically at the same time.[3] CGA has shown that patients with knee pain have increased knee flexion compared with patients who are asymptomatic; this suggests that increased knee flexion combined with inadequate control of hip transverse kinematics may lead to knee joint loading.[44]

ROTATIONAL DEFORMITIES

In patients with myelomeningocele, internal tibial torsion is typically a fixed deformity often associated with clubfoot. The etiology of external tibial torsion is unknown, but dynamic muscle imbalance may be a contributing factor.[45] Internal or external tibial torsion deformity should not be expected to resolve spontaneously without surgical correction. For ambulatory patients, rotational malalignment can substantially alter gait mechanics and velocity, affecting ambulatory efficiency. In an attempt to decrease risk of recurrence, surgical treatment is typically delayed until the age of 5 or 6 years. Prior to that time, AFOs with twister cables can be used to improve ambulatory function, although parents should be counseled not to expect the twister cables to correct the underlying bony torsion.

Surgical correction is recommended for deformity greater than 20° and leads to improved functional outcomes in terms of increased brace tolerance and gait parameters. When planning for correction of external tibial torsion, it is essential to assess for any concomitant hindfoot valgus, which should be addressed at the same time with a medial sliding osteotomy of the calcaneus to achieve a successful result.[3] Tibial derotation osteotomies in patients with myelomeningocele have traditionally been associated with a high rate of complications, including nonunion, delayed union, poor wound healing, and infection. However, the use of technique modifications, including drill corticotomy, rigid compression plating, and meticulous skin closure, has resulted in a substantial decrease in the complication rate.[45]

FOOT DEFORMITY

Foot deformity exists in almost all patients with myelomeningocele and can interfere with brace tolerance, which causes difficulties with ambulation. The goal of treatment is to preserve function and range of motion and avoid pressure sores by maintaining a plantigrade, flexible, and braceable foot.[46] Effort should be made to prevent rigid deformities by early intervention, with bracing or surgical treatment as needed. The principles of surgical treatment include use of tendon excisions rather than transfers or lengthenings to achieve a flail foot, which makes brace fitting easier. For fixed bony deformities, every effort should be made to preserve joint motion with extra-articular osteotomies. Arthrodesis should be avoided because the resulting stiffness combined with an insensate foot leads to a high risk of pressure sores. After surgical treatment, use of an AFO brace helps to maintain correction and prevent recurrence.

Clubfoot

Clubfoot is the most common foot deformity seen in patients with myelomeningocele (**Figure 5**) and is different from idiopathic clubfoot. In patients with myelomeningocele, clubfoot is a severely rigid deformity that is often recalcitrant to treatment and has a propensity for recurrence. The Ponseti method of manipulative treatment combined with Achilles tenotomy has been used to treat patients with myelomeningocele. Early study results show initial correction can be achieved in most patients; however, the recurrence rate is 60% to 70% with a high associated rate of complications, including skin breakdown and fractures.[47,48] A study published in 2018 reviewed average 5-year outcomes of patients with myelomeningocele treated by a single surgeon with the Ponseti method. Although initial correction was achieved in all feet, the authors reported a 58% overall recurrence rate. However, they noted that 100% of patients treated with percutaneous tenotomy had recurrence compared with only 18% of those treated with an open excision of the Achilles tendon. The authors concluded that the Ponseti method leads to reliable initial correction

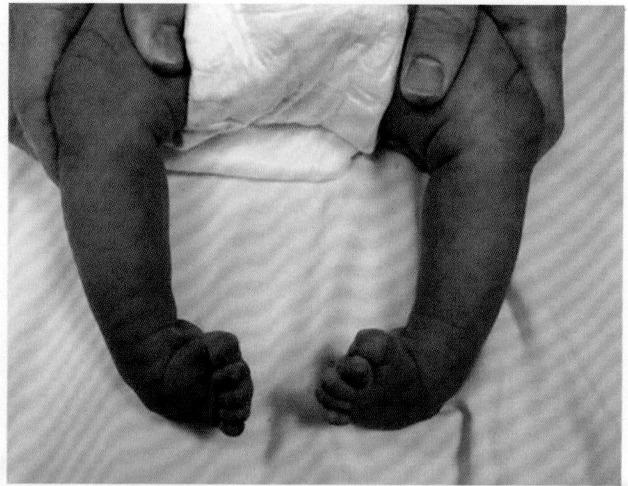

FIGURE 5 Clinical photograph of the lower extremities of a child with bilateral severe, rigid clubfoot. Note the presence of deep medial and posterior creases.

and is useful to decrease extensive soft-tissue release. However, an open excision of the Achilles tendon should be performed.[49]

Although the Ponseti method is useful as a noninvasive method to delay or avoid the need for extensive soft-tissue release, families should be educated about realistic expectations and prepared for the high risk of recurrence, the potential need for further treatment, and the risk of complications. An AFO brace should be used on a full-time basis after casting to prevent recurrence.

Vertical Talus

Vertical talus is a rigid, rocker-bottom flatfoot deformity that occurs in 10% of patients with myelomeningocele. There is extreme, rigid plantar flexion of the talus with dorsolateral dislocation of the talonavicular joint, and the foot is not correctable by manipulation. Correction has traditionally been achieved with complete posteromedial, lateral, and dorsal release when the patient is between 10 and 12 months of age.[46] In 2007, a minimally invasive treatment method was reported consisting of serial manipulation and casting followed by open talonavicular pin fixation and Achilles tenotomy.[50] Initially described for isolated vertical talus, encouraging short-term results have been reported for nonisolated cases as well, including patients with myelomeningocele[51] (**Figure 6**). Although long-term results and recurrence rates are not yet known, this method provides a less invasive option for potentially avoiding the need for extensive soft-tissue release.

TRANSITION/ADULT CARE

A 2016 systematic review examined the influence of myelomeningocele on HR-QOL outcomes. Overall, the authors found a negative impact, with physical HR-QOL being the most affected aspect.[52] In addition, they noted that HR-QOL declines with age, especially after the 13th birthday, and in the domains of psychological well-being,

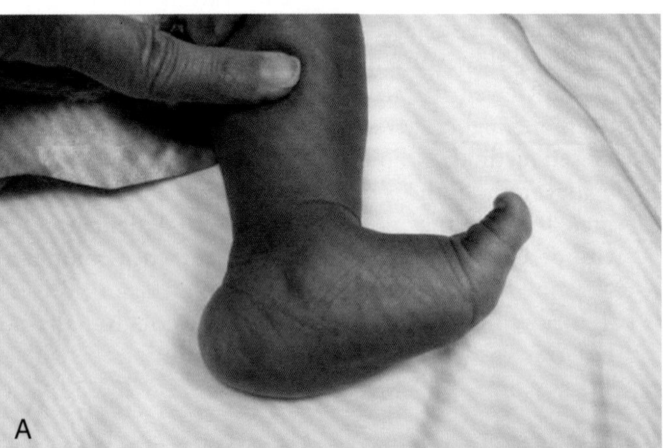

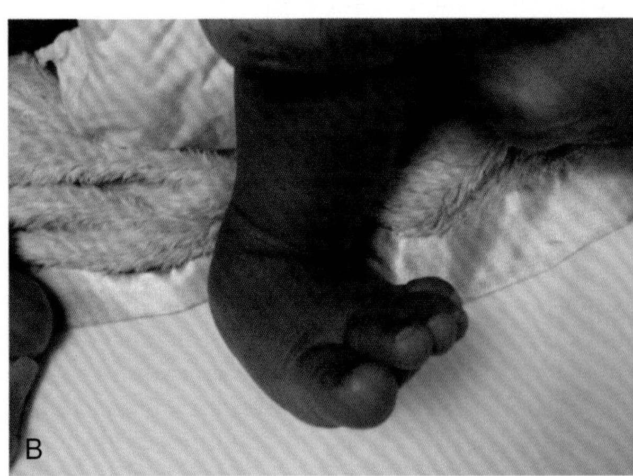

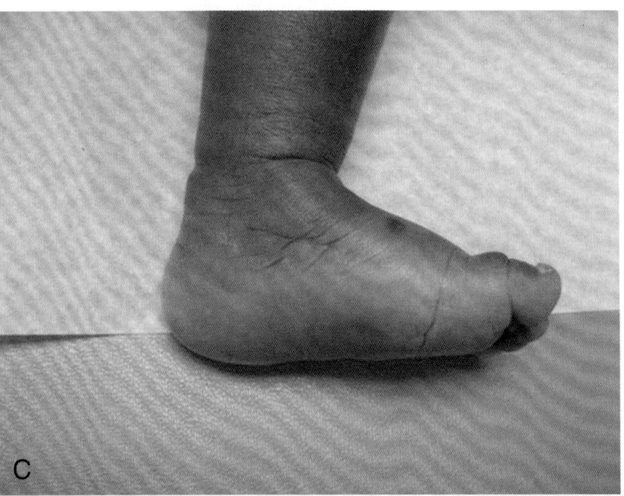

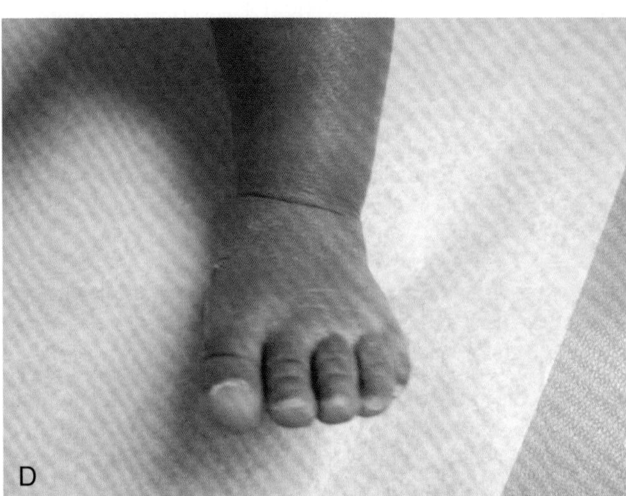

FIGURE 6 Lateral (**A**) and AP (**B**) clinical photographs of the foot of a child with rigid vertical talus. Lateral (**C**) and AP (**D**) clinical photographs of the foot after undergoing a minimally invasive method of treatment.

self-esteem, and peer relations. As such, transition from childhood to young adulthood can be an especially difficult period for those with myelomeningocele.

With an increase in the number of patients surviving into adulthood, many patients with myelomeningocele now require transition to adult medical providers. This presents a challenge because adult providers may lack the expertise necessary to manage the issues unique to adult patients with myelomeningocele. Guiding principles for orthopaedic care include aggressive treatment of tethered cord syndrome, surgical correction of musculoskeletal deformities that have the potential to affect independence, and avoidance of arthrodesis of the foot.[53] Secondary conditions in adults such as obesity and urologic issues have a negative effect on autonomy, function, and the level of community participation. Lymphedema also is common in adult patients and can cause difficulties with brace fitting and lead to functional decline. Pressure sores are another major complication and occasionally require limb amputation.

Multiple large cohort studies have reported on outcome and life satisfaction of adults with myelomeningocele. One study found myelomeningocele did not affect overall reported life satisfaction for adults.[54] Fifty-six percent of the patients completed a technical, associate, or college degree, and 47% were able to maintain employment. Twenty-eight percent had been married, and 18% had biological children. However, the presence of hydrocephalus substantially decreased the likelihood of these outcomes but did not contribute to decreased life satisfaction. Similarly, a 2011 study found adult patients who had never required a VPS placement had higher IQs.[55] All of the patients in that study with neurologic involvement at the thoracic or high lumbar level used wheelchairs; 78% of the patients with low lumbar-level involvement used a wheelchair on a part-time basis. All of the patients with neurologic involvement at the sacral level were ambulatory. In this cohort of patients, spinal fusions protected sitting balance, but hip surgery did not produce congruent hips and occasionally resulted in debilitating stiffness.

SUMMARY

The orthopaedic care of patients with myelomeningocele continues to improve with increased attention to functional outcomes. Ideally, orthopaedic care should be administered as part of a multidisciplinary team approach to optimally manage the complex medical comorbidities of these patients. The goal of the orthopaedic surgeon is to minimize deformity, maximize function and mobility, and limit complications.

KEY STUDY POINTS

- Fetal surgery for myelomeningocele, although associated with serious risks such as preterm delivery and uterine dehiscence, decreases the need for VPS placement and seems to improve lower extremity function and ambulation in short-term follow-up studies.
- The most important factor influencing ambulatory potential in patients with myelomeningocele is the neurologic level of involvement.
- Many factors influence the functional level achieved by patients with myelomeningocele, including spasticity; tethered cord; obesity; neurosurgical complications; poor balance; and musculoskeletal conditions such as hip contractures, scoliosis, and foot deformity.

ANNOTATED REFERENCES

1. Shimoji K, Kimura T, Kondo A, Tange Y, Miyajima M, Arai H: Genetic studies of myelomeningocele. *Childs Nerv Syst* 2013;29(9):1417-1425.
2. Bowman RM, McLone DG, Grant JA, Tomita T, Ito JA: Spina bifida outcome: A 25-year prospective. *Pediatr Neurosurg* 2001;34(3):114-120.
3. Swaroop VT, Dias L: Orthopedic management of spina bifida: Part I. Hip, knee, and rotational deformities. *J Child Orthop* 2009;3(6):441-449.
4. Thomson JD, Segal LS: Orthopedic management of spina bifida. *Dev Disabil Res Rev* 2010;16(1):96-103.
5. Swaroop VT, Dias L: Myelomeningocele, in Weinstein SL, Flynn JM, eds: *Lovell and Winter's Pediatric Orthopaedics*, ed 7. Philadelphia, PA, Lippincott Williams & Wilkins, 2014, pp 555-586.
6. Padmanabhan R: Etiology, pathogenesis and prevention of neural tube defects. *Congenit Anom (Kyoto)* 2006;46(2):55-67.
7. Doran PA, Guthkelch AN: Studies in spina bifida cystica: I. General survey and reassessment of the problem. *J Neurol Neurosurg Psychiatry* 1961;24:331-345.
8. Ingraham FD, Swam H: Spina bifida and cranium bifida: I. A survey of five hundred forty six cases. *N Engl J Med* 1943;228:559.
9. Au KS, Ashley-Koch A, Northrup H: Epidemiologic and genetic aspects of spina bifida and other neural tube defects. *Dev Disabil Res Rev* 2010;16(1):6-15.
10. Copp AJ, Stanier P, Greene ND: Neural tube defects: Recent advances, unsolved questions, and controversies. *Lancet Neurol* 2013;12(8):799-810.
11. Walsh DS, Adzick NS, Sutton LN, Johnson MP: The rationale for in utero repair of myelomeningocele. *Fetal Diagn Ther* 2001;16(5):312-322.

12. Tulipan N, Bruner JP, Hernanz-Schulman M, et al: Effect of intrauterine myelomeningocele repair on central nervous system structure and function. *Pediatr Neurosurg* 1999;31(4):183-188.
13. Adzick NS, Thom EA, Spong CY, et al, MOMS Investigators: A randomized trial of prenatal versus postnatal repair of myelomeningocele. *N Engl J Med* 2011;364(11):993-1004.
14. Moldenhauer JS, Soni S, Rintoul NE, et al: Fetal myelomeningocele repair: The post-MOMS experience at the Children's Hospital of Philadelphia. *Fetal Diagn Ther* 2015;37(3):235-240.
15. Danzer E, Gerdes M, Bebbington MW, et al: Lower extremity neuromotor function and short-term ambulatory potential following in utero myelomeningocele surgery. *Fetal Diagn Ther* 2009;25(1):47-53.
16. Danzer E, Thomas NH, Thomas A, et al: Long-term neurofunctional outcome, executive functioning, and behavioral adaptive skills following fetal myelomeningocele surgery. *Am J Obstet Gynecol* 2016;214(2):269.e1-269.e8.

    Results of fetal myelomeningocele repair at a median follow-up of 10 years showed that fetal surgery improves long-term ambulatory status. Spinal cord tethering is associated with functional loss. A more-than-expected number of children who had fetal repair were continent, but bowel and bladder control continue to be a challenging problem. Level of evidence: III.
17. Farmer DL, Thom EA, Brock JW III, et al: The management of myelomeningocele study: Full cohort 30-month pediatric outcomes. *Am J Obstet Gynecol* 2018;218(2):256.e1-256.e13.

    This study reports the 30-month outcomes for the full cohort of 183 patients enrolled in the MOMS trial and randomized to either prenatal or postnatal repair of myelomeningocele. The authors found prenatal repair significantly improves the composite score of mental development and motor function. In addition, prenatal surgery resulted in improved independent ambulation, functional level at least two better than the anatomic level, and psychomotor development. Level of evidence: I.
18. Seitzberg A, Lind M, Biering-Sørensen F: Ambulation in adults with myelomeningocele. Is it possible to predict the level of ambulation in early life? *Childs Nerv Syst* 2008;24(2):231-237.
19. McDonald CM, Jaffe KM, Mosca VS, Shurtleff DB: Ambulatory outcome of children with myelomeningocele: Effect of lower-extremity muscle strength. *Dev Med Child Neurol* 1991;33(6):482-490.
20. Mazur JM, Shurtleff D, Menelaus M, Colliver J: Orthopaedic management of high-level spina bifida: Early walking compared with early use of a wheelchair. *J Bone Joint Surg Am* 1989;71(1):56-61.
21. Haas RE, Kecskemethy HH, Lopiccolo MA, Hossain J, Dy RT, Bachrach SJ: Lower extremity bone mineral density in children with congenital spinal dysfunction. *Dev Med Child Neurol* 2012;54(12):1133-1137.
22. Szalay EA, Cheema A: Children with spina bifida are at risk for low bone density. *Clin Orthop Relat Res* 2011;469(5):1253-1257.
23. Akbar M, Bresch B, Raiss P, et al: Fractures in myelomeningocele. *J Orthop Traumatol* 2010;11(3):175-182.
24. Bowman RM, McLone DG: Neurosurgical management of spina bifida: Research issues. *Dev Disabil Res Rev* 2010;16(1):82-87.
25. Battibugli S, Gryfakis N, Dias L, et al: Functional gait comparison between children with myelomeningocele: Shunt versus no shunt. *Dev Med Child Neurol* 2007;49(10):764-769.
26. Fiore P, Picco P, Castagnola E, et al: Nutritional survey of children and adolescents with myelomeningocele (MMC): Overweight associated with reduced energy intake. *Eur J Pediatr Surg* 1998;8(suppl 1):34-36.
27. Mueske NM, Ryan DD, Van Speybroeck AL, Chan LS, Wren TA: Fat distribution in children and adolescents with myelomeningocele. *Dev Med Child Neurol* 2015;57(3):273-278.
28. Mita K, Akataki K, Itoh K, Ono Y, Ishida N, Oki T: Assessment of obesity of children with spina bifida. *Dev Med Child Neurol* 1993;35(4):305-311.
29. Mueske NM, Ounpuu S, Ryan DD, et al: Impact of gait analysis on pathology identification and surgical recommendations in children with spina bifida. *Gait Posture* 2019;67:128-132.

    Two pediatric orthopaedic surgeons and two therapists reviewed clinical, video, and gait analysis data from 43 patients. Primary gait pathologies and surgical recommendations were recorded before and after consideration of the gait analysis data. Recognition of excessive hip flexion and abnormal femoral rotation increased significantly after consideration of gait analysis data, and surgical recommendations changed for 44% of patients. Level of evidence: IV.
30. Schoenmakers MA, Gulmans VA, Gooskens RH, Pruijs JE, Helders PJ: Spinal fusion in children with spina bifida: Influence on ambulation level and functional abilities. *Eur Spine J* 2005;14(4):415-422.
31. Mazur J, Menelaus MB, Dickens DR, Doig WG: Efficacy of surgical management for scoliosis in myelomeningocele: Correction of deformity and alteration of functional status. *J Pediatr Orthop* 1986;6(5):568-575.
32. Khoshbin A, Vivas L, Law PW, et al: The long-term outcome of patients treated operatively and non-operatively for scoliosis deformity secondary to spina bifida. *Bone Joint J* 2014;96-B(9):1244-1251.
33. Jain A, Sullivan BT, Kuwabara A, Kebaish KM, Sponseller PD: Sacral-alar-iliac fixation in children with neuromuscular scoliosis: Minimum 5-year follow-up. *World Neurosurg* 2017;108:474-478.

    The authors reviewed a single-surgeon series of 38 patients with neuromuscular scoliosis undergoing spine fusion using sacral-alar-iliac pelvic anchors with minimum 5-year follow-up. Patients had a mean 57% correction of pelvic obliquity, which was maintained at final follow-up. Complications included deep wound infection in 10% patients and screw fracture in one patient. There were no cases of screw displacement, backout, or rod dislodgement. Level of evidence: VI.
34. Garg S, Oetgen M, Rathjen K, Richards BS: Kyphectomy improves sitting and skin problems in patients with myelomeningocele. *Clin Orthop Relat Res* 2011;469(5):1279-1285.

35. Altiok H, Finlayson C, Hassani S, Sturm P: Kyphectomy in children with myelomeningocele. *Clin Orthop Relat Res* 2011;469(5):1272-1278.

36. Bas CE, Preminger J, Olgun ZD, Demirkiran G, Sponseller P, Yazici M, Growing Spine Study Group: Safety and efficacy of apical resection following growth-friendly instrumentation in myelomeningocele patients with gibbus: Growing rod versus Luque trolley. *J Pediatr Orthop* 2015;35(8):e98-e103.

37. Gabrieli AP, Vankoski SJ, Dias LS, et al: Gait analysis in low lumbar myelomeningocele patients with unilateral hip dislocation or subluxation. *J Pediatr Orthop* 2003;23(3):330-334.

38. Swaroop VT, Dias LS: What is the optimal treatment for hip and spine in myelomeningocele?, in Wright JG, ed: *Evidence-Based Orthopaedics*. Amsterdam, the Netherlands, Elsevier Health Sciences, 2008, pp 273-277.

39. Thompson RM, Foley J, Dias L, Swaroop VT: Hip status and long-term functional outcomes in spina bifida. *J Pediatr Orthop* 2019;39(3):e168-e172.

The authors used VR-12 and National Institutes of Health PROMIS outcomes measures to compare functional outcomes across three cohorts of adult patients with myelomeningocele: those with bilateral located hips, unilateral subluxation/dislocation, or bilateral subluxation/dislocation. The authors found no statistically significant difference in any of the outcomes measures between groups. Rather, functional outcomes were correlated with neurologic level and hip range of motion. The authors concluded that efforts to keep myelomeningocele hips reduced are likely without functional benefit and should be avoided in favor of maintaining motion with contracture release as needed. Level of evidence: III.

40. Spiro AS, Babin K, Lipovac S, et al: Anterior femoral epiphysiodesis for the treatment of fixed knee flexion deformity in spina bifida patients. *J Pediatr Orthop* 2010;30(8):858-862.

41. Dias LS: Surgical management of knee contractures in myelomeningocele. *J Pediatr Orthop* 1982;2(2):127-131.

42. Moen TC, Dias L, Swaroop VT, Gryfakis N, Kelp-Lenane C: Radical posterior capsulectomy improves sagittal knee motion in crouch gait. *Clin Orthop Relat Res* 2011;469(5):1286-1290.

43. Dunteman RC, Vankoski SJ, Dias LS: Internal derotation osteotomy of the tibia: Pre- and postoperative gait analysis in persons with high sacral myelomeningocele. *J Pediatr Orthop* 2000;20(5):623-628.

44. Rao S, Dietz F, Yack HJ: Kinematics and kinetics during gait in symptomatic and asymptomatic limbs of children with myelomeningocele. *J Pediatr Orthop* 2012;32(1):106-112.

45. Mednick RE, Eller EB, Swaroop VT, Dias L: Outcomes of tibial derotational osteotomies performed in patients with myelodysplasia. *J Pediatr Orthop* 2015;35(7):721-724.

46. Swaroop VT, Dias L: Orthopaedic management of spina bifida: Part II. Foot and ankle deformities. *J Child Orthop* 2011;5(6):403-414.

47. Dunkley M, Gelfer Y, Jackson D, et al: Mid-term results of a physiotherapist-led Ponseti service for the management of non-idiopathic and idiopathic clubfoot. *J Child Orthop* 2015;9(3):183-189.

48. Gerlach DJ, Gurnett CA, Limpaphayom N, et al: Early results of the Ponseti method for the treatment of clubfoot associated with myelomeningocele. *J Bone Joint Surg Am* 2009;91(6):1350-1359.

49. Arkin C, Ihnow S, Dias L, Swaroop VT: Midterm results of the Ponseti method for treatment of clubfoot in patients with spina bifida. *J Pediatr Orthop* 2018;38(10):e588-e592.

In this retrospective review of 26 clubfeet in patients with spina bifida treated by a single surgeon, the authors report a 58% overall recurrence rate at average 5-year follow-up. Significantly, the authors noted 100% patients treated with percutaneous tenotomy had recurrence compared with only 18% of those treated with an open excision of the Achilles tendon. The authors concluded that in patients with spina bifida, the Ponseti method leads to reliable initial correction and is useful to decrease extensive soft-tissue release. However, an open excision of the Achilles tendon should be performed, and families should be counseled about high risk of recurrence. Level of evidence: III.

50. Dobbs MB, Purcell DB, Nunley R, Morcuende JA: Early results of a new method of treatment for idiopathic congenital vertical talus. Surgical technique. *J Bone Joint Surg Am* 2007;89(suppl 2 pt 1):111-121.

51. Chalayon O, Adams A, Dobbs MB: Minimally invasive approach for the treatment of non-isolated congenital vertical talus. *J Bone Joint Surg Am* 2012;94(11):e73.

52. Bakaniene I, Prasauskiene A, Vaiciene-Magistris N: Health-related quality of life in children with myelomeningocele: A systematic review of the literature. *Child Care Health Dev* 2016;42(5):625-643.

The authors review the existing literature regarding HR-QOL and determinants of HR-QOL in patients with myelomeningocele. They included only studies that used validated HR-QOL instruments. They found that patients with myelomeningocele have overall decreased HR-QOL with physical domains the most affected and discrepancies in psychosocial domains across studies. Level of evidence: V.

53. Selber P, Dias L: Sacral-level myelomeningocele: Long-term outcome in adults. *J Pediatr Orthop* 1998;18(4):423-427.

54. Cope H, McMahon K, Heise E, et al: Outcome and life satisfaction of adults with myelomeningocele. *Disabil Health J* 2013;6(3):236-243.

55. Roach JW, Short BF, Saltzman HM: Adult consequences of spina bifida: A cohort study. *Clin Orthop Relat Res* 2011;469(5):1246-1252.

CHAPTER 16

Arthrogrypotic Syndromes

KATHRYN S. DOUGHTY, MD, MPH, MS • ROBERT H. CHO, MD
CHRISTOPHER M. STUTZ, MD

ABSTRACT

Arthrogryposis refers to a constellation of syndromes characterized by multiple joint contractures. The treatment of any type of arthrogryposis can be challenging, but early intervention and proper nonsurgical and surgical management can achieve improvement in many patients. The goal for any treatment strategy is to maximize function with the minimal amount of hospitalization necessary to achieve that goal. Physical and occupational therapies, as well as bracing, can help improve function in many children so that surgical management can be mitigated or avoided. Surgical treatment should be reserved for enhancing function, not just correcting deformity.

Keywords: amyoplasia; arthrogryposis; Bruck syndrome; contractures; Larsen syndrome

INTRODUCTION

Arthrogryposis multiplex congenita, also known simply as arthrogryposis, is not a diagnosis; rather, arthrogryposis is a generic umbrella term for a heterogeneous group of disorders characterized by multiple congenital joint contractures. Although the exact etiology is usually multifactorial (nerve, muscle, or connective tissue disorders; maternal disease; intrauterine constraint; and vascular compromise), the condition is associated with decreased fetal movement. The earlier the intrauterine insult resulting in fetal akinesis, the more severe the disease at birth. Most deformities are nonprogressive and may improve over time with early treatment. Mental development is usually normal. The most common musculoskeletal deformities associated with arthrogryposis are clubfeet and hip dislocations. The incidence of arthrogryposis is approximately 1 per 3,000 live births.[1]

More than 400 specific conditions are associated with congenital contractures.[2] These conditions are associated with substantial morbidity and economic burden, so understanding the underlying etiology of a child's condition can aid in determining the prognosis and selecting the best treatment options. Approximately 50% of the conditions associated with arthrogryposis have an underlying genetic abnormality. Distal arthrogryposis is one of the most notable conditions, because it can be inherited in an autosomal dominant manner.

Congenital contractures can be categorized as isolated or multiple[3] (**Figure 1**). In a child with multiple congenital contractures, it is necessary to determine whether the neurologic examination has normal or abnormal findings. Amyoplasia and distal arthrogryposis are common types of arthrogryposis that are associated with normal neurologic development. A generalized connective tissue disorder and fetal crowding are less common causes of arthrogryposis that are associated with normal neurologic development. Conversely, an abnormal neurologic examination suggests that in utero movement was diminished as a result of central or peripheral nervous system disorders or intrinsic muscle disease.

Dr. Doughty or an immediate family member serves as a board member, owner, officer, or committee member of the American Academy of Orthopaedic Surgeons. Dr. Cho or an immediate family member serves as a paid consultant to or is an employee of DePuy Spine, NuVasive, OrthoPediatrics, and Prosidyan and serves as a board member, owner, officer, or committee member of the American Academy of Orthopaedic Surgeons, the Pediatric Orthopaedic Society of North America, and the Scoliosis Research Society. Dr. Stutz or an immediate family member is a member of a speakers' bureau or has made paid presentations on behalf of OrthoPediatrics.

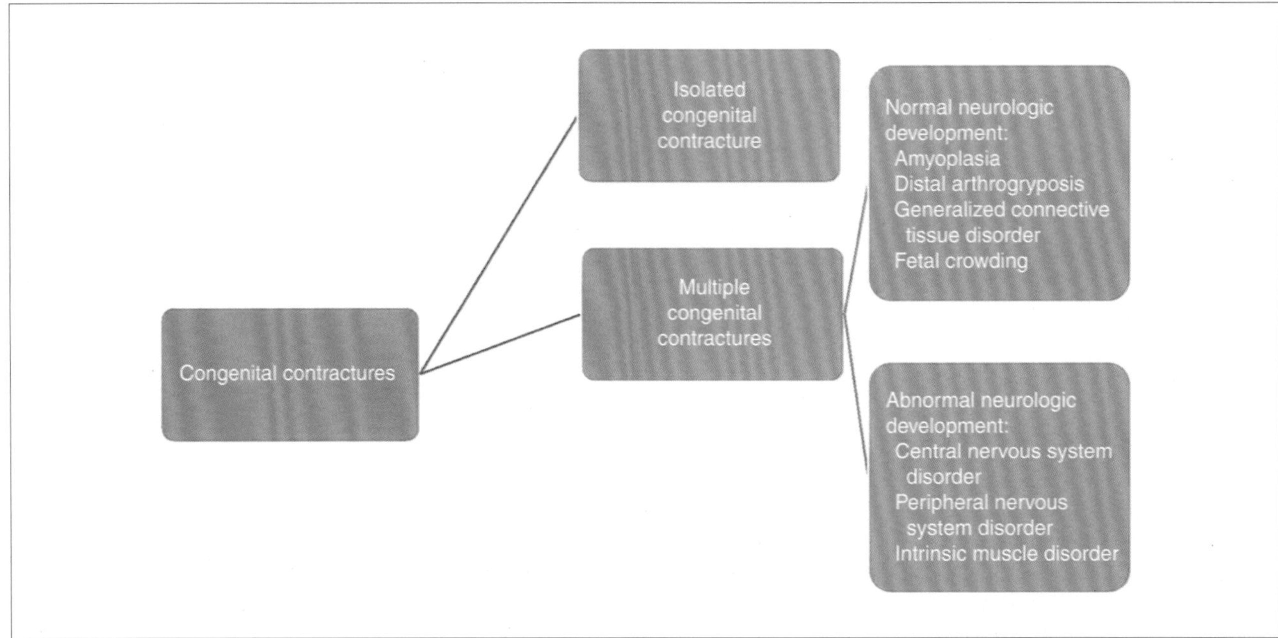

FIGURE 1 Diagram outlining that congenital contractures can be divided into isolated or multiple contractures. Isolated congenital contractures affect only a single area of the body; the most common isolated contracture is congenital clubfoot. Amyoplasia falls under the category of multiple congenital contractures with normal neurologic development.

DIAGNOSIS

Prenatal ultrasonography may be able to document fetal movements and positions that suggest a typically developing fetus versus a fetus affected by multiple joint contractures and akinesis. Genetic testing may be useful; however, only approximately 50% of arthrogrypotic conditions have an identifiable genetic abnormality. Genetic information can be helpful in counseling parents on the risks for future affected pregnancies. Arthrogryposis is not a hereditary condition, whereas distal arthrogryposis is often inherited in an autosomal dominant pattern (**Figure 2**).

Any child with multiple contractures should have a thorough initial history and physical examination, including a family history. Additional studies and consultations with specialists may be warranted if the condition affects the neurologic system or appears to be syndromic. A skeletal survey, including radiographs of the spine, shoulders, elbows, hips, knees, and feet, is usually obtained early in the examination process.

Depending on the results of the skeletal survey, a partial differential diagnosis may include spinal dysraphism, congenital muscular dystrophy, spinal muscular atrophy, structural brain anomalies, chromosomal abnormalities, thrombocytopenia with absent radius syndrome, Möbius syndrome, Larsen syndrome, or Freeman-Sheldon syndrome.[4]

TYPES OF ARTHROGRYPOSIS

Amyoplasia

Amyoplasia is the classic form of arthrogryposis, comprising approximately one-third of all cases. The incidence of amyoplasia is approximately 1 per 10,000 live births.[5] It is not a hereditary condition. All four extremities are affected in approximately 60% of patients. Only the lower extremities are affected in approximately 25% of patients, and only the upper extremities in approximately 15% of patients. Clinical features are often diagnostic, including a midline hemangioma on the forehead, although this usually disappears over time (**Figure 3**).

The lower extremities are usually held in a typical posture—flexed, abducted, and externally rotated hips; rigid knees (flexed or extended); and clubfeet (**Figure 4**). A typical posture, which is described later, also characterizes amyoplasia of the upper extremities. Amyoplasia literally means “without muscle growth,” so muscles are typically hypoplastic or absent; in fact, the skeletal muscle is replaced by dense fibrous tissue and fat. Joints lack flexion creases (**Figure 5**). Intelligence is normal, sensation is intact, and most affected children are able to function independently as adults.[6]

Distal Arthrogryposis

Distal arthrogryposis most notably affects the hands and feet, but may also involve more proximal joints. Distal arthrogryposis is often inherited in an autosomal

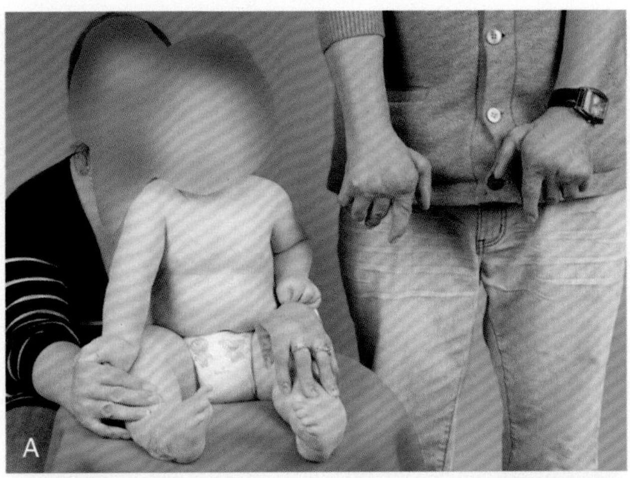

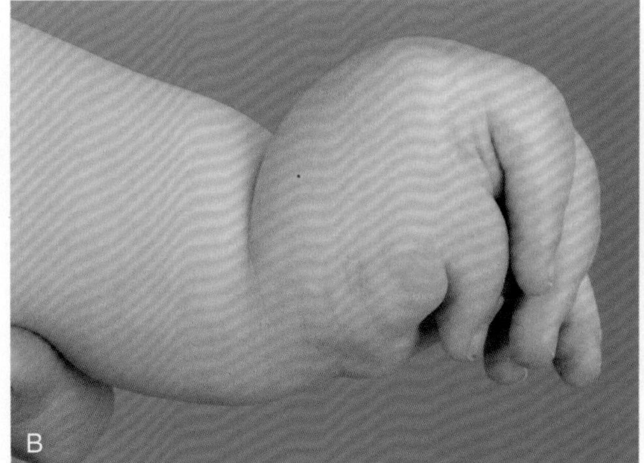

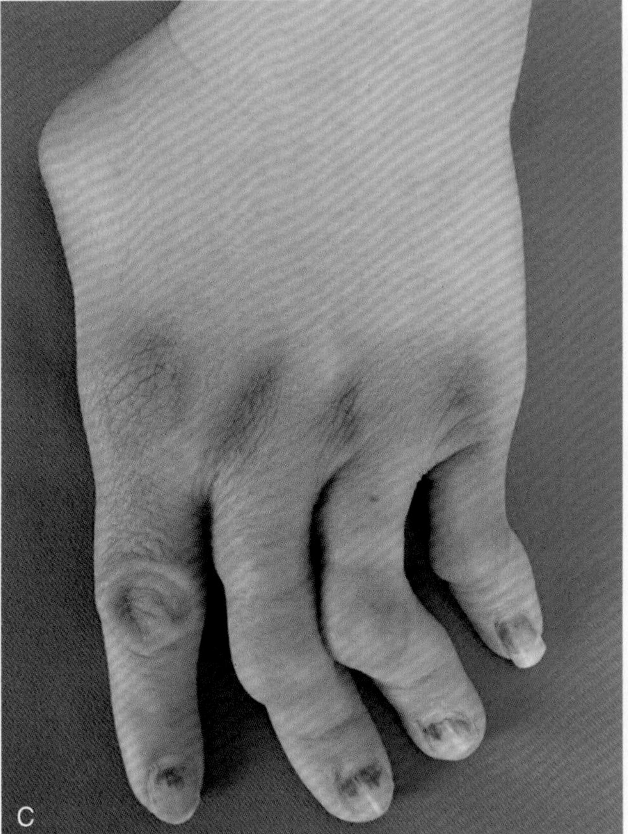

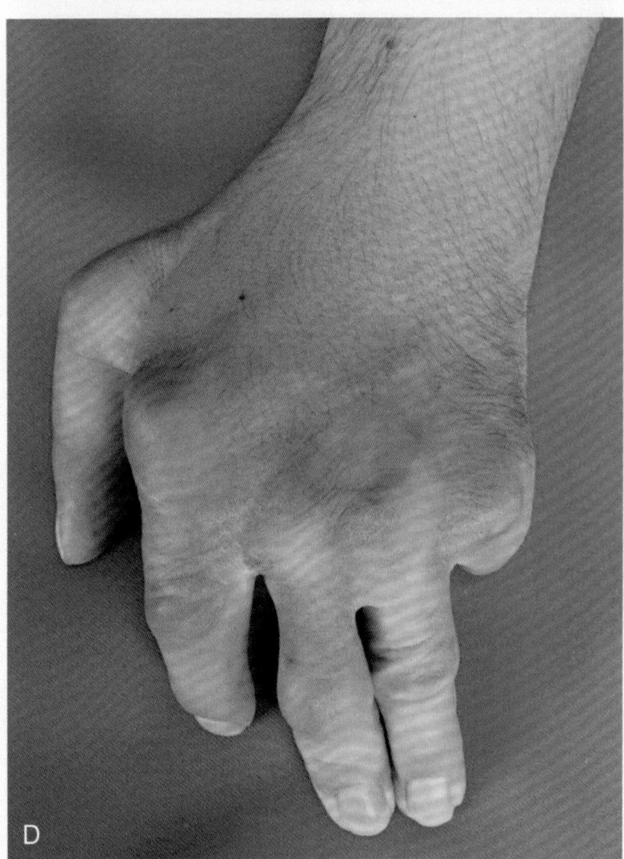

FIGURE 2 **A**, Photograph of a child with distal arthrogryposis with bilateral hand and foot deformities. His mother and uncle (pictured) also are affected, as is his maternal grandmother (not pictured). Photographs of the left hand of the child (**B**), the left hand of the child's mother (**C**), and the left hand of the child's uncle (**D**).

dominant manner. Clinical features are similar to, but less severe than, classic amyoplasia. The hands are usually held in a typical posture with flexed wrists and the thumb in the palm. The lower extremities may exhibit hip dislocations, clubfeet, or congenital vertical tali. Joints are notable for lack of flexion creases. These patients also have normal intelligence and intact sensation, and most can function independently as adults.

Larsen Syndrome

Larsen syndrome, which was originally described in 1950, is a rare hereditary syndrome characterized by multiple

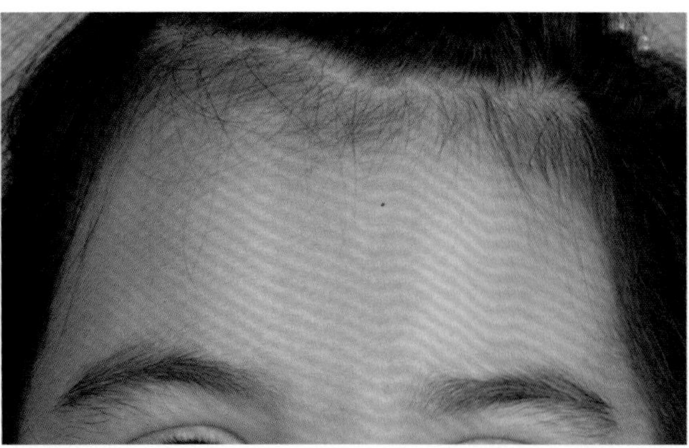

FIGURE 3 Photograph of a 4-year-old girl with a midline hemangioma, which is very common in patients with amyoplasia. Most hemangiomas disappear over time. Although this child's birthmark is vaguely visible, it becomes more prominent when the child is upset.

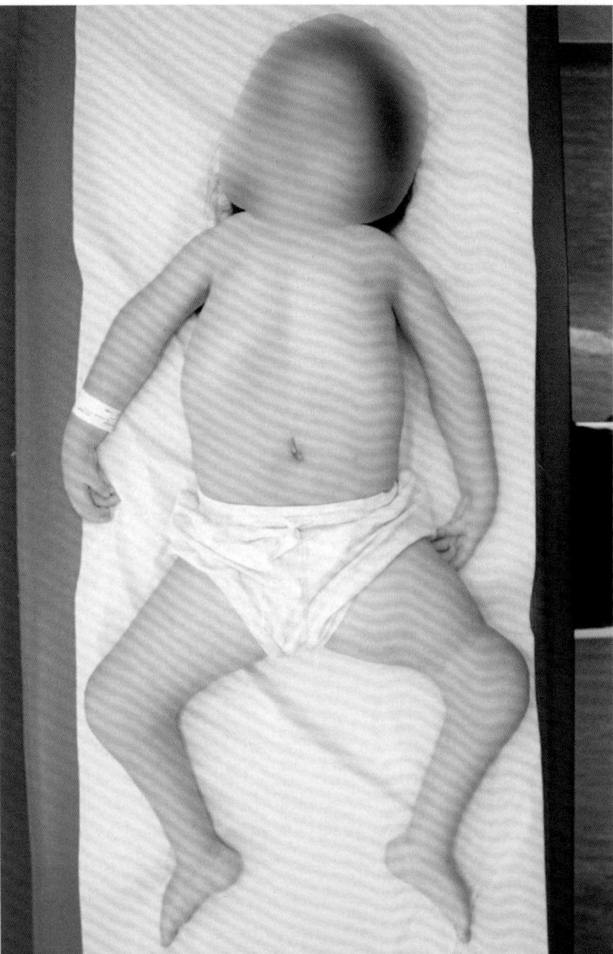

FIGURE 4 Clinical photograph of a child with amyoplasia shows the typical posture: narrow, sloping shoulders; rigid elbows (flexed or extended); flexed, abducted, externally rotated hips; and rigid knees (flexed or extended). This child also has evidence of an amniotic band around the left thigh. Her clubfeet have been surgically treated.

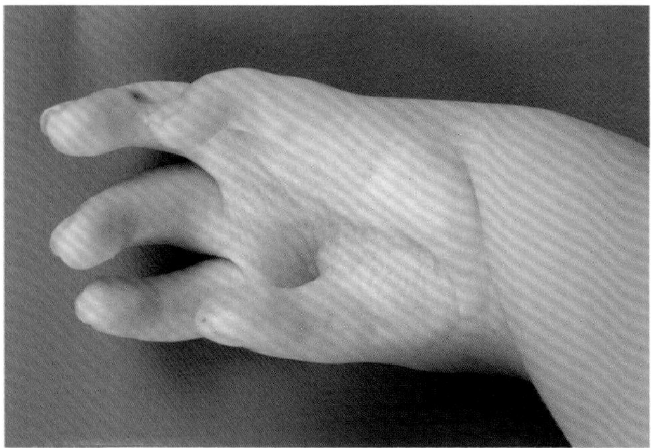

FIGURE 5 Clinical photograph shows the lack of flexion creases in the hand of a child with arthrogryposis.

joint dislocations from birth and characteristic facial features. Characteristics of the syndrome include a flattened dishlike face, bilateral dislocations of multiple joints, and equinovarus deformities of the feet.[7] Mutation occurs in the *FLNB* gene, which encodes for the protein filamin B and acts as a cytoskeletal binder to help chondrocytes differentiate and proliferate during development. The disease is characterized by a combination of laxity and dislocation in large joints that is present from birth (most commonly the cervical spine, hip, knee, and the radiocapitellar joints) and rigid talipes equinovarus deformities of the feet. The cervical spine and knee deformities are particularly challenging to manage, and the goals of treatment are stabilization and prevention of further deformity.[8,9] Unilateral hip dislocations are often managed surgically, but the management of bilateral hip dislocation is controversial and may be best left untreated.[10] Clubfoot deformities also are challenging to treat. Guidelines similar to the management of clubfeet for the other arthrogrypotic syndromes should be followed. Timing of treatment usually involves serial casting for clubfoot, followed by surgical stabilization of the cervical spine if necessary, and then treatment of knee or other joint dislocations.

Multiple Pterygium Syndromes

Multiple pterygium syndromes are a rare spectrum of disorders involving pterygia (skin webbing) of multiple joints, including the elbows and knees; congenital joint contractures; and facial anomalies. Multiple pterygium syndromes are further subcategorized into Escobar syndrome[11] (a milder disorder) and lethal multiple pterygium syndrome, which is often fatal in utero or shortly after birth. Most cases involve a mutation of the *CHRNG* gene, which encodes for the gamma subunit of the fetal acetylcholine receptor protein that allows for neuromuscular signaling. The lethal form involves complete absence of this subunit, whereas the Escobar form involves a decrease in the relative level of this protein. The fetal acetylcholine receptor gene is replaced in utero at approximately 33 weeks of gestation with an adult acetylcholine receptor gene; therefore, most patients with multiple pterygium syndromes have joint contractures without concomitant muscle weakness.

Bruck Syndrome

Bruck syndrome is extremely rare, with approximately 20 patients with this condition reported in the medical literature. This syndrome is a combination of arthrogryposis and osteogenesis imperfecta. Two subtypes have been identified with different gene mutations but similar phenotypic presentations. This condition manifests in neonates with multiple joint contractures and pterygia; fractures are often seen in the postnatal period. Most patients are nonambulatory. Because Bruck syndrome is challenging to treat, realistic goals should be discussed with the patient and the family to achieve satisfactory outcomes (**Figure 6**).

GENERAL MANAGEMENT

Although each child with arthrogryposis is unique and requires a personalized treatment plan and goals, many management principles can be applied to most patients. Clinicians should aim to maximize function while minimizing repeated hospitalizations or medicalization of these children. An accurate diagnosis will help parents understand disease risks in future pregnancies. Some families may require counseling to deal with feelings of guilt (especially if the mother believes the condition is related to the size or shape of her uterus). Local and national arthrogryposis groups can provide valuable support to patients and their families.

Physical therapy and a stretching program done at home should be started as soon as possible. Stretching should be gentle and atraumatic. Stretching can be quite effective in reducing contractures, especially in children younger than 1 year.

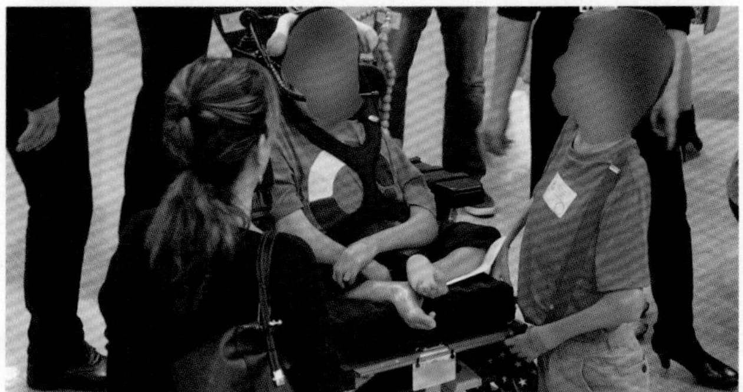

FIGURE 6 Photograph of a boy with Bruck syndrome participating in a publicity event for the hospital where he receives treatment. The patient controls his wheelchair with his lips.

Bracing may be necessary to provide joint stabilization, which can encourage the achievement of normal developmental milestones. Lightweight, nonarticulated ankle-foot and knee-ankle-foot orthoses are often most useful early in development. Bracing is also vital to maintaining any joint range of motion that was obtained through stretching or surgery. For patients with lower extremity or spinal arthrogryposis, adaptive equipment, such as walkers, scooters, and electric wheelchairs, is vital to encourage a child's sense of independence.

Surgical correction should be reserved for enhancing function, not merely correcting deformities. Surgical intervention should be delayed until the child is demonstrating some head and trunk control as well as active hip extension, which are predictors of the future ability to stand. The number of hospitalizations and periods of immobilization should be minimized to allow normal socialization and education. Procedures should be combined whenever possible so that only one recovery period is necessary. Hip extensor strength is mandatory for upright stance, so surgical correction of knee deformities may not be indicated if the child lacks the strength to stand. A 2019 study has attempted to predict a child's ambulation potential at maturity based on the infantile position and muscle strength of the lower extremities.[12]

Surgical intervention for the upper extremities should not be considered until the child demonstrates difficulty with activities of daily living; even then, the child's function may improve more with occupational therapy than with surgery.

The use of anesthesia in patients with arthrogrypotic conditions requires special considerations. Trismus, cervical spine stiffness (or laxity in patients with Larsen syndrome), difficult intravenous access, gastroesophageal reflux disease, and postoperative airway obstruction are common in these patients. One type of pterygium syndrome is associated with malignant hyperthermia.[13] A 2017 study confirmed that there is no increased odds of intraoperative hyperthermia or hypermetabolic response in patients with arthrogrypotic syndromes.[14]

SPINE AND LOWER EXTREMITY

Spine

Scoliosis in arthrogryposis has been reported to have an incidence of up to 70%.[15] Curvatures in these patients may be present at birth and often progress as the child grows. Most curve patterns involve thoracolumbar or lumbar curves with pelvic obliquity, but also can involve the thoracic spine. Most patients with arthrogryposis and scoliosis do not have congenital vertebral anomalies; however, congenital scoliosis with upper extremity arthrogryposis has been described in a small series of patients.[16] Although the use of a thoracolumbar orthosis in these patients is often unsuccessful, it may delay the need for surgical stabilization.

Medical literature provides little guidance for the treatment of children with arthrogryposis and scoliosis. One study found that nonsurgical management of curves may be effective for ambulatory patients who have less than 30° of curvature;[17] however, it is unclear how many of the curves would have progressed without bracing treatment. Of the patients who required spinal fusion from the same study, 80% were nonambulatory and had involvement in all four limbs. Combined anterior and posterior fusion was recommended for this population, but this was before the widespread use of all-pedicle screw constructs and posteriorly based osteotomies, which have much more corrective potential than older technologies.

Traditional spine-based growing rods or rib-based distraction using implants such as the vertical expandable prosthetic titanium rib (VEPTR; DePuy Synthes) are viable alternatives to bracing in patients with progressive early-onset scoliosis. However, in a series of patients with arthrogryposis and early-onset scoliosis who were treated with VEPTR, a 60% incidence of proximal junctional kyphosis was reported. As with all growing spine implant systems, complications were frequent and at least one complication was seen in 40% of the patients.[18]

Newer growth modulation technologies, including the Magnetic Expansion Control (Ellipse Technology) device, are promising because they can be lengthened externally, which decreases the number of surgical procedures that the child must undergo. However, complications can occur. A 2014 study reported a 42% incidence rate of unplanned returns to the operating room in patients without arthrogryposis treated with growing rod surgery.[19]

Hip Dislocation

The management of bilateral hip dislocations remains controversial, because surgical intervention can cause hip stiffness and/or osteonecrosis. Closed reduction is rarely successful. Unilateral dislocation will result in a functional limb-length discrepancy. If surgery is elected, the hips should undergo reduction in infancy, and postoperative immobilization should be limited to 5 weeks to minimize the risk of postoperative stiffness. Although a risk of osteonecrosis exists with medial open reduction, the limited surgical dissection required with this approach compared with an anterior approach minimizes the risk of increasing inherent joint stiffness.[20] In the long term, a stiff hip may be more debilitating than a dislocated hip or a collapsed femoral head. Case reports of total hip arthroplasty in this patient population outline myriad surgical challenges without necessarily an increase in function or range of motion.[21,22]

Hip External Rotation Contracture

External rotation contracture of the hip rarely requires surgical intervention; surgical dissection around the hip should be avoided to minimize the risk of joint stiffness. If the external rotation of the limb is problematic (interfering with gait or wheelchair sitting), it can be addressed using distal femoral derotational osteotomies.

Knee Flexion Contracture

Early stretching may improve the arc of motion in a patient with knee flexion contracture. Casting or bracing should be used to maintain the range of motion. Older children who have not been successfully treated with casting or bracing may require hamstring lengthening, release of the gastrocnemius origin, posterior capsulectomy, and even femoral shortening via a popliteal fossa approach. The goal should be to correct the flexion deformity to approximately 15° to 20°, which can be accommodated in a postoperative knee-ankle-foot orthosis and is compatible with ambulation. Prolonged—essentially indefinite—postoperative bracing is mandatory to prevent recurrent deformity.

Knee Extension Contracture

In a child younger than 1 year, the initial management of knee extension contractures should focus on gentle stretching. Casting, bracing, or a Pavlik harness can be used to maintain knee flexion throughout the process. If the knee is anteriorly dislocated, reduction may be obtained with serial casting or may require surgical quadriceps lengthening and/or femoral shortening. In children older than 1 year, management is more challenging. Quadriceps lengthening, anterior knee releases, or even flexion osteotomies may be required to improve the arc of motion.

Knee extension contractures often allow children to stand without the use of above-knee bracing; however, as the child grows, the knee extension creates sitting challenges in automobiles, at school, and in social settings such as movie theaters. When contemplating surgery for an older child with knee extension contractures, it is important to be aware that increasing the knee range of motion may inhibit the child's ability to stand without above-knee bracing. Knee disarticulation is one surgical option, especially when knee extension (or flexion) contractures are paired with irreparable foot deformities. If the child has good trunk musculature and hip extensor strength, knee disarticulations may allow increased mobility on the distal femoral condyles (**Figure 7**).

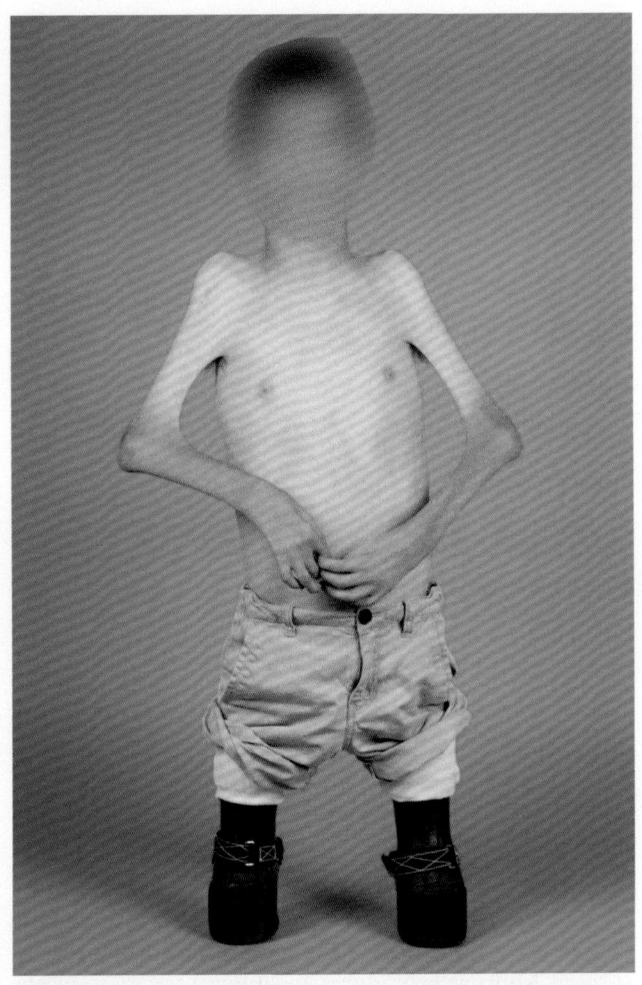

FIGURE 7 Knee disarticulations can allow ambulation in children with excellent trunk and hip extensor strength. Photograph of a child who had undergone multiple surgical procedures to treat rigid, painful knees and feet. After knee disarticulation, he was fitted with prosthetic stubby feet, which improved his independence by allowing him to transfer from wheelchair to bed, to walk in spaces his wheelchair would not fit, to sit more easily in an automobile and at a desk, and to skateboard. Rather than using full-height prostheses, the lower center of gravity of stubby feet helps prevent a head injury in the event of a fall; his upper extremity deformities will not allow him to break a fall.

Talipes Equinovarus

Talipes equinovarus, also known as clubfoot, is one of the most common arthrogrypotic musculoskeletal deformities. Early stretching, casting, percutaneous Achilles tenotomies, bracing, and repeat casting can achieve some correction, although this treatment course is not as successful as in children with idiopathic clubfeet.[23,24] Residual deformity can be corrected with limited posteromedial releases. Prolonged nighttime splinting is mandatory to prevent recurrence. Concomitant hip and knee deformities may preclude the use of traditional boots and bars for clubfoot treatment, so ankle-foot or knee-ankle-foot orthoses may be used. Talectomies may be an appropriate salvage procedure for older children who have substantial residual deformity. This procedure is often delayed until most of the foot growth is completed by approximately 10 years of age.[25]

Congenital Vertical Talus

Congenital vertical talus is the most severe form of pathologic flatfoot. This deformity is usually associated with other conditions such as spina bifida or arthrogrypotic syndromes. As in clubfoot, some correction may be obtained by serial casting; however, many patients with this type of stiff foot will require open reduction, as well as prolonged bracing to maintain the surgical correction.

UPPER EXTREMITY

The findings associated with arthrogryposis in the upper extremity are largely dependent on the underlying cause, with the manifestations of amyoplasia being very different from those of distal arthrogryposis (Freeman-Sheldon or Sheldon-Hall syndromes). Despite the differences in phenotypic presentation, the treatment goals remain largely the same, with a focus on independent accomplishment of the activities of daily living and development of a functional capacity that allows the patient to become a productive member of society. The approach to accomplishing these goals differs based on the presenting limitations. Common objectives include positioning the limb for bimanual use and tabletop activities, facilitating self-care, permitting the use of assistive devices for locomotion if necessary, and enabling the patient to easily interact with communication devices.

Amyoplasia

The typical presentation of amyoplasia in the upper limb consists of a shoulder that is internally rotated and adducted, pronated forearms, flexed and ulnarly deviated wrists, stiff fingers, and clasped thumbs (**Figure 8**). In a patient with upper limb amyoplasia, treatment of the limb begins at an early age with occupational therapy. Stretching and splinting are the mainstays of early intervention. Elbow flexion is the most critical element in obtaining independence in activities of daily living. Stretching exercises to achieve passive elbow flexion past 90° are initiated as early as possible to allow for hand-to-mouth activity. The wrist is splinted to minimize flexion and ulnar deviation deformity that is often present. Passive stretching exercises are used to maximize finger and thumb range of motion. Despite the early initiation of stretching exercises and the diligence of caretakers and therapists, patients with upper limb amyoplasia often require surgery to optimize function. Surgical intervention most often focuses on passive positioning of the upper limb.

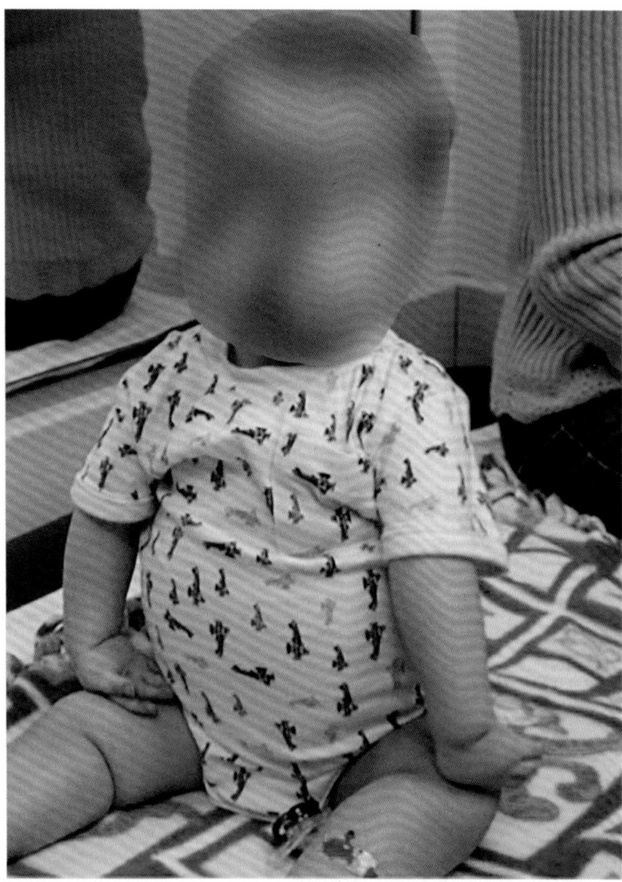

FIGURE 8 Clinical photograph of an infant with upper limb amyoplasia shows the typical appearance of adducted and internally rotated shoulders, extended elbows, flexed and ulnarly deviated wrists, stiff fingers, and clasped thumbs.

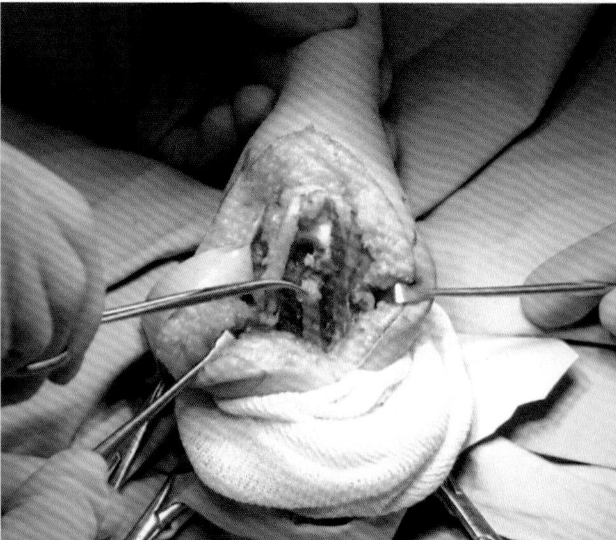

FIGURE 9 Intraoperative photograph shows surgical release of the elbow extension contracture performed through a posterior incision. The triceps tendon is lengthened using W-plasty with the medial and lateral limbs of the tendon remaining attached to the olecranon. Note the complete posterior capsulectomy and visualization of the trochlear cartilage. (Courtesy of Marybeth Ezaki, MD, Dallas, TX.)

Shoulder

An internal rotation deformity of the shoulder may require surgical intervention in more severe cases. An external rotation osteotomy of the humerus will provide an arm position that allows the forearm to clear the abdomen and will facilitate bimanual activities in a palm-facing-palm orientation.[26]

Elbow

Elbow extension contractures that fail to resolve sufficiently to allow for hand-to-mouth activities are managed with surgical release (**Figure 9**). The elbow is approached posteriorly using an extended incision. The ulnar nerve is identified, mobilized, and transposed anteriorly. The triceps tendon is lengthened using W-plasty or a similar technique, and the posterior capsule of the elbow is released. After passive elbow flexion greater than 90° is achieved, the triceps tendon is repaired in its lengthened position. The elbow is splinted at 90° postoperatively for 3 weeks and then placed in a removable splint to allow for mobilization and passive range-of-motion exercises. A subset of children with amyoplasia may be candidates for a muscle transfer to achieve active elbow flexion after the patient has recovered from the release surgery. Multiple procedures, including a triceps to biceps transfer, Steindler flexorplasty, bipolar pectoralis major or latissimus transfer, long head of triceps transfer, or a free-functioning muscle transfer, have been described in an effort to achieve this goal.[27-32] Each technique possesses its own advantages and limitations, with the specific choice of procedure being tailored to the specific needs of the patient as well as the surgeon's preference. Regardless of the selected technique, these procedures are usually performed when the patient is older than 5 years to allow the child to participate in an intensive, active rehabilitation protocol that maximizes the chance for a favorable outcome.

Wrist

The flexed and ulnarly deviated position of the wrist in a patient with upper limb amyoplasia makes hand-to-mouth as well as bimanual activities more difficult. Surgical correction of the wrist is based on the severity of the deformity and the functional capacity of the muscles crossing the joint. Children who demonstrate active extension of the wrist to neutral often respond well to a volar wrist fascial release with or without wrist

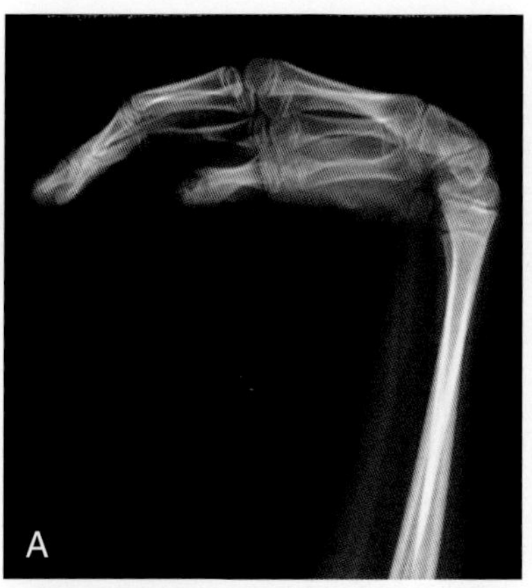

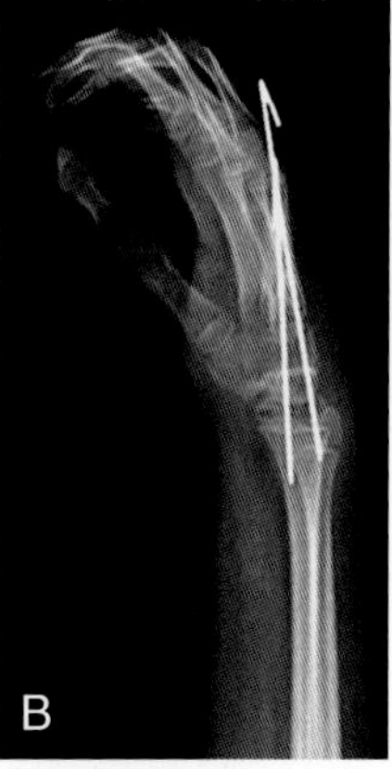

FIGURE 10 **A**, Preoperative lateral radiograph of the wrist of a child with amyoplasia shows the severe flexion deformity. **B**, Lateral radiograph after a dorsal carpal wedge osteotomy for correction of the flexion deformity.

flexor lengthening and/or tenotomy. Centralization of the extensor carpi ulnaris tendon to the anatomic insertion of the extensor carpi radialis brevis can strengthen the power of neutral extension while diminishing the forces of ulnar deviation. Children with a more severe wrist flexion contracture frequently require a bony procedure to attain neutral wrist extension. The procedure is commonly done using a dorsal carpal wedge osteotomy[33-35] (**Figure 10**). It takes advantage of the carpal coalitions often seen in the carpus of children with amyoplasia by obtaining extension and radial deviation through a biplanar wedge resection from the dorsum of the carpus.

Thumb and Fingers

A thumb-in-palm deformity is common in patients with amyoplasia and represents a complex contracture often involving multiple tissues, including skin, muscle, and, occasionally, joint capsule. Surgical correction of the deformity often requires a formal volar thenar release as well as release of the adductor pollicis and first dorsal interossei muscles within the first web space. The skin contracture is commonly present in more than one plane, with shortages being present both within the first web space and over the volar aspect of the thumb metacarpophalangeal joint. Hence, a typical four-flap Z-plasty of the first web space skin is rarely sufficient for correction. Instead, a rotational flap from the radial aspect of the index finger is commonly used to bring needed additional tissue to both areas[36] (**Figure 11**). Occasionally, imbrication or advancement of the dorsal thumb extensor tendons (extensor pollicis longus and brevis) can be helpful in maintaining the thumb in a more extended position. These muscle-tendon units are variably present in the thumbs of children with amyoplasia.

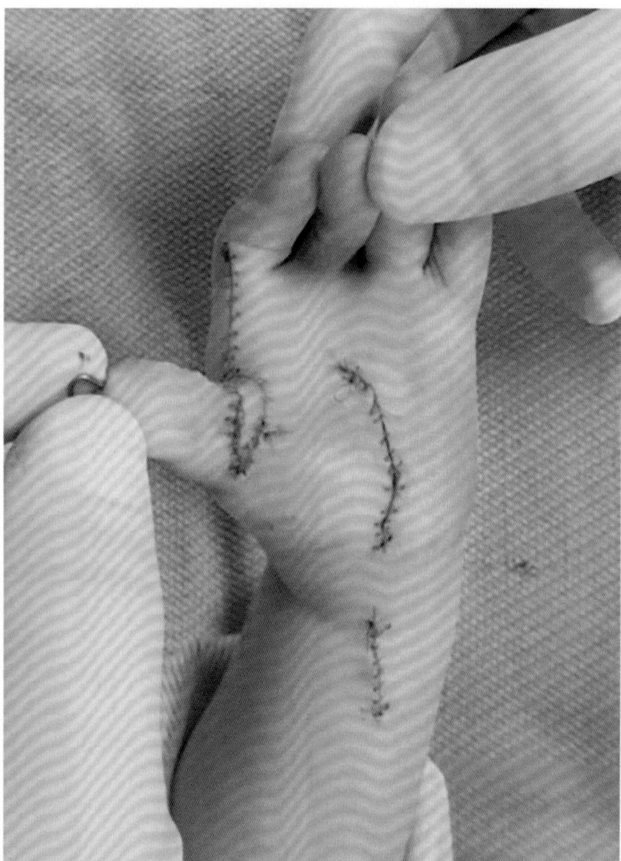

FIGURE 11 Photograph of the hand of a child with a thumb-in-palm deformity who underwent surgical treatment. An index finger rotational flap is used to release the skin contracture within the first web space as well as along the thenar eminence. The donor site is closed primarily.

The function of the fingers can range from a mild degree of stiffness to digits without flexion creases and little interphalangeal joint motion. Passive range-of-motion and stretching exercises can be helpful in the digits that possess some capacity for active digital flexion. In hands without active digital flexion, the fingers are often used as a single unit for gross grasping against an opposed thumb. Currently, surgery plays an extremely limited role in obtaining improved digital function.

Distal Arthrogryposis

In distal arthrogryposis of the upper limb, the shoulders and elbows are largely spared of deformity and dysfunction, wrists are fixed in extension, fingers are flexed and ulnarly deviated, and a substantial thumb-in-palm deformity may exist (**Figure 12**). The first line of treatment is stretching and passive range-of-motion exercises with functional and corrective splinting as an adjunct. Unfortunately, wrist and hand deformities are often recalcitrant to nonsurgical correction.[37]

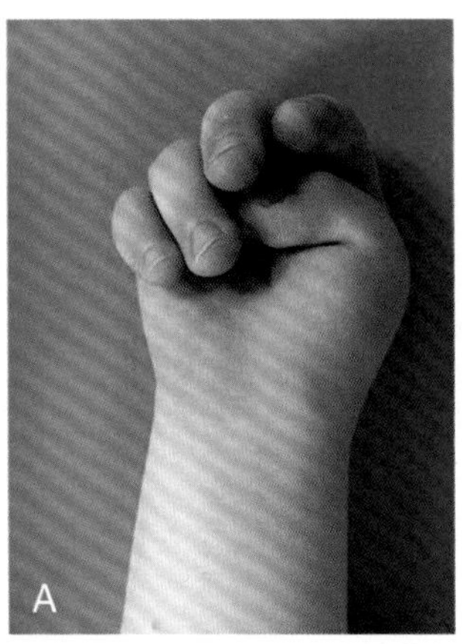

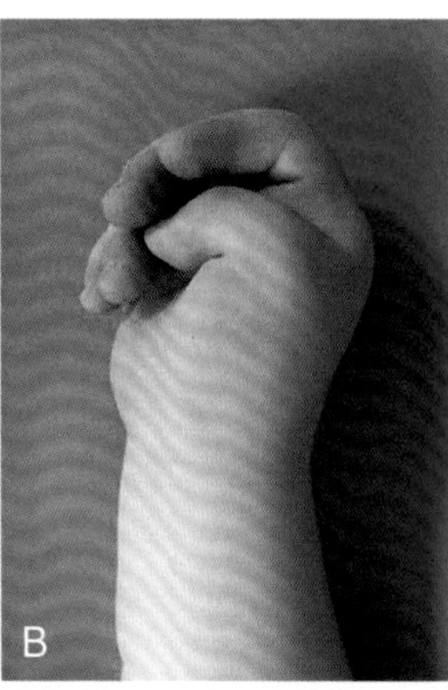

FIGURE 12 PA (**A**) and lateral (**B**) photographs show the typical presentation of the hand of a child with distal arthrogryposis. The wrist is positioned in extension, the fingers are flexed, and the thumb is clasped. (Courtesy of Scott Oishi, MD, Dallas, TX.)

Surgical correction of deformities associated with distal arthrogryposis has not proved particularly successful. A wrist extension contracture is rarely amenable to surgical correction. The abnormalities of the extensor mechanism (ranging from absent to extremely attenuated) also make it difficult to alleviate the flexion deformity of the digits. In rare instances, the extensor tendons are substantial enough that tenolysis and centralization of the tendon over the metacarpophalangeal joint can increase the extensor power and improve digital extension. The thumb-in-palm deformity in distal arthrogryposis is treated in a similar manner to the thumb deformity in amyoplasia. If the primary limitation is a camptodactyly deformity, improvement may be obtained with surgical release to increase proximal interphalangeal joint extension.

SUMMARY

Arthrogryposis refers to a constellation of syndromes characterized by multiple joint contractures. Treatment of arthrogryposis of any type can be challenging, but improvement can be seen in many patients with early intervention and proper nonsurgical and surgical management. The goal for any treatment strategy should be to maximize function with the minimal amount of hospitalization necessary to achieve that goal. Physical and occupational therapy in conjunction with bracing can help improve function in many children, so that surgical management can be mitigated or avoided. Surgical treatment should be reserved for enhancing function, not just improving the appearance of the deformity.

KEY STUDY POINTS

- Arthrogryposis is a constellation of different diseases with a similar phenotype of nonprogressive multiple joint stiffness and contractures.
- Treatment of patients with arthrogryposis focuses on improving a patient's function with as little hospitalization as possible; physical and occupational therapy should be used to minimize or obviate the need for surgery.
- Orthotic devices and surgical treatment should focus on improving function, not necessarily on correcting deformity.
- Both the surgical and nonsurgical management of upper extremity amyoplasia should focus on enhancing the patient's ability to complete hand-to-mouth activities.
- The creation or maintenance of an appropriate thumb-index web space is important for single-handed manipulation of objects.

ANNOTATED REFERENCES

1. Fahy MJ, Hall JG: A retrospective study of pregnancy complications among 828 cases of arthrogryposis. *Genet Couns* 1990;1(1):3-11.
2. Hall JG: Arthrogryposis (multiple congenital contractures): Diagnostic approach to etiology, classification, genetics, and general principles. *Eur J Med Genet* 2014;57(8):464-472.
3. Bamshad M, Van Heest AE, Pleasure D: Arthrogryposis: A review and update. *J Bone Joint Surg Am* 2009;91(suppl 4):40-46.
4. Bernstein RM: Arthrogryposis and amyoplasia. *J Am Acad Orthop Surg* 2002;10(6):417-424.
5. Hall JG: Arthrogryposis multiplex congenita: Etiology, genetics, classification, diagnostic approach, and general aspects. *J Pediatr Orthop B* 1997;6(3):159-166.
6. Dubousset J, Guillaumat M: Long-term outcome for patients with arthrogryposis multiplex congenita. *J Child Orthop* 2015;9(6):449-458.
7. Larsen LJ, Schottstaedt ER, Bost FC: Multiple congenital dislocations associated with characteristic facial abnormality. *J Pediatr* 1950;37(4):574-581.
8. Johnston CE II, Birch JG, Daniels JL: Cervical kyphosis in patients who have Larsen syndrome. *J Bone Joint Surg Am* 1996;78(4):538-545.
9. Munk S: Early operation of the dislocated knee in Larsen's syndrome: A report of 2 cases. *Acta Orthop Scand* 1988;59(5):582-584.
10. Laville JM, Lakermance P, Limouzy F: Larsen's syndrome: Review of the literature and analysis of thirty-eight cases. *J Pediatr Orthop* 1994;14(1):63-73.

11. Escobar V, Bixler D, Gleiser S, Weaver DD, Gibbs T: Multiple pterygium syndrome. *Am J Dis Child* 1978;132(6):609-611.

12. Donohoe M, Pruszczynski B, Rogers K, Bowen JR: Predicting ambulatory function based on infantile lower extremity posture types in amyoplasia arthrogryposis. *J Pediatr Orthop* 2019;39(7):e531-e535.

    The authors propose a five-tiered classification system to predict ambulatory function based on infantile muscle strength and position. Type I: mild ambulatory impairment with infantile position of flexed hips and knees but full range of motion. At maturity, all were community ambulators. Type II: moderate ambulatory impairment having infantile position of hip flexion and external rotation, as well as knee flexion contractures. Hip abductors and external rotators had antigravity strength. All stood and walked during the first decade of life with knee-ankle-foot orthoses. Type III: severe ambulatory impairment having infantile position of hip flexion/abduction/external rotation, and knee flexion contractures, but lacking hip muscle function. All were wheelchair users at maturity. Type IV: mild ambulatory impairment with infantile position of flexed, dislocated hips and extended knees. At maturity, 90% were community ambulators. Type V: variable ambulatory impairment having asymmetric hip and knee alignment with unilateral hip dysplasia with extended knee and opposite limb flexed. Ambulation skill varied at maturity with 27% full-time wheelchair users. Level of evidence: III.

13. Oppitz F, Speulda E, Busley R (English translation): Anesthesia recommendations in patients suffering from arthrogryposis multiplex congenita. Available at: https://www.orphananesthesia.eu/en/rare-diseases/published-guidelines/arthrogryposis-multiplex-congenita/661-arthrogryposis-multiplex-congenita/file.html. Last updated 2019. Accessed August 31, 2020.

    The authors detail the main issues with providing anesthesia to patients with arthrogryposis multiplex congenita, including difficulty in establishing the airway, poor venous circulation, and intraoperative hyperthermia. Regional anesthesia is noted as a good option to minimize these issues for limb surgery. Regional anesthesia for spine surgery tends to be technically difficult to perform and does not provide adequate analgesia. Laryngeal mask airway works well for most patients, but there are case reports of complications related to its use. Blood loss and anticoagulation risks are not increased compared with similar surgeries in the general population.

14. Gleich SJ, Tien M, Schroeder DR, Hanson AC, Flick R, Nemergut ME: Anesthetic outcomes of children with arthrogryposis syndromes: No evidence of hyperthermia. *Anesth Analg* 2017;124(3):908-914.

    The authors hypothesized that children (aged 0 to 25 years) with arthrogryposis multiplex congenita had a greater incidence of intraoperative hyperthermia and more difficulty with airway management and IV access. Charts were reviewed from 1972 to 2013; patients with arthrogryposis multiplex congenita were matched in a 1:2 ratio to patients without arthrogryposis to evaluate the primary outcome of maximum intraoperative temperature. In conclusion, the authors did not find evidence of increased odds of intraoperative hyperthermia or hypermetabolic responses in children with arthrogrypotic syndromes. Level of evidence: IV.

15. Drummond DS, Mackenzie DA: Scoliosis in arthrogryposis multiplex congenita. *Spine (Phila Pa 1976)* 1978;3(2):146-151.

16. Fletcher ND, Rathjen KE, Bush P, Ezaki M: Asymmetrical arthrogryposis of the upper extremity associated with congenital spine anomalies. *J Pediatr Orthop* 2010;30(8):936-941.

17. Yingsakmongkol W, Kumar SJ: Scoliosis in arthrogryposis multiplex congenita: Results after nonsurgical and surgical treatment. *J Pediatr Orthop* 2000;20(5):656-661.

18. Astur N, Flynn JM, Flynn JM, et al: The efficacy of rib-based distraction with VEPTR in the treatment of early-onset scoliosis in patients with arthrogryposis. *J Pediatr Orthop* 2014;34(1):8-13.

19. Cheung KM: Complications of magnetically-controlled growing rod surgery: A prospective multicenter study with minimum 2 year follow-up. *Bone Joint J* 2014;96-B(suppl 15):10. Available at: http://www.bjjprocs.boneandjoint.org.uk/content/96-B/SUPP_15/10. Accessed July 10, 2020.

20. Gardner RO, Bradley CS, Howard A, Narayanan UG, Wedge JH, Kelley SP: The incidence of avascular necrosis and the radiographic outcome following medial open reduction in children with developmental dysplasia of the hip: A systematic review. *Bone Joint J* 2014;96-B(2):279-286.

21. Dalton DM, Magill P, Mulhall KJ: Bilateral total hip replacement in arthrogryposis multiplex congenita. *BMJ Case Rep* 2015;2015:bcr2015212687.

22. Fisher KA, Fisher DA: Total hip and knee replacement in a patient with arthrogryposis multiplex congenita. *Am J Orthop (Belle Mead NJ)* 2014;43(4):E79-E82.

23. Janicki JA, Narayanan UG, Harvey B, Roy A, Ramseier LE, Wright JG: Treatment of neuromuscular and syndrome-associated (nonidiopathic) clubfeet using the Ponseti method. *J Pediatr Orthop* 2009;29(4):393-397.

24. Matar HE, Beirne P, Garg N: The effectiveness of the Ponseti method for treating clubfoot associated with arthrogryposis: Up to 8 years follow-up. *J Child Orthop* 2016;10(1):15-18.

    The Ponseti method was used to treat 17 clubfeet in 10 children with arthrogryposis. The authors reported initial correction in all of the children and satisfactory outcomes for two-thirds of the children at final follow-up. Level of evidence: IV.

25. Iskandar HN, Bishay SN, Sharaf-El-Deen HA, El-Sayed MM: Tarsal decancellation in the residual resistant arthrogrypotic clubfoot. *Ann R Coll Surg Engl* 2011;93(2):139-145.

26. Zlotolow DA, Kozin SH: Posterior elbow release and humeral osteotomy for patients with arthrogryposis. *J Hand Surg Am* 2012;37(5):1078-1082.

27. Chomiak J, Dungl P, Včelák J: Reconstruction of elbow flexion in arthrogryposis multiplex congenita type I: Results of transfer of pectoralis major muscle with follow-up at skeletal maturity. *J Pediatr Orthop* 2014;34(8):799-807.

28. Gogola GR, Ezaki M, Oishi SN, Gharbaoui I, Bennett JB: Long head of the triceps muscle transfer for active elbow flexion in arthrogryposis. *Tech Hand Up Extrem Surg* 2010;14(2):121-124.
29. Goldfarb CA, Burke MS, Strecker WB, Manske PR: The Steindler flexorplasty for the arthrogrypotic elbow. *J Hand Surg Am* 2004;29(3):462-469.
30. Kay S, Pinder R, Wiper J, Hart A, Jones F, Yates A: Microvascular free functioning gracilis transfer with nerve transfer to establish elbow flexion. *J Plast Reconstr Aesthet Surg* 2010;63(7):1142-1149.
31. Stevanovic M, Sharpe F: Functional free muscle transfer for upper extremity reconstruction. *Plast Reconstr Surg* 2014;134(2):257e-274e.
32. Van Heest A, Waters PM, Simmons BP: Surgical treatment of arthrogryposis of the elbow. *J Hand Surg Am* 1998;23(6):1063-1070.
33. Ezaki M, Carter PR: Carpal wedge osteotomy for the arthrogrypotic wrist. *Tech Hand Up Extrem Surg* 2004;8(4):224-228.
34. Foy CA, Mills J, Wheeler L, Ezaki M, Oishi SN: Long-term outcome following carpal wedge osteotomy in the arthrogrypotic patient. *J Bone Joint Surg Am* 2013;95(20):e150-e151.
35. Van Heest AE, Rodriguez R: Dorsal carpal wedge osteotomy in the arthrogrypotic wrist. *J Hand Surg Am* 2013;38(2):265-270.
36. Ezaki M, Oishi SN: Index rotation flap for palmar thumb release in arthrogryposis. *Tech Hand Up Extrem Surg* 2010;14(1):38-40.
37. Smith DW, Drennan JC: Arthrogryposis wrist deformities: Results of infantile serial casting. *J Pediatr Orthop* 2002;22(1):44-47.

CHAPTER 17

Osteogenesis Imperfecta and Metabolic Bone Disease

JARED WILLIAM DANIEL, MD • JENNIFER HARRINGTON, MBBS, PhD
ANDREW W. HOWARD, MD, MSc, FRCSC

ABSTRACT

Osteogenesis imperfecta and metabolic bone diseases are seen with a variety of clinical presentations in pediatric orthopaedic clinics. Basic knowledge is essential for making a diagnosis and managing these conditions. Osteogenesis imperfecta is a group of inherited connective tissue conditions characterized by increased bone fragility and low bone mass. Medical and surgical management of this condition remains an integral part of successful treatment.

Despite many advancements in technology and understanding, rickets continue to affect many children throughout the world. Vitamin D deficiency continues to be the most common cause of calcipenic rickets in children. Prompt treatment is fundamental in the management of rickets and its orthopaedic manifestations. A better understanding of X-linked hypophosphatemia has allowed for improvements in medical and surgical management.

Secondary osteoporosis may be attributable to multiple etiologies; however, glucocorticoid-induced osteoporosis still affects children being treated for a variety of pediatric conditions.

Keywords: calcipenic rickets; glucocorticoid-induced osteoporosis; osteogenesis imperfecta; vitamin D deficiency; X-linked hypophosphatemia

None of the following authors or any immediate family member has received anything of value from or has stock or stock options held in a commercial company or institution related directly or indirectly to the subject of this chapter: Dr. Daniel, Dr. Harrington, and Dr. Howard.

INTRODUCTION

Fundamental knowledge about the underlying conditions and treatment options for osteogenesis imperfecta and metabolic bone diseases is essential for proper management. Advancements in technology and research have provided new treatments and a better understanding of these conditions.

OSTEOGENESIS IMPERFECTA

Osteogenesis imperfecta is a broadly used term to describe a group of inherited connective tissue conditions characterized by increased bone fragility and low bone mass. The estimated prevalence of osteogenesis imperfecta is 1 in 12,000 to 15,000 children.[1] Osteogenesis imperfecta has an expansive clinical phenotype, ranging from perinatal lethality to mild forms without fractures. This condition has substantial heterogeneity, even within affected family members. Patients may have substantial skeletal deformities in long bones, or simple fragility fractures. Scoliosis and joint laxity are orthopaedic conditions seen in patients with osteogenesis imperfecta. Other clinical extraskeletal manifestations include hearing loss, dental abnormalities, blue-gray sclera, hypercalciuria, aortic root dilatation, neurologic conditions (macroencephaly, hydrocephalus, and basilar invagination), and skin hyperlaxity.

Classification

Published in 1979, the Sillence classification described four types of osteogenesis imperfecta: type I, mild nondeforming osteogenesis imperfecta; type II, perinatal lethal osteogenesis imperfecta; type III, severely progressing and deforming osteogenesis imperfecta; and type IV, moderately deforming osteogenesis imperfecta. The most common mutations involve the two genes (*COL1A1* and *COL1A2*) that encode the α chains of type I collagen. With the increased awareness of the genetic complexity and phenotypic heterogeneity of osteogenesis imperfecta, alternative classification schemes such as deforming and nondeforming osteogenesis imperfecta (**Figure 1**) have been proposed. In a practical and functional manner, these schemes help to encompass the ever-expanding list of new genetic mutations leading to osteogenesis imperfecta (**Table 1**).

CHARACTERISTICS OF OSTEOGENESIS IMPERFECTA

Diagnosis of osteogenesis imperfecta typically is made based on family history and associated radiographic and clinical features. Radiographic features include generalized osteopenia and gracile long bones with evidence of bowing. Vertebral fractures are common, with a 71% prevalence rate in patients with type I osteogenesis imperfecta.[1,2] Oblique and transverse fractures of diaphyses are the most frequently seen fractures in long bones.[3] Avulsion-type fractures such as olecranon and patellar fractures are particularly characteristic of osteogenesis imperfecta and occur as a result of the decreased tensile strength of the bone.[1,2] The underlying genetic mutation is more frequently being identified because of the increased ability to test multiple osteogenesis imperfecta–related genes at one time using techniques such as exome sequencing.

In infants, it is essential to differentiate osteogenesis imperfecta from other fracture etiologies, particularly nonaccidental injury. Other causes of fracture in older children include idiopathic juvenile osteoporosis and secondary causes of osteoporosis such as glucocorticoid-induced osteoporosis, hormone deficiency, acute lymphoblastic leukemia, and immobilization.

Low bone mass is a characteristic clinical feature of children with osteogenesis imperfecta.[4] Patients tend to have low bone mineral density (BMD), leading to decreased bone size, decreased volumetric BMD, or both.[5] With decreased bone mass, osteogenesis imperfecta is typically associated with an increased risk of fracture. Newer research is exploring fracture prediction based on mechanical models. Applied finite element models have been used to predict fractures in patients with osteogenesis imperfecta.[2,6] Finite element modeling has been used to estimate the effects of teriparatide treatment on vertebral strength in adults with osteogenesis imperfecta. A finite element model has been used to assess fracture risk at the tibia in children with osteogenesis imperfecta using simulated loading experienced during two-legged hopping, lateral loading, and torsional loading.[2,7] Future finite element modeling may provide quantification of fracture risk in osteogenesis imperfecta and identify activities that pose the greatest risk of fracture. However, given the combination of reduced bone mass and decreased bone quality, bone and/or spinal deformity can occur and further contribute to the risk of fracture.

Treatment and Symptom Management

The goals of management of osteogenesis imperfecta are to maximize a patient's mobility and ability to accomplish the activities of daily living. Treatment also should focus on decreasing bone pain and bone fragility, and correcting deformity. Management typically is multidisciplinary and includes rehabilitation and medical, pharmacologic, and surgical interventions.

Patients with osteogenesis imperfecta usually are seen by an orthopaedic surgeon because of a fracture. It is important to understand that fracture healing time in

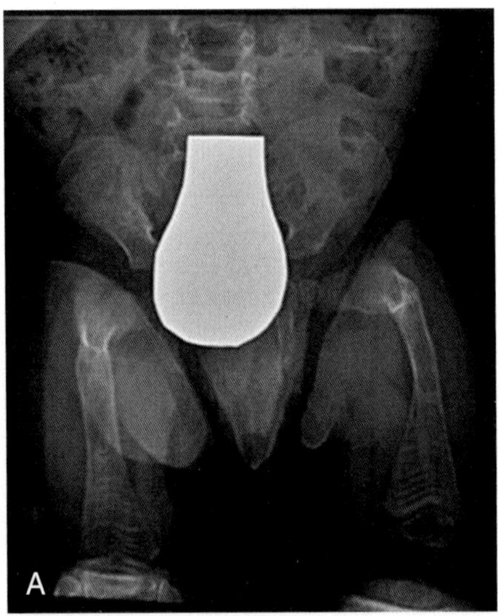

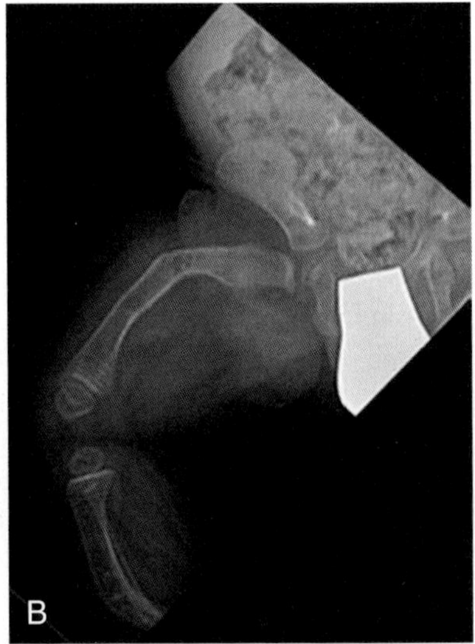

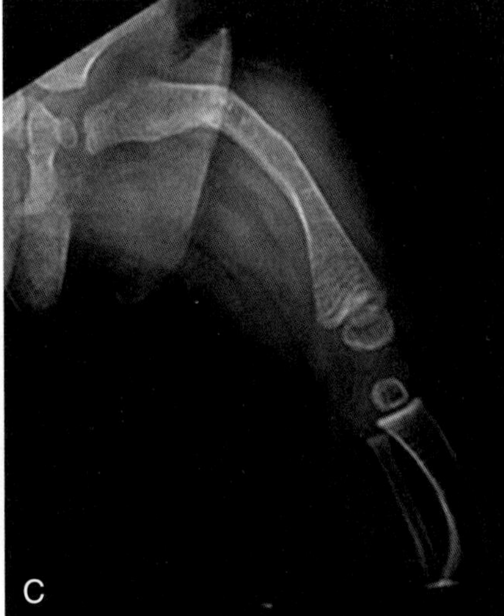

FIGURE 1 AP (**A**) and lateral (**B** and **C**) radiographs from a 20-month-old boy with osteogenesis imperfecta and recurrent femoral fractures.

TABLE 1

Alternative Classification Scheme for Osteogenesis Imperfecta

Phenotype	Gene Involved	Inheritance Pattern
Nondeforming	*COL1A1*	AD
	COL1A2	AD
	CRTAP	AR
	PPIB	AR
	SP7	AR
	PLS3	XL
Progressively deforming	*COL1A1*	AD
	COL1A2	AD
	CRTAP	AR
	LEPRE1(P3H1)	AR
	PPIB	AR
	BMP1	AR
	FKBP10	AR
	PLOD2	AR
	SERPINF1	AR
	SERPINH1	AR
	TMEM38B	AR
	WNT1	AR/AD
	CREB3L1	AR
	SPARC	AR
	FAM46A	AR
	MBTPS2	XL
Osteogenesis imperfecta with calcification of interosseous membranes	*IFITM5*	AD

AD = autosomal dominant, AR = autosomal recessive, XL = X-linked

children with osteogenesis imperfecta is normal, even with diphosphonate treatment.[8] The goals of orthopaedic treatment of osteogenesis imperfecta fractures are to stabilize or protect the whole bone and avoid excessive mobilization. Prolonged immobilization will lead to weak, stiff muscles and secondary disuse osteopenia, which leads to more fractures in this population. Fractures affecting infants are typically treated with the simplest form of immobilization that provides comfort to the limb; 2 to 3 weeks of immobilization is usually required. Toddlers and older children undergo treatment based on the fracture pattern and the amount of deformity present. Treatment with plates should be avoided because of the high risk of subsequent peri-implant fractures. However, transverse fractures of the olecranon or patella (caused by tensile failure) are best treated with tension-band wiring and early motion (**Figure 2**).

Because of the association of osteogenesis imperfecta with potential deformities of the femur and tibia, orthopaedic surgeons must have a full understanding of prior fractures and fixation methods spanning the entire bone length. Deformities can be in a single plane or multiple planes and can be acute or chronic. Preoperative planning is essential to assist with deformity correction. Newer technology allows for full computerized preoperative deformity correction. With the advancement in intramedullary instrumentation, osteogenesis imperfecta long bone deformities can be managed with osteotomies and intramedullary fixation, which maintains straight mechanical alignment and supports the whole bone, allowing for early mobilization, weight bearing, and strengthening.[1] Growing rods provide the mechanical advantages of a rigid nail but reduce the number of revision surgeries needed because of ongoing growth.[1,9] The authors of a 2019 study reported that Fassier-Duvall growing rods had a 90% revision-free survival at 50 months, compared with 50% revision-free survival for static nails.[10]

Children with severe osteogenesis imperfecta often have scoliosis and/or kyphosis. The incidence of scoliosis in osteogenesis imperfecta is between 39% and 80%[10] (**Figure 3**). Up to 60% of patients with osteogenesis imperfecta also have substantial chest wall deformities. Pulmonary compromise is the leading cause of death in adults with osteogenesis imperfecta. Thoracic scoliosis of more than 60° in patients with osteogenesis imperfecta has been associated with adverse effects on pulmonary function.[11] More recent information shows that patients with osteogenesis imperfecta can have substantial restrictive lung disease in the absence of spinal deformity, and that the degree of the curve does not correlate with lung function in these patients.[12] This raises the possibility of underlying direct pulmonary pathology, related to the connective tissue defect. The use of spinal fusion with instrumentation has been reported in selected patients, but it has a high complication rate and is not universally recommended.[1,13] A 2014 study described the surgical technique of using cement augmentation to improve pedicle screw instrumentation and pull-out strength in osteoporotic patients with osteogenesis imperfecta; however, this was a small case series with limited follow-up.[14] In the past 5 years, there have been few advancements in the surgical treatment of spinal deformities in patients with osteogenesis imperfecta.

Patients with osteogenesis imperfecta, particularly those severely affected, have a high rate of anesthesia-related challenges, most commonly higher blood loss, but also challenges related to intravenous access, airway, and neuraxial anaesthesia.[15] Intraoperative fractures occurred in approximately 1% of patients in this large series, related to positioning and not to blood pressure cuff use.

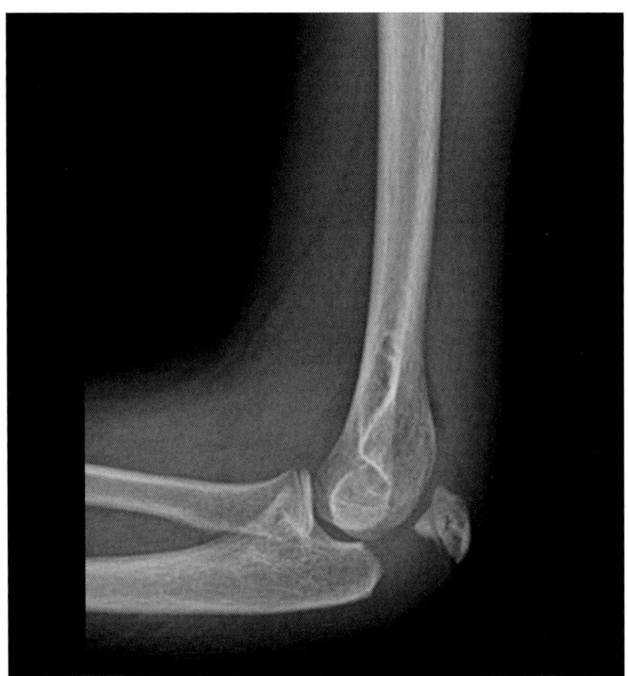

FIGURE 2 Lateral radiograph shows an avulsion fracture of the olecranon in a patient with osteogenesis imperfecta.

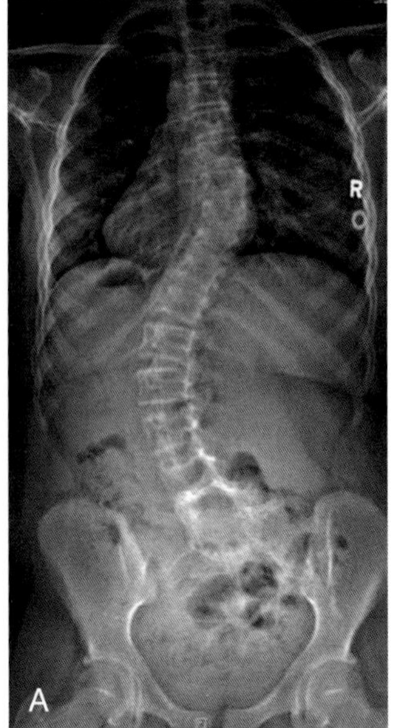

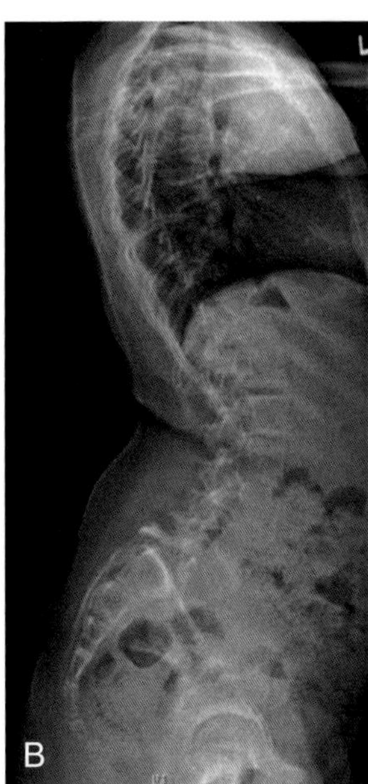

FIGURE 3 PA (**A**) and lateral (**B**) radiographs of the spine in a 13-year-old girl with osteogenesis imperfecta, scoliosis, and spondylolisthesis.

Pediatric patients with osteogenesis imperfecta also have a higher incidence of spondylolysis and spondylolisthesis compared with the normal pediatric population. The authors of a 2011 study retrospectively evaluated radiographs of 110 pediatric patients with osteogenesis imperfecta and concluded that the overall incidence of spondylolysis was 8.2%, with an overall incidence of spondylolisthesis of 10.9%.[16] In contrast, in a normal patient cohort, the incidence of spondylolysis was reported to be 2.6% to 4.0%, with the incidence of spondylolisthesis reported at 4.2%. These findings suggest that it is important to monitor children early in their clinical care to properly manage back pain symptoms.

Physical therapy is important to improve motor skills and maximize the effects of weight-bearing exercises to prevent fracture or facilitate rehabilitation after a fracture. Hydrotherapy can be an important modality to allow for gradual return to weight bearing. Patients with upper limb deformities also may benefit from an occupational therapy evaluation to promote self-care and activities of daily living.

Pharmacologic treatment remains an important aspect in the clinical management of osteogenesis imperfecta. Children should be assessed to ensure sufficient dietary calcium and 25-hydroxyvitamin D intake. The decision to initiate pharmacologic intervention depends on the clinical severity of the disease, not the BMD or collagen mutation. Diphosphonate therapy continues to remain the mainstay of medical treatment for osteogenesis imperfecta and has been shown in observational studies to decrease bone pain, enhance well-being, improve muscle strength and mobility, improve vertebral shape, and decrease fracture rates. Both controlled and observational trials have demonstrated that diphosphonate therapy substantially increases BMD, with most of the clinical gain occurring within the first 2 to 4 years.[1,5] However, two meta-analyses showed that diphosphonate therapy increased BMD in patients with osteogenesis imperfecta but did not show definitive evidence of fracture reduction.[17,18]

Recent literature has described a change in the mechanism and location of femoral fractures in patients with osteogenesis imperfecta receiving diphosphonate therapies.[19,20] The atypical fractures of the femur consist of proximal third femoral fractures involving the subtrochanteric region and more transverse fracture patterns resulting from low-energy injuries. These fractures contrast with the more typically seen high-energy, spiral, middiaphyseal fracture patterns.[19,20] A similar atypical fracture pattern has been described in adults undergoing diphosphonate therapy for osteoporosis. The exact mechanism causing the change in the trend of fracture patterns despite prior intramedullary fixation is unclear, but it may be related to the effects of diphosphonate on bone remodeling and bone stress relationships involving the proximal femur.

Diphosphonate treatment can be associated with flu-like symptoms in up to 85% of children after the first dose and also can lead to transient hypocalcemia.[21] The use of diphosphonates also has been linked to a decrease in bone remodeling and delayed healing of osteotomy sites after intramedullary nailing. Osteonecrosis of the jaw is a described adverse reaction in adults, but it has not been reported in pediatric patients with osteogenesis imperfecta.

Other pharmacologic treatments currently are under trial for the medical management of osteogenesis imperfecta. Teriparatide, an anabolic agent that stimulates bone formation, is being evaluated for the management of adults with osteogenesis imperfecta. Growth hormone has been trialed in patients with osteogenesis imperfecta for its anabolic effects on bone through the stimulation of osteoblasts, collagen synthesis, and bone growth. The current literature is insufficient to support the use of growth hormone as a standard treatment of osteogenesis imperfecta. Denosumab, a monoclonal antibody to receptor activator of nuclear factor kappa B ligand, decreases bone resorption, increases bone density, and reduces fracture rates in postmenopausal women. Several small trials of children with different genetic forms of osteogenesis imperfecta have shown improvements in BMD, vertebral shape, and quality-of-life indices.[22,23] There have, however, been several reports of severe hypercalcemia following denosumab treatment in children, where there is accelerated osteoclast activity when the dose wears off.[24] Larger studies of denosumab use in children with various genetic forms of osteogenesis imperfecta are ongoing. Future therapies include antisclerostin antibodies, transforming growth factor beta antagonism, and gene-based and cell-based therapies. More research is needed, however, before transitioning to new treatment options.

METABOLIC BONE DISEASE

Metabolic bone disease describes a diverse set of conditions that can affect bone health and pediatric growth. Good nutritional status is essential for normal bone growth in pediatric patients. Bone mass can be affected by multiple factors, both modifiable and nonmodifiable[25] (**Table 2**).

Despite medical and nutritional advancements, rickets still exists in various parts of the world. Rickets can be classified into two types: calcipenic and phosphopenic rickets. Secondary causes of osteoporosis are becoming more prevalent and should be considered in the management of pediatric orthopaedic conditions.

Calcipenic Rickets

Vitamin D deficiency is the most common cause of calcipenic rickets in children and osteomalacia in both children and adults. Rickets is characterized by a failure or delay in endochondral ossification at the epiphyseal plate (zone of provisional calcification) of long bones, which can lead to deformities in ambulatory children. Osteomalacia is characterized by defective mineralization of osteoid on the trabecular and cortical surfaces of bone and is associated with widened osteoid seams and the presence of Looser transformation zones. Both conditions can lead to bone pain and muscle weakness in the limbs. Vitamin D deficiency also has been linked to an increased risk of other diseases, including osteoporosis, cardiovascular disease, diabetes, some cancers, and infectious diseases.[26-29]

Vitamin D deficiency continues to be the most common nutritional deficiency worldwide, with children and adults at equal risk. Vitamin D deficiency is defined by the Institute of Medicine as a 25-hydroxyvitamin D level of less than 20 ng/mL (50 nmol/L), whereas vitamin D insufficiency is defined as a 25-hydroxyvitamin D level of 21 to 29 ng/mL (51 to 70 nmol/L). The introduction of food fortification programs and improvements in air quality have substantially reduced the prevalence of rickets in high-income countries. However, in the United States, more than 50% of Hispanic and African-American adolescents in Boston[30] and 48% of white preadolescent girls in Maine had levels below 20 ng/mL.[31] The overall prevalence of rickets has been reported to be up to 70% in developing counties.[32]

Many risk factors predispose the pediatric population to rickets and vitamin D deficiency. Risk factors include poor nutritional intake, premature birth, dark skin, living in areas of limited sun exposure (>37.5° latitude), obesity, taking medications that affect the concentration of vitamin D, and diseases causing nutritional malabsorption (eg, celiac disease and cystic fibrosis). In 2010, the Institute of Medicine published recommendations for administration of vitamin D to healthy children and children at risk for vitamin D deficiency.[33,34] If a pediatric patient has rickets associated with vitamin D deficiency, the American Academy of Pediatrics recommends an initial 2- to 3-month regimen of high-dose vitamin D therapy of 1,000 international units (IU) daily in neonates, 1,000 to 5,000 IU daily in infants 1 to 12 months old, and 5,000 IU daily in patients older than 12 months.[35]

TABLE 2

Factors Affecting Bone Mass

Nonmodifiable	Genetics Sex Ethnicity
Modifiable	Nutrition (calcium, vitamin D, sodium, protein) Exercise and lifestyle Body weight and composition Hormonal status Medication taken

After appropriate levels are obtained, treatment can be adjusted to a maintenance dose of 400 IU of vitamin D daily, depending on the patient's age and risk factors. If a pediatric patient is determined to be at risk for vitamin D deficiency, a maintenance dose (800 IU/day) should be considered. An alternative treatment regimen is providing 50,000 IU of vitamin D_2 once per week for 6 weeks, then transitioning to a maintenance dose of 600 to 1,000 IU daily.[33,34] Supplementation with calcium in conjunction with vitamin D is important for the successful management of rickets; the calcium dosage is based on the patient's age.[25]

Phosphopenic Rickets

Phosphopenic rickets most commonly occurs because of excess urinary phosphate losses, resulting from either genetic mutations leading to isolated phosphaturia or generalized renal tubular dysfunction such as that occurs in Fanconi syndrome. X-linked hypophosphatemic rickets is the most common form of inheritable rickets, with an incidence of 1 in 20,000 live births.[36] X-linked hypophosphatemia (XLH) is inherited in an X-linked dominant fashion, with prominent bowing of the legs, short stature, and medial tibial torsion seen in early childhood. Disease progression may result in progressive bone deformity, dental abscesses, enthesopathy, arthritis, and severe osteomalacia. XLH is caused by mutations in the phosphate-regulating endopeptidase homolog X-linked (*PHEX)* gene, which are expressed in osteocytes. Mutations of the gene result in an increase in fibroblast growth factor-23 (FGF-23), which leads to phosphaturia and inhibition of the activation of 25 hydroxy vitamin D to 1,25 vitamin D.

Medical Management

Early recognition of XLH is essential for appropriate treatment. Early intervention with medical management improves clinical outcomes but does not completely heal the mineralization defect.[37] The current mainstay of treatment is based on phosphate and 1,25-hydroxyvitamin D supplementation. Medical management should begin at the time of the diagnosis in childhood and continue through adolescence until growth has ceased; however, given increasing evidence of disease-related morbidity in adults, many patients continue to require treatment in adulthood. Medical management with supplementation of phosphate and vitamin D has been shown to alleviate bowing, improve attained height, and reduce the need for corrective surgery.[36-40] Recommended treatment is the administration of a 20- to 30-ng/kg dose of calcitriol (split among two to three daily doses), along with 20 to 40 mg/kg of elemental phosphorus (split among three to five daily doses).[39] Multiple daily doses are vital to maintain steady serum levels of phosphorus and reduce adverse gastrointestinal effects. In a developing child, medical therapy should be closely monitored with laboratory values, renal ultrasonography, and radiography.

Newer treatment strategies have been more recently developed to target the excess FGF-23 hormone levels seen in XLH. A randomized clinical trial studied the safety, tolerability, pharmacokinetics, pharmacodynamics, and immunogenicity of an anti-FGF-23 antibody, burosumab versus placebo in 38 adult patients with XLH.[41] The authors reported that the anti-FGF-23 antibody increased the maximum renal tubular threshold for phosphate reabsorption, serum inorganic phosphate, and serum 1,25-dihydroxyvitamin D and had a favorable safety profile. Similarly a randomized trial of burosumab versus conventional therapy in 61 children with XLH demonstrated significantly greater clinical improvements in the rickets severity, growth, and biochemistry in the burosumab-treated children over 64 weeks.[42]

Surgical Management

Although nonsurgical management is the mainstay of XLH management, bone deformities that necessitate surgical intervention can occur. The natural history of bony deformity in XLH makes appropriate treatment in young children challenging because it is unclear when surgical deformity correction is needed. One study reported that deformities of less than 15° frequently correct spontaneously when there is good metabolic control; however, no subsequent study has confirmed these findings.[43] Despite surgical intervention and proper medical management, the rate of deformity recurrence is as high as 90%.[44]

Decisions about surgical care involve anticipating the effects of growth. The understanding of multiapical deformity and preoperative planning has been key to the proper management of the deformities associated with XLH (**Figure 4**).

Guided growth techniques can provide substantial correction of angular deformities with low complication rates and a limited burden of care, whereas complex deformities with multiple apices require multiple levels of correction to achieve an anatomic result. In adults, simultaneous correction of multiple deformities has been advocated with fixator-assisted nailing. Because deformity in children can recur because of growth, it is necessary to plan care based on an analysis of the complete deformity. The timing of surgery, the wisdom of staged correction, and the burden of care also should be considered.

Surgery may be indicated for children with progressive bony deformities that result in substantial gait disturbances, activity limitations, and pain. Various treatment techniques can be used or combined to correct bony deformities, including acute correction and fixation of osteotomies with Kirschner wires, plates, external fixators, and intramedullary nails. Gradual correction of

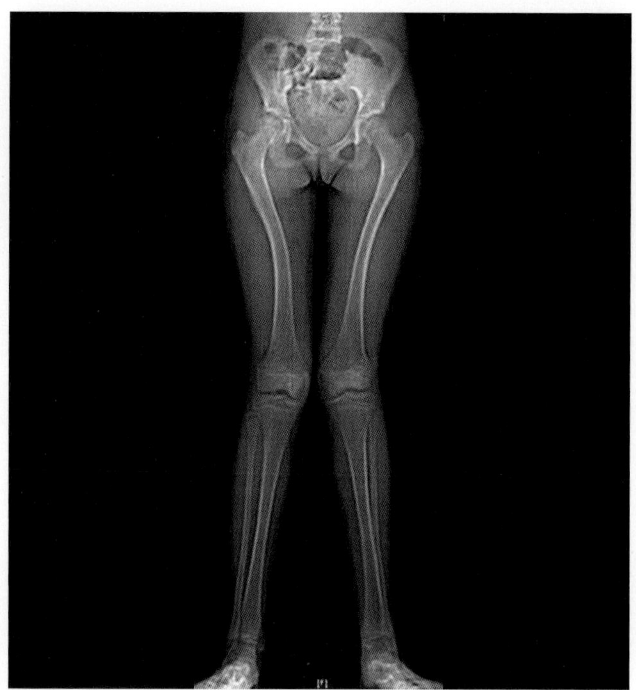

FIGURE 4 Long leg standing AP radiograph from a 12-year-old girl with X-linked hypophosphatemic rickets with a multiapical femoral deformity.

deformities also has been described using an Ilizarov external fixator or a Taylor Spatial Frame (Smith & Nephew). A 2015 review described bone lengthening with corrective osteotomy in a select number of patients who also had been treated with deformity correction. The authors reported that more major complications, including recurrent deformity and refracture, occurred in patients treated with bone lengthening with corrective osteotomy than in patients treated only with deformity correction.[37] Another important advancement has been a return to low-energy, percutaneous, tissue-sparing osteotomies.[37] Because of the concern about recurrent deformity or refracture, intramedullary nailing has been recommended in conjunction with treatment or after treatment with an external fixator because it minimizes the risk of recurrence and refracture.

The use of a minimally invasive technique for guided growth for the management of bone deformity in patients younger than 10 years with XLH has been described.[45,46] This technique corrects the mechanical axis to allow for more normal growth and functioning of the physis and avoids major osteotomy, which could result in early recurrence of a deformity (**Figure 5**). It was found that staples had a higher migration rate and resulted in rebound deformity, but tension-band plates had no hardware migration. Gradual deformity correction maintains alignment, minimizes secondary bony deformity, and avoids the need for future osteotomies for angular correction.

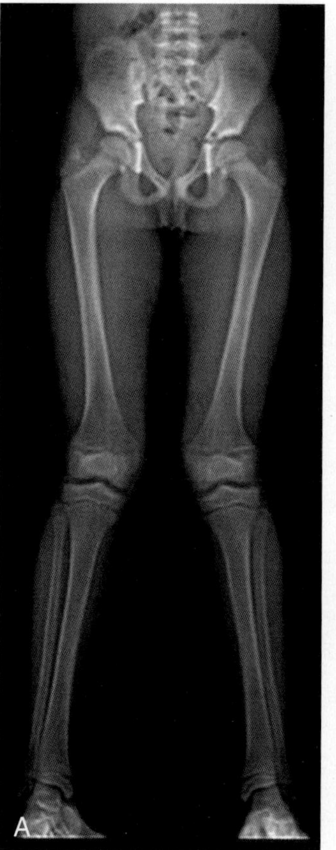

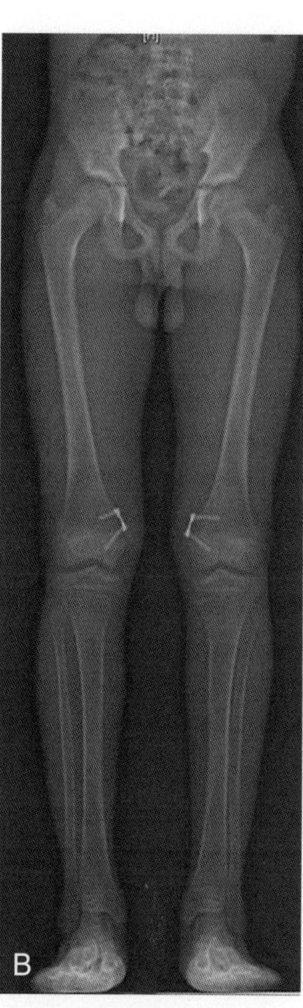

FIGURE 5 **A**, Long leg standing AP radiograph from a 13-year-old boy with X-linked hypophosphatemia with a genu valgus deformity. **B**, Long leg AP radiograph after the patient was treated with a guided growth system for 2 years.

SECONDARY CAUSES OF OSTEOPOROSIS

Osteoporosis is defined as a skeletal disorder characterized by compromised bone strength, which predisposes an individual to an increased risk of fracture. Osteoporosis in children can have many primary and secondary etiologies (**Table 3**). This section focuses on the recent literature regarding glucocorticoid-induced osteoporosis.

Glucocorticoid-induced osteoporosis is the most common form of secondary osteoporosis. Systemic glucocorticoid therapy is associated with an initial increase in bone resorption (especially trabecular bone resorption), which is more pronounced in the first months of therapy. This is followed by decreased bone formation arising from the decreased activity of osteoblasts. A 10% to 20% loss of trabecular bone occurs in the first 6 months of glucocorticoid therapy, followed by a 2% per-year loss in subsequent years.[47] In addition, a 2% to 3% loss of cortical bone occurs in the first year; thereafter, a slow and continuous loss is maintained.[48] The architectural deterioration of bone related to systemic glucocorticoid therapy leads to increased fracture risk.

TABLE 3

Primary and Secondary Etiologies for Osteoporosis in Children

Etiology	
Primary	Structural gene abnormalities (eg, osteogenesis imperfecta, Marfan syndrome, Ehlers-Danlos syndrome, Bruck syndrome, homocystinuria)
	Osteoporosis pseudoglioma
	Spondyloocular syndrome
	Idiopathic juvenile osteoporosis
Secondary	Neuromuscular (eg, Duchenne muscular dystrophy, cerebral palsy, myelomeningocele)
	Endocrine (eg, growth hormone deficiency, hyperthyroidism)
	Infiltrative conditions (eg, leukemia, thalassemia)
	Chronic inflammatory conditions (eg, juvenile idiopathic arthritis, inflammatory bowel disease)
	Nutritional and vitamin deficiencies (eg, celiac disease, anorexia nervosa)
	Drug-related (eg, glucocorticoid, anticonvulsant, methotrexate, cyclosporine)

The risk of chronic glucocorticoid therapy is well established in adults. Several medications are available for the prevention and management of glucocorticoid-induced osteoporosis in adults. However, no evidence-based guideline exists for treating children who require long-term oral glucocorticoid therapy. Glucocorticoid use in growing children may decrease peak bone mass accrual and increase lifelong fracture risk, but the underlying disease process requiring glucocorticoid therapy may also have an adverse effect on the growing skeleton. A 2013 systematic review compared reported bone health outcomes in children treated with systemic glucocorticoid therapy with those of control subjects.[49] Children treated with systemic glucocorticoids had lower spine BMD and high rates of vertebral fractures compared with age-matched and sex-matched healthy control subjects.[49] However, given the paucity of long-term safety and efficacy data regarding the optimal medical treatment of children with glucocorticoid-induced osteoporosis, the use of diphosphonate therapy should be limited in duration and administered only to children with substantial bone fragility.

Osteonecrosis is a devastating consequence of the medical management of several pediatric conditions. Glucocorticoid use is a well-known risk factor for osteonecrosis and there appears to be a dose-related correlation. In a 2013 review of the rate of osteonecrosis in children after chemotherapy and high-dose steroid treatment for hematologic malignancy (acute lymphoblastic leukemia, acute myeloid leukemia, or non-Hodgkin lymphoma), the authors reported that osteonecrosis developed in 7.6% of the patients.[50] It was concluded that osteonecrosis mainly affects the weight-bearing epiphyses, and the risk of osteonecrosis increases with age and higher doses of steroids (mean cumulative dose, 5,967 mg). Early screening for osteonecrosis was recommended in high-risk patients. Dexamethasone is associated with a higher risk of osteonecrosis compared with prednisolone and a higher risk of fractures compared with prednisone.[51,52]

SUMMARY

Bone health is an important aspect of musculoskeletal care. Pediatric patients typically are seen by an orthopaedic surgeon for fracture care; however, it is important to understand the biology of other commonly occurring bone conditions. Future research will continue to provide insight for the nonsurgical and surgical treatment of patients with osteogenesis imperfecta and metabolic bone diseases.

KEY STUDY POINTS

- Osteogenesis imperfecta describes a group of inherited connective tissue conditions characterized by increased bone fragility and low bone mass. A multidisciplinary team should be involved in management.
- The goals of management of osteogenesis imperfecta are to maximize a patient's mobility (decreasing bone pain and preventing or correcting deformity) and ability to accomplish the activities of daily living.
- Rickets can be classified into calcipenic and phosphopenic rickets. Rickets caused by vitamin D deficiency is the most common form of calcipenic rickets worldwide. Medical treatment of patients with rickets is essential.
- X-linked hypophosphatemia is the most common form of inheritable rickets. Mutations of the *PHEX* gene result in an increase in fibroblast growth factor-23 (FGF-23), which leads to phosphaturia. Surgical treatment may be required for correcting angular deformities caused by the condition. Specific treatment with FGF-23 antibodies is now available.

- Glucocorticoid-induced osteoporosis is the most common form of secondary osteoporosis. Systemic glucocorticoid therapy is associated with an initial increase in bone resorption (especially trabecular bone resorption), which is more pronounced in the first months of therapy, then followed by decreased bone formation arising from the decreased activity of osteoblasts.

ANNOTATED REFERENCES

1. Harrington J, Sochett E, Howard A: Update on the evaluation and treatment of osteogenesis imperfecta. *Pediatr Clin North Am* 2014;61(6):1243-1257.
2. Ben Amor IM, Roughley P, Glorieux FH, Rauch F: Skeletal clinical characteristics of osteogenesis imperfecta caused by haploinsufficiency mutations in *COL1A1*. *J Bone Miner Res* 2013;28(9):2001-2007.
3. Peddada KV, Sullivan BT, Margalit A, Sponseller PD: Fracture patterns differ between osteogenesis imperfecta and routine pediatric fractures. *J Pediatr Orthop* 2018;38(4): e207-e212.

   The authors sampled 500 patients with non–osteogenesis imperfecta and compared fracture patterns with those of 52 patients with osteogenesis imperfecta. Patients with osteogenesis imperfecta had more oblique, transverse, and diaphyseal long bone fractures and patients with non-osteogenesis imperfecta had more buckle, metaphyseal, and physeal fractures. Transverse humerus, olecranon, and diaphyseal humerus fractures were the patterns most strongly associated with osteogenesis imperfecta. Level of evidence: III.
4. Shaker JL, Albert C, Fritz J, Harris G: Recent developments in osteogenesis imperfecta. *F1000Res* 2015;4(F1000 Faculty Rev):681.
5. Rauch F, Plotkin H, Zeitlin L, Glorieux FH: Bone mass, size, and density in children and adolescents with osteogenesis imperfecta: Effect of intravenous pamidronate therapy. *J Bone Miner Res* 2003;18(4):610-614.
6. Fritz JM, Guan Y, Wang M, Smith PA, Harris GF: Muscle force sensitivity of a finite element fracture risk assessment model in osteogenesis imperfecta–Biomed 2009. *Biomed Sci Instrum* 2009;45:316-321.
7. Caouette C, Rauch F, Villemure I, et al: Biomechanical analysis of fracture risk associated with tibia deformity in children with osteogenesis imperfecta: A finite element analysis. *J Musculoskelet Neuronal Interact* 2014;14(2): 205-212.
8. Pizones J, Plotkin H, Parra-Garcia JI, et al: Bone healing in children with osteogenesis imperfecta treated with bisphosphonates. *J Pediatr Orthop* 2005;25(3):332-335.
9. Fassier F, Glorieux FH: *Surgical management of osteogenesis imperfecta*, in *Surgical Techniques in Orthopaedics and Traumatology*. Paris, France, Elsevier SAS, 2003.
10. Spahn KM, Mickel T, Carry PM, et al: Fassier-Duval rods are associated with superior probability of survival compared with static implants in a cohort of children with osteogenesis imperfecta deformities. *J Pediatr Orthop* 2019;39(5): e392-e396.

    In a cohort of 21 patients (64 limbs) with osteogenesis imperfecta, the rate of revision surgery was higher for static implants than for Fassier-Duval rods. Level of evidence: II.
11. Widmann RF, Bitan FD, Laplaza FJ, Burke SW, DiMaio MF, Schneider R: Spinal deformity, pulmonary compromise, and quality of life in osteogenesis imperfecta. *Spine (Phila Pa 1976)* 1999;24(16):1673-1678.
12. Bronheim R, Khan S, Carter E, Sandhaus RA, Raggio C: Scoliosis and cardiopulmonary outcomes in osteogenesis imperfecta patients. *Spine (Phila Pa 1976)* 2019;44(15): 1057-1063.

    Among 30 patients with osteogenesis imperfecta aged 12 to 42 years, the pulmonary function was not significantly associated with the magnitude of the scoliosis. This suggests that pulmonary function limitation is intrinsic to osteogenesis imperfecta and/or chest wall deformities, and not secondary to scoliosis. Level of evidence: IV.
13. Topouchian V, Finidori G, Glorion C, Padovani JP, Pouliquen JC: Posterior spinal fusion for kypho-scoliosis associated with osteogenesis imperfecta: Long-term results. *Rev Chir Orthop Reparatrice Appar Mot* 2004;90(6):525-532.
14. Yilmaz G, Hwang S, Oto M, et al: Surgical treatment of scoliosis in osteogenesis imperfecta with cement-augmented pedicle screw instrumentation. *J Spinal Disord Tech* 2014;27(3):174-180.
15. Rothschild L, Goeller JK, Voronov P, Barabanova A, Smith P: Anesthesia in children with osteogenesis imperfecta: Retrospective chart review of 83 patients and 205 anesthetics over 7 years. *Paediatr Anaesth* 2018;28(11): 1050-1058.

    Anesthetic issues in patients with osteogenesis imperfecta included significant blood loss (17%), difficult IV access (4%), difficult airway (1.5%), and perioperative fracture (1%) in a case series at a children's hospital. Severity of osteogenesis imperfecta correlated with complication incidence. Level of evidence: IV.
16. Hatz D, Esposito PW, Schroeder B, Burke B, Lutz R, Hasley BP: The incidence of spondylolysis and spondylolisthesis in children with osteogenesis imperfecta. *J Pediatr Orthop* 2011;31(6):655-660.
17. Phillipi CA, Remmington T, Steiner RD: Bisphosphonate therapy for osteogenesis imperfecta. *Cochrane Database Syst Rev* 2008;4:CD005088.
18. Hald JD, Evangelou E, Langdahl BL, Ralston SH: Bisphosphonates for the prevention of fractures in osteogenesis imperfecta: Meta-analysis of placebo-controlled trials. *J Bone Miner Res* 2015;30(5):929-933.
19. Nicolaou N, Agrawal Y, Padman M, Fernandes J, Bell M: Changing pattern of femoral fractures in osteogenesis imperfecta with prolonged use of bisphosphonates. *J Child Orthop* 2012;6(1):21-27.

20. Hegazy A, Kenawey M, Sochett E, Tile L, Cheung AM, Howard AW: Unusual femur stress fractures in children with osteogenesis imperfecta and intramedullary rods on long-term intravenous pamidronate therapy. *J Pediatr Orthop* 2016;36(7):757-761.

Low-trauma fractures in the subtrochanteric region of the femur were described in six patients with osteogenesis imperfecta and long-term diphosphonate use. These fractures are similar to atypical femoral fractures seen in adults on long-term diphosphonates. Level of evidence: IV.

21. Munns CF, Rajab MH, Hong J, et al: Acute phase response and mineral status following low dose intravenous zoledronic acid in children. *Bone* 2007;41(3):366-370.

22. Trejo P, Rauch F, Ward L: Hypercalcemia and hypercalciuria during denosumab treatment in children with osteogenesis imperfecta type VI. *J Musculoskelet Neuronal Interact* 2018;18(1):76-80.

Four children with osteogenesis imperfecta type VI (SERPINF1 mutation) were treated with denosumab. Hypercalciuria developed in all four patients, two of the four experienced hypercalcemic episodes, and nephrocalcinosis developed in one. The authors suggest combining denosumab with diphosphonate therapy to manage this. Level of evidence: IV.

23. Hoyer-Kuhn H, Stark C, Franklin J, Schoenau E, Semler O: Correlation of bone mineral density on quality of life in patients with osteogenesis imperfectaduring treatment with denosumab. *Pediatr Endocrinol Rev* 2017;15(suppl 1): 123-129.

In a small series of 10 children with osteogenesis imperfecta, denosumab improved bone density but did not improve pain or quality of life. Level of evidence: IV.

24. Hoyer-Kuhn H, Franklin J, Allo G, et al: Safety and efficacy of denosumab in children with osteogenesis imperfect—A first prospective trial. *J Musculoskelet Neuronal Interact* 2016;16(1):24-32.

In a small series of 10 children with osteogenesis imperfecta, 1 year of denosumab improved bone density but did not change mobility parameters or one-minute walking test. Level of evidence: IV.

25. Golden NH, Abrams SA, Committee on Nutrition: Optimizing bone health in children and adolescents. *Pediatrics* 2014;134(4):e1229-e1243.

26. Scientific Advisory Committee on Nutrition: *Scientific Advisory Committee on Nutrition: Update on Vitamin D*. 2016. United Kingdom Government Publication. Available at: https://www.gov.uk/government/publications/sacn-vitamin-d-and-health-report.

27. Bischoff-Ferrari HA, Giovannucci E, Willett WC, Dietrich T, Dawson-Hughes B: Estimation of optimal serum concentrations of 25-hydroxyvitamin D for multiple health outcomes. *Am J Clin Nutr* 2006;84(1):18-28.

28. Lips P: Vitamin D deficiency and secondary hyperparathyroidism in the elderly: Consequences for bone loss and fractures and therapeutic implications. *Endocr Rev* 2001;22(4):477-501.

29. Liu PT, Stenger S, Li H: Toll-like receptor triggering of a vitamin D-mediated human antimicrobial response. *Science* 2006;311(5768):1770-1773.

30. Gordon CM, Feldman HA, Sinclair L, et al: Prevalence of vitamin D deficiency among healthy infants and toddlers. *Arch Pediatr Adolesc Med* 2008;162(6):505-512.

31. Sullivan SS, Rosen CJ, Halteman WA, Chen TC, Holick MF: Adolescent girls in Maine are at risk for vitamin D insufficiency. *J Am Diet Assoc* 2005;105(6):971-974.

32. Prentice A: Vitamin D deficiency: A global perspective. *Nutr Rev* 2008;66(10 suppl 2):S153-S164.

33. Holick MF, Binkley NC, Bischoff-Ferrari HA, et al: Evaluation, treatment, and prevention of vitamin D deficiency: An endocrine society clinical practice guideline. *J Clin Endocrinol Metab* 2011;96(7):1911-1930.

34. Institute of Medicine of the National Academies: *Dietary Reference Intake for Calcium and Vitamin D*. Washington, DC, National Academies Press, 2010.

35. Misra M, Pacaud D, Petryk A, Collett-Solberg PF, Kappy M, Drug and Therapeutics Committee of the Lawson Wilkins Pediatric Endocrine Society: Vitamin D deficiency in children and its management: Review of current knowledge and recommendations. *Pediatrics* 2008;122(2):398-417.

36. Petersen DJ, Boniface AM, Schranck FW, Rupich RC, Whyte MP: X-linked hypophosphatemic rickets: A study (with literature review) of linear growth response to calcitriol and phosphate therapy. *J Bone Miner Res* 1992;7(6):583-597.

37. Sharkey MS, Grunseich K, Carpenter TO: Contemporary medical and surgical management of X-linked hypophosphatemic rickets. *J Am Acad Orthop Surg* 2015;23(7):433-442.

38. Carpenter TO: New perspectives on the biology and treatment of X-linked hypophosphatemic rickets. *Pediatr Clin North Am* 1997;44(2):443-466.

39. Carpenter TO, Imel EA, Holm IA, Jan de Beur SM, Insogna KL: A clinician's guide to X-linked hypophosphatemia. *J Bone Miner Res* 2011;26(7):1381-1388.

40. Tsuru N, Chan JC, Chinchilli VM: Renal hypophosphatemic rickets. Growth and mineral metabolism after treatment with calcitriol (1,25-dihydroxyvitamin D3) and phosphate supplementation. *Am J Dis Child* 1987;141(1):108-110.

41. Carpenter TO, Imel EA, Ruppe MD, et al: Randomized trial of the anti-FGF23 antibody KRN23 in X-linked hypophosphatemia. *J Clin Invest* 2014;124(4):1587-1597.

42. Imel EA, Glorieux FH, Whyte MP, et al: Burosumab versus conventional therapy in children with X-linked hypophosphataemia: A randomised, active-controlled, open-label, phase 3 trial. *Lancet* 2019;393(10189):2416-2427.

43. Rubinovitch M, Said SE, Glorieux FH, et al: Principles and results of corrective lower limb osteotomies for patients with vitamin D-resistant hypophosphatemic rickets. *Clin Orthop* 1988;237:264.

44. Petje G, Meizer R, Radler C, Aigner N, Grill F: Deformity correction in children with hereditary hypophosphatemic rickets. *Clin Orthop Relat Res* 2008;466(12):3078-3085.

45. Novais E, Stevens PM: Hypophosphatemic rickets: The role of hemiepiphysiodesis. *J Pediatr Orthop* 2006;26(2): 238-244.

46. Stevens PM, Klatt JB: Guided growth for pathological physes: Radiographic improvement during realignment. *J Pediatr Orthop* 2008;28(6):632-639.

47. Pereira RM, Carvalho JF, Paula AP, et al: Guidelines for the prevention and treatment of glucocorticoid-induced osteoporosis. *Rev Bras Reumatol* 2012;52(4):580-593.

48. van Staa TP, Leufkens HG, Cooper C: The epidemiology of corticosteroid-induced osteoporosis: A meta-analysis. *Osteoporos Int* 2002;13(10):777-787.

49. Hansen KE, Kleker B, Safdar N, Bartels CM: A systematic review and meta-analysis of glucocorticoid-induced osteoporosis in children. *Semin Arthritis Rheum* 2014;44(1):47-54.

50. Salem KH, Brockert AK, Mertens R, Drescher W: Avascular necrosis after chemotherapy for haematological malignancy in childhood. *Bone Joint J* 2013;95-B(12):1708-1713.

51. Vora A: Management of osteonecrosis in children and young adults with acute lymphoblastic leukaemia. *Br J Haematol* 2011;155(5):549-560.

52. Rayar MS, Nayiager T, Webber CE, Barr RD, Athale UH: Predictors of bony morbidity in children with acute lymphoblastic leukemia. *Pediatr Blood Cancer* 2012;59(1):77-82.

CHAPTER 18

Muscular Dystrophies and Neurodegenerative Conditions

MICHAEL D. SUSSMAN, MD

ABSTRACT

A variety of diseases exist that cause muscle weakness beginning in childhood and are progressive thereafter. These include the muscular dystrophies (specifically, Duchenne muscular dystrophy), spinal muscular atrophy, congenital myotonic dystrophy, and Charcot-Marie-Tooth disease. All of these conditions have a genetic basis, and in many cases, the responsible genes have been identified. Understanding of the genetic basis of these diseases has led to the development of specific medical treatments for several of these conditions. It is essential to be aware of the pathophysiology and clinical course, to provide orthopaedic treatment interventions for these diseases.

Keywords: Charcot-Marie-Tooth disease; congenital myotonic dystrophy; Duchenne muscular dystrophy; spinal muscular atrophy

INTRODUCTION

The most commonly seen progressive neuromuscular diseases in children are diseases of the motor unit, which is defined as the combination of (1) the motor neuron in the anterior horn of the spinal cord, (2) its nerve connecting through the neuromuscular junction to the muscle, and (3) the muscle itself.

Spinal muscular atrophy (SMA) is caused by progressive loss of the motor neurons in the anterior horn of the spinal cord, resulting in progressive paralysis, which in its more severe forms leads to early death from respiratory failure. There is no sensory involvement.

A variety of neuropathies exist that affect the axon between the motor neuron and neuromuscular junction. The most prevalent of these are the group of heritable sensory motor neuropathies known as Charcot-Marie-Tooth (CMT) disease; however, other neuropathies can affect only motor nerves and may be hereditary (such as distal SMA, which may be better referred to as hereditary motor neuropathy and is distinguished from CMT by the lack of sensory involvement on nerve conduction examination) or acquired (such as the inflammatory polyneuropathies).

Duchenne muscular dystrophy (DMD) is the most prevalent of the many childhood-onset diseases of muscle that cause progressive weakness; however, there are other muscular dystrophies and myopathies with onset in childhood. A muscular dystrophy is characterized by a progressive loss of muscle cells and increasing weakness over time, whereas a myopathy will affect the function of a muscle fiber causing weakness, but tends to be nonprogressive. Congenital myotonic dystrophy (CDM) is the second most prevalent muscle disease in pediatric patients. Other muscle diseases exist, such as the congenital muscular dystrophies that manifest early, and the limb-girdle muscular dystrophies that usually do not manifest until later in life.

In many of these progressive neuromuscular diseases, the specific gene abnormality has been identified. This allows for a precise diagnosis and initiation of genetic counselling, and when available, medical treatment interventions specific to the particular gene defect causing the condition, including early treatment in infancy when the disease is identified by newborn screening before symptoms manifest.

Progressive neuromuscular diseases may be inherited in an autosomal dominant, an autosomal recessive, or an X-linked manner. If they are inherited in an autosomal dominant manner, a family history of the disease will

Neither Dr. Sussman nor any immediate family member has received anything of value from or has stock or stock options held in a commercial company or institution related directly or indirectly to the subject of this chapter.

likely exist, whereas this is less likely in an X-linked condition, and unlikely in an autosomal recessive condition, unless there is consanguinity with a common ancestor, or an older involved sibling. Some neuromuscular diseases may manifest early in life, but others may not manifest until the second decade of life or later. The conditions all cause progressive weakness in characteristic patterns. The weakness is not homogeneous and, in general, conditions affecting the muscle tend to manifest first in proximal muscles, whereas those affecting the neuron or axon manifest initially in the distal muscles. Asymmetric muscle weakness can lead to foot deformities, such as equinus, equinovarus, or cavovarus. Conditions causing more proximal weakness and truncal weakness may predispose an affected individual to hip dislocation and scoliosis.

In many neuromuscular diseases, abnormalities of multiple organ systems may be associated, either as part of the underlying genetic abnormality or secondarily. The treatment team may include an orthopaedic surgeon, a neurologist, a geneticist, a physical medicine and rehabilitation specialist, a gastroenterologist, a nutritionist, and a developmental pediatrician, as indicated by organ system involvement. If cardiac and pulmonary dysfunction are involved, these possibly life-threatening conditions will require regular assessment by a pulmonologist and cardiologist. These individuals are best treated in a multidisciplinary clinic, such as the clinics sponsored by the Muscular Dystrophy Association in the United States.

DUCHENNE MUSCULAR DYSTROPHY

DMD is a disease of muscle in which the muscle progressively deteriorates over time and is replaced by fibroadipose tissue. This results in a loss of functional fibers, weakness, scarring, and relative rigidity of the muscles. The incidence of DMD is 1 in 3,500 male births, and it is estimated that there are 15,000 affected males in the United States. Progressive weakness develops, and untreated patients lose the ability to walk by age 8 to 12 years; death usually occurs by age 20 years because of respiratory failure. Although there is no cure for DMD, administration of high-dose corticosteroid markedly ameliorates the degenerative process, leading to an increase of 2 or more years of ambulation, a decreased incidence of scoliosis, and a decrease in cardiac and pulmonary deterioration resulting in a longer life. Respiratory and cardiac interventions also contribute to the longer lifespan. Currently, new molecular and genetically based treatment approaches have been introduced and hold great promise. Comprehensive guidelines for diagnosis and management have been published and are open access.[1-3]

Pathophysiology and Genetics

DMD is caused by the absence of the muscle protein dystrophin, which constitutes only a small portion of the total muscle proteins. Dystrophin plays a critical role in the biophysical stabilization of the myofiber membrane and also provides an attachment site for enzymes (such as nitrous oxide synthetase) that help support muscle function as well as dystrophin-associated proteins that link the actin-myosin network to the extracellular matrix, which are not incorporated into the muscle when dystrophin is absent in DMD. Primary abnormalities in specific dystrophin-associated proteins are the cause of many of the limb-girdle dystrophies, which only occasionally manifest in the pediatric age group, and are not discussed.

The absence of dystrophin is secondary to a mutation in the gene for dystrophin, which is located on the X chromosome. A variety of gene abnormalities can result in the lack of dystrophin production. The most common abnormality (65% of patients) is the deletion of a segment of the gene that interrupts the normal triplet sequence of the DNA, which constitutes the reading frame, so that when the gene is translated into RNA, all of the triplet sequences downstream from the deletion are nonsense. This results in the production of an incomplete protein, which is degraded, and no functional dystrophin is produced.

In 15% of the patients, there is a single nucleotide mutation known as a premature stop codon, which causes the ribosome to stop transcribing the genetic RNA. Any protein that is made up to this point is degraded, so that no dystrophin is produced. A variety of other gene abnormalities, including splice-site mutations and duplications, are responsible for the remainder of the genetic errors. It is important to ascertain the specific gene mutation because there are new treatments being developed that are specific to the type of genetic abnormality present. DNA analysis performed from a cheek swab to determine the gene mutation is available at a reasonable cost, and there are some programs providing free analysis in the United States.

In a similar but milder condition known as Becker muscular dystrophy (BMD), a gene segment deletion also exists, but the deletion does not interrupt the reading frame, and a smaller than normal dystrophin is produced in less than normal quantities. Unlike DMD, which has a relatively homogeneous clinical course, BMD is quite variable, depending on the function of the missing segment. Some affected patients will have a course similar to a mild DMD, whereas others will have much milder involvement and may not manifest until later in life, and show slow deterioration.

Because the gene for dystrophin is located on the X chromosome, DMD and BMD are inherited in an

X-linked fashion. This means that carrier mothers are clinically unaffected, 50% of their daughters will be carriers, and 50% of their sons will be affected with the disease. Given this X-linked inheritance pattern, if the mother had no brothers who were affected and no one in the lineage was previously affected to her knowledge, the gene could still be carried through several generations of females before manifesting in an affected male offspring. This explains why DMD may be a completely unexpected disease. In some instances, there may be a new mutation; this most frequently arises in the germline of the affected patient's maternal grandfather. Because of a variety of factors, even though this is an X-linked recessive trait, some female carriers will also manifest mild signs of muscle disease, including cardiomyopathy, which is dependent on the degree of X inactivation or other genetic factors. Although most affected patients are males, DMD may rarely fully manifest in females for a variety of underlying genetic reasons.

Genetic Modifiers of DMD

It recently has been determined that the severity of the DMD disease process may be modified on the basis of the presence of other inherited gene mutations unrelated to the dystrophin gene. For example, a mutation in LTDP4 leads to a milder clinical course, whereas a mutation in osteopontin leads to more rapid progression of the disease.

Diagnosis

In the future, it is likely that DMD screening will be a part of the standard newborn screening panel. Newborn screening for DMD can be inexpensively performed by measuring the serum creatine kinase level on a neonatal blood spot examination. Because there is normally a transient elevation of the serum creatine kinase level immediately following birth, the recommended threshold for further evaluation for DMD is a neonatal level greater than 1,000 IU/L, which will trigger follow-up creatine kinase testing at 6 weeks. Early diagnosis is important so that the family can be provided with appropriate genetic counseling to allow for future pregnancy planning. Because a diagnosis of DMD is often not made until age 5 years, the affected mother may have other affected boys before she is recognized as a carrier. For known maternal carriers, in vitro fertilization allows preimplantation selection whereby only disease-free embryos are implanted. Prenatal diagnosis of DMD is also possible via amniocentesis or chorionic villus sampling. In addition, early diagnosis also is important because most new treatments will likely be most effective if started early in life before significant muscle damage has occurred.

A diagnosis of DMD, which is often overlooked for years, should be suspected in infant boys who have delayed motor development. It is recommended that any boy who is not walking independently by 16 to 18 months of age (without other reasons for this motor delay) and those with unexplained cognitive delay should be evaluated for DMD (**Table 1**). Affected patients do not run in a completely normal manner and always have difficulty ascending and descending stairs, usually using a handrail and ascending and descending one step at a time rather than reciprocally. Patients with DMD are rarely able to hop on one leg or jump. One of the first obvious changes seen in many but not all patients is calf enlargement, which is specific for DMD and BMD and is rarely seen in any other neuromuscular diseases (**Figure 1**).

TABLE 1

Duchenne Muscular Dystrophy: Clinical Symptoms and Historical Findings

Male sex (boy)
Ambulation begins later than 16 to 18 months of age
Difficulty keeping up with peers
Inability to run normally (excessive use of arms)
Ability to jump and hop is unlikely
Unable to climb stairs reciprocally
Positive finding for Gowers maneuver
Cognitive delay
Easily fatigued
Calf enlargement
Positive family history for Duchenne muscular dystrophy or Becker muscular dystrophy

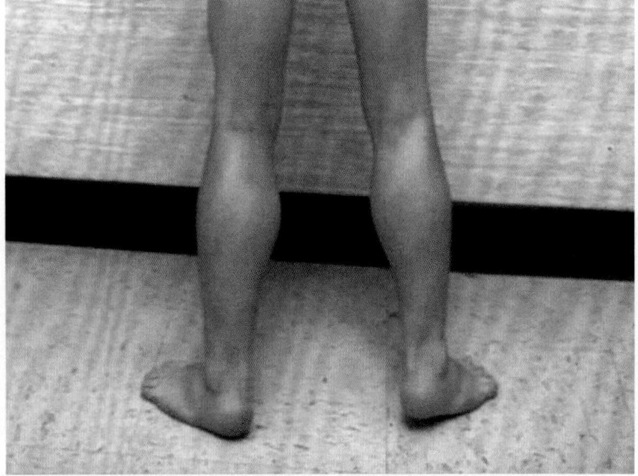

FIGURE 1 Clinical photograph shows calf enlargement in a boy with Duchenne muscular dystrophy.

The Gowers maneuver is a particularly useful clinical finding. Although it occurs in patients with significant weakness of the pelvic girdle musculature from other causes, it is seen in all patients with DMD. The Gowers maneuver describes the method used by a patient to rise from the floor. First, the child will transition from a sitting position on the floor into the prone position on his hands and knees, as if intending to crawl. After assuming this crawling position, the child will then extend the knees into the bear position. The trunk is then brought upright by hip extension, and the child will place the hands on the thighs to assist in the process of getting the trunk in the upright position (**Figure 2**).

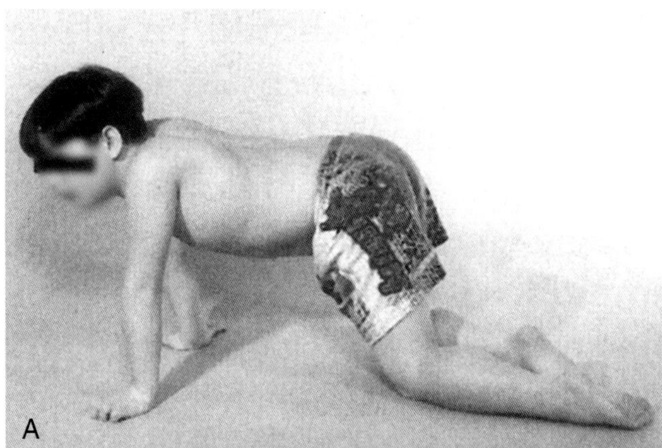

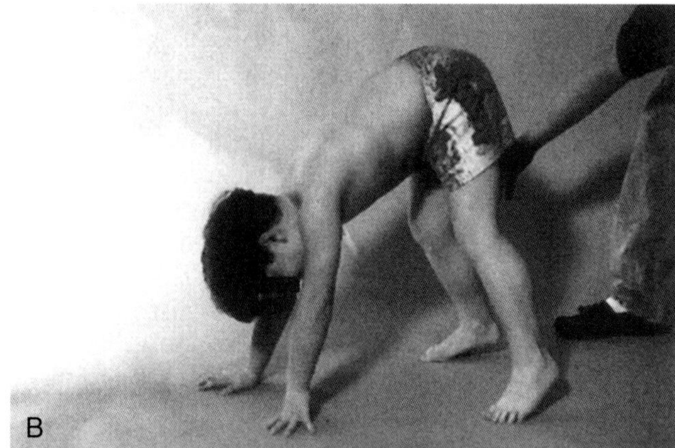

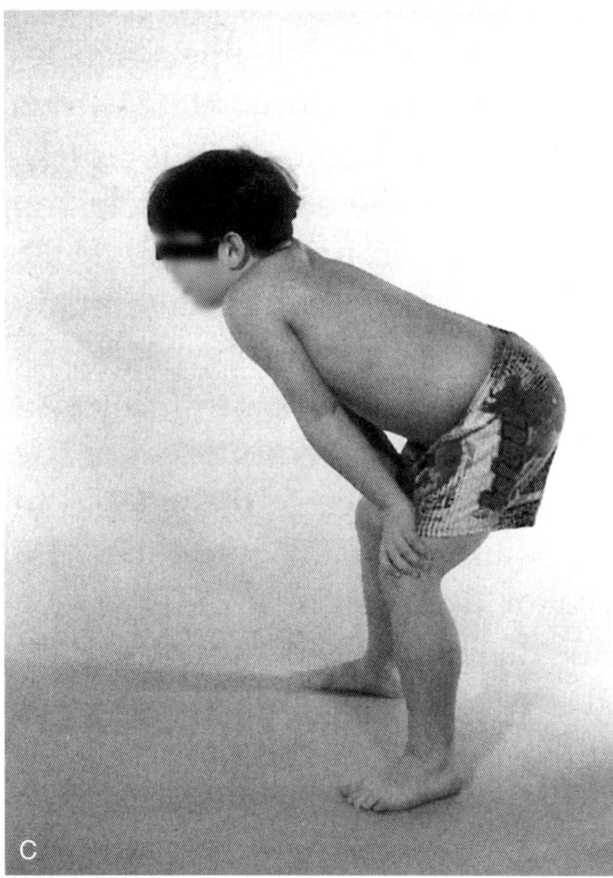

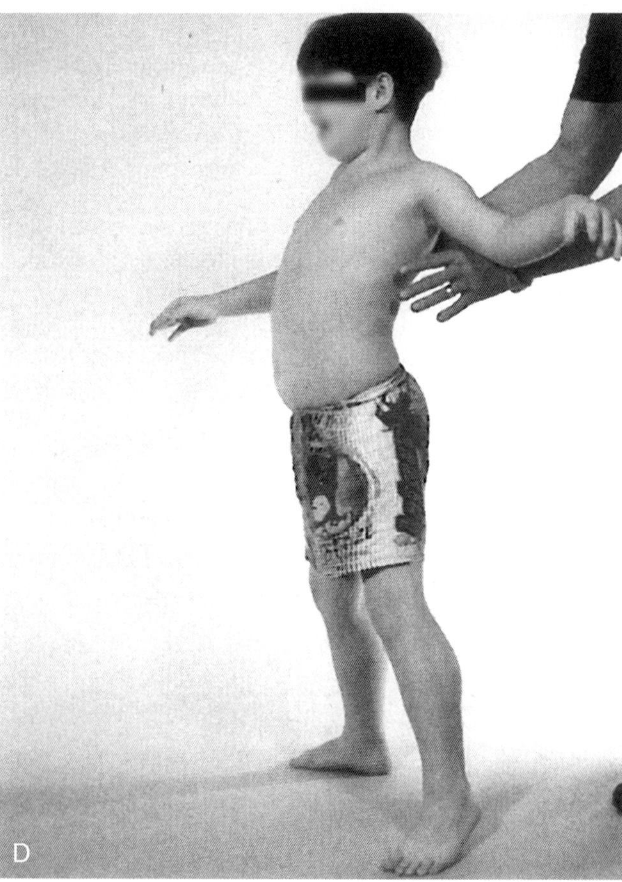

FIGURE 2 Clinical photographs of a child with Duchenne muscular dystrophy demonstrating the Gowers maneuver. **A**, The child moves from sitting on the floor to the prone position on all four limbs. **B**, The child extends the knees and assumes the bear position with all four limbs extended. **C**, The trunk is brought to the upright position using hands and arms on the upper thighs. **D**, The child achieves the upright position. (Reproduced from Sussman M: Duchenne muscular dystrophy. *J Am Acad Orthop Surg* 2002;10[2]:138-151. © 2002 by American Academy of Orthopaedic Surgeons.)

In a study from the United Kingdom, the average age at diagnosis was 5.2 years, and the delay from the time a patient was first seen by an orthopaedic consultant and subsequently referred for DMD testing was 2 years.[4] The delay did not improve over a 10-year period despite a regional educational campaign.

If DMD is suspected, the first diagnostic step is to test for the serum creatine kinase level, which can be ascertained with an inexpensive blood test. The normal level is up to 192 IU/L after 3 months of age; affected patients have levels that are usually greater than 10,000 IU/L. Milder elevations of the serum creatine kinase level (up to 500 units) can occur after strenuous activity or bruising, but also are also persistently seen in other types of muscle disease such as some of the limb-girdle muscular dystrophies. A diagnosis of DMD has been made in some young patients when liver function studies are performed for unrelated reasons, and liver enzymes such as alanine transaminase and aspartate transaminase are elevated along with creatine kinase, which is massively elevated. These other enzymes are typically mildly elevated in patients with DMD and BMD and do not indicate liver disease, and liver biopsy is not indicated.

If after 3 months of age, the serum creatine kinase level is greater than 1,000 IU/L, a cheek swab should be obtained to test for the dystrophin gene. This test is relatively inexpensive, is very specific and reliable, provides a definitive diagnosis, and defines the exact type of abnormality present in the gene in approximately 95% of boys with DMD. Muscle biopsy is rarely indicated and should be performed only in those few patients with an elevated serum creatine kinase level and clinical findings consistent with DMD, but who have negative genetic test results for DMD. Histochemistry for dystrophin and other dystrophin-associated proteins and a Western blot for dystrophin should be performed on the specimen. Muscle biopsy also may be infrequently required to confirm other muscle diseases that cannot be diagnosed based on clinical findings and genetic tests. EMG is infrequently performed, and not indicated if DMD is suspected.

Natural History

In affected patients, muscle weakness is difficult to appreciate in early infancy, but it becomes more apparent as developmental milestones are delayed. Walking is usually delayed until after 16 months of age. When patients begin to walk, the gait is relatively widely based, and increased lumbar lordosis is present. As time progresses, the gait becomes increasingly abnormal.[5] There is improvement in walking speed over the first 5 years, as assessed by the 6-minute timed walk test, until the disease process overwhelms the developmental process between the ages of 5 and 7 years and gait progressively deteriorates. Three-dimensional gait analysis shows that the knee flexion that occurs immediately after weight acceptance is usually lost sometime between the ages of 6 and 8 years. This means in early stance phase the initial wave of knee flexion with loading is lost, and the knee remains in full extension throughout the entire stance phase. By age 6 years, loss of hip extensor moments and power during stance phase occurs.[6] Tightness develops in the triceps surae beginning at age 4 to 5 years or later, and limitation of passive dorsiflexion will be found on physical examination. Loss of dorsiflexion occurs during stance phase, and there is early rise of the heel from the floor in the late stance phase. This progresses to toe walking during all of the stance phase, which is dynamic, and exceeds any fixed ankle contracture, which may also develop at this time. This toe walking helps maintain knee extension as the ground reaction force from the plantarflexed foot forces the knee into extension. Between the ages of 8 and 10 years, gait becomes substantially more labored, with a wider stance base, greater lumbar lordosis, and increased fatigability. Affected patients who receive no treatment will generally stop walking sometime between the age of 8 and 12 years, and the ability to ambulate after the age of 12 years in untreated boys is rare; however, with appropriate corticosteroid treatment, walking can continue for 2 or more additional years, and deflazacort may prolong walking to a greater extent than prednisone.

At approximately the time the ability to ambulate is lost, scoliosis can be clinically and radiologically demonstrated in more than 90% of untreated patients. Curves usually have their apex in the thoracolumbar region and do not respond to brace treatment or adaptive seating, and they continue to progress to a severe magnitude, which interferes with comfort and function during the patients' teenage years unless spinal fusion is undertaken.

An associated decline in pulmonary function begins in the teenage years; however, it appears that the scoliosis is not the major contributor to this decline. The major cause of respiratory decline is weakening of the muscles that support respiration, including the intercostal muscles and the diaphragm. A 2013 study found that stabilization of the scoliosis did not change the rate of respiratory decline based on a comparison with a contemporaneous group who did not undergo surgical correction.[7] Forced vital capacity (FVC) should be measured on a regular basis, which can be done accurately in a clinic by a skilled therapist using a handheld spirometer. If FVC substantially declines, a CoughAssist device (Philips Respironics) should be provided for daily use, and boys should be referred to a pediatric pulmonologist by age 10 years. Patients who have sleeping difficulty should have polysomnography and may benefit from bilevel positive airway pressure ventilation during sleep. The usual cause of death in boys with DMD is respiratory failure, which may be chronic, but also may occur in association with an acquired respiratory infection that has progressed to pneumonia. Death in untreated boys usually occurs by age 20 years, but a patient's lifespan may be extended by artificial ventilation and corticosteroid.

Cardiac function progressively deteriorates because of associated cardiomyopathy. Beginning in the second decade of life, ejection fraction monitoring should be followed by a pediatric cardiologist with echocardiography or cardiac MRI if available, because treatment with angiotensin-converting enzyme inhibitors and beta blockers will help preserve cardiac function.[8]

Medical Treatment With Corticosteroid

The natural history of DMD (and presumably BMD) is dramatically altered by the daily administration of pharmacologic doses of corticosteroid. This treatment has become standard practice and is endorsed by the American Academy of Neurology and is included in care guidelines developed under the guidance of the US Centers for Disease Control and Prevention (CDC).[1-3] Medications used are corticosteroids, either prednisone at 0.75 mg/kg daily or deflazacort at 0.9 mg/kg daily, up to a maximum of 30 mg/day. Therapy is usually initiated between the ages of 5 and 8 years, although some centers are initiating therapy at even younger ages. However, earlier initiation of steroid therapy may result in more severe growth retardation, earlier weight gain, and other adverse effects. Deflazacort, a derivative of prednisolone, has been shown to be associated with less weight gain than prednisone and is thought by some clinicians to be associated with fewer behavioral problems. Deflazacort is available in Europe and is now FDA approved in the United States. The drug is available only through the company PTC as Emflaza, at a cost of approximately $70,000/yr, which is significantly higher than the Canadian or European prices. Although there are reported benefits to deflazacort over prednisone in the area of scoliosis prevention, decreased weight gain, increased age at loss of ambulation, and behavioral issues, many insurance companies are reluctant to cover this cost unless the patient has first demonstrated significant adverse effects from prednisone.

Initial studies of corticosteroid use in patients with DMD published in the early 1990s showed improvement in muscle strength with the initiation of corticosteroid treatment, which was followed by a dramatic deviation from the anticipated loss of muscle strength, as determined by the combined muscle scores over succeeding years. Subsequently functional measures also were shown to be much more stable. A 2006 Canadian study using deflazacort reported dramatic improvements in a variety of functional tests, including walking (at least 2 additional years longer), pulmonary function (at age 18 years, 80% in the group treated with deflazacort versus 33% in the group not treated with corticosteroid), longer maintenance of self-feeding, a decreased need for assisted ventilation during the daytime and nighttime, and longer survival into the fourth decade. In addition, cardiac function deteriorated much less rapidly in patients undergoing corticosteroid therapy.[9]

A very dramatic effect of deflazacort use is a decreased incidence of scoliosis, and therefore decreased need for spinal surgery.[10] Although prednisone may be effective in scoliosis prevention, there are no studies documenting this. However, the effect of both prednisone and deflazacort have been replicated in other centers, including worldwide multicenter studies, in maintenance of ambulation, as well as pulmonary and cardiac function.

Patients who do not undergo spinal fusion usually have an associated total thoracolumbar kyphosis, which, in conjunction with osteopenia, results in a high incidence of vertebral compression fractures (VCFs) frequently at the thoracolumbar junction (**Figure 3**). These fractures may be painful but are not associated with neurologic damage. In patients with substantial pain, the administration of oral diphosphonate (off-label use of alendronate at 5 mg/day) has led to a rapid resolution of pain. This improvement occurs too rapidly to be the result of a change in bone density and may occur because of decreased bone turnover. The exact duration of diphosphonate treatment is unclear. Although it is unknown whether spinal bone density improves, femoral bone density does not improve. In a 2012 study, seven boys with DMD who had painful VCFs were treated with intravenous pamidronate or zoledronic acid infusions.[11] Pain improved in four of the patients and completely resolved in the other three patients. The vertebral height of the affected vertebrae either remained the same or improved and lumbar spine dual-energy X-ray absorptiometry Z-scores improved, although new compression fractures occurred. Further studies are needed in this area.

Although long-term corticosteroid use has adverse effects[12] (**Table 2**), corticosteroid should be continued for the patient's lifetime, even after ambulation ceases, to help preserve pulmonary, cardiac, and upper extremity functions.[1-3]

Orthopaedic and Rehabilitation Treatment

Guidelines for orthopaedic care have been published separately from the overall report, which were developed by a group of experts convened by the US CDC and based on the literature as well as expert opinion.[13]

Pharmacologic dosing of corticosteroid ameliorates the clinical progression, so that treated patients experience much the same milestones as those who are untreated, albeit at a slower rate, so orthopaedic treatment is based on the clinical manifestations.

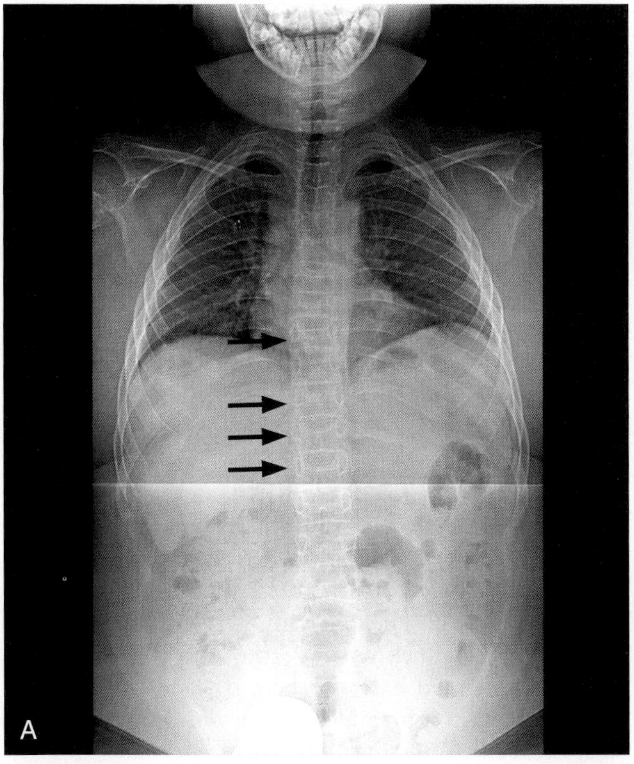

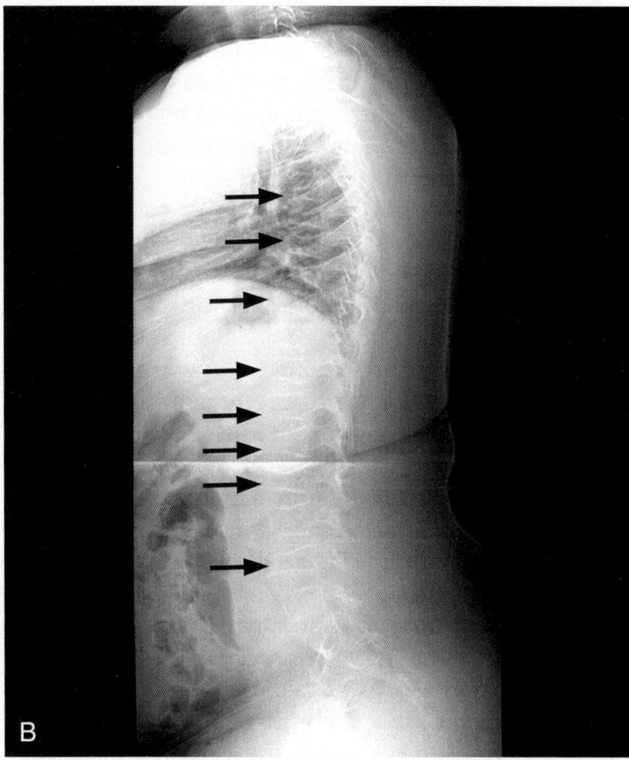

FIGURE 3 AP (**A**) and lateral (**B**) standing spinal radiographs of a 10-year-old boy with Duchenne muscular dystrophy who reported back pain. Multiple vertebral compression fractures can be seen (arrows). (Copyright Shriners Hospitals for Children, Portland, OR.)

No orthopaedic intervention is indicated in the first 5 years. At approximately age 5 or 6 years when tightness of the Achilles tendon develops as evidenced by limitation of passive dorsiflexion to 5° or less, an ankle-foot orthosis (AFO) used at nighttime, which has been custom-molded in a neutral position, is recommended to help prevent progression of the Achilles tightness. However, AFOs should not be used during the daytime because they make ambulation more difficult. Even in the absence of contractures, patients will begin walking on their toes, which is an adaptation (known as the plantar flexion–knee extension couple) that creates a moment to help support the knee in extension. Gait analysis has shown that the hip extensors weaken

TABLE 2

Adverse Effects of Corticosteroid Use

Moon facial features, as seen in Cushing syndrome, may occur.
Puberty may be delayed into late teens, including delayed development of facial and body hair.
Potential height may be lost (as much as 10 to 12 inches if medication is started at age 7 years).
Cataracts may develop, although treatment is rarely needed.
Substantial weight gain may occur (less weight gain with deflazacort than prednisone).
Behavioral problems may occur, including aggressive behavior toward classmates and siblings. Overt behavior problems may be less frequent with deflazacort use compared with prednisone. Depression is more prevalent with deflazacort.
Osteopenia may worsen, although this has not been definitively proven.
Vertebral compression fractures may occur when the spine is not fused because of scoliosis.
There is an increased risk of long-bone fractures.

early, before changes in hip motion can be appreciated. Because patients with DMD are unable to propel their center of mass forward using their weak hip extensor muscles, the triceps surae are used to compensate by helping to propel the center of mass forward during the stance phase of gait.[6]

In 20% or fewer patients, the Achilles contracture is severely progressive, and patients walk completely on their toes with no heel contact. When the contracture reaches approximately 30° or more of fixed equinus, walking becomes unstable. If the patient is a strong ambulator, has full knee extension against gravity, and has the ability to handle some resistance with knee extension (grade 4), a careful Achilles tendon lengthening (TAL) using an open sliding technique to avoid inadvertent complete tenotomy may be undertaken. Short leg casts are placed, and standing and walking are initiated on the first postoperative day. Short leg casts are continued for 4 weeks, and a custom-molded posterior leaf spring AFO is then placed to provide support in the stance phase of gait and control footdrop in swing. After this procedure, some patients will choose to use their AFOs for ambulation; however, AFOs should be used only at night to prevent contracture recurrence if the patient can achieve stability during ambulation without AFOs. Although foot flat gait can be achieved following TAL, walking velocity may be reduced, and gait appears more labored, so this procedure should not be undertaken lightly. However, there are a few boys in whom severe equinus develops who will benefit from a TAL, and when this is accompanied by varus, posterior tibial and toe flexor tenotomies will also be required.

As the disease progresses, contractures develop in most patients because of prolonged sitting and muscle imbalance. Tightness in the hip flexors and the tensor fasciae lata develops in all patients and results in abduction and flexion contractures, which contribute to the adoption of a wide-based, lordotic gait. Knee flexion contractures also may develop and can progress to 80° to 90° in some nonambulatory patients. If knee flexion contracture develops while the patient is still ambulating, the weak quadriceps will be unable to support knee extension, and this may lead to the inability to continue ambulation. However, outcomes following surgical hamstring lengthening for established knee flexion contracture in DMD are disappointing. Prophylactic multilevel tendon release in the lower extremity is advocated by some surgeons, but this technique is not generally recommended. The data supporting this approach are relatively weak. When walking ceases, full-time AFO use is recommended to slow progression of the equinovarus deformity, which will inevitably occur. If severe equinovarus develops, it is rarely uncomfortable and does not require treatment unless the patient desires more stylish shoe wear. In these instances, simple tenotomies of the Achilles tendon can be performed, and, if substantial varus exists, tenotomies of the posterior tibial toe flexor tendons just above the ankle can be added. If there is a significant varus component and marked correction is obtained, this may result in stretching of the posterior tibial nerve and cause pain, and may result in long-term dysesthesia if correction is not moderated by reapplying a cast with less correction. After surgery, short leg casts are placed, kept in place for 3 weeks, followed by the continuous use of a well-molded AFO, molded at the time of surgery, which secures the foot in the corrected position. Releasing hip flexors and abductors and hamstrings in nonambulatory patients with DMD is not performed because correction is minimal after such surgery. Prophylactic stretching has been advocated to control hip and knee flexion contractures, but no evidence exists that this offers any benefits, and stretching may cause discomfort. Night extension orthoses for the knees are not recommended because their efficacy is unproven, they can be uncomfortable, and they may interfere with sleep. Knee flexion contracture can approach 90°, but rarely exceeds 90°, and it does not interfere with sitting but will make positioning for sleep difficult. In some patients with lower extremity contractures, moving or even touching the legs may cause extreme discomfort.

Occupational and Physical Therapy

During the first decade of life, regular physical or occupational therapy is not usually necessary, although a therapist may provide the patient's school with recommendations regarding activities to be performed within the daily school setting. Although stretching exercises are frequently advocated and prescribed, there is no evidence for their efficacy, and they may place an additional burden on patients and their families. Adaptive recreation may be beneficial, and adaptation of a school's physical education program is important because patients with DMD will not be able to perform at the level of their peers. An independent education program should be instituted.

Experimental studies in animals have shown that eccentric muscle activity hastens muscle deterioration in DMD (but not other neuromuscular diseases);[14] therefore, activities that have a large eccentric component, such as weight lifting or walking on soft sand, should be avoided. When walking becomes difficult, patients will require powered devices for mobility. In patients with good upper limb function, a powered scooter may be an appropriate device, particularly for patients taking corticosteroids who can expect a reasonably long period of upper limb function. In those with poor upper limb function, a powered wheelchair with a variety of components, such as the tilt-in-space function (to allow differential pressure relief) and an elevating seat (to bring patients to the level of their peers), should be prescribed. When upper limb function becomes compromised, occupational therapy can help the patient to master the use of adaptive equipment. A computer or tablet with voice-recognition software may be particularly helpful for completing schoolwork.

When ambulation ceases, a pneumatic standing device can provide good support for the trunk and lower extremities to allow standing for up to 30 minutes. Ultimately, standing in this device will become impractical because of the progression of hip, knee, and ankle contractures. In the past, knee-ankle-foot orthoses (KAFOs) were recommended to help prolong ambulatory ability, but it is now apparent that these devices are quite cumbersome, do not allow functional walking, and interfere with toileting. KAFOs are no longer recommended.

In addition to motor delays, cognitive impairment is common in DMD, with the mean IQ of approximately 90. Because a large component of this impairment occurs in the area of expressive language, processing of information may be relatively better than its translation into expressive speech. Some patients may be severely cognitively impaired, but others may be very intelligent. Furthermore, some patients are considered to be in the autism spectrum. Cognitive differences should be considered when establishing an independent education program.

With age and as muscle weakness increases, the patient may be unable to change positions while sleeping. A hospital bed with side rails may allow the patients to turn themselves, but ultimately caregivers may need to turn the patient in bed several times a night. Enuresis is common in patients taking corticosteroids and more prevalent in those taking prednisone than in those taking deflazacort.[12]

Spinal Deformity

Progressive scoliosis develops in 90% of untreated patients and has its onset at approximately 10 to 12 years of age in untreated patients. In the 10% of patients in whom scoliosis does not develop, total thoracolumbar lordosis seems to prevent scoliosis. This is a naturally occurring phenomenon. Although a variety of seating and bracing treatment techniques have been tried to induce this lordotic pattern, they have not been successful. No orthotic devices or seating adaptations have proven to be beneficial in controlling scoliosis in patients with DMD. After a curve reaches 20° to 30°, it is always continually and relentlessly progressive. Spinal instrumentation and fusion from the upper thoracic spine to L5 or the sacrum is recommended as soon as curves reach this magnitude. Performing the surgery at this stage of the disease is advantageous because patients have better pulmonary and cardiac function and are likely to have an easier recovery, and curves are more easily correctable.[15]

At the time of surgery, the surgeon is likely to find hypertrophic rigid fibrofatty tissue replacing the paraspinal muscles, which may require horizontal relaxing incisions to obtain exposure. The preferred treatment for scoliosis is posterior instrumentation with segment fixation. Anterior spinal surgery is contraindicated. Extending the fusion to the sacrum may not be necessary if pelvic obliquity is mild, but fusion should extend distally at least to L5. All patients being considered for spinal fusion should have a thorough preoperative evaluation, including pulmonary and cardiac assessments. Usually the first postoperative night should be spent in an intensive care unit for respiratory care; however, in most instances, extubation is possible on the first postoperative night, and return to a standard nursing care environment can occur thereafter. A total intravenous anesthetic technique should be used in all patients with DMD to avoid anesthesia-induced rhabdomyolysis.

Although correction and stabilization of scoliosis is essential to maintain comfort and function in patients with spinal deformity, spinal stabilization may decrease but not eliminate the progressive decline in pulmonary function. A 2011 study reported a loss of pulmonary function in the immediate postoperative period, followed by a rate of decline similar to the preoperative trajectory;[16] however, other authors have reported that spinal fusion reduces the rate of pulmonary decline.[17] With careful perioperative management, patients with severe curves and pulmonary compromise can undergo successful surgical correction. A Japanese group reported that, in 14 patients with DMD and severe scoliosis (mean curve, 98°) and poor pulmonary function (mean FVC, 22%), FVC improved to 26% after a 6-week pulmonary training program before surgery.[18] Following surgery, all the patients were extubated on the same day and had no decline in pulmonary function at 6 weeks postoperatively but had the expected level of pulmonary decline 2 years after surgery. A Cochrane collaboration report on scoliosis surgery for patients with DMD concluded that because no randomized trials were available to evaluate the effectiveness of scoliosis surgery, no conclusion was possible regarding the efficacy of surgery.[19] However, a published clinical care guideline sponsored by the US CDC strongly recommended that spinal fusion be provided for patients with DMD and progressive curves.[1,14] In a review of 58 patients with progressive neuromuscular scoliosis, 27 of whom had DMD, a Korean group reported substantial improvements in sitting balance, body pain, and social functioning after spinal fusion, although parents did not report improvement in quality of life.[20] In addition, some patients experience greater difficulty with self-feeding after spinal stabilization because they can no longer bend their trunk forward to meet their hand. Patients should be informed of this possible adverse effect before surgery.

Daily use of corticosteroid, particularly deflazacort, has been shown in several studies to result in a dramatic decrease in the incidence of scoliosis. In a careful retrospective study from 2013, the incidence was reduced from 90% in boys with untreated DMD to 20% in those on deflazacort. Half of those developing curves in the treatment group (2/4 patients) had discontinued their medication after skeletal maturity and rapidly developed curves thereafter.[10] This history of rapid development of curves after discontinuing the medication was also noted in other studies, so that once on medication, this should be continued indefinitely, or risk of the development of scoliosis may be high.

Bone Health and Fracture

Boys with DMD are known to have a higher incidence of long bone fractures than able-bodied peers, and dual-energy X-ray absorptiometry has shown that osteopenia associated with DMD occurs early in life.[21] Aggressive treatment may be needed to prevent periods of no ambulation following fracture, which leads to a more marked progression of weakness. Depending on the degree of preexisting weakness, patients may lose the ability to ambulate after a lower limb fracture. Upper limb fractures can cause balance problems and impair ambulatory ability, so physiotherapy to maintain ambulation may be useful. In poor ambulators and nonambulators, casts may be used to treat lower limb fractures. Nonambulatory patients commonly sustain distal femoral fractures in the metaphyseal area in falls during wheelchair transfers. These fractures can be managed with long leg casts or an articulated knee orthosis for comfort. Although, healing is usually rapid, marked flexion at the fracture site should be avoided because it can limit the patient's ability to extend the knee and stand for transfers. Fixation methods for lower limb fractures should allow minimal interruption of ambulation. For distal metaphyseal fractures in ambulatory boys, retrograde intramedullary fixation should be considered.

It appears that corticosteroid further increases the fracture incidence, and deflazacort may be associated with a higher risk of fracture than other corticosteroid regimens. In one large study of 143 patients with DMD, the fracture rate for long bones in patients treated with corticosteroids was 2.6 times greater than in patients who did not receive steroid treatment. In a 2019 study, boys taking deflazacort had a 16-fold increase in time to first fracture compared with steroid-naïve boys with DMD, whereas there was no difference in boys on other corticosteroid regimens.[22] The most common sites for long bone fractures in boys on corticosteroid in another multicenter study were the femur and tibia, and in this series, there were only a few forearm fractures.[23]

Fat embolism, which may be lethal, may occur even in minimally displaced femoral fractures in DMD and should be suspected if there is hypoxia and tachycardia after fracture of a long bone, even a nondisplaced femoral metaphyseal fracture. If hypoxia is present, immediate aggressive pulmonary management is essential.

VCFs are also common in boys with DMD treated with corticosteroid. These may be asymptomatic or may become painful and contribute to a kyphotic deformity, but are not known to result in neurologic impairment. In one study, 91% of patients on deflazacort had VCF by the age of 15 years.[24]

The role of diphosphonates or other medications that may improve bone density and decrease fracture rate has not been established in this patient group by controlled studies, although there is interest in this among pediatric endocrinologists.[25] However, long-term administration of diphosphonates may inhibit bone formation; therefore discontinuation of these drugs is recommended after 5 years of treatment.

Anesthesia-Induced Rhabdomyolysis

Anesthesia-induced rhabdomyolysis is an unusual but frequently fatal reaction to general anesthetic. Triggering agents such as succinylcholine and halogenated hydrocarbon anesthetic gases have been implicated and neither should be used in patients with DMD. A total intravenous technique is recommended for any patient with DMD undergoing a surgical procedure, including spinal fusion. Anesthesia-induced rhabdomyolysis differs from malignant hyperthermia and, although it is not absolutely known, probably does not respond to intravenous dantrolene. In a typical scenario, as the patient is emerging from anesthesia, cardiac arrhythmia and tachycardia occur, followed by cardiac collapse associated with ventricular fibrillation. Most cases are associated with significant hyperkalemia. Rescue treatment should include rapid assessment and reduction of elevated potassium levels, usually by the administration of insulin, glucose, and bicarbonate, and the use of hyperventilation therapy. Younger patients seem most susceptible to anesthesia-induced rhabdomyolysis.[26] Families should be counseled that children with DMD should not receive general anesthesia outside of major hospitals where anesthesiologists are aware of anesthesia-induced rhabdomyolysis and have the resources to provide a rapid response.

Novel New Therapies

An exciting development in the treatment of DMD is the potential availability of a variety of innovative therapies that may arrest or slow disease progression with fewer adverse effects than corticosteroids. Some of these treatments are based on a specific gene defect and are applicable only to patients with that specific abnormality.

The first broad group of potential new treatments is gene-based therapy. Antisense oligonucleotides are compounds that attach to the pre-messenger RNA of dystrophin and mask the deletion that alters the downstream reading frame, and thereby establishes a normal reading frame to allow production of a truncated dystrophin. This abnormal dystrophin is produced in smaller quantities, similar to the dystrophin in patients with BMD. Because antisense oligonucleotides are specific for each deletion, these compounds are being developed for several of the most common deletions in DMD. This treatment will not cure DMD, but the goal is to slow the loss of functional skills. Currently, the first of this class that blocks the expression of exon 51 and allows resplicing of the pre-RNA and resumption of synthesis of a smaller dystrophin has been approved by the FDA as Exondys-51 (eteplirsen). The medication is given by intravenous infusion, and the cost is approximately $125,000 per infusion, which is given six times per year for the first year and four times thereafter, and price varies by weight. Approximately 15% of patients with DMD have deletions that are amenable to the partial correction provided by this first antisense oligonucleotide; however, 80% of patients with deletions (who account for 65% of all patients with DMD) have deletions that are likely to be amenable to this exon-skipping approach. Clinical trials are underway for similar drugs directed at other mutations. Each additional exon-skipping agent requires its own clinical trial. The initial trials have shown modest clinical benefit, with an increase to 7% to 11% dystrophin synthesis (which increases the amount of dystrophin from roughly 0.15% to 1%) and small, but significant delay in deterioration of functional assessment measures such as 6-minute walk test, timed supine to stand, pulmonary function measures, and others. The lack of more dramatic results may be due to the fact that treatment was not initiated until the patient's age was 6 years or older, at which time substantial loss of healthy muscle tissue had already occurred. It is likely that the earlier these medications are started, the greater will be the benefits.[27,28]

In the future, it is possible that the use of CRISPR/Cas9 technology for editing DNA may supersede the antisense oligonucleotide approach by editing the abnormal gene to yield a normal, functional dystrophin gene. This targeted genome editing technology is in the laboratory stage where it has shown success in mice with both deletions and premature termination codons.[29] Satellite cells, from which the muscle originates, also could be removed from the patient, have the normal gene inserted in vitro, and then be injected back into the patient. This approach also should immortalize the correction.

Another treatment approach is applicable to approximately 15% of patients with DMD in whom the defect is the result of a single nucleotide change in the DNA, which results in an abnormal premature termination codon that stops synthesis of pre-RNA dystrophin. This partially synthesized chain is degraded, and no dystrophin is produced. There is normally a stop codon at the end of each protein sequence, but not within the protein sequence where synthesis of dystrophin is interrupted. Translarna, previously known as Ataluren, has been conditionally approved in some European countries but has been denied approval by the US FDA. With a cost of approximately $400,000 to $700,000 per year, the British National Health Service initially decided that the clinical benefit of the drug did not merit the cost and would not pay for the drug for patients in the United Kingdom. This decision was reversed after lobbying by advocacy groups, and the National Health Service agreed to a 5-year trial period and negotiated cost with the company that produces the drug.

Another approach is to introduce a mini-gene using a viral vector. Because the dystrophin gene is too large to be fully inserted by a viral vector, several different mini-genes containing the critical active sites have been developed, which appear to be beneficial in animal models, and are in clinical trials.[30]

Other Innovative Nonspecific Therapies

Other therapies are being investigated, which may be applicable to all patients with DMD, regardless of the genetic defect. CAT-1004 (Catabasis, or Edasalonexent), an anti-inflammatory drug, which is an nuclear factor kappa B inhibitor, has shown promise in animal models. This drug is alleged to have the positive anti-inflammatory effects of corticosteroid without the major adverse effects. A clinical trial has been underway in multiple centers, but no results are available as yet.

Another approach is inhibition of myostatin, which is a normal circulating protein that inhibits muscle growth and regeneration. Myostatin is suppressed during fetal development but is expressed after birth. Inhibition of the circulating myostatin protein by antimyostatin antibodies or other strategies should reduce the effect of circulating myostatin, thereby increasing muscle regeneration. There are several drugs that have been tried based on this principle, but as yet none has shown clinically meaningful efficacy. Facilitating a greater degree of muscle regeneration may enhance the action of other genetically based therapies because the regenerated muscle produced by those therapies is likely to be produced with genetically modified dystrophin.

Several other approaches including upregulation of utrophin, use of tadalafil to increase nitric oxide in muscle, and others, which have shown promise in the laboratory, have had clinical trials but have failed to show clinical benefit.

Treatment with stem cells has a large online presence, but no positive clinical data have been demonstrated. Despite this, there are many clinics, mainly abroad, that have aggressive marketing campaigns using a variety of approaches without any objective evidence of clinical benefit, and high financial cost, so families should be cautioned to assess carefully before subjecting their child to this expensive, unproven approach.

As these various clinical trials are completed and analyzed, it is likely that patients may benefit from a cocktail of several of these medications, which may have complementary effects. Treating physicians should be aware of these trials so that families who want to participate can be informed and counseled.

SPINAL MUSCULAR ATROPHY

SMA is an inherited autosomal recessive disease in which there is progressive loss of the motor neurons (anterior horn cells) of the spinal cord. The loss of motor neurons results in progressive weakness and, ultimately, paralysis of the limbs and trunk and the bulbar enervated muscles (with the exception of the extraocular muscles). SMA is the most common genetic disease that causes childhood mortality. The incidence of SMA ranges from 4 per 100,000 individuals in England to 10 per 100,000 individuals in the United States and Germany. The carrier state of SMA ranges from 1 in 50 to 1 in 90 individuals, depending on the country being studied.[31] Affected patients have normal intelligence.

Classification

SMA is divided into three major subtypes[32] (**Table 3**). The first type, known as SMA type 1 or Werdnig-Hoffman disease, has very early onset, with weakness seen at birth or before age 6 months in a child who seemed to be developing normally. In these children, gross motor skills such as rolling over will begin to develop, but independent sitting is never achieved. Acquired skills begin to be lost. Sucking ability may be deficient from birth, and feeding impairment is a predominant feature of SMA type 1. Tongue fasciculations are frequently seen, which represent spontaneous activity of sick motor neurons. Weakness, including weakness of the muscles that support respiratory function, rapidly progresses. Children also demonstrate a marked drooping of the ribs, which results in a small pear-shaped chest. Death by the age of 2 years occurs in 90% of patients because of pulmonary failure. In a natural history study, the median age at death or of respirator use greater than 16 hr/day was 13.5 months.[33] If patients are provided with artificial ventilation via a tracheostomy, they may survive for many decades. However, full-time care will be needed because the patient will have minimal motor function, with the exception of the eye musculature. If patients survive with full-time assisted ventilation, severe scoliosis and dislocated hips will develop in all of them.

SMA type 2 has an onset between 6 months and 3 years of age and is distinguished by children who are able to sit independently, but never achieve the ability

TABLE 3

Characteristics of the Types of Spinal Muscular Atrophy

Type 1: Werdnig-Hoffman

Onset: 0-6 months of age

Absent deep tendon reflexes

Tongue fasciculations

Highest attainable function: Never able to sit independently

Life expectancy: <2 years

Death caused by pulmonary insufficiency; with newer molecular treatments, function may be preserved, and lifespan increased. However, scoliosis and dislocated hips may still develop, similar to type 2 disease.

Type 2: Intermediate (most commonly seen by orthopaedic surgeons)

Onset: 6+ months of age, with loss of previously acquired skills

Absent deep tendon reflexes

Tongue fasciculations

Highest attainable function: sits unassisted, but no independent standing

Life expectancy: 15+ years

Death caused by pulmonary insufficiency

Scoliosis: almost universal

Dislocated hips: almost universal

Type 3: Kugelberg-Welander

Onset: after age 10 months; may not appear until teenage years

Highest attainable function: walking more than 25 m unassisted

Life expectancy: 25 years to normal

Scoliosis: possible

Dislocated hips: uncommon, but possible

to stand independently. Progression is less rapid than in SMA type 1, and survival is variable depending on the severity of involvement, with life expectancy between 15 and 30 years. These patients have similar orthopaedic problems as those with SMA type 1, including dislocated hips and scoliosis in all patients, usually during the first decade of life. Tongue fasciculation is seen, as is a fine tremor in the fingers. Patients with more severe disease will have marked drooping of the ribs, which results in a pear-shaped chest. Most patients with SMA breathe primarily with their diaphragm, so abdominal expansion is observed on inspiration. Scoliosis also begins in the first decade of life and as early as the first several years of life. If untreated, scoliosis will progress to severe degrees. During the first or second decade of life, a decline in pulmonary function will require varying degrees of respiratory support; pulmonary medicine is a critical need. Feeding difficulties develop in many patients, and they may have difficulty maintaining adequate caloric intake and will require a gastrostomy tube to maintain nutrition and prevent aspiration.

SMA type 3, also known as Kugelberg-Welander syndrome, has a later onset (usually after 2 years of age), and progression is slower than in patients with SMA type 2. These patients will achieve independent standing and walking, although they may lose the ability to walk by the end of the first decade or early into the second decade of life. In patients who lose the ability to walk before skeletal maturity, scoliosis may occur and will require treatment. In addition, hip dislocation also may occur, but may not occur until the second decade of life. Hip pain is seen in some patients, particularly if hip dislocation occurs in the teen years. Respiratory function declines slowly and may not manifest as a problem until the second decade of life or later. Many patients have a relatively normal life span, but will become substantially disabled as adults.

Type 4 SMA (adult-onset) also exists, but it is not seen in the pediatric population.

Genetic Basis

SMA is caused by a deficiency in the survival motor neuron (SMN) protein that results from an abnormality in the *SMN1* gene (located on chromosome 5), which is responsible for producing this protein. Each parent will have one mutated and nonfunctional allele of the *SMN1* gene. There are no clinical abnormalities associated with this heterozygous state; however, each child who is born to a set of parents who are carriers has a 25% chance of receiving two nonfunctional alleles, one from each parent, and will be affected. Children with SMA have no functional SMN protein produced by the *SMN1* gene; however, a second gene, *SMN2*, of which there may be two to five copies, also located on chromosome 5, also produces some complete SMN protein. This *SMN2* gene has an alteration in a single base pair in exon 7, so an incomplete, nonfunctional, SMN protein missing exon 7 is produced. However, each *SMN2* gene also produces approximately 10% of the normal quantity of full-length and fully functional SMN protein. Therefore, the number of *SMN2* genes, which is variable, determines how much fully functional SMN protein is produced. The severity of the disease is determined by the number of *SMN2* genes in the patient. If there are no functional *SMN2* genes, the condition is lethal. With two functional *SMN2* genes present, the child will have the more severe SMA1 phenotype, whereas children with four or five copies of the *SMN2* gene have a much milder form of the disease, probably SMA type 3. Although the number of gene copies of *SMN2* can be determined by genetic testing and is relatively predictive of the type of SMA, the classification of SMA is determined not by genotyping, but by assessing the child's age of onset and functional deficits. However, this classification scheme will become obsolete because the natural history is dramatically altered by new genetically based treatments, and a genetically based classification may become the standard.

The SMN protein is apparently involved in messenger and ribosomal RNA transcription and processing, and it is reduced from 5% up to 95% in patients with SMA. The defect manifests mainly in anterior horn cells, but may be responsible for abnormalities in other organ systems, including the chest deformity.

In autosomal recessive conditions such as SMA, there is usually no family history unless the parents share a common ancestor. In populations where consanguinity is relatively high, such as Saudi Arabia, the prevalence of SMA also will be high if there is an abnormal gene in the lineage.[32] If a common ancestor carried one copy of the abnormal gene, the chance of offspring in subsequent generations also carrying this gene will be high. If two carriers have a common ancestor from whom they both inherited the carrier state, there is a 25% chance that each of their children will have SMA.

Diagnosis

A diagnosis of SMA should be suspected if an infant has obvious weakness, sucking problems, and difficulty breathing at birth or if the child starts to lose acquired motor skills at any time during growth and development. Children may begin to crawl, sit, and even walk and then lose those abilities. The limbs become atrophic and, unlike DMD, calf hypertrophy is not seen.

If SMA is suspected, the child is usually referred to a child neurologist. The clinical examination will reveal weakness throughout and the absence of deep tendon reflexes, and tongue fasciculations and finger tremors at rest, particularly in younger children, will be present.

In the past, electromyography was used to provide diagnostic information, and spontaneous potentials known as fibrillation potentials and giant potentials were noted. Electromyography is no longer used as a diagnostic test in children with suspected SMA; genetic testing for the *SMN* gene deletion, which is positive in 98% of patients, is now favored. Muscle biopsy also is no longer indicated.

Newborn screening by DNA analysis is possible, but is currently only mandated in a few states in the United States. Now that there is a proven treatment for SMA, which is most effective if started before motor neuron loss, there is a strong effort being mounted by advocacy and physician groups to mandate that this be added to the newborn screening examination. If the family has one affected child, chorionic villus sampling or amniocentesis can be done in utero to detect SMA in the developing embryo. Preimplantation selection of eggs fertilized in vitro also can be done, although this procedure may not be covered by insurance providers.

Orthopaedic Issues

In all patients with SMA type 1, most patients with SMA type 2, and some patients with SMA type 3, bilateral hip subluxation, which progresses to dislocation, will occur. However, hip dislocation is rarely symptomatic, and no preventive interventions such as abduction bracing treatment or surgical correction are effective. Surgical procedures to prevent or correct the progressive dislocation usually are unsuccessful, in that although reduction may be achieved, in most cases the hips re-dislocate with time.[34] Unlike patients who have cerebral palsy with muscle spasticity that pulls the femoral head against the pelvis, the muscles are flaccid, and pain is usually not problematic in patients with SMA. As subluxation progresses, there is associated acetabular dysplasia. During a transitory period, a positive Barlow sign may be present, and it will be possible to feel the hip going in and out of the acetabulum. This is not painful for the patient, and instability will disappear over time as the hip becomes completely dislocated. Dislocations are most frequently bilateral. In instances in which only one hip becomes dislocated, pelvic obliquity is usually present. However, in the rare patient, usually where the hip becomes significantly subluxated late in the first decade or later, hip pain may develop, and if nonsurgical measures are unsuccessful, surgical intervention may be considered. It is unclear how the new genetic treatments will influence this progressive hip dysplasia, and what interventions may be successful.

Contractures at the hip (flexion and abduction) and knee (flexion) will develop in nonambulatory patients but usually do not develop in patients who are still walking. Contractures may interfere with the child's ability to stand in a standing frame. Surgical treatment of contractures is not usually indicated in children with SMA unless the contractures interfere with function. Unilateral hip abduction contractures will make standing difficult, and this can be corrected by surgical treatment. Release of the anterior part of the gluteus medius and tensor fasciae femoris from the pelvis along with sectioning of the proximal fascia lata (Ober-Yount procedure) will allow contracture relief and provide a level pelvis in standing and thereby make standing much easier. In a child with severe hip flexion contracture that affects the ability to stand, anterior hip release may be performed to allow continued standing; tenotomies of the anterior gluteus medius, the tensor fascia femoris, the sartorius, and the direct head of the rectus femoris may be included in the surgery. Hamstring lengthening is not usually successful for knee flexion deformity. An alternative approach for knee flexion deformity is an anterior distal femoral hemiepiphysiodesis, although this should be performed before the deformity becomes severe, because a maximum of only 20° to 30° of correction is possible with this procedure.

In the foot, equinus occurs infrequently; however, varus or valgus deformities may occur and can be treated with tenotomy if this is a functional problem.

The upper extremities will also become weak, but surgical interventions are rarely indicated; however, splints to support the wrist in neutral may be helpful, and adaptive technology is critical to maintain function.

Scoliosis will develop in all patients with SMA type 1 and SMA type 2 and many patients with SMA type 3, especially those who manifest substantial weakness before the early teenage years. Curves may develop before 2 years of age in SMA type 1 and SMA type 2 patients with more severe involvement. Although there have been no controlled studies in the use of spinal orthotics to slow curve progression, a progressive curve can be stabilized for a period with a well-molded custom thoracolumbosacral orthosis (TLSO). This orthosis also provides sitting stability and increases comfort. The TLSO must be custom molded and have an extremely large abdominal opening because these patients are abdominal breathers. The abdominal hole should not be covered with fabric, and the abdomen should protrude substantially through the opening. Consultation with the orthotist who is fabricating the TLSO is recommended because the belly hole must extend laterally at least to the anterior axillary line (**Figure 4**). The TLSO may compromise the patient's ability to eat, even with a large belly hole, and may need to be loosened during feedings. In general, the TLSO should be worn whenever the patient is sitting; however, the wearing schedule should be adjusted based on the patient's tolerance for the device, and wearing time

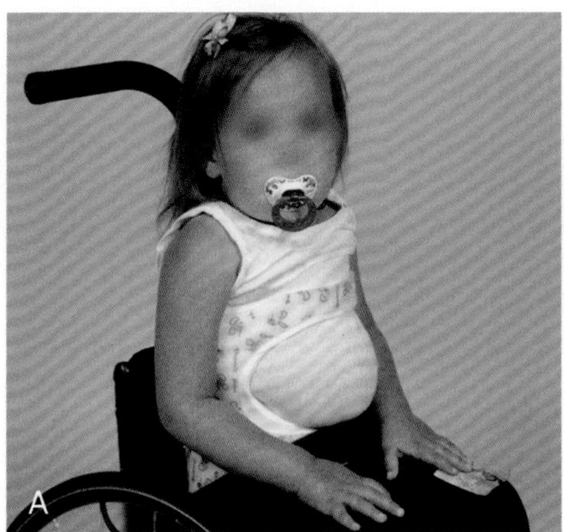
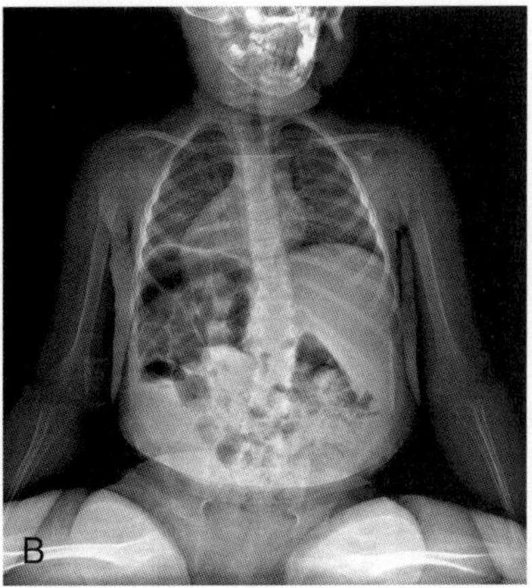
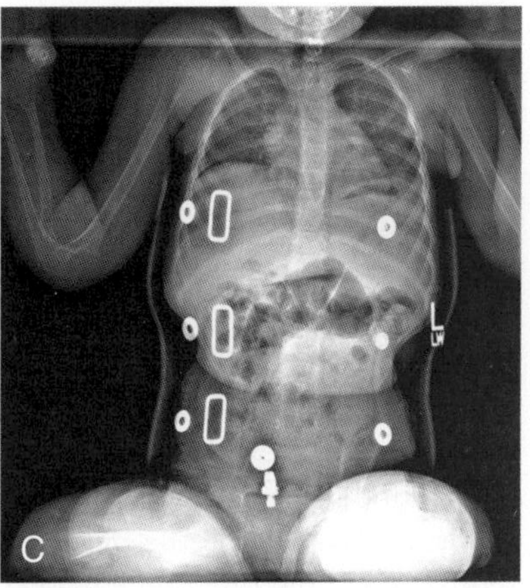

FIGURE 4 A, Photograph of a 2-year-old girl with spinal muscular atrophy wearing a thoracolumbosacral orthosis. The abdomen should be allowed to protrude through the abdominal opening in the orthosis to reduce abdominal compression. B, Radiograph of the girl's spine before bracing treatment shows a Cobb angle of 30°. C, Radiograph after 6 months of brace treatment shows no curvature. (Copyright Shriners Hospitals for Children, Portland, OR.)

can be gradually increased. If there is concern about the effect of the TLSO on respiration, vital capacity can be assessed in and out of the orthosis by a therapist with a handheld spirometer.

Surgical management of a spinal deformity is indicated when the curves can no longer be controlled by the TLSO and cannot be passively corrected to less than 50°. Because patients may be osteopenic and have very small bones, the size of instrumentation is a consideration. In the past, growing rods and the Vertical Expandable Prosthetic Titanium Rib (VEPTR; DePuy Synthes) have been used, but the MAGEC system (Ellipse Technologies), which can be extended without the need for subsequent surgeries, is currently preferred using pedicle screws for fixation. The MAGEC rods are extended in an outpatient clinic by placing an external controller over the rod; incremental extension is produced through a magnetic signal[35,36] (**Figure 5**).

If severe spinal deformity occurs, either in the coronal or sagittal plane, preoperative halo-gravity traction may provide correction to facilitate surgical correction. Attention should be paid to the sagittal plane where severe kyphosis may exist. Once growth is completed with a MAGEC system in place, a decision will have to be made as to whether a definitive fusion is indicated. Some surgeons have chosen to leave the instrumentation in place and perform no additional surgery, unless there is instrument failure, whereas others advocate MAGEC removal and definitive fusion with a pedicle screw construct. When a definitive fusion is done, appropriate lumbar levels must be left unfused to allow spinal access for intrathecal medication administration. Patients who

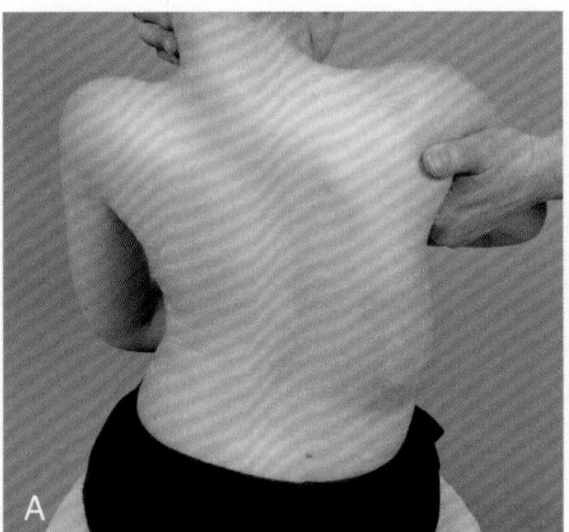
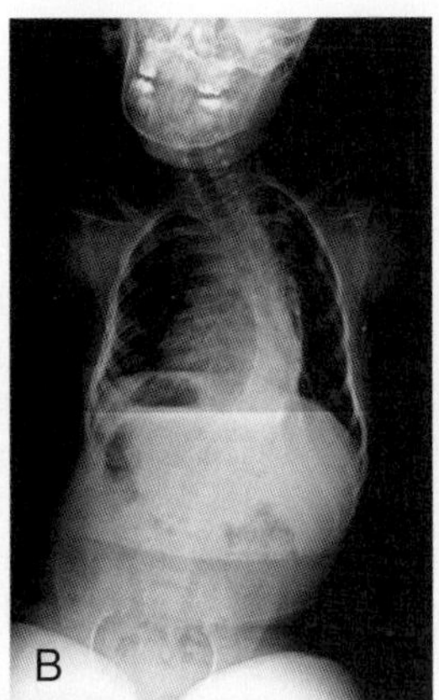
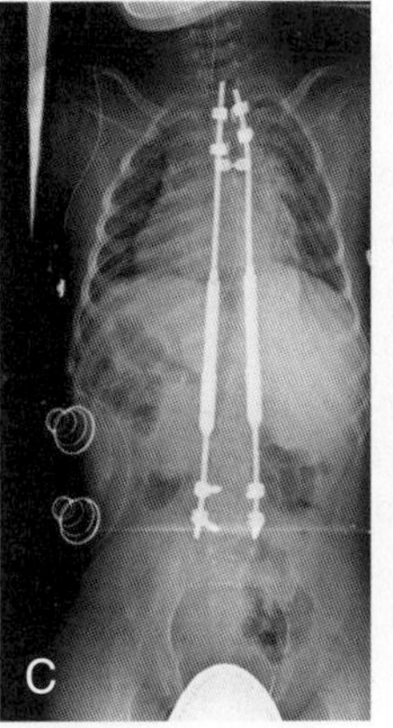
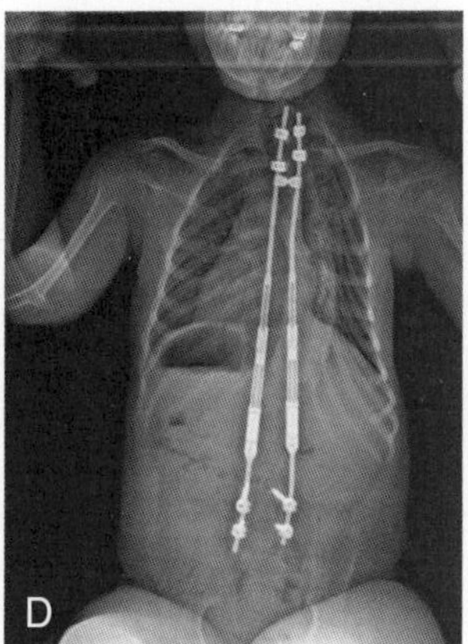

FIGURE 5 Images of a patient with spinal muscular atrophy and scoliosis. A, Clinical photograph of the child's spine before surgery. B, Preoperative radiograph shows a 70° Cobb angle. C, Radiograph immediately after the surgical insertion of a MAGEC rod shows a Cobb angle of 43°. D, Radiograph at the 18-month follow-up shows a Cobb angle of 40°. (Courtesy of Charles R. D'Amato, MD, Portland, OR and copyright Shriners Hospitals for Children, Portland, OR.)

have had a previous fusion to include the lumbar spine may require a procedure to allow access for intrathecal medication administration with fat implantation to prevent bony ingrowth.

Physical and Occupational Therapy and Adaptive Equipment

As the disease progresses, there is a concomitant process of normal growth and development and organization of motor skills as the child ages, which is modified by progressive muscle weakness. Because these two processes occur simultaneously, the progression of the disease will eventually overcome the developmental acquisition of motor skills, and function will begin to decline. Children who are more severely affected may have difficulty sitting and maintaining head support, so having an appropriate adaptive seat with a headrest is beneficial for environment interaction and feeding. Although a seating device will not prevent scoliosis, lateral pad stabilizers help keep the trunk and head centered and allow for better function. A powered wheelchair should be provided for nonambulatory children by the age of 2 years to allow independent mobility. As children age, special controls may be needed for their wheelchairs, depending on the child's level of weakness. Wheelchairs should be equipped with a tilt-in-space function and an attachment for a tablet or computer for schoolwork and/or communication.

For patients who are unable to stand independently, standing devices that control the lower extremities and trunk may provide supported standing. Standing has psychological and physical benefits, particularly in younger children with SMA who have reasonable trunk control. A one-piece custom-molded KAFO with no knee articulation may make it easier for a patient to be placed in the standing position. If reasonable knee stability can be obtained without a KAFO, a custom-molded rigid AFO will also facilitate the ability to stand. Regardless of the child's ambulatory status, if Achilles tightness (<10° of dorsiflexion) begins to develop, custom AFOs should be provided and used full time to slow the progression of foot deformity, and will provide stability for standing.

Strength training may be useful in patients with SMA, and resistance strength training has been shown to improve strength and motor function in children with SMA type 2 and SMA type 3.[37] As in other pediatric disabling conditions, adaptive recreation is very important to the well-being of affected children because most of these patients do not have recreational and social outlets. Many patients with SMA seem to enjoy swimming because it allows movement and limb use.

Other Systemic Problems

Cardiac problems are not associated with SMA, and patients have normal intelligence. Eating becomes difficult because of chewing and swallowing difficulty. As the disease progresses, maintaining an adequate caloric intake may be problematic, so a gastrostomy may be necessary. However, it can be difficult to ascertain whether patients are actually undernourished. The standard body mass index is not relevant in these patients because of diminished muscle mass in the limbs.

Occasionally, patients may experience a metabolic crisis with tachycardia and hypotension after a mild systemic illness or if they become dehydrated. If the patient has metabolic acidosis and hypoglycemia, a rapid intervention with rehydration and correction of hypoglycemia and acidosis should be done in a hospital to allow careful monitoring. Because this problem is prone to recurrence, arrangements should be made to allow rapid hospitalization when early symptoms occur. It has been suggested that the reduced muscle mass in these patients may be a contributing factor.[31] Gastrostomy may be indicated to prevent dehydration and allow rapid home hydration if repeated episodes occur.

Pulmonary function is a major issue as muscle weakness progresses. Patients should be followed up by a pediatric pulmonary specialist on a regular basis, including sleep studies when indicated. Bilevel positive airway pressure ventilation support during sleep will eventually be indicated. When pulmonary function begins to decline, patients should be provided with a CoughAssist device, which should be used on a regular basis (and even more often at the first sign of a respiratory infection). As respiratory function declines, assisted ventilation via a face mask may be required for portions of the day as well as at night, and this will eventually lead to full-time assisted ventilation. In late stages of the disease, a tracheostomy for full-time ventilator support may be chosen by the patient and family, although this is a difficult decision because the patient at this point is very disabled and requires full-time care.

Medical Treatment

Exciting and innovative developments have occurred in the field of medical therapy for SMA with the introduction of certain drugs, which increase the cellular production of SMN protein. Two new medications have been approved by the FDA after extensive clinical testing. The first, nusinersen (Spinraza), uses an antisense oligonucleotide that blocks the abnormal sequence that causes skipping of exon 7 in the *SMN2* gene, thereby allowing the *SMN2* gene to synthesize a full-length SMN protein. In clinical trials of infants with SMA type 1 younger than 1 year treated with this therapy, maintenance of motor function and development of motor milestones have been achieved. Based on the natural history of the disease, untreated patients would be expected to deteriorate quite rapidly, and 90% are either on assisted ventilation or die by age 2 years. Multiple studies of this therapy are ongoing, including a study of presymptomatic infants with genetically confirmed SMA, as well as older patients with milder forms of SMA.[38] Older patients report an increase in strength providing increased function.

Intrathecal injection of the medication with the antisense oligonucleotide attached to a ligand allows it to be taken into the anterior horn cell. Increased circulating levels of SMN protein occur, and instead of deterioration in young children, there is progressive development of motor function with continuing treatment. Treatment will preserve neurons, but because neurons do not regenerate, those that have been lost are not replaced. Therefore, early treatment, including in babies or children in whom a diagnosis was made through screening but who are not yet showing any signs of disease, is essential. Intrathecal injections are given six times during the first year of treatment, and four times a year thereafter at a cost (for the drug alone) of $125,000 per dose. Although expensive, the results are dramatic, and thus far persistent as long as the medication is continued.[39] This medication, known as Spinraza, is FDA approved and is covered by most insurance companies in the United States, but in some European countries the expense is prohibitive, and the drug is not offered, although the company does provide free treatment to a limited number of patients through a lottery program.

In addition, there is an orally administered drug, risdiplam, which has a similar mode of action as Spinraza, has completed clinical trials, and was approved in the summer of 2020. There have been no direct comparison trials of these two drugs, so parents with children on intrathecal Spinraza will be faced with a difficult decision as to whether switch their children to the oral medication.

A second treatment approach inserts a full-length *SMN1* gene using an adeno-associated viral vector AAV9, known as Zolgensma. This treatment is administered intravenously only one time since the inserted gene is incorporated into the genome of the neuron and other cells, and therefore should be immortalized. Infants treated within a short time of disease onset have shown significant resolution of weakness and reestablishment of close to normal development, depending on how much function has been lost before institution of treatment.[40] In the children who have been treated, it has been noted that the earlier the treatment is instituted after a diagnosis of SMA, the more effective the therapy has been. Children may have a fever and transient elevation of liver enzymes after drug administration due to the viral vector, as well as reduction in platelet count, and are treated with a course of corticosteroid. The cost of this medication, which is FDA approved at this point for children younger than 2 years, is $2.1 million, which makes it the most expensive drug on the market, but presumably one injection will be sufficient for life. Older children are not eligible because the dose of drug is adjusted by body weight, and concomitant viral load may be too great with systemic administration, and older children may have developed antibodies to the vector. Intrathecal administration may be possible in the future for older children.[41]

It is possible that in addition to these dramatically effective medications, administration of other agents, such as antimyostatin antibodies to increase muscle regeneration, and agents to improve the efficiency of neuronal function, may further potentiate the treatment effects.

These developments are very exciting and, when combined with newborn (or possibly carrier) screening, will allow treatment to be started early, before neurons are lost, and will totally change the lives of patients with SMA. Although these treatments provide tremendous reduction in morbidity of SMA, they are not likely to be a total cure, and patients may still have some deficits. The patterns of weakness of treated children may be different, and orthopaedic interventions, as described previously, may still be necessary and will be based on individual patient need. However, these new medical treatments lead to many questions for the orthopaedic treatment, such as whether hip dysplasia will occur in fully treated patients and if it does, whether surgical intervention for hip dysplasia should be undertaken. Similarly, will spinal deformity occur, and if so, should early bracing treatment be instituted to delay curve progression? These critical questions will be answered with time, but until then careful assessments will need to be done, and hopefully multicenter studies will reveal useful information on the altered natural history, and indications for interventions will be developed. Furthermore, until newborn screening is fully implemented, and rapid early treatment instituted, there will continue to be partially treated patients for whom concrete guidelines will be difficult to set.

Positive results also have been reported in animal studies using the DNA editing enzyme CRISPR-Cas9, which can alter the DNA of experimental animals that manifest the genetic defect of SMA. The earlier after birth the therapy is initiated, the more likely is a positive response. In a 2020 study, mice with a severe form of SMA that were expected to die within 2 weeks have survived for more than 1 year and have exhibited few deficits using this approach.[42]

CONGENITAL MYOTONIC DYSTROPHY

Myotonic dystrophy is a muscle disease that causes weakness, primarily distally, and is associated with myotonia, which is the inability of muscles to relax after a strong contraction (particularly in the hands). The milder adult-onset form of this disease is the most prevalent progressive neuromuscular disease in adults. A severe form of the disease that affects children, known as CDM, has an incidence of 2/100,000 live births. Newborn infants exhibit weakness, which may be profound, and in some cases require ventilator support from the time of delivery; however, improvement occurs in the first year of life, and most infants are able to be weaned from the ventilator but is followed by a slow loss of strength, primarily distally, beginning during the teenage years. CDM is also characterized by delayed motor development, cognitive impairment, potentially lethal cardiac issues in adulthood, and a very typical facial appearance (**Figure 6**).

CDM is classified as type I or type II based on the underlying genetic defect. Because type I myotonic dystrophy accounts for 95% of the patients with the disease, only type I disease is discussed here.

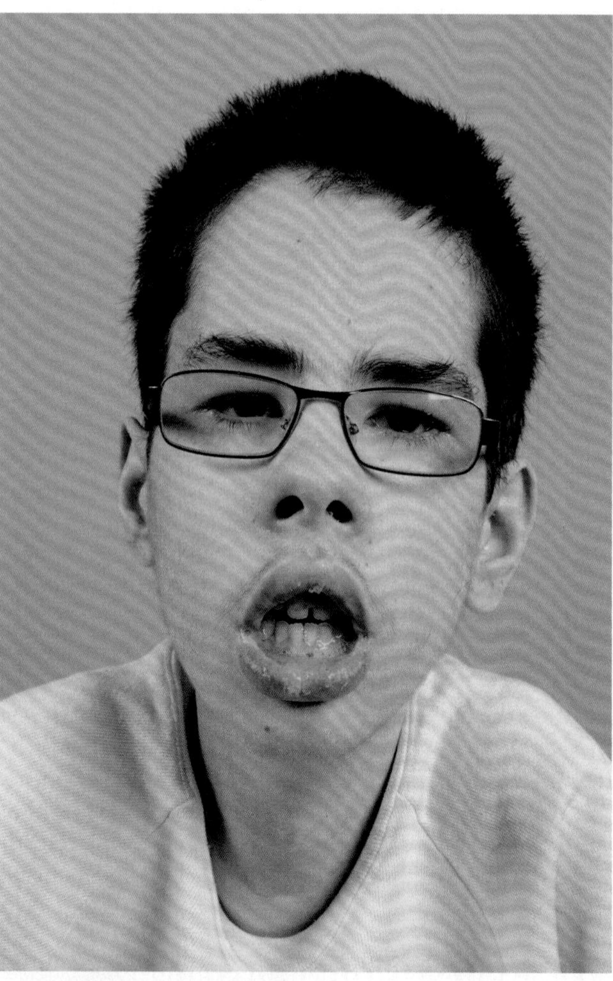

FIGURE 6 Clinical photograph of a patient with congenital myotonic dystrophy shows the typical facial appearance with a head that is elongated and narrowed in the coronal plane and a tented upper lip. (Copyright Shriners Hospitals for Children, Portland, OR.)

Genetics

CDM is inherited in an autosomal dominant fashion and has some interesting genetic characteristics. When the male parent is affected and the child receives the abnormal gene from the father, the child usually has the same degree of disease severity as the father. However, when the mother is affected, even with mild unrecognized disease, the child may be severely affected and require immediate, full-time ventilator support. The disease is caused by an expansion of a CTG trinucleotide sequence on chromosome 9 near the *MPK* gene, and the severity of disease is proportional to the number of trinucleotide repeat sequences, which increase during oogenesis but not spermatogenesis.

The classification is based on the clinical picture, and the limits are approximate. This trinucleotide insertion results in the synthesis of an elongated and toxic messenger RNA that accumulates in the cells. The normal *MPK* gene alters the function of RNA-binding proteins. Other adjacent genes also may be affected, which explains the early onset of cataracts seen in this disease.

Natural History and Orthopaedic Treatment

Newborns with CDM may have profound weakness and require intubation and full-time ventilator support to survive. However, during the first few months of life, infants gain strength and are usually able to be weaned from the ventilator by the time they are a few weeks to a few months old. Over the next few years, generalized muscle strength increases, and most affected children become strong enough to stand and walk by age 5 years (at the latest) if foot deformities are not present. Some children are strong enough to stand but are unable to stand independently because of contracture of the Achilles tendon or fully developed talipes equinovarus. The Achilles tendon tightness should be surgically corrected with TAL to achieve a plantigrade foot to facilitate standing and walking. After surgery, patients should begin standing in short leg casts on the first postoperative day. This cast treatment is continued for 4 weeks, then followed by the use of a custom-molded AFO, which will be needed for standing and walking. If a patient develops sufficient strength and balance, the AFOs may be discontinued; however, the AFO should be worn at nighttime to prevent contracture recurrence.

In a study of 30 children and adolescents with CDM treated at the Muscular Dystrophy Association clinic at the Shriners Hospital for Children in Portland, Oregon, the mean age of ambulation was 30 months and the latest age was 5 years, with the exception of 1 of the 30 patients who was unable to walk.[43] Seventy percent of the patients (22 of 30) required orthopaedic surgery during the study period. Ten patients had one surgical procedure, eight patients had two surgical procedures, and four patients had three or more surgical procedures. These procedures involved the lower extremities and spine; no upper extremity surgery was indicated. None of the patients had hip subluxation, dislocation, or fixed adduction; however, two patients had unilateral abduction contractures that interfered with standing and walking. These patients had a good response to abductor release consisting of an Ober-Yount bipolar release of the tensor fascia femoris, wherein the anterior portion of the gluteus medius and the tensor fascia femoris were released and stripped from the iliac crest. In addition, tenotomy of the proximal iliotibial band in the upper thigh just below the insertion of the tensor fascia femoris muscle was performed. One patient had knee flexion contracture, which was treated by distal femoral extension osteotomy. Five patients had congenital clubfoot, and all of these patients underwent surgery before referral to the clinic. None of the patients were treated with the Ponseti method; however, this would be the currently preferred method. Five patients had TAL only to correct rigid equinus, which interfered with standing. Serial casting was not attempted, but possibly could be successful. Most of these patients were unable to stand independently or walk before the lengthening procedure, but rapidly gained ambulation skills after the procedure. Other surgeries included rotational osteotomies of the tibia or femur, subtalar or triple arthrodesis for severe planovalgus deformity, and correction of miscellaneous toe deformities.

Spinal deformities, including midthoracic to upper thoracic kyphosis and scoliosis, occurred in approximately 30% of patients and frequently were seen in the first decade of life.[43] Spinal bracing treatment was attempted in most of the patients, but it is not clear that bracing treatment was helpful, although it may have slowed curve progression. Surgical correction was done in three patients in this series and can be done safely and successfully. The guidelines for kyphosis surgery have not been well established. Some patients seem to tolerate the kyphosis well during childhood and adolescence, but stand with compensatory excessive cervical lordosis to maintain an upright head, as well as increased lumbar lordosis to maintain sagittal balance.[43] A 2013 study reported similar findings.[44]

Gross motor skills and strength continue to improve over the first decade of life. However, toward the end of the second decade of life, hand weakness and myotonia begin to develop.

Other Systemic Issues

Cognitive delay occurs in most patients and generally parallels the severity of the motor impairment, which is secondary to the number of trinucleotide repeat sequences present in the gene. Patients also have a typical myopathic facial appearance, with the head elongated and narrowed in the coronal plane and a tented upper lip (**Figure 6**). Because the facial appearance is so characteristic of the disease, a diagnosis can be strongly suspected based only on facial appearance. The speech of these patients also has a very nasal tone.

Even with mild involvement, patients have a high sensitivity to opiates and may experience excessive and prolonged sedation, including profound respiratory depression, after administration. Opiates should be avoided or used sparingly. If administered, close monitoring of the patient is required. In some patients with mild degrees of involvement, a diagnosis of CDM is made only after a surgical procedure in which opiates are administered. These patients may require full-time ventilator assistance for several days.

Cardiac involvement includes arrhythmia or conduction disturbances, which can progress to ventricular fibrillation that leads to sudden death in a substantial number of adult affected individuals. Cardiac problems usually are seen beginning in the third decade of life and thereafter. Arrhythmia can be assessed with 24-hour Holter monitoring. Simple electrocardiography and echo examinations are insufficient for assessing arrhythmia. Cardiac arrhythmia also may occur in parents with milder degrees of involvement, so parents should be counseled to have their cardiac status assessed on a regular basis. If evidence of rhythm problems is found, insertion of a demand pacemaker reduces the risk of sudden cardiac death. Hypertrophic cardiomyopathy also may be a problem.[45]

Feeding may be a problem, particularly in infants, who may require a gastrostomy; however, most patients acquire the ability to eat and graduate to oral feeding. Constipation remains a lifetime problem because of bowel dysmotility. Other systemic problems include cataracts, premature male-pattern baldness, insulin resistance, hypersomnolence, and sterility in males.[46]

In a study of 150 parents of children with CDM who were surveyed regarding the biggest issues for their children, the most frequently reported symptomatic themes were issues of communication (82%) and problems with the hands and fingers (80%). Other important issues involved fatigue (77%), cardiac disorders (24%), and anesthesia-associated problems (24%).[47]

Medical Treatment

Because CDM is caused by an elongated trinucleotide segment known as DMPK, it potentially is amenable to treatment with antisense oligonucleotides such as those being investigated in patients with DMD and SMA. A clinical trial was done for a drug called Ionis-dmpk.2.5_{Rx} (Ionis Pharmaceuticals), but the drug was subsequently withdrawn from further development.

CHARCOT-MARIE-TOOTH DISEASE

CMT is a group of more than 60 hereditary motor-sensory neuropathies, which are distinguished by different underlying gene defects and clinical manifestations.[48]

As in most neuropathies, there is initial distal weakness, which manifests in the foot and ankle usually during the second decade, as foot deformity caused by muscle weakness and imbalance, leading to contracture, with later involvement of the of the hands. In addition, an increased incidence of both scoliosis and hip dysplasia has been associated with CMT. Except in patients with unusually severe involvement, independent ambulation continues into adulthood; however, treatment may be needed to prevent the development of severe foot deformities that could affect the ability to ambulate. Deep tendon reflexes are absent. Patients also may have sensory deficits, including a proprioceptive deficit leading to a positive Romberg test. Some patients may experience dysesthesia, particularly in the feet, and this condition may be exacerbated after foot surgery and manifest similar to complex regional pain syndrome, and this may be their major complaint. Other abnormalities, such as optic atrophy and hearing loss, may accompany the primary condition and may help distinguish the specific genetic subtype, but the specific diagnosis is ascertained by genetic testing.

Classification and Diagnosis

CMT is separated into four broad groups on the basis of nerve electrodiagnostic studies, inheritance pattern, and the specific genetic mutation.[49] In general, the diagnostic strategy should be to classify the condition based on the inheritance pattern and electrodiagnostic studies, and then focus is on the specific genetic mutations for testing. Panels that assess multiple gene candidates are available to provide accurate diagnosis. However, genetic testing may be expensive and not covered by insurance providers. Nerve biopsy is not indicated for diagnosing this condition. Identification of the specific type of CMT disease is important for determining a prognosis, potential interventions as they become available, associated problems, and accurate genetic counseling. Identification of the specific gene abnormality will become essential when gene-based therapies are developed. Ninety percent of CMT patients will have a positive family history. CMT is relatively common, and the prevalence in a Norwegian population is 1 in 1, 214.

CMT type 1 disease comprises five subtypes (1A through 1E), all of which are autosomal dominant and characterized by decreased motor and sensory nerve conduction velocity (<50 m/s). The basis of the disease in CMT type 1 is demyelination of nerve axons. Large myelinated sensory nerves are also affected, which may explain the symptoms of pain and dysesthesia in some patients. Seventy percent of all patients with CMT disease have CMT type 1 disease, and 70% of type 1 patients have type 1A; therefore 50% of all CMT patients are type 1A.

CMT type 2 disease is autosomal dominant and includes 18 subtypes. CMT type 2 is distinguished by normal or slightly slowed motor nerve conduction velocity and a substantial decrease in the amplitude of the compound motor action potential. This type of CMT disease is caused by neuronal/axonal abnormalities.

CMT type X is the X-linked form of the disease, and CMT type X1 accounts for 10% of the overall cases of CMT. In this form, which is also called intermediate-type CMT, there is mild slowing of the motor nerve conduction.

CMT type 4 includes 11 autosomal recessive forms, some of which are associated with severe generalized involvement that results in loss of ambulation in the first or second decade of life.

Orthopaedic Treatment

CMT type 1A is the type of CMT disease most frequently seen by pediatric orthopaedic surgeons because the onset of foot deformity usually occurs in the early to middle part of the second decade of life. CMT type 1A accounts for approximately 50% of all patients with the diagnosis of CMT disease. The genetic defect in this type of CMT is a complete duplication of *PMP-22* gene on chromosome 17, and an accurate genetic test is available. Because it has not been demonstrated that genetic confirmation will influence treatment, genetic testing may not be covered by insurance providers. Some variability exists in the expressivity and severity of progression even within families, presumably resulting from the modification of the basic abnormality by other genes. Hand weakness, which begins with an intrinsic minus pattern, may occur, but it usually is not clinically important until the third decade of life in CMT 1A, but may occur earlier in other types of CMT. An occupational therapist may provide adaptive devices, such as pencil grips, special utensils, and computer devices to facilitate schoolwork. Voice-recognition software for dictation also may be indicated for some patients with more severe hand involvement.

The major musculoskeletal deformity associated with CMT type 1A in the teenage years is foot deformity. In the first decade of life, patients may have flexible, flat feet, and some present with toe walking. Subsequently, cavus posturing of the foot develops and progresses to a cavovarus deformity. Manual muscle testing demonstrates weakness of eversion as the first finding, which may precede the development of the cavovarus deformity. An early synonym of CMT was peroneal muscular atrophy.

Cavus deformity can be radiographically measured on standing lateral radiographs of the feet by measuring the Meary angle, which is the angle between the longitudinal axis of the talus and the long axis of the first metatarsal. This measurement may be difficult to obtain in some patients because the first metatarsal may be difficult to distinguish, but generally it is the shortest and broadest of the metatarsals. In milder deformities, the Meary angle is probably reasonably accurate, but in feet with more severe deformity, particularly forefoot adduction, a great deal of variation in measurements of the Meary angle may occur depending on whether the X-ray beam is aligned perpendicular to the forefoot or perpendicular to the hindfoot. In some instance, two lateral views (one aligned to the midfoot and one aligned to the hindfoot) should be obtained to allow better assessment of the deformity. The calcaneal pitch also is increased in patients with CMT type 1A, indicating an elongated Achilles tendon allowing the calcaneus to go into dorsiflexion. Although the foot clinically appears to be in equinus, radiographs will demonstrate that the foot is not in equinus. The appearance of equinus when looking at the foot is actually a manifestation of the cavus deformity, with flexion of the midfoot on the hindfoot with associated dorsiflexion of the calcaneus, which is seen radiographically as increased calcaneal pitch. The Achilles tendon is actually elongated, so it is important not to confuse this cavus with equinus, because lengthening of the Achilles tendon will potentially aggravate the deformity and weaken the triceps surae.[50] As the disease progresses, hindfoot varus increases, and clinical evidence of excessive weight bearing can be seen on the lateral side of the midfoot and forefoot as manifested by callosities, which develop at the head of the first metatarsal, which becomes plantarflexed, and the head and base of the fifth metatarsal. This is also nicely demonstrated on foot pressure studies.

Although the deformities are initially dynamic and relatively flexible, over time they become more fixed. Flexibility can be assessed by evaluating subtalar motion with the patient prone and the hip and the knee flexed to 90° so that the hindfoot varus can be observed.

Studies of foot pressure (pedobarographs) using a dynamic foot pressure measurement system are helpful in monitoring the progression of the foot deformity and will initially show increased pressure at the fifth metatarsal head, and as the disease progresses, concentrated pressure is also seen at the base of the fifth metatarsal. Manual muscle testing will show weak peroneal muscles, whereas the posterior tibial, toe flexors, extensors, and anterior tibial tendons maintain good strength. Although the literature has suggested that the tibialis anterior muscle is weak, this assumption may be incorrect, because testing for active dorsiflexion often demonstrates a strong anterior tibial tendon by palpation during active dorsiflexion. As a manifestation of this weakness, and probably in an effort to overcome the equinus positioning of the forefoot, the toe extensors are often overactive during gait, causing the toes to dorsiflex during swing phase to assist in foot clearance. This has the effect of tightening the plantar fascia, which is contiguous with the fascia of the toes, and this tightness further increases the cavus deformity. Toe dorsiflexion during initiation of the swing phase is an early sign of CMT disease.

Treatment

When the Meary angle is greater than 20° and the clinical examination and foot pressure show palpable plantar fascia tightness and cavus, a plantar fascia release, with stripping of the plantar muscles from the calcaneus (Steindler stripping), can be performed. This is done through an incision on the plantarmedial aspect of the foot at the proximal end of the arch. The skin and fibrofatty tissue are incised down to the fascia, which is then exposed by sweeping attached tissue off the thick fascia with a Cobb elevator; the plantar fascia is then completely incised from lateral to medial. The short plantar muscles are then teased off the calcaneus with the Cobb elevator, taking care to stay superficial to the deep fascia to avoid injury to the lateral plantar branch of the posterior tibial nerve. Postoperatively, the patient is allowed full weight bearing in a walking boot for 3 weeks; this is followed by nightly wear of AFOs. The AFO should be molded with the foot at 90° of dorsiflexion; amounts greater than 90° should not be attempted because this will lead to discomfort and rejection of the AFO. This approach appears to reduce cavus and slow the progression of the deformity (**Figure 7**).

The deformity, however, will ultimately recur and progress. When this occurs and the heel is clearly in varus but is still passively correctable to or past neutral, a number of procedures are used for rebalancing the muscles. It is preferred to perform the following procedures at a single setting, followed by 6 weeks in a non–weight-bearing short leg cast, and then followed by use of a posterior leaf spring AFO. A plantar fascia release as described previously should be performed, if it has not already been done. It may be useful to mobilize all the transfers first and fix the ankle temporarily in dorsiflexion with a Steinmann pin through the heel up across the ankle joint, before inserting them into the bone. (1) The tibialis anterior tendon is transferred to the lateral cuneiform. The tendon is released from its insertion on the navicular, preserving as much length as possible; brought up to the extensor retinaculum, which may be released 1 to 2 cm; then tunneled subcutaneously to its new location on the lateral cuneiform; and then fixed into the bone with moderate tension and the foot

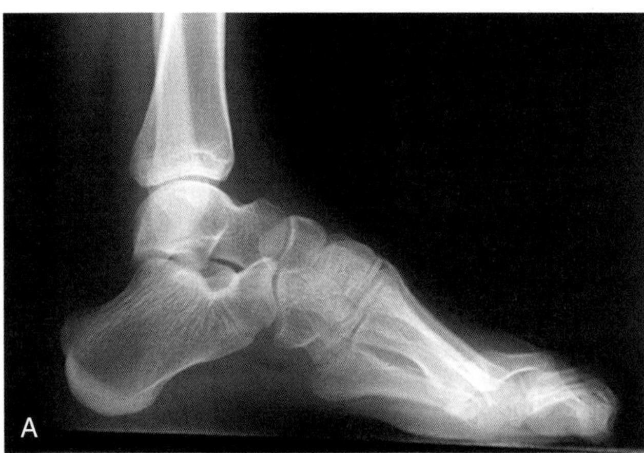

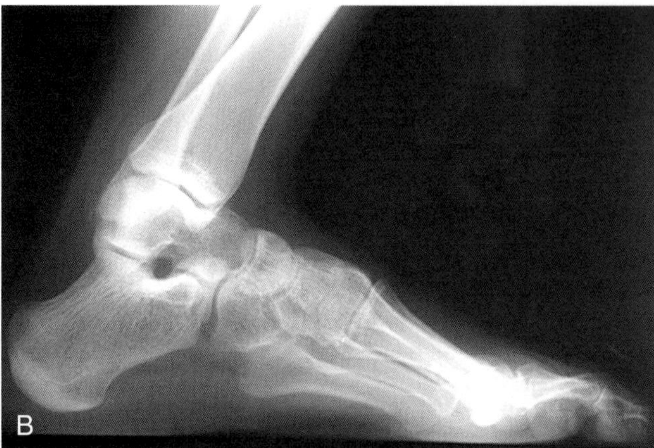

FIGURE 7 Lateral radiographs of the foot of a patient with type 1 Charcot-Marie-Tooth disease before surgery (**A**) and after a plantar fasciotomy, demonstrating a reduction in the Meary angle (**B**). (Copyright Shriners Hospitals for Children, Portland, OR.)

in maximum dorsiflexion, using an interference screw. (2) The toe extensors II through V are transferred as a bundle to the lateral cuneiform using an interference screw for tendon fixation. (3) The tibialis posterior tendon is transferred through the interosseous membrane to the lateral cuneiform using an interference screw for tendon fixation.[51] Once the posterior tibial tendon is detached, the increased mobility of the foot out of varus can be appreciated. If a large amount of varus is present, the tendon will not be long enough to attach into the bone. In these instances, 2 to 3 cm of length can be added by creating a distally based flap of tendon and taking half of the tendon and folding it down. If the tendon is taken off the navicular at the level of the bone, the distal end of the tendon will have a fibrocartilaginous structure; therefore, a distally placed flap of half of the tendon will tend not to separate from the body of the tendon. A suture placed through both sides of the tendon flap will help reinforce and secure it. (4) In addition, a Jones transfer of the extensor hallucis longus to the first metatarsal neck through a drill hole in the metatarsal neck is performed and the tendon is sewn back onto itself.[52] (5) If a Jones transfer is performed, the interphalangeal joint of the great toe should be fused because when the long toe extensor is removed from its insertion on the distal phalanx and transferred to the metatarsal neck, the interphalangeal joint of the great toe will go into flexion. However, in a skeletally immature patient, the surgeon may not want to fuse the interphalangeal joint and instead can perform a tenodesis of the stump of the extensor hallucis longus to the extensor hallucis brevis.[53] (6) If the heel remains in varus after these procedures are performed, a lateral slide of the calcaneal tuberosity with screw fixation can be added.[53] (7) If residual cavus exists, a dorsal closing wedge osteotomy of the first metatarsal also can be performed.[52] If the first metatarsal head remains prominent in the sole because the shaft remains prominent, then a proximal dorsal closing wedge can be done to lift it up. The Jones transfer should not be completed until the osteotomy is done, or it will be flaccid. (8) Transfer of the peroneus longus into the peroneus brevis can be performed to remove the deforming force on the first ray to reduce cavus and supplement the weak eversion strength[52] (**Figure 8**).

The extensor digitorum communis and posterior tibial and anterior tibial transfers should all be inserted into the lateral cuneiform because of its central location in the foot. If the transfer were to be attached into the cuboid, too great of a pronating force may be exerted, and a pronated flatfoot will occur over time. After the surgery, an AFO should be molded and a short leg, non–weight-bearing cast should be worn for 6 weeks. After healing and cast removal, patients should be fitted with a posterior leaf spring AFO. This type of AFO will stabilize the foot and allow some dorsiflexion during the second rocker phase of stance gait. As the disease progresses, the transfers will weaken, and the patient will require an AFO to control foot drop and medial-lateral instability; however, deformity should not recur because the transfers were placed centrally (so as the foot weakens there is no muscle imbalance).

In almost all patients with CMT type 1A, the Achilles tendon should **not** be lengthened, because it is elongated rather than shortened, and lengthening will cause weakness and increase the calcaneal pitch. In rare instances of true equinus, in which equinus of the hindfoot can be radiographically documented, the Achilles tendon should be lengthened.

If the foot deformity is rigid and not passively correctable after release of the posterior tibial tendon, the transfers will be unable to correct the deformity and a Lambrinudi-type triple arthrodesis will be needed to achieve a plantigrade foot (**Figure 9**).

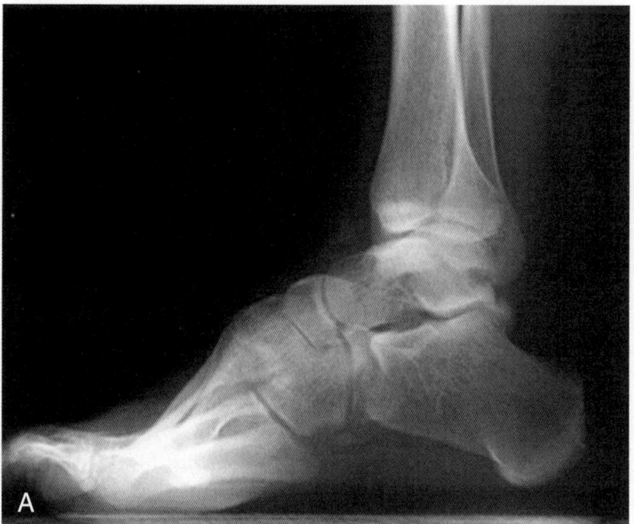

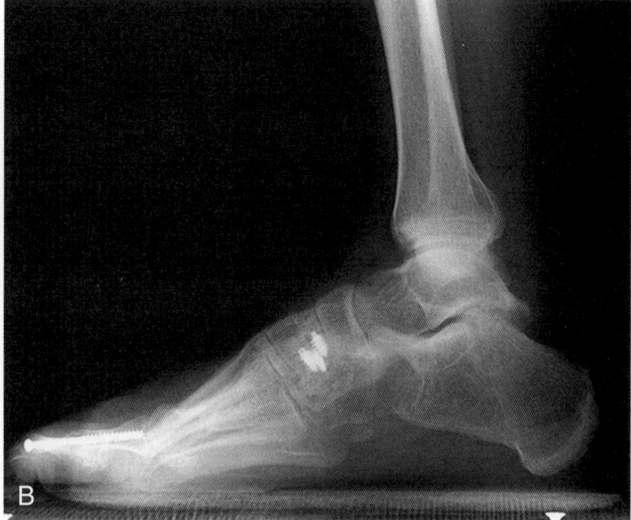

FIGURE 8 Lateral radiographs of the foot of a 17.5-year-old patient with type 1 Charcot-Marie-Tooth disease before surgery (**A**) and after multiple tendon transfers (**B**). (Copyright Shriners Hospitals for Children, Portland, OR.)

Because patients with CMT have protective sensation, pressure sores rarely develop, but a thick callus may develop over pressure points. A molded sole insert can be used to redistribute pressure more evenly. If the foot is plantigrade, most patients will continue to ambulate well into middle age. After middle age, more generalized weakness may develop and the need for assisted mobility will progress. In patients with proprioceptive deficits, an AFO will provide stability.

Although CMT type 2 disease is heterogeneous, in general cavovarus does not develop and hand weakness is more prominent. Frequently, patients will have generalized weakness of all the muscles controlling the foot and ankle, resulting in a flail but plantigrade foot or flatfoot. These patients will benefit from a posterior leaf spring AFO to control footdrop in swing and provide stability in stance. Some subtypes of CMT type 2 disease are associated with severe proprioceptive sensory loss. Affected patients may lose the ability to walk in their second decade of life, but the use of an AFO may be helpful. With other types of CMT disease a variety of foot deformities may develop; however, more proximal deformities of the knee are not seen.

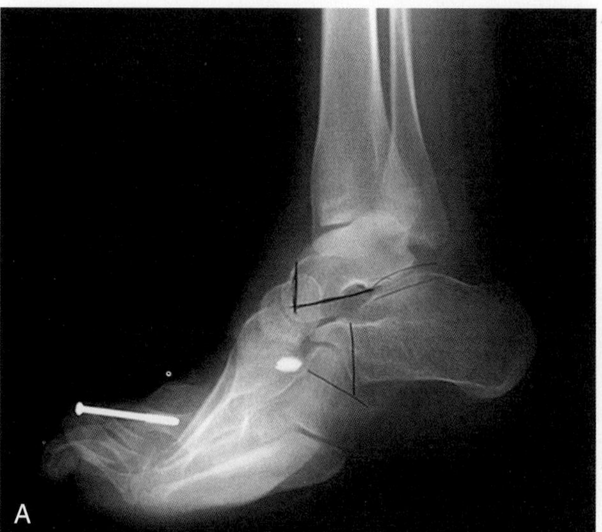

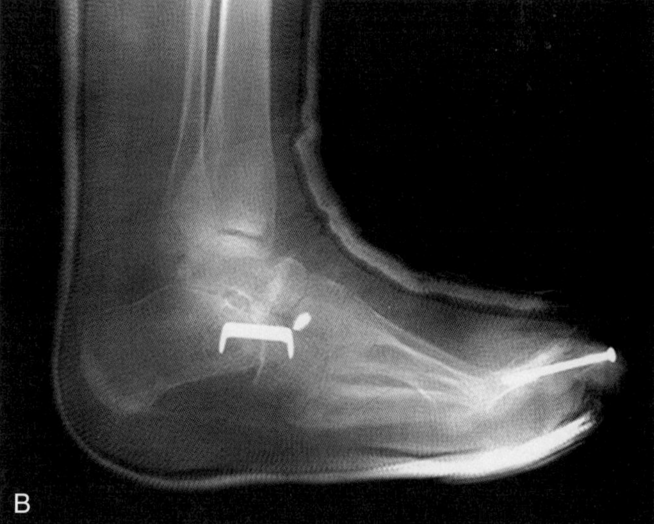

FIGURE 9 **A**, Lateral radiograph of the foot of a patient with Charcot-Marie-Tooth disease with incomplete correction after tendon transfers. **B**, Lateral radiograph of the foot after a Lambrinudi triple arthrodesis. (Copyright Shriners Hospitals for Children, Portland, OR.)

Hip Dysplasia in CMT Disease

Patients with CMT disease are predisposed to the development of acetabular dysplasia with hip subluxation at a much higher rate than the unaffected population. This may lead to degenerative arthritis in adulthood. Dysplasia may become severe, with coxa valga and acetabular dysplasia associated with increased acetabular anteversion, which leads to decreased acetabular containment (**Figure 10**). In a study of 74 patients with CMT, hip radiographs showed hip dysplasia in 6 patients (8%).[54] The age of onset of the dysplasia is unclear. Hip dysplasia during childhood and adolescence is generally asymptomatic, and unless severe cannot be detected on physical examination. Because symptoms do not manifest until degenerative arthritis develops later in life, AP pelvic radiographs for surveillance should be obtained for all patients with CMT. Radiographs should be obtained at the time of the CMT diagnosis and every several years thereafter until skeletal maturity. The cause of this dysplasia is unknown and has not been correlated with any pattern of weakness, and in the case of a family with many affected members, usually affects only one family member. When acetabular dysplasia is severe, surgical correction of the acetabulum and the proximal femur may be required. Good coverage was reported in a group of patients treated with Bernese periacetabular osteotomy.[55]

Scoliosis in CMT Disease

Scoliosis may occur in many types of CMT disease. In a study of 298 patients with CMT disease, scoliosis was radiographically identified in 45 patients.[56] In this study, CMT type 1 was the most prevalent type of disease. In the patients with scoliosis, 18 were females and 27 were males, which is a reversal of the sex ratio seen in idiopathic scoliosis in which more females than males are affected. Twenty-nine of 47 curves were thoracic and 50% of those were left thoracic curves, which also is unusual. Forty-nine percent of the curvatures were associated with increased kyphosis. During the term of the study, curve progression occurred in 70% of the patients. Bracing treatment was attempted in 16 patients but appeared to be successful in only 3 patients. In this group of patients, 14 had posterior spinal instrumentation and fusion without complications. Although intraoperative somatosensory-evoked potential monitoring was attempted in 12 patients, adequate signals were obtained only in 3 patients. Although the age of scoliosis onset was not defined, it is clear that all patients with CMT should have a yearly clinical assessment for scoliosis until skeletal maturity, and radiographic studies should be obtained when indicated. Scoliosis is particularly common in patients with CMT type 4C[49] and is also seen in CMT1A and other subtypes. As with hip dysplasia, cases are sporadic, and usually affect just one member of an affected family. The cause is unknown.

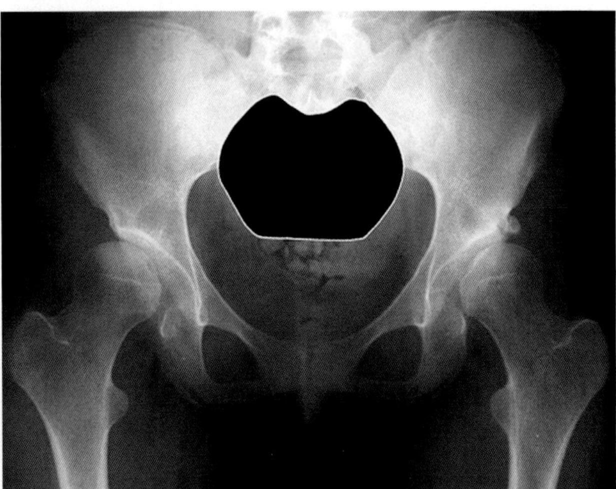

FIGURE 10 Radiograph of the pelvis of a 13-year-old girl with type 1A Charcot-Marie-Tooth disease shows bilateral hip dysplasia. (Copyright Shriners Hospitals for Children, Portland, OR.)

SUMMARY

Children affected by any of the progressive neuromuscular diseases of childhood and adolescence will benefit from care by an orthopaedic surgeon as part of the multidisciplinary team. A predictable set of orthopaedic deformities is associated with each of the neuromuscular diseases. The management of these conditions, which all have a genetic basis, is advancing rapidly. It is hoped that new treatments will ameliorate or eliminate the deterioration associated with these diseases in the future.

KEY STUDY POINTS

- Orthopaedic surgeons should be part of the multidisciplinary clinic team involved in the care of patients with progressive neuromuscular disorders. They are able to recognize evolving deformities and can help to control them (primarily in the lower extremities and spine) with bracing treatment and surgery, when indicated.
- Most of the neuromuscular diseases of childhood associated with weakness are the result of genetic mutations; however, in some instances, the disease may not manifest until later in life. The genetic mutations allow for precise diagnosis by genetically based studies using blood or cheek swabs through DNA analysis.

- The orthopaedic surgeon should be aware of the early clinical signs of DMD to make an early diagnosis, which will allow proper genetic counseling for the family. In addition, this will allow early institution of pharmacologic treatment as newer treatments become available.
- In patients with DMD, progressive weakness, functional loss, and deformity can be delayed, and the need for scoliosis surgery can be reduced, by the pharmacologic daily administration of corticosteroid, although the adverse effects are significant.
- New treatments for DMD and SMA have been developed based on correction of the specific genetic defect. These treatments have totally changed the clinical course and prognosis for patients with SMA and ameliorated the progression of deterioration for boys with DMD.

ANNOTATED REFERENCES

1. Birnkrant DJ, Bushby K, Bann CM, et al: Diagnosis and management of Duchenne muscular dystrophy. Part 2: Respiratory, cardiac, bone health, and orthopaedic management. *Lancet Neurol* 2018;17(4):347-361.

   Updated guidelines from an international group based on literature and expert opinion for all aspects of care of patients with DMD are provided. Level of evidence: V.

2. Birnkrant DJ, Bushby K, Bann CM, et al: Diagnosis and management of Duchenne muscular dystrophy. Part 1: Diagnosis, and neuromuscular, rehabilitation, endocrine, and gastrointestinal and nutritional management. *Lancet Neurol* 2018;17(3):251-267.

   Updated guidelines are provided. Level of evidence: V.

3. Birnkrant DJ, Bushby K, Bann CM, et al: Diagnosis and management of Duchenne muscular dystrophy. Part 3: Primary care, emergency management, psychosocial care, and transitions of care across the lifespan. *Lancet Neurol* 2018;17(5):445-455.

   Updated guidelines are provided. Level of evidence: V.

4. Marshall PD, Galasko CS: No improvement in delay in diagnosis of Duchenne muscular dystrophy. *Lancet* 1995;345(8949):590-591.
5. Case LE, Apkon SD, Eagle M, et al: Rehabilitation management of the patient with Duchenne muscular dystrophy. *Pediatrics* 2018;142(Suppl 2):S17-S33.
6. Heberer K, Fowler E, Staudt L, et al: Hip kinetics during gait are clinically meaningful outcomes in young boys with Duchenne muscular dystrophy. *Gait Posture* 2016;48:159-164.

   This gait laboratory study demonstrated the early loss of hip extensor moment and power, which was normalized after administration of corticosteroid. Level of evidence: I.

7. Alexander WM, Smith M, Freeman BJ, Sutherland LM, Kennedy JD, Cundy PJ: The effect of posterior spinal fusion on respiratory function in Duchenne muscular dystrophy. *Eur Spine J* 2013;22(2):411-416.
8. Duboc D, Meune C, Pierre B, et al: Perindopril preventive treatment on mortality in Duchenne muscular dystrophy: 10 years' follow-up. *Am Heart J* 2007;154(3):596-602.
9. Biggar WD, Harris VA, Eliasoph L, Alman B: Long-term benefits of deflazacort treatment for boys with Duchenne muscular dystrophy in their second decade. *Neuromuscul Disord* 2006;16(4):249-255.
10. Lebel DE, Corston JA, McAdam LC, Biggar WD, Alman BA: Glucocorticoid treatment for the prevention of scoliosis in children with Duchenne muscular dystrophy: Long-term follow-up. *J Bone Joint Surg Am* 2013;95(12):1057-1061.
11. Sbrocchi A, Rauch F, Jacob P, et al: The use of intravenous bisphosphonate therapy to treat vertebral fractures due to osteoporosis among boys with Duchenne muscular dystrophy. *Osteoporos Int* 2012;23(11):2703-2711.
12. Sienko S, Buckon C, Fowler E, et al: Prednisone and deflazacort in Duchenne muscular dystrophy: Do they play a different role in child behavior and perceived quality of life? *PLoS Curr* 2016;8. doi:10.1371/currents.md.7628d9c014bfa29f821a5cd19723bbaa.

    An assessment using standardized behavior measures of boys with DMD and their families showed an increase in aggressive behavior in patients taking prednisone and an increase in depression in those taking deflazacort. Level of evidence: I.

13. Apkon SD, Alman B, Birnkrant DJ, et al: Orthopedic and surgical management of the patient with Duchenne muscular dystrophy. *Pediatrics* 2018;142(suppl 2):S82-S89.

    This article provides orthopaedic guidelines for care of patients with Duchenne muscular dystrophy. Level of evidence: V.

14. Proske U, Morgan DL: Muscle damage from eccentric exercise: Mechanism, mechanical signs, adaptation and clinical applications. *J Physiol* 2001;537(pt 2):333-345.
15. Sussman MD: Advantage of early spinal stabilization and fusion in patients with Duchenne muscular dystrophy. *J Pediatr Orthop* 1984;4(5):532-537.
16. Roberto R, Fritz A, Hagar Y, et al: The natural history of cardiac and pulmonary function decline in patients with Duchenne muscular dystrophy. *Spine (Phila Pa 1976)* 2011;36(15):E1009-E1017.
17. Chua K, Tan CY, Chen Z, et al: Long-term follow-up of pulmonary function and scoliosis in patients with Duchenne's muscular dystrophy and spinal muscular atrophy. *J Pediatr Orthop* 2016;36(1):63-69.

    The authors reported a substantial decline in the loss of pulmonary function in patients with DMD and in those with SMA after spinal fusion. Level of evidence: III.

18. Takaso M, Nakazawa T, Imura T, et al: Surgical management of severe scoliosis with high risk pulmonary dysfunction in Duchenne muscular dystrophy: Patient function, quality of life and satisfaction. *Int Orthop* 2010;34(5):695-702.
19. Cheuk DK, Wong V, Wraige E, Baxter P, Cole A: Surgery for scoliosis in Duchenne muscular dystrophy. *Cochrane Database Syst Rev* 2015;(10):CD005375.

20. Suk KS, Baek JH, Park JO, et al: Postoperative quality of life in patients with progressive neuromuscular scoliosis and their parents. *Spine J* 2015;15(3):446-453.

21. Larson CM, Henderson RC: Bone mineral density and fractures in boys with Duchenne muscular dystrophy. *J Pediatr Orthop* 2000;20(1):71-74.

22. Joseph S, Wang C, Bushby K, et al: Fractures and linear growth in a nationwide cohort of boys with Duchenne muscular dystrophy with and without glucocorticoid treatment: Results from the UK NorthStar database. *JAMA Neurol* 2019;76(6):701-709.

    The authors have documented decreased linear growth and increased fracture rate in DMD boys treated with corticosteroid. Level of evidence: III.

23. Joseph S, Wang C, Di Marco M, et al: Fractures and bone health monitoring in boys with Duchenne muscular dystrophy managed within the Scottish Muscle Network. *Neuromuscul Disord* 2019;29(1):59-66.

    Further documentation of increased fracture rate in DMD boys treated with corticosteroid has been done in this article. Level of evidence: III.

24. Singh A, Schaeffer EK, Reilly CW: Vertebral fractures in Duchenne muscular dystrophy patients managed with deflazacort. *J Pediatr Orthop* 2018;38(6):320-324.

    The incidence of VCFs increases with age and time on deflazacort in boys with DMD. Level of evidence: III.

25. Wong SC, Straub V, Ward LM, Quinlivan R, on behalf of the 236th ENMC Workshop Participants: 236th ENMC International Workshop, Hoofddorp, The Netherlands, 1-3 June 2018. Bone protective therapy in Duchenne muscular dystrophy: Determining the feasibility and standards of clinical trials. *Neuromuscul Disord* 2019;29(3):251-259.

    Strategies to prevent bone loss in DMD are discussed. Level of evidence: V.

26. Hayes J, Veyckemans F, Bissonnette B: Duchenne muscular dystrophy: An old anesthesia problem revisited. *Paediatr Anaesth* 2008;18(2):100-106.

27. Khan N, Eliopoulos H, Han L, et al: Eteplirsen treatment attenuates respiratory decline in ambulatory and non-ambulatory patients with Duchenne muscular dystrophy. *J Neuromuscul Dis* 2019;6(2):213-225.

    Use of the first antisense oligonucleotide slows the loss of vital capacity in boys with DMD. Level of evidence: I.

28. Mendell JR, Goemans N, Lowes LP, et al: Longitudinal effect of eteplirsen versus historical control on ambulation in Duchenne muscular dystrophy. *Ann Neurol* 2016;79(2):257-271.

    This is the first demonstration of clinical efficacy of an antisense oligonucleotide in treatment of DMD in 12 patients. Level of evidence: III.

29. Ousterout DG, Kabadi AM, Thakore PI, Majoros WH, Reddy TE, Gersbach CA: Multiplex CRISPR/Cas9-based genome editing for correction of dystrophin mutations that cause Duchenne muscular dystrophy. *Nat Commun* 2015;6:6244.

30. Mendell J, Rodino-Klapac L, Walker C: Gene therapy clinical trials for Duchenne and limb girdle muscular dystrophies: Lessons learned, in Duan D, Mendell J, eds: *Muscle Gene Therapy*. Cham, Switzerland, Springer, 2019, pp 709-725.

    The possible role for gene therapy by insertion of mini genes for muscle disease is discussed.

31. Prior T, Russman B: Spinal muscular atrophy, in Adam MP, Ardinger HH, Pagon RA, et al, eds: *Gene Reviews*. Seattle, WA, University of Washington, Seattle, 1993.

32. Al-Jumah M, Majumdar R, Al-Rajeh S, et al: Molecular analysis of the spinal muscular atrophy and neuronal apoptosis inhibitory protein genes in Saudi patients with spinal muscular atrophy. *Saudi Med J* 2003;24(10):1052-1054.

33. Finkel RS, McDermott MP, Kaufmann P, et al: Observational study of spinal muscular atrophy type I and implications for clinical trials. *Neurology* 2014;83(9):810-817.

34. Sporer SM, Smith BG: Hip dislocation in patients with spinal muscular atrophy. *J Pediatr Orthop* 2003;23(1):10-14.

35. Lorenz HM, Badwan B, Hecker MM, et al: Magnetically controlled devices parallel to the spine in children with spinal muscular atrophy. *JB JS Open Access* 2017;2(4):e0036.

    Use of the MAGEC rod system for skeletally immature patients with SMA is discussed. Level of evidence: IV.

36. Mesfin A, Sponseller PD, Leet AI: Spinal muscular atrophy: Manifestations and management. *J Am Acad Orthop Surg* 2012;20(6):393-401.

37. Lewelt A, Krosschell KJ, Stoddard GJ, et al: Resistance strength training exercise in children with spinal muscular atrophy. *Muscle Nerve* 2015;52(4):559-567.

38. Darras BT, Chiriboga CA, Iannaccone ST, et al: Nusinersen in later-onset spinal muscular atrophy: Long-term results from the phase 1/2 studies. *Neurology* 2019;92(21):e2492-e2506.

    This study shows a clinically significant response to an oligonucleotide administered intrathecally to increase levels of SMN protein in patients with type II SMA. Level of evidence: IV.

39. Gidaro T, Servais L: Nusinersen treatment of spinal muscular atrophy: Current knowledge and existing gaps. *Dev Med Child Neurol* 2019;61(1):19-24.

    Review of studies of SMA patients treated with nusinersen for SMA shows positive responses in all types. Level of evidence: IV.

40. Al-Zaidy SA, Kolb SJ, Lowes L, et al: AVXS-101 (Onasemnogene Abeparvovec) for SMA1: Comparative study with a prospective natural history cohort. *J Neuromuscul Dis* 2019;6(3):307-317.

    This is a prospective, cohort, nonrandomized study of 12 infants with proven SMA-I compared with a historical group of 16 untreated babies showing a robust positive effect of gene therapy on motor milestones and survival. Level of evidence: III.

41. Lowes LP, Alfano LN, Arnold WD, et al: Impact of age and motor function in a phase 1/2A study of infants with SMA type 1 receiving single-dose gene replacement therapy. *Pediatr Neurol* 2019;98:39-45.

    Dramatic results of gene transfer in infants with SMA are shown. Level of evidence: I.

42. Li J-J, Lin X, Tang C, et al: Disruption of splicing-regulatory elements using CRISPR/Cas9 to rescue spinal muscular atrophy in human iPSCs and mice. *Natl Sci Rev* 2020;7(1):92-101.

43. Canavese F, Sussman MD: Orthopaedic manifestations of congenital myotonic dystrophy during childhood and adolescence. *J Pediatr Orthop* 2009;29(2):208-213.

44. Schilling L, Forst R, Forst J, Fujak A: Orthopaedic disorders in myotonic dystrophy type 1: Descriptive clinical study of 21 patients. *BMC Musculoskelet Disord* 2013;14:338.

45. Lau JK, Sy RW, Corbett A, Kritharides L: Myotonic dystrophy and the heart: A systematic review of evaluation and management. *Int J Cardiol* 2015;184:600-608.

46. Campbell C: Congenital myotonic dystrophy. *J Neurol Neurophysiol* 2012;S7.

47. Johnson NE, Ekstrom AB, Campbell C, et al: Parent-reported multi-national study of the impact of congenital and childhood onset myotonic dystrophy. *Dev Med Child Neurol* 2016;58(7):698-705.

    The authors report on the overall effect of congenital myotonic dystrophy on children and their families. Level of evidence: IV.

48. Mathis S, Goizet C, Tazir M, et al: Charcot-Marie-Tooth diseases: An update and some new proposals for the classification. *J Med Genet* 2015;52(10):681-690.

49. Harel T, Lupski JR: Charcot-Marie-Tooth disease and pathways to molecular based therapies. *Clin Genet* 2014;86(5):422-431.

50. Aktas S, Sussman MD: The radiological analysis of pes cavus deformity in Charcot Marie Tooth disease. *J Pediatr Orthop B* 2000;9(2):137-140.

51. Williams PF: Restoration of muscle balance of the foot by transfer of the tibialis posterior. *J Bone Joint Surg Br* 1976;58(2):217-219.

52. Ward CM, Dolan LA, Bennett DL, Morcuende JA, Cooper RR: Long-term results of reconstruction for treatment of a flexible cavovarus foot in Charcot-Marie-Tooth disease. *J Bone Joint Surg Am* 2008;90(12):2631-2642.

53. Hansen SJ: *Functional Reconstruction of the Foot and Ankle.* Philadelphia, PA, Lippincott Williams & Wilkins, 2000.

54. Walker JL, Nelson KR, Heavilon JA, et al: Hip abnormalities in children with Charcot-Marie-Tooth disease. *J Pediatr Orthop* 1994;14(1):54-59.

55. Novais EN, Kim YJ, Carry PM, Millis MB: Periacetabular osteotomy redirects the acetabulum and improves pain in Charcot-Marie-Tooth hip dysplasia with higher complications compared with developmental dysplasia of the hip. *J Pediatr Orthop* 2016;36(8):853-859.

    The outcomes of patients with hip dysplasia caused by CMT disease and treated with Bernese osteotomy with and without femoral osteotomy are discussed. Level of evidence: IV.

56. Karol LA, Elerson E: Scoliosis in patients with Charcot-Marie-Tooth disease. *J Bone Joint Surg Am* 2007;89(7):1504-1510.

CHAPTER 19

Arthritis

ROBERT M. SHEETS, MD • JOHANNA CHANG, MD • SUHAS M. RADHAKRISHNA, MD

ABSTRACT

Arthritis in children encompasses a wide variety of diseases. Reactive arthritis can include arthritis that lasts less than 6 weeks and includes transient arthritis, poststreptococcal arthritis, and postinfectious arthritis. Chronic arthritis includes various subtypes of juvenile idiopathic arthritis and the arthritis that can be associated with a wide variety of vasculitic diseases as well as juvenile dermatomyositis. In addition, chronic recurrent multifocal osteomyelitis can mimic bacterial osteomyelitis and a bone tumor. Consultation with a pediatric rheumatologist early in a child's disease course can be helpful in making a diagnosis.

Keywords: chronic recurrent multifocal osteomyelitis (CRMO); enthesitis-related arthritis; juvenile arthritis; psoriatic arthritis; transient synovitis

INTRODUCTION

An orthopaedic surgeon often is the first specialist consulted to evaluate a child with persistent but nontraumatic joint pain. Although many such children will have benign conditions, it is essential to consider juvenile arthritis and other systemic rheumatic diseases that occur along with arthritis in the differential diagnosis.

It is important to be familiar with juvenile arthritis and its subtypes, including details about how these disorders are managed. Information about reactive arthritis, which includes transient synovitis; postinfectious arthritis; Lyme disease arthritis; chronic recurrent multifocal osteomyelitis (CRMO); and the arthritis that accompanies granulomatosis with polyangiitis, Kawasaki disease, Henoch-Schönlein purpura, sarcoidosis, and Behçet syndrome, is presented. Key points are the emphasis on a broad differential diagnosis of joint pain and swelling along with an understanding of how these diseases can mimic septic arthritis, osteomyelitis, and benign and malignant diseases of both blood and bone.

JUVENILE ARTHRITIS

Juvenile arthritis is a diagnosis of exclusion based on the patient's history, physical examination, and supportive laboratory and imaging results. An understanding of the subtypes of juvenile arthritis enables timely referral to a pediatric rheumatologist for definitive evaluation and early treatment. The classification nomenclature for the subtypes of juvenile arthritis is based on specific patterns of joint involvement, laboratory prognostic markers, and systemic features such as the presence of a psoriatic rash or inflammatory bowel disease.[1] Fortunately, with the advent of early treatment strategies using targeted biologic medications, long-term outcomes have improved greatly, and the need for surgical intervention is far less than in previous generations.[2]

Immune-mediated arthritis is defined by the presence of chronic synovial inflammation in the absence of another etiology, such as infection. Immune-mediated

None of the following authors or any immediate family member has received anything of value from or has stock or stock options held in a commercial company or institution related directly or indirectly to the subject of this chapter: Dr. Sheets, Dr. Chang, and Dr. Radhakrishna.

This chapter is adapted from Sheets R, Chang J, Radhakrishna S: Arthritis, in Martus JE, ed: *Orthopaedic Knowledge Update®: Pediatrics*, ed 5. Rosemont, IL, American Academy of Orthopaedic Surgeons, 2016, pp 203-213.

arthritis is clinically manifested by either swelling, mild warmth, pain, or decreased range of movement or a combination of these findings. Joint swelling must be continuously present for a minimum of 6 weeks in the same joint. Synovitis of shorter duration is considered viral or postinfectious (reactive) until the 6-week threshold is reached. Erythema and significant tenderness are unusual and suggest infection or malignancy. The degree of pain can vary; most patients have more stiffness than pain. Joint pain alone—in the absence of other inflammatory signs—is defined as arthralgia, not arthritis. Imaging, such as ultrasonography or MRI, may be required to demonstrate synovitis in equivocal cases.[3,4]

Because pathognomonic laboratory tests or clinical findings do not exist for juvenile arthritis, it is imperative to exclude all other etiologies before establishing the diagnosis. Joint swelling has a broad differential diagnosis, including injury, infection, malignancy, foreign body, hemophilia, and rare entities such as pigmented villonodular synovitis. Pathologies in close proximity to the joint space, such as osteomyelitis, bone lesions, hemangiomas, and arteriovenous malformations, may be mistaken for joint swelling. Joint pain without swelling has a more extensive differential diagnosis, including other entities such as benign limb pain of childhood, known colloquially as growing pains; benign joint hypermobility; pes planus; osteochondroses; amplified pain syndrome; and genetic disorders of both connective tissue and metabolism.

History

Several historical clues point toward arthritis. The gel phenomenon of morning and cold-induced stiffness is typical. Synovial fluid becomes more viscous with rest and cold and more fluid with movement and warmth. Parents often will notice a limp present in the morning when their child first arises or after naps. Conversely, a noninflammatory etiology is characterized by intermittent pain with activity and is primarily present in the evening and relieved by rest. Red flag symptoms prompting a broad workup for malignancy or infection include awakening from sleep because of pain, weight loss, fever, and pain disproportionate to any clinical findings.

Physical Examination

The physical examination should entail a brief but comprehensive assessment of range of motion, swelling, pain with motion, and tenderness in all joints. Special attention should be given to the neck's range of motion, the temporomandibular joint (assessed by opening the mouth), and the proximal interphalangeal (PIP) joints. Asking a patient to flex the PIP joints while keeping the metacarpophalangeal joints in extension (allowing the fingertips to touch the palm) is a quick assessment of PIP joint range of motion. Sometimes indirect observation is most helpful. Observation of gait as well as a child's movement on the examination table and in the room is essential. Younger children may be assessed through play or reaching for toys. Children may have had long-standing arthritis, which could be missed without a thorough examination.

Laboratory Tests

Laboratory tests cannot be used to diagnose or rule out arthritis. They are used mainly as supportive data and to exclude other etiologies. Inflammatory markers may be normal, especially in arthritis affecting only a few joints. Highly elevated inflammatory markers with minimal arthritis suggest another etiology. Rheumatoid factor, anti-cyclic citrullinated peptide antibody, and antinuclear antibody screening tests are not helpful, because these substances are present in only a minority of patients with juvenile arthritis and have low specificity. These tests may be obtained in patients with known arthritis, and the rheumatoid factor and cyclic citrullinated peptide may be helpful in polyarticular disease because a high titer suggests a poor prognosis. Antinuclear antibodies can be helpful in screening for systemic lupus erythematosus. An antistreptolysin O titer (blood test) may be useful for screening for poststreptococcal disease. Human leukocyte antigen B27 may be helpful in defining spondyloarthritis. The history and physical examination, rather than laboratory tests, are the main criteria for making a diagnosis of juvenile arthritis.[5,6]

Imaging

Imaging helps establish the presence of synovitis. At the time of the initial clinical visit, radiographs often lack the sensitivity to detect a joint effusion, but they can be helpful in excluding other etiologies. Radiographs in early arthritis typically show only periarticular osteopenia. In advanced arthritis, radiographs can delineate the extent of joint space narrowing, advancement of bone age, erosions, subluxation, and ankylosis (fusion).

MRI is the preferred imaging modality for defining synovitis, with intravenous contrast used to demonstrate synovial hyperemia. Noncontrast MRI with a high T2 signal still can be diagnostic.[3,4] Early arthritis is characterized on MRI by joint effusion, synovial proliferation, and enhancement; later disease is characterized by cartilage thinning and joint erosions (**Figure 1**).

Ultrasonography is emerging as an excellent modality for joint assessment.[3,4] Imaging also is used to monitor radiographic disease progression across time, which may occur even in clinically quiet disease.

Epidemiology

The incidence of juvenile arthritis is approximately 5 to 10 per 100,000 children. In general, it is more common

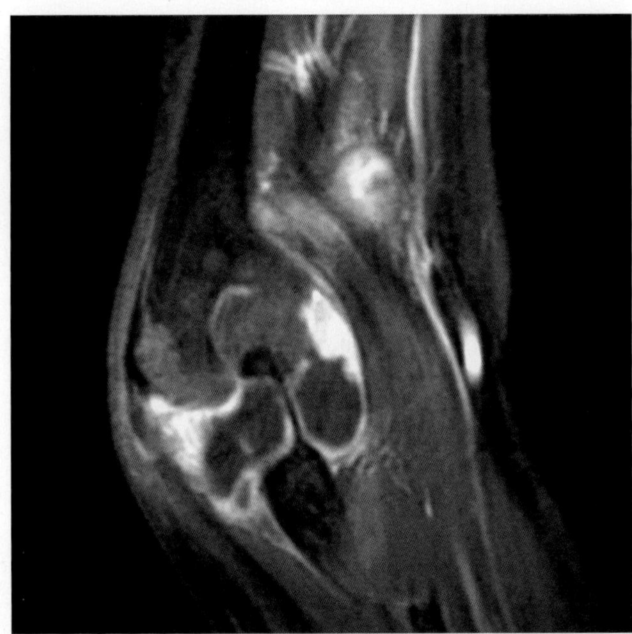

FIGURE 1 Magnetic resonance image shows oligoarticular juvenile idiopathic arthritis of the right elbow.

in Caucasian children than in ethnic minorities, and it is seen in girls more often than in boys.[7] The etiology is multifactorial, with genetic contributions from immune genes, particularly in antigen presentation and cytokine pathways, and still undefined environmental and hormonal influences.

Treatment

The prompt diagnosis of juvenile arthritis enables the pediatric rheumatologist to institute aggressive therapy aimed at achieving early clinical remission. Long-term outcomes are greatly improved by using anti–tumor necrosis factor (anti-TNF) and other biologic medications.[2] However, if arthritis remains active, long-term sequelae include joint contracture, muscular atrophy, bone overgrowth, limb-length discrepancy, subluxation, micrognathia, short stature, and loss of function. Both physical and occupational therapy are vital adjunctive services in the management of these complications. Orthopaedic reconstructive surgery is warranted in patients with advanced arthritis if medical therapy has been unsuccessful. Such procedures include total joint arthroplasty, synovectomy, arthrodesis, and soft-tissue release.

Subtypes of Juvenile Arthritis

The nomenclature for juvenile arthritis continues to evolve. The 1977 American College of Rheumatology criteria defined three forms of juvenile rheumatoid arthritis: systemic, polyarticular, and pauciarticular. The classification used most commonly today is the 2001 International League of Associations for Rheumatology criteria,[1] which has seven subtypes of juvenile idiopathic arthritis (JIA), including oligoarticular JIA, polyarticular JIA (rheumatoid factor positive or negative), psoriatic arthritis, enthesitis-related arthritis, systemic juvenile idiopathic arthritis (sJIA), and undifferentiated arthritis. All subtypes are characterized by the presence of arthritis in one or more joints of at least 6 weeks' duration in a child younger than 16 years in the absence of another etiology. The exception is sJIA, which is diagnosed based on fever, rashes, and a marked systemic inflammatory response rather than the duration or pattern of arthritis.

Oligoarticular JIA is typically diagnosed in toddlers, who have fewer than five involved joints during the first 6 months after diagnosis. These children are generally afebrile, are well appearing, and have large lower limb joint effusions of insidious onset. Distinctive features of other subtypes will develop in many children during the aging process. Uveitis, or ocular inflammation, is clinically silent and may lead to irreversible vision loss in up to 30% of these children, necessitating close monitoring by an ophthalmologist. However, oligoarticular JIA can occur in older children. The maximum age of onset of JIA is 16 years. By definition, adult rheumatoid arthritis has its onset at 16 years of age or older.

Psoriatic arthritis can appear either oligoarticularly or polyarticularly and with or without psoriasis. However, a substantial family history of psoriasis exists in the families of children in whom psoriatic arthritis eventually develops. Blepharitis and nail pits as well as changes of the nails (ie, onycholysis) are common findings with psoriatic arthritis. Enthesitis, dactylitis, and arthritis of the distal interphalangeal joints are also potential hallmarks.[8]

Two categories for polyarticular JIA have been defined based on the involvement of five or more joints and the presence or absence of rheumatoid factor. The joint pattern is typically symmetric, often involving small joints, such as the metacarpophalangeal and PIP joints, the cervical spine, and the temporomandibular joint. Rheumatoid factor–negative polyarticular JIA is typical in preschool children, whereas rheumatoid factor–positive polyarticular JIA more often is seen in adolescents. A positive rheumatoid factor indicates a higher likelihood of erosive arthritis. Cyclic citrullinated peptide antibodies are likely to replace rheumatoid factor, because these are more specific for arthritis. Adolescents with arthritis should be evaluated for other systemic diseases, such as systemic lupus erythematosus.

Although the term spondyloarthropathy was not defined in the juvenile arthritis criteria, it still is used clinically to refer to a constellation of disease manifestations that tend to be associated with arthritis involving the sacroiliac joints and the vertebrae. These manifestations include inflammatory bowel disease, acute symptomatic anterior uveitis, psoriasis, and enthesitis (inflammation at the insertion point of tendons). In the International

League of Associations for Rheumatology criteria, juvenile psoriatic arthritis and enthesitis-related arthritis are separate entities.

Undifferentiated arthritis encompasses arthritis that has overlapping criteria or is not well defined in other criteria, such as arthritis associated with inflammatory bowel disease and juvenile ankylosing spondylitis. In the International League of Associations for Rheumatology criteria, enthesitis-related arthritis is the preferred designation for patients who previously may have been deemed to have juvenile spondyloarthritis and who now have enthesitis. This designation draws attention to the fact that the earliest manifestation for many children is enthesitis, particularly of the Achilles insertion point on the calcaneus. Enthesitis-related arthritis should be considered in children with Sever disease that is not responding to nonsurgical therapy. Most children with juvenile ankylosing spondylitis have enthesitis and thus are classified as having enthesitis-related arthritis. In the International League of Associations for Rheumatology criteria, psoriatic arthritis is distinguished from enthesitis-related arthritis based on a family history of psoriasis, dactylitis, or nail pitting.[9] Given the hereditary pattern of psoriasis and inflammatory bowel disease, knowledge of the family history is important when evaluating a child with arthritis.

Although sJIA is a subtype of JIA, its clinical and immunologic features suggest that it may, in fact, be part of a different disease spectrum. Many rheumatologists consider sJIA part of the autoinflammatory disorders that include familial Mediterranean fever and cryopyrin-associated periodic syndromes.[10,11]

Unlike other forms of JIA, patients with sJIA typically have a high fever accompanied by rash, with laboratory testing showing elevated inflammatory markers. Diagnosis requires the presence of arthritis for a minimum of 2 weeks and quotidian (daily) fevers for at least 3 days accompanied by at least one of the following: an evanescent, nonfixed, erythematous rash; generalized lymphadenopathy; hepatomegaly or splenomegaly; or serositis.[12] Although patients with sJIA often have symmetric, polyarticular arthritis, some children may not exhibit arthritis until later in the disease course.

The incidence of sJIA is 4% to 17% in patients with JIA and accounts for 5% to 10% of cases in the United States and Europe.[11] Although no peak onset has been established, children aged 1 to 5 years are the most frequently affected. Males and females are affected equally. Forty percent of patients with sJIA have a monophasic disease course characterized by variable disease severity and duration, and 50% of patients have disease that is refractory to treatment, with persistent inflammation and arthritis. The remaining 10% of patients have a polycyclic course with episodes of inflammation alternating with disease remission. A life-threatening complication known as macrophage activation syndrome, also known as secondary hemophagocytic lymphohistiocytosis, develops in approximately 10% of children with sJIA. Possible triggers for macrophage activation syndrome include viral illness and the addition of or a change in medication. Clinically, patients appear severely ill and have a persistent fever accompanied by rash, hepatosplenomegaly, lymphadenopathy, liver failure, and neurologic changes. Laboratory testing shows disproportionately low acute phase reactants, cytopenia, elevated ferritin (≥500 μg/L), coagulopathy, elevated liver enzymes, hypofibrinogenemia, and hypertriglyceridemia. A bone marrow biopsy can show phagocytosis of other hematopoietic cells by macrophages or histiocytes.[12,13]

The overall prognosis depends on the disease type and response to drug therapy, although sJIA often is considered the most severe of all JIA subtypes and has a reported disease-related mortality rate ranging from 0.5% to 1%.[11] Treatment-related adverse effects account for a substantial part of disease morbidity. Chronic steroid use results in Cushing syndrome, decreased bone health, and increased risk of infection.

Therapeutic Management of JIA

The main objectives for the management of JIA are pain relief, disease control, and the prevention of damage and disability. Because a standardized approach to the management of the various subtypes of juvenile arthritis is lacking, rheumatologists are working to establish evidence-based guidelines for the medical management of JIA. The Childhood Arthritis and Rheumatology Research Alliance recently published consensus treatment plans for new-onset polyarticular JIA and sJIA.[13,14] The medications described in these consensus treatment plans as well as other medications used in the treatment of JIA are discussed in this section.

NSAIDs, such as ibuprofen and naproxen, are arguably considered first-line therapy, but the development of more effective medications has limited the use of NSAID monotherapy to no more than 2 months in patients who have persistently active arthritis.[15] Aspirin is generally not used. The average time to symptomatic improvement from an NSAID is 1 month; however, 25% of children do not demonstrate clinical improvement until 8 to 12 weeks have passed. NSAIDs are well tolerated, with the most common adverse effects being abdominal pain and anorexia. Patients experiencing substantial gastritis can benefit from using antacids, histamine-2 blockers, or proton pump inhibitors or from switching to a cyclooxygenase-2 inhibitor. A complete blood count, liver enzyme levels, and serum creatinine levels should be checked before or soon after the initiation of routine NSAID use, with repeat laboratory testing every 6 months for long-term daily use.[15]

Intra-articular steroid injections provide quick symptomatic relief while waiting for systemic medications to take effect and can be done with or without additional therapy in patients, especially those with monoarticular or oligoarticular arthritis. However, one study described weak evidence for decreased clinical symptoms of arthritis in patients who had received intra-articular steroid injections in a lower limb.[16] Although intra-articular steroid injections are rarely curative, rapid pain relief can encourage normal activity and prevent the formation of joint contractures.[12,17] Triamcinolone hexacetonide has been shown to be more effective than triamcinolone acetonide, but the former is no longer available, so the acetonide formulation is what is commonly used. Clinical improvement for at least 4 months is expected, and intra-articular steroid injections can be repeated as needed.[15]

Disease-modifying antirheumatic drugs (DMARDs), a large category that includes methotrexate (MTX), sulfasalazine, leflunomide, azathioprine, cyclosporine, and hydroxychloroquine, are steroid-sparing medications that have been shown to reduce joint damage. These medications are immunosuppressants. MTX, a folic acid analogue and inhibitor of enzymes in the folate pathway that leads to anti-inflammatory effects, is the most commonly prescribed DMARD for JIA. MTX can be given either orally or subcutaneously; some studies have shown increased bioavailability of the subcutaneous pathway compared with oral MTX at higher doses. MTX is thought to be an efficacious and safe medication that has been used effectively since the beginning of the practice of pediatric rheumatology.[18] Concomitant use of daily folic acid helps decrease the frequency and severity of MTX adverse effects, including oral ulcers, decreased appetite, and nausea. A complete blood count with differential, hepatic enzyme levels, and serum creatinine level is recommended to be checked before initiation, approximately 1 month after initiation, and then every 3 to 4 months in patients with stable doses and normal prior laboratory results.[15]

Sulfasalazine is another DMARD that previously was used frequently to treat JIA. It is an analogue of 5-aminosalicylic acid linked to sulfapyridine and is both antibacterial and anti-inflammatory. However, current guidelines support its use in only enthesitis-related arthritis, not in other JIA subtypes.[15] Sulfasalazine may trigger macrophage activation syndrome in patients with sJIA and has been shown to cause increased toxicity in adult-onset Still disease.[2,18]

Leflunomide inhibits pyrimidine synthesis and may have similar effects as MTX. It often is used as an alternative medication for patients who cannot tolerate MTX. Cyclosporine is more frequently used in patients with sJIA and features of macrophage activation syndrome.

The main risk associated with using DMARDs is the increased risk of infection. In addition, patients treated with DMARDs should have various laboratory tests checked at monthly intervals. Many DMARDs, including MTX, leflunomide, and sulfasalazine, have bone marrow-suppressing effects. These medications also may have gastrointestinal adverse effects. In particular, sulfasalazine has been reported to have complications that are more serious, such as Stevens-Johnson syndrome.[19]

If substantial synovitis or other signs of active disease persist despite the addition of nonbiologic DMARDs, many rheumatologists consider additional treatment with biologic agents. This relatively new category of medications includes TNF inhibitors, interleukin (IL)-1 inhibitors, tocilizumab, abatacept, rituximab, ustekinumab, and tofacitinib. Only a few of these medications are approved by the FDA for the treatment of JIA, but many are used off-label in patients with refractory JIA.

The TNF cytokine has been implicated in the inflammatory cascade leading to the development of JIA. The three most commonly used anti-TNF medications for JIA treatment are etanercept (a fusion protein consisting of the extracellular domain of the p75 TNF receptor linked to the Fc region of human immunoglobulin-1), adalimumab (a humanized monoclonal antibody to TNF), and infliximab (a chimeric mouse/human monoclonal antibody to TNF). The FDA approved etanercept for the management of polyarticular JIA in May 1999 and adalimumab for the treatment of polyarticular JIA in February 2008. Etanercept is administered as a once-weekly or twice-weekly subcutaneous injection, whereas adalimumab is administered every 1 to 2 weeks. Infliximab is administered intravenously on a monthly basis. Anti-TNF medications are usually combined with MTX or other nonbiologic medications when tolerated. One study showed that children treated with etanercept plus MTX had improved treatment responses compared with etanercept alone, without an increase in adverse events.[2] Because the use of TNF-α inhibitors is associated with reactivated tuberculosis, a negative quantiferon or purified protein derivative skin test should be demonstrated in patients who will be treated with TNF-α inhibitors before starting anti-TNF therapy, and then repeated annually. A complete blood count, hepatic enzyme levels, and serum creatinine level should be obtained before initiating therapy and then repeated every 3 to 6 months.[15]

In 2009, the FDA required that a boxed warning be added to all anti-TNF therapies, highlighting the increased risk of cancer in children receiving these drugs to treat JIA. However, subsequent studies, including several randomized controlled studies, have not demonstrated any important safety concerns of these medications or any other biologic medication. Although some studies showed an increased risk of lymphoma or other malignancy in children treated with anti-TNF therapies, other studies have shown an increased baseline incidence of malignancy in children with JIA.[19] Again, most complications arising from anti-TNF therapies are caused by increased infectious risks, although studies have claimed that the risk is not greater when using anti-TNF therapy compared with use of MTX alone.[19]

IL-1 is an inflammatory cytokine most notably implicated in autoinflammatory syndromes and sJIA. The three commercially available IL-1 antagonists used in the treatment of sJIA are administered subcutaneously and include anakinra (IL-1 receptor antagonist), rilonacept (soluble fusion protein of human immunoglobulin-1 linked to the IL-1 receptor), and canakinumab (monoclonal antibody to IL-1β). All three medications are recommended for the management of sJIA in the consensus treatment plans from the Childhood Arthritis and Rheumatology Research Alliance; anakinra monotherapy can be considered an initial treatment in patients with sJIA who have physical findings that raise concern for active disease.[20] The FDA approved canakinumab for the management of sJIA in May 2013.

Tocilizumab is a monoclonal antibody to the IL-6 receptor and the only biologic agent that is FDA approved for use in both sJIA and polyarticular JIA. IL-6 is a proinflammatory cytokine. Tocilizumab is available as both an infusion and a subcutaneous injection.

Abatacept is a soluble fusion protein that consists of cytotoxic T cell lymphocyte antigen-4 fused with the Fc region of human immunoglobulin and blocks signal transduction between T cells and antigen-presenting cells. It is an infused medication administered on a monthly basis or more recently as a subcutaneous injection and was FDA approved for the management of polyarticular JIA in April 2008. However, it is also considered effective maintenance therapy in patients with sJIA who do not have physical findings concerning for active disease.[20]

Rituximab is a chimeric monoclonal antibody to the CD20 receptor that is present only on B cells. The FDA has approved rituximab combined with MTX in adults with rheumatoid arthritis who have not had adequate response with anti-TNF therapies. Studies in adults with rheumatoid arthritis suggest that the presence of an rheumatoid factor may lead to better response with rituximab therapy,[21] but these studies have not been performed in children. It seems to have some effectiveness in patients with various JIA subtypes, although studies are limited.

The number of biologic medications being developed for the management of inflammatory arthritis continues to grow, although studies for safety and efficacy in JIA have not yet been published. Ustekinumab, a human monoclonal antibody targeting the p40 subunit of IL-12/23, was FDA approved for the treatment of psoriatic arthritis in September 2013 but has not yet been studied in juvenile psoriatic arthritis. However, a randomized phase III trial of ustekinumab in adolescents with plaque psoriasis showed substantially improved signs and symptoms of psoriasis without any unexpected adverse events.[22] Tofacitinib is a Janus-kinase inhibitor that is approved by the FDA for the treatment of adults with rheumatoid arthritis but also seems to be efficacious in managing psoriasis and inflammatory bowel disease. Unlike other biologic medications, tofacitinib is administered orally. A randomized withdrawal, double-blind, placebo-controlled study of this medication in patients with JIA is ongoing.

The last category of medications used in the management of JIA is corticosteroids. Although systemic steroids work quickly to decrease inflammation, they have a limited role in the management of JIA. Steroids have never been proved to be disease modifying and have serious toxic adverse effects with long-term use. Low doses (5 to 15 mg/d) are helpful in cases of severe arthritis in patients with polyarticular JIA and enthesitis-related arthritis. In sJIA and patients with severe uveitis, moderate to high doses (>1 mg/kg/d) are used to control underlying inflammation. The toxicities of steroids include immunosuppression, hypertension, diabetes, cataracts, osteoporosis, osteonecrosis, obesity, and many others.[12,17] In the modern practice of rheumatology, steroids are mainly used as a bridging therapy until the effects of the more slowly acting DMARDs or biologic medications take place.

REACTIVE ARTHRITIS

In pediatric rheumatology, specialists usually use the term reactive arthritis to describe a transient arthritis of any joint lasting less than 6 weeks, thus differentiating this diagnosis from JIA. In adults, the term is usually used in reference to transient arthritis that is linked to spondyloarthritis.

Transient Synovitis

The term transient synovitis often is applied to arthritis of the hip that follows a recent viral upper respiratory tract infection or viral intestinal disease. However, transient synovitis can involve other joints, usually a large joint and often only a single joint. The symptoms are usually acute, and a fever may be present. Inflammatory markers also may be elevated.[23] The major differential diagnosis is septic arthritis, but JIA also can appear in this fashion. Frequently, transient arthritis will respond within 1 or 2 days to an NSAID, such as naproxen. Most patients improve within days rather than weeks, so it becomes a diagnosis of exclusion. The workup consists of a complete blood count, the erythrocyte sedimentation rate, and the C-reactive protein level; joint aspiration is considered to rule out infection. Initial treatment with antibiotics may be warranted based on the erythrocyte sedimentation rate, C-reactive protein level, and joint aspiration.[24,25]

Poststreptococcal Arthritis

The primary difference between transient synovitis, which is considered a postviral disease, and poststreptococcal arthritis is simply the documentation of a recent strep infection. However, this determination is not always simple because symptoms of a prior sore throat may be lacking. A prior sore throat and a positive culture for strep usually have an onset of arthritis in 1 to 2 weeks. However, titers for antistreptolysin O and anti–DNAase-B should be done to confirm that the culture was not a false-positive or an indicator of a streptococcal carrier. The interpretation of streptococcal antibody titers also can be difficult and is, at best, 90% sensitive. The course of poststreptococcal arthritis is more variable than transient synovitis. The streptococcal infection should be treated, and NSAIDs may be needed for a longer term course.[26] A streptococcal infection also needs to be distinguished from rheumatic fever, which often is manifested by migratory, very painful arthritis of large joints, and the Jones criteria would need to be fulfilled[27] (**Table 1**).

Lyme Disease Arthritis

In many but not all parts of the United States, Lyme disease arthritis has been well documented.[28] The diagnosis must be suspected clinically by a careful history and fulfillment of the diagnostic criteria from the Centers for Disease Control and Prevention[29] (**Table 2**). Lyme disease arthritis often occurs in the knee and initially may be indistinguishable from other forms of reactive arthritis or juvenile arthritis and may be self-limited or persistent. A history of exposure in an endemic area, a tick bite, flulike symptoms, and an erythema chronicum migrans rash make the diagnosis much more likely, but one or more of these elements may not be present.[30-34] Misdiagnosis is a common problem if the serology criteria are not applied appropriately.

TABLE 1

Jones Criteria for the Diagnosis of Acute Rheumatic Fever[a]

Major Criteria	Minor Criteria
Carditis	Fever
Arthritis	Arthralgia
Erythema marginatum	Elevated erythrocyte sedimentation rate or C-reactive protein level
Subcutaneous nodules	Prolonged PR interval or other heart block
Sydenham chorea	

[a]To make a diagnosis of rheumatic fever, two major and one minor criteria or one major and two minor criteria must be present, along with evidence of a recent streptococcal infection as evidenced by a positive throat culture or increasing or elevated streptococcal antibody titers.

TABLE 2

CDC Criteria for Lyme Disease

Positive ELISA or immunofluorescence assay test

If symptoms present for <30 d: Positive Western blot IgM with 2 of 3 bands positive, or Western blot IgG with ≥5 of 10 bands positive

If symptoms present for >30 d: Western blot with ≥5 of 10 bands positive

CDC = Centers for Disease Control and Prevention, ELISA = enzyme-linked immunosorbent assay, IgG = immunoglobulin G, IgM = immunoglobulin M

Chronic Recurrent Multifocal Osteomyelitis

The presentation of CRMO, although a rare disease, is extremely important to the orthopaedic surgeon. CRMO can include osteomyelitis that mimics bacterial osteomyelitis with bony changes and periosteal elevation, osteitis of a long bone, osteolytic lesion of a bone, or a mixed picture of any of these with arthritis.[33,34] The pathophysiology of CRMO is considered immune mediated.[35,36]

Radiographic evidence can be very helpful, and some features suggest the diagnosis early in the course. Radiography, bone scans, and MRI have all been used, but MRI seems to be particularly helpful.[37-40] Persistence of a bony lesion, negative bone cultures, a negative bone biopsy for malignancy or other bone tumor, and a lack of response to antibiotics are all useful in developing a suspicion of CRMO. In addition to mimicking infection, the lesions also can have the characteristics of a bone

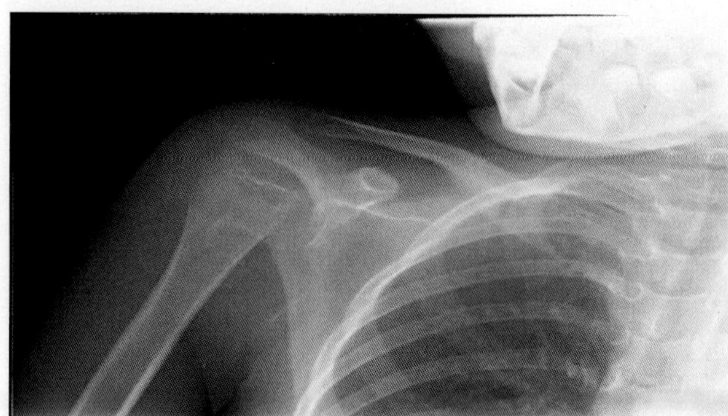

FIGURE 2 AP radiograph shows chronic recurrent multifocal osteomyelitis in the right clavicle.

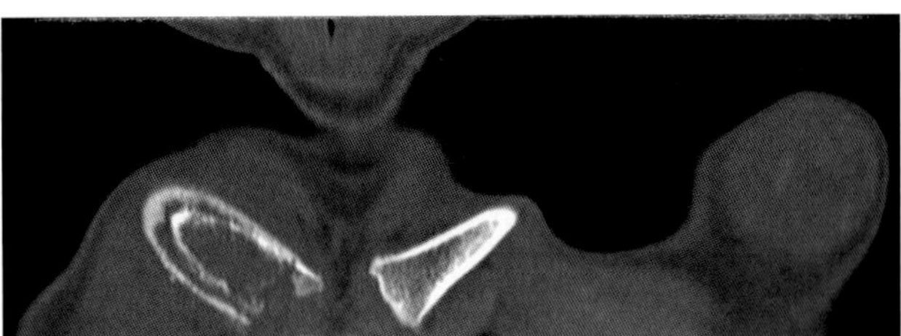

FIGURE 3 CT scan shows chronic recurrent multifocal osteomyelitis in the right clavicle.

tumor.[41] Recurrence of what seems to be osteomyelitis in the same or, more importantly, in a new area is highly suspicious for CRMO (**Figures 2** through **4**). Laboratory testing shows persistent elevation of inflammatory markers if the patient is symptomatic, but these markers may resolve completely if the CRMO remits.

The treatment of CRMO is complicated, and a highly variable response can be seen. Medications may include NSAIDs, MTX, or a biologic medication.[42]

Arthritis in Other Systemic Rheumatic Diseases

Arthritis can occur in children with more complex rheumatic disease, such as systemic lupus erythematosus, juvenile dermatomyositis, sarcoidosis, and in some of the vasculitic diseases, including granulomatosis with polyangiitis, Henoch-Schönlein purpura, Kawasaki disease, eosinophilic granulomatosis with polyangiitis, and polyarteritis nodosa. The history and physical examination are usually able to differentiate these diseases from an orthopaedic etiology toward a rheumatic etiology.

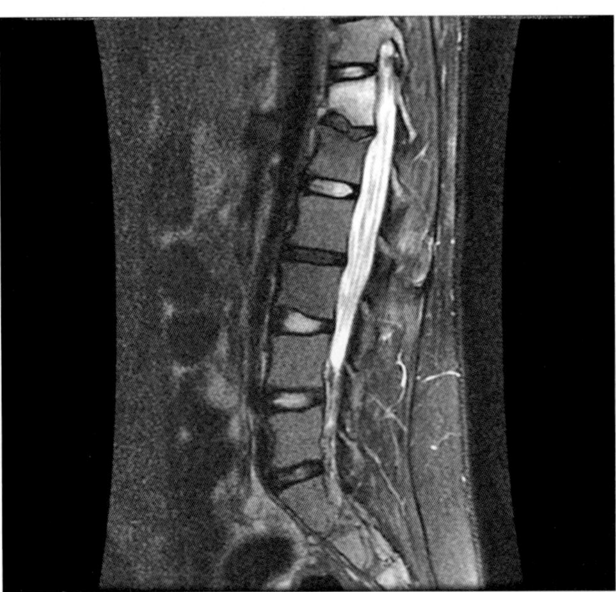

FIGURE 4 Magnetic resonance image shows chronic recurrent multifocal osteomyelitis in the spine.

Systemic lupus erythematosus is diagnosed in a preteen or teenage patient and includes one or more of the following symptoms: fever, fatigue, hair loss, the Raynaud phenomenon, a malar rash, weight loss, pericarditis, pneumonitis, and a pleural effusion.[43,44]

Juvenile dermatomyositis often occurs as proximal muscle weakness and frequently will have a characteristic rash on the face, extensor elbows, and knee, as well as the dorsum of the hands with lesions that are called Gottron papules. Patients frequently also have changes of the nail fold capillary bed that are visible with a magnifier.[45]

The characteristics of Kawasaki disease typically are a high daily fever with injected sclera; a red tongue; dry, red, vertically fissured lips; polymorphous dermatitis of the body; and lymphadenopathy. Patients are usually very irritable and have a marked increase in inflammatory markers as well as in alanine aminotransferase and γ-glutamyltransferase. Most importantly, coronary artery disease may develop in patients.[46]

Henoch-Schönlein purpura usually starts with a petechial or palpable purpuric rash of the distal lower legs that usually spreads to involve most of both legs and the buttocks. The arthritis can follow the onset of the rash within several days, occur at the same time as the purpura, or precede any other symptoms. Abdominal pain that may be severe frequently develops. The arthritis is usually a large-joint arthritis of the ankles and/or knees.[47]

Granulomatosis with polyangiitis (formerly known as Wegener granulomatosis) may include arthritis but usually includes other symptoms, notably significant pneumonitis, sinusitis, or nephritis. Many patients will have a positive antineutrophil cytoplasmic antibody test.[48]

In younger children, sarcoidosis usually manifests as multiple, very swollen joints and may include dermatitis and uveitis. In older children, pulmonary involvement is a more common indication.[49] Behçet syndrome can occur with arthritis, but it usually occurs with recurrent aphthous ulcers, dermatitis, fever, or intestinal symptoms.

SUMMARY

Arthritis in children encompasses a wide variety of diseases ranging from brief forms of reactive arthritis to various forms of juvenile arthritis. Symptoms and clues to the diagnosis vary with the disease subtype. The patient's history and physical examination are still the most important components of the diagnosis; however, laboratory and imaging studies can be helpful in differentiating these disorders from other orthopaedic conditions. Because the treatment of arthritis has changed dramatically in the past 15 years, making a correct diagnosis is very important. Involvement of a pediatric rheumatologist early in the course of a child's disease can help in determining an accurate diagnosis and selecting the proper treatment.

KEY STUDY POINTS

- Postviral reactive arthritis is fairly common in children and can be difficult to differentiate from orthopaedic disorders and chronic rheumatic diseases.
- Chronic forms of juvenile arthritis can present with either systemic features or one or more joints that are typically associated with morning stiffness and pain.
- MRI, with and without contrast, can be helpful in differentiating orthopaedic disorders from various forms of childhood arthritis.

ANNOTATED REFERENCES

1. Petty RE, Southwood TR, Manners P, et al: International League of Associations for Rheumatology classification of juvenile idiopathic arthritis: Second revision, Edmonton, 2001. *J Rheumatol* 2004;31(2):390-392.
2. Stoll ML, Cron RQ: Treatment of juvenile idiopathic arthritis: A revolution in care. *Pediatr Rheumatol Online J* 2014;12:13.
3. Lanni S, Martini A, Malattia C: Heading toward a modern imaging approach in juvenile idiopathic arthritis. *Curr Rheumatol Rep* 2014;16(5):416.
4. Restrepo R, Lee EY, Babyn PS: Juvenile idiopathic arthritis: Current practical imaging assessment with emphasis on magnetic resonance imaging. *Radiol Clin North Am* 2013;51(4):703-719.
5. Saikia B, Rawat A, Vignesh P: Autoantibodies and their judicious use in pediatric rheumatology practice. *Indian J Pediatr* 2016;83(1):53-62.

   The latest guidelines for the use of laboratory tests in pediatric patients with arthritis are presented. Level of evidence: V.
6. Spencer CH, Patwardhan A: Pediatric rheumatology for the primary care clinicians: Recognizing patterns of disease. *Curr Probl Pediatr Adolesc Health Care* 2015;45(7):185-206.
7. Krause ML, Crowson CS, Michet CJ, Mason T, Muskardin TW, Matteson EL: Juvenile idiopathic arthritis in Olmsted County, Minnesota, 1960-2013. *Arthritis Rheumatol* 2016;68(1):247-254.

   This article discusses epidemiology data for JIA in one county in Minnesota.
8. Stoll ML, Nigrovic PA, Gotte AC, Punaro M: Clinical comparison of early-onset psoriatic and non-psoriatic oligoarticular juvenile idiopathic arthritis. *Clin Exp Rheumatol* 2011;29(3):582-588.
9. Ramanathan A, Srinivasalu H, Colbert RA: Update on juvenile spondyloarthritis. *Rheum Dis Clin North Am* 2013;39(4):767-788.
10. Nirmala N, Grom A, Gram H: Biomarkers in systemic juvenile idiopathic arthritis: A comparison with biomarkers in cryopyrin-associated periodic syndromes. *Curr Opin Rheumatol* 2014;26(5):543-552.
11. Bruck N, Schnabel A, Hedrich CM: Current understanding of the pathophysiology of systemic juvenile idiopathic arthritis (sJIA) and target-directed therapeutic approaches. *Clin Immunol* 2015;159(1):72-83.
12. Cassidy J, Petty R: *Textbook of Pediatric Rheumatology Expert Consult*, ed 6. London, UK, Elsevier Health Sciences, 2010, pp 236-248.
13. Ringold S, Weiss PF, Colbert RA, et al: Childhood Arthritis and Rheumatology Research Alliance consensus treatment plans for new-onset polyarticular juvenile idiopathic arthritis. *Arthritis Care Res (Hoboken)* 2014;66(7):1063-1072.
14. DeWitt EM, Kimura Y, Beukelman T, et al: Consensus treatment plans for new-onset systemic juvenile idiopathic arthritis. *Arthritis Care Res (Hoboken)* 2012;64(7):1001-1010.
15. Beukelman T, Patkar NM, Saag KG, et al: 2011 American College of Rheumatology recommendations for the treatment of juvenile idiopathic arthritis: Initiation and safety monitoring of therapeutic agents for the treatment of arthritis and systemic features. *Arthritis Care Res (Hoboken)* 2011;63(4):465-482.
16. Jennings H, Hennessy K, Hendry GJ: The clinical effectiveness of intra-articular corticosteroids for arthritis of the lower limb in juvenile idiopathic arthritis: A systematic review. *Pediatr Rheumatol Online J* 2014;12:23.
17. Szer I: *Arthritis in Children and Adolescents: Juvenile Idiopathic Arthritis.* Oxford, England, Oxford University Press, 2006.
18. Coulson EJ, Hanson HJ, Foster HE: What does an adult rheumatologist need to know about juvenile idiopathic arthritis? *Rheumatology (Oxford)* 2014;53(12):2155-2166.
19. Kessler EA, Becker ML: Therapeutic advancements in juvenile idiopathic arthritis. *Best Pract Res Clin Rheumatol* 2014;28(2):293-313.
20. Ringold S, Weiss PF, Beukelman T, et al: 2013 update of the 2011 American College of Rheumatology recommendations for the treatment of juvenile idiopathic arthritis: Recommendations for the medical therapy of children with systemic juvenile idiopathic arthritis and tuberculosis screening among children receiving biologic medications. *Arthritis Rheum* 2013;65(10):2499-2512.
21. Chatzidionysiou K, Lie E, Nasonov E, et al: Highest clinical effectiveness of rituximab in autoantibody-positive patients with rheumatoid arthritis and in those for whom no more than one previous TNF antagonist has failed: Pooled data from 10 European registries. *Ann Rheum Dis* 2011;70(9):1575-1580.
22. Landells I, Marano C, Hsu MC, et al: Ustekinumab in adolescent patients age 12 to 17 years with moderate-to-severe plaque psoriasis: Results of the randomized phase 3 CADMUS study. *J Am Acad Dermatol* 2015;73(4):594-603.
23. Nouri A, Walmsley D, Pruszczynski B, Synder M: Transient synovitis of the hip: A comprehensive review. *J Pediatr Orthop B* 2014;23(1):32-36.
24. Liberman B, Herman A, Schindler A, Sherr-Lurie N, Ganel A, Givon U: The value of hip aspiration in pediatric transient synovitis. *J Pediatr Orthop* 2013;33(2):124-127.

25. Taekema HC, Landham PR, Maconochie I: Towards evidence based medicine for paediatricians: Distinguishing between transient synovitis and septic arthritis in the limping child. How useful are clinical prediction tools? *Arch Dis Child* 2009;94(2):167-168.
26. Shulman ST, Ayoub EM: Poststreptococcal reactive arthritis. *Curr Opin Rheumatol* 2002;14(5):562-565.
27. van der Helm-van Mil AHM: Acute rheumatic fever and poststreptococcal reactive arthritis reconsidered. *Curr Opin Rheumatol* 2010;22(4):437-442.
28. Mead PS: Epidemiology of Lyme disease. *Infect Dis Clin North Am* 2015;29(2):187-210.
29. Sood SK: Lyme disease in children. *Infect Dis Clin North Am* 2015;29(2):281-294.
30. Oliveira CR, Shapiro ED: Update on persistent symptoms associated with Lyme disease. *Curr Opin Pediatr* 2015;27(1):100-104.
31. Esposito S, Bosis S, Sabatini C, Tagliaferri L, Principi N: Borrelia burgdorferi infection and Lyme disease in children. *Int J Infect Dis* 2013;17(3):e153-e158.
32. O'Connell S: Lyme borreliosis: Current issues in diagnosis and management. *Curr Opin Infect Dis* 2010;23(3):231-235.
33. Walsh P, Manners PJ, Vercoe J, Burgner D, Murray KJ: Chronic recurrent multifocal osteomyelitis in children: Nine years' experience at a statewide tertiary paediatric rheumatology referral centre. *Rheumatology (Oxford)* 2015;54(9):1688-1691.
34. Wipff J, Costantino F, Lemelle I, et al: A large national cohort of French patients with chronic recurrent multifocal osteitis. *Arthritis Rheumatol* 2015;67(4):1128-1137.
35. Scianaro R, Insalaco A, Bracci Laudiero L, et al: Deregulation of the IL-1β axis in chronic recurrent multifocal osteomyelitis. *Pediatr Rheumatol Online J* 2014;12:30.
36. Ferguson PJ, Sandu M: Current understanding of the pathogenesis and management of chronic recurrent multifocal osteomyelitis. *Curr Rheumatol Rep* 2012;14(2):130-141.
37. von Kalle T, Heim N, Hospach T, Langendörfer M, Winkler P, Stuber T: Typical patterns of bone involvement in whole-body MRI of patients with chronic recurrent multifocal osteomyelitis (CRMO). *Rofo* 2013;185(7):655-661.
38. Falip C, Alison M, Boutry N, et al: Chronic recurrent multifocal osteomyelitis (CRMO): A longitudinal case series review. *Pediatr Radiol* 2013;43(3):355-375.
39. Guérin-Pfyffer S, Guillaume-Czitrom S, Tammam S, Koné-Paut I: Evaluation of chronic recurrent multifocal osteitis in children by whole-body magnetic resonance imaging. *Joint Bone Spine* 2012;79(6):616-620.
40. Fritz J, Tzaribachev N, Thomas C, et al: Magnetic resonance imaging-guided osseous biopsy in children with chronic recurrent multifocal osteomyelitis. *Cardiovasc Intervent Radiol* 2012;35(1):146-153.
41. Jibri Z, Sah M, Mansour R: Chronic recurrent multifocal osteomyelitis mimicking osteoid osteoma. *JBR-BTR* 2012;95(4):263-266.
42. Eleftheriou D, Gerschman T, Sebire N, Woo P, Pilkington CA, Brogan PA: Biologic therapy in refractory chronic nonbacterial osteomyelitis of childhood. *Rheumatology (Oxford)* 2010;49(8):1505-1512.
43. Santiago MB, Galvão V: Jaccoud arthropathy in systemic lupus erythematosus: Analysis of clinical characteristics and review of the literature. *Medicine (Baltimore)* 2008;87(1):37-44.
44. Tucker LB: Making the diagnosis of systemic lupus erythematosus in children and adolescents. *Lupus* 2007;16(8):546-549.
45. Quartier P, Gherardi RK: Juvenile dermatomyositis. *Handb Clin Neurol* 2013;113:1457-1463.
46. Gong GW, McCrindle BW, Ching JC, Yeung RS: Arthritis presenting during the acute phase of Kawasaki disease. *J Pediatr* 2006;148(6):800-805.
47. Yang YH, Yu HH, Chiang BL: The diagnosis and classification of Henoch-Schönlein purpura: An updated review. *Autoimmun Rev* 2014;13(4-5):355-358.
48. Twilt M, Benseler S, Cabral D: Granulomatosis with polyangiitis in childhood. *Curr Rheumatol Rep* 2012;14(2):107-115.
49. Wouters CH, Maes A, Foley KP, Bertin J, Rose CD: Blau syndrome: The prototypic auto-inflammatory granulomatous disease. *Pediatr Rheumatol Online J* 2014;12:33.

SECTION 4

Upper Extremity

Section Editor:
Charles A. Goldfarb, MD, FAAOS

CHAPTER 20

Congenital Upper Limb Differences

LINDLEY B. WALL, MD, MSc • CHARLES A. GOLDFARB, MD, FAAOS

ABSTRACT

Congenital upper limb anomalies are uncommon and treatment advances have progressed slowly using information gained from retrospective analyses and reports of evolving surgical techniques. Subjective outcome information is becoming more readily available and will help understand the best treatment for both function and aesthetics moving forward.

Keywords: congenital; limb development; upper extremity; upper limb

INTRODUCTION

The upper limbs develop within the first 2 months of gestation. The upper limb buds begin to emerge at 4 weeks of gestation and achieve final formation at approximately 8 weeks. As the fetus continues to grow, the hands double in size by the time of birth, and the hands again double in size from birth to 2 years of age and then nearly again from 2 years of age to skeletal maturity. The upper limbs develop by a complex interaction of multiple factors along three axes: proximal-distal, anterior-posterior (radioulnar), and dorsal-ventral. Proximal-distal development results from signaling between the apical ectodermal ridge and the underlying mesoderm, primarily through the secretion of fibroblast growth factors. Anterior-posterior development, which results in differentiation between the radial and ulnar aspects of the upper limb, is guided by the release of Sonic Hedgehog morphogen from the zone of polarizing activity located on the posterior aspect of the limb bud. Dorsal-ventral differentiation occurs through signaling of WNT-7a, which allows for development of dorsal structures such as nails.[1]

A better understanding of developmental biology has influenced the classification of congenital upper limb anomalies. In 2013, the Oberg, Manske, and Tonkin (OMT) scheme has been used to classify congenital upper limb anomalies using current knowledge of limb development.[2] In 2014, a modified OMT classification system was accepted by the International Federation of Societies for Surgery of the Hand.

Using the OMT classification system, recent studies have reported both the prevalence and the epidemiology of congenital upper limb anomalies. Two studies from Scandinavia reported an incidence ranging from 5.25 to 21.5 per 10,000 live births;[3,4] the difference between the studies was based on inclusion criteria. Failure of differentiation was the most common pattern, followed by duplication and failure of formation. Radial ray deficiencies were the most common anomaly identified in the Finnish study.[4] A US study reported limb malformations as the most common type of anomaly, specifically those affecting the hand plate, with radial polydactyly being the most frequently reported.[5] More recently, hand plate malformations were also found to be the most common congenital upper limb anomaly in a large multicenter US registry. Continued research efforts will likely contribute to a better understanding of upper limb discrepancies and a more accurate determination of their prevalence.[6]

Dr. Goldfarb or an immediate family member is a member of a speakers' bureau or has made paid presentations on behalf of Arthrex, Inc. and serves as a board member, owner, officer, or committee member of the American Orthopaedic Association. Neither Dr. Wall nor any immediate family member has received anything of value from or has stock or stock options held in a commercial company or institution related directly or indirectly to the subject of this chapter.

MALFORMATIONS

Entire Limb

Transverse Deficiency

A transverse deficiency most commonly relates to a diagnosis of symbrachydactyly. The proposed etiology for symbrachydactyly is a prenatal vascular insult.[7] An insufficient vascular supply to the progress zone of the growing limb results in a truncated limb. This mesodermal insult results in a truncated limb, often with the presence of small nubbins of ectodermal origin (including nails and small tufts of bone). The proximal third of the forearm is the most common level of deficiency. The level of truncation varies and may also occur through the elbow, or more distally.

Historically, treatment of children with this deficiency included prosthetic fitting at approximately 6 months of age or when the child had achieved sitting balance. However, because prosthetic limbs are heavy and can interfere with sensory input, the philosophy concerning the fitting of an upper limb prosthesis has changed. Currently, it has been shown that upper limb prostheses do not improve function or quality of life, although they may be useful for specific tasks or functions.[8] Therefore, upper limb prosthetic fitting should not be universally performed, but should be provided when requested by the patient or family.

Radial Longitudinal Deficiency

A radial longitudinal deficiency (RLD) results from a failure of formation of the radial aspect of the forearm and hand. Historically, classification systems concentrated on the presence and length of the radius, whereas newer classification modifications include the carpus and proximal limb.[9,10] An RLD is often associated with other medical conditions and syndromes such as thrombocytopenia absent radius syndrome, Holt-Oram syndrome, Fanconi anemia, and vertebral-anal-cardiac-tracheal-esophageal-renal-limb association.

Pediatric orthopaedic surgeons and hand surgeons play a critical role in evaluating children with RLD for associated medical conditions because they may be the first physicians to examine these patients. Spinal radiographs, cardiac and renal ultrasonography studies, and a complete blood count with differential are recommended for children with RLD. Smaller children with atypical facial features and café-au-lait spots should be evaluated for Fanconi anemia; the chromosomal challenge test is most commonly used for confirmation.

RLD of the forearm results in hypoplasia or aplasia of the radius. This anomaly results in a short forearm and radial deviation of the wrist (**Figure 1**). In a young child, radial deviation is initially treated with stretching and splinting. As the child ages, wrist deformities can be surgically treated to improve the position of the hand in relation

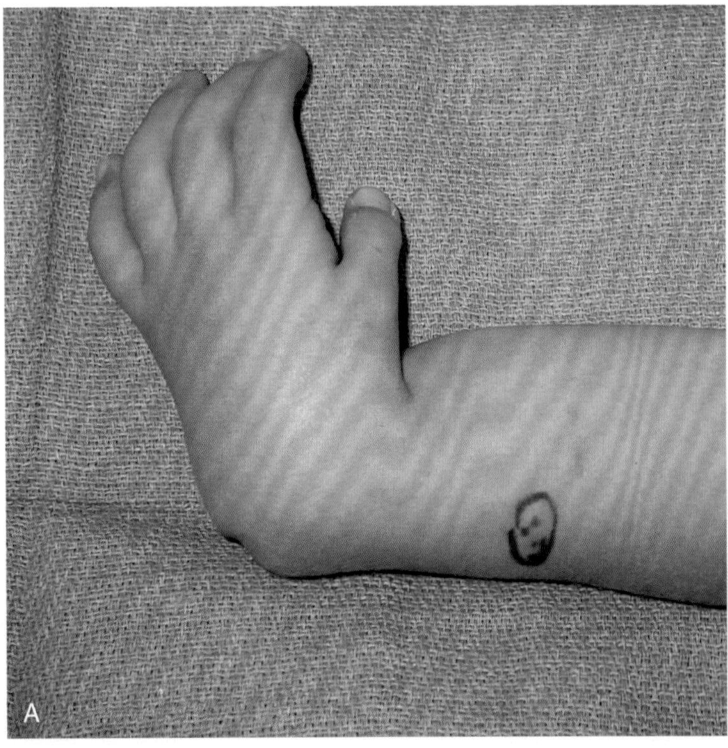

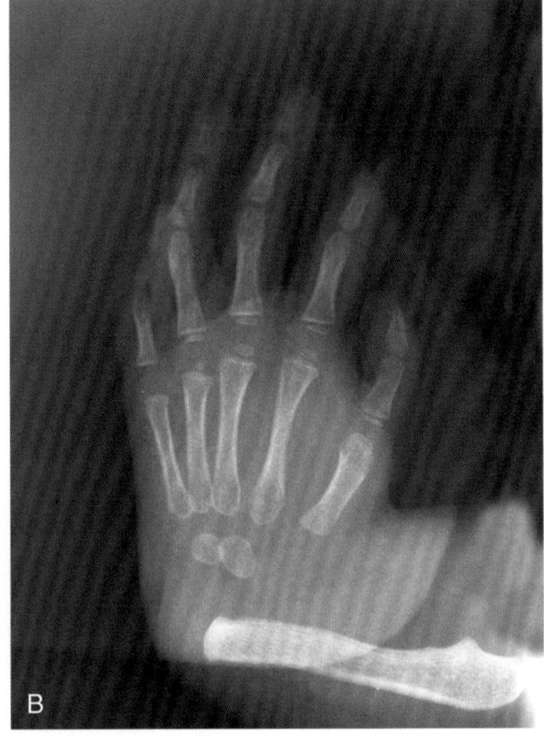

FIGURE 1 Clinical (**A**) and radiographic (**B**) images of a radial longitudinal deficiency.

to the forearm. Classically, these children were treated with an acute centralization of the wrist, which involved an extensive soft-tissue release and placement of the hand on top of the distal ulna with pin fixation. Radialization is a variation of centralization in which tendons are transferred to the ulnar wrist at the time of wrist centralization.[11] More than 20 years of long-term follow-up of patients treated with centralization/radialization compared with those who were treated nonsurgically showed that the surgically treated patients had better cosmetic outcomes along with improved finger and wrist motion, grip strength, and increased ease in performing functional daily activities.[12]

More recently, the use of soft-tissue distraction followed by a staged centralization procedure has been described.[13-16] This technique allows for less extensive soft-tissue release and easier wrist positioning. During centralization, the surgeon must take care to prevent injury to the distal ulna physis to prevent additional shortening of an already short forearm.

An alternative approach uses a volar bilobed flap with soft-tissue release to maintain motion of the wrist and decrease radial deviation.[17] If desired, this procedure may be followed by a free vascularized metatarsophalangeal joint transfer to stabilize the radial aspect of the wrist.[18] Currently, the optimal treatment of radial deviation of the wrist in patients with RLD is debatable, and some surgeons advocate for observation alone.

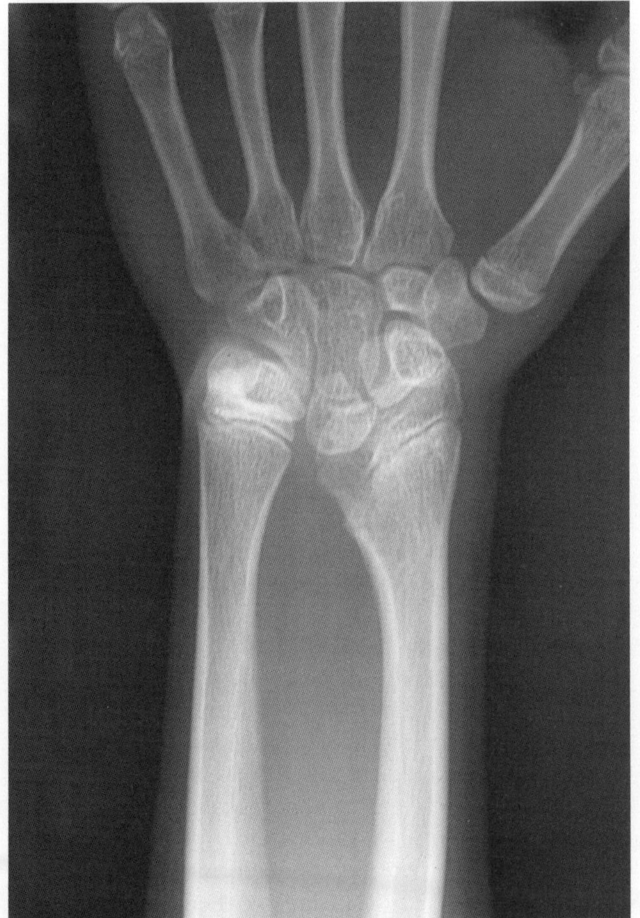

FIGURE 2 AP radiograph shows typical appearance of a Madelung deformity, with increased radial tilt, ulnar translation of the carpus, and triangulation of the carpus.

Ulnar Longitudinal Deficiency

Ulnar longitudinal deficiency (ULD) results from failure of formation of the ulnar aspect of the forearm and hand. Unlike RLD, ULD is not associated with internal organ anomalies, but it can be associated with fibular hemimelia and proximal focal femoral deficiency. ULD also can extend proximally and affect the elbow, including radiohumeral synostosis. Classically, children with ULD are described as having a hand that seems to rest in a backward position; however, these children typically have high functional ability. The performance of daily tasks may become more challenging with growth because children may no longer be able to reach their hands to their mouth. If necessary, an osteotomy of the synostosis and repositioning of the limb may improve function. Alternatively, surgery may focus primarily on the hand.

Madelung Deformity

Madelung deformity is a condition involving abnormal growth of the distal radial physis. The condition can be idiopathic or can result from an autosomal dominant trait with variable penetrance. When associated with Léri-Weill dyschondrosteosis, a form of mesomelic dwarfism, Madelung deformity is associated with a *SHOX* gene (short stature homeobox gene) deficiency.[19] Clinically and radiographically, the wrist is translated volarly and ulnarly. There is limited growth at the volar ulnar aspect of the distal radial physis, which results in an increase in radial tilt, ulnar translation of the carpus, triangulation of the carpus, and a prominent dorsal distal ulna[20] (**Figure 2**). Often, there is a thick volar ligament (Vickers ligament) that tethers the lunate to the distal radial metaphysis and is believed by some to contribute to the deformity. The severity of Madelung deformity varies. In some patients, the entire length of the radius is affected, whereas in others it is only the distal aspect of the radius.[21]

Madelung deformity typically presents in early adolescence and is characterized by the wrist deformity, mild limitation of wrist and forearm motion, and variable wrist pain. Treatment of the deformity may subsequently improve range of motion and reduce pain. The recommended treatment includes excision of the Vickers ligament and a dome osteotomy of the distal radius, which corrects the distal radial deformity in multiple planes.[22] Results of this treatment at an average 11-year follow-up showed maintenance of motion and deformity correction. Patients with more severe deformity had worse functional and radiographic outcomes.[23] In young patients without pain, who have mild deformity and growth remaining, ligament release may be considered to minimize the development of wrist deformity,[24] maintain motion, and limit future pain.

Hand Plate Only

Symbrachydactyly

Symbrachydactyly affecting the hand plate can have a range of presentations from shortened to absent digits.[25] Short-finger symbrachydactyly varies in severity and may occur with or without syndactyly. Although patients with symbrachydactyly often do not need treatment, deepening of the web spaces may be considered. Short-finger symbrachydactyly may be associated with Poland syndrome, with hypoplasia of the ipsilateral chest wall muscles and thorax.

Cleft-type symbrachydactyly is characterized by an ulnar-sided digit and thumb; nubbins may be present within the U-shaped cleft. The severity of thumb involvement is predictive of the child's ability to use the hand. If the thumb can be opposed to the ulnar-sided digit, function can be excellent. If the thumb is positioned in the plane of the hand, side-to-side pinch is used and function is more limited. The thumb position and function can be improved with an osteotomy for length and rotational realignment.

Monodactylous symbrachydactyly is the presence of a single digit, a thumb. Although most children with this type of symbrachydactyly have good hand function, some patients will benefit from the creation or lengthening of an ulnar-sided digit to provide a post for thumb pinch.[26-28] Peromelic symbrachydactyly is a hand with or without nubbins and with varying levels of deficiency (metacarpal, carpal, or through the radiocarpal joint). No true digits exist.

Overall, the goals of symbrachydactyly treatment are to improve a child's functional ability and optimize his or her independence and hand use. Frequently, these children have good functional abilities, because symbrachydactyly is a unilateral condition.

Radial Longitudinal Deficiency

RLD affecting the hand plate results in carpal hypoplasia and/or thumb hypoplasia or aplasia. Children with RLD are medically evaluated as previously detailed. Typically, carpal anomalies do not require treatment. Thumb involvement in RLD ranges from a small thumb to complete thumb aplasia as classified by the Blauth classification system.[29] The authors of a 1995 study[30] modified the Blauth classification based on the stability of the thumb carpometacarpal joint. This modification has implications with regard to the treatment of hypoplastic thumbs.

Blauth type I thumbs are small but have well-developed structures and do not need treatment. Type II thumbs have hypoplastic intrinsic thenar muscles and thumb metacarpophalangeal (MCP) joint laxity and often are improved by either a Huber or flexor digitorum superficialis opponensplasty. The Huber opponensplasty is a rotational flap of the adductor digiti minimi muscle to the radial side of the thumb. This flap must often be supplemented by capsular imbrication of the ulnar side of the MCP joint to manage instability. The flexor digitorum superficialis opponensplasty uses the flexor digitorum superficialis tendon from the ring finger, transferring it across the palm to the thumb MCP joint; the extra tendon length is used to reconstruct the ulnar collateral ligament. Similar reconstruction is applied to type IIIA hypoplastic thumbs. Type III thumbs also demonstrate hypoplasia of the thumb extrinsic muscles, which may need to be treated with tendon transfers. In the Western world, thumbs classified as Blauth types IIIB, IV, or V are treated with index finger pollicization. The hypoplastic thumb is removed (types IIIB and IV), and the index finger is shortened through the metacarpal and repositioned 90° to 110° from the middle finger and abducted out of the plane of the hand.[30] In contrast, Eastern cultures are most likely to reconstruct types IIIB and IV thumbs rather than pollicize.

Ulnar Longitudinal Deficiency

ULD of the hand includes hypoplasia or absence of the ulnar-sided structures. There are two commonly used classification systems for ULD of the hand. ULD of the hand was originally classified according to the number of absent digits.[31] Alternatively, the authors of a 1997 study[32] classified ULD based on the degree of narrowing of the first web space, which directly correlates with functional use of the hand. Management of the ulnar-deficient hand includes deepening of a narrowed first web space and rotational osteotomy of the thumb to improve pinch and grasp as indicated.

Radial Polydactyly

Radial polydactyly or preaxial polydactyly is the presence of an additional thumb. The classification of thumb polydactyly is based on the level of duplication, starting with the distal phalanx and extending to the metacarpal level.[33] A Flatt type IV thumb, with duplication at the level of the MCP joint, is the most common type (**Figure 3**).

Patients with thumb polydactyly often have reasonable function, but the additional thumb is aesthetically abnormal. Reconstruction procedures depend on the level of duplication but include removal of the more hypoplastic thumb, typically the more radial thumb, and reconstruction of the remaining thumb to provide a straight and stable thumb. In selected types, including Flatt types I and II, reconstruction includes either excision of the smaller thumb and stabilization of the remaining thumb or surgical combination of the thumbs, which is technically more challenging.[34-36] To achieve a stable thumb in

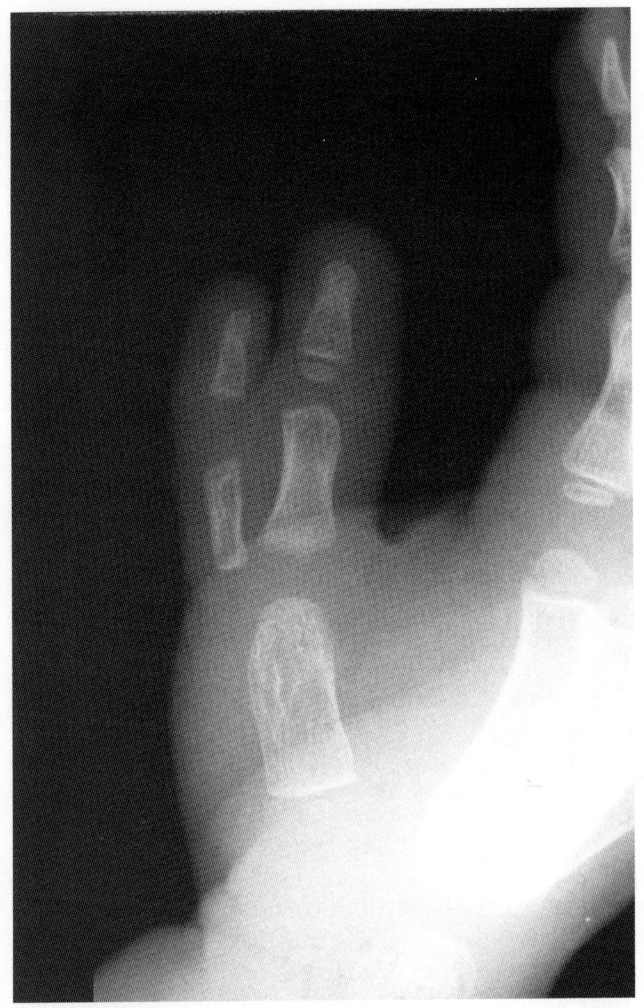

FIGURE 3 Radiograph shows a Flatt type IV radial polydactyly with duplication at the level of the proximal phalanx.

Flatt type IV thumbs, the radial collateral ligament of the MCP joint is re-created with a periosteal sleeve from the excised radial thumb, which it typically the smaller thumb. Residual deformity is treated with an osteotomy to correct angulation. Eccentric insertion of the flexor and/or the extensor tendons may be present and create an abnormal line of pull contributing to angulation. For correction, the tendons can be elevated and reinserted to direct the tendon force more centrally.

Clinical outcomes assessments report that remaining thumb angulation and reduced nail width are associated with decreased patient satisfaction.[37] Long-term follow-up results from polydactyly reconstructions were reported at an average follow-up of more than 10 years. A revision rate of 19% was reported, and in 50% of these revisions, arthrodesis for joint instability and pain was performed. Flatt type III and IV thumbs had weaker pinch than the contralateral side. All of the patients were satisfied with their surgical outcomes.[38]

Ulnar Polydactyly

Ulnar polydactyly (postaxial polydactyly) is duplication of the small finger. This is one of the most common congenital anomalies and is predominantly seen in individuals of African descent. The level of duplication ranges from a small taglike digit (type B) to a complete duplication of the small finger ray (type A), as classified by the authors of a 1969 study.[39] The type B fingers are often tied off in the nursery and may never be evaluated by a surgeon.

In 2013, type A polydactyly has been further classified according to the level of duplication.[40] An associated syndrome or additional congenital anomaly was reported in 24% of the individuals evaluated; however, there is no standard recommendation for syndromic workup in these patients. Type A polydactyly is equally seen in Caucasian patients and those of African descent in contrast to type B polydactyly.

Reconstruction of ulnar polydactyly is a more straightforward procedure than radial polydactyly reconstruction. Type B digits can be tied off with suture or clipped at the base of the stalk. If the base is greater than 1 cm in width, surgical excision is the most reliable treatment. Type A digits are removed surgically, and the ulnar collateral ligament of the small finger MCP joint may be reconstructed with a periosteal flap from the excised digit. Stability is less of a concern with the small finger compared with the thumb.

Syndactyly

Syndactyly results from incomplete recession of the interdigital skin during limb development—a failure of apoptosis. Syndactyly is classified by the extent of involvement and presence of an osseous connection. Syndactyly that extends the entire length of the digits is called complete syndactyly, whereas lesser involvement is termed partial or incomplete syndactyly. Cutaneous syndactyly describes digits that are connected simply by skin. In contrast, a complex syndactyly consists of a bony bridge between the two digits, typically seen at the distal phalanges. When syndactyly is associated with a syndrome, it is classified as complicated. Bilateral involvement is often observed. Involvement of the third web, between the long and ring fingers, is the most common presentation. When ulnar-sided syndactyly involving the small and ring finger is present, the possible association with oculodentodigital dysplasia syndrome should be evaluated[41] (**Figure 4**). In addition to hand involvement, this autosomal dominant condition may include dental and urologic abnormalities as well as progressive neurologic problems including paraparesis and cognitive difficulties. Patients with oculodentodigital dysplasia syndrome should be referred to appropriate subspecialists to identify and treat the associated conditions in a timely manner.

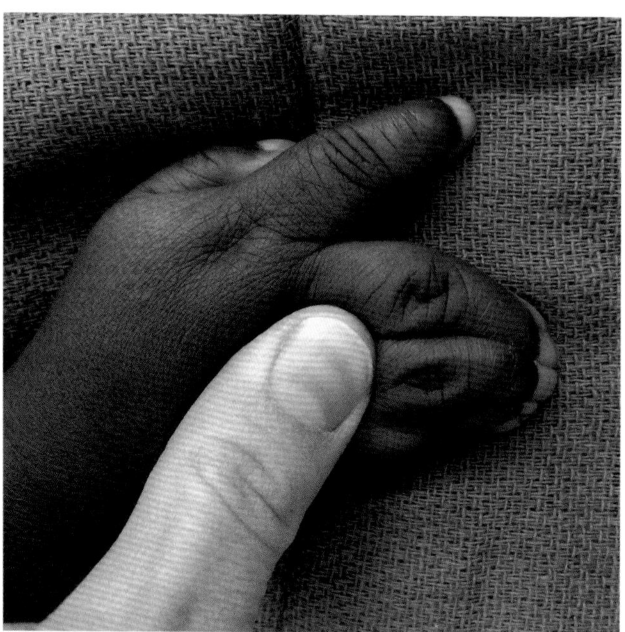

FIGURE 4 Clinical image of the hand of a child with oculodentodigital dysplasia. Note the ulnar-sided syndactyly.

Syndactyly reconstruction of central web spaces is recommended for children at 18 months to 2 years of age.[42,43] If there is syndactyly involving the border digits, earlier reconstruction, before 1 year of age, is advised to prevent contractures or deviation of the tethered digits.

Numerous techniques for syndactyly treatment have been described, including reconstruction with or without skin grafting.[44-47] Techniques that do not use skin grafts require less surgical time and have no donor-site morbidity. Skin grafts can also have a less than optimal aesthetic appearance because of darkening over time and the potential for hair growth if skin is harvested from the groin. The advantages of skin grafting include decreasing the dorsal scar, providing complete wound coverage, and minimizing creep. If skin grafting is used, it can be harvested from the antecubital fossa or wrist flexion crease. In 2014, the use of synthetic matrix has been reported in place of skin grafts for open areas after reconstruction.[48] This technique minimizes surgical time, morbidity, and scarring. Outcome evidence is limited at this time.

DEFORMATIONS

Amniotic Band Syndrome

Amniotic band syndrome (ABS) is a condition characterized by circumferential bands around the limbs, acrosyndactyly (fenestrated syndactyly), and amputated digits (**Figure 5**). The etiology of ABS is still unknown, but there are two prevailing theories: intrinsic and extrinsic.[49] The intrinsic theory hypothesizes that there is a genetic

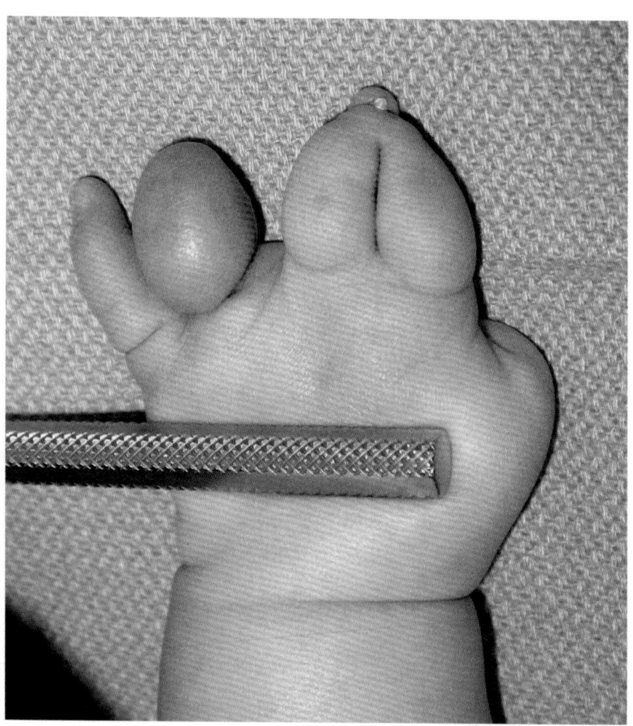

FIGURE 5 Clinical image of the hand of an infant with amniotic band syndrome. Note the constrictive band around the ring finger with distal amputation and acrosyndactyly between the index and middle digits.

etiology for the bands. The common association of ABS with cleft palate supports this theory. In contrast, the extrinsic theory states that bands of amnion form and then wrap around the limbs and digits. This theory is supported by the presence of bands seen at birth and fused distal segments of digits with developed web spaces (acrosyndactyly).

Reconstruction of hands affected by ABS includes release of the fused digits, with skin grafting as needed, and release of bands. Band reconstruction is performed by full-thickness band excision and repair with Z-plasty to break up the resulting scar.

DYSPLASIAS

Amniotic Band Syndrome

Osteochondromatosis or multiple hereditary exostosis is a condition affecting the entire skeletal system. The condition results from mutations in the exostosin (*EXT*) genes (specifically *EXT1* or *EXT2* genes) and is autosomal dominant. Benign bony growths occur as the child grows, primarily at the ends of long bones or on flat bones, such as the scapula. The exostoses appear in childhood and then stop growing after the individual reaches skeletal maturity. If the exostoses continue to grow after skeletal maturity, evaluation for malignant transformation is needed.

With increasing size, the exostoses can cause pain or limb deformity, irritate adjacent structures including nerves, or limit joint motion. In any of these instances, surgery is indicated. Within the upper limbs, forearm exostoses can alter the growth and relationship of the radius and the ulna. Notably, distal ulnar exostoses can tether the distal radius and, over time, lead to radial head dislocation.[50] In addition, it has been shown that both decreased ulnar length and radial head dislocation are risk factors for limited forearm motion.[51]

Varied surgical approaches are available to treat forearm exostoses, with the goals of maintenance of forearm rotation and avoidance of radial head dislocation. One approach is the excision of exostoses and lengthening or corrective osteotomy of the radius or ulna. Alternatively, the radius and ulna can be untethered to allow continued but independent growth. The ideal timing for surgical treatment is currently unknown. Children can be monitored with serial radiographic studies; however, some investigators have found that simple excision of the exostoses is the optimal treatment of forearm exostoses.[52]

SUMMARY

Congenital upper limb anomalies are uncommon. Efforts continue to determine the actual prevalence and effects of these conditions on the global population. The functional and aesthetic implications of each anomaly are unique, and surgical intervention is dependent on the needs of the child and perspective of his or her family. Unfortunately, most research concerning surgical treatment is currently limited to small retrospective studies. There is a need for large, multicenter, prospective studies to advance the care of patients with congenital upper limb anomalies.

KEY STUDY POINTS

- The OMT classification is accepted for classifying congenital upper limb anomalies and is based on the developmental biology of the upper limb.
- Unilateral anomalies are often well tolerated; the child is able to compensate with the well-developed limb for function.
- The surgeon may be the first physician to identify a specific congenital anomaly in a child and therefore must be aware of associated conditions and syndromes and recommend appropriate testing or referral.

ANNOTATED REFERENCES

1. Sammer DM, Chung KC: Congenital hand differences: Embryology and classification. *Hand Clin* 2009;25:151-156.
2. Tonkin MA, Tolerton SK, Quick TJ, et al: Classification of congenital anomalies of the hand and upper limb: Development and assessment of a new system. *J Hand Surg Am* 2013;38:1845-1853.
3. Ekblom AG, Laurell T, Arner M: Epidemiology of congenital upper limb anomalies in Stockholm, Sweden, 1997 to 2007: Application of the Oberg, Manske, and Tonkin classification. *J Hand Surg Am* 2014;39:237-248.
4. Koskimies E, Lindfors N, Gissler M, Peltonen J, Nietosvaara Y: Congenital upper limb deficiencies and associated malformations in Finland: A population-based study. *J Hand Surg Am* 2011;36:1058-1065.
5. Goldfarb CA, Wall LB, Bohn DC, Moen P, Van Heest AE: Epidemiology of congenital upper limb anomalies in a midwest United States population: An assessment using the Oberg, Manske, and Tonkin classification. *J Hand Surg Am* 2015;40:127-132.e121-122.
6. Bae DS, Canizares MF, Miller PE, Waters PM, Goldfarb CA: Functional impact of congenital hand differences: Early results from the Congenital Upper Limb Differences (CoULD) Registry. *J Hand Surg Am* 2018;43:321-330.

   This study includes a description of the Congenital Upper Limb Differences Registry and early results based on the OMT. Level of evidence: III.
7. Bavinck JN, Weaver DD: Subclavian artery supply disruption sequence: Hypothesis of a vascular etiology for Poland, Klippel-Feil, and Mobius anomalies. *Am J Med Genet* 1986;23:903-918.
8. James MA, Bagley AM, Brasington K, et al: Impact of prostheses on function and quality of life for children with unilateral congenital below-the-elbow deficiency. *J Bone Joint Surg Am* 2006;88:2356-2365.
9. James MA, Green HD, McCarroll HR Jr, Manske PR: The association of radial deficiency with thumb hypoplasia. *J Bone Joint Surg Am* 2004;86:2196-2205.
10. Goldfarb CA, Manske PR, Busa R, et al: Upper-extremity phocomelia reexamined: A longitudinal dysplasia. *J Bone Joint Surg Am* 2005;87:2639-2648.
11. Buck-Gramcko D Radialization as a new treatment for radial club hand. *J Hand Surg Am* 1985;10:964-968.
12. Kotwal PP, Varshney MK, Soral A: Comparison of surgical treatment and nonoperative management for radial longitudinal deficiency. *J Hand Surg Eur Vol* 2012;37:161-169.
13. Damore E, Kozin SH, Thoder JJ, Porter S: The recurrence of deformity after surgical centralization for radial clubhand. *J Hand Surg Am* 2000;25:745-751.
14. Goldfarb CA, Murtha YM, Gordon JE, Manske PR: Soft-tissue distraction with a ring external fixator before centralization for radial longitudinal deficiency. *J Hand Surg Am* 2006;31:952-959.
15. Sabharwal S, Finuoli AL, Ghobadi F: Pre-centralization soft tissue distraction for Bayne type IV congenital radial deficiency in children. *J Pediatr Orthop* 2005;25:377-381.
16. Taghinia AH, Al-Sheikh AA, Upton J: Preoperative soft-tissue distraction for radial longitudinal deficiency: An analysis of indications and outcomes. *Plast Reconstr Surg* 2007;120:1305-1312, discussion 1313-1304.

17. Vuillermin C, Wall L, Mills J, et al: Soft tissue release and bilobed flap for severe radial longitudinal deficiency. *J Hand Surg Am* 2015;40:894-899.
18. de Jong JP, Moran SL, Vilkki SK: Changing paradigms in the treatment of radial club hand: Microvascular joint transfer for correction of radial deviation and preservation of long-term growth. *Clin Orthop Surg* 2012;4:36-44.
19. Leri-Weill. Dyschondrosteosis. Online Mendelian Inheritance in Man. Available at: http://omim.org/entry/127300. 2016.
20. McCarroll HR Jr, James MA, Newmeyer WL III, Molitor F, Manske PR: Madelung's deformity: Quantitative assessment of x-ray deformity. *J Hand Surg Am* 2005;30:1211-1220.
21. Zebala LP, Manske PR, Goldfarb CA: Madelung's deformity: A spectrum of presentation. *J Hand Surg Am* 2007;32:1393-1401.
22. Harley BJ, Brown C, Cummings K, Carter PR, Ezaki M: Volar ligament release and distal radius dome osteotomy for correction of Madelung's deformity. *J Hand Surg Am* 2006;31:1499-1506.
23. Steinman S, Oishi S, Mills J, et al: Volar ligament release and distal radial dome osteotomy for the correction of Madelung deformity: Long-term follow-up. *J Bone Joint Surg Am* 2013;95:1198-1204.

    Six patients (12 wrists) with Madelungs were treated with Vickers ligament release and physiolysis between 7 to 9 years of age. The surgery was safe and improved radial inclination was noted in most patients. Level of evidence: IV.
24. Otte JE, Popp JE, Samora JB: Treatment of Madelung deformity with Vicker ligament release and radial physiolyses: A case series. *J Hand Surg Am* 2019;44:158 e151-158 e159.

    Level of evidence: V.
25. Ogino T, Minami A, Kato H: Clinical features and roentgenograms of symbrachydactyly. *J Hand Surg Br* 1989;14:303-306.
26. Dhalla R, Strecker W, Manske PR: A comparison of two techniques for digital distraction lengthening in skeletally immature patients. *J Hand Surg Am* 2001;26:603-610.
27. Goldberg NH, Watson HK: Composite toe (phalanx and epiphysis) transfers in the reconstruction of the aphalangic hand. *J Hand Surg Am* 1982;7:454-459.
28. Kay SP, Wiberg M: Toe to hand transfer in children. Part 1: Technical aspects. *J Hand Surg Br* 1996;21:723-734.
29. Blauth W: The hypoplastic thumb. *Arch Orthop Unfallchir* 1967;62:225-246.
30. Manske PR, McCarroll HR, Jr, James M: Type III-A hypoplastic thumb. *J Hand Surg Am* 1995;20:246-253.
31. Ogino T, Kato H: Clinical and experimental studies on ulnar ray deficiency. *Handchir Mikrochir Plast Chir* 1988;20:330-337.
32. Cole RJ, Manske PR: Classification of ulnar deficiency according to the thumb and first web. *J Hand Surg Am* 1997;22:479-488.
33. Wassel HD: The results of surgery for polydactyly of the thumb: A review. *Clin Orthop Relat Res* 1969;64:175-193.
34. Tonkin MA, Bulstrode NW: The Bilhaut-Cloquet procedure for Wassel types III, IV and VII thumb duplication. *J Hand Surg Eur Vol* 2007;32:684-693.
35. Baek GH, Gong HS, Chung MS, et al: Modified Bilhaut-Cloquet procedure for Wassel type-II and III polydactyly of the thumb. Surgical technique. *J Bone Joint Surg Am* 2008;90(suppl 2, pt 1):74-86.
36. Baek GH, Gong HS, Chung MS, et al: Modified Bilhaut-Cloquet procedure for Wassel type-II and III polydactyly of the thumb. *J Bone Joint Surg Am* 2007;89:534-541.
37. Goldfarb CA, Patterson JM, Maender A, Manske PR: Thumb size and appearance following reconstruction of radial polydactyly. *J Hand Surg Am* 2008;33:1348-1353.
38. Stutz C, Mills J, Wheeler L, Ezaki M, Oishi S: Long-term outcomes following radial polydactyly reconstruction. *J Hand Surg Am* 2014;39:1549-1552.
39. Temtamy S, McKusick V: Synopsis of hand malformations with particular emphasis on genetic factors. *Birth Defects* 1969;3:125-184.
40. Pritsch T, Ezaki M, Mills J, Oishi SN: Type A ulnar polydactyly of the hand: A classification system and clinical series. *J Hand Surg Am* 2013;38:453-458.
41. Jones C, Baldrighi C, Mills J, et al: Oculodentodigital dysplasia: Ulnar-sided syndactyly and its associated disorders. *J Hand Surg Am* 2011;36:1816-1821.
42. Hutchinson DT, Frenzen SW: Digital syndactyly release. *Tech Hand Up Extrem Surg* 2010;14:33-37.
43. Dao KD, Shin AY, Billings A, Oberg KC, Wood VE: Surgical treatment of congenital syndactyly of the hand. *J Am Acad Orthop Surg* 2004;12:39-48.
44. Aydin A, Ozden BC: Dorsal metacarpal island flap in syndactyly treatment. *Ann Plast Surg* 2004;52:43-48.
45. Wafa AM: Hourglass dorsal metacarpal island flap: A new design for syndactylized web reconstruction. *J Hand Surg Am* 2008;33:905-908.
46. Greuse M, Coessens BC: Congenital syndactyly: Defatting facilitates closure without skin graft. *J Hand Surg Am* 2001;26:589-594.
47. Withey SJ, Kangesu T, Carver N, Sommerlad BC: The open finger technique for the release of syndactyly. *J Hand Surg Br* 2001;26:4-7.
48. Landi A, Garagnani L, Leti Acciaro A, et al: Hyaluronic acid scaffold for skin defects in congenital syndactyly release surgery: A novel technique based on the regenerative model. *J Hand Surg Eur Vol* 2014;39:994-1000.
49. Goldfarb CA, Sathienkijkanchai A, Robin NH: Amniotic constriction band: A multidisciplinary assessment of etiology and clinical presentation. *J Bone Joint Surg Am* 2009;91(suppl 4): 68-75.

50. Gottschalk HP, Kanauchi Y, Bednar MS, Light TR: Effect of osteochondroma location on forearm deformity in patients with multiple hereditary osteochondromatosis. *J Hand Surg Am* 2012;37:2286-2293.
51. Clement ND, Porter DE: Forearm deformity in patients with hereditary multiple exostoses: Factors associated with range of motion and radial head dislocation. *J Bone Joint Surg Am* 2013;95:1586-1592.
52. Akita S, Murase T, Yonenobu K, et al: Long-term results of surgery for forearm deformities in patients with multiple cartilaginous exostoses. *J Bone Joint Surg Am* 2007;89:1993-1999.

CHAPTER 21

Brachial Plexus Birth Injuries

ANN E. VAN HEEST, MD • DAVID M. MATSON, MD

ABSTRACT

During the birthing process, injuries can occur to the brachial plexus, which affect both motor and sensory functions of the upper limb. These injuries can be classified based on the anatomic characterization of the neurologic deficit. The patient evaluation primarily relies on serial physical examinations to track neurologic recovery, which is commonly documented using validated assessment tools such as the Active Movement Scale. Ancillary evaluations, including nerve conduction velocity studies, electromyography, MRI, CT, and ultrasonography, may be needed to further assess the extent of the neurologic injury and the prognosis for recovery. Neurosurgical treatment options include primary nerve surgery and/or nerve transfers. The shoulder is the most common site of chronic sequelae, including internal rotation contractures and the possible development of glenohumeral dysplasia.

Keywords: brachial plexus palsy; glenohumeral dysplasia; Narakas classification; primary nerve surgery

Dr. Van Heest or an immediate family member serves as a board member, owner, officer, or committee member of the American Academy of Orthopaedic Surgeons, the American Board of Orthopaedic Surgery, Inc., the American Orthopaedic Association, the American Society for Surgery of the Hand, and the Ruth Jackson Orthopaedic Society. Neither Dr. Matson nor any immediate family member has received anything of value from or has stock or stock options held in a commercial company or institution related directly or indirectly to the subject of this chapter.

INTRODUCTION

Brachial plexus birth injury (BPBI) is a neurologic injury occurring during the birthing process that results in paralysis and/or paresis and a variable loss of sensation in the affected limb. BPBI occurs in approximately 0.2 to 2.6 per 1,000 live births in the United States.[1,2] With the increasing number of cesarean deliveries, the incidence of BPBI decreased over a 15-year period from 1.7 per 1,000 live births in 1997 to 0.9 per 1,000 live births in 2012.[1] Risk factors for this neurologic injury include babies of abnormally large size (macrosomia); previous deliveries resulting in BPBI; prolonged labor, with vacuum or forceps delivery assistance; shoulder dystocia; hypotonia; and multiparous deliveries.[1,3] Although delivery via cesarean section does not eliminate the possibility of BPBI, the likelihood declines to 0.02% compared with 0.2% for a vaginal delivery.[2]

Approximately 75% of infants with BPBI will recover, leaving up to 25% of children with long-term deficits.[4] The reported degrees of clinical recovery may vary based on the time of treatment referral, the type of injury pattern, and subsequent treatment.

EVALUATION

Classification

The original Seddon and Sunderland descriptions of nerve injuries are commonly used to classify peripheral nerve injuries in patients with BPBI.[5] Seddon described patterns of peripheral nerve injury as neurapraxia, axonotmesis, and neurotmesis. Sunderland expanded this classification to include neurapraxia (degree I), axonotmesis (degrees II and III), neuroma in continuity (degree IV), and neurotmesis (degree V). The Seddon and Sunderland

This chapter is adapted from Van Heest AE, Partington MD: Brachial plexus birth injuries, in Martus JE, ed: *Orthopaedic Knowledge Update®: Pediatrics*, ed 5. Rosemont, IL, American Academy of Orthopaedic Surgeons, 2016, pp 227-234.

TABLE 1

Seddon and Sunderland Classification of Nerve Injury

Degree of Injury	Recovery	Rate of Recovery	Surgical Management
I, Neurapraxia	Complete	Up to 12 wk	None
II, Axonotmesis	Complete	1 inch/mo	None
III, Axonotmesis	Partial	1 inch/mo	None or neurolysis
IV, Neuroma in continuity	None	None	Nerve repair, graft, or transfer
V, Neurotmesis	None	None	Nerve repair, graft, or transfer

classifications evaluate postganglionic peripheral nerve injuries and aid in predicting the prognosis for neurologic recovery and the need for surgical intervention[5] (**Table 1**).

Avulsion is another type of injury occurring as a subset of BPBI. This preganglionic injury occurs at the spinal cord origin of the nerve roots. Avulsion injuries have the worst prognosis because spontaneous recovery is not possible, and such injuries cannot be surgically repaired. BPBI can include different types of preganglionic or postganglionic injury for each of the involved nerve roots, trunks, or divisions.

The Narakas classification is the most commonly used classification system for BPBI.[6] The author of a 1987 study[7] subdivided these injuries based on the extent of plexus involvement, with type I involving the typical upper trunk (C5 and C6), type II including C5 and C6 with the addition of C7, type III being a pan-plexus injury, and type IV being a pan-plexus injury with associated Horner syndrome. Differentiating these types of injuries in a newborn is based on physical examination findings. The Narakas classification provides prognostic information that can help guide treatment. Patients with Narakas types I and II nerve injuries have substantially higher rates of recovery than those with Narakas types III or IV nerve injuries.[4,8] In the past, terminology has included terms such as Erb palsy; however, it is now preferable to describe the anatomic lesion (eg, upper trunk BPBI or pan-plexus BPBI).

Patient Evaluation

Making a diagnosis of BPBI requires a careful patient history, physical examination, and often radiographic studies. No other specific diagnostic testing is required if the history and physical examination are consistent with the characteristic features of BPBI. Most commonly, BPBI is diagnosed at the time of delivery. Most children with BPBI are large for their gestational age and are delivered after prolonged labor, often requiring the use of vacuum or forceps assistance. A known shoulder dystocia is common. After birth, abnormal movement of one upper limb is frequently noted. The muscle tone in the affected arm is usually flaccid or limp.

A radiograph may be taken to assess for fracture; radiography is mandated if the limb is painful with palpation. Initial management includes fracture management if a fracture is present; in these situations, it is difficult to discern whether the loss of normal movement of the arm is associated with pain from the fracture or concomitant BPBI. If loss of normal arm movement persists after the fracture heals, the diagnosis of BPBI is made.

The type of Narakas nerve injury is determined based on the physical examination of the newborn using active range of motion of the shoulder, elbow, forearm, wrist, and hand. All patients with Narakas type III or IV nerve injuries are referred directly to a center dedicated to treatment of BPBI. For patients with signs of recovery from Narakas type I or II nerve injuries, referral often is made at 2 to 4 weeks after birth if recovery is not complete. Some BPBI are transient, and resolution is seen by the first checkup; these patients do not require referral. In infants who recover antigravity upper muscle strength in the first 2 months of life, a full and complete neurologic recovery can be expected.[9]

Each infant is examined for passive range of motion, active range of motion, and strength testing. Determining the presence or absence of Horner syndrome is important because it is associated with a worse prognosis.[6,8] Horner syndrome is characterized by miosis (constricted pupils), partial ptosis (drooping eyelids), and anhidrosis (loss of hemifacial sweating).

Particular attention is given to assessing passive range of motion of the shoulder into external rotation with the arm at the side because loss of shoulder external rotation is associated with shoulder subluxation or dislocation and may predict the success of closed treatment for infants.[10,11] It also is necessary to assess the infant's ability to bring his or her hand to his or her mouth against gravity (commonly called the cookie test) because absence of this ability has been used as an indication for surgical intervention.[12] In children with a pan-plexus injury, including Horner syndrome, phrenic nerve function is carefully assessed. Involvement can be assessed with ultrasonography or chest radiographs and is important if general anesthesia is planned.[13]

Serial examinations of infants with BPBI allow tracking of neurologic recovery and determination of the need for surgery. For infants at a center dedicated to the treatment of BPBI, the Active Movement Scale (AMS) is the most commonly used and validated physical examination tool for tracking neurologic recovery.[11] The AMS gives an objective and validated measure to assess nerve deficits and subsequent recovery. Strength is graded on a 0 to 7 scale, with grades 0 to 4 as active movement with gravity eliminated and grades 5 to 7 as active movement against gravity; each level requires a demonstration of motion at the previous level.[6,11,14] The presence of any contracture is recorded, monitored, and treated with physical therapy interventions. For infants with a loss of shoulder external rotation, further evaluation with radiographic imaging or ultrasonography is indicated.

Evaluation Methods

A meta-analysis of 307 articles examining BPBI found that the four most commonly used modalities for the diagnostic assessment of BPBI are electromyographic evaluations (standard and intraoperative), MRI, CT, and radiography.[6] Ultrasonography is an important tool in screening patients with BPBI and allows for dynamic assessment of the glenohumeral joint without the need for general anesthesia.[15,16] The most common methods for physically assessing the extent of BPBI are measurements of active and passive range of motion, modified Mallet scale, Toronto Test Score, AMS, the Medical Research Council scale for muscle strength,[17] and the Narakas Motor Scale.[6,18] The AMS, modified Mallet scale, Toronto Test Score, and the Narakas Motor Scale have been validated in the BPBI population. In addition, performance-based functional outcome measures, such as the Assisting Hand Assessment, have been standardized and validated (per reports) within the BPBI population.[19]

MANAGEMENT

Early Therapy

Therapy starts immediately at the time of diagnosis, usually at birth, unless a concomitant fracture is present. If fracture is excluded and BPBI is diagnosed, initial management includes a supervised home therapy program to maintain passive range of motion. During the period of infancy, neurologic return is potentially occurring. Because the infant is not able to actively carry out certain movements because of paresis or paralysis, the caregiver must perform those movements for the infant to prevent contracture and promote awareness for neurologic return. Therapists monitor motor recovery and age-appropriate functional use of the limb. Cortical recognition and awareness of the affected limb is promoted using methods such as sensory stimulation. When neurologic return is imbalanced across a joint, the risk of contracture exists. This is particularly true in the shoulder. Because of the risk of internal rotation contracture, scapular stabilization and passive glenohumeral mobilization are frequently necessary. Instruction in performing a home therapy program and supervised professional monitoring are recommended.

Botulinum Toxin Injections: Techniques and Outcomes

Botulinum toxin injections have been described for use in BPBI for children with dynamic imbalance across a joint caused by disparate levels of neurologic return. The most common indications for botulinum toxin injections in BPBI are (1) neurologic return to the shoulder internal rotator muscles that overpowers weak neurologic return to the shoulder external rotator muscles and (2) neurologic return to the triceps that overpowers poor neurologic return to the biceps. For both clinical scenarios, botulinum toxin has been described for injection into the overpowering muscle (eg, the elbow extensor muscles or the shoulder internal rotator muscles) to facilitate functional use of the weak antagonist muscle. In a report of 1-month and 1-year results after the injection of botulinum toxin into the shoulder internal rotator muscles in 19 children with shoulder imbalance and into the elbow extensor muscles in eight children with elbow imbalance, there was initial improvement in AMS scores in those with shoulder imbalance at 1 month; however, this improvement was not sustained at 1 year. The AMS scores of patients with elbow imbalance improved slightly at 1 month, and even greater improvement was found at 1 year because of the ongoing return of biceps neurologic function.[20] Botulinum toxin has also been used as an adjunct to closed reduction and casting in infants with shoulder subluxation and BPBI and may help to avoid open surgical procedures.[21] A recent systematic review of botulinum toxin use in BPBI found an overall beneficial effect for its use in shoulder internal rotation contractures, elbow contractures, and forearm pronation contractures, particularly in younger patients.[22] Botulinum toxin injections may be a useful temporizing measure and area treatment option in select children with muscle imbalance associated with BPBI.[20-22]

Primary Nerve Surgery: Technique and Outcomes

Most patients with BPBI recover spontaneously; however, for those who do not recover or those who have an incomplete recovery, surgical intervention is warranted. The indications for surgery are varied, but in infants with Narakas types III and IV pan-plexus injuries, the consensus is that surgery is indicated at 3 months of age. The rationale for surgery is that studies have consistently

Section 4: Upper Extremity

shown that all these children will have profound neurologic deficits without intervention.[9,11,12] Early surgical intervention in pan-plexus lesions may help minimize motor end plate loss and provide sufficient time for the return of neurologic function to the forearm and the hand. The three preferred options for primary nerve surgery in a patient with a pan-plexus lesion are plexus exploration with neurolysis, neuroma excision with sural nerve grafting, and outside-the-plexus reconstruction with nerve transfer procedures. Nerve transfer procedures include transferring the terminal motor branches of the spinal accessory nerve to the suprascapular nerve or transferring the thoracic intercostal nerves to the musculocutaneous nerve for preganglionic avulsions.[3,9,11,23,24] Neurolysis alone has been shown to be ineffective in patients with pan-plexus injuries.[25]

The indications for and timing of treatment for infants with Narakas types I and II injuries are more controversial. Historically, it had been recommended that the absence of return of biceps function by 3 months of age was an indication for microsurgical intervention.[26] Later, a failure to demonstrate elbow flexion as evaluated by the cookie test at 6 months of age has been advocated as an indication for microsurgical intervention.[11,12] However, a large meta-analysis reported that delaying surgery (even beyond 6 months of age) for this patient group may yield better outcomes.[27] Currently, the inability to bring the hand to the mouth against gravity by 6 months of age is an accepted indication for surgical intervention.[3,17]

The preferred primary nerve surgery for patients with Narakas types I and II also is controversial. Although plexus exploration and neurolysis with excision of a nonconducting neuroma and nerve grafting are commonly used,[3,13] neurolysis alone for conducting neuromas in the upper trunk also has been described.[23,25,28]

Nerve Transfers: Techniques and Outcomes

Innovations in the treatment of infants with BPBI have included the increased use of nerve transfers, which also is known as secondary nerve surgery. Although the results of nerve transfer procedures have been increasingly reported in the adult population, such procedures in the treatment of infants remains unclear. A 2015 report by the International Federation of Societies for Surgery of the Hand stated that no existing evidence is available for using nerve transfers for primary nerve surgery in patients with BPBI. However, nerve transfers have been reported to be effective in infants with BPBI in specific clinical circumstances, including late presentation, isolated deficits, failed primary reconstruction, and the presence of multiple nerve root avulsions.[24] Two nerve transfer procedures for secondary nerve reconstruction to provide elbow flexion (the Oberlin procedure) and shoulder abduction (the Leechavengvongs procedure) have garnered notable attention.[29]

Transfer of the ulnar and/or median nerve fascicles to the musculocutaneous nerve to provide elbow flexion is commonly termed the Oberlin procedure. Because this procedure has been used primarily in adult brachial plexus injuries, reports regarding results in children with BPBI are limited, but increasing.[30] A 2012 study reported on 17 infants treated with an Oberlin transfer at an average age of 12 months for absent elbow flexion caused by nerve root avulsion or failed primary nerve reconstruction.[31] At a mean follow-up of 31 months, the authors reported good to excellent results, with 3 patients achieving a modified British Medical Research Council scale grade of 2, 3 patients achieving a grade of 3, and 11 patients achieving a grade of 4. A 2014 study reported on 31 infants with BPBI treated with an Oberlin nerve transfer at 8 months of age.[32] At a mean follow-up of 35 months, 27 of the patients had an AMS score of 6 or 7, which is considered functional use of the elbow. In this study, four patients did not regain functional use of the elbow (final AMS score of less than 5). In these two reports, one patient had a transient anterior interosseous nerve deficit; no other donor deficit was noted.[24,31] More recently, a 2018 report comparing 19 babies with Oberlin transfer with 31 patients with nerve grafting at 1-year follow-up reported equivalent elbow flexion return in both groups, and superior supination return in the Oberlin group.[33]

The Leechavengvongs procedure transfers one branch of the radial nerve from the triceps muscle to the axillary nerve (deltoid muscle).[34] When combined with other shoulder stabilization procedures, improved shoulder function can be achieved with no weakness in elbow extension.[35]

Shoulder Techniques and Outcomes

A residual shoulder deficit is the most common chronic sequelae of BPBI. The authors of a 2014 study reviewed 69 children (median age, 14 years) to determine outcomes of BPBI. Reduced shoulder external rotation was found to be the most common deficit.[36] Early identification and treatment of glenohumeral dysplasia is a key factor in preventing chronic shoulder deficits.

The shoulder joint is particularly at risk for poor neurologic return, functional weakness, and skeletal deformity because of several neurologic factors. The upper trunk is most at risk for injury during the birthing process. In infants with Narakas type I injuries, the suprascapular nerve is at the greatest risk for injury because it is the first branch off the upper trunk, and it is tethered in its distal course into the suprascapular notch, which subjects it to the greatest stretch during shoulder dystocia during delivery. Across the shoulder joint, the internal rotator muscles (subscapularis, pectoralis major, latissimus dorsi, and teres major) often have excellent neurologic return and good functional strength in an isolated upper truck lesion. In contrast, the shoulder external rotator muscles (supraspinatus, infraspinatus, and teres minor) often have poor neurologic return and limited functional strength because of substantial injury to the suprascapular nerve and the axillary nerve in an upper trunk lesion. The strong internal rotators overpower the weak external rotators, leading to a power imbalance. A long-standing imbalance between the two muscle groups can lead to internal rotation shoulder contractures and, eventually, shoulder subluxation and dislocation with the secondary skeletal changes of glenohumeral dysplasia.

Ultrasonography has been used extensively at most BPBI centers to diagnose glenohumeral subluxation or dislocation in infants during their first 12 months of life, before ossification of the humeral head. Ultrasonography has been used in the diagnosis of hip dysplasia for decades, but its use in the shoulder for the diagnosis and treatment of glenohumeral dysplasia has been described and validated, in 2007, in comparison with the contralateral side to verify normal values based on patient age.[37] Multiple studies have identified ultrasonography as a reliable and valuable tool that can be used for screening and dynamic evaluation of the glenohumeral joint without the need for anesthesia.[15,16,38] The most common sonographic measurements for assessing glenohumeral development are the alpha (α) angle and the percentage of humeral head dysplasia. Ultrasonography can be performed in patients as young as 6 weeks. Normal values for the α angle are 30° or less, with the percentage of humeral head dysplasia less than 10% different from the contralateral (normal) side. The α angle is formed by the posterior scapular margin and a line tangent to the humeral head passing through the posterior osseous lip of the glenoid (**Figure 1**).

The second measurement is the percentage of humeral head displacement that is posterior to the posterior scapular margin. This measurement is determined from the ratio of the distance from the posterior scapular line to the posterior margin of the humeral head divided by the greatest diameter of the humeral head and then multiplied by 100 (**Figure 2**).

Shoulder Management

In a newborn, it is imperative to begin passive range of motion for all joints that are affected by a neurologic injury. In the shoulder, loss of shoulder external rotation is an indication that shoulder internal rotation contracture is developing, and the child is at risk for shoulder subluxation or dislocation. Before ossification, ultrasonography can be used to diagnose subluxation or dislocation (**Figure 3**). MRI is an alternative advanced imaging option, but it requires general anesthesia for patients in this age group.

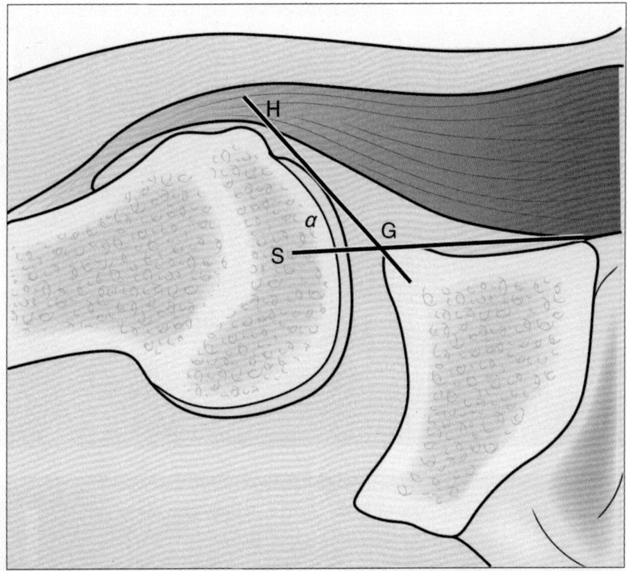

FIGURE 1 Illustration shows the method for calculating the α angle. The posterior osseous lip of the glenoid is identified (point G). A reference line (S) is drawn along the posterior scapular margin through point G. A tangential reference line (H) is drawn from the humeral head through point G.

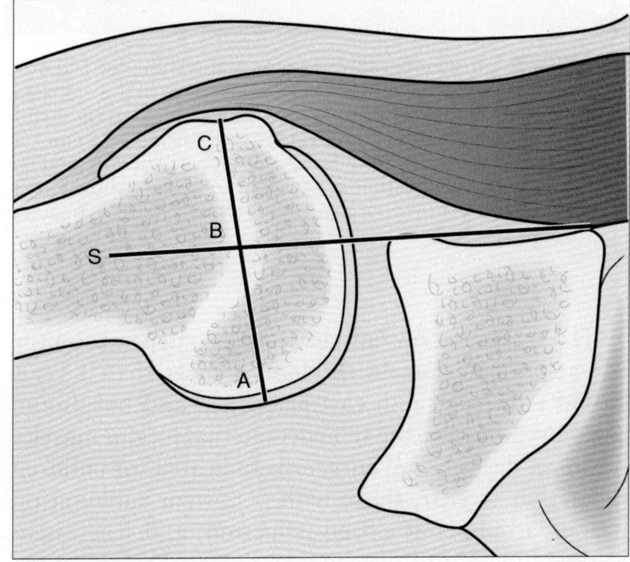

FIGURE 2 Illustration demonstrating the elements needed to calculate the percentage of humeral head displacement. A reference line (S) is drawn along the posterior scapular margin through the posterior osseous lip of the glenoid. Line AC is drawn at the greatest diameter of the humeral head. Point B is the intersection of line AC and line S. The humeral head displacement equals BC divided by AC multiplied by 100.

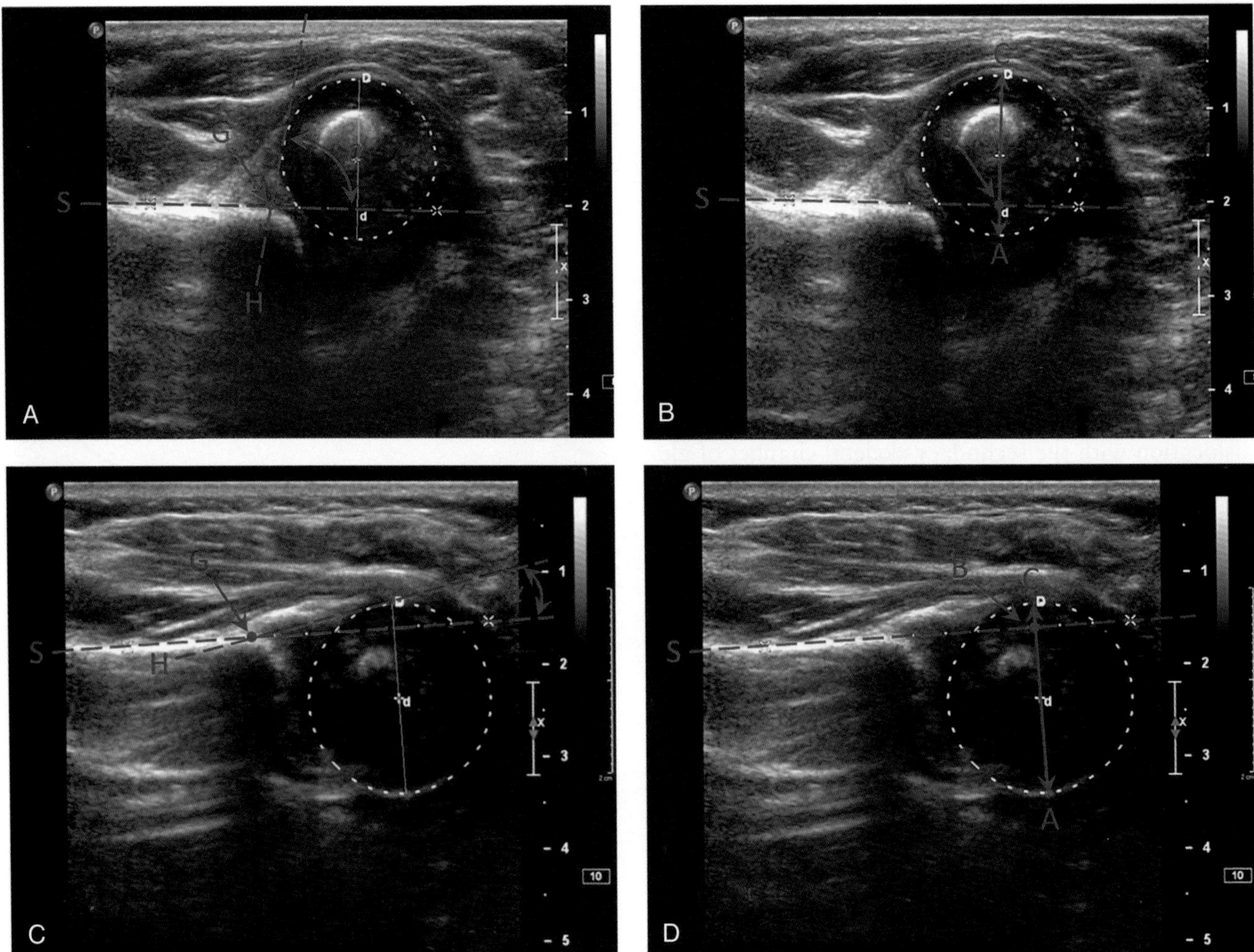

FIGURE 3 Ultrasonographic images of the shoulder of a 6-month-old infant who had loss of passive shoulder external rotation. Superimposed lines allow calculation of the α angle (see **Figure 1**) and the percentage of humeral head coverage (see **Figure 2**). **A**, Preoperative image shows a dislocated right shoulder in neutral position with a preoperative α angle of 81°. **B**, The preoperative humeral head coverage was calculated to be 19%. **C**, The patient was treated with a closed reduction while under general anesthesia. A shoulder spica cast was applied, and botulinum toxin was injected into the shoulder internal rotator muscles. Ultrasonographic image after treatment shows the reduced right shoulder in the neutral position with a postoperative α angle of 14°. **D**, Postoperative image shows humeral head coverage of 87%.

The treatment of shoulder dysplasia depends on the age at presentation. In children younger than 1 year, closed reduction with cast placement and botulinum toxin injection into the shoulder internal rotator muscles has been described.[21] Surgery is indicated for children older than 1 year, those with persistent subluxation despite attempts at closed reduction, and when neurologic function of the shoulder external rotator muscles fails to return. A tendon transfer of the latissimus dorsi and/or teres major is most commonly performed.[39] Elongation of the subscapularis muscle with or without transfer of the latissimus dorsi has also been described with improved glenohumeral congruency and long-term functional outcomes.[40] Loss of midline function with weak internal rotation is a known sequela of many of the surgical options for shoulder dysplasia in BPBI; attention to maintaining internal rotation function needs to be prioritized to avoid this sequela.[41] Concomitant open or arthroscopic anterior release or open reduction with posterior capsulorrhaphy may be considered. Controversy exists in the literature regarding the timing and indications for these procedures.[3] In children younger than 18 months, remodeling of the glenohumeral joint after extra-articular procedures has been reported.[42] In children older than 7 years with a fixed glenohumeral dysplasia, treatment with derotation osteotomy of the proximal humerus may be considered[2] (**Figure 4**).

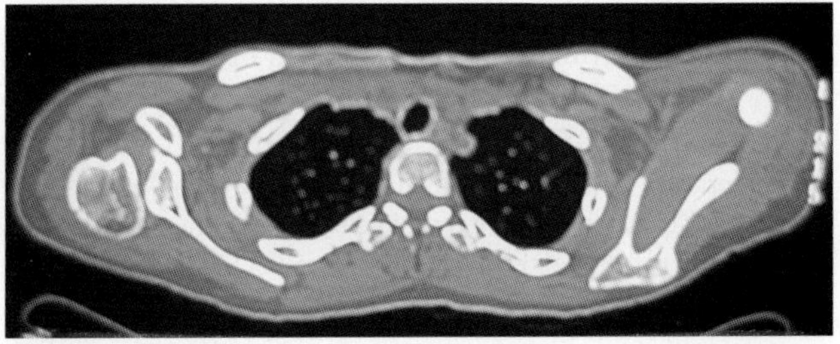

FIGURE 4 CT of the left shoulder of a 16-year-old patient with fixed glenohumeral dysplasia shows a flattened humeral head, retroversion of the glenoid, and posterior subluxation of the humeral head.

SUMMARY

The ultimate goal of patient care during the birthing process is to prevent all birth injuries. The appropriate management of second-stage delivery, the appropriate use of forceps or vacuum suction, work on evidence-based guidelines for preventing shoulder dystocia in the delivery of large or hypotonic infants, and guidelines for proceeding to cesarean section may help decrease the number of infants with BPBI.

Although most infants with BPBI recover, approximately 25% of children have long-term deficits, primarily associated with shoulder limitations. Early therapy is important in the treatment of these patients and often leads to favorable outcomes. In those patients who do not have neurologic recovery or have only an incomplete recovery, surgical intervention is warranted. Prioritization of maintaining shoulder joint development and improving shoulder joint function is necessary, particularly in the most common pattern of upper trunk Narakas I type injuries.

KEY STUDY POINTS

- During the birthing process, shoulder dystocia most commonly leads to injury of the upper trunk of the brachial plexus (C5-C6), which is a Narakas type I injury. The next most common injury occurs in the upper and middle trunk of the brachial plexus (C5 through C7), which is a Narakas type II injury.
- If a patient with a Narakas type I or II injury does not show sufficient neurologic return by 6 months of age (allowing the child to bring his or her hand to the mouth), surgical exploration with neurolysis or nerve resection and grafting is indicated.
- If a pan-plexus injury exists with no neurologic return by 3 months of age, brachial plexus exploration with nerve grafting is indicated, provided nerve root avulsions are not present.
- Nerve root avulsions are not surgically repairable and require alternative strategies such as nerve transfer to provide neurologic return.

ANNOTATED REFERENCES

1. Abzug JM, Mehlman CT, Ying J: Assessment of current epidemiology and risk factors surrounding brachial plexus birth palsy. *J Hand Surg Am* 2019;44(6):515.e1-515.e10.

   The authors reviewed a large database from 1997 to 2012 to identify the incidence of BPBI over this period as well as any risk factors associated with the development of BPBI. The incidence of BPBI has decreased over the years, with an incidence of 0.9 per 1,000 live births in 2012, largely attributed to the increase in cesarean deliveries over that period. Multiple risk factors were identified including shoulder dystocia, large baby, and specific delivery methods such as forceps and vacuum-assisted delivery, among others. Level of evidence: II.

2. Foad SL, Mehlman CT, Ying J: The epidemiology of neonatal brachial plexus palsy in the United States. *J Bone Joint Surg Am* 2008;90(6):1258-1264.
3. Hale HB, Bae DS, Waters PM: Current concepts in the management of brachial plexus birth palsy. *J Hand Surg Am* 2010;35(2):322-331.
4. Andersen J, Watt J, Olson J, Van Aerde J: Perinatal brachial plexus palsy. *Paediatr Child Health* 2006;11(2):93-100.
5. Sunderland S. *Nerves and Nerve Injuries*. ed 2. London, England, Churchill Livingstone, 1978.
6. Chang KW, Justice D, Chung KC, Yang LJ: A systematic review of evaluation methods for neonatal brachial plexus palsy: A review. *J Neurosurg Pediatr* 2013;12(4):395-405.
7. Narakas AO: Injuries of the brachial plexus and neighboring peripheral nerves in vertebral fractures and other trauma of the cervical spine [German]. *Orthopade* 1987;16(1):81-86.
8. Foad SL, Mehlman CT, Foad MB, Lippert WC: Prognosis following neonatal brachial plexus palsy: An evidence-based review. *J Child Orthop* 2009;3(6):459-463.
9. Waters PM: Comparison of the natural history, the outcome of microsurgical repair, and the outcome of operative reconstruction in brachial plexus birth palsy. *J Bone Joint Surg Am* 1999;81(5):649-659.
10. Greenhill DA, Wissinger K, Trionfo A, Solarz M, Kozin SH, Zlotolow DA: External rotation predicts outcomes after closed glenohumeral joint reduction with botulinum toxin type A in brachial plexus birth palsy. *J Pediatr Orthop* 2018;38(1):32-37.

    The authors evaluated the outcome of 49 patients with BPBI who underwent closed reduction and botulinum toxin injection at an average age of 11.5 months to determine the success of treatment and identify pretreatment predictors of success. Sixty-five percent of patients required repeat reduction (closed or open). Pretreatment AMS score and passive external rotation >30° predicted success of treatment. Level of evidence: IV.

11. Clarke HM, Curtis CG: An approach to obstetrical brachial plexus injuries. *Hand Clin* 1995;11(4):563-580, discussion 580-581.
12. Michelow BJ, Clarke HM, Curtis CG, Zuker RM, Seifu Y, Andrews DF: The natural history of obstetrical brachial plexus palsy. *Plast Reconstr Surg* 1994;93(4):675-680, discussion 681.

13. Al-Qattan MM, Clarke HM, Curtis CG: The prognostic value of concurrent phrenic nerve palsy in newborn children with Erb's palsy. *J Hand Surg Br* 1998;23(2):225.

14. Curtis C, Stephens D, Clarke HM, Andrews D: The active movement scale: An evaluative tool for infants with obstetrical brachial plexus palsy. *J Hand Surg Am* 2002;27(3):470-478.

15. Donohue KW, Little KJ, Gaughan JP, Kozin SH, Norton BD, Zlotolow DA: Comparison of ultrasound and MRI for the diagnosis of glenohumeral dysplasia in brachial plexus birth palsy. *J Bone Joint Surg Am* 2017;99(2):123-132.

Four independent evaluators reviewed the magnetic resonance and ultrasonographic images of 39 patients with BPBI (age 4 to 54 months) for a variety of measurements. The authors found good to excellent inter-rater reliability for MRI. Ultrasonography was found to underestimate alpha angle and glenoid version and significant differences between MRI and ultrasonography were identified for alpha angle. Although both techniques were found to be reliable measures, ultrasonography may be better suited as a screening tool as opposed to a stand-alone modality. Level of evidence: I.

16. Bauer AS, Lucas JF, Heyrani N, Anderson RL, Kalish LA, James MA: Ultrasound screening for posterior shoulder dislocation in infants with persistent brachial plexus birth palsy. *J Bone Joint Surg Am* 2017;99(9):778-783.

The authors evaluated 66 infants to determine the prevalence of shoulder dislocation using ultrasonography and to identify physical examination findings that correlate with dislocation. Twenty-nine percent of patients demonstrated dislocation. Passive external rotation in adduction was the best physical examination finding at discriminating shoulder dislocation. Level of evidence: IV.

17. Frese E, Brown M, Norton BJ: Clinical reliability of manual muscle testing. Middle trapezius and gluteus medius muscles. *Phys Ther* 1987;67(7):1072-1076.

18. Bae DS, Waters PM, Zurakowski D: Reliability of three classification systems measuring active motion in brachial plexus birth palsy. *J Bone Joint Surg Am* 2003;85-A(9):1733-1738.

19. Holmefur M, Krumlinde-Sundholm L, Eliasson AC: Interrater and intrarater reliability of the assisting hand assessment. *Am J Occup Ther* 2007;61(1):79-84.

20. Arad E, Stephens D, Curtis CG, Clarke HM: Botulinum toxin for the treatment of motor imbalance in obstetrical brachial plexus palsy. *Plast Reconstr Surg* 2013;131(6):1307-1315.

21. Ezaki M, Malungpaishrope K, Harrison RJ, et al: OnabotulinumtoxinA injection as an adjunct in the treatment of posterior shoulder subluxation in neonatal brachial plexus palsy. *J Bone Joint Surg Am* 2010;92(12):2171-2177.

22. Buchanan PJ, Grossman JAI, Price AE, Reddy C, Chopan M, Chim H: The use of botulinum toxin injection for brachial plexus birth injuries: A systematic review of the literature. *Hand (NY)* 2019;14(2):150-154.

The authors reviewed studies published between 2000 and 2017 on the use of botulinum toxin for patients with BPBI. Ten studies, which included 325 patients, demonstrated overall beneficial effect of botulinum toxin on contractures of the shoulder, elbow, and forearm. Level of evidence: II, IV, and V.

23. Lin JC, Schwentker-Colizza A, Curtis CG, Clarke HM: Final results of grafting versus neurolysis in obstetrical brachial plexus palsy. *Plast Reconstr Surg* 2009;123(3):939-948.

24. Tse R, Kozin SH, Malessy MJ, Clarke HM: International Federation of Societies for Surgery of the Hand committee report: The role of nerve transfers in the treatment of neonatal brachial plexus palsy. *J Hand Surg Am* 2015;40(6):1246-1259.

25. Clarke HM, Al-Qattan MM, Curtis CG, Zuker RM: Obstetrical brachial plexus palsy: Results following neurolysis of conducting neuromas-in-continuity. *Plast Reconstr Surg* 1996;97(5):974-982, discussion 983-984.

26. Gilbert A, Tassin JL: Surgical repair of the brachial plexus in obstetric paralysis [French]. *Chirurgie* 1984;110(1):70-75.

27. Ali ZS, Bakar D, Li YR, et al: Utility of delayed surgical repair of neonatal brachial plexus palsy. *J Neurosurg Pediatr* 2014;13(4):462-470.

28. Andrisevic E, Taniguchi M, Partington MD, Agel J, Van Heest AE: Neurolysis alone as the treatment for neuroma-in-continuity with more than 50% conduction in infants with upper trunk brachial plexus birth palsy: Clinical article. *J Neurosurg Pediatr* 2014;13(2):229-237.

29. Oberlin C, Beal D, Leechavengvongs S, Salon A, Dauge MC, Sarcy JJ: Nerve transfer to biceps muscle using a part of ulnar nerve for C5-C6 avulsion of the brachial plexus: Anatomical study and report of four cases. *J Hand Surg Am* 1994;19(2):232-237.

30. Al-Qattan MM, Al-Kharfy TM: Median nerve to biceps nerve transfer to restore elbow flexion in obstetric brachial plexus palsy. *Biomed Res Int* 2014;2014:854084.

31. Siqueira MG, Socolovsky M, Heise CO, Martins RS, Di Masi G: Efficacy and safety of Oberlin's procedure in the treatment of brachial plexus birth palsy. *Neurosurgery* 2012;71(6):1156-1160, discussion 1161.

32. Little KJ, Zlotolow DA, Soldado F, Cornwall R, Kozin SH: Early functional recovery of elbow flexion and supination following median and/or ulnar nerve fascicle transfer in upper neonatal brachial plexus palsy. *J Bone Joint Surg Am* 2014;96(3):215-221.

33. Chang KWC, Wilson TJ, Popadich M, Brown SH, Chung KC, Yang LJS: Oberlin transfer compared with nerve grafting for improving early supination in neonatal brachial plexus palsy. *J Neurosurg Pediatr* 2018;21(2):178-184.

The authors compared 19 babies with Oberlin transfer with 31 patients with nerve grafting with 1-year follow-up. They demonstrated equivalent elbow flexion return in both groups and superior supination return in the Oberlin group. Level of evidence: III.

34. Leechavengvongs S, Witoonchart K, Uerpairojkit C, Thuvasethakul P: Nerve transfer to deltoid muscle using the nerve to the long head of the triceps, part II: A report of 7 cases. *J Hand Surg Am* 2003;28(4):633-638.

35. Leechavengvongs S, Witoonchart K, Uerpairojkit C, Thuvasethakul P, Malungpaishrope K: Combined nerve transfers for C5 and C6 brachial plexus avulsion injury. *J Hand Surg Am* 2006;31(2):183-189.

36. Hulleberg G, Elvrum AK, Brandal M, Vik T: Outcome in adolescence of brachial plexus birth palsy. 69 individuals re-examined after 10-20 years. *Acta Orthop* 2014;85(6):633-640.

37. Vathana T, Rust S, Mills J, et al: Intraobserver and interobserver reliability of two ultrasound measures of humeral head position in infants with neonatal brachial plexus palsy. *J Bone Joint Surg Am* 2007;89(8):1710-1715.

38. Pöyhiä TH, Lamminen AE, Peltonen JI, Kirjavainen MO, Willamo PJ, Nietosvaara Y: Brachial plexus birth injury: US screening for glenohumeral joint instability. *Radiology* 2010;254(1):253-260.

39. Greenhill DA, Smith WR, Ramsey FV, Kozin SH, Zlotolow DA: Double versus single tendon transfers to improve shoulder function in brachial plexus birth palsy. *J Pediatr Orthop* 2019;39(6):328-334.

The authors performed a retrospective analysis of combined latissimus dorsi and teres major compared with isolated teres major transfers external rotation deficits in patients with BPBI. Combined latissimus dorsi and teres major transfers produced greater gains in Mallet score external rotation but was associated with greater loss of midline function. Level of evidence: III.

40. Hultgren T, Jönsson K, Roos F, Järnbert-Pettersson H, Hammarberg H: Surgical correction of shoulder rotation deformity in brachial plexus birth palsy: Long-term results in 118 patients. *Bone Joint J* 2014;96-B(10):1411-1418.

41. Greenhill DA, Trionfo A, Ramsey FV, Kozin SH, Zlotolow DA: Postoperative loss of midline function in brachial plexus birth palsy. *J Hand Surg Am* 2018;43(6):565.e1-565.e10.

The authors retrospectively reviewed 172 patients who underwent a procedure for BPBI with at least 1-year follow-up to evaluate the rate of limited internal rotation postoperatively and risk factors associated with this sequela. 19.8% of patients ultimately developed loss of internal rotation (Mallet internal rotation score <3). Patients with a more severe initial palsy, those with poor spontaneous recovery of upper trunk function before surgery, and those who ultimately required open surgical reduction were at higher risk for loss of midline function. Level of evidence: IV.

42. Van Heest A, Glisson C, Ma H: Glenohumeral dysplasia changes after tendon transfer surgery in children with birth brachial plexus injuries. *J Pediatr Orthop* 2010;30(4):371-378.

CHAPTER 22

Limb Deficiency and Prosthetics

APURVA S. SHAH, MD, MBA

ABSTRACT

Transverse deficiency (or peromelia) is a rare congenital anomaly that is typically sporadic and unilateral. This deficiency reflects the failure of embryonic limb development in the proximodistal axis and results in the absence of the distal limb but with proximal structures essentially spared. The treatment of a patient with a transverse deficiency involves function optimization as well as patient and family education to improve the child's quality of life.

Keywords: congenital hand; prosthesis; transverse deficiency

INTRODUCTION

A transverse deficiency is a rare congenital anomaly that occurs in approximately 1 in 12,300 live births.[1] The most common form is a congenital proximal forearm (below-elbow) amputation that is typically sporadic and unilateral (70% to 96% of all instances) and rarely associated with other congenital anomalies.[1,2]

INCIDENCE AND EMBRYOLOGY

Transverse deficiency reflects the failure of embryonic limb development in the proximodistal axis and results in the absence of the distal limb but with proximal structures essentially spared (**Figure 1**). The limb bud appears during the fourth week of gestation, with growth and development occurring in three planes: proximodistal, ventrodorsal, and anterior-posterior (radioulnar). The apical ectodermal ridge (AER), a rim of epithelial cells at the distal extent of the limb bud, has been shown to be critical for outgrowth of the limb. AER function is mediated through fibroblast growth factor signaling to the underlying mesenchymal cells, thus preventing cell death and maintaining mesenchymal cell proliferation.[3,4] In animal models, injury to the AER results in transverse deficiency.[5] Traditionally, the area of proliferating mesenchymal cells underlying the AER was characterized by the progress zone model, where the fate of these pluripotent cells depended on their time of exit from the influence of the AER, with later exit giving rise to more distal elements. Some authors have recently questioned the time-dependent nature of this model and rather propose the prespecified model,[3,4,6,7] in which all the precursor cells are present early in the limb bud, with cells contributing to the proximal limb elements proliferating earlier than cells contributing to distal elements (**Figure 2**).

In most patients, transverse deficiency is unilateral and affects the upper limb two to three times more commonly than the lower limb.[8,9] One study noted that 93% of patients with a transverse deficiency have soft-tissue nubbins, skin invaginations, or hypoplasia of the proximal radius and ulna on the residual limb[10] (**Figure 3**). These findings support the concept that transverse deficiency and symbrachydactyly represent a continuum of a single disease process.[10]

The exact mechanism or teratogens through which transverse deficiency occurs are unknown, although an impediment in the vascular supply of the limb during development is thought to contribute to the

Dr. Shah or an immediate family member serves as a board member, owner, officer, or committee member of the American Society for Surgery of the Hand and the Pediatric Orthopaedic Society of North America.

This chapter is adapted from Shah AS, Thibaudeau S: Congenital transverse deficiency of the upper limb, in Martus JE, ed: *Orthopaedic Knowledge Update®: Pediatrics*, ed 5. Rosemont, IL, American Academy of Orthopaedic Surgeons, 2016, pp 235-241.

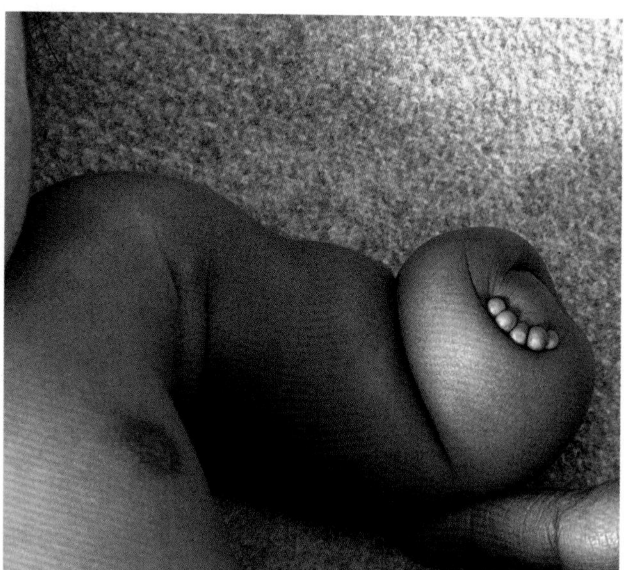

FIGURE 1 Photograph of the limb of a child with transverse deficiency of the upper limb. (Courtesy of Charles Goldfarb, MD, St. Louis, MO.)

pathophysiology.[11] This theory arose from associating symbrachydactyly with Poland syndrome, which, along with the Klippel-Feil and Möbius syndromes, is grouped under the subclavian disruption sequence hypothesis.[12] Approximately 40% of patients with Poland syndrome, which is an absence of the pectoralis major muscle, also have symbrachydactyly.[13] Adams-Oliver syndrome often occurs in conjunction with aplasia cutis congenita and may indicate a vascular pathway as an etiology of transverse deficiency.[14] Maternal misoprostol ingestion also has been associated with transverse deficiency (odds ratio of 11.9).[15]

The pathophysiology and characteristics of transverse deficiency are important to recognize to differentiate transverse deficiency from other congenital limb anomalies that also may appear to have a transverse loss. The differential diagnoses include amniotic band syndrome (1 in 16,100 live births), longitudinal deficiency (1 in 3,700 live births), and hypodactyly/undergrowth (1 in 8,400 live births).[1] Longitudinal deficiencies affect anterior-posterior growth, resulting in the absence of radial or ulnar structures. In contrast, in transverse deficiency or symbrachydactyly, where the ectodermal elements (nails, distal phalanges) are preserved, hypodactyly results in the loss of all ectodermal elements.[16] Amniotic band syndrome can be differentiated by other associated features, such as multiple limb involvement, cleft lip, lymphedema, acrosyndactyly, and lower limb constriction bands or amputations.[17]

EVALUATION: UPPER LIMB FUNCTION AND QUALITY OF LIFE

In congenital hand deficiencies, clinicians often disproportionately focus on physical domains, such as body structure and function, because they are more tangible and easier to measure objectively compared with psychosocial issues. To integrate the psychosocial effects of health status on an individual, the World Health Organization created the International Classification of Functioning, Disability, and Health (WHO-ICF), which describes a health state by four domains: body structure, body function, environmental factors, and activity and participation.[18] Ideally, patient-reported outcome measures (PROMs) should address all WHO-ICF domains. A 2015 comprehensive review of the literature evaluated whether PROMs used to evaluate the management of congenital hand deficiency captured WHO-ICF domains.[19] PROMs covered a mean of 1.3 WHO-ICF domains when evaluating the management of congenital hand deficiency. The Prosthetic Upper Limb Functional Index was the only PROM in the review that was specifically validated for children with transverse deficiencies. Further development of PROMs that specifically address congenital hand deficiency and its subclassifications is required.

Importantly, patients' and parents' perception of the disability may be discordant, reflecting the importance of collecting information from both patients and parents.[20] A group of 439 children and adolescents with congenital below-elbow transverse deficiency and their parents were administered the Pediatric Outcomes Data Collection Instrument and the Pediatric Quality of Life Inventory.[21] High social functioning and upper limb function were reported within the normal range by both children and their parents. However, the children reported better upper limb function on the Pediatric Outcomes Data Collection Instrument and better social functioning on the Pediatric Quality of Life Inventory compared with the reports of their parents. However, the parents overestimated the scores for comfort in the pain-comfort domain of the Pediatric Outcomes Data Collection Instrument.[21] As the child ages, clinicians may need to pay particular attention to physical domains, such as bodily pain and comfort, because these have been correlated with lower health-related quality-of-life scores in adults.[22] It is hypothesized that chronic compensatory behaviors and prosthetic use can lead to increased strain and pain that are eventually manifested as decreased health-related quality-of-life scores.[22] However, early psychosocial support and a multidisciplinary team approach in treating children with complex limb deformities may facilitate acceptance and improved self-esteem.[23]

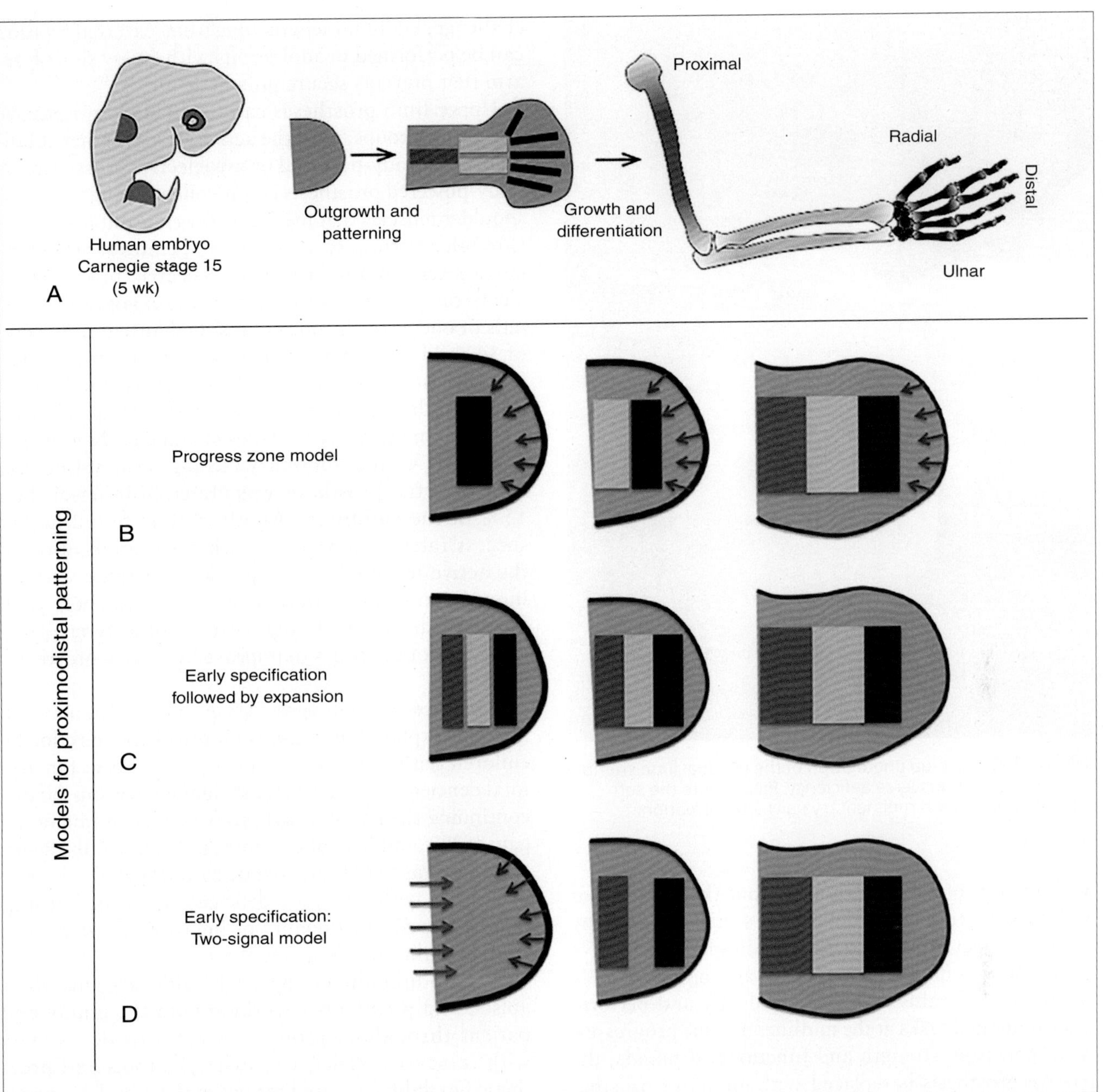

FIGURE 2 Illustration of embryology of proximodistal limb development. **A**, The limb bud emerges as a bud of mesenchymal cells encased in an ectodermal hull. Patterning (indicated by the color coding) is needed to establish the different proximodistal compartments of the limb. Three models (**B** through **D**) have been proposed to describe how this patterning arises. The validity of the progress zone model has recently been questioned. (Reprinted from *J Hand Surg Am* 39[4]. Vogeli KM, Mariani FV, Lightdale N: Updated embryology of the upper limb, 811-812. Copyright © 2014 American Society for Surgery of the Hand.)

Recent prospective data of 586 children with congenital upper limb differences from two pediatric hospitals in the United States suggest that children with congenital hand and upper limb anomalies in general report decreased upper limb function, but better peer relationships, less anxiety, and less depression.[24]

TREATMENT AND UPPER LIMB PROSTHESES

The treatment of patients with transverse deficiency involves function optimization as well as patient and family education to improve the child's quality of life. Surgery is infrequently needed. Historically, many

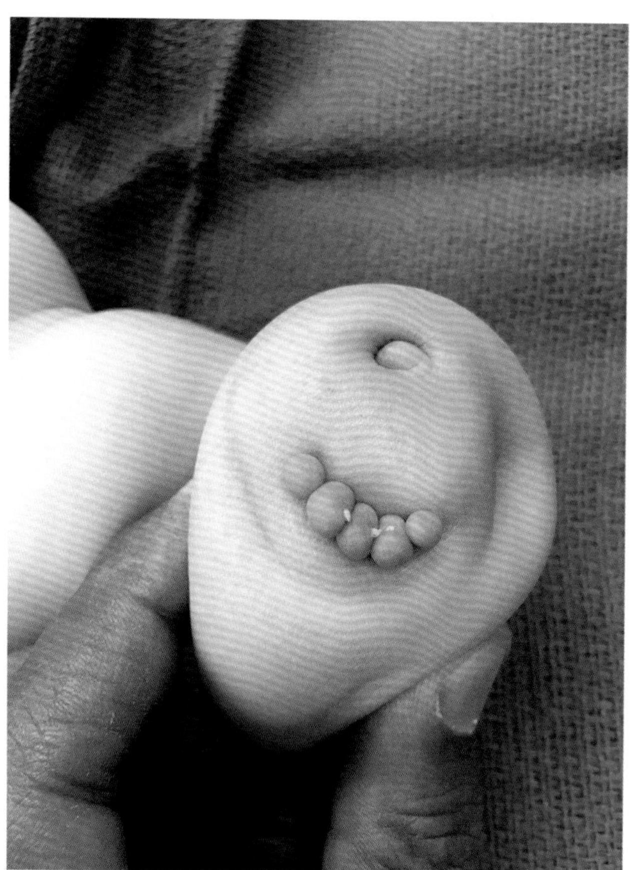

FIGURE 3 Close-up photograph of the residual limb stump in a child with transverse deficiency. Please note the soft-tissue nubbins with rudimentary nail plate formation.

healthcare professionals thought that the function of a child with transverse deficiency would improve by using an upper limb prosthesis. Traditionally, a passive prosthesis was fitted at 6 months of age, approximately when a child begins to sit independently and perform basic bimanual tasks at the midline. As time progresses, with increasing strength and functional demands, the passive prosthesis is replaced with an active prosthesis, often between the ages of 2 and 5 years. However, prosthesis rejection rates have been reported to range from 10% to 49%, and the optimal timing and use of prostheses in children with congenital transverse deficiency is controversial.[25-30] In a large cohort study of 256 patients, 49% of the patients were noncompliant in prosthesis use.[25] Fitting a child before 3 years of age improved long-term compliance, although there was no difference in compliance if a child was fitted before 1 year of age. Prosthetic fitting before 1 year of age may inhibit neurosensory input during the learning of bimanual activities and may delay the achievement of developmental milestones such as crawling. Achieving an acceptable prosthetic fit during childhood remains a challenge, but ulnar lengthening using external fixation can be performed in adolescents with a very short forearm that prevents secure prosthetic fitting.[31]

Upper limb prostheses can be divided into passive and active groups, with the active group further subdivided into body-powered or myoelectric prostheses. A body-powered prosthesis is controlled through residual shoulder muscles that mechanically transmit movement through a harness to a voluntary opening or voluntary closing terminal device. A myoelectric prosthesis is electrically powered through electromyographic signals of one or two groups of residual muscles. A group of 34 children from the Shriners Hospital for Children in Minnesota was given multiple prosthetic choices; these children most often selected a simple cosmetic passive hand (passive prosthesis) and a body-powered prosthesis with a voluntary closing terminal device. A myoelectric prosthesis was preferred in fewer than 15% of the children.[32] Another study found higher success rates with active prostheses if application of the active terminal device was accompanied with an intensive training program that involved short-term hospitalization.[25] Offering a variety of different prosthetic options appears to improve long-term prosthetic use.[25,32,33]

A multicenter study across Shriners Hospitals in North America explored the reasons for prosthetic rejection by children with unilateral congenital transverse forearm total deficiency.[29] The two most common reasons for discontinuing the use of prosthesis were lack of functional gain (53%) and lack of comfort (49%). Overall, the literature seems to indicate that traditional prosthetic wear in children with transverse deficiency does not translate into improved functionality or improvement in health-related quality-of-life scores.[34]

A multidisciplinary approach, with surgeons, therapists, and prosthetists working with the family and patient throughout growth, might provide patients with transverse deficiencies with the tools and prosthetic flexibility required for optimal use and cosmesis. Cost, limited funding, and the need for frequent prosthetic adjustments in a growing child can further contribute to prosthetic rejection rates.[33] A body-powered prosthesis for a below-elbow amputation ranges from $4,000 to $8,000, whereas a myoelectric prosthesis ranges between $25,000 and $50,000.[35] The process of three-dimensional printing of upper limb prostheses may soon become streamlined. Increased access to advanced computer imaging, the decreased cost of three-dimensional printed prostheses, and the ability to allow remote fitting of a prosthesis may allow more children access to prosthetic devices.[36,37] In a case study for an adult patient with a transradial amputation, the cost of a three-dimensional printed myoelectric prosthesis was $300.[36] Nonprofit organizations, such as Enabling the Future, which provides free three-dimensional printed upper limb prostheses for children in need, may further help the medical community improve and tailor prostheses for the specific needs of children.[38]

Loss of sensory feedback from prosthetic wear is arguably the primary reason for limited functional gains and low compliance. Technologic advances in prosthetics, such as targeted muscle reinnervation and sensory biofeedback through neural interfaces, may overcome these obstacles. Targeted muscle reinnervation consists of transferring nerves from the nonfunctional limb segment to the chest wall or upper arm musculature (pectoralis major) to provide additional electromyographic output signals, thus refining the control and complexity of prosthetic actions.[39] The efficacy of targeted muscle reinnervation in children with transverse deficiency has not been determined.[40] Targeted sensory nerve transfers provide reinnervated areas on the chest wall that represent the amputated hand.[41] Sensory input through direct peripheral nerve interfaces (ie, intraneural electrodes) and regenerative peripheral nerve interfaces (muscle neurotized through a sensory nerve fascicle) are under investigation and have a promising future for real-time sensory feedback, obviating the need for visual cues.[42] Brain-machine interfaces are another novel method to control a prosthesis through electroencephalography and bypass the peripheral nervous system. The development of hybrid brain-machine interfaces with multiple inputs, including electroencephalography, electromyography, and electrooculography, will improve the ability of patients to perform functional tasks through brain control.[43]

Further treatment options may arise from the microsurgical reconstruction of transverse deficiencies. The success of a pediatric hand transplant in the United States, for a young child already receiving immunosuppression therapy for a kidney transplant and with below-elbow amputations secondary to sepsis, may open the door for future applications of vascularized composite allotransplantation.[44] Careful candidate selection cannot be overemphasized, because vascularized composite allotransplantation requires lifelong immunosuppression therapy; its side effects have important ethical implications and potentially serious health repercussions in pediatric patients. Future advances in immunosuppression therapy and regeneration may broaden the indications for vascularized composite allotransplantation.[45]

Organ regeneration may present additional opportunities in the distant future. Organ regeneration requires three steps: (1) the formation of all cell types comprising the organ, (2) tissue organization, and (3) the creation of a three-dimensional morphology of the organ.[46] Major strides in molecular biology and genetics have helped in the better understanding of limb regeneration in vertebrate models, such as the zebra fish and the axolotl.[46,47] Amputation of the limb is followed by epithelization from cells at the circumference of the stump. These epithelial cells then proliferate to form the apical epithelial cap. The blastemal cells, which are undifferentiated mesenchymal cells, proliferate under the apical epithelial cap and contribute to limb regeneration. Most interestingly, these cells maintain positional memory of their proximodistal location and thus allow for maintenance of the three-dimensional morphology of the regenerating limb.[46] Maintenance of the apical epithelial cap and blastemal cell formation is dependent on peripheral nerve innervation.[48] Further characterization of these events, in particular the ability of blastemal cells to maintain positional memory, may allow researchers to develop blastemal cells for mammalian embryos and eventually limb regeneration.

SUMMARY

Congenital transverse deficiency results from the failure of embryonic limb development in the proximodistal axis. Injury, whether mechanical or vascular, to the AER in utero is thought to result in transverse deficiency. Because of shared clinical features, transverse deficiency appears to represent the proximal continuum of symbrachydactyly. The use of prosthetics in patients with transverse deficiency remains controversial, but providing patients and families with multiple options appears to maximize adoption rates for prosthesis use. Technologic advances in engineering and computing have allowed for technologic advances in prostheses, including targeted muscle reinnervation and three-dimensional printed prostheses. Future advances in molecular biology and genetics may allow for limb regeneration and/or immune tolerance for vascularized composite allotransplantation.

KEY STUDY POINTS

- Congenital transverse deficiency results from the failure of embryonic upper limb development in the proximodistal axis.
- Patients with transverse deficiency and their parents report social functioning and upper limb function within normal ranges.
- Pediatric prosthesis rejection ranges from 10% to 49%. Two main reasons for prosthetic discontinuation are a lack of functional gains and discomfort.

ANNOTATED REFERENCES

1. Koskimies E, Lindfors N, Gissler M, Peltonen J, Nietosvaara Y: Congenital upper limb deficiencies and associated malformations in Finland: A population-based study. *J Hand Surg Am* 2011;36(6):1058-1065.
2. Jain SK: A study of 200 cases of congenital limb deficiencies. *Prosthet Orthot Int* 1994;18(3):174-179.
3. Dudley AT, Ros MA, Tabin CJ: A re-examination of proximodistal patterning during vertebrate limb development. *Nature* 2002;418(6897):539-544.
4. Sun X, Mariani FV, Martin GR: Functions of FGF signalling from the apical ectodermal ridge in limb development. *Nature* 2002;418(6897):501-508.
5. Oberg KC, Feenstra JM, Manske PR, Tonkin MA: Developmental biology and classification of congenital anomalies of the hand and upper extremity. *J Hand Surg Am* 2010;35(12):2066-2076.
6. Duboule D: Making progress with limb models. *Nature* 2002;418(6897):492-493.
7. Saunders JW Jr: Is the progress zone model a victim of progress? *Cell* 2002;110(5):541-543.
8. Ephraim PL, Dillingham TR, Sector M, Pezzin LE, Mackenzie EJ: Epidemiology of limb loss and congenital limb deficiency: A review of the literature. *Arch Phys Med Rehabil* 2003;84(5):747-761.
9. Gold NB, Westgate MN, Holmes LB: Anatomic and etiological classification of congenital limb deficiencies. *Am J Med Genet A* 2011;155A(6):1225-1235.
10. Kallemeier PM, Manske PR, Davis B, Goldfarb CA: An assessment of the relationship between congenital transverse deficiency of the forearm and symbrachydactyly. *J Hand Surg Am* 2007;32(9):1408-1412.
11. Bavinck JN, Weaver DD: Subclavian artery supply disruption sequence: Hypothesis of a vascular etiology for Poland, Klippel-Feil, and Mobius anomalies. *Am J Med Genet* 1986;23(4):903-918.
12. Buckwalter JA V, Shah AS: Presentation and treatment of Poland anomaly. *Hand (NY)* 2016;11(4):389-395.

    Nonsystematic review of Poland anomaly which examines the etiology, presentation, natural history and treatment. Level of evidence: V.
13. Woodside JC, Light TR: Symbrachydactyly – Diagnosis, function, and treatment. *J Hand Surg Am* 2016;41(1):135-143, quiz 143.

    This article reviews the morphologic forms of symbrachydactyly, which presents with a shorter and smaller hand with underdeveloped short or webbed digits, digital nubbins or digital absence. Level of evidence: V.
14. Snape KM, Ruddy D, Zenker M, et al: The spectra of clinical phenotypes in aplasia cutis congenita and terminal transverse limb defects. *Am J Med Genet A* 2009;149A(8):1860-1881.
15. da Silva Dal Pizzol T, Knop FP, Mengue SS: Prenatal exposure to misoprostol and congenital anomalies: Systematic review and meta-analysis. *Reprod Toxicol* 2006;22(4):666-671.
16. Knight JB, Pritsch T, Ezaki M, Oishi SN: Unilateral congenital terminal finger absences: A condition that differs from symbrachydactyly. *J Hand Surg Am* 2012;37(1):124-129.
17. Ogino T: Clinical features and teratogenic mechanisms of congenital absence of digits. *Dev Growth Differ* 2007;49(6):523-531.
18. World Health Organization: *Towards a Common Language for Functioning, Disability and Health ICF. The International Classification of Functioning, Disability and Health.* Available from: http://www.who.int/classifications/icf/icfbeginnersguide.pdf?ua=1. Accessed March 31, 2016.
19. Adkinson JM, Bickham RS, Chung KC, Waljee JF: Do patient- and parent-reported outcomes measures for children with congenital hand differences capture WHO-ICF domains? *Clin Orthop Relat Res* 2015;473(11):3549-3563.
20. Ardon MS, Selles RW, Roebroeck ME, Hovius SE, Stam HJ, Janssen WG: Poor agreement on health-related quality of life between children with congenital hand differences and their parents. *Arch Phys Med Rehabil* 2012;93(4):641-646.
21. Sheffler LC, Hanley C, Bagley A, Molitor F, James MA: Comparison of self-reports and parent proxy-reports of function and quality of life of children with below-the-elbow deficiency. *J Bone Joint Surg Am* 2009;91(12):2852-2859.
22. Johansen H, ØstlieK, AndersenLØ, Rand-HendriksenS: Health-related quality of life in adults with congenital unilateral upper limb deficiency in Norway. A cross-sectional study. *Disabil Rehabil* 2016;38(23):2305-2314.

    The authors report on the outcomes of 131 children, 116 with congenital deficiencies, who were fitted with upper limb prostheses at the Ontario Crippled Children's Centre between 1965 and 1975. The level of deficiency was a key factor in long-term compliance, with longer forearms having decreased compliance. Fifty percent of the children older than 2 years who were fitted with prostheses abandoned them. Level of evidence: III.
23. Andersson GB, Gillberg C, Fernell E, Johansson M, Nachemson A: Children with surgically corrected hand deformities and upper limb deficiencies: Self-concept and psychological well-being. *J Hand Surg Eur Vol* 2011;36(9):795-801.
24. Bae DS, Canizares MF, Miller PE, Waters PM, Goldfarb CA: Functional impact of congenital hand differences: Early results from the congenital upper limb differences (CoULD) registry. *J Hand Surg Am* 2018;43(4):321-330.

    The congenital hand and upper limb registry characterizes both upper extremity function and psychosocial function in 586 children with congenital upper limb differences. The registry demonstrates that children with congenital hand differences report decreased upper limb function but superior peer relationships and positive emotional states in comparison with population norms. Level of evidence: I.

25. Davids JR, Wagner LV, Meyer LC, Blackhurst DW: Prosthetic management of children with unilateral congenital below-elbow deficiency. *J Bone Joint Surg Am* 2006;88(6):1294-1300.
26. Glynn MK, Galway HR, Hunter G, Sauter WF: Management of the upper-limb-deficient child with a powered prosthetic device. *Clin Orthop Relat Res* 1986;209:202-205.
27. Postema K, van der Donk V, van Limbeek J, Rijken RA,Poelma MJ: Prosthesis rejection in children with a unilateral congenital arm defect. *Clin Rehabil* 1999;13(3):243-249.
28. Scotland TR, Galway HR: A long-term review of children with congenital and acquired upper limb deficiency. *J Bone Joint Surg Br* 1983;65(3):346-349.
29. Wagner LV, Bagley AM, James MA: Reasons for prosthetic rejection by children with unilateral congenital transverse forearm total deficiency. *J Prosthet Orthot* 2007;19(2):51-54.
30. Farr S, Catena N, Martinez-Alvarez S, Soldado F, EPOS Upper Limb Study Group: Peromelia–congenital transverse deficiency of the upper limb: A literature review and current prosthetic treatment. *J Child Orthop* 2018;12(6):558-565.

    The authors present a nonsystematic review of congenital transverse deficiency summarizing the etiology, pathogenesis and treatment alternatives. Level of evidence: V.
31. Klein C, Ferrari V, Deroussen F, Juvet-Segarra M, Gouron R: Forearm lengthening and prosthetic management in children with transverse congenital forearm deficiency. *Hand Surg Rehabil* 2019;38(2):129-134.

    This is a retrospective review of four children with transverse deficiency who underwent ulnar lengthening to improve prosthetic fitting. The mean length gain was 21 mm in this cohort. Level of evidence: IV.
32. Crandall RC, Tomhave W: Pediatric unilateral below-elbow amputees: Retrospective analysis of 34 patients given multiple prosthetic options. *J Pediatr Orthop* 2002;22(3):380-383.
33. Krebs DE, Edelstein JE, Thornby MA: Prosthetic management of children with limb deficiencies. *Phys Ther* 1991;71(12):920-934.
34. James MA, Bagley AM, Brasington K, Lutz C, McConnell S, Molitor F: Impact of prostheses on function and quality of life for children with unilateral congenital below-the-elbow deficiency. *J Bone Joint Surg Am* 2006;88(11):2356-2365.
35. Resnik L, Meucci MR, Lieberman-Klinger S, et al: Advanced upper limb prosthetic devices: Implications for upper limb prosthetic rehabilitation. *Arch Phys Med Rehabil* 2012;93(4):710-717.
36. Gretsch KF, Lather HD, Peddada KV, Deeken CR, Wall LB, Goldfarb CA: Development of novel 3D-printed robotic prosthetic for transradial amputees. *Prosthet Orthot Int* 2016;40(3):400-403.

    This article is a case report of a three-dimensional printed prosthesis for a transradial amputee. Level of evidence: IV.
37. Zuniga J, Katsavelis D, Peck J, et al: Cyborg beast: A low-cost 3d-printed prosthetic hand for children with upper-limb differences. *BMC Res Notes* 2015;8:10.
38. E-Nable Community: *Enabling the Future*. Available from: http://enablingthefuture.org/about/. Accessed November 2, 2015.
39. Kuiken TA, Li G, Lock BA, et al: Targeted muscle reinnervation for real-time myoelectric control of multifunction artificial arms. *J Am Med Assoc* 2009;301(6):619-628.
40. Zuo KJ, Willand MP, Ho ES, Ramdial S, Borschel GH: Targeted muscle reinnervation: Considerations for future implementation in adolescents and younger children. *Plast Reconstr Surg* 2018;141(6):1447-1458.

    The authors present a nonsystematic review of targeted muscle reinnervation and its potential application in a pediatric population with congenital or acquired proximal upper limb absence. Level of evidence: V.
41. Kuiken TA, Marasco PD, Lock BA, Harden RN, Dewald JPA: Redirection of cutaneous sensation from the hand to the chest skin of human amputees with targeted reinnervation. *Proc Natl Acad Sci USA* 2007;104(50):20061-20066.
42. Nghiem BT, Sando IC, Gillespie RB, et al: Providing a sense of touch to prosthetic hands. *Plast Reconstr Surg* 2015;135(6):1652-1663.
43. McMullen DP, Hotson G, Katyal KD, et al: Demonstration of a semi-autonomous hybrid brain-machine interface using human intracranial EEG, eye tracking, and computer vision to control a robotic upper limb prosthetic. *IEEE Trans Neural Syst Rehabil Eng* 2014;22(4):784-796.
44. Scudder L, Levin LS: *World's First Pediatric Bilateral Hand Transplant*, 2015. Available from: http://www.medscape.com/viewarticle/848727. Accessed November 2, 2015.
45. Leonard DA, Kurtz JM, Cetrulo CL Jr: Achieving immune tolerance in hand and face transplantation: A realistic prospect? *Immunotherapy* 2014;6(5):499-502.
46. Tamura K, Ohgo S, Yokoyama H: Limb blastema cell: A stem cell for morphological regeneration. *Dev Growth Differ* 2010;52(1):89-99.
47. Monaghan JR, Maden M: Cellular plasticity during vertebrate appendage regeneration. *Curr Top Microbiol Immunol* 2013;367:53-74.
48. Stocum DL: The role of peripheral nerves in urodele limb regeneration. *Eur J Neurosci* 2011;34(6):908-916.

SECTION 5

Lower Extremity

Section Editor:

Vishwas R. Talwalkar, MD, FAAP, FAAOS

CHAPTER 23

Developmental Dysplasia of the Hip

WILLIAM Z. MORRIS, MD • DANIEL J. SUCATO, MD, MS

ABSTRACT

Developmental dysplasia of the hip (DDH) represents a broad spectrum of disease from mild dysplasia through frank dislocation. Early diagnosis and treatment is of paramount importance to favorably alter the natural history of DDH. Early treatment of an unstable hip with a Pavlik harness is generally safe and effective in patients younger than 6 months. In older patients or those in whom a Pavlik harness fails to achieve reduction, closed or open reduction can be used to obtain a stable, congruent joint. Osteotomy of the femur or pelvis may be needed to augment an open reduction. Osteonecrosis and redislocation are two complications associated with closed or open reduction. High rates of residual dysplasia and need for secondary surgery underscore the importance of continued hip surveillance through skeletal maturity. In adolescence, acetabular dysplasia is characterized by increased inclination in the coronal and sagittal planes and a lateralized hip joint center. Treatment is dependent on the severity of dysplasia and symptoms. Restoration of a normal hip joint center with improved/normalized acetabular coverage is achieved with triple innominate osteotomies in those with open triradiate cartilage or a periacetabular osteotomy in the skeletally mature patient.

Neither of the following authors nor any immediate family member has received anything of value from or has stock or stock options held in a commercial company or institution related directly or indirectly to the subject of this chapter: Dr. Morris and Dr. Sucato.

Keywords: developmental dysplasia of the hip (DDH); diagnosis; treatment

INTRODUCTION

Developmental dysplasia of the hip (DDH) is one of the most common abnormal conditions present at birth, affecting up to 15% of infants based on ultrasonographic findings.[1] DDH represents a broad spectrum of disease affecting the femoral head, the acetabulum, or both and ranges from physiologic immaturity of the hip to frank dislocation. Referral for evaluation is frequently triggered by an abnormal newborn hip examination (eg, hip click, instability, limited abduction), which may be present in 4% to 5% of newborns, or because of risk factors (eg, breech position or family history).[2] Although the precise prevalence is difficult to determine, approximately 5 in 1,000 newborns are ultimately treated for neonatal hip dysplasia.[2] Large cross-sectional studies report the prevalence of hip dysplasia in the adult population is between 3% and 5%.[3,4] Identification and early management of DDH has gained increased attention as a recent retrospective study reported that almost half of patients undergoing total hip arthroplasty before 50 years of age have osteoarthritis associated with acetabular dysplasia.[5] However, despite this association, fewer than 10% of young adults requiring arthroplasty for dysplasia-associated osteoarthritis had hip instability at birth.[6] Treatment options are directly related to the severity of the condition and the patient's age at the time of initial treatment. The best results and long-term outcomes occur in patients who are treated earlier in the neonatal period with the least residual dysplasia.[7]

This chapter is adapted from Castañeda P: Developmental dysplasia of the hip, in Martus JE, ed: *Orthopaedic Knowledge Update®: Pediatrics*, ed 5. Rosemont, IL, American Academy of Orthopaedic Surgeons, 2016, pp 245-257.

ETIOLOGY

The etiology of DDH is multifactorial, affected by both intrinsic and environmental factors.[8-17] Traditional risk factors associated with DDH include being female, a firstborn child, a breech presentation, and having a positive family history of dysplasia, oligohydramnios, or foot deformity.[9,10] A murine model of acetabular development revealed that the femoral head must be positioned against the acetabulum for normal development to occur.[18] Similarly, many of the risk factors for DDH reflect an abnormal position of the fetus in the womb during development (eg, breech position, oligohydramnios, or foot deformity), which did not allow the femoral head and acetabulum to maintain a normal relationship during development. The increased incidence of left hip involvement is also thought to be related to positioning as in the left occiput anterior positioning of the newborn the left hip is positioned against the spine, possibly limiting abduction of the hip.[11] Numerous studies have also identified susceptible genes associated with the development of dysplasia, and this genetic component is likely reflected in the risk factor of female sex, with an increased incidence up to 10:1 compared with males,[12] and family history.[13] In fact, one historical series reported that, in co-twins where one twin has congenital dislocation of the hip, the incidence of involvement of the second twin rose from 3% in dizygotic twins to 34% in monozygotic twins.[14] Positioning after birth, such as tightly swaddling the infant with hips and knees in extension and adduction, has also been shown to influence the ongoing hip development and incidence of DDH.[15,16] Cultural differences in the use of swaddling after birth have been shown to influence rates of dysplasia, and in one retrospective study, the incidence of dysplasia decreased after a national campaign sought to change swaddling practices to avoid hip and knee extension.[17]

PATHOLOGIC ANATOMY

Three major pathoanatomic factors in DDH—capsular laxity, acetabular dysplasia, and femoral anteversion—tend to be found in varying degrees in most patients.[19] These factors are present in varying severities based on the spectrum of disease (mild instability to subluxation to frank dislocation) and occur as the femoral head displaces. With continued displacement, the labrum becomes deformed as greater pressure is applied by the femoral head; when the head dislocates, a pseudoacetabulum is formed superior to the true acetabulum. The acetabulum is filled with fibroadipose tissue known as pulvinar, which fills the void left by the femoral head. The joint capsule becomes constricted, and the transverse acetabular ligament is pulled laterally, obstructing the inferior acetabulum. The ligamentum teres is hypertrophic, and with the hip in extension, the iliopsoas tendon constricts the capsule (**Figure 1**). With continued subluxation/dislocation of the femoral head, the stimulus for ongoing development of the cartilaginous acetabulum is lost and relative acetabular dysplasia can persist or worsen.[20]

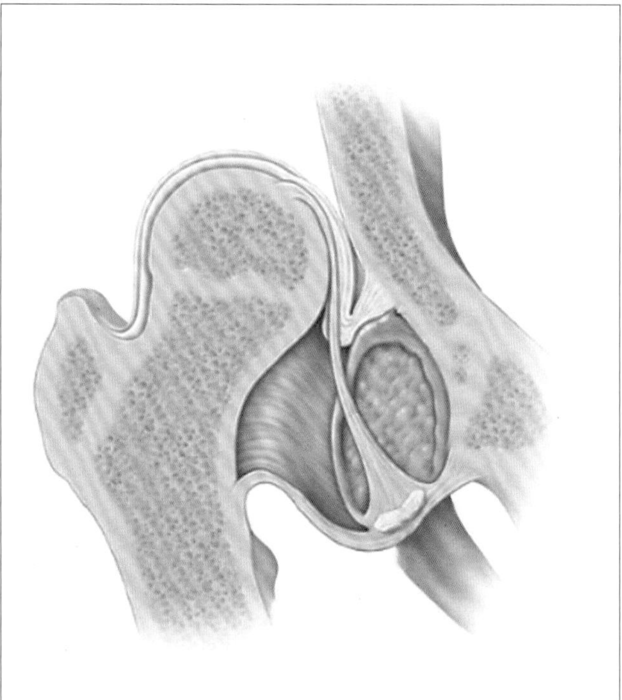

FIGURE 1 Illustration shows pathoanatomy of developmental dysplasia of the hip, including femoral anteversion, acetabular insufficiency, and capsular laxity, which are always present in varying degrees. Hypertrophy of the ligamentum teres, the transverse ligament, and an hourglass constriction of the capsule are present. In a dislocated hip, the so-called pulvinar tissue fills the empty acetabulum. (Adapted with permission from Herring JA: *Tachdjian's Pediatric Orthopedics: from the Texas Scottish Rite Hospital for Children*, ed 5. Copyright Elsevier 2014.)

Strategies for reducing the incidence of DDH have focused on newborn screening and postnatal positioning (safe swaddling) that avoids knee and hip extension.[17]

SCREENING

In 2000, the American Academy of Pediatrics (AAP) released a Clinical Practice Guideline for Early Detection of Developmental Dysplasia of the Hip.[11] They advocated for universal screening with physical examination by the pediatrician. Referral for imaging (ultrasonography or radiography) or evaluation by an orthopaedic surgeon was based on the presence of abnormal/equivocal examination findings or risk factors for DDH including female sex, breech position, and/or family history (**Figure 2**). Several studies have determined that routine neonatal examination combined with selective screening with ultrasonography is the optimal method for early detection.[21-23]

In the first months of life, physical examination screening of infants may reveal signs of dysplasia/dislocation including limited hip abduction, asymmetric thigh folds, an apparent limb-length discrepancy with the hips and knees flexed (the Galeazzi sign), and the

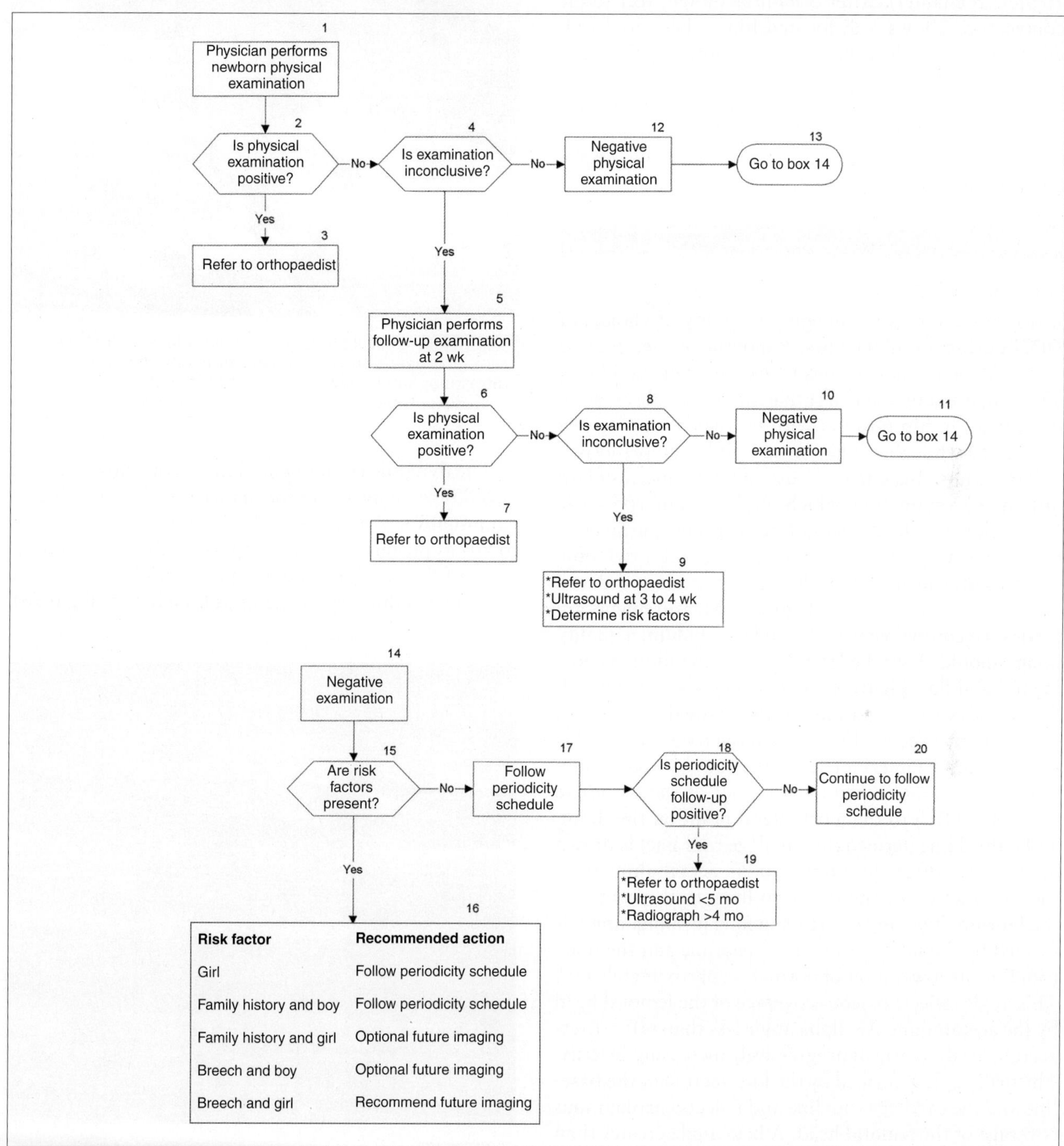

FIGURE 2 Clinical algorithm for screening for developmental dysplasia of the hip. (Reproduced with permission from American Academy of Pediatrics, Committee on Quality Improvement, Subcommittee on Developmental Dysplasia of the Hip: Clinical practice guideline: Early detection of developmental dysplasia of the hip. *Pediatrics* 105[4]:896-905. Copyright © 2000 AAP.)

classic signs of hip instability: a positive Barlow maneuver (hip in place at rest but dislocatable with posteriorly directed stress on the knee with the hip flexed and adducted) or a positive Ortolani maneuver (hip dislocated at rest but reducible with hip flexion, abduction, and an anteriorly directed force on the posterior greater trochanter). After 3 months of age, soft-tissue contracture allows a dislocated hip to become fixed, which may limit the utility of the Barlow and Ortolani tests in that population. As reflected in the Clinical Practice Guidelines, patients with abnormal or equivocal examinations may be further studied with imaging examinations, which generally include ultrasonography and radiography.[11]

IMAGING

Ultrasonography

Ultrasonography is the imaging modality of choice for DDH during an infant's first 6 months of life, because it can define the nonosseous components of the hip. In addition, it is a dynamic test that allows the observation of changes in hip position with movement and can be performed while the child is awake and in an orthosis.[24]

Most clinicians currently use the dynamic standard minimum examination, which combines a morphologic approach using the measurement of specific parameters on a coronal ultrasonographic image, and a dynamic component, which assesses the hip in positions produced by physical maneuvers[24,25] (**Figure 3**). Measurements are made on a coronal view in the midacetabulum; a quality image should show the lateral wall of the ilium as horizontal and flat (**Figure 4**). Three lines are constructed: a baseline is drawn parallel to the ossified lateral wall of the ilium; a second line (termed the bony roof line) is drawn from the inferior edge of the osseous acetabulum (the inferior iliac margin) at the roof of the triradiate cartilage (TRC) to the most lateral point on the ilium; and a third line (termed the cartilage roof line) is drawn along the roof of the cartilaginous acetabulum from the intersection of the first two lines to the center of the labrum. Two angles are created. The alpha angle is formed by the intersection of the baseline and the bony roof line; its lower limit of normal is approximately 60°. This angle reflects osseous coverage of the femoral head by the acetabulum. An alpha angle less than 60° reflects acetabular dysplasia of progressively increasing severity. The beta angle is formed by the intersection of the baseline and the cartilage roof line and reflects cartilaginous coverage of the femoral head. A beta angle greater than 55° represents an increasing degree of subluxation or dislocation and is used less often in the evaluation and treatment than the alpha angle[24] (**Figure 5**).

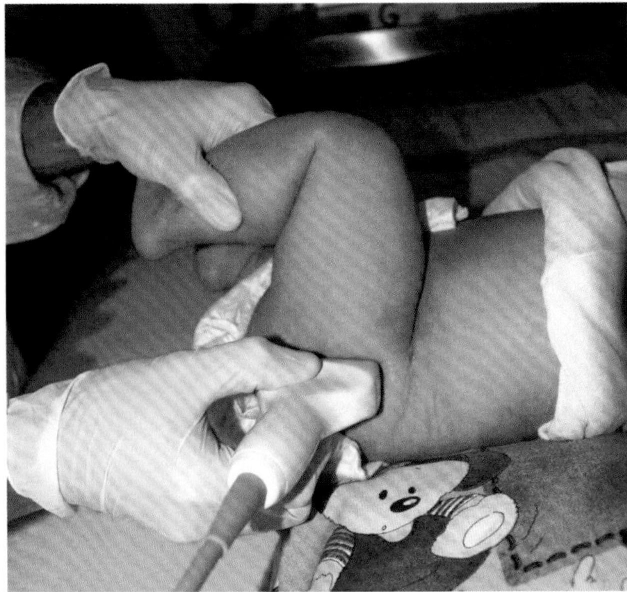

FIGURE 3 Clinical photograph shows placement of the clinician's hands and the transducer to obtain a coronal ultrasonographic view of an infant's hip. Note that the transducer is perpendicular to the femoral axis.

The dynamic component of hip ultrasonography is a visual representation of the maneuvers done on clinical examination. An image is obtained with the hip flexed to 90° as posterior stress is applied to the knee with the palm of the hand, reproducing the Barlow provocative test; any resultant subluxation is then noted (**Figure 6**).

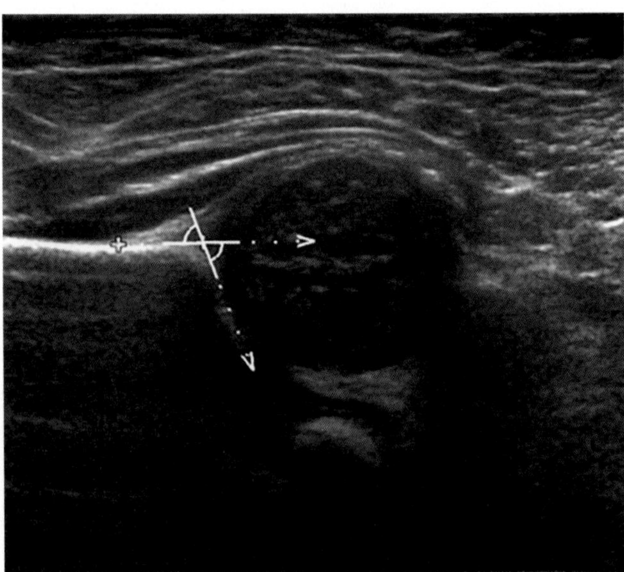

FIGURE 4 Coronal ultrasonogram of an infant's hip shows the ilium on the left and the femoral head, which is the hypoechoic circle in the middle. The lines indicate measurement of the alpha angle.

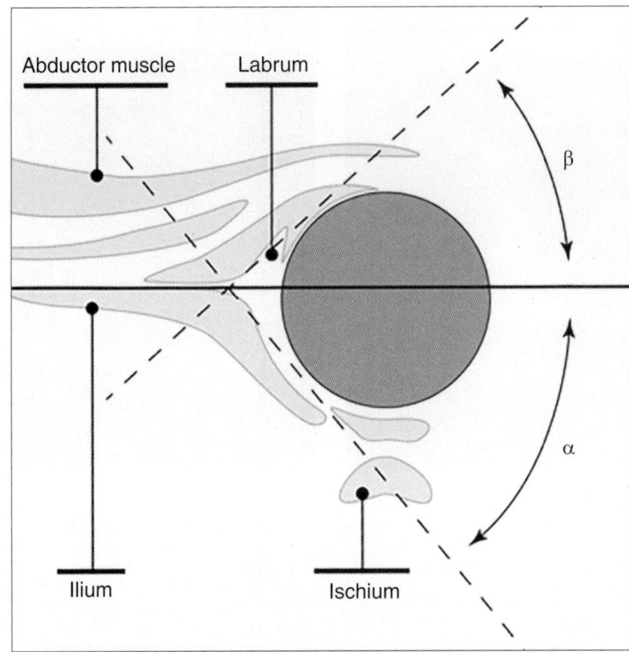

FIGURE 5 Illustration shows the parameters used with measurements on a coronal ultrasonogram to determine the alpha angle and the beta angle.

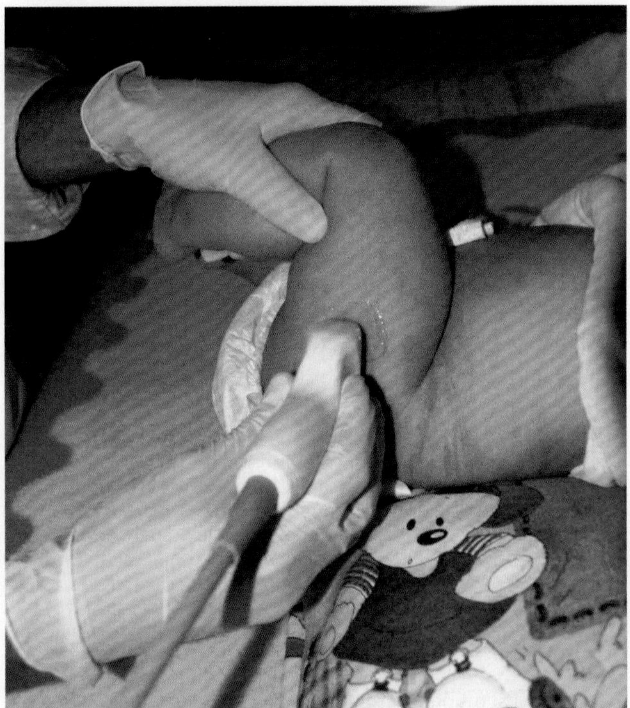

FIGURE 6 Clinical photograph shows placement of the clinician's hands and the transducer to obtain a transverse ultrasonographic view of an infant's hip. Note that the transducer is parallel to the femoral axis.

During the first 4 weeks of life, the femoral head may be reduced in the acetabulum at rest, but up to 4 mm of displacement (physiologic laxity) may be seen under stress. In infants older than 4 weeks, more than 2 mm of subluxation of the femoral head on the transverse view or less than 50% coverage of the femoral head on the longitudinal view is considered abnormal[24] (**Figure 7**).

Universal screening of newborns for DDH has the risks of overdiagnosis and unnecessary treatment. Consequently, the American Academy of Orthopaedic Surgeons (AAOS) released evidence-based guidelines in 2015[26] reporting moderate evidence recommending against universal screening of newborns. However, both the AAOS and AAP guidelines[11,26,27] recommend further evaluation with ultrasonography in infants with one or more risk factors for DDH including breech presentation, family history, or history of clinical hip instability. The ultrasonography is generally performed between 2 and 6 weeks after birth on any newborn with a questionable physical examination finding. When the physical examination is normal but risk factors are present, an ultrasonography should be obtained at 5 to 6 weeks after birth (but not sooner to avoid overdiagnosis and overtreatment).[28]

Radiography

As the ossification center grows and matures (typically beginning by 4 to 6 months of age), radiography can be used to assess the hip joint for signs of DDH. When the hip is dislocated or subluxated, the femoral head is displaced laterally and proximally. Based on the Tönnis system, this displacement can be classified according to the level of the ossific nucleus relative to the lateral margin of the acetabulum (**Figure 8**). Lesser Tönnis grades of dysplasia correlate with an improved prognosis for satisfactory long-term outcomes. Each increase in the Tönnis grade at the time of diagnosis doubles the likelihood of failure of nonsurgical treatment.[29,30] One shortcoming of this classification is that it relies on the presence of a femoral head ossification center, whose appearance is frequently delayed in DDH. The International Hip Dysplasia Institute recently introduced a classification system that accounts for this obstacle by basing the severity of subluxation on the position of the center of the metaphysis relative to a horizontal line connecting the two TRCs (Hilgenreiner line) and a vertical line at the lateral border of the ossified acetabulum (Perkin line, **Figure 9**). This classification system has since been demonstrated to be both reliable and prognostic for success of closed reduction and need for late pelvic osteotomy.[31,32]

A useful radiographic measurement in children younger than 8 years is the acetabular index.[29] It is a

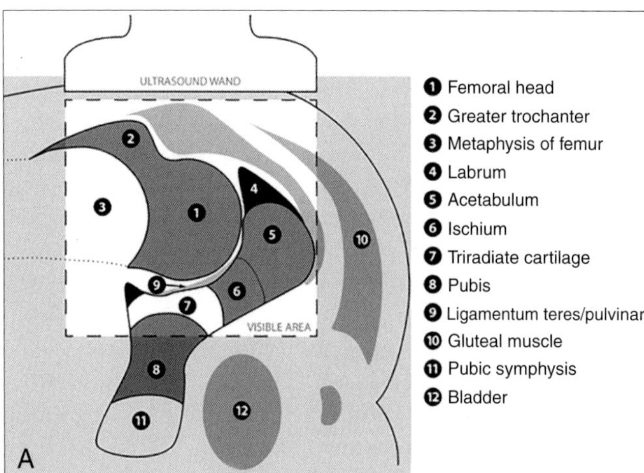

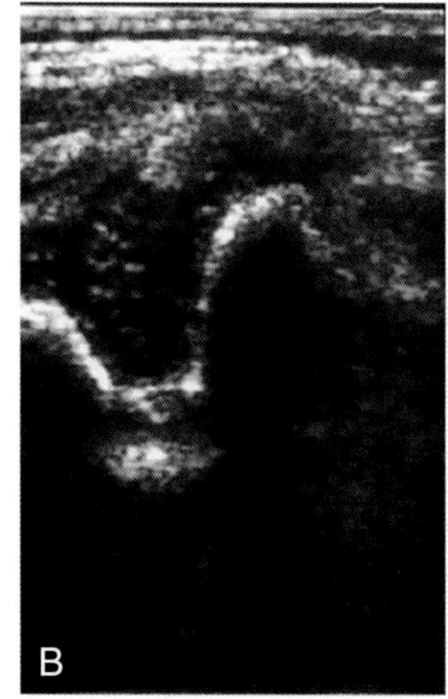

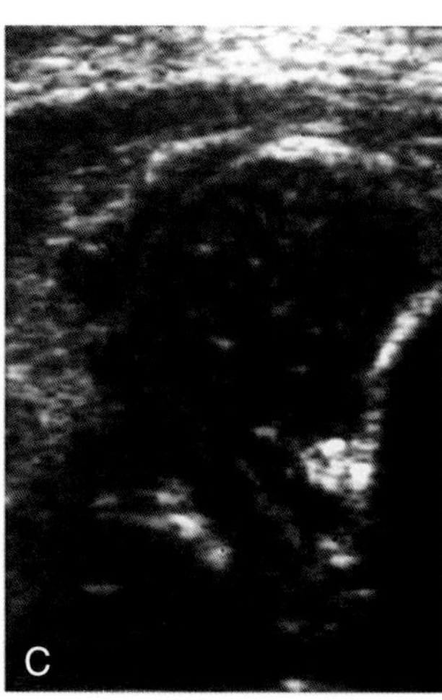

FIGURE 7 **A**, Diagram describes the anatomy seen on a longitudinal ultrasonogram of an infant's hip. Ultrasonograms of an unstable hip demonstrate that the distance from the femoral head to the acetabulum (**B**) increases (**C**) when posterior stress is applied.

measure of the inclination of the ossified acetabulum as determined by the angle formed between a horizontal line connecting the TRCs (Hilgenreiner line) and a line drawn from the iliac margin at the upper edge of the TRC to the most lateral edge of the ossified acetabulum (**Figure 10**). The acetabular index progressively

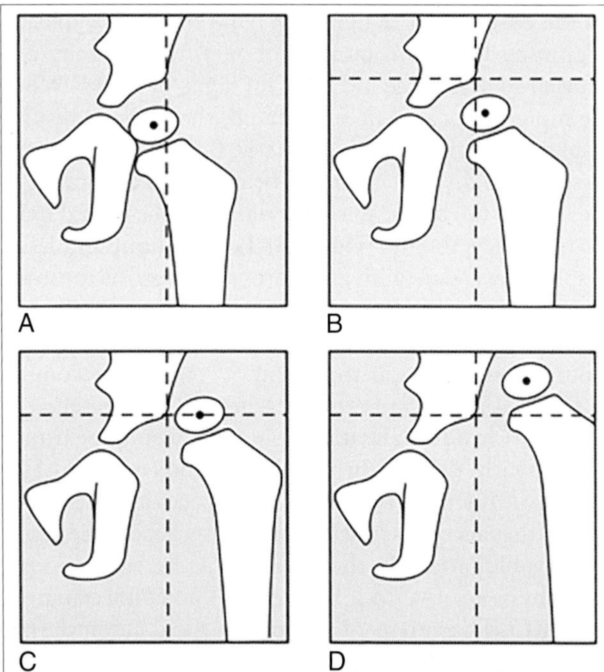

FIGURE 8 Illustrations of grade I (**A**), grade II (**B**), grade III (**C**), and grade IV (**D**) of the Tönnis classification of developmental dysplasia of the hip, in which femoral head displacement is determined based on the level of the ossific nucleus relative to the lateral margin of the acetabulum.

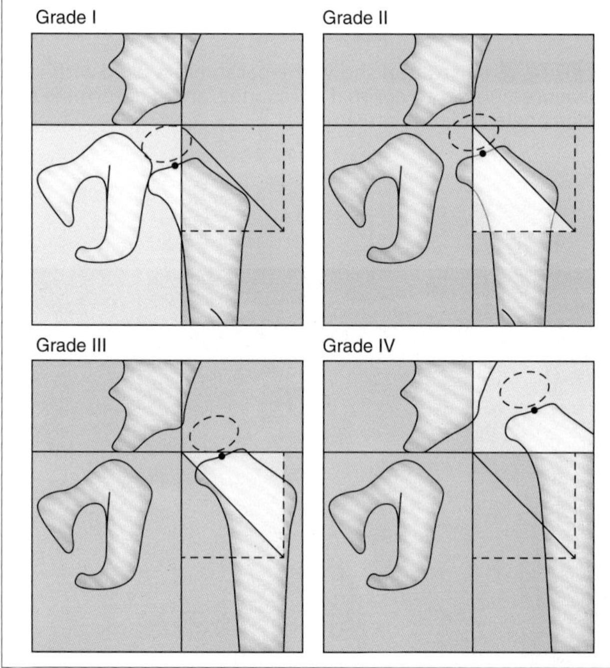

FIGURE 9 Illustration showing the International Hip Dysplasia Institute classification for developmental dysplasia of the hip (not requiring the presence of an ossific nucleus). H-line is Hilgenreiner line drawn through the top of the triradiate cartilages bilaterally. P-line is Perkin line drawn perpendicular to the H-line at the superolateral margin of the acetabulum. D-line is diagonal line drawn 45° from the junction of H-line and P-line. H-point is the midpoint of the superior margin of the ossified metaphysis. Grade I: the H-point is at or medial to the P-line. Grade II: the H-point is lateral to the P-line and at or medial to the D-line. Grade III: the H-point is lateral to the D-line and at or inferior to the H-line. Grade IV: the H-point is superior to the H-line. (Reproduced with permission from Narayanan U, Mulpuri K, Sankar WN, Clarke NM, Hosalkar H, Price CT, International Hip Dysplasia Institute: Reliability of a new radiographic classification for developmental dysplasia of the hip. *J Pediatr Orthop* 2015;35[5]:478-484.)

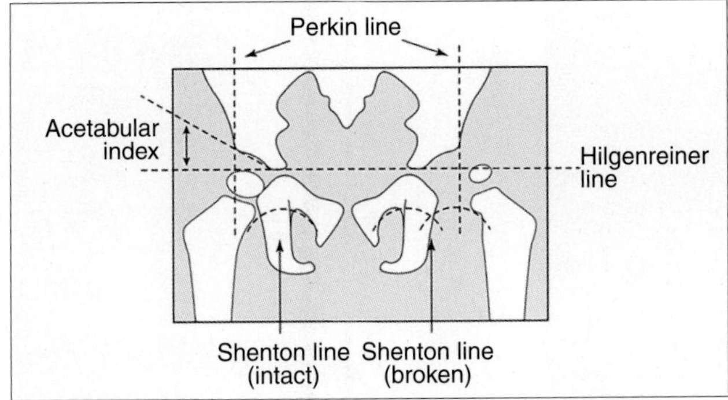

FIGURE 10 Illustration shows basic radiographic parameters used in determining the acetabular index.

decreases with age but will remain abnormally high in a dysplastic hip. The range for normal acetabular indices has been defined in a 1976 study[29] (**Figure 11**).

In adolescents and young adults, measurement of acetabular dysplasia is most commonly measured through the lateral center-edge angle (LCEA), anterior center-edge angle, and Tönnis angle[33] (**Figure 12**). The LCEA of Wiberg reflects lateral acetabular coverage and is measured on the AP radiograph as the angle subtended between a vertical line and a line from the center of the femoral head to the lateral border of the sourcil (the weight-bearing portion of the acetabulum). A normal value is greater than 25°. The anterior center-edge angle reflects anterior acetabular coverage and is measured on the false-profile view as the angle formed between a vertical line and a line from the center of the femoral head to the anterior border of the sourcil. A normal value is greater than 20°. The Tönnis angle reflects acetabular inclination and is determined from an AP radiograph as the angle formed between a horizontal line connecting the radiographic teardrops and a line connecting the medial and lateral edges of the sourcil. A normal value is less than 10°.

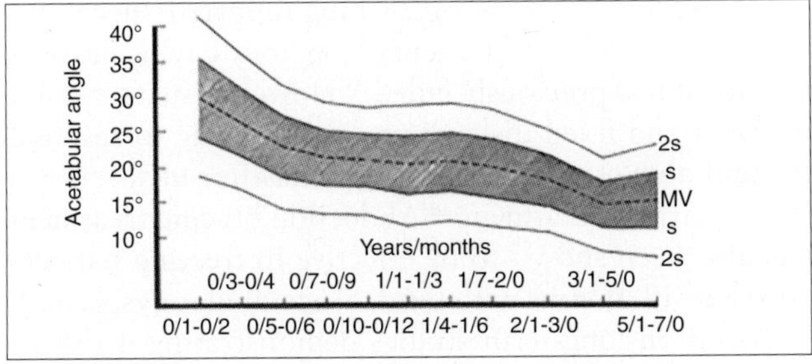

FIGURE 11 Nomogram shows means and standard deviations for the acetabular index based on the patient's age. (Reproduced with permission from Tönnis D: Normal values of the hip joint for the evaluation of X-rays in children and adults. *Clin Orthop Relat Res* 1976;119:39-47.)

INFANTS YOUNGER THAN 6 MONTHS

Treatment

Treatment is indicated at the time a dislocation is noted or when sonographic instability or significant dysplasia persist beyond 6 weeks of age. In cases of mild dysplasia (eg, Graf IIa hips) or in cases of physiologic immaturity associated with premature infants, close surveillance with serial ultrasonography may be used to monitor for resolution before committing to treatment. Clinical instability, which is determined by the presence of a positive Barlow sign, should be treated if it persists beyond the second week of extrauterine life. Before this time, it may be acceptable to wait, because some hips resolve spontaneously. However, if the instability is present after the second extrauterine week, it is generally agreed that most hips should receive treatment because spontaneous resolution is unlikely. The definition of instability or dysplasia is not universal.[34] Instability is considered to be present when the femoral head displaces more than 4 mm from the acetabulum on ultrasonography in an infant older than 6 weeks. Dysplasia is considered to be present when the bony coverage of the femoral head is less than 50% or the α-angle is less than 50°. Because these parameters change with increasing age, more than 2 mm of displacement is considered abnormal in a child older than 3 months, and the mean alpha angle also should be substantially higher than 60° in a child older than 3 months.[24,25]

Of the multiple devices available for treatment of DDH, the most commonly used in North America is the Pavlik harness. The method developed by Pavlik consists of obtaining dynamic abduction while allowing the child to move freely within the confines of the harness, which consists of a chest strap that provides sites of attachment for two lower extremity straps. These straps prevent hip extension and allow dynamic abduction while avoiding adduction and maintaining flexion, generally between 90° and 110°. Avoiding forced abduction decreases the risk for the development of osteonecrosis. The harness should be worn for 23 hours a day to allow for baths, and recent retrospective studies demonstrated no difference in clinical or radiographic short-term outcomes between 23-hour and 24-hour use.[35,36] The initial weekly visit should include an ultrasonography with the Pavlik harness on to demonstrate a good reduction, which may take a few weeks. Following an adequate reduction, the ultrasonography evaluations can take place with the Pavlik harness off and do not require weekly checks.[37,38] In almost 98% of patients, reduction is achieved within the first 3 weeks in the harness.[37] Treatment of a persistently dislocated hip with a Pavlik harness beyond 3 to 4 weeks has traditionally not been recommended because of potential damage to the posterior wall of the acetabulum, which leads

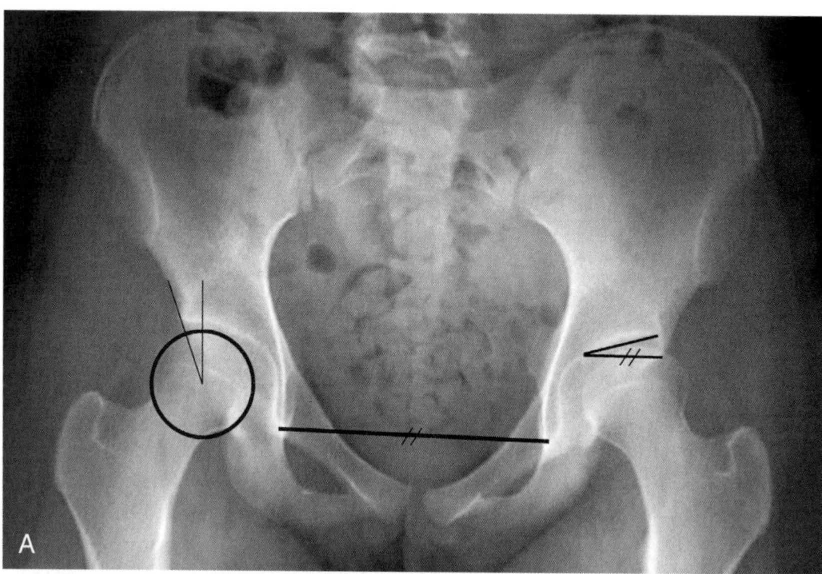

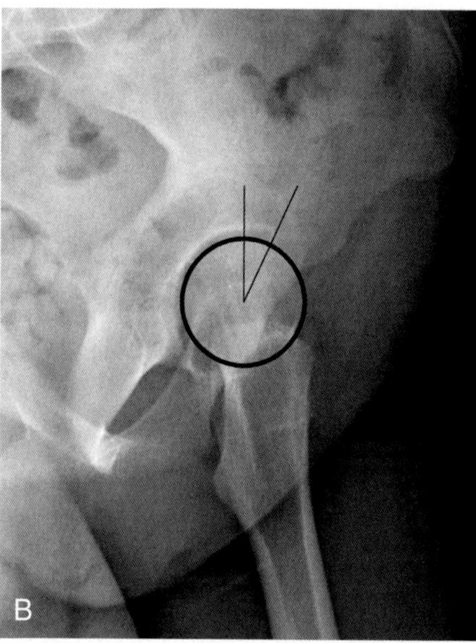

FIGURE 12 The lateral center-edge angle of Wiberg reflects lateral acetabular coverage and is measured on the AP radiograph (**A**, left) as the angle subtended between a vertical line and a line from the center of the femoral head to the lateral border of the sourcil (the weight-bearing portion of the acetabulum). A normal value is greater than 25°. The anterior center-edge angle reflects anterior acetabular coverage and is measured on the false-profile view (**B**) as the angle formed between a vertical line and a line from the center of the femoral head to the anterior border of the sourcil. A normal value is greater than 20°. The Tönnis angle (**A**, right) reflects acetabular inclination and is determined from an AP radiograph as the angle formed between a horizontal line connecting the radiographic teardrops and a line connecting the medial and lateral edges of the sourcil. A normal value is less than 10°.

to worsening dysplasia and instability.[39,40] The harness should be worn until the hip is sonographically normal and stable within the acetabulum and has bony coverage of at least 50% and an alpha angle of at least 60°. In general, full-time harness wear is prescribed for 6 weeks followed by a 6-week period of part-time wear (nights and naps) with excellent clinical and radiographic results.

Complications

Complications, which can include transient femoral nerve palsy caused by hyperflexion of the hips and osteonecrosis caused by excessive abduction, are rare and usually originate in physician or parental misunderstanding regarding proper application of the harness. A report of 30 cases of femoral nerve palsy identified an incidence of 2.5%.[38] Femoral nerve palsy is more likely to occur in larger infants with more severe dislocations. Most nerve palsies occur in the first week after application of the harness, and recovery always occurs with harness removal. Resuming harness wear with less hip flexion following nerve function return will help to prevent further nerve palsy and provide the best opportunity for successful dysplasia treatment. Osteonecrosis of the femoral epiphysis has been reported in the normal and abnormal hips of infants treated with a Pavlik harness.[41] A 2013 systematic review summarized reported rates of osteonecrosis between 1% and 30% with increased risk associated with increased severity of dysplasia/dislocation.[42]

Outcomes

The success rates with the Pavlik method are varied and dependent on the severity of the dysplasia and the definition of success. A systematic review reported that between 80% and 100% of dislocated hips are successfully reduced with Pavlik harness wear.[42] The success rate decreases substantially with higher grades of dislocation and increasing patient age, with the lowest success rates seen in dislocated hips and in patients in whom Pavlik harness wear is initiated at 4 months of age or later.[43,44] If reduction is not obtained within 3 to 4 weeks but the hip can be reduced by manipulation (Ortolani positive), rigid abduction bracing treatment can be of value as a second-line treatment in patients younger than 6 months. A retrospective review of 28 hips reported successful reduction in 82% of patients in whom Pavlik harness treatment had previously failed.[45] However, success is not uniform and fixed dislocations are unlikely to respond to rigid abduction bracing treatment after unsuccessful Pavlik harness treatment.[46] Abduction bracing treatment has also been shown to be effective in treating patients aged 6 to 12 months with residual acetabular dysplasia.[47]

Based on long-term studies demonstrating a risk of development of secondary dysplasia following successful treatment of DDH in infancy, radiographic surveillance of acetabular development until skeletal maturity is currently recommended for all patients with DDH.[48,49] Radiographic signs of improving acetabular development include a decreasing acetabular index, the development of a smooth horizontal sourcil (dense bone on the weight-bearing surface of the acetabulum), and the development of a narrow U-shaped radiographic teardrop lateral to the ilio-ischial line. Radiographic signs of persistent acetabular dysplasia include an acetabular index greater than 24° by the age of 2 years, an acetabular index higher than 2 SDs above the mean,[50] or no improvement over a substantial period of time. MRI also has been used to predict the presence of residual dysplasia[51,52] (**Figure 13**).

CHILDREN OF WALKING AGE

Treatment

The treatment of DDH becomes increasingly challenging as a child ages. The ideal treatment obtains a timely, stable reduction while minimizing the need for further surgery and the risk for development of complications such as redislocation or osteonecrosis. After the age of approximately 4 to 6 months or when orthotic treatment has failed, other treatments should be considered.

Closed reduction is indicated for two groups of children: (1) those with a dislocated hip in whom orthotic treatment has failed and (2) those with a late-presenting dislocated hip for whom primary Pavlik harness treatment is not suitable. These children generally range from 4 to 18 months of age. Imaging should be obtained to determine the severity of the dislocation and rule out the presence of a so-called teratologic hip (a hip that has been dislocated since a very early time in embryonic development), which is not amenable to closed reduction.

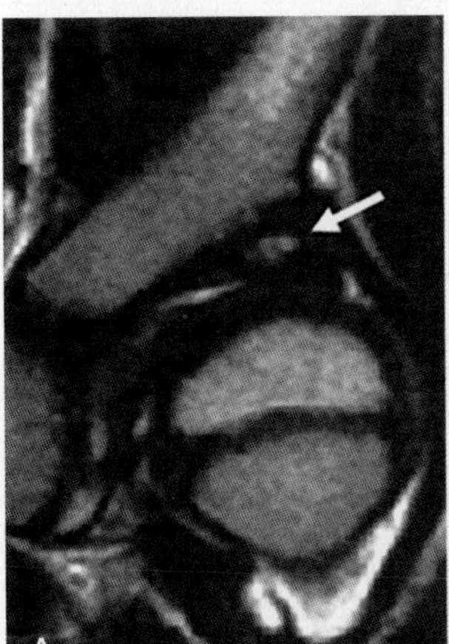

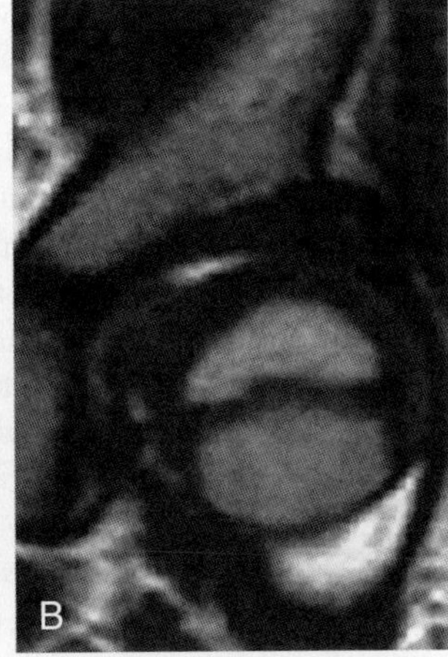

FIGURE 13 Magnetic resonance images of the hips of infants with a positive high signal intensity area (white arrow, **A**) and negative high signal intensity area (**B**). A high signal intensity area correlates with an increased likelihood of residual dysplasia after a closed reduction. (Reproduced with permission from Wakabayashi K, Wada I, Horiuchi O, Mizutani J, Tsuchiya D, Otsuka T: MRI findings in residual hip dysplasia. *J Pediatr Orthop* 2011;31[4]:381-387.)

Teratologic dislocations tend to show very marked and advanced changes in the hip joint and can be associated with various conditions, including arthrogryposis multiplex congenita, lumbosacral agenesis, chromosomal abnormalities, diastrophic dwarfism, and Larsen syndrome. Teratologic hips can be difficult to distinguish radiographically; however, these hips tend to have certain characteristics such as the absence of a sulcus seen on the lateral border of the acetabulum caused by the mechanical effect of the femoral head sliding out of the acetabulum. In teratologic dislocations, this phenomenon is not seen because the femoral head has never been in the acetabulum. The ilium also tends to be smaller, and the degree of dysplasia tends to be greater than in typical dysplasia. A teratologic hip is best managed with open reduction at a minimum age of 8 to 9 months. Relative contraindications for closed reduction are the existence of an important medical problem or evidence of a failure to thrive. Treatment can be delayed until the child's medical condition has improved.

A closed reduction is performed under general anesthesia with hip abduction and an anteriorly directed force on the posterior aspect of the greater trochanter to obtain reduction. The use of preoperative overhead traction has recently been demonstrated to offer no advantage to achieving a successful reduction or avoiding osteonecrosis in a large series of patients.[53] Once reduction is obtained, assessment of the safe zone determines the range of hip abduction and adduction at 90° of flexion through which the reduction is maintained. In hips with adduction contracture creating a narrow safe zone, an adductor tenotomy can be used to widen the safe zone so that forced abduction is not required to maintain the hips in 40° to 60° of abduction. Arthrography is used to evaluate the reduction intraoperatively with a medial dye pool ≤6 mm or 16% of the femoral head diameter both shown to be predictive of a successful reduction.[54,55] Advanced imaging may also be obtained to confirm reduction. MRI is commonly the modality of choice because of the lack of radiation and greater ability to visualize the cartilaginous femoral head and other soft tissues. Gadolinium can be added to the study to evaluate perfusion of the femoral head after the reduction, with preliminary data suggesting that perfusion MRI may be predictive of osteonecrosis and allow the surgeon to revise the reduction/cast positioning at the same visit.[56,57] However, recent recognition of deposition of gadolinium-based contrast agents in the basal ganglia (with undetermined long-term consequences) has increased concern about their use in the developing brain.[58] CT can be of use, with limited cut sequences developed to reduce the radiation required. A cast change can be performed if the hip is not reduced, but the goal is maintenance of the human position of at least 90° of flexion and the least amount of necessary abduction to retain a stable hip while avoiding the risk of osteonecrosis.

Open reduction should be considered if an acceptable closed reduction is unobtainable or would require excessive force. An open reduction can be performed through a medial or anterior approach. In both cases, the open reduction allows the surgeon to address the impediments to reduction: the joint capsule, inverted labrum/limbus, hypertrophied ligamentum teres, pulvinar, and transverse acetabular ligament. However, a capsulorrhaphy can only be performed through an anterior approach. The timing of open reduction and the use of a medial or anterior approach has been studied extensively given concerns that earlier open reduction (particularly before the appearance of femoral head ossification center) may be associated with the development of osteonecrosis. However, a 2016 meta-analysis found no association between closed or open reduction before or after 12 months of age and the development of osteonecrosis. They similarly found no association between medial or anterior surgical approach and the development of osteonecrosis, but noted that many of the studies were level III or IV evidence.[59]

In children younger than 18 months, substantial remodeling of the acetabulum can occur after a closed or open reduction without bony surgery. Pelvic or femoral osteotomies are rarely required in these younger children. In addition, the bone in the pelvis of children younger than 18 months is too soft to allow optimal correction or maintain correction with an innominate osteotomy. After 18 months of age, there is an increased likelihood of either femoral or pelvic osteotomy. A femoral shortening osteotomy may be indicated if soft-tissue contractures result in excessive pressure on the femoral head in the acetabulum following open reduction. The osteotomy also allows for derotation as increased femoral anteversion is frequently present in a dislocated hip.

In patients older than 18 months with severe dysplasia or in patients for whom an open reduction with or without femoral osteotomy does not provide a stable reduction, a pelvic osteotomy may augment acetabular coverage and improve hip stability. Pelvic osteotomies may be performed to either reorient the acetabulum (eg, innominate/Salter, triple osteotomies) or to change the shape of the acetabulum (eg, Pemberton or Dega acetabuloplasties). An innominate osteotomy is most commonly used in patients between 18 months and 3 years of age. It allows for redirection of the acetabulum to improve anterolateral coverage of the hip and reliably obtains 15° of anterior and 25° of lateral coverage if performed properly. Technical errors such as pulling up on the proximal iliac fragment, allowing the posterior aspect of the osteotomy to open, or allowing the distal fragment to fall posteriorly will not allow anterolateral rotation of the acetabular fragment in the correct plane.[19,60]

In patients with severe acetabular dysplasia in whom instability persists after open reduction, capsulorrhaphy, innominate osteotomy, femoral shortening osteotomy (to decrease the tension across the hip joint), and the resolution of all technical issues, the use of a transarticular fixation pin has been shown to be safe and effective.[61] The pin is removed through a window in the spica cast after 4 weeks. The hip should never be left subluxated at the conclusion of the primary procedure because redislocation will invariably occur, and any revision will be considered salvage surgery. A well-reduced hip following an open reduction frequently appears as though the femoral head is partially subluxated inferiorly with a break in the Shenton line, because this confirms removal of the obstacles to reduction including the transverse acetabular ligament.

Following open or closed reduction, the patient is generally treated in a spica cast for approximately 3 months (based on surgeon preference) while the soft tissues and possible osteotomies heal, cementing the stability of the reduction.

Complications

The two most serious and common complications in the surgical management of DDH are osteonecrosis and redislocation. Osteonecrosis is an iatrogenic complication because it does not occur as part of the natural history of DDH, but it can occur even when treatment is performed by an experienced orthopaedic surgeon. Osteonecrosis can affect the long-term function of a hip and has been reported to occur in up to approximately 40% of hips after open reduction based on the stringency used to define the condition.[59] Osteonecrosis may be compatible with satisfactory function until the teenage years, at which point the hip may become symptomatic with stiffness, pain, and degenerative changes. Although open reduction and the use of an anterior approach before the age of 12 months have been traditionally associated with osteonecrosis, a 2016 meta-analysis revealed no association between surgical approach (medial or anterior) or reduction before 12 months of age and the development of osteonecrosis.[59] However, technical factors such as avoiding excessive tension across the hip joint, damage to the circulation to the femoral head, and excessive abduction in the spica cast clearly have a role in reducing the rate of osteonecrosis.[19]

Redislocation usually results from a technical failure on the part of the operating surgeon. The most common cause of redislocation is failure to identify the true acetabulum. This failure may occur because established dislocations often have a well-formed pseudoacetabulum located superolateral to the true acetabulum. The first attempt at surgical reduction of a dislocated hip has the best chance for achieving a satisfactory result. Secondary procedures on a redislocated hip are technically challenging and the results are far less ensured than those of a primary open reduction; therefore, revision procedures are considered salvage procedures.

The treatment of redislocation varies depending on when it is identified; in the immediate postoperative period, the issue is likely a technical surgical failure. All steps in the surgical procedure should be reviewed to identify the primary problem. CT can help identify structural problems such as inadequate correction by pelvic osteotomy or excessive derotation of the femur. Revision surgery is appropriate in these cases to correct problems, and the addition of a transfixation pin can be considered for persistent instability. A less-than-satisfactory result can be expected if hip subluxation is present in the immediate postoperative period, because the hip will not stabilize spontaneously.

If redislocation is identified at a later stage (eg, after removal of the hip spica cast), early revision surgery is not recommended, because the hip will be stiff and osteopenic. These factors make surgery far more challenging, and the risk of further complications, including pathologic fracture, is more likely. A prerequisite for any osteotomy is an adequate range of motion in the adjacent joints. In this situation, a delay in open reduction revision is indicated after a rehabilitation period of approximately 3 months with weight bearing as tolerated to allow range of motion of the hip to return and promote strengthening of bone stock. During this time, the technical reasons for dislocation should be assessed, essential imaging such as CT should be obtained, and the revision should be planned.

Outcomes and Residual Dysplasia

Historical long-term results for patients undergoing closed or open reductions for DDH have shown good, but guarded outcomes. A retrospective study of closed reductions with mean 30-year follow-up reported good or excellent functional outcomes in 90% of patients, but residual radiographic dysplasia in over half of the patients.[62] A retrospective study of patients undergoing open reduction and innominate osteotomy with mean 43-year follow-up reported hip survivorship of 99% at 30 years, but only 54% by 45 years after initial treatment. Successful primary surgery correlated with better long-term outcomes while risk factors for poor outcomes include bilateral surgery (a 2.9 times greater risk of needing a subsequent hip replacement than those who initially underwent unilateral surgery) and the need for revision surgery.[63]

Contemporary studies of midterm outcomes following closed and open reduction highlight the need for continued surveillance of the hip through skeletal maturity. Two recent retrospective studies reported rates of secondary surgery for residual dysplasia following closed reduction between 35% and 58% while 19% of patients who underwent open reduction required secondary surgery.[64,65] Given these findings, continued clinical and radiographic follow-up is essential as secondary acetabular dysplasia may necessitate additional surgical intervention in adolescence or young adulthood.

ADOLESCENT HIP DYSPLASIA

Adolescent hip dysplasia can be defined radiographically as a hip with an abnormally inclined acetabulum. Several other radiographic findings can be associated with this to include decreased joint space, a lateralized joint center, an abnormally shaped femoral head, and sclerotic margins of the sourcil with subchondral cysts. A careful history with specific details of the presence and location of symptoms is critically important when radiographic dysplasia is seen because this will help to develop the ideal game plan for treatment of each patient.

The history is important and should include whether symptoms are present, because often patients may have radiographic dysplasia without associated pain or discomfort. The location of symptoms generally distinguishes between lateral hip pain, which is most often attributed to decreased hip abductor muscle strength, and deep anterior groin pain, which generally indicates pain originating from the joint itself. This latter pain can occur from joint overload, edge-loading of the acetabulum, labral irritation or injury, or labral chondral injury. These symptoms provide a more direct relationship linking the symptoms to the hip pathology. Lateral hip pain is most often the initial symptom, occurring later in the day as fatigue develops, and is due to altered biomechanics leading to a greater force required to maintain normal walking. This initial symptom is often missed because it is mild compared with the deep groin pain. Deep groin pain occurs later, is reported to be more common, is activity-related, and improves when activity restriction is instituted.[66]

The physical examination should include observation of ambulation to assess for an antalgic gait (decreased stance phase, which is uncommon in the adolescent) and/or a subtle Trendelenburg gait (centering body weight over the hip as a protective mechanism to avoid pain or to offset the relatively weak abductors). The hip range of motion should be examined for restriction in motion as well as to determine relative femoral version. An important maneuver is the impingement test that assesses the status of pain with flexion, internal rotation, and adduction and should be performed to determine the likelihood of true symptomatic labral pathology. Labral tears may occur because of joint overload and rim-loading, femoroacetabular impingement related to concurrent cam morphology (an asphericity of the femoral head-neck junction), or a combination of the two.

Imaging of the patient with adolescent hip dysplasia should include a well-centered AP pelvis radiograph to determine the radiographic parameters previously outlined and can be done standing (our preferred technique) or supine. Assessment of the degree of early osteoarthritis should be determined using the Tönnis grading system (1, slight joint space narrowing, lipping, sclerosis; 2, subchondral cysts, further joint space narrowing, loss of femoral head sphericity; 3, large cysts, severe joint space narrowing, femoral head deformity) because advanced degeneration is widely associated with poor outcomes following surgery. An abduction-internal rotation view, known as the Von Rosen view, is used to determine whether the hip reduces concentrically—a prerequisite for a rotational acetabular osteotomy. The false-profile radiograph is used to determine the anterior coverage of the femoral head by the acetabulum and also provides an understanding of the width of the posterior column for planning osteotomies, which travel down this structure. A 45° or 90° Dunn lateral view is used to determine whether there is concurrent presence of cam morphology, an asphericity of the femoral head-neck junction, which can lead to femoroacetabular impingement and chondrolabral injury even in the presence of acetabular dysplasia. Objective measurement of cam morphology is most frequently determined by the alpha angle. The alpha angle is measured by placing a best-fit circle over the femoral head and determining the angle subtended by a line from the center of the head along the femoral neck axis and a line from the center of the femoral head and the point where the anterosuperior head-neck junction exits from the best-fit circle (**Figure 14**). Although the precise threshold to define cam morphology is variable, an alpha angle >42° suggests some femoral head-neck offset deformity.[33] More recently, the osseous anatomy has been assessed with a CT scan to determine femoral and acetabular version, evaluate for possible cam morphology, and assess overall acetabular morphology, but is not a routine study for most cases.[67] The indication for a magnetic resonance arthrogram in the adolescent patient population to assess labral and labral-chondral abnormalities is controversial but is generally indicated for severe groin pain with a positive impingement sign even at mild arcs of flexion/internal rotation/adduction. The incidence of labral pathology in patients with hip dysplasia is reported to occur in two-thirds of patients,[68] which should be weighed against the approximately 40% incidence found in an asymptomatic young adults.[69] Although there are limited data on imaging findings in the adolescent population, other findings in adult hip dysplasia include acetabular cartilage lesions (69%) and combined labral/cartilage lesions (59%) most commonly seen on the anterior and superolateral acetabulum.

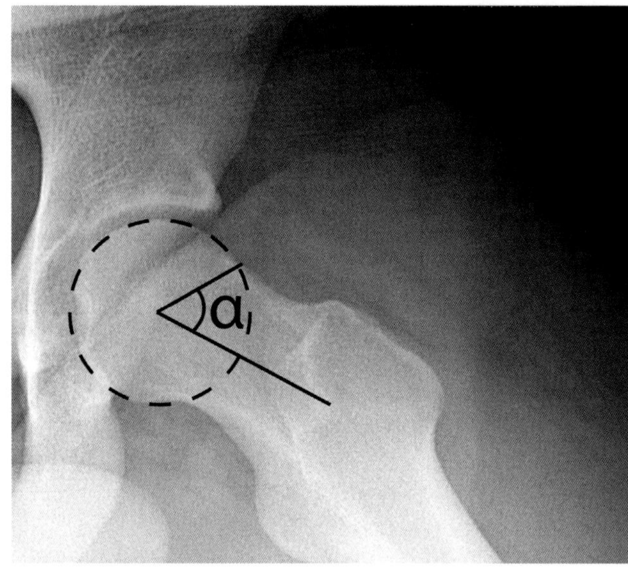

FIGURE 14 The alpha angle is measured from a 45° or 90° Dunn lateral view. Measurement is performed by placing a best-fit circle over the femoral head and determining the angle subtended by a line from the center of the head along the femoral neck axis and a line from the center of the femoral head and the point where the anterosuperior head-neck junction exits from the best-fit circle. Although the precise threshold to define cam morphology is variable, an alpha angle >42° suggests some femoral head-neck offset deformity.

Treatment of the asymptomatic patient with hip dysplasia is controversial. Observation with maintenance or improvement in hip abductor and flexor strength is generally recommended with continued clinical and radiographic surveillance. Nonsurgical management is primarily recommended because of the lack of a long-term comparative study demonstrating a significant change in the natural history of the condition with surgical treatment. In patients who initially present with symptoms, hip abductor and flexor strengthening should be initiated to improve symptoms and facilitate more rapid recovery if surgical treatment is ultimately performed.

Surgical management is the mainstay of treatment in the adolescent age group and addresses the acetabular position within the pelvis to improve the typical biomechanical deficiencies: a lateralized hip joint center, decreased anterior and lateral coverage of the femoral head by the acetabulum, and abnormal version of the acetabulum. Indication for surgery is a symptomatic patient with radiographic findings of hip dysplasia using the radiographic parameters noted earlier. Controversy exists regarding the borderline dysplasia in which the center edge angle is 20° to 25° or even as low as 18°. However, early literature suggests the benefits of a periacetabular osteotomy (PAO) with improved pain and function at short-term follow-up in this patient population.[70]

The reorientation of the acetabulum can be performed with either a triple innominate osteotomy if the TRC is open, or a PAO if the TRC is closed (or closing). All triple osteotomies share two of the three cuts of the pelvis: the superior ramus osteotomy (beginning medial to the anterior limb of the TRC extending into the obturator foramen) and the innominate osteotomy (beginning just distal to the anterior superior iliac spine and extending into the sciatic notch). The differences between versions of triple osteotomies are present in the location of the ischial cut. The Steel involves a vertical cut in the ischial tuberosity and the Carliosz involves a horizontal osteotomy starting inferior to the acetabulum and extending distal to the ischial spine. A preferred version of the triple osteotomy is the Tönnis because the ischial cut begins just distal to the acetabulum but travels proximal to the ischial spine so that the sacrospinous ligament remains with the pelvis and does not restrict the rotation of the acetabular fragment (**Figure 15**). This osteotomy provides nearly the same mobility as the PAO while avoiding the open TRC. It is more unstable following positioning of the fragment (because of the discontinuity of the posterior column of the acetabulum) and requires more fixation than a PAO. Long-term outcomes (mean follow-up of 15 years) following Tönnis triple osteotomy demonstrate 88% survival with good to excellent results in 64%.[71]

Currently, the most common osteotomy to correct acetabular dysplasia in the adolescent or young adult is the Bernese PAO (**Figure 16**). Advantages of this osteotomy over others include the following: it is performed through a single incision and an abductor muscle-sparing approach; it results in a stable osteotomy (because of an intact posterior column) to allow early rehabilitation; the approach allows for access to the hip joint for intra-articular work; and it has little effect on the pelvic outlet to allow for subsequent normal childbearing in female patients. The prerequisites for treatment with PAO are hip dysplasia with the ability for the hip to reduce concentrically on the abduction-internal rotation view without radiographic evidence of significant osteoarthritis. Outcomes are dependent on proper positioning of the acetabular fragment, and assessment of correction should consequently focus on four primary measurements: lateral coverage aiming for an LCEA of 25°, anterior coverage with an anterior center edge angle of 25°, medialization of the hip joint center with restoration of Shenton line, and normal acetabular version based on the anterior and posterior walls meeting laterally at the same position. Correction can be assessed using intraoperative fluoroscopic imaging, which has been shown to correlate with postoperative plain radiographs with only small differences noted for the LCEA (−0.38°) and the acetabular index (−0.84°).[72] The learning curve for the PAO seems to be realized after 20 procedures, and a recent study of outcomes in adolescent and young adult patients demonstrated 10-year survival of 93%, with success dependent on excellent joint congruency and proper orientation of the acetabulum with a center edge angle between 20° and 40°.[73] A long-term outcome study demonstrates a 30-year survival of 29% with recommendations not to perform the procedure for patients with

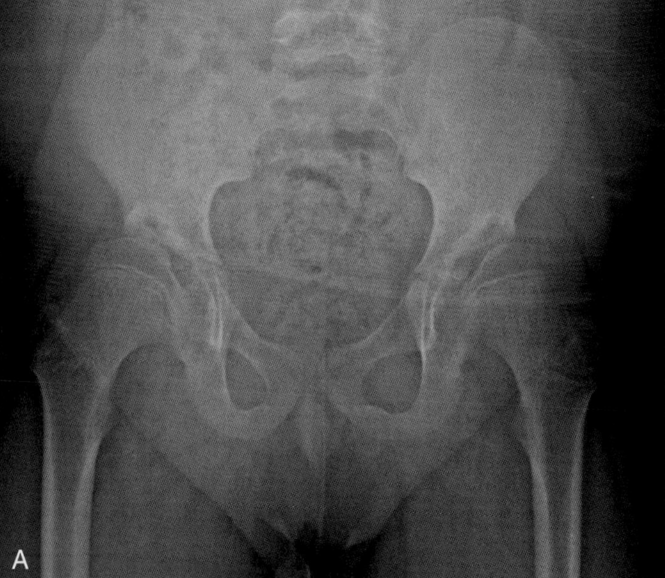

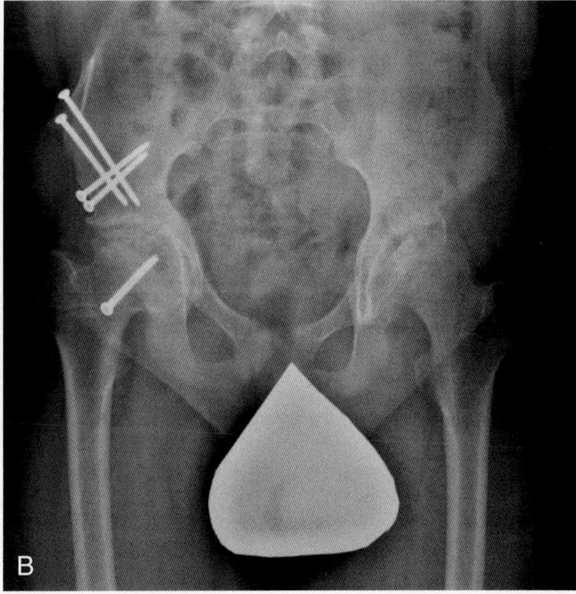

FIGURE 15 Tönnis triple osteotomy. **A**, The preoperative standing AP pelvis radiograph from a 7-year-old boy with an unknown mild developmental delay and bilateral hip dysplasia that is symptomatic on the right. **B**, The standing AP pelvis radiograph 2 years following a Tönnis triple osteotomy with excellent correction of the acetabulum with good lateral an anterior coverage with a medialized joint center. The subchondral cyst that was present preoperatively is no longer seen.

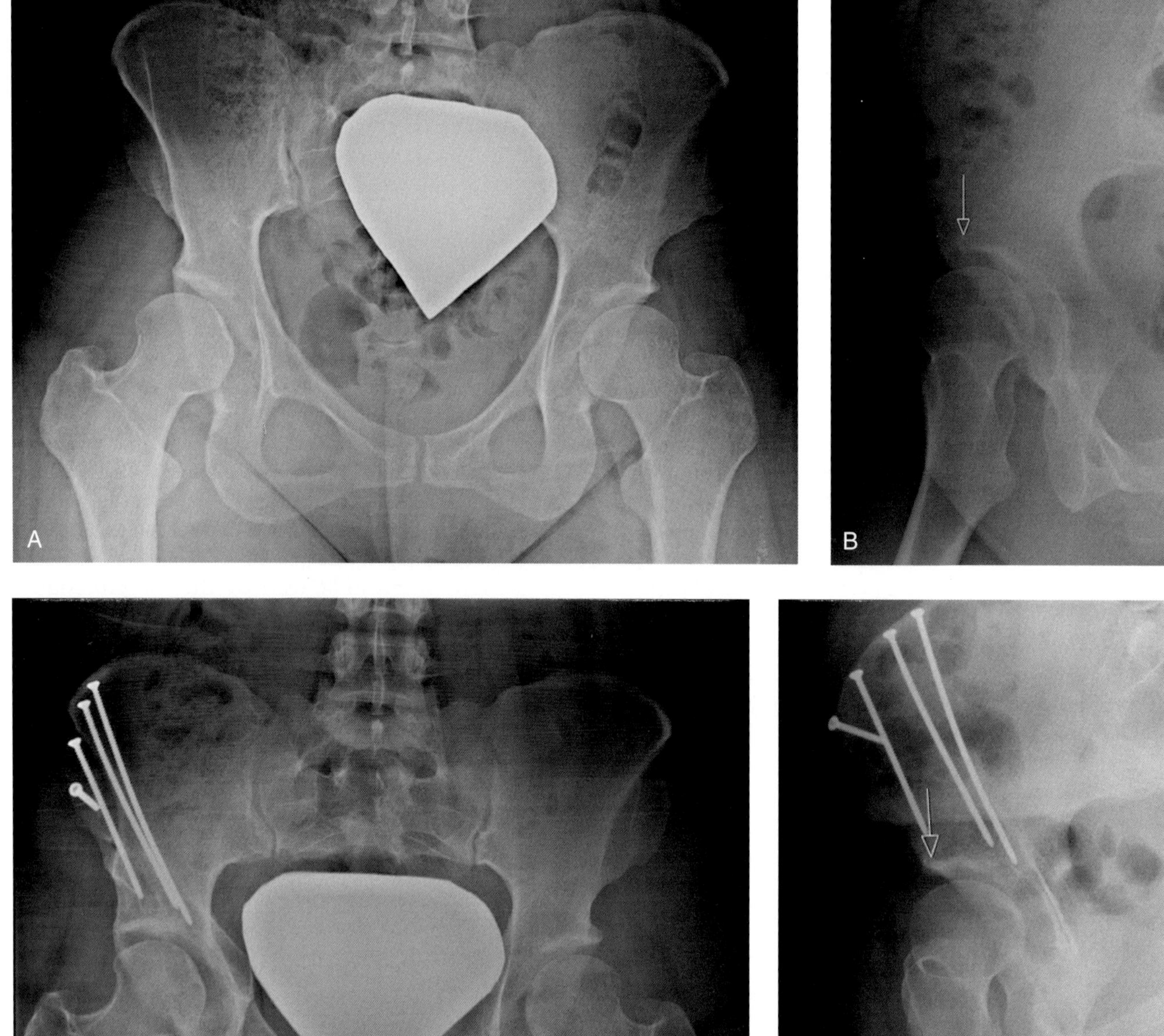

FIGURE 16 Bernese periacetabular osteotomy (PAO). **A** and **B**, The preoperative AP and false-profile views of a 19-year-old patient with symptomatic right hip dysplasia. The AP view demonstrates severe hip dysplasia but a maintained joint space, whereas the false-profile view demonstrates moderately poor anterior coverage (arrow points to the anterior coverage). **C** and **D**, Two years following a Bernese PAO without labral surgery or femoral osteochondroplasty, the AP pelvis view demonstrates excellent lateral coverage and medialization of the acetabulum with the false-profile view demonstrating significantly improved anterior coverage. The patient's painful symptoms have completely resolved.

advanced degenerative changes (Tönnis grade ≥2) and to avoid excessive anterior coverage and retroversion of the acetabulum.[74] Others have used the rotational acetabular osteotomy with similarly good 20-year survival of 96% for those without preoperative early osteoarthritic changes. Risk factors associated with poor outcome included fair postoperative joint congruency and age at surgery older than 46 years.[75]

SUMMARY

DDH represents a broad spectrum of disease from mild dysplasia through frank dislocation. Early diagnosis and treatment is of paramount importance to favorably alter the natural history of DDH. Most patients in whom a diagnosis is made within 6 months of age are successfully treated with a Pavlik harness. In refractory cases or late detection of DDH, a stable, concentrically reduced hip can be achieved with closed or open reduction, with femoral or pelvic osteotomies used selectively in older patients to augment stability. Residual dysplasia is common following closed or open reduction as is the need for secondary surgery. In adolescents, acetabular dysplasia is characterized by increased inclination in the coronal and sagittal planes and a lateralized hip joint center. Treatment is dependent on the severity of dysplasia, symptoms, and triradiate cartilage status. Restoration of a normal hip joint center with improved/normalized acetabular coverage is achieved with triple innominate osteotomies in those with open TRC or a periacetabular osteotomy in the skeletally mature patient.

KEY STUDY POINTS

- Hip dysplasia is one of the most prevalent conditions seen in musculoskeletal pathology.
- Early detection of DDH is paramount for good results.
- Nonsurgical treatment in infants has provided excellent results.
- Follow-up until skeletal maturity is warranted because the rates of adolescent and adult dysplasia have been underestimated in the past.
- Adolescent hip dysplasia is most commonly treated with PAO with excellent intermediate and long-term outcomes in hips without prior degenerative changes.

ANNOTATED REFERENCES

1. Rosendahl K, Markestad T, Lie RT: Developmental dysplasia of the hip: Prevalence based on ultrasound diagnosis. *Pediatr Radiol* 1996;26(9):635-639.
2. Boeree NR, Clarke NM: Ultrasound imaging and secondary screening for congenital dislocation of the hip. *J Bone Joint Surg Br* 1994;76(4):525-533.
3. Gosvig KK, Jacobsen S, Sonne-Holm S, Palm H, Troelsen A: Prevalence of malformations of the hip joint and their relationship to sex, groin pain, and risk of osteoarthritis: A population-based survey. *J Bone Joint Surg Am* 2010;92(5):1162-1169.
4. Jacobsen S, Sonne-Holm S: Hip dysplasia: A significant risk factor for the development of hip osteoarthritis. A cross-sectional survey. *Rheumatology (Oxford)* 2005;44(2):211-218.
5. Clohisy JC, Dobson MA, Robison JF, et al: Radiographic structural abnormalities associated with premature, natural hip-joint failure. *J Bone Joint Surg Am* 2011;93(suppl 2):3-9.
6. Engesaeter IO, Lie SA, Lehmann TG, Furnes O, Vollset SE, Engesaeter LB: Neonatal hip instability and risk of total hip replacement in young adulthood: Follow-up of 2,218,596 newborns from the Medical Birth Registry of Norway in the Norwegian Arthroplasty Register. *Acta Orthop* 2008;79(3):321-326.
7. Albinana J, Dolan LA, Spratt KF, Morcuende J, Meyer MD, Weinstein SL: Acetabular dysplasia after treatment for developmental dysplasia of the hip. Implications for secondary procedures. *J Bone Joint Surg Br* 2004;86(6):876-886.
8. Kenanidis E, Gkekas NK, Karasmani A, Anagnostis P, Christofilopoulos P, Tsiridis E: Genetic predisposition to developmental dysplasia of the hip. *J Arthroplasty* 2019;35:P291-P300.

   This is a meta-analysis of 45 studies investigating gene associations with DDH. They report candidate gene associations but no firm correlation between genotype and DDH phenotype. Level of evidence: I.
9. Paton RW, Hinduja K, Thomas CD: The significance of at-risk factors in ultrasound surveillance of developmental dysplasia of the hip. A ten-year prospective study. *J Bone Joint Surg Br* 2005;87(9):1264-1266.
10. Schams M, Labruyere R, Zuse A, Walensi M: Diagnosing developmental dysplasia of the hip using the Graf ultrasound method: Risk and protective factor analysis in 11,820 universally screened newborns. *Eur J Pediatr* 2017;176(9): 1193-1200.

    A retrospective analysis of 11,820 universally screened newborns confirms the traditional risk factors for DDH including female sex, family history, and breech presentation. Level of evidence: III.
11. American Academy of Pediatrics, Committee on Quality Improvement, Subcommittee on Developmental Dysplasia of the Hip: Clinical practice guideline: Early detection of developmental dysplasia of the hip. *Pediatrics* 2000;105(4 pt 1):896-905.
12. Carter CO, Wilkinson JA: Genetic and environmental factors in the etiology of congenital dislocation of the hip. *Clin Orthop Relat Res* 1964;33:119-128.
13. Zamborsky R, Kokavec M, Harsanyi S, Attia D, Danisovic L: Developmental dysplasia of hip: Perspectives in genetic screening. *Med Sci (Basel)* 2019;7(4):59.

    This is a review article of advances in identifying genetic contribution to DDH. Many candidate/susceptible genes have been identified, which may contribute to the DDH phenotype.
14. Wilkinson JA: Etiologic factors in congenital displacement of the hip and myelodysplasia. *Clin Orthop Relat Res* 1992;281:75-83.
15. Kutlu A, Memik R, Mutlu M, Kutlu R, Arslan A: Congenital dislocation of the hip and its relation to swaddling used in Turkey. *J Pediatr Orthop* 1992;12(5):598-602.
16. Kremli MK, Alshahid AH, Khoshhal KI, Zamzam MM: The pattern of developmental dysplasia of the hip. *Saudi Med J* 2003;24(10):1118-1120.

17. Yamamuro T, Ishida K: Recent advances in the prevention, early diagnosis, and treatment of congenital dislocation of the hip in Japan. *Clin Orthop Relat Res* 1984;184: 34-40.
18. Harrison TJ: The influence of the femoral head on pelvic growth and acetabular form in the rat. *J Anat* 1961;95:12-24.
19. Salter RB: Etiology, pathogenesis and possible prevention of congenital dislocation of the hip. *Can Med Assoc J* 1968;98(20):933-945.
20. Li LY, Zhang LJ, Li QW, Zhao Q, Jia JY, Huang T: Development of the osseous and cartilaginous acetabular index in normal children and those with developmental dysplasia of the hip: A cross-sectional study using MRI. *J Bone Joint Surg Br* 2012;94(12):1625-1631.
21. Sink EL, Ricciardi BF, Torre KD, Price CT: Selective ultrasound screening is inadequate to identify patients who present with symptomatic adult acetabular dysplasia. *J Child Orthop* 2014;8(6):451-455.
22. Shorter D, Hong T, Osborn DA: Screening programmes for developmental dysplasia of the hip in newborn infants. *Cochrane Database Syst Rev* 2011;(9):CD004595.
23. Mahan ST, Katz JN, Kim YJ: To screen or not to screen? A decision analysis of the utility of screening for developmental dysplasia of the hip. *J Bone Joint Surg Am* 2009;91(7): 1705-1719.
24. Graf R: Fundamentals of sonographic diagnosis of infant hip dysplasia. *J Pediatr Orthop* 1984;4(6):735-740.
25. Clarke NM, Harcke HT, McHugh P, Lee MS, Borns PF, MacEwen GD: Real-time ultrasound in the diagnosis of congenital dislocation and dysplasia of the hip. *J Bone Joint Surg Br* 1985;67(3):406-412.
26. Mulpuri K, Song KM, Gross RH, et al: The American Academy of Orthopaedic Surgeons evidence-based guideline on detection and nonoperative management of pediatric developmental dysplasia of the hip in infants up to six months of age. *J Bone Joint Surg Am* 2015;97(20):1717-1718.
27. Shaw BA, Segal LS, Section on Orthopaedics: Evaluation and referral for developmental dysplasia of the hip in infants. *Pediatrics* 2016;138(6):e20163107.
28. Clarke NM, Castaneda P: Strategies to improve nonoperative childhood management. *Orthop Clin North Am* 2012;43(3):281-289.
29. Tönnis D: Normal values of the hip joint for the evaluation of X-rays in children and adults. *Clin Orthop Relat Res* 1976;119:39-47.
30. Rosen A, Gamble JG, Vallier H, Bloch D, Smith L, Rinsky LA: Analysis of radiographic measurements as prognostic indicators of treatment success in patients with developmental dysplasia of the hip. *J Pediatr Orthop B* 1999;8(2): 118-121.
31. Narayanan U, Mulpuri K, Sankar WN, Clarke NM, Hosalkar H, Price CT, International Hip Dysplasia Institute: Reliability of a new radiographic classification for developmental dysplasia of the hip. *J Pediatr Orthop* 2015;35(5):478-484.
32. Ramo BA, De La Rocha A, Sucato DJ, Jo CH: A new radiographic classification system for developmental hip dysplasia is reliable and predictive of successful closed reduction and late pelvic osteotomy. *J Pediatr Orthop* 2018;38(1):16-21.

    This is a retrospective review of 235 hips that underwent attempted closed reduction for DDH. This study validated the reliability of the International Hip Dysplasia Institute Classification with independent observers and revealed that this classification system was prognostic for success of closed reduction and need for late osteotomy. Level of evidence: III.
33. Clohisy JC, Carlisle JC, Beaule PE, et al: A systematic approach to the plain radiographic evaluation of the young adult hip. *J Bone Joint Surg Am* 2008;90(suppl 4):47-66.
34. Roposch A, Liu LQ, Protopapa E: Variations in the use of diagnostic criteria for developmental dysplasia of the hip. *Clin Orthop Relat Res* 2013;471(6):1946-1954.
35. Hines AC, Neal DC, Beckwith T, Jo C, Kim HKW: A comparison of Pavlik harness treatment regimens for dislocated but reducible (Ortolani+) hips in infantile developmental dysplasia of the hip. *J Pediatr Orthop* 2019;39(10):505-509.

    A retrospective review of 62 patients with Ortolani positive hips (dislocated but reducible) revealed no difference in treatment success with Pavlik harness based on 23-hour versus 24-hour wear or frequency of clinical/ultrasonography follow-up. Level of evidence: III.
36. Neal D, Beckwith T, Hines A, et al: Comparison of Pavlik harness treatment regimens for reduced but dislocatable (Barlow positive) hips in infantile DDH. *J Orthop* 2019;16(5):440-444.

    A retrospective review of 65 patients with Barlow positive hips (reduced but dislocatable) treated with Pavlik harness revealed no difference in outcomes between 23-hour versus 24-hour harness wear or frequency of clinical follow-up. Level of evidence: III.
37. Malkawi H: Sonographic monitoring of the treatment of developmental disturbances of the hip by the Pavlik harness. *J Pediatr Orthop B* 1998;7(2):144-149.
38. Murnaghan ML, Browne RH, Sucato DJ, Birch J: Femoral nerve palsy in Pavlik harness treatment for developmental dysplasia of the hip. *J Bone Joint Surg Am* 2011;93(5):493-499.
39. Jones GT, Schoenecker PL, Dias LS: Developmental hip dysplasia potentiated by inappropriate use of the Pavlik harness. *J Pediatr Orthop* 1992;12(6):722-726.
40. Viere RG, Birch JG, Herring JA, Roach JW, Johnston CE: Use of the Pavlik harness in congenital dislocation of the hip. An analysis of failures of treatment. *J Bone Joint Surg Am* 1990;72(2):238-244.
41. Pap K, Kiss S, Shisha T, Marton-Szucs G, Szoke G: The incidence of avascular necrosis of the healthy, contralateral femoral head at the end of the use of Pavlik harness in unilateral hip dysplasia. *Int Orthop* 2006;30(5):348-351.
42. Tibrewal S, Gulati V, Ramachandran M: The Pavlik method: A systematic review of current concepts. *J Pediatr Orthop B* 2013;22(6):516-520.

43. Novais EN, Kestel LA, Carry PM, Meyers ML: Higher Pavlik harness treatment failure is seen in Graf type IV Ortolani-positive hips in males. *Clin Orthop Relat Res* 2016;474(8):1847-1854.

    This study is a retrospective review of 150 patients with DDH treated with a Pavlik harness. Multivariate analysis revealed that male sex and Graf IV hips (dislocated with alpha angle <43°) were independent risk factors for failure of treatment. Level of evidence: III.

44. Omeroglu H, Kose N, Akceylan A: Success of Pavlik harness treatment decreases in patients ≥ 4 months and in ultrasonographically dislocated hips in developmental dysplasia of the hip. *Clin Orthop Relat Res* 2016;474(5):1146-1152.

    A retrospective study of 153 children younger than 6 months treated with Pavlik harness for DDH reported that age at harness initiation was the only patient-related variable influencing success of treatment. Statistical modeling with a receiver operating characteristic curve demonstrated 4 months to be the most specific and sensitive threshold for treatment with Pavlik harness with a higher risk of failure after that age. Level of evidence: III.

45. Sankar WN, Nduaguba A, Flynn JM: Ilfeld abduction orthosis is an effective second-line treatment after failure of Pavlik harness for infants with developmental dysplasia of the hip. *J Bone Joint Surg Am* 2015;97(4):292-297.

46. Ibrahim DA, Skaggs DL, Choi PD: Abduction bracing after Pavlik harness failure: An effective alternative to closed reduction and spica casting? *J Pediatr Orthop* 2013;33(5):536-539.

47. Gans I, Flynn JM, Sankar WN: Abduction bracing for residual acetabular dysplasia in infantile DDH. *J Pediatr Orthop* 2013;33(7):714-718.

48. Modaressi K, Erschbamer M, Exner GU: Dysplasia of the hip in adolescent patients successfully treated for developmental dysplasia of the hip. *J Child Orthop* 2011;5(4):261-266.

49. Shaw KA, Moreland CM, Olszewski D, Schrader T: Late acetabular dysplasia after successful treatment for developmental dysplasia of the hip using the Pavlik method: A systematic literature review. *J Orthop* 2019;16(1):5-10.

    This is a systematic review of the literature investigating long-term outcomes of DDH treated with Pavlik harness. This study reported an incidence of late dysplasia in 280 of 6,029 hips (4.6%) and demonstrates that late dysplasia is not an uncommon clinical entity. Level of evidence: IV.

50. Novais EN, Pan Z, Autruong PT, Meyers ML, Chang FM: Normal percentile reference curves and correlation of acetabular index and acetabular depth ratio in children. *J Pediatr Orthop* 2018;38(3):163-169.

    This is a contemporary case series of 1,152 patients used to develop modern reference values for acetabular index and acetabular depth ratio in the normally developing hip through 14 years of age. Level of evidence: IV.

51. Wakabayashi K, Wada I, Horiuchi O, Mizutani J, Tsuchiya D, Otsuka T: MRI findings in residual hip dysplasia. *J Pediatr Orthop* 2011;31(4):381-387.

52. Douira-Khomsi W, Smida M, Louati H, et al: Magnetic resonance evaluation of acetabular residual dysplasia in developmental dysplasia of the hip: A preliminary study of 27 patients. *J Pediatr Orthop* 2010;30(1):37-43.

53. Sucato DJ, De La Rocha A, Lau K, Ramo BA: Overhead Bryant's traction does not improve the success of closed reduction or limit AVN in developmental dysplasia of the hip. *J Pediatr Orthop* 2017;37(2):e108-e113.

    A retrospective study of 342 hips that underwent attempted closed reduction revealed that overhead Bryant traction did not improve rates of successful closed reduction or rates of osteonecrosis. Level of evidence: III.

54. Gans I, Sankar WN: The medial dye pool revisited: Correlation between arthrography and MRI in closed reductions for DDH. *J Pediatr Orthop* 2014;34(8):787-790.

55. Race C, Herring JA: Congenital dislocation of the hip: An evaluation of closed reduction. *J Pediatr Orthop* 1983;3(2):166-172.

56. Gornitzky AL, Georgiadis AG, Seeley MA, Horn BD, Sankar WN: Does perfusion MRI after closed reduction of developmental dysplasia of the hip reduce the incidence of avascular necrosis? *Clin Orthop Relat Res* 2016;474(5):1153-1165.

    This is a retrospective cohort study investigating the use of postreduction perfusion MRI as a means of avoiding osteonecrosis. Although underpowered, the study suggests there may be a role for immediate perfusion MRI following closed reduction to identify impaired perfusion and adjust the spica cast. Level of evidence: III.

57. Tiderius C, Jaramillo D, Connolly S, et al: Post-closed reduction perfusion magnetic resonance imaging as a predictor of avascular necrosis in developmental hip dysplasia: A preliminary report. *J Pediatr Orthop* 2009;29(1):14-20.

58. Malayeri AA, Brooks KM, Bryant LH, et al: National Institutes of Health perspective on reports of gadolinium deposition in the brain. *J Am Coll Radiol* 2016;13(3):237-241.

    This is a review article from the National Institutes of Health summarizing the literature on gadolinium-based contrast agent deposition in the brain.

59. Novais EN, Hill MK, Carry PM, Heyn PC: Is age or surgical approach associated with osteonecrosis in patients with developmental dysplasia of the hip? A meta-analysis. *Clin Orthop Relat Res* 2016;474(5):1166-1177.

    A meta-analysis of the literature regarding closed and open reduction reveals that neither open reduction before 12 months of age nor medial/anterior surgical approach was associated with an increased risk of the development of osteonecrosis. Level of evidence: III.

60. Salter RB: The classic. Innominate osteotomy in the treatment of congenital dislocation and subluxation of the hip. *Clin Orthop Relat Res* 1978;137:2-14. Reprinted from Salter RB: *J Bone Joint Surg Br* 1961;43B(3):518.

61. Castaneda P, Tejerina P, Nualart L, Cassis N: The safety and efficacy of a transarticular pin for maintaining reduction in patients with developmental dislocation of the hip undergoing an open reduction. *J Pediatr Orthop* 2015;35(4):358-362.

62. Malvitz TA, Weinstein SL: Closed reduction for congenital dysplasia of the hip. Functional and radiographic results after an average of thirty years. *J Bone Joint Surg Am* 1994;76(12):1777-1792.

63. Thomas SR, Wedge JH, Salter RB: Outcome at forty-five years after open reduction and innominate osteotomy for late-presenting developmental dislocation of the hip. *J Bone Joint Surg Am* 2007;89(11):2341-2350.

64. Bolland BJ, Wahed A, Al-Hallao S, Culliford DJ, Clarke NM: Late reduction in congenital dislocation of the hip and the need for secondary surgery: Radiologic predictors and confounding variables. *J Pediatr Orthop* 2010;30(7):676-682.

65. Luhmann SJ, Bassett GS, Gordon JE, Schootman M, Schoenecker PL: Reduction of a dislocation of the hip due to developmental dysplasia. Implications for the need for future surgery. *J Bone Joint Surg Am* 2003;85(2):239-243.

66. Nunley RM, Prather H, Hunt D, Schoenecker PL, Clohisy JC: Clinical presentation of symptomatic acetabular dysplasia in skeletally mature patients. *J Bone Joint Surg Am* 2011;93(suppl 2):17-21.

67. Wells J, Nepple JJ, Crook K, et al: Femoral morphology in the dysplastic hip: Three-dimensional characterizations with CT. *Clin Orthop Relat Res* 2017;475(4):1045-1054.

A retrospective review of 100 patients who underwent PAO for acetabular dysplasia revealed that cam deformity or reduced femoral head-neck offset was present in 42% and 82% of hips, respectively. This study highlights the frequency of concurrent femoral-sided pathology in patients presenting with symptomatic acetabular dysplasia. Level of evidence: IV.

68. Ross JR, Zaltz I, Nepple JJ, Schoenecker PL, Clohisy JC: Arthroscopic disease classification and interventions as an adjunct in the treatment of acetabular dysplasia. *Am J Sports Med* 2011;39(suppl):72S-78S.

69. Lee AJ, Armour P, Thind D, Coates MH, Kang AC: The prevalence of acetabular labral tears and associated pathology in a young asymptomatic population. *Bone Joint J* 2015;97-B(5):623-627.

70. McClincy MP, Wylie JD, Kim YJ, Millis MB, Novais EN: Periacetabular osteotomy improves pain and function in patients with lateral center-edge angle between 18° and 25°, but are these hips really borderline dysplastic? *Clin Orthop Relat Res* 2019;477(5):1145-1153.

This retrospective study of 91 patients with borderline acetabular dysplasia (LCEA of 18° to 25°) who underwent PAO reported excellent short-term outcomes (94% survival at 2 years) and improved functional outcomes scores. Furthermore, advanced preoperative imaging confirmed that most patients with borderline dysplasia based on LCEA had other markers of dysplasia such as anterior undercoverage, retroversion, or acetabular inclination. Level of evidence: IV.

71. van Hellemondt GG, Sonneveld H, Schreuder MHE, Kooijman MAP, de Kleuver M: Triple osteotomy of the pelvis for acetabular dysplasia: Results at a mean follow-up of 15 years. *J Bone Joint Surg Br* 2005;87(7):911-915.

72. Wylie JD, Ross JA, Erickson JA, Anderson MB, Peters CL: Operative fluoroscopic correction is reliable and correlates with postoperative radiographic correction in periacetabular osteotomy. *Clin Orthop Relat Res* 2017;475(4):1100-1106.

In a retrospective review of 121 patients who underwent PAO, the authors demonstrated excellent accuracy and reliability of intraoperative fluoroscopic images for assessment of surgical correction of acetabular dysplasia. Level of evidence: III.

73. Grammatopoulos G, Wales J, Kothari A, Gill HS, Wainwright A, Theologis T: What is the early/mid-term survivorship and functional outcome after Bernese periacetabular osteotomy in a pediatric surgeon practice? *Clin Orthop Relat Res* 2016;474(5):1216-1223.

A retrospective review of 68 consecutive periacetabular osteotomies revealed excellent long-term outcomes with 93% 10-year survivorship. Level of evidence: III.

74. Lerch TD, Steppacher SD, Liechti EF, Tannast M, Siebenrock KA: One-third of hips after periacetabular osteotomy survive 30 years with good clinical results, no progression of arthritis, or conversion to THA. *Clin Orthop Relat Res* 2017;475(4):1154-1168.

A retrospective study of 75 hips in 63 patients that underwent PAO revealed survivorship of almost one-third of hips. Advanced joint degeneration (Tönnis grade ≥2) was associated with increased risk of failure. Level of evidence: III.

75. Yasunaga Y, Ochi M, Yamasaki T, Shoji T, Izumi S: Rotational acetabular osteotomy for pre- and early osteoarthritis secondary to dysplasia provides durable results at 20 years. *Clin Orthop Relat Res* 2016;474(10):2145-2153.

A retrospective study of 159 patients who underwent rotational acetabular osteotomy revealed excellent long-term outcomes with osteoarthritis-free survival in 96% of prearthritic hips and 78% of early arthritic hips at 20 years. Level of evidence: IV.

CHAPTER 24

Slipped Capital Femoral Epiphysis and Femoroacetabular Impingement

RACHEL MEDNICK THOMPSON, MD • DAVID A. PODESZWA, MD

ABSTRACT

Slipped capital femoral epiphysis (SCFE) is one of the most common and most challenging hip disorders affecting adolescents. Although the etiology is unknown, obesity may be a modifiable risk factor for SCFE. In situ pinning remains the preferred treatment for stable and unstable SCFE. However, even with relatively minimal displacement, the residual deformity has been shown to lead to a high rate of subsequent disability. Open reduction and fixation of unstable SCFE using the modified Dunn procedure can restore normal hip motion with very low rates of associated osteonecrosis when highly trained surgeons administer treatment.

Femoroacetabular impingement is another common diagnosis in adolescents and young adults who have hip pain with an unclear etiology. This disorder has a likely association with high-level athletic participation and cam lesions in males. Femoroacetabular impingement can be treated through either open or arthroscopic approaches, with excellent clinical outcomes and return to sports.

Dr. Thompson or an immediate family member serves as a board member, owner, officer, or committee member of the Pediatric Orthopaedic Society of North America and the American Academy for Cerebral Palsy and Developmental Medicine. Dr. Podeszwa or an immediate family member serves as an unpaid consultant to OrthoPediatrics and serves as a board member, owner, officer, or committee member of the American Academy of Orthopaedic Surgeons and the Pediatric Orthopaedic Society of North America.

Keywords: femoroacetabular impingement (FAI); hip arthroscopy; slipped capital femoral epiphysis (SCFE); surgical hip dislocation

INTRODUCTION

Slipped capital femoral epiphysis (SCFE) is one of the most common hip disorders affecting adolescents, and although it is ubiquitous, treatment remains a challenge. Epiphysiolysis and the subsequent displacement of the proximal femoral epiphysis relative to the metaphysis result in a three-dimensional deformity that most commonly involves varus, extension, and external rotation. Even when relatively minimal displacement is present, the residual deformity has been shown to lead to a high rate of subsequent disability. Although a proportion of femoroacetabular impingement (FAI) results from SCFE, FAI is a distinct clinical entity whose etiology varies. Ultimately, the surgical management of SCFE-related deformity and FAI is complementary and will be reviewed.

SLIPPED CAPITAL FEMORAL EPIPHYSIS

Epidemiology

The incidence of SCFE is regional, ranging from 0.2 per 100,000 children in eastern Japan to 17.15 children in the northeastern United States,[1] with an overall US incidence of approximately 10.8 per 100,000 children. The increasing incidence in certain regions correlates with the rise in obesity. Children who are obese have an earlier onset of SCFE than children who are not obese, and the age at initial presentation has decreased substantially in the past 20 years, because obesity has become increasingly more common in younger children. The mean age at presentation is 12 years in boys and 11.2 years in girls. SCFE affects boys more often than girls.

The incidence of SCFE varies not only by region but also with race and ethnicity. However, numerous epidemiologic studies contradict one another in regard to the influence of race, and the reported variability may actually be reflective of differences between typical body mass indices (BMIs) in certain ethnic and racial groups.[1]

Etiology

The underlying causality in SCFE has not been definitively established and is likely multifactorial. No established genetic predilection for SCFE exists, regardless of the marked variability between different regions and races.

More than 50% of children with SCFE are classified as being in greater than the 95th percentile for weight, and the average BMI in children with SCFE is 25 to 30 kg/m^2 (>85th percentile).[1] Furthermore, obesity at the age of 5 to 6 years, before the onset of SCFE, is strongly associated with a subsequent slip such that for every integer increase in BMI *z*-score, the risk of SCFE increases by a factor of 1.7.[2] Serum leptin levels may, in part, explain this correlation. A 2017 case-control study revealed that serum leptin levels increase with obesity and that elevated leptin levels increase the risk of SCFE by a factor of 4.9 even after controlling for BMI.[3]

Furthermore, changes in the proximal femoral physis associated with obesity may biomechanically predispose children who are obese to SCFE. Increased femoral retroversion, which is common in these children, results in elevated physeal shear stress, which is then compounded by the shear stress associated with elevated proximal femoral physeal inclination seen in children with SCFE. Decreased epiphyseal tubercle height has additionally been associated with SCFE.[4] Whether this is a predisposing anatomical variant or a response to increased shear forces remains unclear.

Classification

SCFE can be classified based on the duration of symptoms, the degree of radiographic displacement, or the patient's ability for mobilization. Perhaps the most clinically relevant classification is that of functional stability,[5] in which a slip is defined as stable if a patient is able to bear weight with or without crutches. Unstable SCFEs are classically associated with much higher rates of osteonecrosis compared with stable slips (4.7% to 58% versus zero to 1.4%, respectively). However, two high-volume centers reported poor sensitivity (39%) and moderate specificity (76%) of the functional stability classification scheme compared with an intraoperative evaluation of physeal stability.[6] Because this classification scheme largely drives treatment decisions, a more comprehensive scheme that better reflects stability status and the risk of osteonecrosis is needed.

Treatment

Stable SCFE

The goals of initial surgical management for all slips are the prevention of further slips and the avoidance of osteonecrosis. A systematic review of the literature confirmed that a single central screw placed in situ perpendicular to the physis is the best method of treatment and has the lowest incidence of associated complications in stable slips.[7] Although the modified Dunn technique has been popularized for the management of unstable slips, the risk of osteonecrosis is significantly higher when applied to stable slips (6% versus 29.4%, $P = 0.027$)[8] and less commonly used in this population.

Unstable SCFE

In situ pinning remains the preferred treatment, with the treating surgeon determining the need to add a decompressive arthrotomy. However, a systematic literature review suggests that gentle urgent reduction with internal fixation and a decompressive arthrotomy results in the lowest risk of osteonecrosis (excluding those treated with surgical dislocation), but this conclusion was based on level IV evidence.[7] Conversely, a 2006 meta-analysis failed to demonstrate a statistically significant reduction in osteonecrosis rates with the addition of a decompressive arthrotomy (27% without versus 17% with arthrotomy, OR = 0.80, CI: 0.48 to 1.35).[9] However, even this meta-analysis was underpowered, highlighting the need for large, prospective, comparative studies. In addition, biomechanical studies have shown that a two-screw construct provides greater stability than one screw for unstable slips.[10]

Alternatively, there has been great enthusiasm for open reduction and fixation of unstable SCFE using the modified Dunn procedure.[11] Anatomic reduction with resultant restoration of normal hip motion is a preferred outcome, but it is a technically demanding procedure. Early reports suggested very low rates of associated osteonecrosis when highly trained surgeons performed the procedure; however, the actual rate of osteonecrosis may be substantially higher when the procedure is attempted in lower volume centers. A multicenter prospective series of 27 unstable slips with an average 22-month follow-up revealed that, although near-anatomic correction can be achieved with this approach (average slip angle = 6°), the rate of osteonecrosis remains high (26%).[12] This series also reported a 15% rate of broken hardware that required revision fixation. In those patients in whom osteonecrosis did not develop, excellent clinical outcomes were reported at nearly 2 years postoperatively. All outcomes scores were substantially lower in the patients with osteonecrosis. In addition to osteonecrosis, there is an associated 4% risk of postoperative iatrogenic hip instability, regardless of Loder classification; however, this complication has only been associated with chronic and acute-on-chronic cases.[13]

Contralateral Prophylactic Pinning

A contralateral slip will subsequently develop in 11% to 24% of patients with SCFE.[14-16] The relatively high risk of a contralateral slip has prompted many surgeons to recommend prophylactic pinning in all children presenting with unilateral SCFE; however, the possible consequences of this additional procedure must be considered. With a minimum follow-up of 12 months after prophylactic pinning, a multicenter retrospective case series reported a 2% risk of osteonecrosis, a 2% risk of peri-implant fracture, and a 3% risk of symptomatic hardware.[17] A subsequent contralateral slip was prevented in the 99 patients in the study.

A review of 260 patients initially treated for a unilateral SCFE who were followed up to skeletal maturity or until the development of a contralateral slip demonstrated that demographic factors were not predictive of a contralateral slip, but the modified Oxford bone score provides probability data for predicting a contralateral slip.[15] The positive predictive value for a modified Oxford bone score between 16 and 18 is 96%, and the negative predictive value is 92%. In addition, a 2019 retrospective analysis of 318 patients with unilateral SCFE found a correlation between the unaffected side's proximal femoral morphology and risk of contralateral slip.[18] For each additional degree of posterior tilt, the odds of contralateral slip increased by 8%; for each 0.01 increase in superior epiphyseal extension ratio, the odds of contralateral slip increased by 6%.

Reconstruction of Residual Deformity

Even with relatively minimal displacement, the residual deformity after in situ fixation of SCFE results in an increased risk of osteoarthritis. A series of 92 hips treated with in situ fixation had an average α angle of 72.7°, which is a radiographic finding associated with symptomatic FAI.[19] In addition, a linear relationship existed between the degree of deformity and subsequent degenerative changes.

Historically, osteotomy at the intertrochanteric level has been the preferred procedure for moderate or severe slips, because it provides adequate deformity correction with a low risk of osteonecrosis. A review of 32 symptomatic patients treated with a flexion osteotomy templated from preoperative CT scans showed excellent clinical outcomes. Hip flexion was greater than 90° in more than 90% of the patients, and the anterior impingement sign had resolved in 75% of the patients at the most recent follow-up.[20] A similar review of eight patients treated with an Imhäuser osteotomy demonstrated substantial improvement in postoperative hip range of motion, gait deviation index, Pediatric Outcomes Data Collection Instrument scores, and radiographic measures of FAI.[21] The addition of a concomitant proximal femoral osteochondroplasty (open or arthroscopic) may offer improved outcomes without a substantial increase in associated complications[22,23] (**Figure 1**). Long-term results of this combined approach were published in 2017, reporting a 68.5% survivorship free from conversion to arthroplasty at 39 years.[24] Advanced age at surgery, osteonecrosis, and chondrolysis were associated with worse outcomes. There were two instances of osteonecrosis and two of chondrolysis in this cohort of 45 patients.

A more powerful deformity correction can be achieved with subcapital osteotomy performed through a surgical hip dislocation approach. This technically demanding procedure may substantially improve hip function, but it is associated with a high complication rate (25%).[25]

Outcomes

Osteonecrosis is one of the most concerning outcomes associated with the management of SCFE. A systematic literature review of unstable SCFE showed an overall osteonecrosis rate of 21%.[26] A 2013 literature review (excluding surgical hip dislocation) reported an overall osteonecrosis rate of 23.9%. No correlation was found between the osteonecrosis rate and the method of fixation, the use of capsulotomy, or attempted reduction.[27] When comparing the management of surgical hip dislocation by using a modified Dunn procedure with in situ pinning in 88 patients with unstable SCFE, the results showed a 43% rate of osteonecrosis with in situ pinning and a 29% rate with a modified Dunn procedure.[28] For patients with stable SCFE, no instances of osteonecrosis occurred with in situ pinning, but the modified Dunn procedure had a 20% rate of osteonecrosis.

The preferred treatment for SCFE is still considered to be in situ screw fixation. However, recent midterm and long-term clinical studies have reported that in situ screw fixation leads to high rates of residual deformity and moderate rates of associated pain and osteoarthritis. A review of 176 hips treated with in situ fixation resulted in an 89.5% fixation survival rate (no corrective osteotomy or conversion to arthroplasty) at 10 years.[29] In 105 patients not treated with additional reconstruction surgery and who were available for evaluation with outcome measures, 33% of the patients reported pain (more than 3 on a 10-point visual analog scale) at an average of 23 years after initial treatment. Similar 20-year outcomes

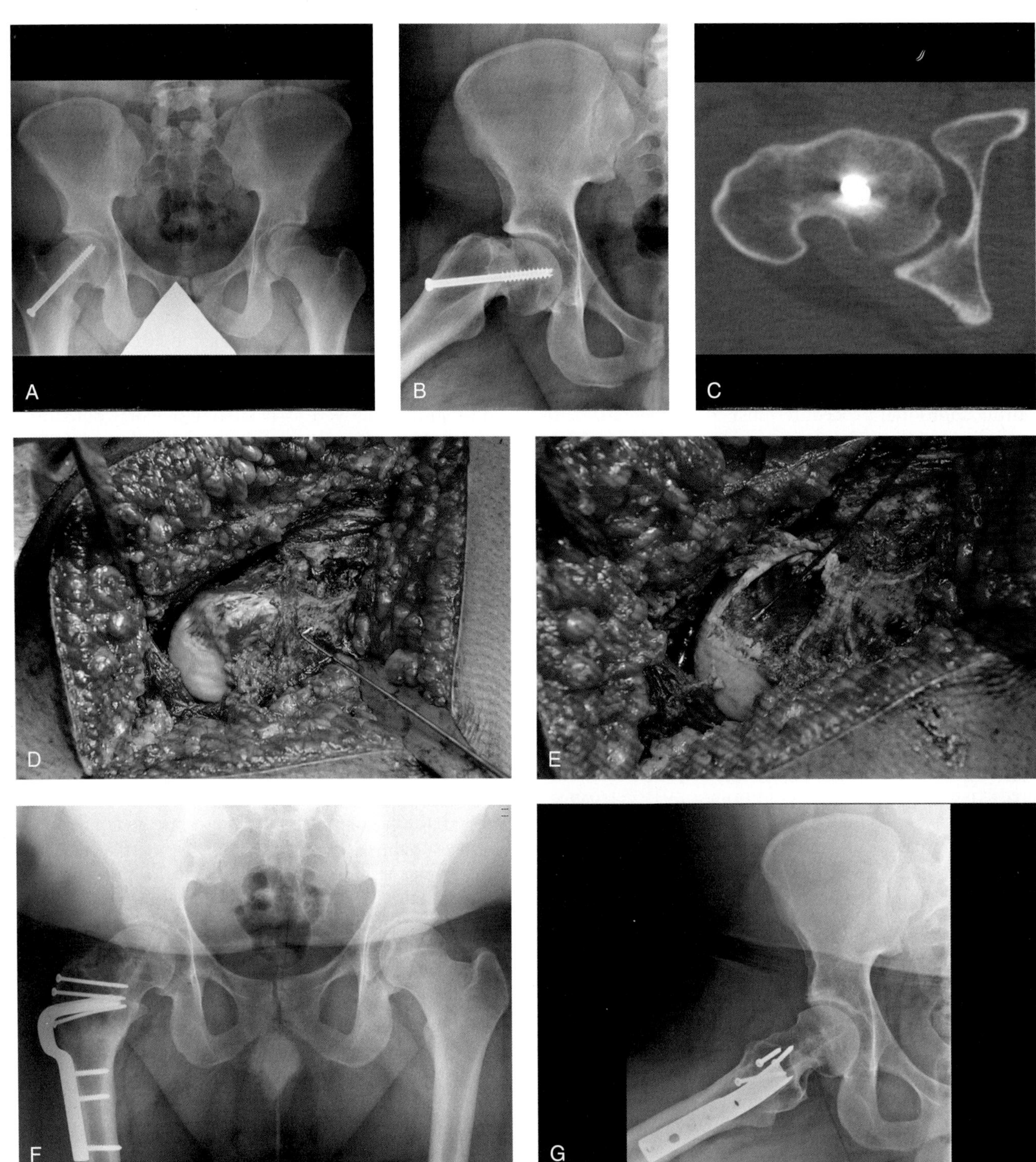

FIGURE 1 Standing AP pelvic (**A**) and lateral (**B**) radiographs of the right hip of a symptomatic 17-year-old adolescent boy with severe deformity secondary to a slipped capital femoral epiphysis. **C**, Axial CT scan demonstrates severe posterior displacement of the femoral epiphysis and metaphyseal prominence. Typical intraoperative photographs of a femoral head-neck junction before (**D**) and after (**E**) resection of the metaphyseal prominence. Standing AP pelvic (**F**) and lateral (**G**) radiographs of the right hip 2 years postoperatively show correction of the trochanteric height and the head-neck offset.

were reported from a tertiary care center in Mexico. Of 121 patients, 96 had clinical (positive impingement sign) and radiographic (α angle >55°) evidence of impingement, and all patients had radiographic evidence of osteoarthritis.[30] Of the patients with FAI, the mean Harris hip score was 75.4, which was substantially lower than the mean Harris hip score of patients without FAI (89.3). Similarly, at an average follow-up of 37 years, patients with SCFE had higher α angles compared with age-matched and sex-matched control subjects. Higher α angles correlated with worse outcomes, as quantified by the Harris hip score.[31]

Long-term follow-up of the modified Dunn procedure is limited, but a 10-year follow-up study reported a 93% survival rate (no progression in Tonnis score, no conversion to arthroplasty, and no significant decrease in outcomes scores) in the setting of high-volume, experienced surgeons.[32]

FEMOROACETABULAR IMPINGEMENT

Epidemiology

FAI is a clinical diagnosis supported by radiographic findings of proximal femoral or acetabular dysmorphology (decreased femoral head-neck offset and/or increased acetabular coverage or depth). This condition typically manifests as anterior hip and/or groin pain with flexion-related activities. Radiographic findings in the absence of symptoms are common. A review of 473 CT scans showed that 40% of asymptomatic hips had radiographic findings associated with FAI,[33] with these findings more common in men than in women. Similar findings were reported in a review of hip CT scans in otherwise healthy asymptomatic adolescents. The study demonstrated a 16.8% rate of cam deformity in asymptomatic adolescents (defined as an α angle ≥55°), a 32.4% rate of pincer deformity (defined as a lateral center edge angle ≥40°), and a 6.1% rate of mixed-type deformity.[34] Cam morphology was substantially more common in males, and pincer deformities were equally distributed among males and females.

A high prevalence of radiographic findings is consistent with FAI, but poor correlation exists between radiographic FAI and degenerative radiographic changes. One study evaluated 96 asymptomatic hips with radiographic findings consistent with FAI. The patients had been treated with arthroplasty of the contralateral hip. Because 82.3% of the patients had remained free of radiographic arthritic changes at a mean follow-up of 18.5 years, the authors recommend against treatment of asymptomatic radiographic FAI.[35]

A multicenter prospective study of patients undergoing surgical treatment for symptomatic FAI reported that 55% of the patients were female, 88% were Caucasian, the average age was 28.4 years, and the average BMI was 25.1 kg/m^2.[36] Cam-type FAI was most common (47.6%), followed by mixed type (44.5%) and pincer type (7.9%).

Etiology

Pincer-type deformities are generally thought to be idiopathic morphologic differences in acetabular ossification, but cam lesions may result from multiple etiologies, including SCFE, Legg-Calvé-Perthes disease, infection, trauma, or increased repetitive loading. However, most lesions do not have a direct cause and are deemed idiopathic.

In males, a likely association exists between participation in high-level athletic activities and the presence of cam lesions. In a case-control study that compared 72 hips in elite-level basketball players with 76 hips in age-matched control subjects, the athletes had a 10-fold increased likelihood of having a cam lesion, which was defined as an α angle greater than 55° measured on MRI. Although there was a definitive propensity toward an increased α angle in athletes at all ages, the differences were magnified after physeal closure.[37] It was hypothesized that the repetitive stress of loading coupled with the directional change of loading through the proximal femur may alter growth patterns, resulting in a cam deformity at skeletal maturity. A radiographic review of 96 adolescents found a direct relationship between increased α angle and increased epiphyseal extension ratio,[38] which has previously been associated with activities that increase shear force on the physis.

Four hundred two adolescents (446 hips, age range 13.6 to 19.0 years) undergoing hip arthroscopy were studied using a matched case-control analysis to identify radiographic predictors of pathologic acetabular cartilage lesions. Increased α angle increased the likelihood of acetabular cartilage changes, whereas the presence of a crossover sign decreased the likelihood of degenerative changes. Older age, male sex, and higher BMI were further predictive of acetabular cartilage lesions.[39]

Assessment

In a patient with signs and symptoms of FAI, radiographic examination will likely confirm the diagnosis. The initial imaging should include a standing AP pelvic radiograph and a lateral projection of the affected hip. A 2011 retrospective review comparing lateral radiographs with radial MRIs in 60 patients who received a clinical diagnosis of FAI reported sensitivity for cam deformity of 96.4% with the 45° Dunn view compared with 70.6% for the cross-table lateral view. The specificity for cam deformity was 90% and 100%, respectively.[40] Dunn lateral views were recommended over cross-table lateral views for FAI evaluation. The Dunn lateral view also has a relatively low effective radiation dose compared with cross-table lateral and single frog-lateral views, and the need for repeated exposure is lowest with a Dunn lateral radiograph.[41]

Management

Conservative, nonsurgical management should be attempted before considering surgical intervention. Nonsurgical strategies include rest, nonsteroidal anti-inflammatory medications, activity modification or restriction, and physical therapy. A prospective study of 76 adolescents (93 hips, average age 15.3 years) using a nonsurgical protocol consisting of a trial of rest, physical therapy, and activity modification demonstrated that 82% of the patients could be treated nonsurgically with significant improvements in outcome scores at a mean follow-up of 2 years. Patients with cam or combined cam and pincer deformities were 4.4 times more likely to subsequently seek and receive surgical intervention than patients with pincer deformities alone.[42]

Hip arthroscopy is now the most widely used surgical procedure to address the proximal femoral deformity and intra-articular pathology associated with FAI. The first national consensus-based best practice guidelines for hip arthroscopy in FAI using the Delphi and nominal group technique have been published and include preoperative recommendations, intraoperative practices, and postoperative protocols. This best practice guideline is intended to serve as a tool to reduce the variability in preoperative, intraoperative. and postoperative practices.[43]

Despite the popularity of hip arthroscopy, the surgical hip dislocation approach for the management of symptomatic FAI enables all osseous and soft-tissue abnormalities to be addressed as needed. A matched cohort of 60 consecutive patients treated surgically for FAI by either surgical hip dislocation or arthroscopy reported similar improvement in all radiographic measures of FAI except the AP α angle, which was treated more effectively with surgical hip dislocation.[44] The study authors recommended surgical hip dislocation for treating patients with superolateral or posterosuperior loss of femoral offset, because an arthroscopic approach is limited in its ability to fully access and address cam-type deformities in these anatomic regions.

A similar retrospective review of patients treated for cam-type or mixed-type FAI found statistically comparable improvement in radiographic parameters with open or arthroscopic treatment.[45] However, the authors reported a 2.2% rate of nonunion of the greater trochanter in the cohort treated with surgical hip dislocation. In addition, the need for arthroscopic lysis of adhesions was substantially higher in the surgical hip dislocation cohort than in the arthroscopically treated cohort (12% versus 6.1%, respectively).[45]

Athletes undergoing a surgical dislocation can be reassured that they will be able to return to their sport. A study of 24 athletes who underwent open treatment of FAI reported that 21 (87.5%) returned to play at a median 7 months postoperatively. Of those patients, 19 (90%) returned at an equivalent or greater level of play. The three that failed to return to play did so for reasons unrelated to their hip.[46]

An alternative approach uses a modified Smith-Peterson interval in a mini-open approach. A prospective case series reviewed 49 hips at an average follow-up of 22 months. Substantial improvements in the Harris hip score, the Western Ontario and McMaster Universities Index, and the Medical Outcomes Study 36-Item Short Form measures were reported, with return to preinjury activity levels. Of note, a 20% rate of meralgia paresthetica was reported in this cohort.[47]

A similar minimally invasive approach used an anterolateral approach in 118 hips. At a mean follow-up of 26 months, similar improvements in functional outcomes were reported as assessed by the Harris hip score, Western Ontario and McMaster Universities Index, and the Nonarthritic Hip score.[48] However, a 6.8% revision rate, a 3.5% rate of conversion to total hip arthroplasty (THA), and a 15% rate of increased Tönnis stage within 1 year were reported.[48] Long-term comparative studies are required to further evaluate the efficacy of minimally invasive approaches and define their role in treating FAI compared with surgical hip dislocation and arthroscopic approaches.

Outcomes

Adolescent-specific outcome studies evaluating the use of hip arthroscopy in the management of FAI are becoming more common. One study evaluated 122 consecutive hips in 108 adolescents with symptomatic FAI and compared the arthroscopic findings and outcomes with those of 122 adult hips. The duration of symptoms averaged 16.6 months, and 95.9% participated in athletic activities. Thirty-six cam, 17 pincer, and 69 combined lesions were identified. One hundred eleven labral tears underwent 85 refixations and 26 débridements. There were 101 acetabular chondral lesions (51 grade 3 or 4), with four microfractures and three femoral chondral lesions. At an average of 30 months postoperatively, the average modified Harris Hip Score improved 25.4 points, from 68.3 preoperatively to 93.6 postoperatively. Four patients subsequently underwent a revision arthroscopy.[49]

Adolescents undergoing revision arthroscopy for the management of FAI may not have the same outcomes as those undergoing primary arthroscopy. A study of 42 adolescents (all aged 18 years or younger) who underwent revision arthroscopy were compared with

84 adolescents who underwent primary arthroscopy. Those undergoing revision arthroscopic surgery showed significant improvement in patient-reported outcomes, but their final scores were lower for sport activity, general health, and satisfaction as compared with those undergoing primary arthroscopy. Outcome scores were poorer for those who required more than one revision surgery when compared with those who required only one revision.[50]

Surgical hip dislocation is a powerful tool for correcting cam-type and pincer-type deformities. A review of 75 patients (minimum 5-year follow-ups) showed a 91% hip preservation survival rate (no conversion to THA, progression of osteoarthritis, or a Meryl d'Aubigné-Postel score <15).[51] Excessive acetabular rim trimming, preoperative arthritic changes, older age at surgery, and increased weight were predictive of failure. At the 10-year follow-up of this cohort, the hip preservation survival rate was 80%.[52]

A direct comparison between open and arthroscopic techniques found no difference between techniques in preoperative (48 versus 53, respectively) and postoperative (83 versus 82) nonarthritic hip scores at a mean follow-up of 59 months.[53] However, despite these promising clinical results, a prospective analysis of delayed gadolinium-enhanced MRI of cartilage (dGEMRIC) indices in patients with FAI who did not have surgery compared with those with both arthroscopic and open surgery found that while all patients with FAI have diminishing dGEMRIC indices, the decline was more pronounced in surgical patients 1-year postoperatively.[54] Long-term follow-up studies are needed to evaluate the arch of recovery and/or degeneration in these populations.

Regardless of the treatment method, whether open or arthroscopic, the failure of hip preservation surgery is most commonly associated with residual intra-articular impingement (74.8% of all revision cases) followed by extra-articular impingement (9.5% of cases). The rate of revision surgery was comparable in patients who were initially treated by arthroscopy or surgical hip dislocation (7.01% versus 7.25%, respectively), and most revisions could be accomplished arthroscopically.[55]

SUMMARY

Both SCFE and FAI remain difficult entities to treat. Although recently reported radiographic and clinical results of newer surgical approaches are encouraging, the inexperienced practitioner should approach these patients with caution and should recognize the risks and nuances associated with the more advanced surgical management of these conditions.

KEY STUDY POINTS

- The modified Dunn osteotomy is a powerful tool for the management of unstable SCFE, but the learning curve is steep. The procedure should be reserved for surgeons with specific training in this approach.
- Prophylactic contralateral in situ pinning is not without risks and should be reserved for patients with substantial risks for a contralateral slip based on the modified Oxford bone score or those with an underlying endocrinopathy.
- FAI is a clinical diagnosis. A high prevalence of radiographic findings is consistent with FAI, but poor correlation exists between the radiographic findings and ultimate degenerative radiographic changes. Therefore, treatment should be reserved for patients with symptomatic FAI.
- For many patients with FAI, nonsurgical treatment is effective. For those in whom nonsurgical treatment fails, FAI can be managed with either an arthroscopic approach or a surgical hip dislocation with similarly reliable results.

ANNOTATED REFERENCES

1. Loder RT, Skopelja EN: The epidemiology and demographics of slipped capital femoral epiphysis. *ISRN Orthop* 2011;2011:486512.
2. Perry DC, Metcalfe D, Lane S, Turner S: Childhood obesity and slipped capital femoral epiphysis. *Pediatrics* 2018;142:e20181067.

   A nationwide cohort series of 597,017 children found that among obese children at 5 to 6 years old, 75% remained obese at age 11 to 12 years and that there was a strong correlation between BMI at age 5 to 6 years and SCFE, with an odds ratio of 1.7 (95% confidence interval 1.5 to 1.9) for each integer increase in BMI score. Level of evidence: III.
3. Halverson SJ, Warhoover T, Mencio GA, Lovejoy SA, Martus JE, Schoenecker JG: Leptin elevation as a risk factor for slipped capital femoral epiphysis independent of obesity status. *J Bone Joint Surg Am* 2017;99:865-872.

   A case-control study of 40 patients with SCFE and 30 control patients matched for BMI found that patients with elevated leptin levels were 4.9 times more likely to develop SCFE as compared with those without elevated leptin levels regardless of BMI, sex, or race (95% confidence interval, 1.31 to 18.49, $P < 0.02$). These authors further demonstrated a direct correlation between BMI and leptin levels. Level of evidence: III.
4. Novais EN, Maranho DA, Vairagade A, Kim YJ, Kiapour A: Smaller epiphyseal tubercle and larger peripheral cupping in slipped capital femoral epiphysis compared with healthy hips: A 3-dimensional computed tomography study. *J Bone Joint Surg Am* 2020;102:29-36.

An analysis of 3D CT scans of the proximal femur in 51 children with SCFE and 80 children without hip symptoms found that hips with SCFE have a smaller epiphyseal tubercle and larger peripheral cupping, regardless of slip severity. These authors hypothesized that the larger cupping was an adaptive response to perceived instability. Level of evidence: III.

5. Loder RT, Richards BS, Shapiro PS, Reznick LR, Aronson DD: Acute slipped capital femoral epiphysis: The importance of physeal stability. *J Bone Joint Surg Am* 1993;75(8):1134-1140.
6. Ziebarth K, Domayer S, Slongo T, Kim YJ, Ganz R: Clinical stability of slipped capital femoral epiphysis does not correlate with intraoperative stability. *Clin Orthop Relat Res* 2012;470(8):2274-2279.
7. Loder RT, Dietz FR: What is the best evidence for the treatment of slipped capital femoral epiphysis? *J Pediatr Orthop* 2012;32(suppl 2):S158-S165.
8. Davis RL II, Samora WP III, Persinger F, Klingele KE: Treatment of unstable versus stable slipped capital femoral epiphysis using the modified Dunn procedure. *J Pediatr Orthop* 2019;39(8):411-415.

   A retrospective chart review of 44 consecutive patients who underwent a modified Dunn procedure for SCFE found that unstable slips resulted in improved radiographic outcomes with less major complications as compared with stable slips. Of the 29 stable slips, two (6%) developed osteonecrosis, and of the 15 stable slips, five (29.4%) developed osteonecrosis. Three patients in the stable group developed postoperative instability, all of which developed osteonecrosis. Level of evidence: III.
9. Kaushal N, Chen C, Agarwal KN, Schrader T, Kelly D, Dodwell ER: Capsulotomy in unstable slipped capital femoral epiphysis and the odds of AVN: A meta-analysis of retrospective studies. *J Pediatr Orthop* 2019;39:e406-e411.

   A meta-analysis including 453 hips from 17 retrospective studies found 34/201 (17%) of hips with decompressive capsulotomy developed osteonecrosis while 67/252 (27%) without developed osteonecrosis. This difference did not reach statistical significance. Level of evidence: III.
10. Kishan S, Upasani V, Mahar A, et al: Biomechanical stability of single-screw versus two-screw fixation of an unstable slipped capital femoral epiphysis model: Effect of screw position in the femoral neck. *J Pediatr Orthop* 2006;26(5):601-605.
11. Leunig M, Slongo T, Kleinschmidt M, Ganz R: Subcapital correction osteotomy in slipped capital femoral epiphysis by means of surgical hip dislocation. *Oper Orthop Traumatol* 2007;19(4):389-410.
12. Sankar WN, Vanderhave KL, Matheney T, Herrera-Soto JA, Karlen JW: The modified Dunn procedure for unstable slipped capital femoral epiphysis: A multicenter perspective. *J Bone Joint Surg Am* 2013;95(7):585-591.
13. Upasani VV, Birke O, Klingele KE, Millis MB, International SCFE Study Group: Iatrogenic hip instability is a devastating complication after the modified Dunn procedure for severe slipped capital femoral epiphysis. *Clin Orthop Relat Res* 2017;475:1229-1235.

   Out of 406 patients who underwent modified Dunn procedure, 17 (4%) developed iatrogenic hip instability postoperatively, 14 of which developed osteonecrosis and three required THA at an average of 2-year follow-up. Level of evidence: III.
14. Baghdadi YM, Larson AN, Sierra RJ, Peterson HA, Stans AA: The fate of hips that are not prophylactically pinned after unilateral slipped capital femoral epiphysis. *Clin Orthop Relat Res* 2013;471(7):2124-2131.
15. Popejoy D, Emara K, Birch J: Prediction of contralateral slipped capital femoral epiphysis using the modified Oxford bone age score. *J Pediatr Orthop* 2012;32(3):290-294.
16. Swarup I, Williams BA, Talwar D, Sankar WN: Rates of contralateral SCFE in the United States: Analysis of the Pediatric Health Information System. *J Pediatr Orthop* 2020;40(7):e58 7-e591.

   Utilizing the Pediatric Health Information System database, 9755 patients who underwent in situ pinning for unilateral SCFE between 2004 and 2016 were identified, of which 11% developed a contralateral slip at an average of 277 days after the index procedure. The odds of contralateral SCFE decreased by 20% with each increasing year of age. Level of evidence: III.
17. Sankar WN, Novais EN, Lee C, Al-Omari AA, Choi PD, Shore BJ: What are the risks of prophylactic pinning to prevent contralateral slipped capital femoral epiphysis? *Clin Orthop Relat Res* 2013;471(7):2118-2123.
18. Maranho DA, Ferrer MG, Kim YJ, Miller PE, Novais EN: Predicting risk of contralateral slip in unilateral slipped capital femoral epiphysis: Posterior epiphyseal tilt increases and superior epiphyseal extension reduces risk. *J Bone Joint Surg Am* 2019;101:209-217.

   After controlling for triradiate cartilage status, lateral tilt angle and superior epiphyseal extension ratio were found to be independently associated with risk of contralateral slip in 318 patients treated for unilateral slip at a single institution. A higher posterior tilt was associated with increased risk, while increased superior extension was associated with reduced risk of contralateral slip. Level of evidence: IV.
19. Kamegaya M, Saisu T, Nakamura J, Murakami R, Segawa Y, Wakou M: Drehmann sign and femoro-acetabular impingement in SCFE. *J Pediatr Orthop* 2011;31(8):853-857.
20. Saisu T, Kamegaya M, Segawa Y, Kakizaki J, Takahashi K: Postoperative improvement of femoroacetabular impingement after intertrochanteric flexion osteotomy for SCFE. *Clin Orthop Relat Res* 2013;471(7):2183-2191.
21. Caskey PM, McMulkin ML, Gordon AB, Posner MA, Baird GO, Tompkins BJ: Gait outcomes of patients with severe slipped capital femoral epiphysis after treatment by flexion-rotation osteotomy. *J Pediatr Orthop* 2014;34(7):668-673.
22. Bali NS, Harrison JO, Bache CE: A modified Imhäuser osteotomy: An assessment of the addition of an open femoral neck osteoplasty. *Bone Joint J* 2014;96-B(8):1119-1123.
23. Chen A, Youderian A, Watkins S, Gourineni P: Arthroscopic femoral neck osteoplasty in slipped capital femoral epiphysis. *Arthroscopy* 2014;30(10):1229-1234.

24. Trisolino G, Pagliazzi G, Di Gennaro GL, Stilli S: Long-term results of combined epiphysiodesis and imhauser intertrochanteric osteotomy in SCFE: A retrospective study on 53 hips. *J Pediatr Orthop* 2017;37:409-415.

A retrospective review of 53 consecutive hips treated with combined epiphysiodesis and Imhäuser osteotomy with a mean follow-up of 21 ± 11 years found a cumulative 39-year survivorship free from conversion to THA of 68.5% (95% confidence interval, 42.4% to 84.7%). Postoperative osteonecrosis or chondrolysis significantly worsened long-term outcomes. Level of evidence: IV.

25. Anderson LA, Gililland JM, Pelt CE, Peters CL: Subcapital correction osteotomy for malunited slipped capital femoral epiphysis. *J Pediatr Orthop* 2013;33(4):345-352.

26. Loder RT: What is the cause of avascular necrosis in unstable slipped capital femoral epiphysis and what can be done to lower the rate? *J Pediatr Orthop* 2013;33(suppl 1):S88-S91.

27. Zaltz I, Baca G, Clohisy JC: Unstable SCFE: Review of treatment modalities and prevalence of osteonecrosis. *Clin Orthop Relat Res* 2013;471(7):2192-2198.

28. Souder CD, Bomar JD, Wenger DR: The role of capital realignment versus in situ stabilization for the treatment of slipped capital femoral epiphysis. *J Pediatr Orthop* 2014;34(8):791-798.

29. Larson AN, Sierra RJ, Yu EM, Trousdale RT, Stans AA: Outcomes of slipped capital femoral epiphysis treated with in situ pinning. *J Pediatr Orthop* 2012;32(2):125-130.

30. Castañeda P, Ponce C, Villareal G, Vidal C: The natural history of osteoarthritis after a slipped capital femoral epiphysis/the pistol grip deformity. *J Pediatr Orthop* 2013;33(suppl 1):S76-S82.

31. Wensaas A, Gunderson RB, Svenningsen S, Terjesen T: Femoroacetabular impingement after slipped upper femoral epiphysis: The radiological diagnosis and clinical outcome at long-term follow-up. *J Bone Joint Surg Br* 2012;94(11):1487-1493.

32. Ziebarth K, Milosevic M, Lerch TD, Steppacher SD, Slongo T, Siebenrock KA: High survivorship and little osteoarthritis at 10-year followup in SCFE patients treated with a modified Dunn procedure. *Clin Orthop Relat Res* 2017;475:1212-1228.

Forty-three consecutive patients with SCFE including stable and unstable slips were treated with modified Dunn osteotomy, had a resultant cumulative survivorship of 93% at 10 years with significant, and sustained improvement in Merle d'Aubigne and Postel scores at long-term follow-up. Level of evidence: IV.

33. Kim J, Choi JA, Lee E, Lee KR: Prevalence of imaging features on CT thought to be associated with femoroacetabular impingement: A retrospective analysis of 473 asymptomatic adult hip joints. *AJR Am J Roentgenol* 2015;205(1):W100-W105.

34. Li Y, Helvie P, Mead M, Gagnier J, Hammer MR, Jong N: Prevalence of femoroacetabular impingement morphology in asymptomatic adolescents. *J Pediatr Orthop* 2017;37(2):121-126.

An analysis of pelvic CT scans from 558 asymptomatic patients aged 10 to 18 years revealed that the prevalence of cam morphology in asymptomatic adolescents (16.8%) was comparable to what has been reported in adult populations, while pincer prevalence was more common (32.4%). Cam morphology was found more commonly in males, while pincer and mixed-type were equally common in males and females. Level of evidence: III.

35. Hartofilakidis G, Bardakos NV, Babis GC, Georgiades G: An examination of the association between different morphotypes of femoroacetabular impingement in asymptomatic subjects and the development of osteoarthritis of the hip. *J Bone Joint Surg Br* 2011;93(5):580-586.

36. Clohisy JC, Baca G, Beaulé PE, et al, ANCHOR Study Group: Descriptive epidemiology of femoroacetabular impingement: A North American cohort of patients undergoing surgery. *Am J Sports Med* 2013;41(6):1348-1356.

37. Siebenrock KA, Ferner F, Noble PC, Santore RF, Werlen S, Mamisch TC: The cam-type deformity of the proximal femur arises in childhood in response to vigorous sporting activity. *Clin Orthop Relat Res* 2011;469(11):3229-3240.

38. Morris WZ, Weinberg DS, Gebhart JJ, Cooperman DR, Liu RW: Capital femoral growth plate extension predicts cam morphology in a longitudinal radiographic study. *J Bone Joint Surg Am* 2016;98:805-812.

Analysis of historical, longitudinal radiographs of 96 healthy adolescents revealed a direct relationship between increased α angle and increased epiphyseal extension ratio, which has previously been associated with activities that increase shear force on the physis. These authors postulate that this is an adaptive mechanism to stabilize the physis against SCFE. Level of evidence: III.

39. McClincy MP, Lebrun DG, Tepolt FA, Kim YJ, Yen YM, Kocher MS: Clinical and radiographic predictors of acetabular cartilage lesions in adolescents undergoing hip arthroscopy. *Am J Sports Med* 2018;46(13):3082-3089.

A cohort of 446 hip in 402 adolescents undergoing hip arthroscopy were analyzed. Older age, male sex, and higher BMI were predictive of acetabular cartilage lesions. Level of evidence: IV.

40. Domayer SE, Ziebarth K, Chan J, Bixby S, Mamisch TC, Kim YJ: Femoroacetabular cam-type impingement: Diagnostic sensitivity and specificity of radiographic views compared to radial MRI. *Eur J Radiol* 2011;80(3):805-810.

41. Young M, Dempsey M, Rocha DL, Podeszwa DA: The cross-table lateral radiograph results in a significantly increased effective radiation dose compared with the Dunn and single frog lateral radiographs. *J Pediatr Orthop* 2015;35(2):157-161.

42. Pennock AT, Bomar JD, Johnson KP, Randich K, Upasani VV: Nonoperative management of femoroacetabular impingement: A prospective study. *Am J Sports Med* 2018;46(14):3415-3422.

Eighty-two percent of adolescent patients presenting with symptomatic FAI were managed nonsurgically and demonstrated significant improvements in outcome scores at a mean follow-up of 2 years. Level of evidence: II.

43. Lynch TS, Minkara A, Aoki S, et al: Best practice guidelines for hip arthroscopy in femoroacetabular impingement: Results of a Delphi process. *J Am Acad Orthop Surg* 2020;28(2):81-89.

    This is the first national consensus-based best practice guideline for the surgical and nonsurgical management of FAI. Level of evidence: V.

44. Bedi A, Zaltz I, De La Torre K, Kelly BT: Radiographic comparison of surgical hip dislocation and hip arthroscopy for treatment of cam deformity in femoroacetabular impingement. *Am J Sports Med* 2011;39(suppl 1):20S-28S.

45. Büchler L, Neumann M, Schwab JM, Iselin L, Tannast M, Beck M: Arthroscopic versus open cam resection in the treatment of femoroacetabular impingement. *Arthroscopy* 2013;29(4):653-660.

46. Novais EN, Mayo M, Kestel LA, Carry PM, Mayer SW: Return to play following open treatment of femoroacetabular impingement in adolescent athletes. *J Am Acad Orthop Surg* 2016;24(12):872-879.

    Twenty-one of 24 (87.5%) adolescent athletes returned to play at the same or greater level at a median 7 months after open treatment of their FAI. Level of evidence: III.

47. Cohen SB, Huang R, Ciccotti MG, Dodson CC, Parvizi J: Treatment of femoroacetabular impingement in athletes using a mini-direct anterior approach. *Am J Sports Med* 2012;40(7):1620-1627.

48. Chiron P, Espié A, Reina N, Cavaignac E, Molinier F, Laffosse JM: Surgery for femoroacetabular impingement using a minimally invasive anterolateral approach: Analysis of 118 cases at 2.2-year follow-up. *Orthop Traumatol Surg Res* 2012;98(1):30-38.

49. Byrd JW, Jones KS, Gwathmey FW: Arthroscopic management of femoroacetabular impingement in adolescents. *Arthroscopy* 2016;32(9):1800-1806.

    One hundred twenty-two hips in 108 adolescents were evaluated at an average of 30 months following hip arthroscopy. There was a significant improvement in the modified Harris Hip Score from 68.3 preoperatively to 93.6 postoperatively. Level of evidence: III.

50. Newman JT, Briggs KK, McNamara SC, Phillippon M: Outcomes after revision hip arthroscopic surgery in adolescent patients compared with a matched cohort undergoing primary arthroscopic surgery. *Am J Sports Med* 2016;44(12):3063-3069.

    Those undergoing revision arthroscopic surgery showed significant improvement in patient-reported outcomes, but their final scores were lower for sport activity, general health, and satisfaction as compared with those undergoing primary arthroscopy. Level of evidence: III.

51. Steppacher SD, Huemmer C, Schwab JM, Tannast M, Siebenrock KA: Surgical hip dislocation for treatment of femoroacetabular impingement: Factors predicting 5-year survivorship. *Clin Orthop Relat Res* 2014;472(1):337-348.

52. Steppacher SD, Anwander H, Zurmühle CA, Tannast M, Siebenrock KA: Eighty percent of patients with surgical hip dislocation for femoroacetabular impingement have a good clinical result without osteoarthritis progression at 10 years. *Clin Orthop Relat Res* 2015;473(4):1333-1341.

53. Rego PA, Mascarenhas V, Oliveira FS, Pinto PC, Sampaio E, Monteiro J: Arthroscopic versus open treatment of cam-type femoro-acetabular impingement: Retrospective cohort clinical study. *Int Orthop* 2018;42:791-797.

    A retrospective cohort study of 198 patients treated with hip arthroscopy or surgical hip dislocation for symptomatic FAI with a minimum follow-up of 2 years found a significant improvement in alpha angle (71.5° to 40.8°) and mean nonarthritic hip score (50 to 83) with no difference between groups. Level of evidence: III.

54. Schmaranzer F, Haefeli PC, Hanke MS, et al: How does the dGEMRIC index change after surgical treatment for FAI? A prospective controlled study: Preliminary results. *Clin Orthop Relat Res* 2017;475:1080-1099.

    A prospective analysis of dGEMRIC indices in patients with FAI who did not have surgery (20 hips) compared with those with either arthroscopic and open surgery (20 hips) found that while all patients with FAI have diminishing dGEMRIC indices, the decline is more pronounced in surgical patients 1-year postoperatively despite comparable baseline Tonnis osteoarthritic scores, patient-reported outcome measures, and baseline dGEMRIC indices. Level of evidence: II.

55. Ricciardi BF, Fields K, Kelly BT, Ranawat AS, Coleman SH, Sink EL: Causes and risk factors for revision hip preservation surgery. *Am J Sports Med* 2014;42(11):2627-2633.

CHAPTER 25

Legg-Calvé-Perthes Disease

HOLLY B. LESHIKAR, MD, MPH • JONATHAN G. SCHOENECKER, MD, PhD

ABSTRACT

Legg-Calvé-Perthes disease is a disruption of the normal physiology of the capital femoral epiphysis, physis, and metaphysis. Although its exact pathophysiology remains uncertain, strong associations between the development of this condition in late childhood and an ischemic etiology have been demonstrated. The unique vascularity of the pediatric hip likely plays a role in the development of the condition. The goals of treatment in Legg-Calvé-Perthes disease are focused on maintaining containment and motion of the femoral head within the acetabulum as the disease progresses through the characteristic stages, with the femoral head initially more susceptible to deformation until blood flow returns. Outcomes vary, with some patients having no subsequent difficulty with the affected hips and other patients ultimately requiring total hip arthroplasty because of early degenerative changes.

Keywords: femoroacetabular impingement; Legg-Calvé-Perthes disease; osteonecrosis; physeal bar

Dr. Schoenecker or an immediate family member serves as a paid consultant to or is an employee of OrthoPediatrics; serves as an unpaid consultant to Orthopediatrics Foundation for Education and Research; has received research or institutional support from IONIS, Ionis Pharmaceuticals, OrthoPediatrics, and PXE International; and serves as a board member, owner, officer, or committee member of the Pediatric Orthopaedic Society of North America. Neither Dr. Leshikar nor any immediate family member has received anything of value from or has stock or stock options held in a commercial company or institution related directly or indirectly to the subject of this chapter.

INTRODUCTION

Legg-Calvé-Perthes disease (LCPD) is an ailment of skeletal immaturity that manifests as idiopathic necrosis of the proximal femoral epiphysis, physis, and, in severe cases, the metaphysis. The segregation of the epiphyseal vasculature from the metaphyseal vasculature of the proximal femur during development and the relatively feeble epiphyseal vasculature make the epiphysis uniquely susceptible to osteonecrosis. The disease follows a protracted course, which is readily observed by plain radiography, and is characterized by sclerosis, fragmentation, reossification, and remodeling. The predominant feature of sclerosis is avascular necrotic bone. The fragmentation stage of LCPD features bone resorption and metaplastic development of a neocartilage anlage, which promotes subsequent revascularization and ossification.

The overwhelmingly benign course of the disease in children younger than 6 years suggests that the age of the patient is the single most important factor in disease severity. In older children, disease severity is initially correlated with the extent of proximal femoral involvement, but the outcome is ultimately associated with the resultant geometry and condition of the articular cartilage of the hip. Loss of containment and the development of a physeal bar contribute to poor hip geometry. Femoroacetabular impingement, subluxation, and the extent of revascularization of the epiphysis are among the factors that influence the health of the articular cartilage. Therefore, the optimal treatment is to minimize geometric deformity of the proximal femur and acetabulum, promote complete revascularization, and avoid the development of a physeal bar. Because no current therapies that alter the extent of revascularization of the epiphysis or physeal bar development exist, containment is the only factor associated with outcome that is treatable. Initially, containment is treated by any combination of range-of-motion therapy, bracing treatment, activity modification, and anti-inflammatory drugs. Surgical management may be considered if containment cannot be maintained. Proposed surgical containment methods range from adductor tenotomy and casting to femoral and pelvic osteotomies. Better outcomes are achieved if containment occurs early in the disease process. Late LCPD deformity, especially in the setting of a physeal bar, characteristically includes coxa magna, a short femoral neck, and a high-riding greater trochanter with variable acetabular dysplasia. These deformities can cause impingement between the anterior head-neck junction and the anterior aspect of the acetabular rim and external impingement of the posterosuperior greater trochanter and ischium. In severe LCPD, propagated acetabular dysplasia also may include paradoxic joint instability transposed on femoroacetabular impingement. These geometric deformities instigate degradation of the chondrolabral junction and articular cartilage. The goal of addressing these late deformities is to achieve impingement-free and stable, normal hip range of motion in an effort to delay the development of osteoarthritis.

EPIDEMIOLOGY

LCPD is a unique process of osteonecrosis of the proximal femur that typically involves the capital epiphysis and physis and, variably, the metaphysis. LCPD occurs in skeletally immature patients, with the typical onset occurring from 4 to 8 years of age. This condition has even been recently described in the remains of a skeleton from the third century BCE.[1] The incidence tends to increase with closer proximity to Northern Europe and is highest in Caucasians, although it ranges widely from 0.4 to 29.0 children per 100,000.[2] Children with LCPD have a short stature. Most epidemiologic studies show delay in bone maturation of more than 1 year, suggesting that the disease is likely more systemic and not limited to the proximal femur.[3] Although LCPD had previously been described as affecting children with short stature and lower weights, a recent case series of 150 patients showed 48% of patients were obese or overweight at the time of presentation, and these patients had more severe disease at presentation.[4] Affected patients are disproportionately male by a 4:1 ratio.[2,5] A large case series reported no important difference in the age of presentation between female and male patients.[6] Because the natural history differs substantially, it is important to highlight the distinction between LCPD and osteonecrosis of the femur, which occurs in older children, adolescents, and adults.

Pathophysiology

A 1957 study demonstrated that the epiphyseal vascularity is segregated from the metaphysis in the growing skeleton by the avascular physis.[7] At skeletal maturity, resorption of the physis allows blood vessels from the metaphysis to form anastomoses with those of the epiphysis. With a less redundant vasculature, the capital femoral epiphysis in children is a watershed area of bone and is susceptible to pathologies different from those of adults (**Figure 1**). This unique aspect of the vascular anatomy, the relatively feeble epiphyseal vasculature, and the timing of the onset of LCPD suggest that the condition is caused, at least in part, by insufficient vascularity at a particular point in skeletal development when the epiphysis is most susceptible to osteonecrosis. This theory of an insufficient blood supply to the proximal femoral epiphysis is reinforced by the universal involvement of the anterior aspect of the femoral head, which is most susceptible because of its vascular supply. Osteologic specimens show a vascular watershed anteriorly in the femoral epiphysis, potentially predisposing it to collapse despite similar trabecular architecture in comparison to the surrounding bone.[8]

A sudden or catastrophic loss of perfusion to the femoral head seems a less likely cause given the rare history of injury in patients with LCPD and the insidious onset of symptoms.[9] Instead, a vascular mechanism is supported, but the exact underlying pathology remains unknown. In

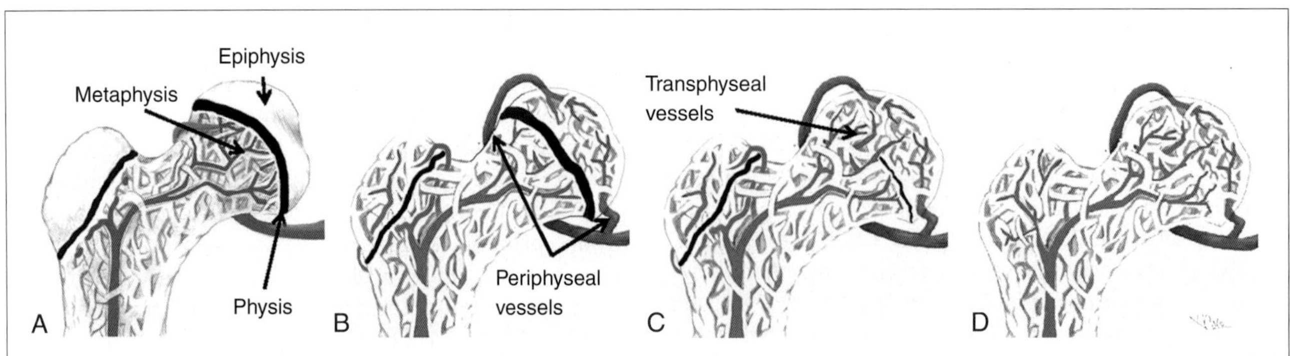

FIGURE 1 Illustrations show the development of the proximal femur in humans. **A**, Initially, the proximal femoral epiphysis in humans consists of avascular cartilage. **B**, At approximately 6 months of age, a secondary ossification center develops as a result of a vascular system that does not cross the physis (arrows indicate periphyseal vessels). At skeletal maturity (**C**), transphyseal vessels (indicated by the arrow shown crossing the physis) develop that result in physeal closure (**D**).

a study that examined the brachial arteries of children, those with LCPD tended to have smaller caliber arteries and impaired arterial function compared with the healthy counterparts.[5] This microvascular dysfunction, which is known to play a role in cardiovascular disease, may help explain the increased prevalence of ischemic heart disease and hypertension in young adults with a prior diagnosis of LCPD.[10] Environmental risk factors for vascular dysfunction, such as exposure to tobacco smoke, have also been associated with higher rates of LCPD.[11-13] These findings suggest an underlying vascular mechanism.

A thrombotic etiology also has been proposed. In a large case-control study of 169 patients with LCPD and 474 control subjects, a higher incidence of factor V Leiden mutation, protein S deficiency, elevated factor VIII, and prothrombin G20210A mutations were found in the children with LCPD.[14] Leptin, which is an angiogenic factor and positive vascular endothelial growth factor regulator known to affect bone metabolism, has been considered as a factor in the pathogenesis of the disease.[15,16] A case-control study reported that leptin resistance was elevated in children with LCPD compared with control subjects. The authors hypothesized that the increased leptin resistance may contribute to the pathology of the disease.[15-17] The authors of a 2015 study suggested that elevated interleukin 6 levels, which were found to be high in patients with LCPD during the initial and fragmentation phases of the disease, may result in a portion of the osteoclastic activity.[18] The prolonged injury to the physis and epiphysis that occurs in LCPD may act as a potent instigator that induces an acute-phase response. It is premature to assign causation of the disease course to these mediators (even when elevated) because they may represent only the downstream outcomes of the course of the condition.

NATURAL HISTORY

The initial radiographic observations of LCPD progression described by Waldenström have continued to frame the stages of the disease process (**Figure 2**). An inciting event occurs during stage I with observable sclerosis followed by subsequent fragmentation of the epiphysis in stage II and reossification in stage III. Remodeling may occur in stage IV. Disease severity is initially correlated with the extent of proximal femoral involvement during stage II. The predominant feature of sclerosis is osteonecrosis. Unlike adult forms of osteonecrosis, the fragmentation stage features bone resorption and

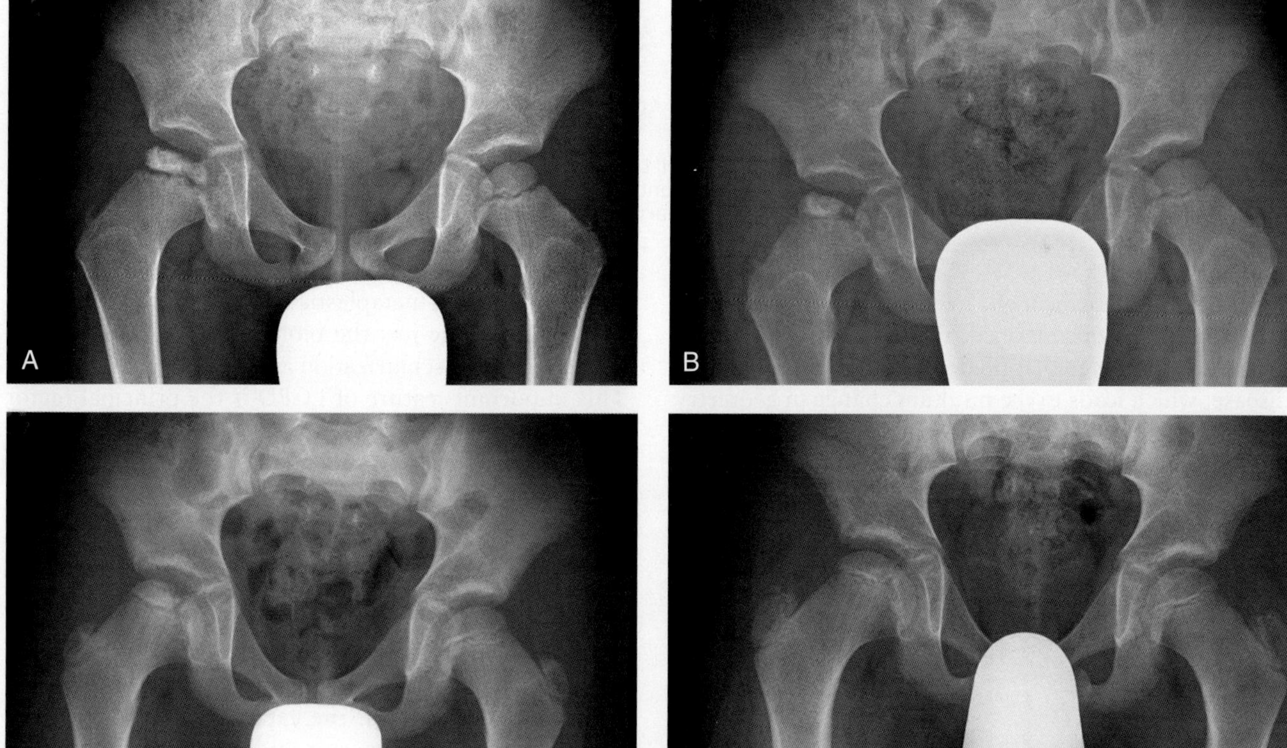

FIGURE 2 AP radiographs show the four stages of Legg-Calvé-Perthes disease described by Waldenström: **A**, Sclerosis. **B**, Fragmentation. **C**, Reossification. **D**, Remodeling.

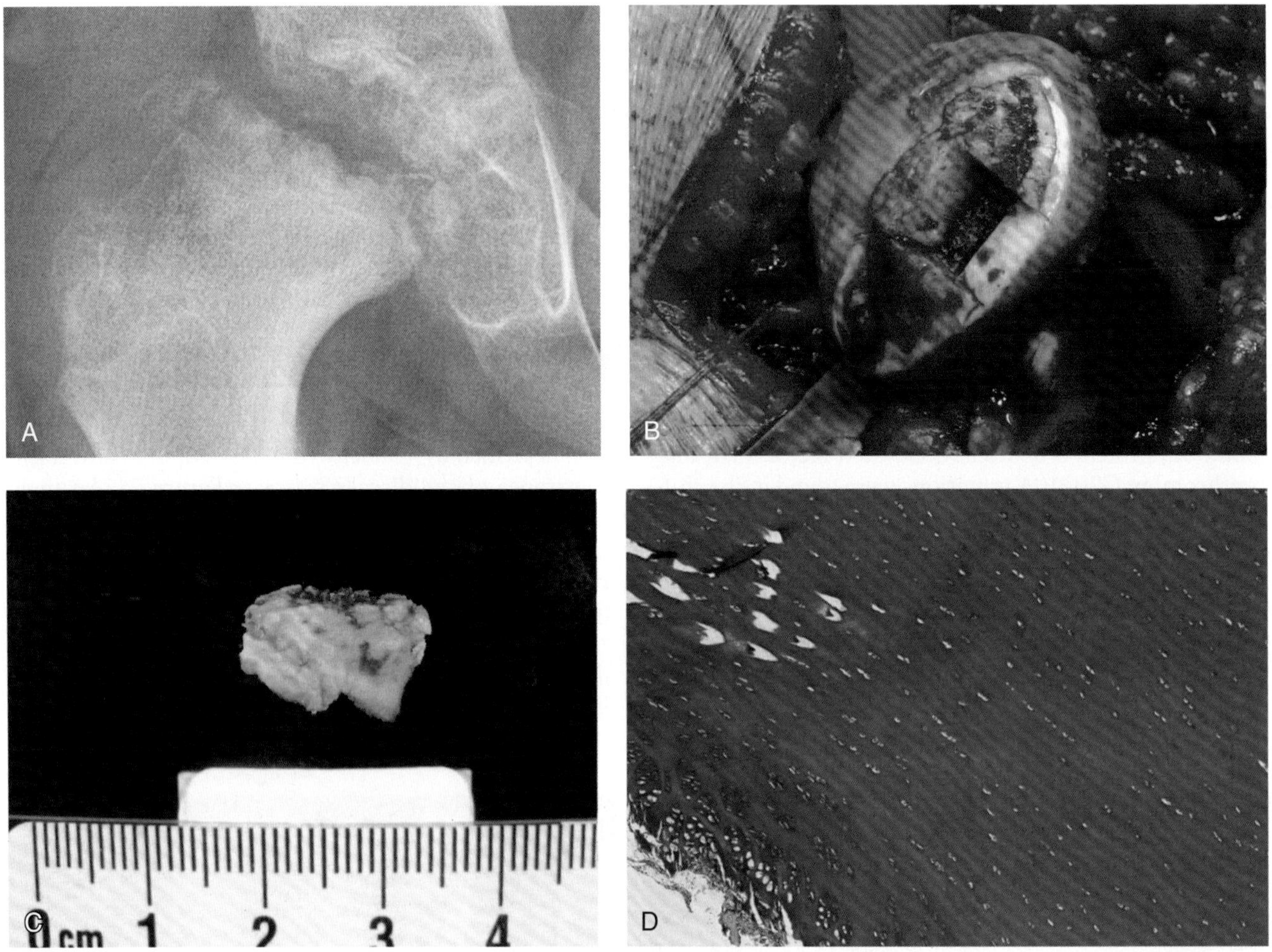

FIGURE 3 **A**, Radiograph of the femur in a patient with stage II Legg-Calvé-Perthes disease. **B**, Intraoperative photograph showing the femoral head during surgical hip dislocation for containment. **C**, Photograph of a specimen removed during femoral head reshaping. **D**, Histologic analysis of the specimen found cartilage instead of necrotic bone.

Section 5: Lower Extremity

metaplastic development of a neocartilage anlage (**Figure 3**). Especially if uncontained, the deforming forces act on the soft cartilage that predominates this stage of the disease, which leads to the resultant change in geometry of the femoral head (**Figure 4**).

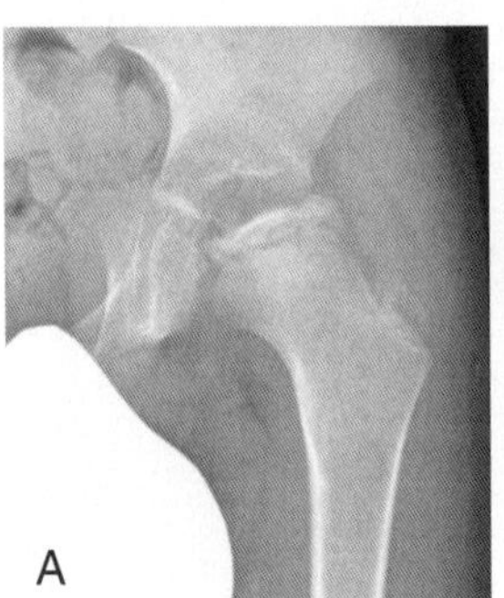

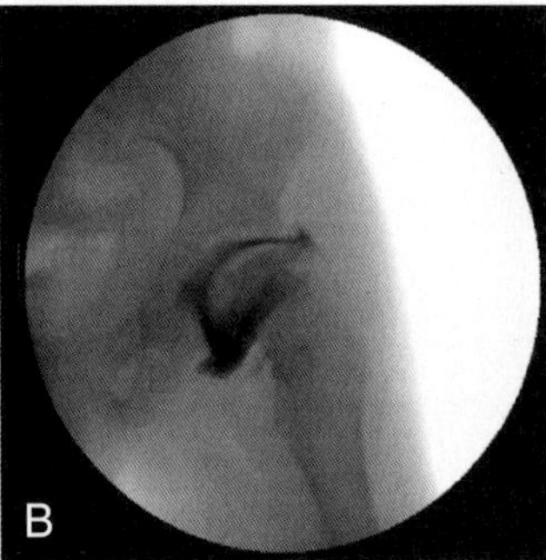

FIGURE 4 **A**, Radiograph of the femoral head in an 8-year-old boy with stage II Legg-Calvé-Perthes disease. **B**, Arthrogram demonstrating the cartilage anlage.

By undergoing metaplastic change, the resultant cartilaginous anlage has the biologic capacity to initiate endochondral vascularization and ossification (stage III). This important feature of LCPD is the principal factor that differentiates it from less efficient and often futile revascularization and ossification through the process of creeping substitution, which is observed in osteonecrosis without metaplasia and is seen in older children and adults. Thus, the pediatric hip has a substantially greater potential for revascularization of avascular areas, which effectively resets the hip back to a stage in development at which the epiphysis was largely a cartilaginous anlage, before ossification. Reossification (stage III) is directed by revascularization of the capital epiphysis, and the method by which this occurs and whether it is complete direct the disease severity.

The following three main outcomes exist regarding revascularization: (1) revascularization without consequence, (2) revascularization with consequence, and (3) incomplete revascularization. Anatomically, restoration of the blood flow to the epiphysis may occur through creation of periphyseal vessels, which spare the physis, maintain segregation of the metaphyseal and epiphyseal blood flow, and lead to the maintenance of the characteristic proximal femoral geometry. Alternatively, injury to the physis during the first two stages of the disease can promote channels of vascularity through the physis, leading to premature ossification across the physis and physeal bar formation.[19,20] With a healthy physis and periphyseal revascularization, the hip may remodel (stage IV) in the plane of motion, which results in a hip with relatively little deficiency in motion. Alternatively, revascularization via physeal bar formation impedes the ability of the hip to remodel and may instead propagate further geometric changes in the proximal femur. The role of physeal bar formation in the overall deformity has been described and suggests a poorer outcome with characteristic residual post-LCPD deformities, including femoral head widening (coxa magna) and flattening (coxa plana), a shortened neck (coxa breva), and relative overgrowth of the greater trochanter.

The outcome is ultimately associated with the resultant geometry of the femoral head and the condition of the articular cartilage of the hip[21,22] (**Figure 5**). Although healing occurs in many patients with little or no permanent change in the morphology of the femoral head and acetabulum, long-term studies have shown that a substantial change develops in approximately 50% of patients, which leads to premature degenerative joint disease and disability.[23,24] Factors that are known to negatively influence the resultant hip geometry are a loss of containment and the development of a physeal bar. Factors that are known to negatively influence the health of the articular cartilage are femoroacetabular impingement and/or subluxation and the extent of revascularization of the epiphysis. More recently, patient-reported outcomes have allowed for recognition of the natural history of this disease as it pertains to the patient's quality of life. In an effort to be better able to report these health-related outcomes, the authors of 2020 study[25] validated the use of Patient-Reported Outcomes Measurement Information System in LCPD. Additionally, through a systematic review, Delphi method, and consensus, the authors of a 2020 study[26] defined a core outcome set with domains defined in parts by affected families.

CLASSIFICATION AND IMAGING

Classification systems are based on the radiographic course of the femoral head in LCPD. As previously discussed, Waldenström divided the disease course into four stages based on radiographic characteristics. Other classifications include the Catterall, Salter-Thompson, and Herring lateral pillar systems. The lateral pillar classification was suggested in 1992 and then modified in 2004. It is based on the height of the lateral epiphysis and the extent of the collapse in the fragmentation stage[27] (**Figure 6**). Many studies have shown the excellent interobserver and intraobserver reliability of this classification system.[28] Although widely used, it should be applied cautiously in the early fragmentation stage because progression to a group other than the previously assigned group can occur in up to 75% of hips initially classified as Herring lateral pillar group A. Twenty-one percent to 33% of hips are ultimately assigned a more severe group later in the fragmentation stage.[29,30] Additionally, a height-width ratio of the proximal femur has been suggested for use

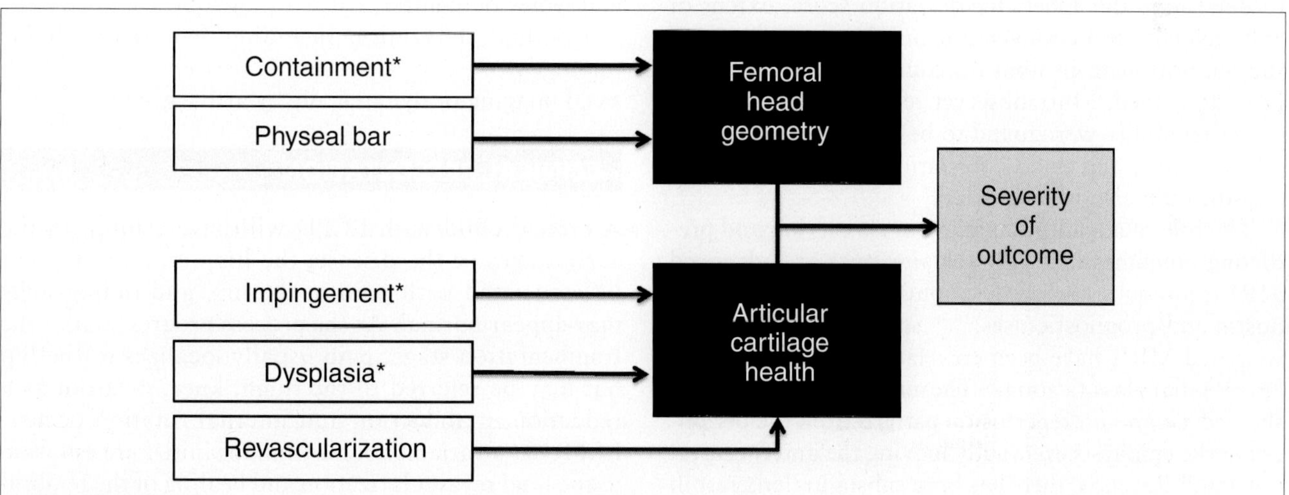

FIGURE 5 Algorithm of factors that contribute to the severity of the outcome in Legg-Calvé-Perthes disease. Outcome is associated with the resultant geometry of the femoral head and the health of the articular cartilage at the end of the disease process. The asterisks indicate factors that currently can be treated.

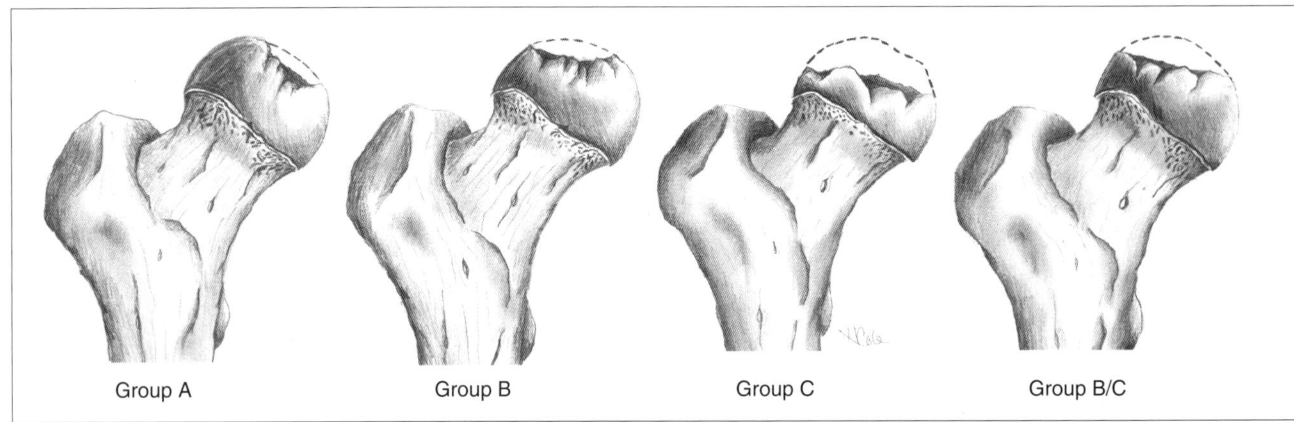

FIGURE 6 Illustrations of the Herring lateral pillar classification of Legg-Calvé-Perthes disease. The lateral one-third of the epiphysis, usually located lateral to the central sequestrum, is compared with the contralateral hip and measured for grading during the fragmentation stage. The epiphysis is considered group A if the height is equal to the contralateral epiphysis, group B if there is partial collapse but the height is greater than 50% of the contralateral epiphysis, and group C if there is greater collapse and the height is less than 50% of the contralateral epiphysis. A fourth type, called B/C, is a borderline group that was included to categorize hips with a thin or poorly ossified lateral pillar and loss of exactly 50% of the original height of the lateral pillar.

in bilateral disease when the contralateral side cannot be used for comparison. Good correlation has been found with the lateral pillar classification.[31]

The most widely used system for outcome measurements in LCPD is the Stulberg classification, which categorizes the mature hip into one of five classes. The Stulberg system is based on the shape of the femoral head and its congruency and has been shown to predict degeneration.[32] The reproducibility of this classification was improved by pooling class I and II hips and class III and IV hips.[33]

Visual assessment of the degree of femoral head deformity in LCPD is unreliable, and most authors have advocated for a more objective classification.[34] A new classification that relies on digitalized imaging to determine the sphericity deviation score, extent of enlargement, and composite femoral congruity arc of the femoral head in final outcome classifications has been developed.[35] Intraobserver reliability and interobserver reliability were found to be good to excellent for all measures, and good correlation with the Stulberg classification also was reported.

The role of advanced imaging in classifying and predicting outcomes in LCPD remains unclear. Advanced MRI techniques have been popularized for both diagnostic and prognostic uses.[36-38] Specifically, diffusion-weighted MRIs have been correlated with the Herring lateral pillar classification.[39] The authors of a 2016 study showed a common reperfusion pattern from the periphery of the epiphysis eventually moving the anterocentral portion.[40] Recently, there has been substantial interest in the use of early diffusion MRI for making a prognosis. In a 2014 study, 31 hips were imaged and classified using the Herring lateral pillar system. A diffusion MRI was obtained when the patient was first treated and again when the fragmentation stage was reached.[39] The apparent diffusion coefficient of the metaphysis correlated with the Herring lateral pillar classification as early as the condensation (sclerotic) phase, but more studies to elucidate its role in prognosis beyond plain radiography remain unsupported. Interestingly, the authors of a 2011 study suggested that diffusion MRI may play a role later in the disease process to illustrate a pattern of reperfusion during the reossification stage.[36] In this study, substantial differences in metaphyseal diffusion ratios between hips were reported, with the hips having the higher ratios being statistically more likely to have transphyseal reperfusion and focal physeal irregularity. This finding was suggestive of physeal bar formation and worse outcomes.

Residual deformity, including femoroacetabular impingement, can occur and is best characterized on axial imaging or dynamically by arthrography.

CLINICAL PRESENTATION

A typical child with LCPD will have a limp. In the early stages of the disease, the limp may or may not be associated with pain in the hip, and radiographs may appear normal. As the process progresses into the fragmentation stage, pain usually localizes to the hip but may be referred to the thigh, knee, or groin as a reduction in abduction and internal rotation occurs. LCPD has a variable course from the initial presentation to the final revascularization and healing of the femoral epiphysis, with the disease process lasting between 2 and 5 years. The inflammatory stage of fragmentation is characterized by a decrease in motion but an improvement in pain. During the reossification stage, there is little pain, but improvement in motion depends on the residual deformity.

Musculoskeletal infections, including proximal femoral osteomyelitis, septic arthritis, and pyomyositis, should be ruled out by clinical examination, imaging, and laboratory analysis. Slipped capital femoral epiphysis may also be included in the differential diagnosis in older children. Bilaterality suggests the possibility of epiphyseal dysplasia, sickle cell disease, or other conditions with greater systemic manifestations such as Meyer dysplasia, Gaucher disease, or hypothyroidism. It is important to recognize that LCPD may involve bilateral disease, but different stages of the disease are likely to be seen in each hip.

MANAGEMENT AND OUTCOMES

The goal of treatment in LCPD is to minimize geometric deformity and maintain congruency of the hip as revascularization occurs and the hip progresses through the stages of this condition. The biologic plasticity suggested by the author of a 1980 study[41] creates a condition of malleable cartilage. It follows that the shape of the cartilaginous epiphysis governs the shape of the ossified femoral head at the completion of the disease course. Therefore, containment of the femoral head within the acetabulum is most important during the early disease stages (I and II) when the femoral head is most susceptible to deforming forces. Although no current treatments that can influence the rate of revascularization or prevent physeal bar formation exist, methods are available to maintain containment. At each stage of the disease, treatment should be directed by the underlying occurring physiology.

The hip is painful early in the disease process. The loss of vascularity to the epiphysis is accompanied by synovitis of the joint.[11] Limited range of motion is often a clinical sign of pain, which is caused by irritability of the hip more than deformity or subluxation of the joint. Treatment is aimed at minimizing pain by the administration of anti-inflammatory medications, activity restrictions, and periods of non–weight bearing. The range of motion directs therapy. If the child's motion is excellent, there is no need for further treatment other than observation. When range of motion cannot be maintained or dramatically diminishes, dynamic observation with arthrography and clinical examination under anesthesia can be helpful in defining the problem and assessing congruity.

When lateral subluxation is present but joint congruity has been maintained, multiple treatment strategies have been suggested; these strategies range from bracing treatment to osteotomies of both the femur and the acetabulum. These treatments help to contain the hip and prevent subluxation, which may prevent further deformity by promoting congruity.

Bracing Treatment

A 2013 study suggested that a well-developed approach that uses soft-tissue releases (adductor tenotomy to achieve abduction), Petrie casting (to achieve containment), and an A-frame orthosis (to maintain containment) can achieve excellent outcomes. These outcomes can be achieved even in children with Herring lateral pillar B or B/C hips and are equivalent to outcomes reported after osteotomy containment techniques.[42] This technique avoids osteotomies, which may lead to abnormal force distribution across the epiphyseal cartilage and possibly further flattening of the femoral head. The unsuccessful maintenance of femoral head containment with nonsurgical management may be an indication for surgical intervention.

Femoral or Acetabular Osteotomy

A prospective multicenter study of LCPD treatment, which included patients older than 6 years, reported good radiographic results (Stulberg class I or II) in 61% of hips treated surgically with femoral or acetabular osteotomy and in 46% of hips treated nonsurgically.[43] In patients with onset of LCPD after 8 years of age who had Herring lateral pillar B and B/C hips, a higher rate of good results was reported with surgical treatment than with nonsurgical treatment. However, Herring lateral pillar C hips frequently had poor radiographic results, and outcomes were similar in the surgically treated and nonsurgically treated groups. This highlights the challenge of obtaining optimal containment in patients with extensive lateral ischemic changes. A review of the results of femoral osteotomy from the study resulted in a recommendation that caution be exercised in creating more than 15° of varus correction of the proximal femur, which often fails to remodel.[44]

Various acetabular osteotomies to achieve containment also have been reported. A shelf osteotomy was described for treatment in the early stages of LCPD; however, it did not show clear superiority over femoral osteotomy or nonosteotomy techniques in terms of radiographic markers of containment or the final Stulberg classification.[19] These procedures have been performed alone or in conjunction with other procedures such as iliopsoas and adductor tenotomies[45] or femoral osteotomies.[46] In the later study, despite good radiographic outcomes at skeletal maturity in only 59% of the 69 hips, 86% had excellent or good outcomes as defined by Harris hip score.[46]

Although early surgery has not been definitively shown to prevent deformity in all patients, it is logical that containment of the femoral head within the acetabulum is most important during the early disease stages when the femoral head is most susceptible to deforming forces. A recent multicenter prospective study, treated with early proximal femoral varus osteotomy during Waldenström stage 1, showed some patients who underwent this treatment had a shorter fragmentation phase and ultimately less collapse at final follow-up. Unfortunately, only 19% of the patients treated benefited, whereas others who underwent the surgical procedure followed a similar progression as those with no intervention.[47,48] Other procedures such as arthrodiastasis also have been used to contain the hip while preventing weight bearing through the soft epiphysis; however, this procedure is used less frequently because there is insufficient evidence to support or refute its efficacy as a treatment method. Drilling of the epiphysis in early stages to stimulate vascular ingrowth has been advocated by some surgeons, but the potential to create a physeal bar with revascularization from the metaphysis to the epiphysis suggests that this treatment should be studied further before being widely accepted.

In a child younger than 6 years with little or no involvement of the lateral epiphysis, the prognosis and outcome tends to be favorable regardless of the chosen treatment. The consensus among authors is for nonosteotomy treatment protocols, with emphasis on range of motion and symptom management.

When deformity occurs quickly in stages 1 and 2, femoral head extrusion may occur where the anterolateral portion of the femoral head is unable to roll under the acetabulum with abduction. This creates impingement of the lateral portion of the femoral head with the lateral acetabulum, resulting in pain and loss of motion. This phenomenon has been termed hinged abduction and is best demonstrated with arthrography. With this dynamic deformity, containment of the hip may not be achieved through abduction alone. This is further challenged by the fact that only moderate interobserver agreement has been shown for recognizing and defining hinged abduction by fluoroscopic examination, highlighting the difficulty of using this as an indication for further surgical intervention.[49] Studies suggest that there is little advantage to treatment to contain the femoral head when hinged abduction exists; therefore, many surgeons prefer a salvage procedure to improve a mechanically disadvantaged situation.[24] The goal of a valgus osteotomy is to reorient the medial femoral head superiorly so that it becomes load bearing. Although a full arc of motion is not restored, the more congruent medial head is able to roll under the acetabulum without hinging.

The authors of a 2013 study reported on 25 patients (18 Herring lateral pillar C and 7 lateral pillar B hips) in the late fragmentation stage or early reossification stage with hinged abduction who were treated with valgus femoral osteotomy.[50] At a mean follow-up of 6.3 years (range, 3.1 to 11.2 years), the mean Iowa hip score improved from 71 to 90. Some authors advise that valgus femoral osteotomy should be performed when reossification has occurred so that further deformity will not develop in the reoriented head.[51]

On the acetabular side, hinged abduction has been addressed with a Chiari or shelf osteotomy, with the goal of alleviating impingement by extending the effective edge of the acetabulum over the extruded portion of the femoral head. In a study of 27 consecutively treated hips with hinged abduction, which was demonstrated by arthrography, substantial improvements in pain scores and abduction were reported after shelf osteotomy (even in Catterall III and IV grade hips at the time of surgery).[52,53]

RESIDUAL DEFORMITY AT SKELETAL MATURITY

At skeletal maturity, the incongruent hip with substantial residual deformity represents a complex treatment challenge. The constellation of acetabular and femoral deformities causes pain and functional deficits and eventually progresses to osteoarthritis. Long-term outcomes reported in a 2012 study suggested that impingement plays an important role in the frequency of pain and is associated with lower hip scores in mature patients with LCPD.[24] Joint preservation surgery addresses the femoral and acetabular deformities that lead to impingement. An aspheric femoral head, a shortened and wide femoral neck, coxa vara, and a high-riding greater trochanter are commonly present following the disease course. These residual deformities may lead to joint incongruity, with abnormal loading of the chondrolabral junction and the resultant complex labral and cartilage pathologies.

A 2013 study reported abnormalities of the labrum in 44 of 59 post-LCPD hips (75%).[54] These abnormalities most commonly occurred in the anterolateral aspect of the joint and were highly correlated with cartilaginous abnormalities. Labral abnormalities were found in 97% of patients with an elevated alpha angle, which suggests a loss of sphericity. Treatment should be individualized based on the existing pathology, with the goals of restoring motion and decreasing pain. Surgical dislocation allows for the assessment and treatment of labral pathology and femoral head deformity and for relative femoral neck lengthening via trochanteric advancement to improve the biomechanical efficiency of the abductor muscles. Greater trochanteric apophyseodesis or greater trochanteric descent when used alone do not improve the gluteal muscle strength or ultimate Stulberg type, suggesting these are surgical techniques to be used in combination with those that change the intra-articular geometry.[55]

Femoral head abnormalities can be managed with a variety of techniques. Osteochondroplasty can be used to manage peripheral impingement lesions, although the extent of the resection may be limited by the entrance of the blood supply into the femoral head-neck junction. Central lesions may still be present.[56] Surgical hip dislocation can be used to address osteochondral defects through either osteochondral autologous transplant or fixation.[57] These techniques have been shown to be effective in small case series and should be replicated on a larger scale if possible for more rigorous evaluation. Osteochondral autologous transplantation can assist in managing central osteocartilaginous lesions, although this has not been rigorously evaluated, and further studies are needed[58] (**Figure 7**). The central head reduction procedure, which is technically challenging and has evolving indications, may be used to improve sphericity and containment. The central portion of the femoral head is removed, and the lateral column is reduced to the medial column with the articular cartilage approximated. Femoral head perfusion is maintained by metaphyseal blood flow to the stable medial portion of the head and flow from the inferior retinacular arteries through the retinacular flap to the lateral column.[59] Short-term studies have reported improvements in sphericity and Harris hip scores, even in hips in advanced Stulberg classes.[22,60]

If instability is present preoperatively or is created by concurrent femoral head-neck osteochondroplasty or central head reduction, a periacetabular osteotomy can be performed to maintain reduction. The authors of a 2015 study reported significant clinical improvement when combined procedures were performed.[61] The median Harris hip score improved from 64 preoperatively to 92 postoperatively ($P < 0.0001$).

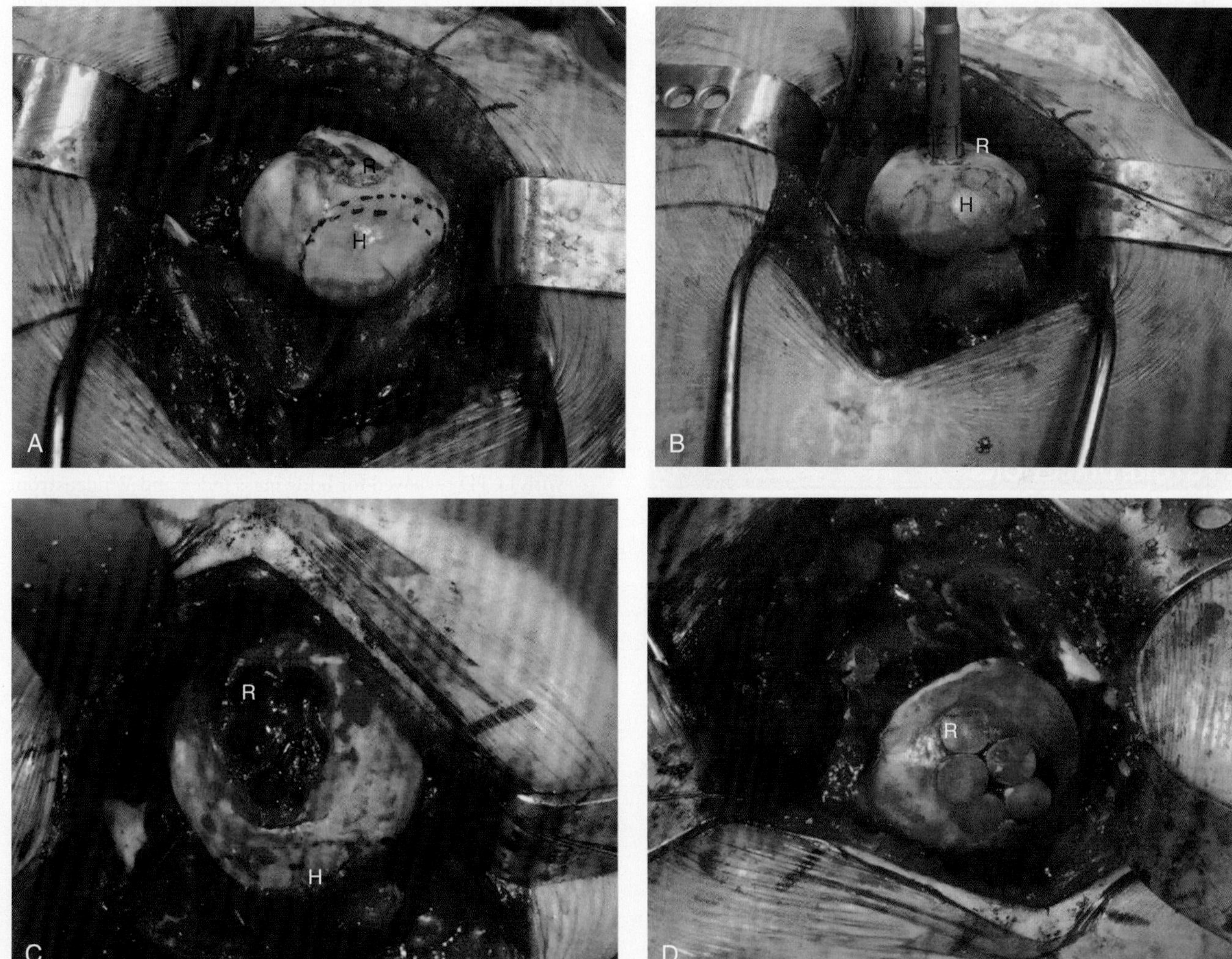

FIGURE 7 Intraoperative photographs of osteochondral autologous transplantation performed for a large central necrotic defect in a patient with Legg-Calvé-Perthes disease during stage IV. **A**, Healthy osteochondral plugs are transplanted from the anterior impingement region into the central area of necrosis. **B**, The recipient site is prepared by removing necrotic cartilage and bone. **C**, The recipient site after preparation. **D**, The recipient site after transplantation. H = harvest site, R = recipient site

In a systematic review that included 138 patients with residual LCPD deformities, the most commonly performed procedures were femoral head-neck osteochondroplasty and relative femoral neck lengthening.[62,63] An intertrochanteric osteotomy was performed in 22.5% of the patients. The complication rate was low (6%), and 75% of patients showed an improvement in symptoms, although 10% of patients still progressed to total hip arthroplasty. Multiplanar deformities resulting from the disease process or hip preservation surgeries create a technical challenge for surgeons who undertake total hip arthroplasty in this population. The use of custom implants or modular stems has been discussed.[64,65]

Hip arthroscopy is likely to play an increasing role in the management of LCPD. Osteochondroplasty as well as labral débridement and loose body removal can be successfully performed. Good short-term improvement in hip scores has been reported.[52]

If osteoarthritis develops, total hip arthroplasty remains the mainstay of treatment. Large registry series suggest similar survival rates for implants performed in patients younger than 40 years with all pathologies and older patients treated with arthroplasty for osteoarthritis.[66,67] In a smaller study specific to LCPD, the cumulative implant survival rate was 96.9% at 15 years.[68] All patients had substantial postoperative improvement in the Harris hip scores. It is important to understand and address the complex deformity innate to the disease and also secondary to previous treatments. Studies within the arthroplasty literature suggest excellent results when modular or custom implants are used to manage a metaphyseal-diaphyseal mismatch.[64,69]

FUTURE DIRECTIONS

Biologic treatments are currently being investigated in animal models of LCPD, but human clinical evidence is not yet available. The use of diphosphonates to theoretically inhibit initial bone resorption and collapse as well as the use of recombinant human bone morphogenetic protein to augment this process is an appealing treatment approach. However, the biologic mechanisms, safety of the systemic effects, and adverse effects such as local heterotopic ossification must be explored more thoroughly before clinical implementation.

SUMMARY

Because LCPD is ultimately a vascular disease, the ability to shorten the course of the disease and lessen the sequela depends on innovative techniques of promoting efficient revascularization of the epiphysis. Future treatment must be aimed at increasing the speed of revascularization to prevent or decrease damage to the femoral head.

KEY STUDY POINTS

- The etiology of LCPD is likely caused by the unique characteristics of the blood supply of the femoral head in children and a multifactorial localized ischemia.
- The goal of treatment in LCPD is to minimize geometric deformity and maintain congruency of the hip as revascularization occurs and the hip progresses through the stages of this condition.
- The chronic deformity associated with LCPD represents a complex problem that often eventually progresses to osteoarthritis.

ANNOTATED REFERENCES

1. Manzon VS, Ferrante Z, Giganti M, Gualdi-Russo E: On the antiquity of Legg-Calvé-Perthes disease: Skeletal evidence in iron age Italy. *Homo* 2017;68(1):10-17.

   This is a case report giving skeletal evidence of the oldest known record of LCPD dating back to the sixth to third century BCE.

2. Loder RT, Skopelja EN: The epidemiology and demographics of Legg-Calvé-Perthes' disease. *ISRN Orthop* 2011;2011:504393.
3. Lee ST, Vaidya SV, Song HR, Lee SH, Suh SW, Telang SS: Bone age delay patterns in Legg-Calvé-Perthes disease: An analysis using the Tanner and Whitehouse 3 method. *J Pediatr Orthop* 2007;27(2):198-203.
4. Neal DC, Alford TH, Moualeu A, Jo CH, Herring JA, Kim HK: Prevalence of obesity in patients with Legg-Calvé-Perthes disease. *J Am Acad Orthop Surg* 2016;24:660-665.

   This is a retrospective case series of 150 patients (172 hips) with LCPD reviewed for body mass index and Waldenström stage at presentation. Sixteen percent of patients were overweight and 32% were obese at presentation. Obesity correlated with advanced Waldenström stage at presentation ($P = 0.003$) as well as known social determinants of health, such as lower median household income by ZIP code ($P < 0.001$) and greater use of government-funded health insurance ($P < 0.001$). Level of evidence: III.

5. Perry DC, Bruce CE, Pope D, Dangerfield P, Platt MJ, Hall AJ: Perthes' disease of the hip: Socioeconomic inequalities and the urban environment. *Arch Dis Child* 2012;97(12):1053-1057.
6. Georgiadis AG, Seeley MA, Yellin JL, Sankar WN: The presentation of Legg-Calvé-Perthes disease in females. *J Child Orthop* 2015;9(4):243-247.
7. Trueta J: The normal vascular anatomy of the human femoral head during growth. *J Bone Joint Surg Br* 1957;39-B(2):358-394.
8. Morris WZ, Liu RW, Chen E, Kim HK: Analysis of trabecular microstructure and vascular distribution of capital femoral epiphysis relevant to Legg-Calve-Perthes disease. *J Orthop Res* 2019;37(8):1784-1789.

Thirty-two hips from 17 subjects belonging to the Hamann-Todd osteologic collection were analyzed. Subjects ranged in age from 4 to 16 years with open proximal femoral physes. Analysis involved vascular channel mapping and tomographic imaging of the trabeculae and microarchitecture. Findings suggest that the two main blood supplies from the medial femoral circumflex artery and the artery to the ligamentum teres enter posteriorly leaving a vascular watershed area anteriorly potentially predisposing it to collapse, although its trabecular architecture was similar to other parts of the epiphysis.

9. Holdsworth FW: Epiphyseal growth: Speculations on the nature of Perthes's disease. *Ann R Coll Surg Engl* 1966;39(1):1-16.

10. Hailer YD, Montgomery SM, Ekbom A, Nilsson OS, Bahmanyar S: Legg-Calve-Perthes disease and risks for cardiovascular diseases and blood diseases. *Pediatrics* 2010;125(6):e1308-e1315.

11. Atsumi T, Yamano K, Muraki M, Yoshihara S, Kajihara T: The blood supply of the lateral epiphyseal arteries in Perthes' disease. *J Bone Joint Surg Br* 2000;82(3):392-398.

12. Daniel AB, Shah H, Kamath A, Guddettu V, Joseph B: Environmental tobacco and wood smoke increase the risk of Legg-Calvé-Perthes disease. *Clin Orthop Relat Res* 2012;470(9):2369-2375.

13. Bahmanyar S, Montgomery SM, Weiss RJ, Ekbom A: Maternal smoking during pregnancy, other prenatal and perinatal factors, and the risk of Legg-Calvé-Perthes disease. *Pediatrics* 2008;122(2):e459-e464.

14. Vosmaer A, Pereira RR, Koenderman JS, Rosendaal FR, Cannegieter SC: Coagulation abnormalities in Legg-Calvé-Perthes disease. *J Bone Joint Surg Am* 2010;92(1):121-128.

15. Sezgin H, Gülman B, Çıraklı A, et al: Effects of circulating endothelial progenitor cells, serum vascular endothelial growth factor and hypogammaglobulinemia in Perthes disease. *Acta Orthop Traumatol Turc* 2014;48(6):628-634.

16. Talavera-Adame D, Xiong Y, Zhao T, Arias AE, Sierra-Honigmann MR, Farkas DL: Quantitative and morphometric evaluation of the angiogenic effects of leptin. *J Biomed Opt* 2008;13(6):064017.

17. Lee JH, Zhou L, Kwon KS, Lee D, Park BH, Kim JR: Role of leptin in Legg-Calvé-Perthes disease. *J Orthop Res* 2013;31(10):1605-1610.

18. Kamiya N, Yamaguchi R, Adapala NS, et al: Legg-Calvé-Perthes disease produces chronic hip synovitis and elevation of interleukin-6 in the synovial fluid. *J Bone Miner Res* 2015;30(6):1009-1013.

19. Bowen JR, Schreiber FC, Foster BK, Wein BK: Premature femoral neck physeal closure in Perthes' disease. *Clin Orthop Relat Res* 1982;171:24-29.

20. Jaramillo D, Kasser JR, Villegas-Medina OL, Gaary E, Zurakowski D: Cartilaginous abnormalities and growth disturbances in Legg-Calvé-Perthes disease: Evaluation with MR imaging. *Radiology* 1995;197(3):767-773.

21. Shah H, Siddesh ND, Joseph B: To what extent does remodeling of the proximal femur and the acetabulum occur between disease healing and skeletal maturity in Perthes disease? A radiological study. *J Pediatr Orthop* 2008;28(7):711-716.

22. Tannast M, Hanke M, Ecker TM, Murphy SB, Albers CE, Puls M: LCPD: Reduced range of motion resulting from extra- and intraarticular impingement. *Clin Orthop Relat Res* 2012;470(9):2431-2440.

23. Froberg L, Christensen F, Pedersen NW, Overgaard S: The need for total hip arthroplasty in Perthes disease: A long-term study. *Clin Orthop Relat Res* 2011;469(4):1134-1140.

24. Larson AN, Sucato DJ, Herring JA, et al: A prospective multicenter study of Legg-Calvé-Perthes disease: Functional and radiographic outcomes of nonoperative treatment at a mean follow-up of twenty years. *J Bone Joint Surg Am* 2012;94(7):584-592.

25. Matsumoto H, Hyman JE, Shah HH, et al: Validation of pediatric self-report Patient-Reported Outcomes Measurement Information System (PROMIS) measures in different stages of Legg-Calvé-Perthes disease. *J Pediatr Orthop* 2020;40(5):235-240.

    This is a multicenter study to report validity of Patient-Reported Outcomes Measurement Information System (PROMIS) for LCPD. Authors reported on cross-sectional analysis of 190 patients with 81% males and an average age of 10.4 ± 3.1 years (range, 4 to 18 years). Authors reported the worst PROMIS scores in all domains in those patients with early-stage disease and that additionally scores between domains were correlated, demonstrating construct validity of the PROMIS for patients with LCPD. Level of evidence: III.

26. Leo DG, Jones H, Murphy R, et al: The outcomes of Perthes' disease. *Bone Joint J* 2020;102-B:611-617.

    This article describes the technique used to identify a core outcome set for LCPD. This was performed using a combination of a systematic review of the literature and a Delphi survey method of parents, surgeons, and patients. Consensus was reviewed at the International Perthes Study Group and outcome sets were created with 14 individual outcomes identified.

27. Herring JA, Kim HT, Browne R: Legg-Calve-Perthes disease: Part I. Classification of radiographs with use of the modified lateral pillar and Stulberg classifications. *J Bone Joint Surg Am* 2004;86(10):2103-2120.

28. Rajan R, Chandrasenan J, Price K, Konstantoulakis C, Metcalfe J, Jones S: Legg-Calvé-Perthes: Interobserver and intraobserver reliability of the modified Herring lateral pillar classification. *J Pediatr Orthop* 2013;33(2):120-123.

29. Lappin K, Kealey D, Cosgrove A: Herring classification: How useful is the initial radiograph? *J Pediatr Orthop* 2002;22(4):479-482.

30. Park MS, Chung CY, Lee KM, Kim TW, Sung KH: Reliability and stability of three common classifications for Legg-Calvé-Perthes disease. *Clin Orthop Relat Res* 2012;470(9):2376-2382.

31. Woratanarat P, Lorungroj K, Dechosilpa C, et al: Height-width ratio of proximal femoral epiphysis: Estimation of lateral pillar involvement in bilateral Perthes disease. *J Pediatr Orthop* 2018;38(10):e577-e583.

    A cross-sectional study of children aged 2 to 15 years with and without LCPD was conducted between 2009 and 2015. Lateral pillar height and metaphyseal width were independently measured, and there was strong intraobserver and interobserver reliability noted and good correlation with lateral pillar classification. Authors suggested its use in case of bilateral disease, where the contralateral hip could not be used as a control. Level of evidence: III.

32. Stulberg SD, Cooperman DR, Wallensten R: The natural history of Legg-Calvé-Perthes disease. *J Bone Joint Surg Am* 1981;63(7):1095-1108.

33. Wiig O: Perthes' disease in Norway. A prospective study on 425 patients. *Acta Orthop Suppl* 2009;80(333):1-44.

34. Ross JR, Nepple JJ, Baca G, Schoenecker PL, Clohisy JC: Intraarticular abnormalities in residual Perthes and Perthes-like hip deformities. *Clin Orthop Relat Res* 2012;470(11):2968-2977.

35. Shah H, Siddesh ND, Pai H, Tercier S, Joseph B: Quantitative measures for evaluating the radiographic outcome of Legg-Calvé-Perthes disease. *J Bone Joint Surg Am* 2013;95(4):354-361.

36. Yoo WJ, Kim YJ, Menezes NM, Cheon JE, Jaramillo D: Diffusion-weighted MRI reveals epiphyseal and metaphyseal abnormalities in Legg-Calvé-Perthes disease: A pilot study. *Clin Orthop Relat Res* 2011;469(10):2881-2888.

37. Laine JC, Martin BD, Novotny SA, Kelly DM: Role of advanced imaging in the diagnosis and management of active Legg-Calvé-Perthes disease. *J Am Acad Orthop Surg* 2018;26:526-536.

This review article provides a thorough examination of the role of different imaging modalities in the diagnosis, staging, and management of LCPD. The authors discuss relevant evidence and guidance on use of each modality. In addition, the authors introduce areas of potential for future study for newer modalities such as dynamic gadolinium-enhanced subtraction and diffusion-weighted MRI.

38. Kim HK, Kaste S, Dempsey M, Wilkes D: A comparison of non-contrast and contrast-enhanced MRI in the initial stage of Legg-Calvé-Perthes disease. *Pediatr Radiol* 2013;43:1166-1173.

39. Baunin C, Sanmartin-Viron D, Accadbled F, et al: Prognosis value of early diffusion MRI in Legg Perthes Calvé disease. *Orthop Traumatol Surg Res* 2014;100(3):317-321.

40. Kim HK, Burgess J, Thoveson A, Gudmundsson P, Dempsey M, Jo CH: Assessment of femoral head revascularization in Legg-Calve-Perthes disease using serial perfusion MRI. *J Bone Joint Surg Am* 2016;98:1897-1904.

In a retrospective review of 29 hips that had undergone serial perfusion MRI, revascularization was observed to occur in a common pattern from the lateral, posterior, and medial periphery and then toward the center region and anteriorly. The rate of revascularization was independent of age, sex, and lateral pillar classification. Level of evidence: IV.

41. Salter RB: Legg-Perthes disease: The scientific basis for the methods of treatment and their indications. *Clin Orthop Relat Res* 1980;150:8-11.

42. Rich MM, Schoenecker PL: Management of Legg-Calvé-Perthes disease using an A-frame orthosis and hip range of motion: A 25-year experience. *J Pediatr Orthop* 2013;33(2):112-119.

43. Herring JA, Kim HT, Browne R: Legg-Calve-Perthes disease: Part II. Prospective multicenter study of the effect of treatment on outcome. *J Bone Joint Surg Am* 2004;86-A(10):2121-2134.

44. Kim HK, da Cunha AM, Browne R, Kim HT, Herring JA: How much varus is optimal with proximal femoral osteotomy to preserve the femoral head in Legg-Calvé-Perthes disease? *J Bone Joint Surg Am* 2011;93(4):341-347.

45. Park KS, Cho KJ, Yang HY, Eshnazarov KE, Yoon TR: Long-term results of modified Salter innominate osteotomy for Legg-Calvé-Perthes disease. *Clin Orthop Surg* 2017;9(4):397-404.

Thirty hips with LCPD, which had previously underwent a modified Salter innominate osteotomy, were retrospectively reviewed. In addition, hips also underwent iliopsoas and adductor tenotomies when flexion contracture or limitation of abduction was noted. The mean age at the time of surgery was 7.1 years (range, 4.3 to 11.0 years), and the mean follow-up was 12.9 years (range, 9.1 to 16.0 years). Surgery was performed when there was loss of containment of the femoral head or involvement of more than half of the femoral epiphysis. Harris hip scores improved from a mean of 80.2 points (range, 70 to 92 points) before surgery to 96.2 points (range, 93 to 100 points) at the final follow-up ($P = 0.001$).

46. Mosow N, Vettorazzi E, Breyer S, Ridderbusch K, Stücker R, Rupprecht M: Outcome after combined pelvic and femoral osteotomies in patients with Legg-Calve-Perthes disease. *J Bone Joint Surg Am* 2017;99:207-213.

This is a case series of 69 patients followed up for mean of 10.8 years who underwent double osteotomy for LCPD. Only 59% had good radiographic outcome (Stulberg I or II) at skeletal maturity; however, 71% had an excellent outcome, and 15% had a good result as defined by Harris hip score. There was a strong correlation between younger age at diagnosis of LCPD and higher Harris hip score at the time of follow-up ($P < 0.001$). Level of evidence: IV.

47. Sankar WN, Lavalva SM, Mcguire M, et al: Does early proximal femoral varus osteotomy shorten the duration of fragmentation in Perthes disease? Lessons from a prospective multicenter cohort. *J Pediatr Orthop* 2020;40(5):e322-e328.

In this prospective study, 46 patients with LCPD who were identified during Waldenström stage I were followed up with serial radiographs. Eight of 46 patients (17%) demonstrated partial bypass of fragmentation with evidence of early fissuring (stage IIa) but never advanced fragmentation or collapse (stage IIb). One patient showed no evidence of either phase suggesting complete bypass. Authors suggested that an early proximal femoral varus osteotomy could shorten the fragmentation phase in some patients, and in those that did, the patients may experience a milder form of fragmentation and subsequent femoral head deformity. Level of evidence: IV.

48. Shohat N, Copeliovitch L, Smorgick Y, et al: The long-term outcome after varus derotational osteotomy for Legg-Calve-Perthes disease: A mean follow-up of 42 years. *J Bone Joint Surg Am* 2016;98:1277-1285.

In a retrospective case series of 37 hips with prior varus derotational osteotomy between 1953 and 1989 followed up for a mean of 42.5 years, 17% of the original cohort of hips had undergone total hip arthroplasty. Of those hips that had not undergone arthroplasty, 64.5% had no or slight occasional pain without limitation in activity, 22.6% had moderate pain, and

12.9% had marked pain with serious limitation in activities. Patients with Stulberg I or II hips were more likely to have had varus derotational osteotomy at a younger age (6.88 years versus 8.76 years) and were associated with better Harris hip scores (93.2 versus 56.5) and Medical Outcomes Study 36-Item Short Form scores (85.5 versus 55.4). Level of evidence: IV.

49. Shore BJ, Miller PE, Zaltz I, Schoenecker PL, Sankar WN: Determining hinge abduction in Legg-Calvé-Perthes disease: Can we reliably make the diagnosis? *J Pediatr Orthop* 2019;39:e95-e101.

 AP and abduction fluoroscopic images were reviewed from 30 cases of LCPD to determine hinged abduction. Interobserver agreement for presence of hinged abduction was noted to be moderate ($\kappa = 0.54$ to 0.56), whereas intraobserver agreement was better ranging from 0.59 to 1.0. Level of evidence: III.

50. Kim HT, Gu JK, Bae SH, Jang JH, Lee JS: Does valgus femoral osteotomy improve femoral head roundness in severe Legg-Calvé-Perthes disease? *Clin Orthop Relat Res* 2013;471(3):1021-1027.

51. Bankes MJ, Catterall A, Hashemi-Nejad A: Valgus extension osteotomy for 'hinge abduction' in Perthes' disease. Results at maturity and factors influencing the radiological outcome. *J Bone Joint Surg Br* 2000;82(4):548-554.

52. Freeman CR, Jones K, Byrd JW: Hip arthroscopy for Legg-Calvè-Perthes disease: Minimum 2-year follow-up. *Arthroscopy* 2013;29(4):666-674.

53. Freeman RT, Wainwright AM, Theologis TN, Benson MK: The outcome of patients with hinge abduction in severe Perthes disease treated by shelf acetabuloplasty. *J Pediatr Orthop* 2008;28(6):619-625.

54. Maranho DA, Nogueira-Barbosa MH, Zamarioli A, Volpon JB: MRI abnormalities of the acetabular labrum and articular cartilage are common in healed Legg-Calvé-Perthes disease with residual deformities of the hip. *J Bone Joint Surg Am* 2013;95(3):256-265.

55. Haskel JD, Feder OI, Mijares J, Castañeda P: Isolated trochanteric descent and greater trochanteric apophyseodesis are not effective in the treatment of post-Perthes deformity. *Clin Orthop Relat Res* 2020;478(1):169-175.

 This is a retrospective case-control study of 89 children treated during reossification stage with greater trochanteric transfer, greater trochanteric apophyseodesis, or conservative management. Treatment was based on surgeon and family preference. Follow-up ranged from 6.0 to 9.2 years. Patients who underwent surgical treatments were not found to have significant differences in median abductor strength ($P = 0.34$), neck-shaft angle, or number of patients with Stulberg class II heads at final follow-up ($P = 0.46$) compared with those in the nonsurgical group. Authors concluded therefore that these surgical techniques were ineffective.

56. Risto O, Sandquist S, Lind S, Madan S: Outcome after osteochondroplasty and relative neck lengthening for patients with healed Legg-Calvé-Perthes disease: A retrospective cohort study of patients with hip-deformities treated with osteochondroplasty and relative neck lengthening. *Hip Int* 2019;1120700019896767.

 The authors evaluated the effect of surgery using self-assessed health scores. Outcome was correlated with grade of deformity or age at surgery in order to determine whether periacetabular osteotomy is the best treatment for concurrent acetabular dysplasia.

57. Lamplot JD, Schoenecker PL, Pascual-Garrido C, Nepple JJ, Clohisy JC: Open reduction and internal fixation for the treatment of symptomatic osteochondritis dissecans of the femoral head in patients with sequelae of Legg-Calvé-Perthes disease. *J Pediatr Orthop* 2020;40(3):120-128.

 This is a case series of seven patients treated with surgical hip dislocation and open reduction and internal fixation of femoral head osteochondritis dissecans fragments in setting of LCPD. There was a statistically significant ($P = 0.002$) improvement in Harris hip score from 47.8 ± 13.6 preoperatively to 82.7 ± 18.4 at final follow-up. Additionally, there was no radiographic progression of osteoarthritis as defined by Tönnis grade. Level of evidence: IV.

58. Khanna V, Tushinski DM, Drexler M, et al: Cartilage restoration of the hip using fresh osteochondral allograft: Resurfacing the potholes. *Bone Joint J* 2014;96-B(11 suppl A):11-16.

59. Kalhor M, Horowitz K, Gharehdaghi J, Beck M, Ganz R: Anatomic variations in femoral head circulation. *Hip Int* 2012;22(3):307-312.

60. Burian M, Dungl P, Nanka O, et al: Anteromedial wedge reduction osteotomy for the treatment of femoral head deformities. *Hip Int* 2013;23(3):281-286.

61. Clohisy JC, Nepple JJ, Ross JR, Pashos G, Schoenecker PL: Does surgical hip dislocation and periacetabular osteotomy improve pain in patients with Perthes-like deformities and acetabular dysplasia? *Clin Orthop Relat Res* 2015;473(4):1370-1377.

62. Novais EN: Application of the surgical dislocation approach to residual hip deformity secondary to Legg-Calvé-Perthes disease. *J Pediatr Orthop* 2013;33(suppl 1):S62-S69.

63. Shore BJ, Novais EN, Millis MB, Kim YJ: Low early failure rates using a surgical dislocation approach in healed Legg-Calvé-Perthes disease. *Clin Orthop Relat Res* 2012;470(9):2441-2449.

64. Al-Khateeb H, Kwok IH, Hanna SA, Sewell MD, Hashemi-Nejad A: Custom cementless THA in patients with Legg-Calve-Perthes disease. *J Arthroplasty* 2014;29(4):792-796.

65. Suzuki K, Kawachi S, Matsubara M, Morita S, Jinno T, Shinomiya K: Cementless total hip replacement after previous intertrochanteric valgus osteotomy for advanced osteoarthritis. *J Bone Joint Surg Br* 2007;89(9):1155-1157.

66. Lehmann TG, Engesaeter IØ, Laborie LB, Lie SA, Rosendahl K, Engesaeter LB: Total hip arthroplasty in young adults, with focus on Perthes' disease and slipped capital femoral epiphysis: Follow-up of 540 subjects reported to the Norwegian Arthroplasty Register during 1987-2007. *Acta Orthop* 2012;83(2):159-164.

67. Sedrakyan A, Romero L, Graves S, et al: Survivorship of hip and knee implants in pediatric and young adult populations: Analysis of registry and published data. *J Bone Joint Surg Am* 2014;96(suppl 1):73-78.

68. Traina F, De Fine M, Sudanese A, Calderoni PP, Tassinari E, Toni A: Long-term results of total hip replacement in patients with Legg-Calvé-Perthes disease. *J Bone Joint Surg Am* 2011;93(7):e25.

69. Seufert CR, McGrory BJ: Treatment of arthritis associated with Legg-Calve-Perthes disease with modular total hip arthroplasty. *J Arthroplasty* 2015;30(10):1743-1746.

CHAPTER 26

Congenital Dislocation of the Knee and Congenital Patellar Dislocations

AMY L. MCINTOSH, MD

ABSTRACT

Congenital dislocation of the knee is a rare condition that is apparent at birth. The usual presentation is a dramatic hyperextension deformity. Ultrasonography is used for prenatal diagnosis. Female sex, premature birth, and breech delivery are risk factors associated with the condition. Treatment should begin in infancy as soon as possible. Long leg plaster casting is preferred and performed on a serial basis every 7 to 10 days. A trial of nonsurgical treatment is appropriate until 12 months of age. Surgical treatment is indicated in patients not responding to casting. It includes lengthening of the quadriceps mechanism via either V-Y quadricepsplasty or a relative lengthening via an acute femoral shortening (2 to 3 cm). Congenital patellar dislocation is defined as a laterally displaced, hypoplastic patella with severe trochlear dysplasia/absent trochlea that often presents at birth; diagnosis may occur years later. It is associated with knee flexion contracture and valgus/external rotation deformity of the tibia. It is often associated with Down syndrome, Rubinstein-Taybi syndrome, nail-patella syndrome, Larsen syndrome, arthrogryposis, diastrophic dysplasia, and Ellis-Van Creveld syndrome. Congenital patellar dislocation must be differentiated from the more common obligatory subluxation, a condition that occurs later in childhood and adolescence. Nonsurgical treatment cannot correct the congenital patellar dislocation. If the child has progressive functional decline or inability to gain milestones, then surgical treatment should be considered.

Dr. McIntosh or an immediate family member is a member of a speakers' bureau or has made paid presentations on behalf of Nuvasive.

Keywords: congenital dislocation of the knee; congenital patellar dislocation; quadricepsplasty

INTRODUCTION

Congenital dislocation of the knee (CDK) and congenital patellar dislocation are rare conditions that are often associated with underlying syndromes or neuromuscular conditions. CDK is quite obvious at birth, and the patient's foot is often touching their face or shoulder. It is classified based on severity of the quadriceps contracture. Grades 1 and 2 are treated with weekly serial long leg plaster casting, followed by transition into a Pavlik harness when the knee can be flexed to 90°. Grade 3 often requires surgical treatment. Congenital patellar dislocations are not apparent at birth and often do not present until the child has gained walking ability. The child may present with a knee flexion contracture, delayed walking, genu valgum, and/or external tibial torsion. Nonsurgical treatment cannot correct the congenital patellar dislocation. If the child has progressive functional decline or inability to gain milestones, then surgical treatment should be considered.

CONGENITAL DISLOCATION OF THE KNEE

CDK is a rare condition with an incidence of ≤0.1%.[1,2] It is apparent at birth, and infants usually present with a dramatic hyperextension deformity (**Figure 1**). It can be diagnosed prenatally with ultrasonography.[3] It is most commonly associated with female sex, premature birth, and breech delivery. Ipsilateral hip dysplasia and clubfoot are present 70% and 50% of the time, respectively.[4,5] Bilateral CDK is almost always syndromic, with related laxity conditions (Larsen, Beals, Ehlers-Danlos) or neuromuscular conditions such as

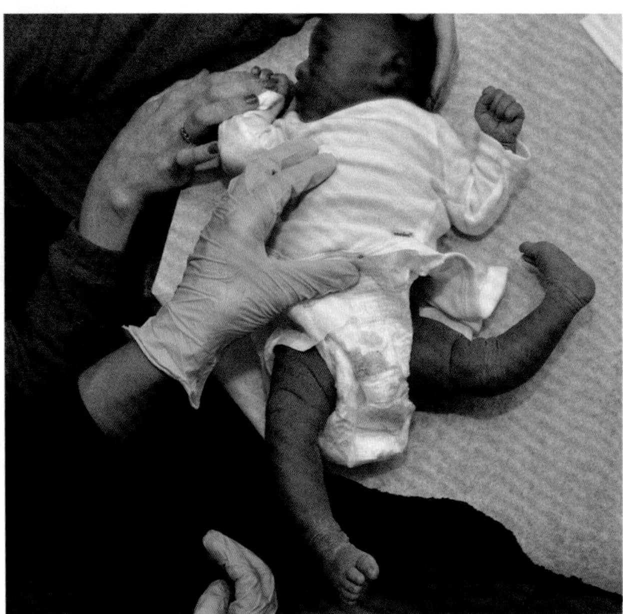

FIGURE 1 Clinical photograph of an infant with a grade 1 congenital dislocation of the left knee. Note the dramatic hyperextension of the knee. (© 2020, Texas Scottish Rite Hospital for Children, Dallas, Texas, All Rights Reserved.)

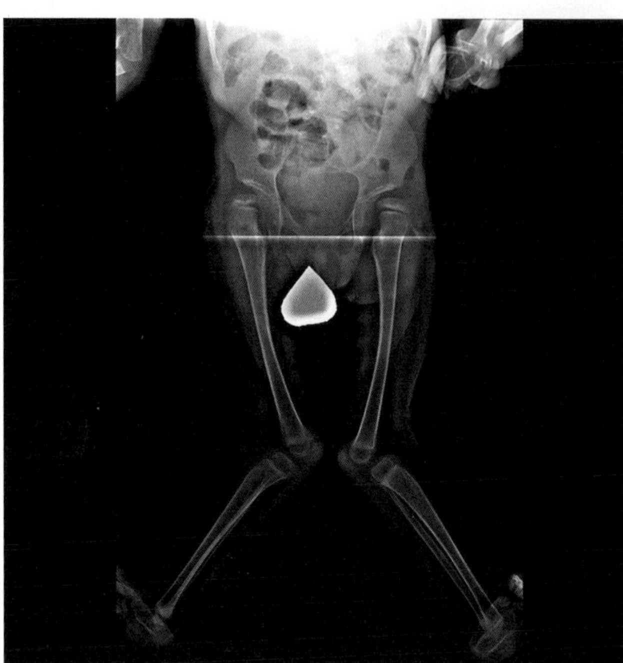

FIGURE 2 Radiograph of a child with a bilateral grade 2 congenital dislocation of the knee demonstrating that the tibial and femoral epiphyses are in contact with anterior translation of the tibia on the femur. (© 2020, Texas Scottish Rite Hospital for Children, Dallas, Texas, All Rights Reserved.)

arthrogryposis or myelodysplasia. If such conditions are suspected, then a genetics and/or neurology referral is necessary.

Clinically, the femoral condyles are prominent posteriorly in the popliteus fossa. The foot may be touching the infant's face or shoulder with marked hyperflexion of the hip. The flexibility of the quadriceps contracture is assessed by applying gentle traction to the tibia while attempting flexion of the knee. They are classified based on severity. Grade 1 (hyperextension) is defined as hyperextension greater than 15° with full flexion and normal radiographs. Grade 2 (subluxated) occurs when the knee is in hyperextension greater than 15°, it will not flex beyond neutral extension, and radiographs demonstrate the tibial and femoral epiphyses are in contact with anterior translation of the tibia on the femur (**Figure 2**). Grade 3 (dislocated) occurs when the knee is hyperextended, and any flexion is impossible. On radiographs, the tibial and femoral epiphyses are not in contact. The tibia lies anterior to the femur.

In grade 3 CDK, the anatomic findings include a shortened and fibrotic quadriceps mechanism, anterior displacement of the hamstring tendons and iliotibial band, contracted anterior capsule, loss of the suprapatellar pouch, redundancy of the posterior capsule, and absence/abnormality of the cruciate ligaments.

Treatment should begin in infancy as soon as possible. Long leg plaster casting is preferred and performed on a serial basis every 7 to 10 days. This is repeated until the knee will flex more than 90°. Associated clubfoot deformities are managed simultaneously with the Ponseti method.[6] When 90° of knee flexion has been achieved, then a plastic splint or Pavlik harness can be used until all tendencies for recurrence are overcome. In the knees with more severe quadriceps contracture that prevents effective gradual flexion, a femoral nerve block or botulinum toxin (Botox) can be a helpful adjunct. Botox has the advantage of longer term quadriceps paralysis allowing gradual stretching to occur.[7] A trial of nonsurgical management is appropriate until 12 months of age. Closed treatment is stopped if anatomic reduction of the tibia cannot be confirmed radiographically and knee flexion >90° cannot be achieved.[6]

Surgical management is indicated in patients not responding to casting. It includes lengthening of the quadriceps mechanism via either V-Y quadricepsplasty or a relative lengthening via an acute femoral shortening (2 to 3 cm).[1,8,9] Femoral shortening is preferred because it minimizes the quadriceps dissection and weakening. It also decompresses the anterior skin, thus reducing skin necrosis. The iliotibial band is often released from its distal insertion, and the anterior capsule/suprapatellar pouch is completely mobilized. Posterolateral and posteromedial capsulorrhaphy should be performed after excision of the redundant capsule. Following these capsulorrhaphies, the knee should lack 30° or more from full extension. At this point, the knee must be assessed for ligamentous laxity/instability of the anterior cruciate ligament with an anterior drawer test performed with the knee flexed. If the anterior drawer is unacceptable, then the anterior cruciate ligament should be reconstructed with a medial hamstring autograft. The knee should be casted in 45° to 60° of flexion for 8 weeks and then braced to limit full extension for the first 4 months postoperatively.[1]

Minimally invasive treatment for CDK (mini-open and percutaneous quadricepsplasty) has been described with good short-term results.[6,10-12] The percutaneous quadricepsplasty was performed with a needle at an average of 14.5 days of life. All of the patients had idiopathic CDK without underlying syndromic or neuromuscular conditions.[12] The mini-open quadricepsplasty is performed under general anesthesia. A short 2-cm midline incision is made over the superior pole of the patella. The quadriceps tendon is transected completely under direct vision 1 cm proximal to its insertion on the superior pole of the patella. After the tenotomy, the anterior capsule and lateral retinaculum are released through the same incision until 90° of knee flexion is obtained. The knee is then casted in 90° of knee flexion for 6 weeks.[6] The mini-open quadricepsplasty was performed at a mean age of 10 weeks.

CONGENITAL PATELLAR DISLOCATION

Congenital patellar dislocation is defined as a laterally displaced, hypoplastic patella with severe trochlear dysplasia/absent trochlea (**Figure 3**). It is often present at birth but may not be diagnosed until years later. It is associated with knee flexion contracture and valgus/external rotation deformity of the tibia.[13,14] It is often associated with Down syndrome, Rubinstein-Taybi syndrome, nail-patella syndrome, Larsen syndrome, arthrogryposis, diastrophic dysplasia, and Ellis-Van Creveld syndrome. Congenital patellar dislocation must be differentiated from the more common obligatory subluxation, which develops later in childhood and adolescence.[15]

Anatomic findings include a thickened, tight lateral retinaculum and iliotibial band; thinned and stretched medial retinaculum and medial patellofemoral ligament; and a quadriceps that is lateralized and shortened.[16]

Clinically, the child may present with a knee flexion contracture, delayed walking, genu valgum, external tibial torsion, or an associated syndrome/condition. On physical examination, the femoral condyles appear prominent anteriorly. The patella is small and laterally dislocated throughout the knee range of motion. Radiographs often demonstrate an empty intercondylar space on merchant views and are often unreliable in patients younger than 3 years because of lack of patellar ossification. MRI or ultrasonography may be necessary to confirm the diagnosis.[17]

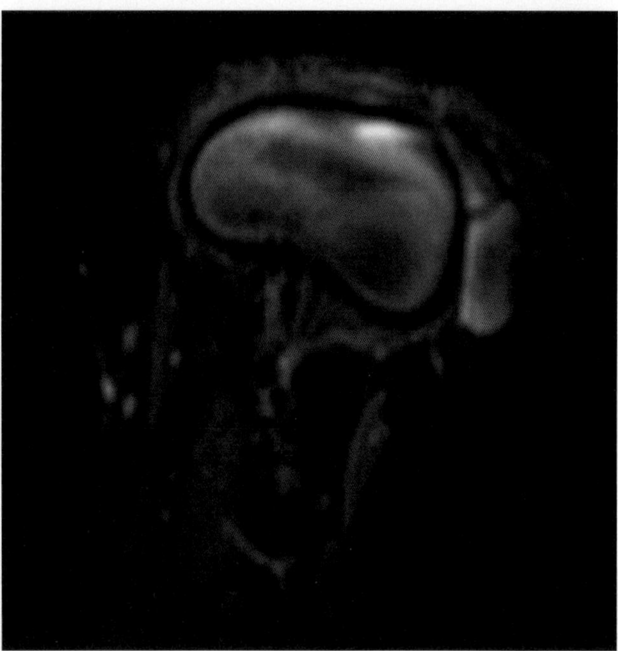

FIGURE 3 Magnetic resonance image of a congenital patellar dislocation in a 3-year-old girl. Note the laterally displaced, hypoplastic patella with severe trochlear dysplasia/absent trochlea.

Nonsurgical treatment cannot correct the congenital patellar dislocation. If the child has progressive functional decline or inability to gain appropriate milestones, then surgical treatment should be considered. Extensive lateral release with release of the iliotibial band and occasionally the biceps femoris should be performed. If this does not allow for centralization of the patella and quadriceps mechanism, then a V-Y quadricepsplasty versus an acute femoral shortening should be performed. A medial imbrication is then necessary to maintain reduction. A medial patellofemoral ligament reconstruction can be performed to augment the medial imbrication. There is no need to close/repair the extensive lateral release.[1] Last, assessment of the distal patellar tendon insertion should be performed. If distal realignment is deemed necessary, then a Goldthwait transfer versus patellar tendon periosteal sleeve medialization can be performed.[18,19]

SUMMARY

Congenital knee dislocation can be treated early with serial casting; if unsuccessful, then surgical intervention is necessary. Congenital patellar dislocation is a condition that requires surgical intervention.

KEY STUDY POINTS

- Grade 1 and grade 2 CDK are managed with weekly serial long leg plaster casting, followed by transition into a Pavlik harness when the knee can be flexed to 90°.
- Grade 3 CDK often requires surgical treatment. The mini-open quadricepsplasty has shown good short-term results when performed around 3 months of age.
- Nonsurgical treatment cannot correct a congenital patellar dislocation. Surgical treatment consists of an extensive lateral release with medical imbrication with or without medial patellofemoral ligament reconstruction. To regain full knee extension, an acute femoral shortening osteotomy is preferred. If distal realignment is also necessary, then a Goldthwait transfer versus a patellar tendon periosteal sleeve medialization can be performed.

ANNOTATED REFERENCES

1. Johnston CE II, Oetgen ME: Congenital deformities of the knee, in Scott WN, ed: *Insall & Scott Surgery of the Knee*, ed 5. Philadelphia, PA, Elsevier, 2012.
2. Charif P, Reichelderfer TE: Genu recurvatum congenitum in the newborn: Its incidence, course, treatment, prognosis. *Clin Pediatr (Phila)* 1965;4:587-594.
3. Monteagudo A, Kudla MM, Essig M, Santos R, Timor-Tritsch IE: Real-time and 3-dimensional sonographic diagnosis of postural congenital genu recurvatum. *J Ultrasound Med* 2006;25(8):1079-1083.
4. Johnson E, Audell R, Opeenheim WL: Congenital dislocation of the knee. *J Pediatr Orthop* 1987;7:194-200.
5. Bensahel H, Dal Monte A, Hjelmstedt A, et al: Congenital dislocation of the knee. *J Pediatr Orthop* 1989;9:174-177.
6. Youssef AO: Limited open quadriceps release for treatment of congenital dislocation of the knee. *J Pediatr Orthop* 2017;37:192-198.

   Treatment began with gentle manipulation and serial weekly long leg plaster casting in the outpatient clinic. Limited open quadriceps release was performed after failure of nonsurgical treatment or in patients who presented late (>12 weeks). Sixteen knees were treated by limited open quadriceps release. The age of the patients at the time of surgery ranged between 8 and 16 weeks with a mean age of 10 weeks. The mean postoperative passive arc of range of motion of the affected knees was 110° (range: 95° to 145°). Minor degrees of flexion deformity at the knee were encountered frequently (mean: 8.5°). Slight instability was observed in six patients. At final follow-up, the knee outcome was excellent in 6 knees and good in 10 knees. Level of evidence: IV.

7. Kaissi AA, Ganger R, Klaushofer K, Grill F: The management of knee dislocation in a child with Larsen syndrome. *Clinics (Sao Paulo)* 2011;66(7):1295-1299.
8. Oetgen ME, Walick KS, Tulchin K, Karol LA, Johnston CE: Functional results after surgical treatment for congenital knee dislocation. *J Pediatr Orthop* 2010;30(3):216-223.
9. Johnston CE II: Simultaneous open reduction of ipsilateral congenital dislocation of the hip and knee assisted by femoral diaphyseal shortening. *J Pediatr Orthop* 2011;31(7):732-740.
10. Abdelaziz TH, Samir S: Congenital dislocation of the knee: A protocol for management based on degree of knee flexion. *J Child Orthop* 2011;5:143-149.
11. Shah NR, Limpaphayom N, Dobbs MB: A minimally invasive treatment protocol for the congenital dislocation of the knee. *J Pediatr Orthop* 2009;29(7):720-725.
12. Patwardhan S, Shah K, Shyam A, Sancheti P: Assessment of clinical outcome of percutaneous needle quadriceps tenotomy in the treatment of congenital knee dislocation. *Int Orthop* 2015;39(8):1587-1592.
13. Stanisavljevic S, Zemenick G, Miller D: Congenital, irreducible, permanent lateral dislocation of the patella. *Clin Orthop Relat Res* 1976;116:190-197.
14. Gao GX, Lee EH, Bose K: Surgical management of congenital and habitual dislocation of the patella. *J Pediatr Orthop* 1990;10:255-260.
15. Weeks KD III, Fabricant PD, Ladenhauf HN, Green DW: Surgical options for patellar stabilization in the skeletally immature patient. *Sports Med Arthrosc Rev* 2012;20(3):194-202.
16. Ghanem I, Wattincourt L, Seringe R: Congenital dislocation of the patella. Part II: Orthopedic management. *J Pediatr Orthop* 2000;20:817-822.
17. Koplewitz BZ, Babyn PS, Cole WG: Congenital dislocation of the patella. *AJR Am J Roentgenol* 2005;184:1640-1646.
18. Langenskiold A, Ritsilä V: Congenital dislocation of the patella and its operative treatment. *J Pediatr Orthop* 1992;12:315-323.
19. Sever R, Fishkin M, Hemo Y, Wientroub S, Yaniv M: Surgical treatment of congenital and obligatory dislocation of the patella in children. *J Pediatr Orthop* 2019;39:436-440.

    The study group included 12 patients, 9 females and 3 males (15 knees), whose mean age was 5 years 2 months at diagnosis and 7 years 5 months at surgery. Nine patients had an underlying diagnosed genetic background (Down syndrome [$n = 6$], Larsen syndrome [$n = 2$], nail-patella syndrome [$n = 1$]). The mean follow-up was 46.2 months. Eleven patients gained stable patella with no recurrence of dislocation. Postoperative knee active extension was improved significantly ($P < 0.0001$) for all patients. The average postoperative Pediatric International Knee Documentation Committee and Pediatric Outcomes Data Collection Instrument scores were significantly higher ($P < 0.001$) among the idiopathic group. Level of evidence: IV.

CHAPTER 27

Tibial Deformities

ERIK C. B. KING, MD, MS • JOHN J. GRAYHACK, MD, MS

ABSTRACT

Orthopaedic surgeons who care for children should be familiar with recent literature published regarding the etiology, clinical features, and management of tibia vara, congenital pseudarthrosis of the tibia, and congenital posteromedial bowing of the tibia.

Keywords: anterolateral tibial bowing; Blount disease; congenital posteromedial bowing of the tibia; congenital pseudarthrosis of the tibia; tibia vara; tibial dysplasia

INTRODUCTION

The recent literature addressing the etiology, clinical features, and management of tibia vara, congenital pseudarthrosis of the tibia (CPT), and congenital posteromedial bowing of the tibia (CPMBT) is reviewed. In some situations, successful treatment remains challenging. An expanded understanding of tibial deformities may lead to better outcomes for patients.

Dr. Grayhack or an immediate family member has stock or stock options held in DePuy, a Johnson & Johnson, and Medtronic Sofamor Danek and serves as a board member, owner, officer, or committee member of the Pediatric Orthopaedic Society of North America. Neither Dr. King nor any immediate family member has received anything of value from or has stock or stock options held in a commercial company or institution related directly or indirectly to the subject of this chapter.

TIBIA VARA

Etiology and Clinical Features

Tibia vara is characterized by varus deformity of the proximal tibia. Tibia vara historically has been classified as infantile, juvenile, or adolescent, based on the patient's age at the time of diagnosis. Infantile tibia vara occurs in children younger than 4 years, juvenile in children aged 4 to 10 years, and adolescent in those older than 10 years.[1] Some authors have used the terms early-onset and late-onset, with late-onset tibia vara referring to both the juvenile and adolescent forms. Infantile tibia vara corresponds to the classic description of Blount disease. However, in published studies, the terms tibia vara and Blount disease are sometimes used interchangeably, including in patients older than those in the infantile age range.

Infantile tibia vara is bilateral in 50% of patients. Although in all age ranges tibia vara is more likely to affect black children, patients with early-onset tibia vara are more likely to have bilateral involvement and are less likely to be black or male compared with patients with late-onset tibia vara.[2] This disease is usually progressive, although spontaneous regression has been noted.[3] The differential diagnosis includes physiologic genu vara, metaphyseal chondrodysplasia, renal osteodystrophy, vitamin D–deficiency rickets, vitamin D–resistant rickets (hypophosphatemic rickets), and focal fibrocartilaginous dysplasia.

The cause of tibia vara is not known. Histologic studies have demonstrated disruption of the normal columnar architecture of the physis, replacement of physeal cartilage by fibrous tissue, and osseous bridging between the epiphysis and metaphysis in patients with advanced disease.[1] Children who have tibia vara are typically overweight or obese. Given the role of vitamin D in bone and epiphyseal plate mineralization and regulation, research has been performed to clarify the relationship between tibia vara and vitamin D deficiency; however, the results are mixed. A 2010 study found tibia vara to be more likely in patients with low levels of vitamin D.[4] In contrast, a 2016 study found that the mean vitamin D level in Blount children was lower than in normal healthy children, but this difference was not statistically significant.[5]

Tibia vara is associated with childhood obesity. This finding may be the result of increased compressive forces and growth inhibition at the proximal tibia physis.[6] A 2014 study investigated whether children with tibia vara had a lower body mass index after gradual correction with an external fixator.[7] Of 47 patients, 36 (76%) had an increase in the body mass index at an average follow-up of 48 months, despite successful correction of varus deformity and limb-length discrepancy along with nutritional counseling. Thus, other strategies are needed to address obesity in these children.

In addition, compared with the peers, children with tibia vara have advanced skeletal maturity.[8] Because advanced skeletal maturity affects the strategy for surgical realignment and the magnitude of planned overcorrection of lower limb deformity, preoperative assessment of bone age should be considered.

Both tibia vara and slipped capital femoral epiphysis (SCFE) are obesity-related bone diseases, but the relationship, if any, between the two entities is unclear. Children with both tibia vara and subsequent SCFE have been reported in the literature.[9] Hypertension also has been shown to be more prevalent in patients with both tibia vara and SCFE. In most patients, hypertension was previously undiagnosed. Because hypertension is a modifiable risk factor, it is plausible that hypertension may represent a modifiable risk factor for both tibia vara and SCFE.[10]

The classic radiographic features of infantile tibia vara are varus angulation at the epiphyseal-metaphyseal junction, a widened and irregular physeal line medially, a medially sloped and irregularly ossified epiphysis, prominent beaking of the medial metaphysis with lucent cartilage islands within the beak, and lateral subluxation of the proximal end of the tibia.[11] The Langenskiöld classification describes the severity and progression of pathologic changes to the proximal tibia epiphysis and metaphysis as seen on radiographs.[3] The authors of a 2019 study have proposed a modified Langenskiöld classification for infantile tibia vara, consisting of three stages[12] (**Figure 1**). Type A has a partially lucent medial metaphyseal defect, with or without beaking; type B deformity has downward-sloping curvature of the lateral and inferior rim of a completely lucent metaphyseal defect, which then has an upslope at the medial rim, resembling a ski jump, with no epiphyseal downward slope; and type C has vertical, downsloping deformity of both the epiphysis and metaphysis, with no upward curvature projecting medially at the inferior extent, while the epiphysis slopes downward into the metaphyseal defect. In patients younger than 3 years, it can be difficult to distinguish infantile tibia vara from physiologic genu varum because the classic radiographic features may not yet be present. Although historically a metaphyseal-diaphyseal angle greater than 11° on plain radiographs was deemed predictive of an increased risk for the subsequent development of radiographic changes characteristic of infantile tibia vara,[13] later consensus among most authors was that metaphyseal-diaphyseal angles less than 9° suggest physiologic genu vara, angles between 9° and 16° are indeterminate and should be monitored, and angles greater than 16° likely indicate infantile tibia vara and should be treated.[14]

Tibia vara characteristically includes procurvatum deformity in the sagittal plane. However, the authors of a 2014 study reported that clinical evaluation of procurvatum deformity tends to underestimate the true deformity as measured on radiographs.[15] Thus, in planning correction of the three-dimensional deformity, attention should be paid to findings on both coronal and sagittal radiographs.

In addition to bone deformities, abnormalities of the intra-articular structures of the knee occur in tibia vara. As demonstrated in MRI studies, the most severe of these abnormalities occur in the medial compartment of the knee, including increased thickness of the epiphyseal cartilage of the proximal medial aspect of the tibia, increased height and width of the medial meniscus, and abnormal signal in the posterior horn of the medial meniscus.[16,17] These morphologic changes may compensate for, or be a consequence of, the diminished height of the ossified portion of the medial proximal aspect of the tibia.

Treatment

Bracing treatment remains the first line of treatment in children when a diagnosis of tibia vara is made before the age of 4 years. It is most likely to be effective in children with mild deformity (Langenskiöld stage I and II) and in children younger than 3 years. It is especially effective in patients with unilateral involvement. In children aged 4 years or older, surgery should be considered. Multiple studies have demonstrated that the rate of deformity recurrence after osteotomy is greater when performed after the age of 4 years. In addition, extreme vertical sloping of the medial metaphyseal defect may carry a poor prognosis for successful correction by high tibial osteotomy alone or in combination with epiphysiolysis.[12]

Traditional surgical techniques include proximal tibial-fibular osteotomy, acute or gradual correction, and hemiepiphysiodesis. In patients with severe or recurrent deformity, epiphysiolysis (physeal bar resection) and medial tibial plateau elevation may be considered. A recent

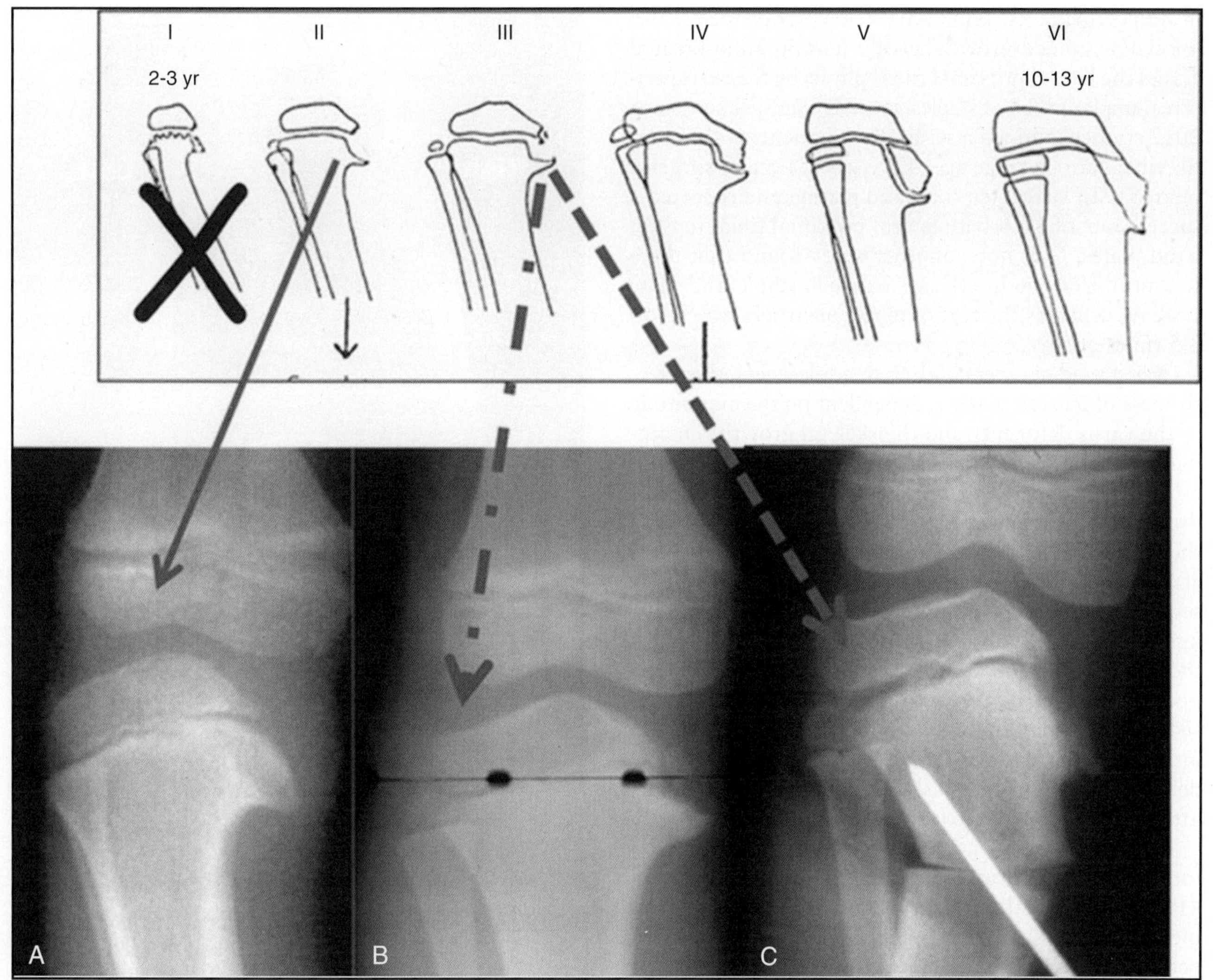

FIGURE 1 Correlation of original Langenskiöld diagrams with the new modified classification. Note the partial lucency of the metaphyseal defect in type A, compared with the complete lucency of type B. The upsloping rim of the inferior margin of the defect in type B is absent in type C. Traces of epiphyseal bone sliding into the metaphyseal defect (as in Langenskiöld III) may or may not be present in types B and C. (Reproduced with permission from LaMont L, McIntosh A, Jo C, Birch J, Johnston C: Recurrence after surgical intervention for infantile tibia vara: Assessment of a new modified classification. *J Pediatr Orthop* 2019;39[2]:65-70.)

study reports good to excellent outcomes for a single-stage double osteotomy performed proximal to the tibial tubercle for the late-presenting infantile tibia vara for children 7 years of age or older, combined with lateral proximal tibial hemiepiphysiodesis to minimize recurrence.[18]

Intraoperative neurophysiologic monitoring has been shown to be a useful adjunct in tibial osteotomy surgery, potentially preventing irreversible neurologic damage.[19] A 2013 study confirmed that osteotomy with gradual correction with an external fixator is successful, even in patients who are obese.[20] Patients and families should be counseled before treatment that more modest complications, such as pin tract infections, are commonplace and that more difficult complications often must be identified and managed during the treatment course.[21]

Both uniplanar external fixators and circular external fixators are safe and effective.[22] Hexapod external fixators, such as the Taylor Spatial Frame, are currently the most popular external fixation devices. A recent study demonstrated equivalent outcomes for infantile and adolescent patients with Blount disease treated with either Ilizarov external fixator or Taylor Spatial Frame.[23] If minimal lengthening is needed in addition to angular correction, then osteotomy of the fibula is unnecessary.[24]

Growth modulation techniques, previously reserved for adolescent patients, have been shown to be effective in younger patients. Temporary hemiepiphysiodesis, also known as guided growth, uses a tension band created across the lateral proximal tibial physis by the extraperiosteal implantation of staples, tension plates, or screws. A 2012 study examined a series of 12 patients with infantile tibia vara (average age, 4.8 years at time of surgery) treated with lateral tension band plating and reported a success rate of 89% with lateral proximal tibial tension band plates.[25] Of note, another study found that there was no difference in efficacy between staple and plate systems, whereas the cost of plate constructs was 1.5 to 3.5 times greater.[26]

When used in older children or adolescents, the effectiveness of tension plates is dependent on the magnitude of the varus deformity and the skeletal growth remaining.[27] A 2010 study found that the eight-Plate (Orthofix) effectively treats angular deformities in growing children and is less likely to extrude spontaneously than the Blount staple.[28] Failures and delayed correction were attributed to broken screws and wound infection that required plate removal. Some recurrence of varus deformity occurred in a few patients. After removal of plates, the risk of recurrent varus deformity is attributed to the poor growth potential of the proximal medial tibial physis. Growth modulation does not correct the associated internal tibial rotational deformity in all patients, but this deformity has spontaneously resolved in many patients after coronal plane correction.

Multiple recent studies have investigated risk factors for failure of growth modulation. One study found 41% (25/61) overall surgical failure rate and 11% (7/61) mechanical failure rate[29] (**Figure 2**). In addition to patient-related risk factors, such as obesity and deformity, titanium instrumentation seems to be an independent risk factor for failure compared with stainless steel. Two literature analyses have been published. The first study concluded that guided growth is a moderately complex technique and that outcomes are variable. Nonetheless, guided growth is reasonable as an initial treatment, and osteotomies should be considered the salvage procedures.[30] The second study found that neither age at index surgery nor the type of implant correlated with the need for unplanned additional surgeries.[31]

It has been clearly established that titanium cannulated screws are prone to breakage in patients with infantile or adolescent tibia vara because of the high body mass index of these patients. A 2012 study used biomechanical testing of cyclic loading to failure to compare the strength of two guided growth devices. With the use of titanium cannulated screws, one guided growth device was found to be significantly stronger than the other ($P = 0.036$).[32] Solid stainless steel screws were shown to be substantially stronger than cannulated screws in both devices. Some authors now recommend implants such as parallel eight-Plates and solid noncannulated stainless steel screws for plate fixation.[33,34] Techniques for solid screw insertion using cannulated drilling have been described.[35]

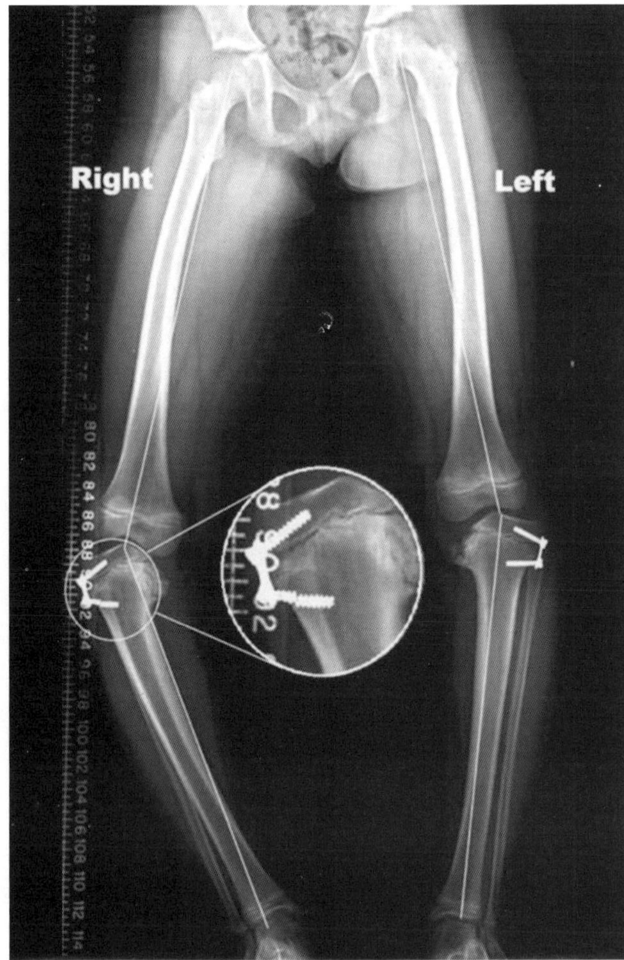

FIGURE 2 Radiograph showing the surgical failure case in Blount disease. Right: Mechanical failure in the form of screw breakage (magnified view). Left: Incomplete correction, which may lead to functional failure at skeletal maturity. (Reproduced with permission from Jain MJ, Inneh IA, Zhu H, Phillips WA: Tension band plate (TBP)-guided hemiepiphysiodesis in Blount disease: 10-year single-center experience with a systematic review of literature. *J Pediatr Orthop* 2020;40[2]:e138-e143.)

A recent article is the first report in the literature of plate failure in a guided growth implant. Scanning electron microscopy demonstrated that the cause of failure was cyclical compression and relaxation.[36] In view of these issues, surgeons may need to consider stronger plates or multiple implants in obese patients.

Medial tibial plateau elevation should be considered in older patients who walk with a large varus thrust and have advanced depression of the medial tibial plateau. Delay in ossification of the medial epiphysis may make the magnitude of medial depression appear more significant on plane radiographs than anatomic reality. An intraoperative arthrogram can be useful in determining the true amount of medial plateau depression. Medial tibial plateau elevation can be performed alone or combined with varus correction of the metaphysis (the so-called double osteotomy).[37,38]

CONGENITAL PSEUDARTHROSIS OF THE TIBIA (TIBIAL DYSPLASIA)

Etiology and Clinical Features

CPT is an uncommon disorder that represents a spectrum of disease ranging from anterolateral bowing to fracture pseudarthrosis. Because most patients do not have a true pseudarthrosis at birth, tibial dysplasia is a more accurate term. Approximately 5.7% of children with neurofibromatosis have CPT, whereas up to 55% of children with CPT have neurofibromatosis type 1 (NF1).[39,40] A recent study found a 84% prevalence rate for NF1 in its study population of patients with CPT, suggesting that NFI may be more common in CPT patients than previously believed.[41]

The understanding of CPT etiology is evolving. Histologically, the pseudarthrosis site consists of fibrous hamartoma; thick, abnormal periosteum; and fibrovascular tissue. The double inactivation of the *NF1* gene has been suggested as part of the pathologic mechanism, as reported in two studies.[42,43] The authors theorize that periosteal cells with this double inactivation of the *NF1* gene fail terminal osteoblastic differentiation. These abnormal cells proliferate and form the fibrous hamartoma in the tibia that results in pseudarthrosis. It is unknown why this formation is more common in the tibia.

Treatment

Successful management of anterolateral bowing and CPT is both challenging and unpredictable. The treatment goal in children who have isolated anterolateral bowing is to prevent fracture. To that end, full-time bracing treatment with a custom orthosis during weight-bearing activities should be prescribed until the child reaches skeletal maturity.

After fracture or pseudarthrosis occurs, the treatment goals are to achieve and maintain union while minimizing angular deformity and limb-length discrepancy. Multiple surgeries over many years may be required to achieve these goals. Success is not guaranteed, and amputation remains an alternative choice in the most difficult of cases.

Surgical management should address both the biology of CPT and issues of mechanical stability. Surgical options include combinations of resection of the abnormal pseudarthrosis bone, shortening of the tibial defect, bone grafting or transport, and stabilization of the tibia. Success rates of each technique reported in the literature have varied.

A variety of surgical techniques have been described, including intramedullary nailing, vascularized fibular grafting, external fixation, and bone transport. Using excision of pseudarthrosis, intramedullary rodding, and cortical bone grafting, a 2011 study found union of the pseudarthrosis was achieved in 9 of 11 children (82%) after the index operation and in the 2 remaining children after further surgery.[44] At final follow-up, all 11 children had a soundly united tibia, although persistent fibular pseudarthrosis was present in 10 children. Ten children underwent 21 secondary surgeries for various indications. Recently, Fassier-Duval telescopic rods have been used to manage CPT. The effectiveness of these rods has been demonstrated in osteogenesis imperfecta; however, only one study of its efficacy in CPT has been published.[45] The authors concluded that utilization of the Fassier-Duval rods is demanding and associated with intraoperative and postoperative complications. Supplemental stabilization in a circular external fixator may be beneficial. More studies are needed before the effectiveness of this technique can be determined for patients with CPT.

Several studies reporting management of congenital pseudarthrosis of the tibia with external fixtures have substantiated its efficacy.[46,47] A 2011 study suggested a fibular status–based classification and a multitargeted fibular status–based algorithmic approach for osteosynthesis, ankle stabilization, and limb-length equalization.[48] In addition, the Ilizarov technique can be successfully combined with conventional antegrade intramedullary nailing.[49] After successful bony union through surgical intervention, an unacceptable leg-length discrepancy often remains. To address this leg-length discrepancy, distraction osteogenesis through the physis or through subphyseal osteotomy has been shown to be effective.[50] Another case report describes the successful use of a motorized intramedullary lengthening nail to correct residual limb-length discrepancy and rotational malalignment after management of CPT by Masquelet induced membrane technique and intramedullary fixation.[51]

Bone transport has demonstrated good short-term results; however, the risk of refracture was high. A study of long-term outcomes in 12 patients treated with Ilizarov bone transport found that primary consolidation was achieved in 10 patients (83%) at an average follow-up of 24.5 years.[52] Half of these patients had a refracture. At final follow-up, fracture union was achieved in eight patients and fracture nonunion occurred in four patients, including one patient who underwent amputation. Even healed and united bone is often of inferior biologic and mechanical quality, so lifelong protection with intramedullary devices, braces, or a combination of both is recommended.

Three approaches to vascularized fibular grafting may be used: transfer of ipsilateral fibula on its intact vascular pedicle, transfer of ipsilateral free vascularized fibula, and transfer of contralateral free vascularized fibula. The latter two approaches require microvascular surgical techniques. The use of ipsilateral free vascularized fibula grafts was reported to achieve union in 73% of patients at an average follow-up of 20.1 months.[53] To enhance union of the free vascularized fibular graft technique, a novel split-tibia coaptation technique was used successfully to achieve bone union in two patients[54] (**Figure 3**). In this technique, both the proximal and distal stumps of the tibia are split longitudinally and pivoted open to form gutters. The vascularized fibular graft is placed into the tibial gutters and stabilized by external fixation.

In addition to the usual complications of persistent nonunion, refracture, shortening, and angular deformity, the use of the contralateral fibula is associated with donor leg morbidity, most commonly ankle valgus.[55] To minimize ankle valgus, distal tibiofibular joint arthrodesis is recommended, and a distal fibular remnant greater than 5 cm should be retained.[56]

Two recombinant human bone morphogenetic proteins (rhBMPs) are now available for clinical use: rhBMP-2 and rhBMP-7. rhBMP-2 plays an important role in early differentiation of mesenchymal progenitor cells to preosteoblast cells, whereas rhBMP-7 promotes differentiation of preosteoblast cells to osteoblasts. For management of CPT, it seems likely that rhBMP-2 would be effective in the presence of pluripotent cells, as when autologous bone grafting is performed. In contrast, rhBMP-7 alone would not be as effective until active normal osteoblast cells are present and ready for terminal differentiation. The FDA has not approved labeling rhBMPs for the management of CPT.

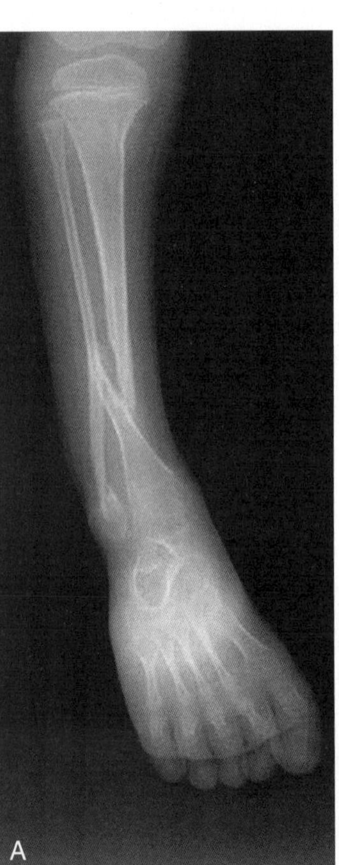

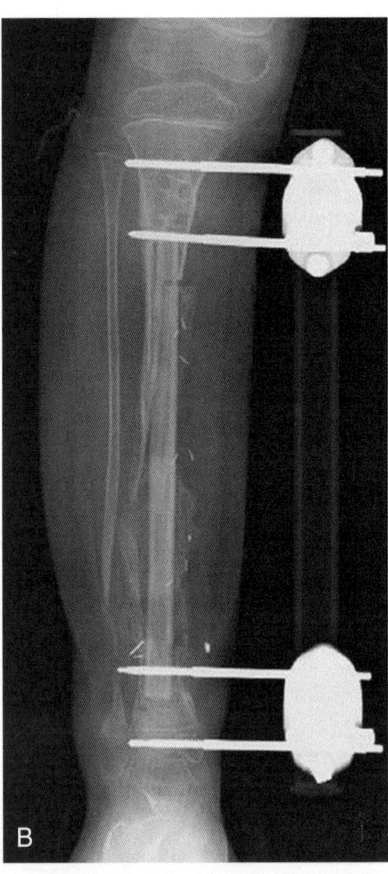

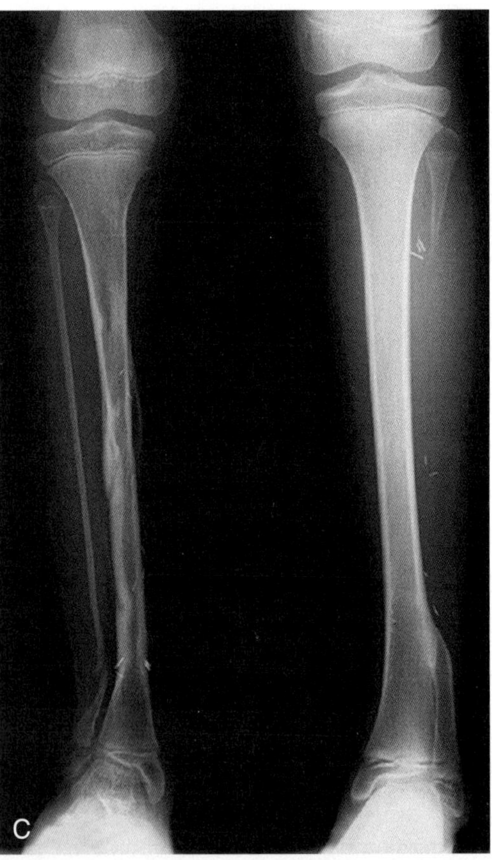

FIGURE 3 Radiographs from a 5-year-old girl with Boyd type II congenital pseudarthrosis of the tibia. **A**, Preoperative AP radiograph of the affected right tibia. **B**, Postoperative AP radiograph of the affected right tibia. **C**, AP radiograph of both legs at 4 years and 1 month after treatment with a free vascularized fibular graft. The diameter of the graft has enlarged to 83% of the contralateral tibia with no refracture. (Reproduced with permission from Takazawa A, Matsuda S, Fujioka F, Uchiyama S, Kato H: Split tibia vascularized fibular graft for congenital pseudarthrosis of the tibia: A preliminary report of 2 cases. *J Pediatr Orthop* 2011;31[4]:e20-24.)

In a case series of seven patients, the use of rhBMP-2 combined with iliac crest and Williams rodding was shown to lead to earlier union in patients with congenital pseudarthrosis and a higher rate of maintenance of union compared with earlier studies.[57] Similarly, the authors of a 2011 study reported a series of five patients with a mean age of 7.4 years who were treated with rhBMP-2 and intramedullary rodding.[58] Circular frame external fixation also was used in four of these patients. Radiologic union of the pseudarthrosis was evident in all of the patients at a mean follow-up of 3.5 months postoperatively.

Surprisingly, in a different 2018 multicenter long-term study, the use of BMP (BMP-7 in 2 children and BMP-2 in 14 children) was associated with a poorer outcome.[59] In addition, the authors found that combining intramedullary nailing with the Ilizarov technique was associated with poor results. In contrast, the authors report that use of the Ilizarov technique, transfixing the ankle and subtalar joints, and use of cortical graft while not operating on the fibula were associated with a better outcome. The authors conclude that these may be inclined to withhold the routine use of BMP, avoid combining Ilizarov technique with intramedullary rodding, and consider including cortical graft when bone grafting is performed. The authors emphasized the ongoing need for an international multicenter registry of CPT to generate good-quality prospective data.

Conversely, rhBMP-7 was evaluated in a 2014 follow-up study in which 20 patients were randomized into two groups.[60] Group 1 received rhBMP-7 along with intramedullary Kirschner wire fixation and autologous bone grafting, and group 2 received only Kirschner wire fixation and grafting. The authors found no substantial difference in healing time between autologous grafting and autologous grafting plus rhBMP-7 at 5 years postoperatively. Similarly, an earlier study reported that the use of rhBMP-7 alone was not sufficient to overcome the poor healing environment associated with CPT.[61]

In 2011, therapy combining rhBMP-2 and a diphosphonate (zoledronic acid) was applied to a mouse model of deficient NF1 fracture repair.[62] Surgical repair of fracture that included rhBMP-2 therapy followed by the systemic postoperative administration of zoledronic acid halved the rate of ununited fractures to 37.5%. Only one clinical study using a combination of rhBMP and diphosphonates in humans has been reported. Eight patients with CPT were administered rhBMP-7 at the time of surgery in addition to receiving bone grafting and stabilization, followed by the administration of either pamidronate or zoledronic acid postoperatively.[63] In six of eight patients, primary healing was achieved at an average of 5.5 months after surgery.

A 2010 study described a two-stage technique in the management of extensive diaphyseal defects by induction of a membrane for bone reconstruction (Masquelet technique, also known as the induced membrane technique).[64] In stage 1, bone débridement is performed, and the defect is filled with bone cement. The cement remains in place for a period of 8 weeks, which allows the formation of induction membrane. In stage 2, the bone cement is gently removed, and the defect is filled with cancellous bone graft. Mixed results have been reported in small case series of patients (including children) with CPT.[65-69] A 2017 study found that the induced membrane technique and the transfer of the contralateral vascularized fibula produced similar outcomes.[70] Although vascularized fibula grafting theoretically involves a single stage, the mean number of surgical procedures was statistically the same.

Amputation is the appropriate treatment of resistant pseudarthrosis when other treatments have not achieved a functional extremity. A 2018 study evaluated the long-term functional, radiographic, and clinical outcomes of patients who underwent amputations as treatment of CPT.[71] Within this study cohort, 76% required secondary procedures after the initial amputation. Successful union was ultimately achieved in 92% of patients, and at most recent follow-up, averaged 11.1 years, all patients were functioning without limitations with the use of prosthetic device (**Figure 4**).

Given the heterogeneity of CPT and the myriad of treatment options, the European Pediatric Orthopaedic Society performed a multicenter study and proposed a stepwise incremental protocol for the management of CPT. This protocol uses bracing treatment, intramedullary rods, circular frame fixation, and rhBMP-2[72] (**Figure 5**). The goal of this stepwise approach is to optimize pseudarthrosis union while avoiding the use of aggressive limb reconstruction techniques at a young age. To compare the current treatments for congenital pseudarthrosis of tibia, a total of 33 studies were reviewed in a 2018 systematic analysis and meta-analysis.[73] The timing of surgery is controversial within the CPT literature. A recent study suggests that there is no need to defer surgery until the child is older than 3 years.[74]

CONGENITAL POSTEROMEDIAL BOWING OF THE TIBIA

Etiology and Clinical Features

CPMBT is a rare condition usually associated with calcaneovalgus foot deformity. Although the deformity in a newborn is distressing to the family, the condition usually resolves spontaneously. CPMBT is most likely caused by intrauterine malpositioning of the leg. In the

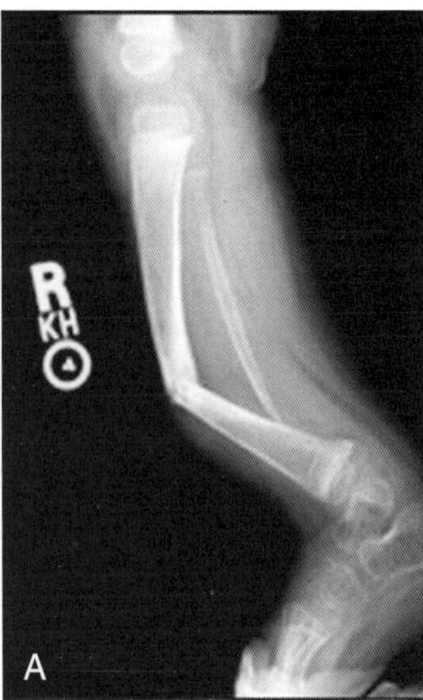

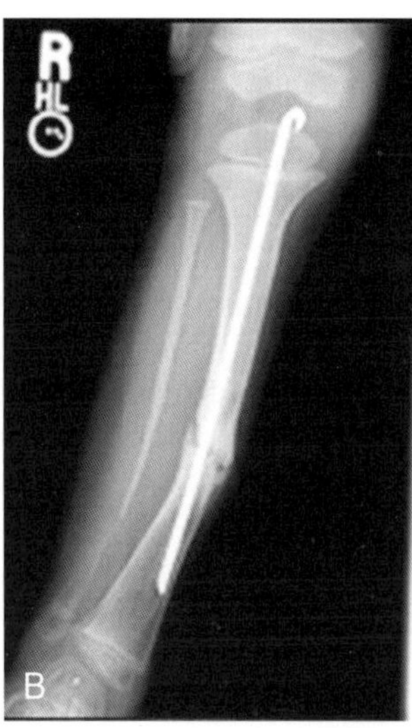

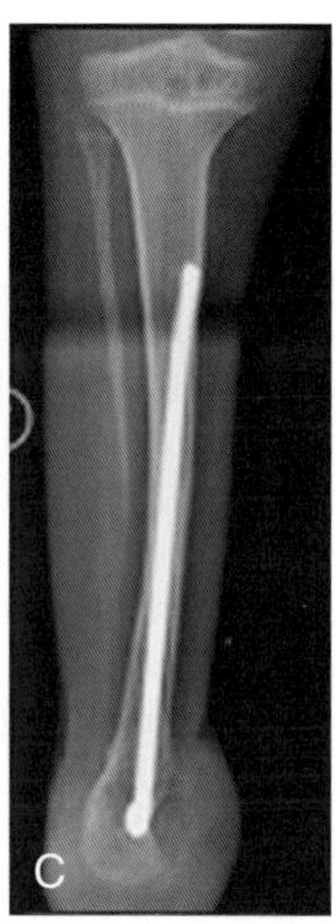

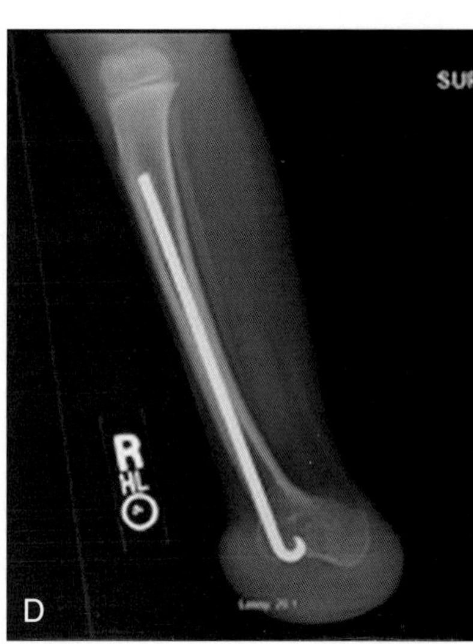

FIGURE 4 **A**, Lateral radiograph of 2-year-old boy with pathologic fracture and pseudarthrosis. **B**, AP radiograph obtained 3 months following treatment with intramedullary rod placement, allograft, and bone morphogenetic protein demonstrating nonunion of pseudarthrosis. **C** and **D**, AP and lateral views at age 6 years with union of the pseudarthrosis following the Boyd amputation. (Reproduced with permission from Westberry DE, Carpenter AM, Tisch J, Wack LI: Amputation outcomes in congenital pseudarthrosis of the tibia. *J Pediatr Orthop* 2018;38[8]:e475-e481.)

first year of life, rapid resolution of angulation is noted (**Figure 6**), but the rate of resolution is reduced substantially thereafter. If complete resolution does not occur, the residual deformity consists of tibial shortening and valgus deformity. The degree of residual shortening is directly related to the initial severity of the posteromedial bowing. As with other congenital shortening disorders, the multiplier method is commonly used to predict CPMT limb-length inequality at skeletal maturity.[75] A 2018 study showed that for several congenital shortening disorders, the relative discrepancy of the short limb to long limb remains static throughout growth beginning in utero and continuing after birth.[76] Knowing that constant inhibition begins in utero allows the use of utero leg-length measurements to predict of the ultimate limb-length discrepancy at birth and at skeletal maturity.

Two distinct mechanisms seem to be responsible for resolution of the deformity in CPMBT. One mechanism involves physeal realignment, and the other involves diaphyseal remodeling. A 2009 study reported that physeal realignment occurred at a faster rate than diaphyseal remodeling.[77]

Wedging of the distal tibial epiphysis and fibular hypoplasia with valgus inclination of the distal tibial articular surface occur in some children with CPMBT. Eccentric ossification of the distal tibial epiphysis in early childhood may be a predictor of wedging of the distal tibial epiphysis when the child is older. Periodic follow-up is recommended in children with CPMBT until skeletal maturity is reached to identify those with residual bowing, ankle deformity, muscle weakness, and limb-length inequality. Active surgical intervention may be needed to correct these conditions.

Treatment

Because few studies have been published on CPMBT, there is no strong basis on which to make a recommendation about the age at which surgery should be performed. When treatment is necessary, it usually is aimed at addressing residual limb-length discrepancy and deformity. If the projected limb-length discrepancy at skeletal maturity is small, then no treatment or contralateral epiphysiodesis should be offered. However, for larger projected limb-length discrepancies, surgical limb lengthening combined with angular correction is indicated.[78]

To correct angulation, single-level tibial and fibular osteotomies may be performed, or multilevel osteotomies may be used if the residual angulation is large or spread over a large segment of bone. A 2014 study reported a series of four patients who were surgically treated for congenital posteromedial bowing of the tibia and congenital posteromedial bowing of the fibula exceeding 35° in the coronal plane.[79] In all of the patients, tibial osteotomy was performed at two or three levels accompanied by fibular osteotomy. Intramedullary stabilization was achieved using Kirschner wires or Rush pins. Follow-up ranged from 3 to 7.7 years. Axis correction and bone healing were achieved in all of the patients. An extensive circumferential periosteal release that accompanied the surgery may have stimulated bone growth, which possibly contributed to limb-length equalization.

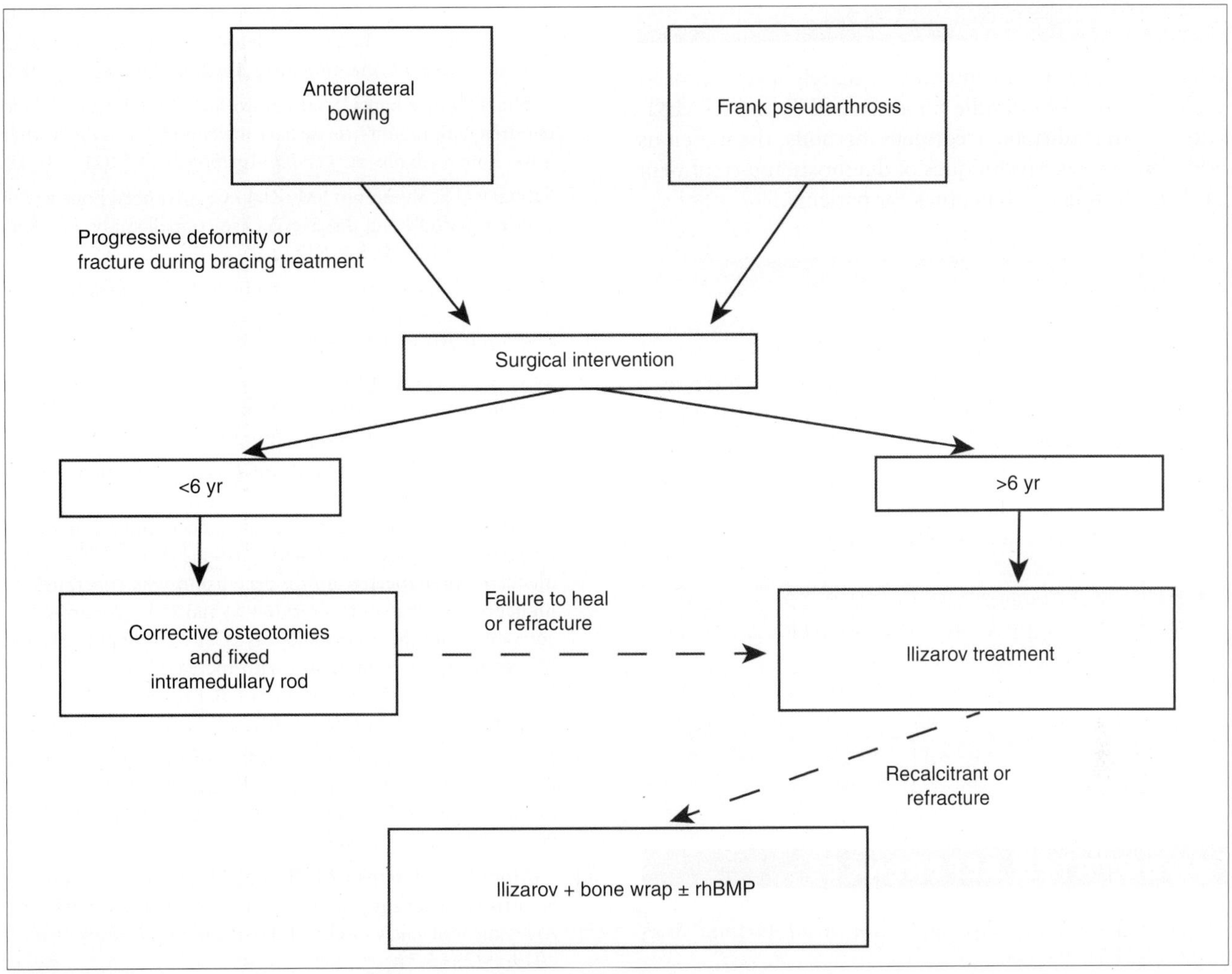

Anterolateral bowing

Frank pseudarthrosis

Progressive deformity or fracture during bracing treatment

Surgical intervention

<6 yr

>6 yr

Corrective osteotomies and fixed intramedullary rod

Failure to heal or refracture

Ilizarov treatment

Recalcitrant or refracture

Ilizarov + bone wrap ± rhBMP

FIGURE 5 Schematic diagram shows the treatment protocol for the management of congenital pseudarthrosis of the tibia. rhBMP = recombinant bone morphogenetic protein. (Adapted with permission of British Editorial Society of Bone & Joint Surgery. Nicolaou N, Ghassemi A, Hill RA: Congenital pseudarthrosis of the tibia: The results of an evolving protocol of management. *J Child Orthop* 2013;7[4]:269-276.)

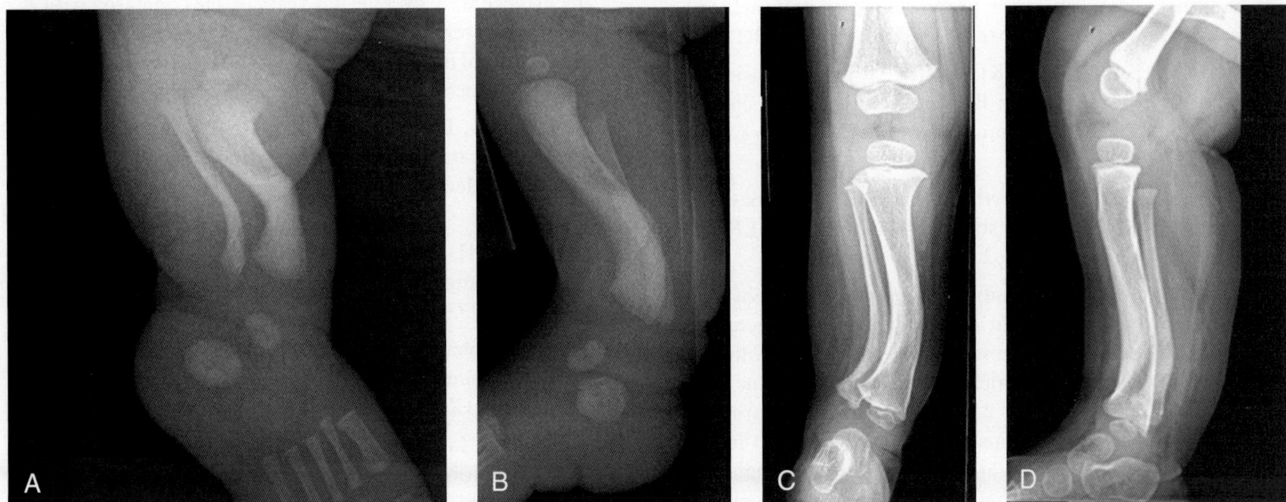

FIGURE 6 AP (**A**) and lateral (**B**) radiographs of a newborn with congenital posteromedial bowing of tibia. AP (**C**) and lateral (**D**) radiographs taken at 18 months of age show partial resolution of angulation.

SUMMARY

Recent preclinical and outcomes research have improved understanding of infantile tibia vara, CPT, and CPMBT. Along with traditional treatment methods, the judicious addition of newer techniques of diagnosis and treatment may result in better outcomes for patients.

KEY STUDY POINTS

- Tibia vara is characterized by epiphyseal and metaphyseal proximal tibia changes, varus deformity, procurvatum deformity in the sagittal plane, and intra-articular abnormalities in the medial compartment of the knee.
- When bracing treatment is unsuccessful, and for children older than 4 years, tibial osteotomy or growth modulation is an effective technique in managing tibia vara.
- Successful management of CPT remains difficult, although a stepwise incremental protocol may be useful in managing CPT.
- CPMBT usually resolves spontaneously. If CPMBT does not resolve adequately, surgical management of angulation and limb-length discrepancy is recommended.

ANNOTATED REFERENCES

1. Birch JG: Blount disease. *J Am Acad Orthop Surg* 2013;21(7):408-418.
2. Rivero SM, Zhao C, Sabharwal S: Are patient demographics different for early-onset and late-onset Blount disease? Results based on meta-analysis. *J Pediatr Orthop B* 2015;24(6):515-520.
3. Langenskiöld A: Tibia vara; (osteochondrosis deformans tibiae): A survey of 23 cases. *Acta Chir Scand* 1952;103(1):1-22.
4. Montgomery CO, Young KL, Austen M, Jo CH, Blasier RD, Ilyas M: Increased risk of Blount disease in obese children and adolescents with vitamin D deficiency. *J Pediatr Orthop* 2010;30(8):879-882.
5. Lisenda L, Simmons D, Firth GB, Ramguthy Y, Kebashni T, Robertson AJ: Vitamin D status in Blount disease. *J Pediatr Orthop* 2016;36(5):e59-e62.

   This is a retrospective study of preoperative and postoperative patients with Blount disease who were screened for vitamin D deficiency. The study patients had the following blood tests performed: calcium, phosphate, alkaline phosphatase, parathyroid, and 25-hydroxyvitamin D hormones. Fifty patients were recruited. The mean vitamin D level in children with Blount disease was low in both females and males; however, these differences were not statistically significant. Level of evidence: III.
6. Sabharwal S, Zhao C, McClemens E: Correlation of body mass index and radiographic deformities in children with Blount disease. *J Bone Joint Surg Am* 2007;89(6):1275-1283.
7. Sabharwal S, Zhao C, Sakamoto SM, McClemens E: Do children with Blount disease have lower body mass index after lower limb realignment? *J Pediatr Orthop* 2014;34(2):213-218.
8. Sabharwal S, Sakamoto SM, Zhao C: Advanced bone age in children with Blount disease: A case-control study. *J Pediatr Orthop* 2013;33(5):551-557.
9. Jamil K, Abdul Rashid AH, Ibrahim S: Tibia vara and slipped upper femoral epiphysis: Is there an association? *J Pediatr Orthop B* 2015;24(1):46-49.
10. Taussig MD, Powell KP, Cole HA, et al: Prevalence of hypertension in pediatric tibia vara and slipped capital femoral epiphysis. *J Pediatr Orthop* 2016;36(8):877-883.

    This study evaluated blood pressure measurements in 44 patients with tibia vara and 127 patients with SCFE. The cohorts were compared with age-matched and sex-matched patients with obesity and without bone disease. The prevalence of prehypertension/hypertension was substantially higher in the tibia vara cohort (64%) and SCFE cohort (64%) compared with the control subjects (43%). The hypothesis that hypertension in conjunction with increased biomechanical forces potentiate the occurrence of SCFE and tibia vara was supported. Level of evidence: III.
11. Johnston CE, Young M: Disorders of the leg, in Herring JA, ed: *Tachdjian's Procedures in Pediatric Orthopaedics: From the Texas Scottish Rite Hospital for Children*, ed 5. Philadelphia, PA, Elsevier, 2014, pp 713-760.
12. LaMont LE, McIntosh AL, Jo CH, Birch JG, Johnston CE: Recurrence after surgical intervention for infantile tibia vara: Assessment of a new modified classification. *J Pediatr Orthop* 2019;39(2):65-70.

    The authors propose a modified three-stage (types A, B, and C) Langenskiöld classification of infantile tibia vara. A retrospective review of 82 patients (115 limbs) who underwent surgery at a single institution was performed. Patients without recurrence were average 4.3 years of age compared with 6.2 years of age for those with recurrence. Extreme vertical sloping of the medial metaphyseal defect (type C) carries a poor prognosis for successful surgical correction. Level of evidence: II.
13. Levine AM, Drennan JC: Physiological bowing and tibia vara: The metaphyseal-diaphyseal angle in the measurement of bowleg deformities. *J Bone Joint Surg Am* 1982;64(8):1158-1163.
14. Feldman MD, Schoenecker PL: Use of the metaphyseal-diaphyseal angle in the evaluation of bowed legs. *J Bone Joint Surg Am* 1993;75(11):1602-1609.
15. Kim SJ, Sabharwal S: Is there a difference in sagittal alignment of Blount's disease between radiographic and clinical evaluation? *Clin Orthop Relat Res* 2014;472(12):3807-3813.
16. Ho-Fung V, Jaimes C, Delgado J, Davidson RS, Jaramillo D: MRI evaluation of the knee in children with infantile Blount disease: Tibial and extra-tibial findings. *Pediatr Radiol* 2013;43(10):1316-1326.

17. Sabharwal S, Wenokor C, Mehta A, Zhao C: Intra-articular morphology of the knee joint in children with Blount disease: A case-control study using MRI. *J Bone Joint Surg Am* 2012;94(10):883-890.
18. Abraham E, Toby D, Welborn MC, Helder CW, Murphy A: New single-stage double osteotomy for late-presenting infantile tibia vara: A comprehensive approach. *J Pediatr Orthop* 2019;39(5):247-256.

    The authors report outcomes of patients with infantile tibial Blount disease treated surgically with a dome-shaped osteotomy proximal to the tibial tubercle using a six-hole lateral tibial plateau plate. The author concludes that this surgery effectively corrects all radiographic components of tibia vara deformity, with good to excellent patient satisfaction. Level of evidence: IV.
19. Jahangiri FR: Multimodality neurophysiological monitoring during tibial/fibular osteotomies for preventing peripheral nerve injuries. *Neurodiagn J* 2013;53(2):153-168.
20. Li Y, Spencer SA, Hedequist D: Proximal tibial osteotomy and Taylor Spatial Frame application for correction of tibia vara in morbidly obese adolescents. *J Pediatr Orthop* 2013;33(3):276-281.
21. Cherkashin AM, Samchukov ML, Birch JG, Da Cunha AL: Evaluation of complications of treatment of severe Blount's disease by circular external fixation using a novel classification scheme. *J Pediatr Orthop B* 2015;24(2):123-130.
22. Oh CW, Kim SJ, Park SK, et al: Hemicallotasis for correction of varus deformity of the proximal tibia using a unilateral external fixator. *J Orthop Sci* 2011;16(1):44-50.
23. Mayer SW, Hubbard EW, Sun D, Lark RK, Fitch RD: Gradual deformity correction in Blount disease. *J Pediatr Orthop* 2016;39(5):257-262.

    The authors conducted a retrospective review of 41 patients (51 limbs) who underwent correction of Blount disease with either an Ilizarov external fixator or a Taylor Spatial Frame by a single surgeon. Following treatment, there was no difference in medial proximal tibial angle and mean axis deviation between the treatment groups. Level of evidence: III.
24. Sachs O, Katzman A, Abu-Johar E, Eidelman M: Treatment of adolescent Blount disease using Taylor Spatial Frame with and without fibular osteotomy: Is there any difference? *J Pediatr Orthop* 2015;35(5):501-506.
25. Scott AC: Treatment of infantile Blount disease with lateral tension band plating. *J Pediatr Orthop* 2012;32(1):29-34.
26. Funk SS, Mignemi ME, Schoenecker JG, Lovejoy SA, Mencio GA, Martus JE: Hemiepiphysiodesis implants for late-onset tibia vara: A comparison of cost, surgical success, and implant failure. *J Pediatr Orthop* 2016;36(1):29-35.

    This is a retrospective review of late-onset tibia vara in 25 patients treated with staple or plate hemiepiphysiodesis. The rate of surgical failure was 58%. Greater body mass index and more severe deformity predicted higher rates of surgical failure. Younger age predicted higher rates of implant failure. There were no differences in surgical or implant failure between staple and plate systems. Hospital costs of plate constructs were 1.5 to 3.5 times greater than for staple constructs. Level of evidence: II.
27. Park SS, Gordon JE, Luhmann SJ, Dobbs MB, Schoenecker PL: Outcome of hemiepiphyseal stapling for late-onset tibia vara. *J Bone Joint Surg Am* 2005;87(10):2259-2266.
28. Burghardt RD, Herzenberg JE: Temporary hemiepiphysiodesis with the eight-plate for angular deformities: Mid-term results. *J Orthop Sci* 2010;15(5):699-704.
29. Jain MJ, Inneh IA, Zhu H, Phillips WA: Tension band plate (TBP)-guided hemiepiphysiodesis in Blount disease: 10-year single-center experience with a systematic review of literature. *J Pediatr Orthop* 2020;40(2):e138-e143.

    This is a single-institution retrospective study and a systematic literature review of patients with Blount disease treated with tension band plate from 2008 to 2017. The odds of surgical failure increased by 1.2 times with severe deformity and 5.9 times with titanium tension band plate. The authors recommend the use of stainless steel plates over titanium and the use of solid screws in all obese and severe deformity patients to reduce the risk of screw mechanical failure. Level of evidence: III.
30. Burghardt RD, Herzenberg JE, Strahl A, Bernius P, Kazim MA: Treatment failures and complications in patients with Blount disease treated with temporary hemiepiphysiodesis: A critical systematic literature review. *J Pediatr Orthop B* 2018;27(6):522-529.

    This systematic review includes 12 studies and reports complications and reasons for failure with temporary hemiepiphysiodesis. The main reported obstacles were under correction and poor predictability of obtainable correction. Obese patients with severe deformity are the most challenging patients. If hemiepiphysiodesis fails, osteotomy remains the preferred salvage procedure. Level of evidence: IV.
31. Fan B, Zhao C, Sabharwal S: Risk factors for failure of temporary hemiepiphysiodesis in Blount disease: A systematic review. *J Pediatr Orthop B* 2020;29(1):65-72.

    The authors performed a systematic review of outcomes for patients with Blount disease treated using either extraperiosteal staples or plates. Eight articles met inclusion criteria. A total of 53 patients (63 bone segments) underwent temporary hemiepiphysiodesis at a mean age of 8.8 years. Overall, 32/63 (51%) segments achieved neutral mechanical axis and 31/63 (49%) underwent unplanned subsequent procedures. Neither age at index surgery nor the type of implant correlated with the need for unplanned additional surgeries. Level of evidence: III.
32. Stitgen A, Garrels K, Kobayashi H, Vanderby R, McCarthy JJ, Noonan KJ: Biomechanical comparison between 2 guided-growth constructs. *J Pediatr Orthop* 2012;32(2):206-209.
33. Schroerlucke S, Bertrand S, Clapp J, Bundy J, Gregg FO: Failure of Orthofix eight-plate for the treatment of Blount disease. *J Pediatr Orthop* 2009;29(1):57-60.
34. Burghardt RD, Specht SC, Herzenberg JE: Mechanical failures of eight-plate guided growth system for temporary hemiepiphysiodesis. *J Pediatr Orthop* 2010;30(6):594-597.
35. Kadhim M1, Hammouda AI, Herzenberg JE: Solid screw insertion for tension band plates: A surgical technique tip. *J Child Orthop* 2016;10(4):307-311.

This study describes a surgical technique to insert solid screws accurately using a standard tension band plate instrumentation set and a tapping screw. Level of evidence: V.

36. Clement AE, Vanderby R Jr, Halanski MA, Noonan KJ: Guided growth implant failure is a result of cyclic fatigue: explant analysis with scanning electron microscopy. *J Pediatr Orthop* 2017;37(1):e37-e42.

This is the first published case report of a fractured plate in guided growth for Blount disease. The patient was 8.3 years old at the time of index surgery, and 10.2 years old at time of determination of fractured plate removal. The implants were analyzed using scanning electron microscopy. The authors concluded that failure was not a result of static tension from growth, but rather cyclic fatigue and then crack propagation across the anterior side of the plate until overload and complete plate failure. Level of evidence: V.

37. Gkiokas A, Brilakis E: Management of neglected Blount disease using double corrective tibia osteotomy and medial plateau elevation. *J Child Orthop* 2012;6(5):411-418.

38. Fitoussi F, Ilharreborde B, Lefevre Y, et al: Fixator-assisted medial tibial plateau elevation to treat severe Blount's disease: Outcomes at maturity. *Orthop Traumatol Surg Res* 2011;97(2):172-178.

39. Crawford AH, Schorry EK: Neurofibromatosis in children: The role of the orthopaedist. *J Am Acad Orthop Surg* 1999;7(4):217-230.

40. Andersen KS: Congenital pseudarthrosis of the leg: Late results. *J Bone Joint Surg Am* 1976;58(5):657-662.

41. Van Royen K, Brems H, Legius E, Lammens J, Laumen A: Prevalence of neurofibromatosis type 1 in congenital pseudarthrosis of the tibia. *Eur J Pediatr* 2016;175(9):1193-1198.

The authors retrospectively analyzed the population of patients (32 patients) with CPT or anterolateral bowing of tibia. Among the patients who had sufficient data, the prevalence of NF1 by National Institutes of Health criteria reported in the literature is 55%. Level of evidence: IV.

42. Lee DY, Cho TJ, Lee HR, et al: Disturbed osteoblastic differentiation of fibrous hamartoma cell from congenital pseudarthrosis of the tibia associated with neurofibromatosis type I. *Clin Orthop Surg* 2011;3(3):230-237.

43. Lee SM, Choi IH, Lee DY, et al: Is double inactivation of the NF1 gene responsible for the development of congenital pseudarthrosis of the tibia associated with NF1? *J Orthop Res* 2012;30(10):1535-1540.

44. Shah H, Doddabasappa SN, Joseph B: Congenital pseudarthrosis of the tibia treated with intramedullary rodding and cortical bone grafting: A follow-up study at skeletal maturity. *J Pediatr Orthop* 2011;31(1):79-88.

45. Birke O, Davies N, Latimer M, Little DG, Bellemore M: Experience with the Fassier-Duval telescopic rod: First 24 consecutive cases with a minimum of 1-year follow-up. *J Pediatr Orthop* 2011;31(4):458-464.

46. Shabtai L, Ezra E, Wientroub S, Segev E: Congenital tibial pseudarthrosis, changes in treatment protocol. *J Pediatr Orthop B* 2015;24(5):444-449.

47. Choi IH, Lee SJ, Moon HJ, et al: "4-in-1 osteosynthesis" for atrophic-type congenital pseudarthrosis of the tibia. *J Pediatr Orthop* 2011;31(6):697-704.

48. Choi IH, Cho TJ, Moon HJ: Ilizarov treatment of congenital pseudarthrosis of the tibia: A multi-targeted approach using the Ilizarov technique. *Clin Orthop Surg* 2011;3(1):1-8.

49. Agashe MV, Song SH, Refai MA, Park KW, Song HR: Congenital pseudarthrosis of the tibia treated with a combination of Ilizarov's technique and intramedullary rodding. *Acta Orthop* 2012;83(5):515-522.

50. Jang WY, Choi YH, Park MS, Yoo WJ, Cho TJ, Choi IH: Physeal and subphyseal distraction osteogenesis in atrophic-type congenital pseudarthrosis of the tibia: Efficacy and safety. *J Pediatr Orthop* 2019;39(8):422-428.

The authors studied radiographic and clinical parameters of five patients who underwent proximal tibial metaphyseal or metadiaphyseal lengthening as a control subject and seven patients who underwent physeal and subphyseal distraction osteogenesis. The authors discuss several advantages and risks of this approach. Level of evidence: III.

51. Pollon T, Sales de Gauzy J, Pham T, Thévenin Lemoine C, Accadbled F: Salvage of congenital pseudarthrosis of the tibia by the induced membrane technique followed by a motorised lengthening nail. *Orthop Traumatol Surg Res* 2018;104(1):147-153.

In this case report, an 18-year-old man with NF-I was treated for CPT using the Masquelet induced membrane technique with a transplantar intramedullary nail and, subsequently, a motorized intramedullary lengthening nail. The rotational malalignment and limb-length discrepancy were successfully corrected. Level of evidence: V.

52. Vanderstappen J, Lammens J, Berger P, Laumen A: Ilizarov bone transport as a treatment of congenital pseudarthrosis of the tibia: A long-term follow-up study. *J Child Orthop* 2015;9(4):319-324.

53. Tan JS, Roach JW, Wang AA: Transfer of ipsilateral fibula on vascular pedicle for treatment of congenital pseudarthrosis of the tibia. *J Pediatr Orthop* 2011;31(1):72-78.

54. Takazawa A, Matsuda S, Fujioka F, Uchiyama S, Kato H: Split tibia vascularized fibular graft for congenital pseudarthrosis of the tibia: A preliminary report of 2 cases. *J Pediatr Orthop* 2011;31(4):e20-e24.

55. Iamaguchi RB, Fucs PM, Carlos da Costa A, Chakkour I, Gomes MD: Congenital pseudoarthrosis of the tibia: Results of treatment by free fibular transfer and associated procedures. Preliminary study. *J Pediatr Orthop B* 2011;20(5):323-329.

56. Iamaguchi RB, Fucs PM, da Costa AC, Chakkour I: Vascularised fibular graft for the treatment of congenital pseudarthrosis of the tibia: Long-term complications in the donor leg. *Int Orthop* 2011;35(7):1065-1070.

57. Richards BS, Oetgen ME, Johnston CE: The use of rhBMP-2 for the treatment of congenital pseudarthrosis of the tibia: A case series. *J Bone Joint Surg Am* 2010;92(1):177-185.

58. Spiro AS, Babin K, Lipovac S, et al: Combined treatment of congenital pseudarthrosis of the tibia, including recombinant human bone morphogenetic protein-2: A case series. *J Bone Joint Surg Br* 2011;93(5):695-699.

59. Shah H, Joseph B, Nair BVS, et al: What factors influence union and refracture of congenital pseudarthrosis of the tibia? A multicenter long-term study. *J Pediatr Orthop* 2018;38(6):e332-e337.

    This is a multicenter study of 119 children who underwent a surgery for Crawford-type IV CPT. Logistic regression and recursive partitioning analyses were used to test associations between several variables and the outcome. On recursive partitioning, use of the Ilizarov technique, transfixing the ankle and subtalar joints, use of cortical graft, and not operating on the fibula were associated with a better outcome. Use of BMP and combining intramedullary nailing with the Ilizarov technique were associated with poor results. Level of evidence: II.

60. Das SP, Ganesh S, Pradhan S, Singh D, Mohanty RN: Effectiveness of recombinant human bone morphogenetic protein-7 in the management of congenital pseudoarthrosis of the tibia: A randomised controlled trial. *Int Orthop* 2014;38(9):1987-1992.

61. Lee FY, Sinicropi SM, Lee FS, Vitale MG, Roye DP Jr, Choi IH: Treatment of congenital pseudarthrosis of the tibia with recombinant human bone morphogenetic protein-7 (rhBMP-7): A report of five cases. *J Bone Joint Surg Am* 2006;88(3):627-633.

62. Schindeler A, Birke O, Yu NY, et al: Distal tibial fracture repair in a neurofibromatosis type 1-deficient mouse treated with recombinant bone morphogenetic protein and a bisphosphonate. *J Bone Joint Surg Br* 2011;93(8):1134-1139.

63. Birke O, Schindeler A, Ramachandran M, et al: Preliminary experience with the combined use of recombinant bone morphogenetic protein and bisphosphonates in the treatment of congenital pseudarthrosis of the tibia. *J Child Orthop* 2010;4(6):507-517.

64. Masquelet AC, Begue T: The concept of induced membrane for reconstruction of long bone defects. *Orthop Clin North Am* 2010;41(1):27-37.

65. Pannier S, Pejin Z, Dana C, Masquelet AC, Glorion C: Induced membrane technique for the treatment of congenital pseudarthrosis of the tibia: Preliminary results of five cases. *J Child Orthop* 2013;7(6):477-485.

66. Gouron R, Deroussen F, Juvet M, Ursu C, Plancq MC, Collet LM: Early resection of congenital pseudarthrosis of the tibia and successful reconstruction using the Masquelet technique. *J Bone Joint Surg Br* 2011;93(4):552-554.

67. Gouron R, Deroussen F, Plancq MC, Collet LM: Bone defect reconstruction in children using the induced membrane technique: A series of 14 cases. *Orthop Traumatol Surg Res* 2013;99(7):837-843.

68. Dohin B, Kohler R: Masquelet's procedure and bone morphogenetic protein in congenital pseudarthrosis of the tibia in children: A case series and meta-analysis. *J Child Orthop* 2012;6(4):297-306.

69. Mansour TM, Ghanem IB: Preliminary results of the induced membrane technique for the reconstruction of large bone defects. *J Pediatr Orthop* 2017;37(1):e67-e74.

    Nine consecutive children with bone defects ranging from 5 to 14 cm were included in the study. There were three congenital pseudarthrosis of the fibula, one congenital pseudarthrosis of the tibia, one Ewing sarcoma of the tibia, 1 Ewing sarcoma of the ulna, 1 tibial osteosarcoma, 1 fibular osteosarcoma, and 1 chronic diffuse tibial osteomyelitis. Among the eight surviving children, six healed uneventfully, and two required revision with additional grafting and/or better internal fixation. Level of evidence: IV.

70. Vigouroux F, Mezzadri G, Parot R, Gazarian A, Pannier S, Chotel F: Vascularised fibula or induced membrane to treat congenital pseudarthrosis of the tibia: A multicentre study of 18 patients with a mean 9.5-year follow-up. *Orthop Traumatol Surg Res* 2017;103(5):747-753.

    This retrospective multicenter study included 18 patients with CPT and NF1, mean age of 2.8 years at surgery. The induced membrane technique was used in 10 patients and vascularized fibula grafting in 8 patients. At mean follow-up was 9.5 years, the two groups showed no significant differences for healing or the occurrence of complications, such as limb-length discrepancy and residual malalignment. Level of evidence: IV.

71. Westberry DE, Carpenter AM, Tisch J, Wack LI: Amputation outcomes in congenital pseudarthrosis of the tibia. *J Pediatr Orthop* 2018;38(8):e475-e481.

    This is a retrospective study of 17 patients with a mean age of 4.5 years (range, 0.7 to 9.2 years) at the time of amputation. The mean number of surgeries before amputation was 2.2 procedures. Thirteen patients underwent Boyd amputation and four underwent transtibial amputation. The authors report that 13 of 17 patients required secondary procedures, and 12 of 13 patients who underwent Boyd amputation achieved radiographic union at last follow-up. Level of evidence: IV.

72. Nicolaou N, Ghassemi A, Hill RA: Congenital pseudarthrosis of the tibia: The results of an evolving protocol of management. *J Child Orthop* 2013;7(4):269-276.

73. Kesireddy N, Kheireldin RK, Lu A, Cooper J, Liu J, Ebraheim NAJ: Current treatment of congenital pseudarthrosis of the tibia: A systematic review and meta-analysis. *Pediatr Orthop B* 2018;27(6):541-550.

    This is a systematic review in which 33 studies met inclusion criteria. Vascularized fibular graft with external fixation or combined fixation had the fastest time until initial union ($P < 0.05$). BMP had no advantage in terms of initial union, time until union, and refracture rates. Fixation with corticocancellous bone autograft using the combined technique of Ilizarov external fixation and intramedullary rod stabilization ensure a statistically significant reduction in the number of refractures compared with standalone fixation methods. Level of evidence: III.

74. Liu Y, Mei H, Zhu G, et al: Congenital pseudarthrosis of the tibia in children: Should we defer surgery until 3 years old? *J Pediatr Orthop B* 2018;27(1):17-25.

This is a retrospective study of 42 patients with Crawford type IV CPT treated with a combined surgical technique to determine relationship between postoperative complications and age of surgery. Patients were divided into two groups according to the age: group A (less than 3 years) and group B (greater than 3 years). The incidence rates of refracture, ankle valgus, tibial valgus, and limb-length discrepancy were evaluated. Level of evidence: III.

75. Paley D, Bhave A, Herzenberg JE, Bowen JR: Multiplier method for predicting limb-length discrepancy. *J Bone Joint Surg Am* 2000;82(10):1432-1446.

76. Tsai A, Laor T, Estroff JA, Kasser JR: Constant inhibition in congenital lower extremity shortening: Does it begin in utero? *Pediatr Radiol* 2018;48(10):1451-1462.

This is a study of in utero developmental pattern of limb-length discrepancy in fetuses with congenital lower extremity shortening disorders. Lower extremity bone lengths were measured on fetal sonograms and postnatal radiographs of 18 patients. The correlations between postnatal and prenatal length ratios were high for the femur, tibia, and fibula. The authors conclude that the postnatal and prenatal length ratios were equivalent, supporting the constant inhibition pattern of limb-length discrepancy in utero. This finding validates the prenatal multiplier method for predicting limb-length discrepancy. Level of evidence: III.

77. Shah HH, Doddabasappa SN, Joseph B: Congenital posteromedial bowing of the tibia: A retrospective analysis of growth abnormalities in the leg. *J Pediatr Orthop B* 2009;18(3):120-128.

78. Kaufman SD, Fagg JA, Jones S, Bell MJ, Saleh M, Fernandes JA: Limb lengthening in congenital posteromedial bow of the tibia. *Strategies Trauma Limb Reconstr* 2012;7(3):147-153.

79. Napiontek M, Shadi M: Congenital posteromedial bowing of the tibia and fibula: Treatment option by multilevel osteotomy. *J Pediatr Orthop B* 2014;23(2):130-134.

CHAPTER 28

Congenital Disorders of the Foot

DAVID D. SPENCE, MD • BENJAMIN W. SHEFFER, MD

ABSTRACT

Congenital deformities of the pediatric foot range in severity from mild, asymptomatic disorders to severe conditions that cause marked functional impairment. The age of affected patients ranges from newborns to adolescents. Nonsurgical treatment is the initial choice for almost all congenital foot deformities and may include NSAIDs, activity modification, stretching, bracing treatment, and casting. Surgical treatment generally is reserved for patients in whom nonsurgical measures fail to relieve symptoms or improve function.

Keywords: accessory navicular; clubfoot; congenital foot disorders; congenital vertical talus; flatfoot; juvenile hallux valgus; osteochondrosis; pediatric foot; tarsal coalition

INTRODUCTION

Deformities of the pediatric foot range from variations in normal anatomy to those causing severe functional impairment. The clinical presentation, diagnosis, and treatment options for the most common pediatric deformities are discussed.

CLUBFOOT

Congenital talipes equinovarus (also known as clubfoot) is an idiopathic foot deformity of unclear etiology more common in males and bilateral in 50% of all patients. It is the most common musculoskeletal birth defect. A genetic etiology has been suggested, with a recent link to the PITX1-TBX4 transcription factor. It is associated with other conditions, including arthrogryposis, myelodysplasia, and tibial hemimelia.

Clubfoot is characterized by numerous bone and soft-tissue abnormalities of variable severity. In general, the major muscle contractures lead to midfoot cavus, forefoot adductus, and relative pronation, in addition to varus and equinus of the hindfoot (**Figure 1**). Specifically, contractures of the Achilles tendon and the posterior tibial tendon lead to hindfoot equinus and varus, with the calcaneus rotated medially around the talus. The posterior tibial contracture also leads to adduction of the forefoot and medial displacement of the navicular with lateral uncovering of the talus. The plantarmedial tissues, including the plantar fascia, the spring ligament, the deltoid ligament, the intrinsic muscles of the foot, and the toe flexors, become contracted, leading to midfoot cavus deformity. Deformities of bone also occur, including plantar flexion and medial deviation of the talar neck, wedging of the navicular, and first ray plantar flexion.

The diagnosis usually is made in infancy or, increasingly, before birth on routine prenatal ultrasonography. The foot should be inspected to determine (1) the presence and severity of bone and soft-tissue abnormalities

Dr. Spence or an immediate family member has received research or institutional support from OrthoPediatrics and serves as a board member, owner, officer, or committee member of the Pediatric Orthopaedic Society of North America. Neither Dr. Sheffer nor any immediate family member has received anything of value from or has stock or stock options held in a commercial company or institution related directly or indirectly to the subject of this chapter.

This chapter is adapted from Spence DD, Bettin CC: Congenital disorders of the foot, in Martus JE, ed: *Orthopaedic Knowledge Update®: Pediatrics*, ed 5. Rosemont, IL, American Academy of Orthopaedic Surgeons, 2016, pp 303-313.

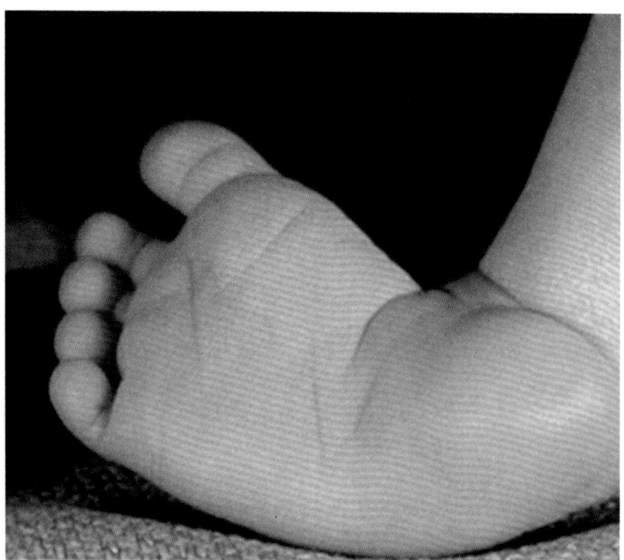

FIGURE 1 Clinical photograph of congenital clubfoot in a newborn. Multiple deformities are evident: inversion, plantar flexion, internal rotation of the calcaneus, and cavus deformity with a transverse plantar crease. (Reproduced with permission from Kelly DM: Congenital anomalies of the lower extremity, in Azar FM, Beaty JH, Canale ST, eds: *Campbell's Operative Orthopaedics*, ed 13. Philadelphia, 2017, pp 1016-1117.)

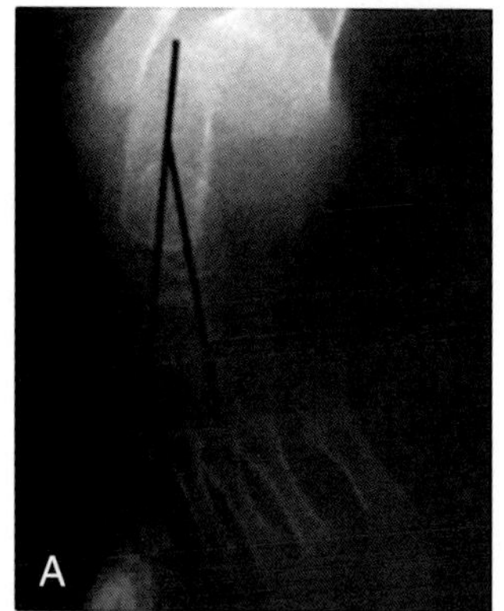

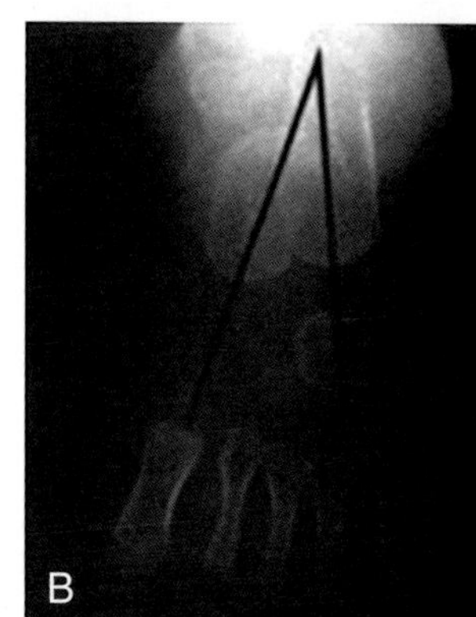

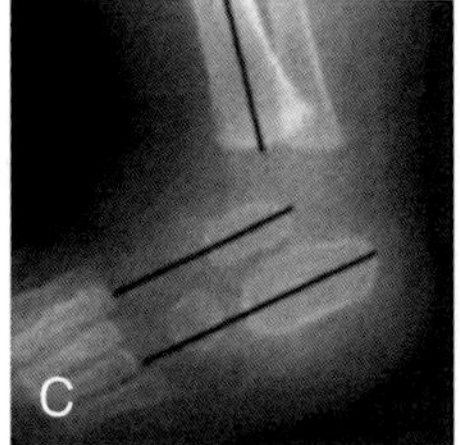

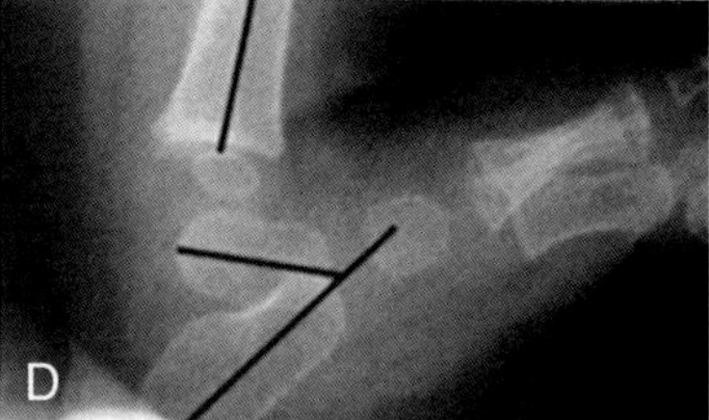

FIGURE 2 Radiographic images of clubfoot. **A**, AP view of a right clubfoot with a decrease in the talocalcaneal angle and a negative talus–first metatarsal angle. **B**, Talocalcaneal angle on the AP view of a normal left foot. **C**, Talocalcaneal angle of 0° and negative tibiocalcaneal angle on dorsiflexion lateral view of a right clubfoot. **D**, Talocalcaneal and tibiocalcaneal angles on dorsiflexion lateral view of a normal left foot. (Reproduced with permission from Kelly DM: Congenital anomalies of the lower extremity, in Azar FM, Beaty JH, Canale ST, eds: *Campbell's Operative Orthopaedics*, ed 13. Philadelphia, 2017, pp 1016-1117.)

and (2) the extent to which these deformities are passively correctable. Skin creases may be noted medially and posteriorly.

The diagnosis of clubfoot is clinical, and radiographs are not routinely obtained. Radiographs may be useful later in the treatment course to confirm that equinus is being corrected at the ankle joint rather than at the midfoot or in cases of recurrence (**Figure 2**).

Treatment options for clubfoot include minimally invasive and extensive surgical methods. There has been a shift away from primary surgical intervention because long-term (>30 years) functional outcomes of extensive soft-tissue releases for idiopathic clubfoot were worse than those reported for patients treated with serial casting with the Ponseti method. A slightly undercorrected casted foot generally has a better functional outcome than a stiff, surgically corrected foot. A survey of 323 members of the Pediatric Orthopaedic Society of North America showed that 96.7% of the members use the Ponseti treatment method. Patients have an average time to correction of 7.1 weeks, and 81% require an Achilles tenotomy.[1] It was estimated from the survey that 22% of the treated patients encountered a relapse and 7% required comprehensive release. Of interest, 75% of the survey respondents reported that the current treatment approaches differed from those presented in the initial training, and 82% had been trained in the Ponseti method within the past few years. The most common nonsurgical techniques are serial casting (the Ponseti method) and daily stretching and taping by a physical therapist (the French method). The superiority of one method over the other has not been established, and the overall quality of evidence in comparative trials is low.

In the Ponseti method, long leg plaster casts are applied with manipulation to rotate the foot laterally around a fixed talus. With the first cast, the cavus deformity and relative pronation of the forefoot are corrected by supinating the forefoot to bring it in line with the hindfoot. The knee is casted in 90° of flexion, and casts are changed weekly. Subsequent casts are applied to correct forefoot adduction and hindfoot varus by rotating the calcaneus and the forefoot around the talus, using the talar head as a fulcrum. When the foot can be abducted 70° and the hindfoot is in valgus, the foot must be dorsiflexed at least 15° in the final cast. In more than 90% of patients, this positioning requires a percutaneous Achilles tenotomy. The final cast remains in place for 3 weeks, which is followed by full-time bracing treatment in a foot abduction orthosis (such as a Denis Browne bar orthosis) that maintains the foot in 70° of external rotation and 15° of dorsiflexion. It is worn 23 hr/d for 3 months after correction, followed by wear during nighttime and naps until the child is 4 years of age.

Poor compliance with brace wear has been correlated with a need for additional surgical procedures.[2] In a 2015 prospective study using a novel pressure sensor to determine actual brace wear, the authors reported decreased actual wear rates for the first, second, and third months of 91.7%, 86.8%, and 77.1%, respectively.[3] At the same time, parents self-reported wear rates of 94.9%, 95.6%, and 94.8%, which calls into question previous assumptions regarding brace compliance. Parents should be instructed on the importance of brace wear in a positive communication style because a physician's communication style affects brace wear and recurrence.[4]

In a prospective randomized study, plaster casts have been demonstrated to have better outcomes than fiberglass casts,[5] and short leg casts have been shown to be inferior to long leg casts;[6] equivalent outcomes have been demonstrated when casts are applied by either physical therapists or orthopaedic surgeons.[7] Although initially described for idiopathic clubfoot, the Ponseti method has been applied to patients with arthrogryposis and myelomeningocele. Short-term outcomes suggest that initial correction may be achieved with a longer period of casting than required for idiopathic clubfoot, although the rates of recurrence may be higher.[8,9]

In the French method, a physical therapist performs daily manipulations, and temporary taping instead of casting is applied between therapy sessions. A comparison between the Ponseti and French methods showed them to be equally effective, with 95% initial correction rates in both groups, with correction maintained at 4 years in 84%.[4] Gait analysis showed distinct gait differences between patients treated with these two methods: patients with the French method had an equinus gait and foot drop, and the Ponseti group had increased dorsiflexion of the stance phase.[10] This difference was likely attributable to using an Achilles tenotomy in the Ponseti method and the absence of tenotomy in the French method. The French method now has been modified to include tenotomy.[11]

Recurrence in children younger than 2 years usually is correlated with an inability to tolerate bracing treatment and is treated with a trial of repeat casting. For recurrence in children older than 2 years, a repeat trial of casting should be attempted, followed by transfer of the anterior tibial tendon to the lateral cuneiform (if ossified) if repeat casting fails. Factors shown to predict increased risk for surgical intervention include brace noncompliance; female sex; and a higher Diméglio score, which correlates with the severity of the clubfoot deformity at the time of the diagnosis and brace application.[2] Surgical intervention generally is reserved for multiple recurrences and residual deformity, typically with dynamic supination and equinus. For dynamic supination, a complete transfer of the anterior tibial tendon to the lateral cuneiform is performed.[12] Anterior tibial tendon transfer has been shown to be effective at preventing additional relapse without affecting long-term foot function.[13]

Lengthening of the Achilles tendon may be required for recurrent equinus. For resistant clubfoot in young children in whom multiple attempts at casting have failed, a posteromedial soft-tissue release with tendon lengthening may be attempted; the extent of soft-tissue release is negatively correlated to long-term foot function. Talonavicular arthrodesis, triple arthrodesis, and talectomy may be required for refractory clubfoot in older patients and as salvage procedures.

FLEXIBLE FLATFOOT

Pes planus, also known as flatfoot, is a common foot deformity in the pediatric cohort. Its prevalence has been reported to be as high as 80% in children, but decreases to 10% to 20% in adults. The prevalence has been shown to decrease substantially from 54% of 3-year-old children to 21% of 6-year-old children and is associated with younger age, male sex, ligamentous laxity, and obesity.[14]

In flexible flatfoot, hindfoot valgus and loss of the normal medial longitudinal arch with standing are evident. The talar head may be palpable medially because of its plantarflexed position, and uncovering of the navicular and associated calluses may be present. The hindfoot shows full passive motion with inversion and eversion; with toe rise, the arch is restored, and the hindfoot rolls into varus to lock the transverse tarsal joints. The range of motion of the tibiotalar joint should be tested, and the Silfverskiöld test should be performed because the condition often is associated with Achilles tendon or gastrocnemius contracture. Many patients are asymptomatic and undergo an orthopaedic evaluation because of parental concerns about the appearance of the foot. Patients who are symptomatic may report medial arch pain, calf pain caused by contracture, and/or lateral sinus tarsi pain caused by calcaneofibular abutment. The entire limb should be inspected for rotational malalignment.

Radiographs should be obtained only if the patient is symptomatic. Weight-bearing AP, lateral, and oblique views are used to evaluate for other potential sources of the planovalgus deformity. On the AP view, the talar head may appear uncovered, and the amount of talonavicular coverage has been shown to be related to the onset of symptoms.[15] On lateral radiographs, the talar declination angle is increased, as is the Meary angle (the angle between the first metatarsal and the axis of the talus). Decreased calcaneal pitch may be observed in patients with contracture of the Achilles tendon.

Nonsurgical measures are the initial treatment choice, beginning with an explanation of the natural history of the condition to both the patient and the family.

In 2013, a study of 580 preschool-aged children with flexible flatfoot demonstrated complete resolution in 38% after 1 year.[16] No high-level studies support the treatment of patients who are asymptomatic. In patients with arch pain, a navicular pad, medial arch support, or a University of California Biomechanics Laboratory orthotic may help with symptoms, but it will not correct the deformity or prevent progression in patients who are asymptomatic. Patients with contractures of the Achilles tendon or gastrocnemius muscle should begin a stretching program to decrease associated calf pain. In the few patients in whom prolonged nonsurgical measures fail, consideration can be given to lateral column lengthening, either through a calcaneal lengthening osteotomy or through a combined calcaneal-cuboid-cuneiform osteotomy.[17] Any surgical intervention needs to be carefully planned to correct all aspects of the deformity. Gastrocnemius recession may be simultaneously considered to manage the associated equinus deformity.[18]

TARSAL COALITION

In patients with a rigid flatfoot, where the arch does not reconstitute with toe rise and the heel does not invert, the most common cause is a tarsal coalition. A tarsal coalition is an abnormal fibrous, cartilaginous, or osseous connection between two bones in the foot that results from abnormal mesenchymal segmentation. This connection blocks normal motion at the subtalar joint and leads to overcompensation by other joints, resulting in a valgus hindfoot, lowering of the arch, and peroneal spasm. The incidence varies between 1% and 5%, and most coalitions are found incidentally, although some are part of genetic syndromes, including Apert syndrome, Muenke syndrome, and fibular deficiency.

Coalitions are most common between the calcaneus and the navicular (age of onset of symptoms is 8 to 12 years) or the talus and the calcaneus (age of onset of symptoms is 12 to 15 years). Patients typically have pain that increases with activity around the age at which coalition begins to ossify. Calf pain may result from peroneal muscle spasms, and recurrent ankle sprains may occur because of impaired subtalar mobility. On physical examination, limited subtalar motion is evident and may be associated with contractures of the gastrocnemius-soleus complex. Toe rise should be closely observed to look for reconstitution of the arch and hindfoot inversion, both of which may be impaired in the presence of a coalition.

Standard radiographic studies should include weight-bearing AP, lateral, 45° oblique, and axial Harris views (**Figure 3**). Cross-sectional imaging with CT or MRI is necessary to evaluate for additional coalitions[19] and guide treatment decisions based on the extent of joint involvement and any signs of surrounding joint degeneration (**Figure 4**). The size of the coalition does not appear to be correlated to the amount of hindfoot valgus or long-term functional outcome.[20]

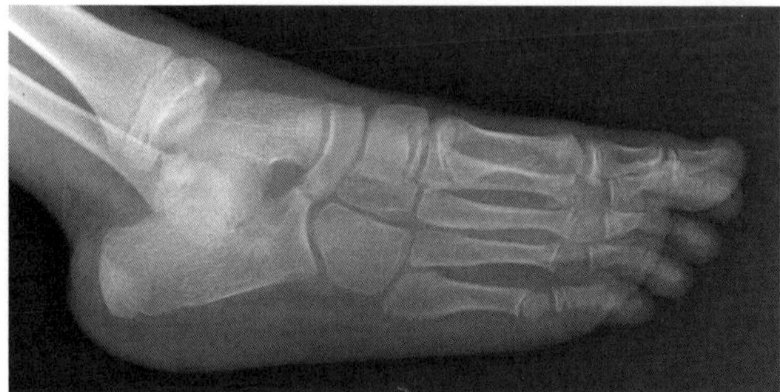

FIGURE 3 Oblique radiograph of a foot with a calcaneonavicular coalition.

Nonsurgical measures should be attempted first because many patients with tarsal coalitions are asymptomatic. A period of immobilization, including a cast or walking boot, may provide symptom relief and avoid surgical intervention. Physical therapy may also play a role in relieving pain from secondary issues such as Achilles tendon contractures. If nonsurgical measures fail, surgical interventions range from excision to arthrodesis. Surgical excision of the coalition is performed through an oblique sinus tarsi incision just distal to the subtalar joint for a calcaneonavicular coalition; for a talocalcaneal coalition, a medial incision between the flexor digitorum longus and the neurovascular bundle is used. The coalition should be completely excised, and adjacent tissue should be interposed. Commonly used tissues include the extensor digitorum brevis and/or fat graft from anterior

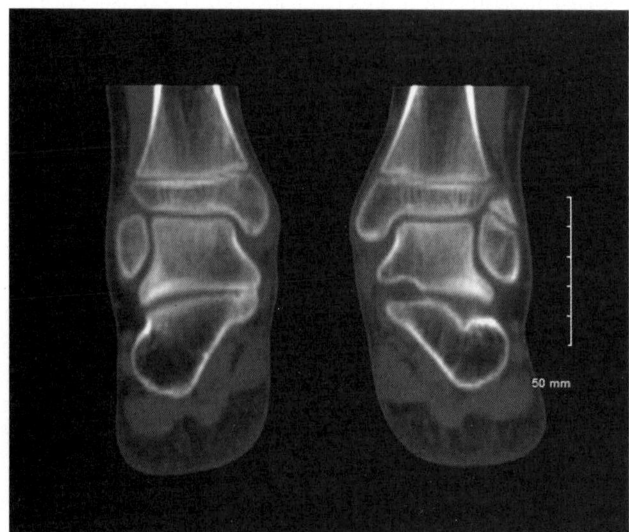

FIGURE 4 CT scan demonstrates joint space narrowing, articular irregularity, and subchondral cyst formation of the posterior facet of the right foot, which is consistent with a nonosseous talocalcaneal coalition.

to the Achilles tendon. It has been demonstrated that the extensor digitorum brevis was able to fill only 65% of the typical resection gap in calcaneonavicular coalitions, and this deficit, combined with cosmetic issues, led to the adoption of the fat graft for all cases.[21] If substantial hindfoot valgus is present preoperatively, a medial displacement calcaneal osteotomy may also be considered.

The role for arthrodesis is controversial. Traditional guidelines included involvement of more than 30% to 50% of the posterior facet and less than 16° to 21° of hindfoot valgus; however, current literature has suggested that good results can be obtained with joint-preserving procedures, including coalition resection and flatfoot reconstruction even in coalitions involving more than 50% of the posterior talocalcaneal facet.[20,22,23] The goal of surgery is to decrease pain and improve function, but numerous studies have found that normal kinematics are not fully restored after surgery. The exact surgical technique should be based on pain location, the size of the coalition, the health of surrounding joints and the medial facet, the degree of deformity, and any excursion of the Achilles tendon.[24] More than 70% of patients with a surgically treated tarsal coalition did not believe that the activities were limited by foot pain at 4.6 years after surgery, and no substantial difference was found between talocalcaneal and calcaneonavicular coalitions.[25]

CONGENITAL VERTICAL TALUS

Congenital vertical talus is a rare foot deformity consisting of a dorsolateral dislocation of the navicular on the talus that is irreducible and produces a rigid flatfoot deformity. The head of the talus is forced plantarly and medially and is palpable on the medial aspect of the foot and produces the rocker-bottom foot deformity. The involved hindfoot shows a fixed equinovalgus posture resulting from contracture of the peroneal and Achilles tendons. Rigid hyperdorsiflexion through the midfoot is caused by the dislocated navicular, and the forefoot is abducted and dorsiflexed by contractures of the anterior tibial, extensor hallucis longus, and extensor digitorum tendons. The talonavicular, posterior ankle, and subtalar joint capsules typically have contractures, and an MRI study showed subtalar joint abnormalities, including lateral translation and eversion of the calcaneus.[26]

One of five patients with congenital vertical talus (**Figure 5**) has a family history of the disorder, and 50% have an associated genetic or neuromuscular disorder. The condition is bilateral in 50% of patients. A mutation has been identified in the homeobox *D10* gene in families with congenital vertical talus, and an autosomal dominant inheritance pattern with incomplete penetrance has been suggested. Associated conditions include chromosomal abnormalities, arthrogryposis, myopathy, and myelodysplasia. Abnormal muscle biopsies are present in 62% of patients, although it is unclear whether this is primary or secondary to the joint deformities.[27]

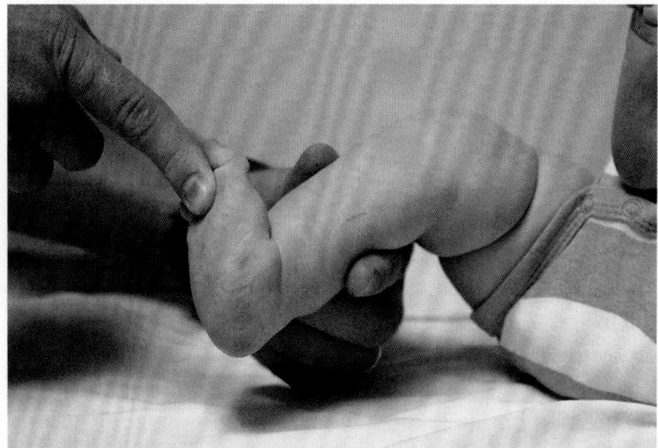

FIGURE 5 Clinical photograph shows the rocker-bottom appearance of the foot of an infant with congenital vertical talus.

On a lateral radiograph, the talus is in a vertical position, and the long axis of the talus is plantar to the axis of the first metatarsal-cuneiform axis because of dorsal dislocation of the navicular. Because the navicular typically does not appear on radiographs until age 3 years, the first metatarsal is referenced instead on imaging. A forced plantar flexion lateral radiograph should be obtained and will show a persistent dorsal dislocation of the talonavicular joint (**Figure 6**). In cases of congenital oblique talus, a reduction will be observed on forced

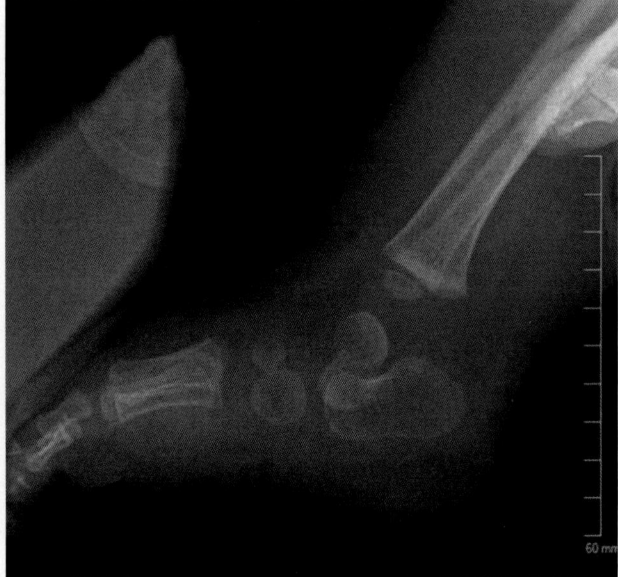

FIGURE 6 A forced, plantar flexion lateral radiograph of the foot of a patient with congenital vertical talus shows a persistent dorsal dislocation of the talonavicular joint.

Section 5: Lower Extremity

plantar flexion lateral radiographs. Cross-sectional imaging of the foot generally is not required; however, additional imaging of the spine may be required if the history and physical examination suggest an associated spinal pathology.

Untreated congenital vertical talus has a poor outcome and is associated with substantial functional deficits because of weak push-off strength, plantar calluses, and difficulty with shoe wear. Initial treatment begins with stretching of the contracted dorsal soft-tissue structures with plantar flexion and inversion of the foot. This can be done with serial casting similar to the management of clubfoot; however, the technique, commonly referred to as the reverse Ponseti, involves applying serial casts in the opposite direction used for clubfoot to reduce the talonavicular joint.[28,29] The casts are followed by pinning the talonavicular joint in a reduced position, with a small arthrotomy if residual reduction is needed, followed by a percutaneous Achilles tenotomy to correct the equinus deformity. Alternatively, a comprehensive release may be performed with open reduction and pinning of the talonavicular joint followed by casting. Regardless of whether a posterior Cincinnati incision or a dorsal approach is used, all contracted tissues must be released, including the peroneal, Achilles, and dorsal extensor tendons. Similar to surgically treated clubfoot, a comprehensive release for congenital vertical talus is associated with stiffness and, in some cases, osteonecrosis of the talus. A recent retrospective study of 27 patients treated for congenital vertical talus reported better range of motion and lower pain scores in patients treated with a minimally invasion approach compared with an extensive soft-tissue release at an average follow-up of 7 years.[30] However, other researchers reported the use of a minimally invasive technique in a prospective cohort of 21 feet with both idiopathic and teratologic etiologies and noted a 48% recurrence rate.[31] Corrective surgery generally is more successful in younger patients. Salvage procedures may require a naviculectomy to shorten the medial column, a triple arthrodesis, or a talectomy.

JUVENILE HALLUX VALGUS

Hallux valgus that occurs in the preteen or teenage years often is associated with a smaller medial eminence prominence, increased magnitude of the first-second intermetatarsal angle, increased hypermobility of the first tarsometatarsal joint, less pronation, and a higher recurrence rate with surgical intervention than in the adult cohort.[32] Juveniles are more likely to have bilateral deformities and a family history of hallux valgus as well. Patients may have difficulty with shoe wear, plantar callosities, and transfer metatarsalgia. Nonsurgical management should be considered first in all patients, especially those with ligamentous laxity or neuromuscular disorders, because of the higher recurrence rate with surgical intervention. Shoes with a wide toe box, toe spacers, and night splints may be used for symptomatic management until physeal closure but are unlikely to correct the deformity. Although patients may dislike the cosmetic deformity, the main indications for surgical intervention are pain and discomfort with shoe wear. Numerous procedures have been described, and determining the appropriate surgical intervention is the subject of much debate. Overarching principles include correcting the associated pathology, including first ray hypermobility with arthrodesis of the proximal first ray, increasing the distal metatarsal articular angle with biplanar or double osteotomies, decreasing the intermetatarsal angle with a proximal osteotomy, and avoiding soft-tissue procedures in isolation for incongruent deformities. Arthrodesis of the metatarsophalangeal joint is appropriate in patients with ligamentous laxity (Ehlers-Danlos syndrome), cerebral palsy, Down syndrome, and rheumatoid arthritis.

METATARSUS ADDUCTUS

Metatarsus adductus (forefoot adduction with normal hindfoot alignment) may occur in children as part of residual clubfoot or as an isolated deformity. Isolated metatarsus adductus has an unclear etiology and likely results from a combination of intrauterine positioning, hereditary/environmental factors, osseous abnormalities, and muscle imbalance. The Ponseti group reported on 45 feet (32-year follow-up) and found that all the patients with mild to moderate deformity who were treated with observation had good outcomes with deformity resolution.[33] A group of patients with moderate to severe deformity were treated with casting and also had good outcomes, with the exception of three patients with mild residual deformity who experienced mild pain with strenuous activity. This study demonstrates deformity correction in patients with mild to moderate metatarsus adductus with observation only. Patients with flexible deformities that can be passively corrected to midline can be treated at home with serial stretching performed by parents. Rigid deformities can be treated with serial casting or a stretching orthotic to obtain a straight lateral foot border. A recent prospective, randomized trial compared the use of Bebax (Trulife) orthoses with serial casting in 27 infants with resistant metatarsus adductus. The authors found that Bebax orthoses achieved greater improvement in the heel bisector measurement and were substantially less expensive than serial casting; however, the orthosis treatment required more active parental involvement.[34]

ACCESSORY NAVICULAR

An accessory navicular is a normal variant seen in 12% to 14% of patients who are asymptomatic. The navicular ossifies at age 3 years in girls and at age 5 years in boys. The navicular tuberosity may have a secondary ossification center (accessory navicular) that begins to ossify at approximately age 8 years and may not fuse to the primary ossification center, leading to symptom development in some patients. The posterior tibial tendon inserts on the navicular tuberosity medially, and the accessory navicular may appear as a sesamoid bone within the tendon itself (type I). A type II accessory navicular is attached to the tuberosity by a synchondrosis, whereas a type III accessory navicular is a complete bony enlargement of the navicular. Patients report medial arch pain with activity, and a physical examination may show swelling at the plantarmedial aspect of the navicular. Fifty percent of patients have a flexible pes planovalgus deformity as well.

In addition to routine weight-bearing radiographs, an external oblique view will more clearly show the accessory navicular. MRI is useful to evaluate the synchondrosis, rule out concomitant pathology, and assist with surgical planning if initial nonsurgical treatment is unsuccessful.

Initial nonsurgical measures should include NSAIDs, activity modification, and orthotics. A medial-posted orthotic may alleviate some symptoms from forced heel inversion and decrease the pull of the posterior tibial tendon in a patient with a flexible flatfoot; however, the prominence for the support often lies directly under the navicular, so the orthotic may be more irritating than helpful to patients. When used, the orthotic should be constructed with pressure relief in the posteromedial navicular region. Stretching of the Achilles tendon complex also should be done in those with an associated contracture. A short period of cast immobilization also may be beneficial if orthotics fail. Most symptoms will abate after the patient reaches skeletal maturity. In recalcitrant cases, surgical intervention for excision of the accessory navicular may be considered. Kidner originally described excision of the ossicle with advancement of the posterior tibial tendon to the medial cuneiform, but most authors now advocate ossicle excision with side-to-side repair rather than tendon advancement in the pediatric cohort.[35,36] A generous resection of bone such that the navicular is flush with the medial cuneiform and talus should be performed because the most common cause of persistent pain is inadequate initial excision. In patients approaching skeletal maturity with hindfoot valgus deformity, a lateral column lengthening or a medial displacement osteotomy of the calcaneus is a useful adjunctive procedure; however, it is unclear in the literature whether additional procedures result in better clinical outcomes because no comparative studies have been performed.

OSTEOCHONDROSIS

Osteochondrosis is an aseptic, ischemic necrosis of bone that can occur in any bone of the foot during childhood or adolescence; however, it is more commonly observed in the navicular and the head of the metatarsal.

Köhler Disease

Osteochondrosis of the navicular, also known as Köhler disease, commonly is seen as limping in a child who reports medial-sided foot pain with associated swelling over the navicular and may be initially misdiagnosed as an infection. First described in 1908, Köhler disease generally occurs in young children and more commonly in boys than girls. Radiographs show flattening of the navicular with sclerotic margins and fragmentation. These findings, along with clinical symptoms that may or may not be associated with fracture at presentation, typically resolve in the long term.[37] Management of this condition includes NSAIDs and activity modification for mild symptoms and immobilization for more severe symptoms. Surgical intervention has no role in this condition as the disease is self-limiting with full resolution of symptoms without foot deformity.

Freiberg Disease

Osteochondrosis of the second metatarsal head is known as Freiberg disease or infraction. It more commonly occurs in adolescent females and may occur in any metatarsal, although the second metatarsal is most common. Patients typically show pain with weight-bearing activities, swelling of the involved area, and exacerbation of symptoms with distraction and compression of the joint. Depending on the chronicity of the problem, radiographs may show subchondral sclerotic changes in early disease, leading to flattening and joint destruction in late presentations. Initial nonsurgical measures include NSAIDs and a Morton extension orthotic, with immobilization in a cast or a walking boot if orthotics fail.

If prolonged nonsurgical management fails, surgical intervention may be considered, with surgical options including joint débridement, a dorsal closing-wedge osteotomy,[38] osteochondral autograft transplantation,[39] and interpositional devices.[40] In early 2016, a group of researchers reported long-term follow-up of 23 years in 20 patients treated with an intra-articular dorsal wedge osteotomy.[41] The clinical outcomes were excellent in 80% of the patients and good in 20%, with better results observed in patients with less collapse at the time of intervention (Smillie stages II and III). Resection of the metatarsal head should be avoided to prevent the development of transfer metatarsalgia and joint instability.

APOPHYSITIS

Apophysitis refers to inflammation and irritation at an apophysis, which is a secondary ossification center that also is the site of a tendon insertion. Although apophysitis technically can occur at any apophysis, it is most common in the calcaneus and the base of the fifth metatarsal. It typically occurs in young males as part of an overuse injury.

Sever Disease

Calcaneal apophysitis (also known as Sever disease) was first described in 1912 and is most common in children aged 9 to 12 years. It typically presents with a waxing and waning course of pain at the insertion of the Achilles tendon on the calcaneus, along the calcaneal apophysis, or near the insertion of the plantar fascia. Although a direct cause has not been established, pedobarographic analysis has shown an association between symptoms of calcaneal apophysis, high plantar pressures, and hindfoot equinus.[42] Activities such as sports that involve repetitive forceful contraction of the Achilles tendon are bothersome; however, symptoms also may occur with walking.

Sever disease is a clinical diagnosis with a differential diagnosis that includes a stress fracture or a benign bone lesion. Radiographs are not essential to the diagnosis because studies have demonstrated only a 1.4% to 5% rate of abnormal radiographic findings in the workup of this apophysitis;[43] however, a single lateral radiograph is logical in the initial evaluation to assess for occult pathology. Treatment is nonsurgical, with heel cushions, activity modification, stretching of the gastrocnemius-soleus complex, and NSAIDs; symptoms typically resolve with closure of the calcaneal apophysis. The natural history of the disease should be explained to parents, with reassurance frequently provided, because the continuation of symptoms until skeletal maturity can be concerning.

Iselin Disease

Iselin disease also was first described in 1912 as an apophysitis of the fifth metatarsal in an adolescent girl. Apophysitis of the fifth metatarsal appeared radiographically in boys at age 12 years and girls at age 10 years, which are the typical ages of presentation for the disease.[44] Patients may have lateral foot pain from an acute inversion injury or chronic overuse activities and have pain with palpation at the base of the fifth metatarsal. Resistance against eversion of the peroneus brevis reproduces the pain. Because the apophysis may be confused with an avulsion fracture, radiographs of the involved foot as well as contralateral radiographs are useful in the workup. Nonsurgical measures, including rest, ice, immobilization, and NSAIDs, generally are successful in managing symptoms.

SUMMARY

Numerous deformities of the pediatric foot with varying clinical presentations have been identified. Understanding the associated conditions, natural history, and outcomes of nonsurgical and surgical intervention are paramount for managing patient and parent expectations and achieving good clinical outcomes.

KEY STUDY POINTS

- Nonsurgical treatment is the initial choice for almost all congenital foot deformities and may include stretching, bracing treatment, and casting.
- Clubfoot is the most common musculoskeletal birth defect and may involve numerous bone and soft-tissue abnormalities of varying severity. Generally, this condition is managed with serial casting (the Ponseti method) or daily stretching and taping (the French method), with comprehensive surgical release reserved for recurrent and residual deformities.
- Flexible flatfoot is asymptomatic in most children. If pain or functional limitations persist after prolonged nonsurgical management, lateral column lengthening may be considered.
- Tarsal coalitions are most common between the calcaneus and the navicular or the talus and the calcaneus. A period of cast immobilization may provide pain relief. Surgical options include excision of the coalition, osteotomy, and arthrodesis, depending on pain location, the size of the coalition, the health of surrounding joints, the degree of deformity, and contracture of the Achilles tendon.
- Untreated congenital vertical talus is associated with substantial functional deficits. A rigorous casting regimen has become the initial mode of treatment, followed by minimally invasive surgery; however, more extensive procedures may be required.
- The primary indications for surgical correction of juvenile hallux valgus are pain and discomfort with shoe wear. Surgery should address all underlying pathology.

ANNOTATED REFERENCES

1. Zionts LE, Sangiorgio SN, Ebramzadeh E, Morcuende JA: The current management of idiopathic clubfoot revisited: Results of a survey of the POSNA membership. *J Pediatr Orthop* 2012;32(5):515-520.

2. Goldstein RY, Seehausen DA, Chu A, Sala DA, Lehman WB: Predicting the need for surgical intervention in patients with idiopathic clubfoot. *J Pediatr Orthop* 2015;35(4):395-402.

3. Morgenstein A, Davis R, Talwalkar V, Iwinski H Jr, Walker J, Milbrandt TA: A randomized clinical trial comparing reported and measured wear rates in clubfoot bracing using a novel pressure sensor. *J Pediatr Orthop* 2015;35(2):185-191.
4. Richards BS, Faulks S, Rathjen KE, Karol LA, Johnston CE, Jones SA: A comparison of two nonoperative methods of idiopathic clubfoot correction: The Ponseti method and the French functional (physiotherapy) method. *J Bone Joint Surg Am* 2008;90(11):2313-2321.
5. Pittner DE, Klingele KE, Beebe AC: Treatment of clubfoot with the Ponseti method: A comparison of casting materials. *J Pediatr Orthop* 2008;28(2):250-253.
6. Maripuri SN, Gallacher PD, Bridgens J, Kuiper JH, Kiely NT: Ponseti casting for club foot: Above- or below-knee? A prospective randomised clinical trial. *Bone Joint J* 2013;95-B(11):1570-1574.
7. Janicki JA, Narayanan UG, Harvey BJ, Roy A, Weir S, Wright JG: Comparison of surgeon and physiotherapist-directed Ponseti treatment of idiopathic clubfoot. *J Bone Joint Surg Am* 2009;91(5):1101-1108.
8. Boehm S, Limpaphayom N, Alaee F, Sinclair MF, Dobbs MB: Early results of the Ponseti method for the treatment of clubfoot in distal arthrogryposis. *J Bone Joint Surg Am* 2008;90(7):1501-1507.
9. Gerlach DJ, Gurnett CA, Limpaphayom N, et al: Early results of the Ponseti method for the treatment of clubfoot associated with myelomeningocele. *J Bone Joint Surg Am* 2009;91(6):1350-1359.
10. El-Hawary R, Karol LA, Jeans KA, Richards BS: Gait analysis of children treated for clubfoot with physical therapy or the Ponseti cast technique. *J Bone Joint Surg Am* 2008;90(7):1508-1516.
11. Steinman S, Richards BS, Faulks S, Kaipus K: A comparison of two nonoperative methods of idiopathic clubfoot correction: The Ponseti method and the French functional (physiotherapy) method. Surgical technique. *J Bone Joint Surg Am* 2009;91(suppl 2):299-312.
12. Gray K, Burns J, Little D, Bellemore M, Gibbons P: Is tibialis anterior tendon transfer effective for recurrent clubfoot? *Clin Orthop Relat Res* 2014;472(2):750-758.
13. Holt JB, Oji DE, Yack HJ, Morcuende JA: Long-term results of tibialis anterior tendon transfer for relapsed idiopathic clubfoot treated with the Ponseti method: A follow-up of thirty-seven to fifty-five years. *J Bone Joint Surg Am* 2015;97(1):47-55.
14. Chen KC, Yeh CJ, Tung LC, Yang JF, Yang SF, Wang CH: Relevant factors influencing flatfoot in preschool-aged children. *Eur J Pediatr* 2011;170(7):931-936.
15. Moraleda L, Mubarak SJ: Flexible flatfoot: Differences in the relative alignment of each segment of the foot between symptomatic and asymptomatic patients. *J Pediatr Orthop* 2011;31(4):421-428.
16. Chen KC, Tung LC, Yeh CJ, Yang JF, Kuo JF, Wang CH: Change in flatfoot of preschool-aged children: A 1-year follow-up study. *Eur J Pediatr* 2013;172(2):255-260.
17. Moraleda L, Salcedo M, Bastrom TP, Wenger DR, Albiñana J, Mubarak SJ: Comparison of the calcaneo-cuboid-cuneiform osteotomies and the calcaneal lengthening osteotomy in the surgical treatment of symptomatic flexible flatfoot. *J Pediatr Orthop* 2012;32(8):821-829.
18. Rong K, Ge WT, Li XC, Xu XY: Mid-term results of intramuscular lengthening of gastrocnemius and/or soleus to correct equinus deformity in flatfoot. *Foot Ankle Int* 2015;36(10):1223-1228.
19. Masquijo JJ, Jarvis J: Associated talocalcaneal and calcaneonavicular coalitions in the same foot. *J Pediatr Orthop B* 2010;19(6):507-510.
20. Khoshbin A, Law PW, Caspi L, Wright JG: Long-term functional outcomes of resected tarsal coalitions. *Foot Ankle Int* 2013;34(10):1370-1375.
21. Mubarak SJ, Patel PN, Upasani VV, Moor MA, Wenger DR: Calcaneonavicular coalition: Treatment by excision and fat graft. *J Pediatr Orthop* 2009;29(5):418-426.
22. Mosca VS, Bevan WP: Talocalcaneal tarsal coalitions and the calcaneal lengthening osteotomy: The role of deformity correction. *J Bone Joint Surg Am* 2012;94(17):1584-1594.
23. Lisella JM, Bellapianta JM, Manoli A II: Tarsal coalition resection with pes planovalgus hindfoot reconstruction. *J Surg Orthop Adv* 2011;20(2):102-105.
24. Mosca VS: Subtalar coalition in pediatrics. *Foot Ankle Clin* 2015;20(2):265-281.
25. Mahan ST, Spencer SA, Vezeridis PS, Kasser JR: Patient-reported outcomes of tarsal coalitions treated with surgical excision. *J Pediatr Orthop* 2015;35(6):583-588.
26. Thometz JG, Zhu H, Liu XC, Tassone C, Gabriel SR: MRI pathoanatomy study of congenital vertical talus. *J Pediatr Orthop* 2010;30(5):460-464.
27. Merrill LJ, Gurnett CA, Connolly AM, Pestronk A, Dobbs MB: Skeletal muscle abnormalities and genetic factors related to vertical talus. *Clin Orthop Relat Res* 2011;469(4):1167-1174.
28. Dobbs MB, Purcell DB, Nunley R, Morcuende JA: Early results of a new method of treatment for idiopathic congenital vertical talus: Surgical technique. *J Bone Joint Surg Am* 2007;89(suppl 2 pt 1):111-121.
29. Chalayon O, Adams A, Dobbs MB: Minimally invasive approach for the treatment of non-isolated congenital vertical talus. *J Bone Joint Surg Am* 2012;94(11):e73.
30. Yang JS, Dobbs MB: Treatment of congenital vertical talus: Comparison of minimally invasive and extensive soft-tissue release procedures at minimum five-year follow-up. *J Bone Joint Surg Am* 2015;97(16):1354-1365.
31. Wright J, Coggings D, Maizen C, Ramachandran M: Reverse Ponseti-type treatment for children with congenital vertical talus: Comparison between idiopathic and teratological patients. *Bone Joint J* 2014;96-B(2):274-278.
32. Agrawal Y, Bajaj SK, Flowers MJ: Scarf-Akin osteotomy for hallux valgus in juvenile and adolescent patients. *J Pediatr Orthop B* 2015;24(6):535-540.

33. Farsetti P, Weinstein SL, Ponseti IV: The long-term functional and radiographic outcomes of untreated and nonoperatively treated metatarsus adductus. *J Bone Joint Surg Am* 1994;76(2):257-265.

34. Herzenberg JE, Burghardt RD: Resistant metatarsus adductus: Prospective randomized trial of casting versus orthosis. *J Orthop Sci* 2014;19(2):250-256.

35. Cha SM, Shin HD, Kim KC, Lee JK: Simple excision vs the Kidner procedure for type 2 accessory navicular associated with flatfoot in pediatric population. *Foot Ankle Int* 2013;34(2):167-172.

36. Pretell-Mazzini J, Murphy RF, Sawyer JR, et al: Surgical treatment of symptomatic accessory navicular in children and adolescents. *Am J Orthop (Belle Mead NJ)* 2014;43(3):110-113.

37. Ippolito E, Ricciardi Pollini PT, Falez' F: Köhler's disease of the tarsal navicular: Long-term follow-up of 12 cases. *Pediatr Orthop* 1984;4(4):416-417.

38. Chao KH, Lee CH, Lin LC: Surgery for symptomatic Freiberg's disease: Extraarticular dorsal closing-wedge osteotomy in 13 patients followed for 2-4 years. *Acta Orthop Scand* 1999;70(5):483-486.

39. Tsuda E, Ishibashi Y, Yamamoto Y, Maeda S, Kimura Y, Sato H: Osteochondral autograft transplantation for advanced stage Freiberg disease in adolescent athletes: A report of 3 cases and surgical procedures. *Am J Sports Med* 2011;39(11):2470-2475.

40. Sansone V, Morandi A, Dupplicato P, Ungaro E: Treatment of late-stage Freiburg's disease using a temporary metal interpositional device. *J Bone Joint Surg Br* 2010;92(6):807-810.

41. Pereira BS, Frada T, Freitas D, et al: Long-term follow-up of dorsal wedge osteotomy for pediatric Freiberg disease. *Foot Ankle Int* 2016;37(1):90-95.

Patients who were treated with a dorsal wedge osteotomy for pediatric Freiberg disease were very satisfied with pain levels and quality of life at a mean follow-up of 23.4 years. Level of evidence: IV.

42. Becerro de Bengoa Vallejo R, Losa Iglesias ME, Rodríguez Sanz D, Prados Frutos JC, Salvadores Fuentes P, Chicharro JL: Plantar pressures in children with and without Sever's disease. *J Am Podiatr Med Assoc* 2011;101(1):17-24.

43. Rachel JN, Williams JB, Sawyer JR, Warner WC, Kelly DM: Is radiographic evaluation necessary in children with a clinical diagnosis of calcaneal apophysitis (Sever disease)? *J Pediatr Orthop* 2011;31(5):548-550.

44. Canale ST, Williams KD: Iselin's disease. *J Pediatr Orthop* 1992;12(1):90-93.

CHAPTER 29

Rotational and Angular Limb Deformity

BRIAN T. MUFFLY, MD • RYAN D. MUCHOW, MD

ABSTRACT

Rotational or angular limb deformities are among the most common pediatric orthopaedic concerns. Because such deformities in children generally can be stratified within a physiologic range, it is important for the physician to have a solid understanding of normal growth patterns. Children with rotational problems most commonly have intoeing that has an age-based etiology: metatarsus adductus at birth to the age of 1 year, internal tibial torsion for toddlers aged 1 to 3 years, and femoral anteversion for children older than 4 years. Children who have angular problems typically have genu varum identified between birth and the age of 18 to 24 months and genu valgum identified at approximately 3 to 4 years of age. In addition to providing the necessary education to parents for the treatment of children with these benign conditions, it is important to provide the context for identifying the pathologic causes of deformity and proper interventions. The history and the physical examination are keys to identifying pathologic deformity and implementing the proper treatment.

Keywords: femoral anteversion; internal tibial torsion; intoeing; outtoeing; physiologic valgus; physiologic varus; rotational profile

Neither of the following authors nor any immediate family member has received anything of value from or has stock or stock options held in a commercial company or institution related directly or indirectly to the subject of this chapter: Dr. Muffly and Dr. Muchow.

INTRODUCTION

Rotational or angular limb deformities are common concerns of parents when children are seen in the office of a pediatric orthopaedic surgeon. Although most of these deformities occur in healthy children and will spontaneously resolve, the art of caring for these families lies in understanding expected development and recognizing conditions that may not be within normal boundaries. The history and the physical examination are the mainstays of the physician's tools to determine underlying structural or neurologic abnormalities that may be contributing to the deformity and to educate and provide reassurance to the families of these children.

ROTATIONAL DEFORMITY

Normal Development of Femoral Rotation

Femoral rotation, either anteversion or retroversion, is defined by the angle of the femoral neck in the axial plane relative to the femoral shaft. Anteversion is the condition most commonly seen in pediatric patients and results from the normal developmental pathway. Femoral anteversion is greatest in infancy, where the average amount of anteversion is 40°. The degree of anteversion steadily decreases throughout a child's growing years to an average of 16° at maturity.[1,2] Females tend to have greater amounts of anteversion than males, anteversion is typically symmetric, and normal children follow the natural course of decreasing anteversion with age.[3]

In children with femoral anteversion and absence of any other condition, the natural history is benign and improves with age. Various studies have placed an upper limit on the age at which anteversion ceases to

This chapter is adapted from Muchow RD: Rotational and angular limb deformity, in Martus JE, ed: *Orthopaedic Knowledge Update®: Pediatrics*, ed 5. Rosemont, IL, American Academy of Orthopaedic Surgeons, 2016, pp 315-322.

improve, which ranges from 8 to 16 years.[1,3-5] When subdivided by children with normal gait, intoeing gait, and outtoeing gait, femoral anteversion decreased at a rate of 1° per year in children with normal gait, decreased 1.6° per year in children with intoeing, and did not change in children with outtoeing.[4] A summary of the literature definitively defines femoral anteversion as a normal developmental finding that improves in most children.[3-9]

Normal Development of Tibial Rotation

Tibial rotation is defined as the inward or outward rotation of the foot relative to the knee. Intrauterine positioning in general forces the hips into an externally rotated position, and the foot is internally rotated relative to the knee, thus producing internal tibial torsion. The natural progression of tibial rotation is from internal at birth to slightly external at maturity.[8,10] The transmalleolar axis, the angle formed in the axial plane from a line connecting the malleoli against a line across the femoral condyles, begins at 4° internal in newborns (lateral malleolus anterior to medial malleolus) and progresses to an average of 23° external in adults (lateral malleolus posterior to medial malleolus).[8,10] Similarly, if using the thigh-foot axis, which is the angle between the thigh and the foot in a prone child with the knee flexed to 90°, infants have, on average, 5° of internal tibial torsion, which changes to 10° external by the age of 10 years.[8,10] In a 2018 study examining the foot progression angle (longitudinal axis of the foot relative to the forward line of progression) of 5,910 children, a shift toward moderate external rotation was seen between 2 and 4 years of age. The authors recommend monitoring those with bilateral intoeing after the age of 4 years, or unilateral intoeing after the age of 7 years.[11] It is important to note that a wide range of tibial torsion has been noted throughout development, and the SDs include both internal and external tibial torsion at any given time.[3,8] The natural history of internal tibial torsion, however, is benign and trends external as a child reaches maturity.

Evaluation of a Patient With a Rotational Deformity

History

The clinical evaluation begins by assessing the child's development and the history of the deformity. The onset of the deformity, its progression or improvement, and the perceived functional limitations of the child are ascertained from the parents. Coupling this information with birth history, family history, and developmental milestones helps the physician place the child's condition in either a normal category or one where underlying pathology is suspected. All information collected is analyzed against the backdrop of variability in normal development, with the goal being to identify any potential pathologic causes of deformity.

Physical Examination and the Rotational Profile

Observing the child play in the examination room, analyzing his or her gait, and performing a thorough neurologic examination will help confirm or refute suspicions gathered during the history regarding the presence of underlying pathology. From there, a specific assessment of the rotational problem that prompted the chief report can be performed. The rotational profile involves examination of gait, the hip, tibia, and feet to identify the location of the torsional abnormality.[8,12]

Gait is observed to note the foot-progression angle, a measure of the degree that the foot turns inward (designated a negative value) or outward (designated a positive value) relative to the axis of the leg. This provides an overview of the rotational deformity and summarizes all the components of the rotational profile. Symmetry and the direction the patellae point also should be noted.

The static evaluation begins with an assessment of hip version. The child is positioned prone on an examination table with the knees bent to 90°. The legs are maximally rotated internally and externally. Internal rotation measuring greater than 70°, with a lesser amount of external rotation, is caused by an increase in femoral anteversion (**Figure 1**). Tibial torsion is assessed with the thigh-foot axis and the transmalleolar axis (**Figure 2**).

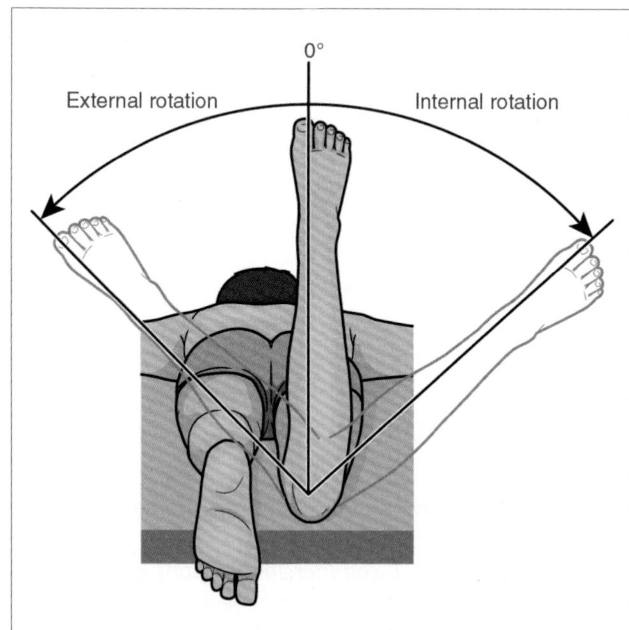

FIGURE 1 Illustration of the assessment of femoral rotation. The child should lie prone on an examination table with the knees flexed at 90°. The feet are rotated maximally internally and externally.

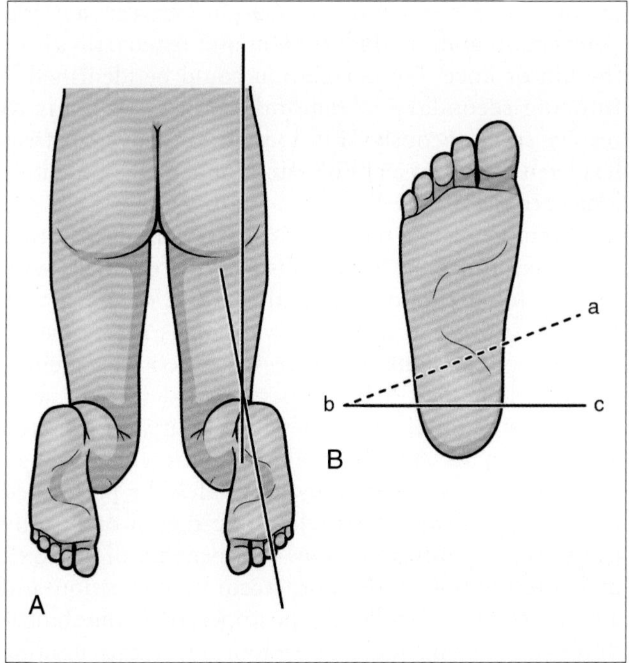

FIGURE 2 Illustrations for assessing tibial torsion. **A**, For the thigh-foot axis, the child should lie prone on an examination table with the knees flexed at 90°. The angle of the axis of the thigh and the axis of the foot determines internal or external tibial torsion. **B**, The transmalleolar axis is the angle between a line drawn connecting the malleoli (line a-b) and the coronal plane of the tibia (line b-c).

The trochanter palpation test is another method of identifying true anteversion.[13] With the child positioned prone and the knee flexed to 90°, the leg is rotated until the prominence of the greater trochanter is palpated most distinctly. Because this represents the most lateral position of the trochanter, the femoral neck is parallel to the floor. Thus, the angle between the vertical and the tibia represents the actual amount of anteversion.

The foot is the final component that contributes to a rotational issue. The heel-bisector line, a line drawn down the axis of the hindfoot through the forefoot, should normally pass through the second web space. Medial or lateral deviations of the line indicate a component of forefoot adduction or abduction, respectively[14] (**Figure 3**).

The results of the rotational profile will allow the physician to identify the location of the rotational deformity. Combining these results with knowledge of normal development, the physician is directed to further evaluate the child radiographically when the deformity exists 2 SDs outside the mean for the child's age.[8] The physical examination will be the key determinant in identifying deformity that requires radiographic evaluation.

Low-dose biplanar radiography has shown promise as an imaging modality in the evaluation of femoral and tibial torsional deformity in this patient population, particularly in its correlation to CT measurements and decreased radiation exposure.[15,16]

Intoeing

The most common age-related causes of intoeing are metatarsus adductus with or without internal tibial torsion from birth to 1 year of age, internal tibial torsion for toddlers aged 1 to 3 years, and femoral anteversion for children older than 4 years. Although intoeing is an extremely common chief report, most cases are benign with the mainstays of treatment involving both education and reassurance.[17]

Metatarsus Adductus

Most cases of metatarsus adductus are postural in nature and resolve spontaneously with time.[18-20] A natural history of metatarsus adductus was published in 1978 and showed 86% of feet as normal or mildly deformed, 10% as moderately deformed but asymptomatic, and 4% as deformed and stiff at an average of 7 years of age.[20] In terms of prognosis and treatment, it may be helpful to classify the deformity as mild (the foot can be passively corrected beyond

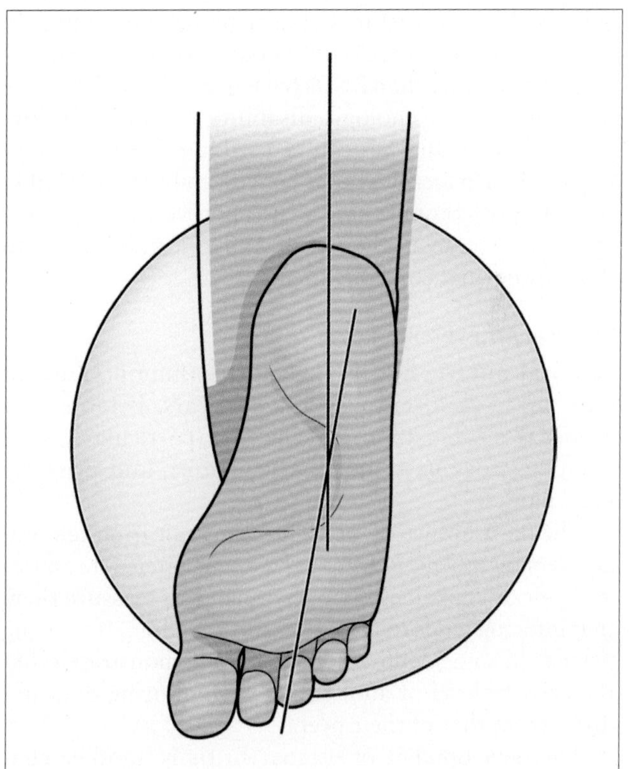

FIGURE 3 Illustration of the heel-bisector line. The axis of the hindfoot should be parallel to the axis of the forefoot. This illustration shows a mild metatarsus adductus deformity.

neutral), moderate (the foot is passively correctable to neutral), and severe (the foot is unable to be passively corrected).[21] Both serial casting and bracing treatment/orthoses have been shown to be effective in the management of metatarsus adductus.[22,23] Surgery is reserved for the most resistant cases of metatarsus adductus. In the literature, viable options with adequate results include lengthening of the abductor hallucis with a medial capsulotomy[24] and an opening wedge osteotomy of the medial cuneiform combined with a closing wedge osteotomy of the cuboid.[25]

Internal Tibial Torsion

Internal tibial torsion is the most common cause of intoeing in children aged 1 to 3 years. Parents may report that the child is clumsy or trips frequently, and the child typically does not have pain. A proper rotational profile confirms the diagnosis, with the thigh-foot axis and the transmalleolar axis demonstrating internal tibial torsion.

Management of the condition predominantly involves education, reassurance, and expectant observation. Special shoes, the Denis Browne bar orthosis, twister cables, and shoe inserts have not demonstrated benefit in the management of internal tibial torsion.[1,26,27]

Surgical management of internal tibial torsion is rare but may be indicated in a child who has not improved or has intoeing progression, is older than 8 years, has deformity greater than 2 SDs from normal, and has some functional or psychologic disability derived from the torsion.[8,9] Gait analysis can be used in this patient population to help identify functional disability.[6] Distal tibia corrective osteotomies are able to improve knee moments and restore many of the kinetic and kinematic values to those of normal control patients.[28]

Femoral Anteversion

Femoral anteversion is the most common cause of intoeing in children older than 4 years. Parents may report W-sitting, abnormal running (particularly with compensatory external tibial torsion), and possibly knee pain.

The natural history of an intoeing gait from femoral anteversion is benign. Although parents often note abnormal gait or clumsiness, the physician can reassure them that intoeing tends to resolve in most children. If intoeing persists in some children, it has been demonstrated that the activity level of adolescents with intoeing does not differ from that of their peers.[7]

The development of osteoarthritis is another concern. It has been proposed that femoral anteversion leads to an increase in osteoarthritis of the hip and knee, but this has been refuted in numerous studies.[29-31] In 2017, researchers studied 1,158 cadaver tibiae and femora to determine an association between femoral anteversion and/or tibial torsion and osteoarthritis of the hip or knee. No correlation could be identified.[29] Intoeing secondary to femoral anteversion tends to resolve spontaneously; if it does not, no adverse effect has been found on a child's functional development or long-term health.

Given the benign natural history, parental education and reassurance are the mainstays of treatment, with no role for orthotics, physical therapy, or restriction from W-sitting. Surgical intervention is a rare event; however, indications for corrective osteotomy include a child older than 8 years, persistent deformity with marked functional or cosmetic disability, anteversion greater than 50°, and internal hip rotation greater than 80°.[8,9] Corrective osteotomy may safely be performed proximally in the intertrochanteric region or distally in the supracondylar region. The benefits of a proximal osteotomy include more accurate correction and a decreased requirement for postoperative immobilization[32] versus being able to use a tourniquet, thus limiting blood loss.[33] Both of these methods report success from a technical and patient-satisfaction perspective and limited complications. A 2018 prospective study demonstrated that diaphyseal osteotomy with fixation using an intramedullary nail provided predictable deformity correction with significant improvements in patient-reported pain and function.[34]

Outtoeing

An external foot-progression angle, also known as outtoeing, occurs less frequently than intoeing, but it may be of no less concern to parents. The benign natural history of this deformity typically allows for treatment that consists of education, reassurance, and expectant observation. However, knowledge of characteristic presentations and a thorough physical examination will allow the physician to differentiate between normal variations and underlying pathology.

Children are typically born with an external rotation contracture of the hip that may exceed the internal rotation from metatarsus adductus present at birth. This is the most common cause of outtoeing in infancy. These children may have an accompanying calcaneovalgus foot, which also will correct itself with time. During the toddler years, children may have external tibial torsion that will trend internal with continued growth. As children get older, they are more likely to have outtoeing secondary to decreased femoral anteversion or planovalgus feet.

Certain conditions occur with outtoeing and should trigger the physician to perform some additional workup. External tibial torsion is associated with cerebral palsy, myelomeningocele, and other neuromuscular disorders.

Decreased femoral anteversion is associated with obesity,[35] slipped capital femoral epiphysis, and coxa vara.

Torsional Malalignment Syndrome

Torsional malalignment syndrome (also called miserable malalignment syndrome) may be present in adolescents as the summation of excessive femoral anteversion combined with external tibial torsion. Because of the biomechanical disadvantage this confers on the patellofemoral joint, adolescents often have anterior knee pain. Typically, treatment involves observation of the malrotation and therapy for anterior knee pain. Patients rarely have persistent symptoms that warrant surgical intervention. In the most severe cases, a double osteotomy of the femur and tibia is warranted to correct femoral anteversion and external tibial torsion. Two reports in the literature encompassing 17 patients demonstrated resolution of knee pain and deformity at an average follow-up of 5 and 16 years, respectively.[36,37] Given the complexity of assessing rotation in both segments of the lower extremity, CT assessment of any rotation is recommended before intervention.[37]

ANGULAR DEFORMITY

Normal Development of Lower Extremity Alignment

Understanding the normal physiologic growth patterns in children is fundamental to the evaluation of children with angular deformity. Symmetric varus is the expected angular pattern of growth in children between birth and 18 to 24 months of age. This growth transitions to a symmetric valgus alignment that is typically maximal at approximately 3 to 4 years of age and ultimately normalizes by the age of 6 to 8 years. Normal alignment of the lower extremity as a child reaches maturity is 5° to 7° of valgus.[38]

The natural history of angular deformity in the lower extremity depends on its etiology. Physiologic deformity, by definition, will resolve spontaneously. Progressive angular deformity will continue to worsen with time, resulting in gait disturbance, limitations in function, and pain. Regarding the effect of malalignment on osteoarthritis, the literature is decidedly unclear on its association. Various biomechanical and gait studies describe increased force through the medial and lateral compartments, with genu varum and genu valgum, respectively. However, this has not been directly linked to osteoarthritis in any study.[39-42]

Differential Diagnoses

The differential diagnoses for angular deformity are presented in **Table 1**.

Evaluation of a Child With Angular Deformity

The history of presentation is key to working through the differential diagnosis to identify a source for a growth abnormality. Most conditions will be categorized as physiologic, so it is very important to rule out other etiologies and gain a perspective of the onset, duration, and progression of the deformity. Specific events, a history of abnormal growth, or other diseases may help guide the questioning into the large

Section 5: Lower Extremity

TABLE 1

The Differential Diagnosis for Angular Deformity

Category	Diagnosis
Physiologic	—
Idiopathic genu valgum	—
Heuter-Volkmann principle	Infantile and adolescent tibia vara
Acquired (insult to the physis)	Trauma, infection, radiation, iatrogenic cause, juvenile inflammatory arthritis, osteochondroma
Congenital (condition affecting the health/growth of the physis)	Skeletal dysplasia, focal fibrocartilaginous dysplasia, osteogenesis imperfecta, multiple hereditary exostosis, Ollier disease, Maffucci syndrome
Metabolic bone disease (the physis is susceptible to the Heuter-Volkmann principle at the age of physiologic angulation: onset earlier than age 2 typically results in varus, and onset after age 4-5 yr typically results in valgus)	Rickets, renal osteodystrophy
Adaptive response to a long bone deformity	—

categories of acquired, congenital, or metabolic deformities, respectively. In addition, it is important to gain a sense of the patient's limitations resulting from the deformity and any symptoms that the child may be experiencing.

The physical examination is used to further precisely determine the diagnosis and specifically identify the location of the deformity. An overall assessment of a child should include the child's height, weight, and development. A 2019 study of 6,992 children found limb defects in 90.2% of obese children and demonstrated that increased body mass index is correlated with a higher risk of developing lower extremity postural defects.[43] The child's gait should be observed for any abnormalities, including the presence of medial or lateral thrust, joint instability, crouch, or equinus. The musculoskeletal examination is used to identify deformity, assess joints, identify sources of pain, perform a rotational profile, and assess for limb-length discrepancy. The neurologic examination should confirm that the child is developing normally and assess for any underlying neural axis abnormality.

Radiographs are indicated whenever the history and the physical examination create suspicion for true bony deformity. Radiographs are not indicated in cases of physiologic patterns of growth. A standing, full-length AP radiograph that includes both lower limbs is the preferred imaging tool for assessing angular alignment and limb length. Additional biplanar imaging of the involved bones or joints may be necessary for diagnostic purposes, and a bone age test may be helpful for assessing growth remaining. Advanced imaging may be used for evaluating pathology related to the physis or assessing rotational anatomy.

Alignment is assessed by determining the anatomic and mechanical axis of the lower extremity. The anatomic axis is the middiaphyseal line of a bone. The mechanical axis represents the weight-bearing alignment of the lower extremity and normally should involve a straight line from the center of the femoral head to the center of the distal tibia passing through the center of the knee. Normal anatomic alignment of the lower extremity produces a femoral-tibial angle of 5° to 7° of valgus at maturity.[44] Normal values of alignment (**Table 2**) are helpful for identifying deformity in a long bone (**Figure 4**).

The center of rotation of angulation is the location of deformity in a long bone. If a single point of deformity exists, the point of intersection between the proximal mechanical axis and the distal mechanical axis is the center of rotation of angulation. Therefore, deformity correction should occur at the center of rotation of angulation to restore the mechanical axis.[44]

TABLE 2

Normal Values of Alignment

Angle Type	Angle Measurement
Hip	
Neck-shaft angle	130°
Knee	
Lateral distal femoral angle	87°
Medial proximal tibial angle	87°
Posterior distal femoral angle	83°
Posterior proximal tibial angle	81°
Ankle	
Lateral distal tibial angle	89°
Anterior distal tibial angle	80°

The physis should be specifically assessed in a growing child, both as a potential etiology of deformity and as a potential solution for correcting the deformity.

Treatment of Angular Deformity

The indications for treating angular deformity include malalignment that results in pain or functional limitation. Physiologic deformity can be managed with expectant observation. Orthotic management of progressive angular deformity has minimal support in the literature, with perhaps infantile Blount disease having the greatest benefit from bracing treatment.[45-47] Surgical intervention is the mainstay treatment of deformity that causes pain or functional limitation, particularly when the deformity is progressive.

The menu of options for the treatment of angular deformity is extensive and involves three general categories: growth modulation, acute correction, and gradual correction through multiplanar external fixation.[48-50] The technique chosen depends on numerous variables, including physeal growth, the location of the deformity, the age of the patient, any underlying conditions, and the amount of deformity.

SUMMARY

There can be much anxiety associated with a clinic visit for rotational or angular deformities in a child. Given the positive natural history of physiologic growth patterns, parents can take much relief in the knowledge that their child will outgrow the current deformity when it is properly identified. The role of the physician is highly

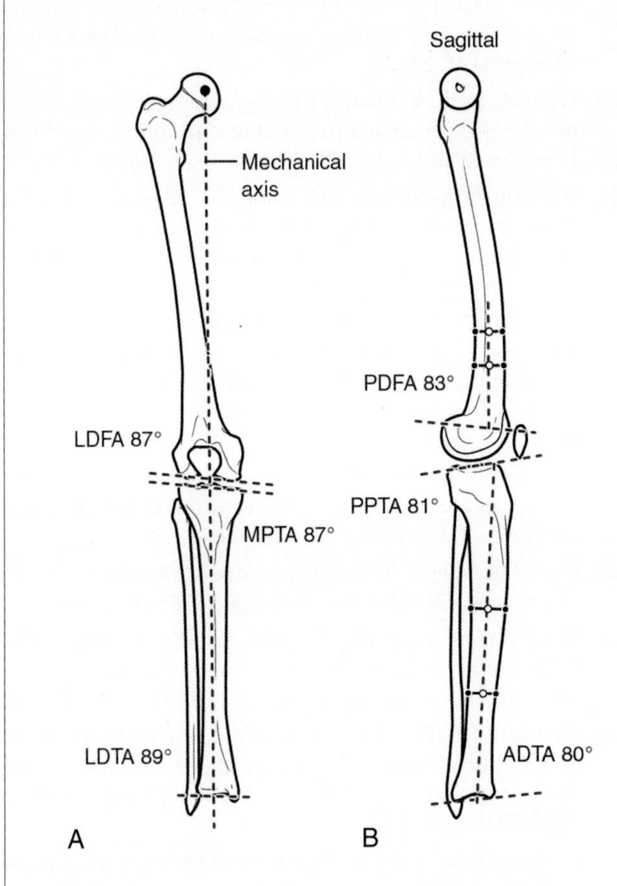

FIGURE 4 Illustrations of the mechanical axis of the lower limb. A straight line drawn connecting the center of the femoral head to the center of the distal tibia. **A**, The normal angles for the lateral distal femoral angle (LDFA), the medial proximal tibia angle (MPTA), and the lateral distal tibia angle (LDTA) will assist in identifying the location of deformity in the coronal plane. **B**, The posterior distal femoral angle (PDFA), the posterior proximal tibia angle (PPTA), and the anterior distal tibia angle (ADTA) assist in locating the deformity in the sagittal plane. The ideal degree measurements for each angle type are provided in **Table 2**.

instrumental in determining whether the child's condition is within the normal range or if the underlying etiology will result in progressive and limiting deformity.

When performed correctly, tension band plating for correction of angular deformity is a successful procedure with low complication rate.[51] The treating surgeon can reasonably expect femoral deformities to correct faster than deformities of the tibia, and valgus to correct faster than varus malalignment.[52] Before undertaking growth modulation procedures, the surgeon should counsel parents/guardians on the importance of frequent postoperative evaluation, as loss to follow-up and subsequent overcorrection is common.[53]

KEY STUDY POINTS

- Most cases of intoeing are benign in etiology and necessitate education/reassurance.
- Femoral anteversion may improve until the age of 8 years. Long-term functional limitation from persistent femoral anteversion is uncommon.
- Internal tibial torsion is the most common cause of intoeing in toddlers aged 1 to 3 years.
- Physiologic varus is present between birth and the age of 18 to 24 months, and physiologic valgus is maximal at the age of 3 to 4 years and should resolve by the age of 7 years.
- Tension band plating is a successful treatment for angular deformity; however, extensive discussion with family regarding importance of follow-up is recommended before surgical intervention.

ANNOTATED REFERENCES

1. Fabry G, MacEwen GD, Shands AR Jr: Torsion of the femur: A follow-up study in normal and abnormal conditions. *J Bone Joint Surg Am* 1973;55(8):1726-1738.
2. Shands AR Jr, Steele MK: Torsion of the femur: A follow-up report on the use of the dunlap method for its determination. *J Bone Joint Surg Am* 1958;40(4):803-816.
3. Jacquemier M, Glard Y, Pomero V, Viehweger E, Jouve JL, Bollini G: Rotational profile of the lower limb in 1319 healthy children. *Gait Posture* 2008;28(2):187-193.
4. Matovinović D, Nemec B, Gulan G, Sestan B, Ravlić-Gulan J: Comparison in regression of femoral neck anteversion in children with normal, intoeing and outtoeing gait: Prospective study. *Coll Antropol* 1998;22(2):525-532.
5. Svenningsen S, Apalset K, Terjesen T, Anda S: Regression of femoral anteversion: A prospective study of intoeing children. *Acta Orthop Scand* 1989;60(2):170-173.
6. Radler C, Kranzl A, Manner HM, Höglinger M, Ganger R, Grill F: Torsional profile versus gait analysis: Consistency between the anatomic torsion and the resulting gait pattern in patients with rotational malalignment of the lower extremity. *Gait Posture* 2010;32(3):405-410.
7. Staheli LT, Lippert F, Denotter P: Femoral anteversion and physical performance in adolescent and adult life. *Clin Orthop Relat Res* 1977;129:213-216.
8. Staheli LT, Corbett M, Wyss C, King H: Lower-extremity rotational problems in children: Normal values to guide management. *J Bone Joint Surg Am* 1985;67(1):39-47.
9. Staheli LT: Torsion: Treatment indications. *Clin Orthop Relat Res* 1989;247:61-66.
10. Staheli LT, Engel GM: Tibial torsion: A method of assessment and a survey of normal children. *Clin Orthop Relat Res* 1972;86:183-186.

11. Verch R, Hirschmüller A, Müller J, Baur H, Mayer F: Is intoing gait physiological in children? – Results of a large cohort study in 5910 healthy (pre-) school children. *Gait Posture* 2018;66:70-75.

Foot progression angle (FPA) measurements from 5,910 healthy children were obtained to establish reference values for children aged 1 to 14 years. Maximum FPA was seen in 2-year-old children and decreased significantly to moderate outtoeing at the age of 4 years. There were no differences in FPA for those aged 5 to 14 years. The authors concluded that a wide FPA range exists in children, and development shows spontaneous shift toward moderate external rotation between the age of 2 and 4 years. Level of evidence: III.

12. Staheli LT: Torsional deformity. *Pediatr Clin North Am* 1977;24(4):799-811.
13. Ruwe PA, Gage JR, Ozonoff MB, DeLuca PA: Clinical determination of femoral anteversion. A comparison with established techniques. *J Bone Joint Surg Am* 1992;74(6):820-830.
14. Smith JT, Bleck EE, Gamble JG, Rinsky LA, Pena T: Simple method of documenting metatarsus adductus. *J Pediatr Orthop* 1991;11(5):679-680.
15. Rosskopf AB, Ramseier LE, Sutter R, Pfirrmann CWA, Buck FM: Femoral and tibial torsion measurement in children and adolescents: Comparison of 3D models based on low-dose biplanar radiography and low-dose CT. *AJR Am J Roentgenol* 2014;202(3):W285-W291.
16. Meyrignac O, Moreno R, Baunin C, et al: Low-dose biplanar radiography can be used in children and adolescents to accurately assess femoral and tibial torsion and greatly reduce irradiation. *Eur Radiol* 2015;25(6):1752-1760.
17. Faulks S, Brown K, Birch JG: Spectrum of diagnosis and disposition of patients referred to a pediatric orthopaedic center for a diagnosis of intoeing. *J Pediatr Orthop* 2017;37(7):e43 2-e435.

This study evaluated the efficacy and parental satisfaction of an Advanced Practice Provider (APP). APPs conducted Intoeing Clinic for initial evaluation of children referred to pediatric orthopaedic center for diagnosis of intoeing. Of the 926 patients seen, 95% had a confirmed diagnosis of benign intoeing/other benign condition. Despite this, 5% of patients requested a reevaluation for the same concern. The authors concluded that such an APP-led clinic is an effective and efficient method of evaluating patients referred for the common diagnosis of intoeing. Level of evidence: IV.

18. Farsetti P, Weinstein SL, Ponseti IV: The long-term functional and radiographic outcomes of untreated and nonoperatively treated metatarsus adductus. *J Bone Joint Surg Am* 1994;76(2):257-265.
19. Ponseti IV, Becker JR: Congenital metatarsus adductus: The results of treatment. *J Bone Joint Surg Am* 1966;48(4):702-711.
20. Rushforth GF: The natural history of hooked forefoot. *J Bone Joint Surg Br* 1978;60(4):530-532.
21. Bleck EE: Metatarsus adductus: Classification and relationship to outcomes of treatment. *J Pediatr Orthop* 1983;3(1):2-9.
22. Katz K, David R, Soudry M: Below-knee plaster cast for the treatment of metatarsus adductus. *J Pediatr Orthop* 1999;19(1):49-50.
23. Herzenberg JE, Burghardt RD: Resistant metatarsus adductus: Prospective randomized trial of casting versus orthosis. *J Orthop Sci* 2014;19:250-256.
24. Asirvatham R, Stevens PM: Idiopathic forefoot-adduction deformity: Medial capsulotomy and abductor hallucis lengthening for resistant and severe deformities. *J Pediatr Orthop* 1997;17(4):496-500.
25. McHale KA, Lenhart MK: Treatment of residual clubfoot deformity – The "bean-shaped" foot – By opening wedge medial cuneiform osteotomy and closing wedge cuboid osteotomy: Clinical review and cadaver correlations. *J Pediatr Orthop* 1991;11(3):374-381.
26. Heinrich SD, Sharps CH: Lower extremity torsional deformities in children: A prospective comparison of two treatment modalities. *Orthopedics* 1991;14(6):655-659.
27. Knittel G, Staheli LT: The effectiveness of shoe modifications for intoeing. *Orthop Clin North Am* 1976;7(4):1019-1025.
28. MacWilliams BA, McMulkin ML, Baird GO, Stevens PM: Distal tibial rotation osteotomies normalize frontal plane knee moments. *J Bone Joint Surg Am* 2010;92(17):2835-2842.
29. Weinberg DS, Park PJ, Morris WZ, Liu RW: Femoral version and tibial torsion are not associated with hip or knee arthritis in a large osteological collection. *J Pediatr Orthop* 2017;37(2):e120-e128.

In this cadaver study, 1,158 femora and tibiae were assessed for femoral anteversion and tibial torsion, and a correlation was made with the development of hip or knee arthritis. The results of multiple regression analysis showed that femoral anteversion and internal tibial torsion were not associated with osteoarthritis. Level of evidence: IV.

30. Hubbard DD, Staheli LT, Chew DE, Mosca VS: Medial femoral torsion and osteoarthritis. *J Pediatr Orthop* 1988;8(5):540-542.
31. Wedge JH, Munkacsi I, Loback D: Anteversion of the femur and idiopathic osteoarthrosis of the hip. *J Bone Joint Surg Am* 1989;71(7):1040-1043.
32. Payne LZ, DeLuca PA: Intertrochanteric versus supracondylar osteotomy for severe femoral anteversion. *J Pediatr Orthop* 1994;14(1):39-44.
33. Hoffer MM, Prietto C, Koffman M: Supracondylar derotational osteotomy of the femur for internal rotation of the thigh in the cerebral palsied child. *J Bone Joint Surg Am* 1981;63(3):389-393.
34. Stambough JB, Davis L, Szymanski DA, Smith JC, Schoenecker PL, Gordon JE: Knee pain and activity outcomes after femoral derotation osteotomy for excessive femoral anteversion. *J Pediatr Orthop* 2018;38:503-509.

This study prospectively evaluated 28 patients to determine clinical and functional outcomes of symptomatic excessive femoral anteversion managed with femoral derotational osteotomy stabilized with an intramedullary nail. At 1-year follow-up, there was significant improvement in all clinical examination measurements. The procedure was deemed a reliable surgical option that provides predictable improvement in deformity correction, as well as significant improvements in function and pain scales. Level of evidence: II.

35. Galbraith RT, Gelberman RH, Hajek PC, et al: Obesity and decreased femoral anteversion in adolescence. *J Orthop Res* 1987;5(4):523-528.
36. Bruce WD, Stevens PM: Surgical correction of miserable malalignment syndrome. *J Pediatr Orthop* 2004;24(4):392-396.
37. Leonardi F, Rivera F, Zorzan A, Ali SM: Bilateral double osteotomy in severe torsional malalignment syndrome: 16 years follow-up. *J Orthop Traumatol* 2014;15(2):131-136.
38. Salenius P, Vankka E: The development of the tibiofemoral angle in children. *J Bone Joint Surg Am* 1975;57(2):259-261.
39. Bruns J, Volkmer M, Luessenhop S: Pressure distribution at the knee joint: Influence of varus and valgus deviation without and with ligament dissection. *Arch Orthop Trauma Surg* 1993;113(1):12-19.
40. McKellop HA, Llinás A, Sarmiento A: Effects of tibial malalignment on the knee and ankle. *Orthop Clin North Am* 1994;25(3):415-423.
41. Morrison JB: The mechanics of the knee joint in relation to normal walking. *J Biomech* 1970;3(1):51-61.
42. Tetsworth K, Paley D: Malalignment and degenerative arthropathy. *Orthop Clin North Am* 1994;25(3):367-377.
43. Brzezinski M, Czubek Z, Niedzielska A, Jankowski M, Kobus T, Ossowski Z: Relationship between lower-extremity defects and body mass among polish children: A cross-sectional study. *BMC Musculoskelet Disord* 2019:20(1):84.

    This study analyzed the prevalence of lower extremity postural defects in 6,992 Polish children aged 8 to 12 years and assessed the probability that these were associated with body mass index. 90.2% of obese, 25.7% of normal weight, and 15.1% of underweight children were found to have limb defects. The authors concluded that increasing prevalence of lower limb defects were seen with increasing body mass index. Level of evidence: III.

44. Paley D: *Principles of Deformity Correction*. Berlin, Germany, Springer, 2002, pp 1-18.
45. Alsancak S, Guner S, Kinik H: Orthotic variations in the management of infantile tibia vara and the results of treatment. *Prosthet Orthot Int* 2013;37(5):375-383.
46. Raney EM, Topoleski TA, Yaghoubian R, Guidera KJ, Marshall JG: Orthotic treatment of infantile tibia vara. *J Pediatr Orthop* 1998;18(5):670-674.
47. Zionts LE, Shean CJ: Brace treatment of early infantile tibia vara. *J Pediatr Orthop* 1998;18(1):102-109.
48. Stevens PM, Maguire M, Dales MD, Robins AJ: Physeal stapling for idiopathic genu valgum. *J Pediatr Orthop* 1999;19(5):645-649.
49. Stevens PM: Guided growth for angular correction: A preliminary series using a tension band plate. *J Pediatr Orthop* 2007;27(3):253-259.
50. Métaizeau JP, Wong-Chung J, Bertrand H, Pasquier P: Percutaneous epiphysiodesis using transphyseal screws (PETS). *J Pediatr Orthop* 1998;18(3):363-369.
51. Shabtai L, Herzenberg JE: Limits of growth modulation using tension band plates in the lower extremities. *J Am Acad Orthop Surg* 2016;24(10):691-701.

    This review article examines the role of tension band plating for growth modulation in the lower extremities. Following a systematic literature review, the authors concluded that growth modulation with tension band plating is a well-established technique with high success rates and should be considered for mild to moderate deformity.

52. Danino B, Rödl R, Herzenberg JE, et al: Growth modulation in idiopathic angular knee deformities: Is it predictable? *J Child Orthop* 2019;13(3):318-323.

    In this study, 372 physes in 206 patients were reviewed to determine the temporal and spatial sequence of events following hemiepiphysiodesis for idiopathic angular knee deformities. The authors found that the femur corrects faster than the tibia and that valgus femoral deformities correct faster than varus deformities. Level of evidence: IV.

53. Lawing C, Margalit A, Ukwuani G, Sponseller PD: Predicting late follow-up and understanding its consequences in growth modulation for pediatric lower limb deformities. *J Pediatr Orthop* 2019;39:295-301.

    The authors retrospectively reviewed 112 patients who underwent procedures with implants for growth modulation of the lower extremities to determine factors associated with late clinical follow-up and overcorrection rates. Late follow-up, obesity, and primary language other than English were found to be associated with overcorrection in guided-growth procedures. Level of evidence: IV.

CHAPTER 30

Limb-Length Discrepancy, Limb Deficiency, and Prosthetics

JANET L. WALKER, MD

ABSTRACT

Children with lower limb-length discrepancy can be treated with epiphysiodesis, limb shortening, and limb lengthening. It is helpful to be familiar with the most common types of lower limb deficiencies and their orthopaedic management along with surgical and prosthetic techniques when lower limb amputation is necessary.

Keywords: amputations in children; congenital limb deficiency; leg length inequality

INTRODUCTION

The general management of limb-length discrepancy, including epiphysiodesis, shortening, and lengthening, is reviewed. The classifications and management of the most common lower limb deficiencies—fibular, femoral, tibial, and transverse—are discussed, and general surgical and prosthetic considerations for children with amputations are presented.

LIMB-LENGTH DISCREPANCY

Length discrepancy in the lower limbs is very common, with some studies demonstrating small degrees of limb-length inequality in more than half of the US population. A limb-length discrepancy of 2 cm or more was found in 7% of typical 8- to 12-year-old children.[1] Gait patterns may be altered when discrepancies are 2 cm or greater. Finite element models show increased sacroiliac joint loading, with peak stresses that progressively increase with discrepancies from 1 to 3 cm.[2] These models propose a mechanism by which limb-length discrepancies may lead to low back pain and may explain the correlation of greater than 5 mm discrepancies with degenerative changes at L4, L5, and S1. Studies looking at the relationship between limb-length discrepancy and osteoarthritis suggest that it is more common in the hip on the long side and the knee on the short side.[3] For children with a limb-length discrepancy, their parents reported no difference in Pediatric Outcomes Data Collection Instrument scores related to the amount of their child's discrepancy.[4] For those with a limb-length discrepancy greater than 2 cm, parents were less satisfied with their child's appearance and more concerned about possible surgery in the future. They thought that the happiness of their child was adversely affected by the limb-length discrepancy, and for larger degrees of discrepancy, parents were more willing to seek surgical treatment.

Neither Dr. Walker nor any immediate family member has received anything of value from or has stock or stock options held in a commercial company or institution related directly or indirectly to the subject of this chapter.

ASSESSMENT

Direct clinical measurement of limb-length inequality with a tape measure, which is designed to measure differences in the distances between bony landmarks, can be performed in both the supine and standing positions. Indirect clinical measurement of limb-length discrepancy can be determined with the patient standing with blocks under the short leg until the iliac crests are level. Radiographic techniques include orthoradiography, scanography, and CT. Scanography measures only limb lengths. Orthoradiography and CT assess both length and limb alignment. CT has a lower radiation dosage than orthoradiography, but it is less accessible at most medical centers.[5-7] Although supine tape measurements of limb lengths have excellent interrater and intrarater reliability compared with CT,[5] most centers rely on some objective form of documentation. Many centers have switched to digital radiography systems because they have been shown to produce reliable measurements that are comparable with hard copy long leg radiographs.[6,8] Low-dose, upright biplanar radiographic imaging using highly sensitive gaseous photon detectors has been shown to produce reliably accurate limb-length measurements compared with teleoroentgenograms and CT scans and has less radiation exposure.[6] Biplanar imaging also allows for measurements of limb alignment and torsion but requires a standing position (**Figure 1**). In all cases, length calculations, especially those methods that require standing, must take into account joint contractures, limb posturing, foot deficiency or deformity, pelvic anomalies, and/or hip dysplasia that might affect overall limb length.

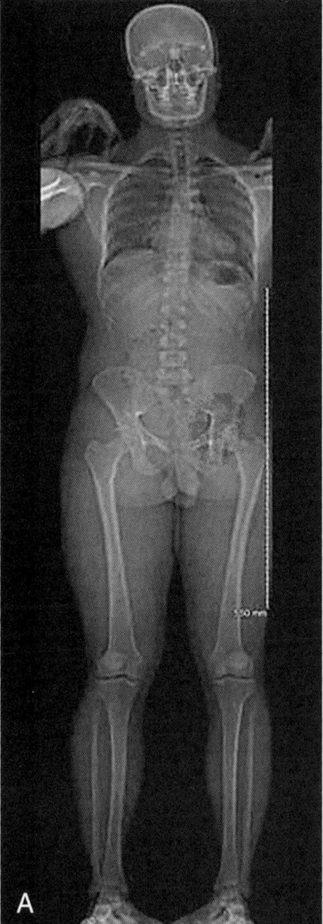

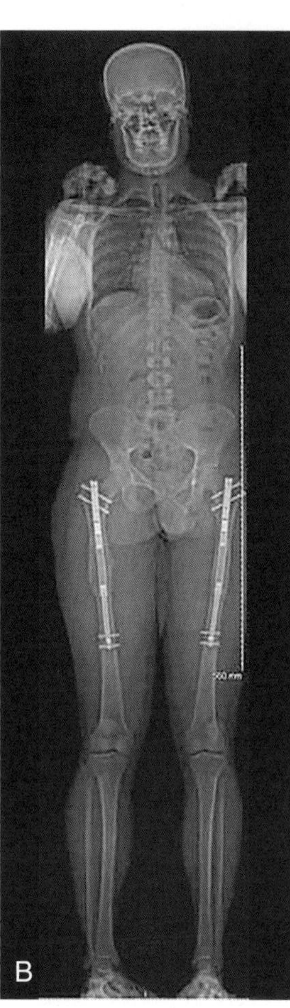

FIGURE 1 EOS radiographic images accurately measure limb length and alignment. **A**, Image before limb lengthening was performed because of the short stature of the patient. **B**, Image after limb lengthening was performed using the PRECICE intramedullary lengthener. (Reproduced with permission from Paley D, Harris M, Debiparshad K, Prince D: Limb lengthening by implantable limb lengthening devices. *Tech Orthop* 2014;29[2]:72-85.)

CLINICAL DECISION MAKING

In general, treatment decisions about limb equalization are based on the projected limb-length discrepancy at maturity. Observation or shoe modification is recommended for discrepancies of 2 cm or less. Discrepancies ranging from 2 to 5 cm are amenable to shortening procedures by either epiphysiodesis before maturity or femoral shortening at maturity. Greater degrees of shortening can result in a disproportionate body appearance. Limb lengthening is used for discrepancies of 5 cm or more. Combining shortening or epiphysiodesis with lengthening can reduce the amount of lengthening needed. For patients with discrepancies greater than 20 cm or those with a limb that cannot tolerate lengthening, amputation and prosthetic fitting should be considered.

Many other factors also need to be considered. A child who is already below typical height may not accept a treatment that results in further loss of stature. Families may not want to consider a surgery on the normal leg. Greater degrees of shortening or epiphysiodesis may be appropriate if the abnormal leg is too long (eg, hemihypertrophy). Associated deformities that require corrective surgery can be combined with lengthening to correct milder degrees of limb-length discrepancy. Limbs with unstable joints, contracted soft tissues, or neurovascular problems may be poor candidates for lengthening; alternatives such as amputation or contralateral shortening may be more acceptable, even if a disproportionate appearance results.

Four widely used methods estimate lower limb growth and predict limb-length inequality. The arithmetic method combines the rate of growth of the distal femur (0.375 inch or 9.5 mm per year) and the proximal tibia (0.25 inch or 6.4 mm per year) with chronologic age and the assumption of maturity at 16 years for boys and 14 years for girls.[9] The growth-remaining method uses growth-remaining graphs and skeletal age.[10] The straight-line graph method[11] simplifies the estimation process of the growth-remaining method.[10] The multiplier method uses chronologic age and data from several limb-length databases.[12] In planning for the timing of epiphysiodesis, the use of skeletal age reduced the prediction error for all methods, and the multiplier method was found to be the least accurate.[13]

EPIPHYSIODESIS OR SHORTENING

Epiphysiodesis is a commonly used procedure to achieve limb-length equalization by maturity and has a low morbidity rate. It is generally recommended for predicted limb-length discrepancies of 2 to 6 cm at maturity. The original technique for epiphysiodesis required an open bone block (Phemister technique) and had predictably good results. Currently, percutaneous techniques have been popularized because of reduced morbidity and scarring.[14] Radiostereometric analysis has demonstrated that growth arrest can be expected within 12 weeks when using percutaneous physeal drilling and curettage.[15] Implants to tether, rather than arrest, growth have been described using transphyseal screws and physeal plates. They are an attractive option when the timing of growth arrest is unpredictable. Implant removal can reverse the tether when length equality is achieved. Recent studies, however, have shown that medial and lateral physeal plates are less effective than epiphysiodesis using drilling and curettage.[16] In addition, transphyseal screws achieved only 66% of the expected growth retardation from the preoperative prediction.[17]

Limb shortening after maturity is most commonly performed in the femoral segment because of fewer neurovascular concerns. Open and closed intramedullary techniques produce shortening of accurately defined amounts of up to 5 cm or 10% of bone length. Greater degrees of shortening produce a disproportionate appearance and excessive weakness, especially of the quadriceps, and are not recommended.

LIMB LENGTHENING

Distraction osteogenesis is the most accepted method of limb lengthening, especially for deficits greater than 2.5 cm.[18] The process consists of a low-energy corticotomy or osteotomy of the bone and a latency period of 5 to 7 days to allow for the early fracture repair process. This process is then followed by a gradual stretching of the distraction gap of 1 mm per day, which is divided into 0.25 mm or smaller increments. External fixators or intramedullary lengthening nails provide relative mechanical stability and facilitate the distraction process. When sufficient distraction has occurred, the regenerated bone is allowed to heal. Lengthening of 3 to 6 cm or 20% of bone length is usually accomplished with few major complications. Greater amounts of lengthening are associated with an exponential increase in complications.

Overall, studies report that limb lengthening is associated with substantial rates of complications that range from 50% to 100%.[18,19] Complications are so frequent that authors have tried to classify them by severity, the need for further surgery, prolongation of treatment, or lasting sequelae. To help assess the complexity of limb lengthening for an individual patient, the Limb Lengthening and Reconstruction Society developed the LLRS AIM Index (a mnemonic indicating seven pretreatment domains: location and number of deformities, leg-length inequality at maturity, risk factors, soft-tissue coverage, angular deformity, infection/bone quality, and motion/stability of the joints above and below),[20] which serves to quantify the severity of lower limb deformities. The index provides a method for communicating the complexity of a deformity by a scale that is reliable and has good interrater and intraobserver validity. However, based on expert opinion, the LLRS AIM Index does not separate congenital versus acquired etiologies and has not yet been tested to prove that it correlates with the difficulty of lengthening. In children, unlike in patients of other ages, concomitant deformity does not always influence the complication rate. In a 2014 study, only the proportion of limb-length discrepancy predicted complications.[19] The techniques of lengthening continue to evolve to address potential complications.

External fixation systems are frequently used to provide distraction in limb lengthening. Lengthening fixators consisting of monolateral frames and lengthening rails are easy to apply and are less cumbersome for patients. However, they have limited ability to progressively correct deformities. Circular external fixator systems, originally popularized for lengthening by Ilizarov, allow the progressive correction of deformities in multiple planes and can be adjusted during the lengthening process. They also can be extended across joints to protect them from subluxation. Originally described with transfixing fine wires, modifications that use half pins have decreased soft-tissue complications and improved frame stability. Distraction and deformity correction occur by adjusting the uprights and hinges attached to the frames in a particular order. Computer-assisted distraction and deformity correction systems use six struts attached to a circular external fixator. The struts can be adjusted, based on computer calculations, to simultaneously correct length, angulation, translation, and rotation about a virtual hinge, thereby reducing the time required for the correction while increasing the correction accuracy.[21]

Pins and wires may cause neurovascular injury when they are placed percutaneously. However, detailed knowledge of the cross-sectional anatomy and the use of nerve stimulators will reduce neurovascular risks. The complications are associated with pin infections and usually can be managed with antibiotics. In the long term, pins and wires may loosen or break if stress levels are exceeded, but sturdy constructs will minimize this risk. In most designs, the fixation system is strong enough to allow for weight bearing, thereby facilitating bone formation.

To address complications of external fixation, the length of time in the external device can be reduced by also using internal fixation with intramedullary nails or plates. Because of the concern about deep infection with such hybrid systems, completely implanted intramedullary lengtheners have been developed. The two FDA-approved devices for intramedullary lengthening are the Intramedullary Skeletal Kinetic Distractor (Orthofix) and the PRECICE nail (Ellipse Technology).[22] The Intramedullary Skeletal Kinetic Distractor has a clutch mechanism that is triggered by limb rotation of 3° to 7° to achieve elongation. Control of distraction has been reported as being inconsistent (either going too fast or too slowly) and cannot be reversed. The PRECICE nail has a magnetic actuator drive that uses an external electromagnetic activator to control the rate and direction of the nail telescoping. Blocking screws are necessary to correct and prevent deformity during lengthening. Both nail systems lengthen along the anatomic axis and have potential mechanical complications. In the femur, where the mechanical axis is substantially different from the anatomic axis, lengthening can result in valgus deformity that may require other corrective procedures. One centimeter of femoral lengthening results in a 1° increase of genu valgum.[23] Results show that the Intramedullary Skeletal Kinetic Distractor may be inferior to lengthening with an external fixator over an intramedullary nail.[24] Compared with monorail fixators, femoral lengthening with the PRECICE nail had fewer complications, was better tolerated, and thought to have a better cosmetic result by patients[25] (**Figure 1**). Joint subluxation with intramedullary lengthening still remains a concern.

Loss of joint motion frequently occurs during limb lengthening. Physical therapy, splinting, and botulinum toxin injections are used to avoid contractures and loss of motion while the soft tissues are being stretched. Loss of motion may signal joint subluxation. Preventing joint subluxation may require preoperative reconstructive surgery to increase the stability of the joints, and external frames may need to be extended, with hinges across the joints. This modification is especially crucial with lengthening of a congenital deficiency. The lengthening process may need to be slowed if loss of motion or joint subluxation occurs. Secondary soft-tissue releases for the hip adductors, the quadriceps, the hamstrings, and the gastrocnemius may be needed. Joint motion may improve up to 2 years after lengthening, but aggressive physical therapy and splinting during the process is required. Recovery of lost muscle strength should also be a major goal of rehabilitation.

In 2013, researchers found electrophysiologic evidence of nerve dysfunction during lengthening in 7 of 36 patients, which also was more common when lengthening was being performed for congenital etiologies.[26] Nerve changes may not be correlated with the amount of lengthening but rather the rate of distraction or double-level lengthening. Neurologic signs were found in three patients with electromyographic changes. The peroneal nerve was more susceptible than the tibial nerve, especially in tibial lengthening. Twenty-five percent of the patients undergoing lengthening after a traumatic event had preoperative electromyographic changes not detected clinically, and the electromyographic changes were found to deteriorate with lengthening. If the distraction is slowed or stopped, nerve symptoms usually are resolved. Nerve decompression before lengthening may prevent complications.

Bone healing complications occur with premature or delayed consolidation, angular displacement, fractures, and bending of the regenerated bone. Fractures occur most often after lengthening for a congenital deficiency in children younger than 9 years with lengthening greater than 15% and a latency period of less than 7 days.[27] Bone consolidation must be followed closely, and the rate of distraction should be adjusted accordingly. Proven techniques do not exist for predicting the strength of the regenerated bone or determining the time for fixator removal, although most look for cortical bone formation on at least three cortices. Intramedullary nails and submuscular plates can provide supplemental stability. Bone formation enhancement techniques have included low-intensity pulsed ultrasound, pulsed electromagnetic fields, and the use of diphosphonates and bone morphogenetic proteins,[28] all of which are off-label uses for pediatric applications. Cultured, expanded bone marrow, stem cells, and platelet-rich plasma injections seem to produce encouraging results, but they require additional surgical procedures and specialized capabilities for processing the cells.

As more aggressive lengthening and reconstruction plans become possible, procedures before skeletal maturity are required. Maintenance of residual growth is paramount for a limb that is already short. Factors that have been found to maintain good residual growth following lengthening include lengthening before the pubertal growth spurt (girls younger than 9 years and boys younger than 12 years), interval between the lengthenings of greater than 3 years, lengthening less than 30% of the initial segment, and no more than two lengthenings during growth.[29]

LIMB DEFICIENCIES

Prenatal ultrasonography can detect most upper and lower limb deficiencies, but they will be undiagnosed in 20% to 25% of prenatal patients.[30] The rate of detection is greatest for those involving the femoral segment. Both femoral and tibial segments should be examined because most mothers surveyed preferred to have prenatal detection to allow for prenatal counseling. Most children with lower limb deficiencies will require orthopaedic surgery.

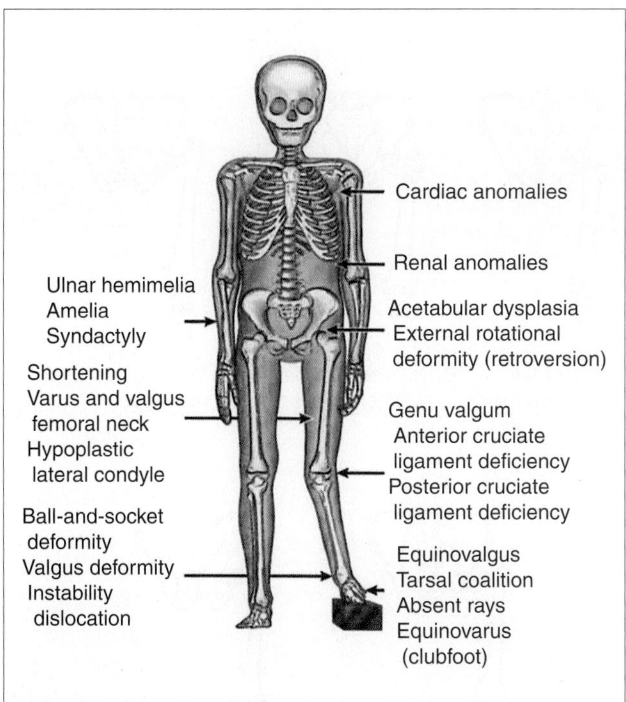

FIGURE 2 Illustration shows fibular deficiency and associated anomalies.

The genetic mechanisms involved in limb deficiencies are areas of active research. From animal studies, the gene *FGF10* is known to be necessary for limb development. *FGF10* induces formation of the apical ectodermal ridge. In a 2012 population-based study of limb deficiencies without known cause, researchers found that, in non-Hispanic Caucasian infants, variants of *FGF10* increased the risk for a wide range of nonsyndromic limb deficiencies.[31] Recent epidemiologic studies have linked slightly increased risks for limb deficiency to maternal active smoking and passive exposure to cigarette smoke, increased nitrates in drinking water, and increased maternal dietary consumption of caffeine.

Fibular Deficiency

Fibular deficiency is the most common lower limb deficiency and has a prevalence of 7 to 20 per 1 million births.[32] Fibular deficiency is part of a spectrum of anomalies thought to be related to a defect in the so-called femoral-fibular-ulnar developmental field.[33] Somatic gene dysfunction, involving WNT7A and sonic hedgehog, is thought to play a role. It is associated with femoral hypoplasia, including proximal femoral focal deficiency (PFFD), genu valgum, lateral femoral condylar hypoplasia, cruciate ligament deficiency, tibial bowing and shortening, ankle instability, tarsal coalition, deficient foot rays, and ulnar deficiency in the upper limb (**Figure 2**). The most common classification is based on the amount of deficient fibula.[33] However, this system has poor correlation with treatment. Other researchers have proposed a classification system based on the clinical deformity, which helps direct treatment[34] (**Figure 3**). Salvage of the foot is considered in patients who have three or more foot rays that are stable enough for weight bearing. Because upper limb anomalies are common, upper limb function also must be considered before foot amputation.

Milder degrees of limb shortening can be managed with epiphysiodesis, although linear growth inhibition patterns are seen in 82% of patients, making such predictions less precise.[32,35] Limb lengthening may be used to correct greater degrees of shortening, but the process is fraught with a high rate of complications, including tibial bowing and ankle displacement. Resection of the fibular anlage has been demonstrated to reduce

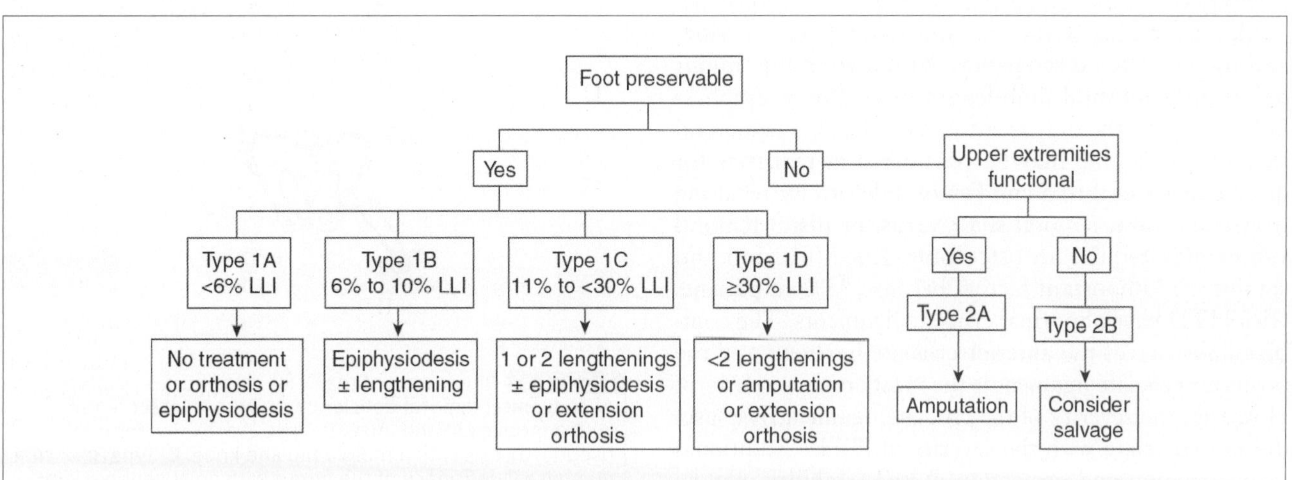

FIGURE 3 Flowchart shows the Birch classification and algorithm for the management of fibular deficiency. LLI = limb-length inequality

the recurrence of genu valgum, valgus tibial deformity, and lateral ankle displacement with lengthening procedures.[36] Reconstruction of the lateral malleolus has been described using the cartilaginous fibular remnant or the contralateral proximal fibula.[37,38] Reorientation of the valgus deformity in the distal tibial epiphysis and/or the subtalar joint can be managed with osteotomies and facilitates a stable weight-bearing ankle with reduced ankle displacement during lengthening.

Regardless of how the limb-length inequality is managed, fibular deficiency is frequently associated with progressive genu valgum that may require additional treatment. If identified and sufficient growth remains, guided growth can correct the deformity.[39] Recurrence after osteotomy or guided growth frequently occurs if growth is remaining, and overcorrection may be appropriate to compensate for the expected recurrence.

Although cruciate ligament deficiency accompanies knee concerns for many patients, a long-term follow-up study showed that only 20% of the patients had occasional instability during sporting activities, and none required bracing treatment or surgery.[40] Previous studies have suggested hypertrophy of the ligament of Humphrey provides extra stability in the absence of the cruciate ligaments.

Femoral Deficiency

As discussed previously, femoral deficiency may be part of a spectrum of disorders with fibular deficiency because they frequently occur together. The classification of PFFD alone has been expanded to include the spectrum of femoral deficiency and is primarily radiographic in design. A 2007 classification system has incorporated this wide spectrum of femoral deficiency with an approach to treatment[41] (**Figure 4**). Considerations for the treatment of limb-length discrepancy depend on the stability and mobility of the hip (either primarily or with reconstruction), the integrity of the foot and ankle, knee function, and the projected discrepancy. With a good hip, minor deformity, and mild limb-length discrepancy, epiphysiodesis may be the only treatment needed. Contralateral femoral shortening may be considered at maturity for discrepancies of 2 to 5 cm. Femoral deformity resulting from coxa vara, femoral shaft varus, or distal femoral valgus may require an osteotomy. Knee function and stability are important factors because 95% of patients with PFFD have abnormal cruciate ligaments. The combined absence of the anterior cruciate ligament and the posterior cruciate ligament is the most common pattern. However, the severity of the cruciate ligament dysplasia did not correlate with the severity of PFFD. Additional reconstruction and protection of knee stability may be needed if femoral lengthening is to be performed.

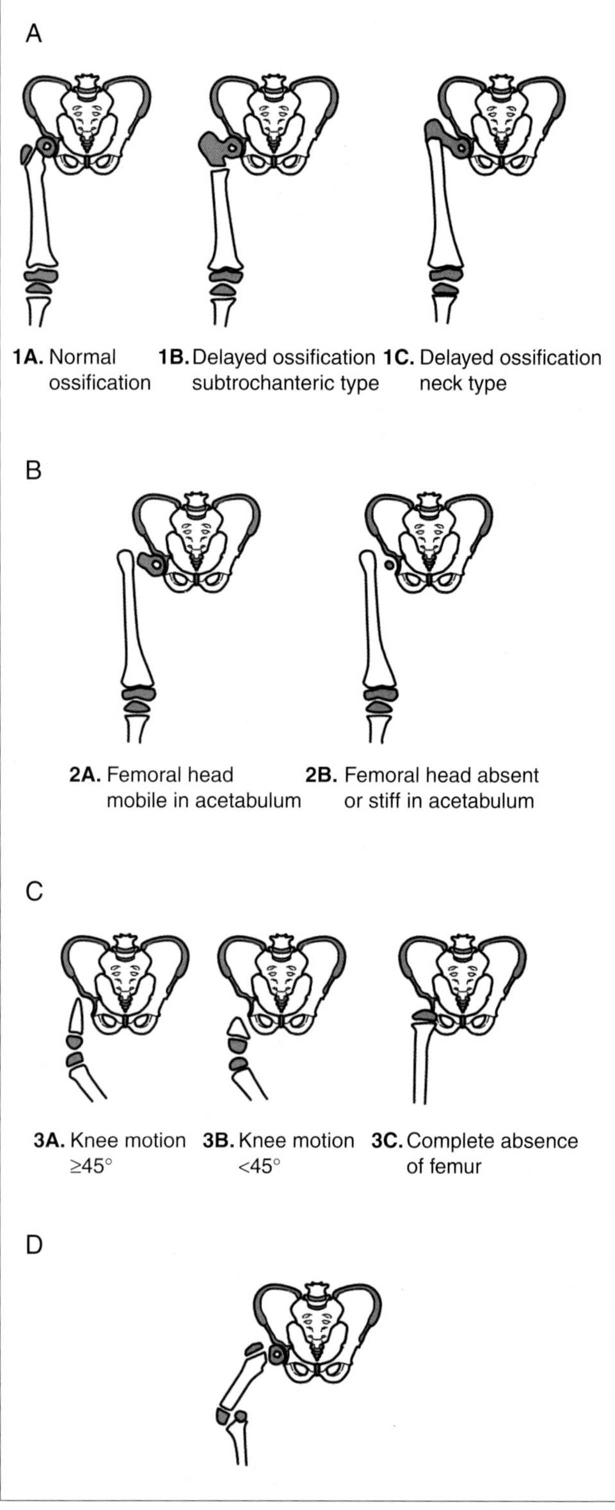

FIGURE 4 Illustration of the Paley classification system of congenital femoral deficiency. **A**, Type 1: intact femur with a mobile hip and knee. **B**, Type 2: proximal femoral pseudarthrosis with a mobile hip and knee. **C**, Type 3: diaphyseal deficiency of the femur with an absent hip joint and a mobile knee. **D**, Type 4: distal femoral deficiency.

A Van Nes rotationplasty is a viable alternative for initial treatment of PFFD or can be used after failed limb reconstruction for PFFD.[42,43] This procedure fuses the short femur to the tibia, thus creating a combined thigh bone, and rotates the ankle 90° into the plane to function as a knee. Despite the unusual appearance of the limb with the foot rotated, no differences were found in the long-term Medical Outcomes Study 36-Item Short Form or other health-related quality-of-life measures.[42] A literature review demonstrated good to excellent results in 56 of 59 patients.[43] Those with poor results had associated fibular deficiency and three foot rays or fewer, thus indicating that good foot and ankle function is necessary for a good outcome.

If the hip in femoral deficiency cannot be stabilized, lengthening and rotationplasty options are rarely considered. Many patients may consider an extension prosthesis that fits over the foot without surgery. Alternatively, surgery with fusion of the residual femur to the tibial segment produces a combined bone that serves as a thigh segment. Amputation of the foot then facilitates prosthetic fitting with a transfemoral prosthesis.

Tibial Deficiency

Tibial deficiency is the least common lower limb deficiency and has a prevalence of one per 1 million births.[44] In some families, tibial deficiencies may be inherited, often as an autosomal dominant trait. Associated anomalies, such as great toe polydactyly, toe syndactyly, absent foot rays, tarsal coalition, hip dysplasia, femoral duplication, cleft hand or foot, radial deficiency, thumb hypoplasia, congenital scoliosis, tethered cord, and spinal dysraphism, occur in 78% of patients with tibial deficiency. Unlike fibular deficiency, other organ systems are frequently involved. Patients may have cardiopulmonary, gastrointestinal, and genitourinary anomalies; hydrocephalus; blindness; and ear malformations.

The four-part Jones classification is the most accepted classification system and is based on the presence or absence of the proximal or distal tibia (**Figure 5, A**). Based on a 2015 review of 95 patients with tibial deficiency, an additional classification (type 5) was proposed, wherein there is hypoplasia of the tibia, but both the proximal and distal tibial physes are present[44] (**Figure 5, B**).

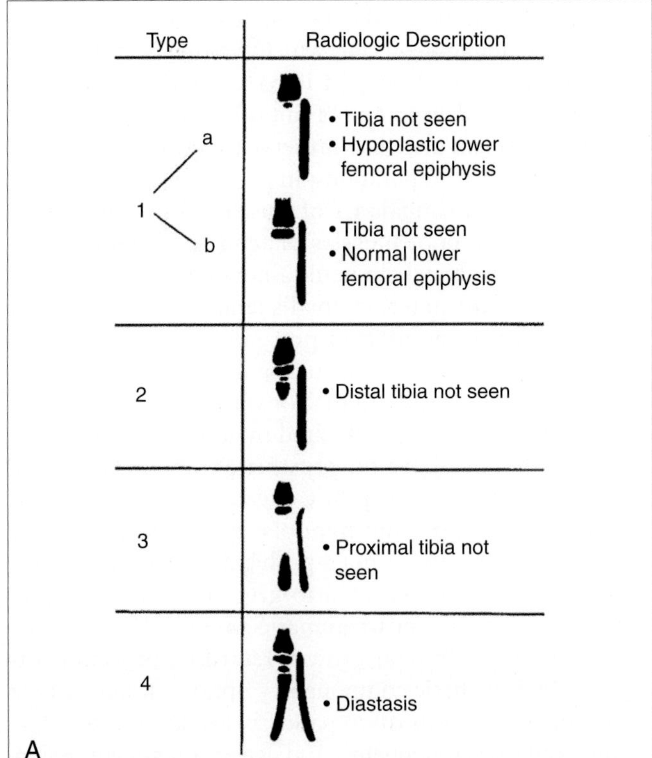

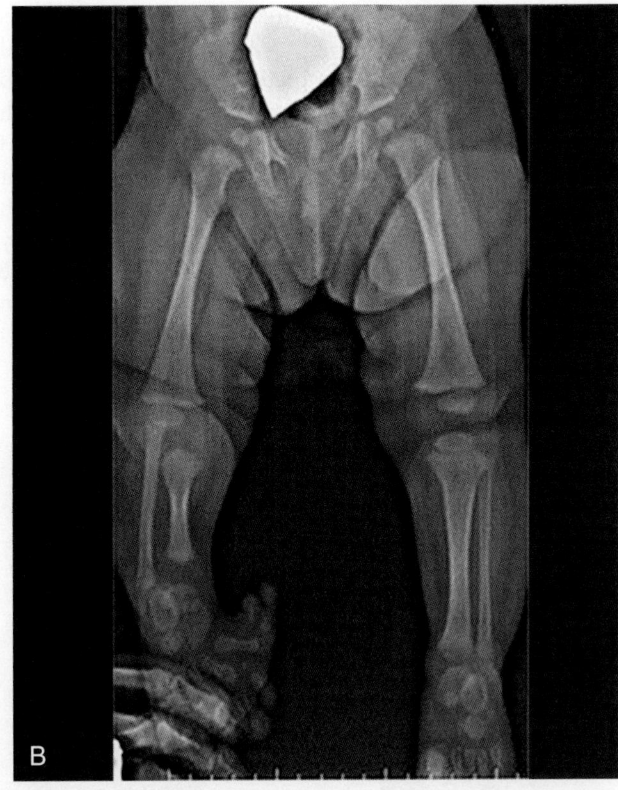

FIGURE 5 **A**, Illustration of the four-part Jones classification of tibial deficiency. **B**, AP radiograph of the tibiae of a patient with the proposed type 5 classification characterized by hypoplasia of the tibia; however, both the proximal and distal tibial physes are present. (Panel **A** republished with permission of British Editorial Society of Bone and Joint Surgery from Jones D, Barnes J, Lloyd-Roberts GC: Congenital aplasia and dysplasia of the tibia with intact fibula: Classification and management. *J Bone Joint Surg Br* 1978;60[1]:31-39, and panel **B** republished with permission from Clinton R, Birch JG: Congenital tibial deficiency: A 37 year experience at one institution. *J Pediatr Orthop* 2015;35[4]:385-390.)

Treatment depends on the presence or absence of active knee extension and knee stability. Reconstruction without active knee extension, by centralizing the fibula (Brown procedure), is unsuccessful, and knee disarticulation is recommended. With active knee extension, a vestigial proximal tibial segment can be elongated by synostosis to the fibula. A modified Syme ankle disarticulation or a Boyd amputation at the end of the fibula can facilitate prosthetic fitting with below-knee prostheses. Patients with some preservation of the distal tibia may be candidates for lengthening and reconstruction of the ankle with preservation of the foot.

Transverse Deficiency

Congenital transverse deficiency is much less common in the lower limbs compared with the upper limbs. It is important to distinguish congenital transverse deficiencies from congenital amputations resulting from amniotic bands. Congenital deficiencies are suspected if nubbins caused by failure formation are present. Nubbins may have an indentation but no band where they attach to the limb and may have small nail remnants (**Figure 6**). Amputations caused by amniotic band syndrome frequently have manifestations of bands elsewhere in the limbs or the body, and the residual skeletal structures are completely normal proximal to the loss. Congenital deficiencies are associated with increased risks for other anomalies, and screening renal ultrasonographs should be obtained to look for silent urogenital anomalies. In addition, terminal overgrowth problems seen with transosseous amputations caused by amniotic bands do not occur in congenital transverse deficiencies. The congenital transverse deficiency can be managed with a prosthetic fitting based on the level of the deficiency.

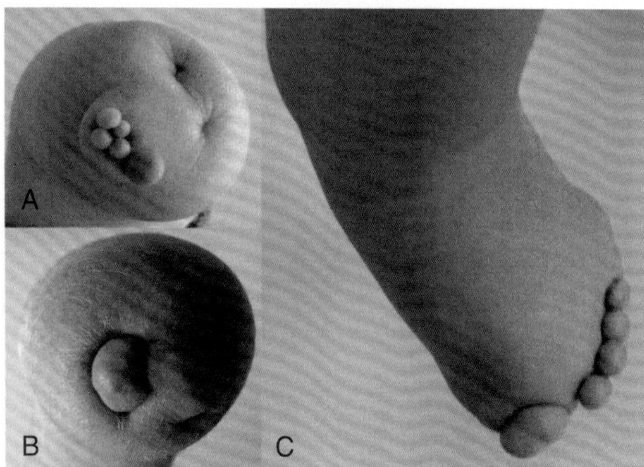

FIGURE 6 **A** through **C**, Clinical photographs of nubbins caused by failure of formation resulting from limb deficiency, not by amputation caused by amniotic bands.

AMPUTATIONS AND PROSTHETICS

Surgical Techniques

In children, amputations through joints are preferred to avoid the complication of terminal or appositional bony overgrowth. The biologically active skeleton of children produces bone spikes and extensions after transosseous amputations, resulting in pain and bony protrusions through the skin. Multiple surgeries may be needed to manage these protrusions throughout the growing years. Why this problem is avoided with disarticulations in children is not completely clear. The concept of a protective cartilage cap is used to manage overgrowth, which may explain why terminal overgrowth does not occur in disarticulations. If a transosseous amputation is needed, using a cartilaginous remnant, such as a metatarsal or a proximal/distal fibula plugged into the distal canal, may reduce overgrowth. The proximal fibula can be used in transtibial amputations as a secondary procedure to reduce the frequency of revisions needed for bony overgrowth.[45]

Although maintaining bone length is important for function, insufficient soft-tissue coverage with skin grafts may result in a limb that cannot tolerate prosthetic wear. The most durable grafts are composed of full-thickness skin and subcutaneous fat, which is mobile. At the ankle, maintaining the heel pad is particularly helpful and allows for end bearing. Maintaining muscle coverage and attachment also may preserve function, particularly in transfemoral amputations. In partial foot amputations, there may be an imbalance of muscle pull. Reattachment of the remnants of muscles or tendons to more proximal locations may help maintain balance. For example, reattaching the anterior tibialis tendon to the talus in a midfoot-level amputation prevents the gastrocnemius from being unopposed, resulting in equinus.

Even though disarticulations are preferred in children, they are poorly tolerated in adults because ample space is not available for prosthetic componentry if the limbs are the same length. Congenital deficiencies usually have enough limb hypoplasia, so space for prosthetic componentry is not a problem. However, children whose bones are expected to grow fully, for example, those sustaining a posttraumatic amputation, may have to undergo additional growth-retarding procedures to enhance prosthetic componentry options at maturity. A 10-cm limb-length discrepancy is needed for standard knee and foot components, and newer component designs may require more space.

Prosthetic Management

Children should be fitted with lower limb prostheses when they begin to pull to stand. Historically, the initial prosthetic knee did not have a joint or the joint was permanently locked to provide stability while the child was learning to ambulate. Early fitting with an articulating knee, however, has been shown to reduce the adoption of clearance adaptations, especially circumduction, as ambulation develops.[46] Most children with lower limb amputations respond to physical therapy and adapt quickly. Those with unilateral lower limb amputation will have diminished walking speed, distance, and functional balance compared with control subjects. Improved postural control and balance are associated with faster walking speeds. Because many children with limb deficiencies have associated deformities, the prosthesis may need to be adjusted to compensate for and maintain appropriate mechanical alignment. Children undergoing guided growth treatment may need prosthetic components that allow for adjustment as bony alignment changes. Radiographs can be helpful in correctly aligning the prosthesis.[47]

Prosthetic designs for adults are rapidly improving, and some of these features are beneficial for the pediatric population. A wide variety of suspension silicone/gel liners, especially those that do not require additional length for prosthetic attachment, have greatly improved prosthetic suspension in this very active population. Increased durability of the components, complex foot systems with vertical loading, energy storage and return, and multiaxial rotation and deflection also are important prosthetic improvements that are applicable for both adult and pediatric patients. Dynamic response and energy return are important for children. Many children participate in high-level physical activities, and prosthetic feet specifically designed for high-level sporting activities are becoming available in pediatric sizes. A 2014 study showed that, although high-performance prosthetic feet may improve gait mechanics, they do not affect patient measurements on sports/physical functioning or happiness scales of the Pediatric Outcomes Data Collection Instrument. Both scales were noted to decline when comparing children 4 to 9 years of age with adolescents 10 to 19 years of age.[48] Microprocessor-controlled components for prosthetic knee and ankle joints are available for the adolescent population and allow greater gait adaptation for a variety of real-world situations.

Outcomes

Amputation often is considered a failure of medical science. In treatment discussions, patients and physicians must carefully weigh all the risks and benefits of amputation versus reconstruction. Children with limb loss have participation and health-related quality-of-life goals equal to children without limb loss.[49] However, adolescents with lower limb loss often have less diverse participation and less interaction in social and skill-based activities. If amputation is required, the family should be advised that children who undergo multiple surgical attempts at reconstruction before amputation have lower global function, more pain, and poorer adjustment to their limitations compared with those having amputation as an initial procedure.[50] Adults who had amputations for fibular deficiency as children have an average to above average quality of life when compared with the able-bodied adult population.[51] Most individuals with a congenital limb deficiency live ordinary lives. However, adults do report increased prevalence of chronic pain and early retirement.

SUMMARY

Lower limb-length discrepancy can be associated with altered gait, increased knee pain, and less parental satisfaction concerning the child's condition. Radiographic assessment methods have improved and now offer reduced radiation exposure. These assessments can aid in measuring and predicting lower limb-length discrepancy. Percutaneous drilling is preferred over implant-only techniques for epiphysiodesis. Techniques for limb lengthening are evolving with the use of intramedullary devices to reduce the high complication rates of limb lengthening. Limb-length equalization techniques are often used in the treatment of lower limb deficiencies. Improvements in ultrasonography have increased the prenatal detection rate of limb deficiencies. Refinements in the classification systems for fibular, femoral, and tibial deficiency are helpful in clinical decision making. In children with congenital limb loss, the presence of nubbins predicts congenital deficiency instead of amputation by amniotic bands. In children who have amputations to manage limb anomalies, tumors, or trauma, disarticulation or cartilage capping procedures should be considered to reduce terminal overgrowth. Children with lower limb amputation can expect a high quality of life because of improving prosthetic designs.

KEY STUDY POINTS

- Skeletal age is important in the accurate estimation of lower limb-length discrepancy and the timing of epiphysiodesis, especially during the adolescent growth spurt.
- Percutaneous drilling techniques are preferred over those with implants only for epiphysiodesis.
- Lower limb lengthening using implantable lengthening nails is still associated with high but improved complication rates compared with external fixation.
- Improving classification systems in fibular, femoral, and tibial deficiencies can help guide clinical decision making.
- The presence of nubbins indicates a congenital deficiency, not amputation caused by amniotic bands.

ANNOTATED REFERENCES

1. Drnach M, Kreger A, Corliss C, Kocher D: Limb length discrepancies among 8- to 12-year-old children who are developing typically. *Pediatr Phys Ther* 2012;24(4):334-337.
2. Kiapour A, Abdelgawad AA, Goel VK, Souccar A, Terai T, Ebraheim NA: Relationship between limb length discrepancy and load distribution across the sacroiliac joint: A finite element study. *J Orthop Res* 2012;30(10):1577-1580.
3. Gordon JE, Davis LE: Leg length discrepancy: The natural history (and what do we really know). *J Pediatr Orthop* 2019;39(6 suppl 1):S10-S13.

   A review of literature found consensus that >2 cm leg-length discrepancy is a problem and some evidence that >5 mm can lead to long-term hip, knee, and lower back problems. Level of evidence: V.
4. Lee KM, Chung CY, Gwon DK, et al: Parental perspectives on leg length discrepancy. *J Pediatr Orthop B* 2012;21(2):146-149.
5. Neelly K, Wallmann HW, Backus CJ: Validity of measuring leg length with a tape measure compared to a computed tomography scan. *Physiother Theory Pract* 2013;29(6):487-492.
6. Khakharia S, Bigman D, Fragomen AT, Pavlov H, Rozbruch SR: Comparison of PACS and hard-copy 51-inch radiographs for measuring leg length and deformity. *Clin Orthop Relat Res* 2011;469(1):244-250.
7. Aaron A, Weinstein D, Thickman D, Eilert R: Comparison of orthoroentgenography and computed tomography in the measurement of limb-length discrepancy. *J Bone Joint Surg Am* 1992;74(6):897-902.
8. Escott BG, Ravi B, Weathermon AC, et al: EOS low-dose radiography: A reliable and accurate upright assessment of lower-limb lengths. *J Bone Joint Surg Am* 2013;95(23):e18 31-e1837.
9. Westh RN, Menelaus MB: A simple calculation for the timing of epiphysial arrest: A further report. *J Bone Joint Surg Br* 1981;63(1):117-119.
10. Anderson M, Green WT, Messner MB: Growth and predictions of growth in the lower extremities. *J Bone Joint Surg Am* 1963;45:1-14.
11. Moseley CF: A straight-line graph for leg-length discrepancies. *J Bone Joint Surg Am* 1977;59(2):174-179.
12. Paley D, Bhave A, Herzenberg JE, Bowen JR: Multiplier method for predicting limb-length discrepancy. *J Bone Joint Surg Am* 2000;82(10):1432-1446.
13. Markov MR, Jackson TJ, Smith CM, Jo CH, Birch JG: Timing of epiphysiodesis to correct leg-length discrepancy: A comparison of prediction methods. *J Bone Joint Surg Am* 2018;100:1217-1222.

    Seventy-seven patients undergoing epiphysiodesis surgery were followed up. Use of skeletal age improved prediction over chronologic age, and the multiplier method was the least accurate method. Level of evidence: III.
14. Canale ST, Christian CA: Techniques for epiphysiodesis about the knee. *Clin Orthop Relat Res* 1990;255:81-85.
15. Horn J, Gunderson RB, Wensaas A, Steen H: Percutaneous epiphysiodesis in the proximal tibia by a single-portal approach: Evaluation by radiostereometric analysis. *J Child Orthop* 2013;7(4):295-300.
16. Bayhan IA, Karatas AF, Rogers KJ, Bowen JR, Thacker MM: Comparing percutaneous physeal epiphysiodesis and eight-plate epiphysiodesis for the treatment of limb length discrepancy. *J Pediatr Orthop* 2017;37(5):323-327.

    This study compared 48 percutaneous epiphysiodeses and 24 dual eight-plate epiphysiodeses about the knee. The percutaneous method resulted in greater correction, fewer complications, and fewer additional procedures. Level of evidence: III.
17. Ilharreborde B, Gaumetou E, Souchet P, et al: Efficacy and late complications of percutaneous epiphysiodesis with transphyseal screws. *J Bone Joint Surg Br* 2012;94(2):270-275.
18. Hasler CC, Krieg AH: Current concepts of leg lengthening. *J Child Orthop* 2012;6(2):89-104.
19. Oostenbroek HJ, Brand R, van Roermund PM, Castelein RM: Paediatric lower limb deformity correction using the Ilizarov technique: A statistical analysis of factors affecting the complication rate. *J Pediatr Orthop B* 2014;23(1):26-31.
20. McCarthy JJ, Iobst CA, Rozbruch SR, Sabharwal S, Eismann EA: Limb Lengthening and Reconstruction Society AIM Index reliably assesses lower limb deformity. *Clin Orthop Relat Res* 2013;471(2):621-627.
21. Solomin LN, Paley D, Shchepkina EA, Vilensky VA, Skomoroshko PV: A comparative study of the correction of femoral deformity between the Ilizarov apparatus and Ortho-SUV Frame. *Int Orthop* 2014;38(4):865-872.
22. Rozbruch SR, Birch JG, Dahl MT, Herzenberg JE: Motorized intramedullary nail for management of limb-length discrepancy and deformity. *J Am Acad Orthop Surg* 2014;22(7):403-409.
23. Burghardt RD, Paley D, Specht SC, Herzenberg JE: The effect on mechanical axis deviation of femoral lengthening with an intramedullary telescopic nail. *J Bone Joint Surg Br* 2012;94(9):1241-1245.
24. Mahboubian S, Seah M, Fragomen AT, Rozbruch SR: Femoral lengthening with lengthening over a nail has fewer complications than intramedullary skeletal kinetic distraction. *Clin Orthop Relat Res* 2012;470(4):1221-1231.
25. Laubscher M, Mitchell C, Timms A, Goodier D, Calder P: Outcomes following femoral lengthening: An initial comparison of Precice intramedullary nail and lengthening with the LRS external fixator monorail system. *Bone Joint J* 2016;98-B(10):1382-1388.

    A comparison of 20 PRECICE and 13 LRS lengthenings showed that the intramedullary technique had fewer complications with better implant tolerance and cosmetic results. Level of evidence: III.

26. Simpson AH, Halliday J, Hamilton DF, Smith M, Mills K: Limb lengthening and peripheral nerve function—Factors associated with deterioration of conduction. *Acta Orthop* 2013;84(6):579-584.

27. Launay F, Younsi R, Pithioux M, Chabrand P, Bollini G, Jouve JL: Fracture following lower limb lengthening in children: A series of 58 patients. *Orthop Traumatol Surg Res* 2013;99(1):72-79.

28. Sabharwal S: Enhancement of bone formation during distraction osteogenesis: Pediatric applications. *J Am Acad Orthop Surg* 2011;19(2):101-111.

29. Journeau P, Lascombes P, Barbier D, Popkov D: Residual bone growth after lengthening procedures. *J Child Orthop* 2016;10:613-617.

    A review of 150 patients with 207 lengthened bone segments demonstrated better growth with surgery before the pubertal growth spurt, more than 3 years between procedures, less than 30% lengthened, and two or less procedures during growth. Level of evidence: IV.

30. Dicke JM, Piper SL, Goldfarb CA: The utility of ultrasound for the detection of fetal limb abnormalities: A 20-year single-center experience. *Prenat Diagn* 2015;35(4):348-353.

31. Browne ML, Carter TC, Kay DM, et al: Evaluation of genes involved in limb development, angiogenesis, and coagulation as risk factors for congenital limb deficiencies. *Am J Med Genet A* 2012;158A(10):2463-2472.

32. Lewin SO, Opitz JM: Fibular a/hypoplasia: Review and documentation of the fibular developmental field. *Am J Med Genet Suppl* 1986;2:215-238.

33. Achterman C, Kalamchi A: Congenital deficiency of the fibula. *J Bone Joint Surg Br* 1979;61(2):133-137.

34. Birch JG, Lincoln TL, Mack PW, Birch CM: Congenital fibular deficiency: A review of thirty years' experience at one institution and a proposed classification system based on clinical deformity. *J Bone Joint Surg Am* 2011;93(12):1144-1151.

35. Hamdy RC, Makhdom AM, Saran N, Birch J: Congenital fibular deficiency. *J Am Acad Orthop Surg* 2014;22(4):246-255.

36. Radler C, Antonietti G, Ganger R, Grill F: Recurrence of axial malalignment after surgical correction in congenital femoral deficiency and fibular hemimelia. *Int Orthop* 2011;35(11):1683-1688.

37. El-Tayeby HM, Ahmed AA: Ankle reconstruction in type II fibular hemimelia. *Strategies Trauma Limb Reconstr* 2012;7(1):23-26.

38. Cavadas PC, Thione A: Reconstruction of the lateral malleolus in a type-Ib fibular hemimelia with a microvascular proximal fibular flap: A case report. *J Pediatr Orthop B* 2015;24(4):370-372.

39. Gyr BM, Colmer HG IV, Morel MM, Ferski GJ: Hemiepiphysiodesis for correction of angular deformity in pediatric amputees. *J Pediatr Orthop* 2013;33(7):737-742.

40. Crawford DA, Tompkins BJ, Baird GO, Caskey PM: The long-term function of the knee in patients with fibular hemimelia and anterior cruciate ligament deficiency. *J Bone Joint Surg Br* 2012;94(3):328-333.

41. Paley D, Standard SC: Lengthening reconstruction surgery: For congenital femoral deficiency, in Rozbruch SR, Ilizarov S, eds: *Limb Lengthening and Reconstruction Surgery*. New York, NY, Informa Healthcare, 2007, pp 393-428.

42. Ackman J, Altiok H, Flanagan A, et al: Long-term follow-up of Van Nes rotationplasty in patients with congenital proximal focal femoral deficiency. *Bone Joint J* 2013;95-B(2):192-198.

43. Canavese F, Samba A, Khan A, Dechelotte P, Krajbich JI: Rotationplasty as a salvage of failed primary limb reconstruction: Up to date review and case report. *J Pediatr Orthop B* 2014;23(3):247-253.

44. Clinton R, Birch JG: Congenital tibial deficiency: A 37-year experience at 1 institution. *J Pediatr Orthop* 2015;35(4):385-390.

45. Fedorak GT, Watts HG, Cuomo AV, et al: Osteocartilaginous transfer of the proximal part of the fibula for osseous overgrowth in children with congenital or acquired tibial amputation: Surgical technique and results. *J Bone Joint Surg Am* 2015;97(7):574-581.

46. Geil M, Coulter C: Analysis of locomotor adaptations in young children with limb loss in an early prosthetic knee prescription protocol. *Prosthet Orthot Int* 2014;38(1):54-61.

47. Mooney R, Carry P, Wylie E, et al: Radiographic parameters improve lower extremity prosthetic alignment. *J Child Orthop* 2013;7(6):543-550.

48. Jeans KA, Karol LA, Cummings D, Singhal K: Comparison of gait after Syme and transtibial amputation in children: Factors that may play a role in function. *J Bone Joint Surg Am* 2014;96(19):1641-1647.

49. Michielsen A, van Wijk I, Ketelaar M: Participation and health-related quality of life of Dutch children and adolescents with congenital lower limb deficiencies. *J Rehabil Med* 2011;43(7):584-589.

50. Dabaghi A, Haces F, Cadevila R: Is there a difference in function, outcome, satisfaction and adjustment to having a prosthesis in primary transtibial amputations versus multiple previous reconstructive procedures prior to amputation? *J Prosthet Orthot* 2015;27(2):40-43.

51. Walker JL, Knapp D, Minter C, et al: Adult outcomes following amputation or lengthening for fibular deficiency. *J Bone Joint Surg Am* 2009;91(4):797-804.

SECTION 6

Spine

Section Editor:
James O. Sanders, MD, FAAOS

CHAPTER 31

Early-Onset Scoliosis and Congenital Spine Disorders

MICHAEL P. GLOTZBECKER, MD • DANIEL J. HEDEQUIST, MD • JOHN B. EMANS, MD

ABSTRACT

Early-onset idiopathic scoliosis and congenital spine anomalies present unique treatment challenges because of the need to balance control of spinal and chest deformities while allowing growth of the spine and chest. To provide optimal care to patients, it is helpful to review treatment principles common to these conditions and understand the natural history, clinical and radiographic evaluations, nonsurgical and surgical treatment options, clinical outcomes, and complications related to these diagnoses.

Keywords: congenital scoliosis; early-onset idiopathic scoliosis; early-onset scoliosis; thoracic insufficiency syndrome

INTRODUCTION

Early-onset scoliosis (EOS) is an all-encompassing term, and it is inclusive of all etiologies of scoliosis in patients younger than 10 years.[1] The use of this age-based separation reflects the potential physiologic consequences of spinal deformity at a young age and the shared goals of treatment. A consideration uniquely important in this age group is the development of the lungs in the setting of a growing and changing thoracic cavity. The most commonly encountered forms of EOS, early-onset idiopathic scoliosis (EOIS) and congenital scoliosis, are discussed.

Dr. Glotzbecker or an immediate family member is a member of a speakers' bureau or has made paid presentations on behalf of Biomet, DePuy, a Johnson & Johnson Company, Medtronic, and Nuvasive; serves as a paid consultant to or is an employee of Nuvasive; and has received research or institutional support from PSSG and HSG. Dr. Emans or an immediate family member has received royalties from VEPTR II – Johnson and Johnson (Synthes spine) and serves as a paid consultant to or is an employee of Zimmer/Biomet. Neither Dr. Hedequist nor any immediate family member has received anything of value from or has stock or stock options held in a commercial company or institution related directly or indirectly to the subject of this chapter.

SPINE GROWTH AND LUNG DEVELOPMENT

The bony anatomy of the spinal column forms in utero at 3 to 5 weeks of gestation, and segmentation occurs between weeks 6 and 8.[2] Other organ systems are formed concurrently, which explains why abnormalities in these organ systems are commonly encountered in patients with congenital scoliosis.

Two-thirds of adult sitting height is achieved by the age of 5 years, 50% of the adult thoracic volume is achieved by the age of 10 years, and the most rapid increase in the number and volume of alveoli occur from birth to the age of 3 years.[3] For this reason, spinal deformity at a young age has been associated with pulmonary dysfunction, which in its most severe form presents as thoracic insufficiency syndrome.[4] Pulmonary function is dependent on adequate thoracic volume (height, width, and depth) and thoracic function (chest expansion and diaphragm contraction). For these reasons, treatment goals and strategies in EOS are directed at preserving growth of the spine and thoracic cavity to maximize lung function.

DEFINITIONS

The use of the term early onset is meant to distinguish patients who have substantial remaining growth of the spine and thorax such that this growth must be accounted for when making treatment decisions. EOS includes all etiologies (congenital, neuromuscular, syndromic, and idiopathic). The traditional classification of idiopathic scoliosis divided patients into groups based on age: infantile, younger than 3 years; juvenile, aged 3 years to younger than 10 years; and adolescent, aged 10 years and older. Although this terminology is still used, the treatment considerations are similar in the first two groups; therefore, it is probably more useful to consider both of these groups as having EOIS. A 2015 position statement grouped all patients younger than 10 years as having EOS.[1] However, because many studies have used the more historical terminology, that terminology will be used in this chapter.

Thoracic insufficiency syndrome is defined as the inability of the thorax to support normal respiration and growth.[4] The most common scenario for this diagnosis is encountered in patients with congenital scoliosis with a shortened spine, fused ribs, and a constricted hemithorax. The shortened spine and fused ribs lead to a reduction in thoracic volume and abnormal thoracic cage motion. However, the term thoracic insufficiency syndrome can be used for any patient with substantial spinal or thoracic deformity leading to inadequate pulmonary function. The thoracic lordosis associated with many types of spinal deformity can lead to a reduction in anterior-posterior chest depth as the spine moves toward the sternum. The clinical signs associated with thoracic insufficiency syndrome include loss of chest wall expansion, failure to thrive (delayed growth and poor weight gain), worsening thoracic deformity based on three-dimensional imaging studies, and a decline in pulmonary function. The patient may have restrictive lung disease, with a reduction in vital capacity and total lung capacity, leading to alveolar hypoventilation, hypoxic vasoconstriction, and eventually pulmonary artery hypertension or cor pulmonale.[5]

Given the heterogeneity of individuals with EOS, in 2014, there have been attempts to create a classification system.[6] The Classification of Early-Onset Scoliosis (C-EOS) system categorizes patients based on age, etiology, major Cobb angle, kyphosis, and progression (**Figure 1**). The C-EOS has excellent interobserver reliability and is being used in current research efforts to standardize communication as well as for correlation of patient characteristics with outcome data. Recent literature has begun to emerge to demonstrate the association of C-EOS and complication risk.[7]

GENERAL PRINCIPLES

Outcome Measures

Choosing the appropriate outcome measures in this patient population is challenging. Most research has focused on reporting changes in spinal and thoracic growth, such as the Cobb angle and the thoracic height before and after treatment.[8] However, it is unclear whether maintaining or improving spinal growth actually leads to better clinical outcomes. The Early-Onset Scoliosis Questionnaire has been developed and can be used as a disease-specific outcome measure.[9,10] It has been validated in several languages so that it can be used to compare outcomes

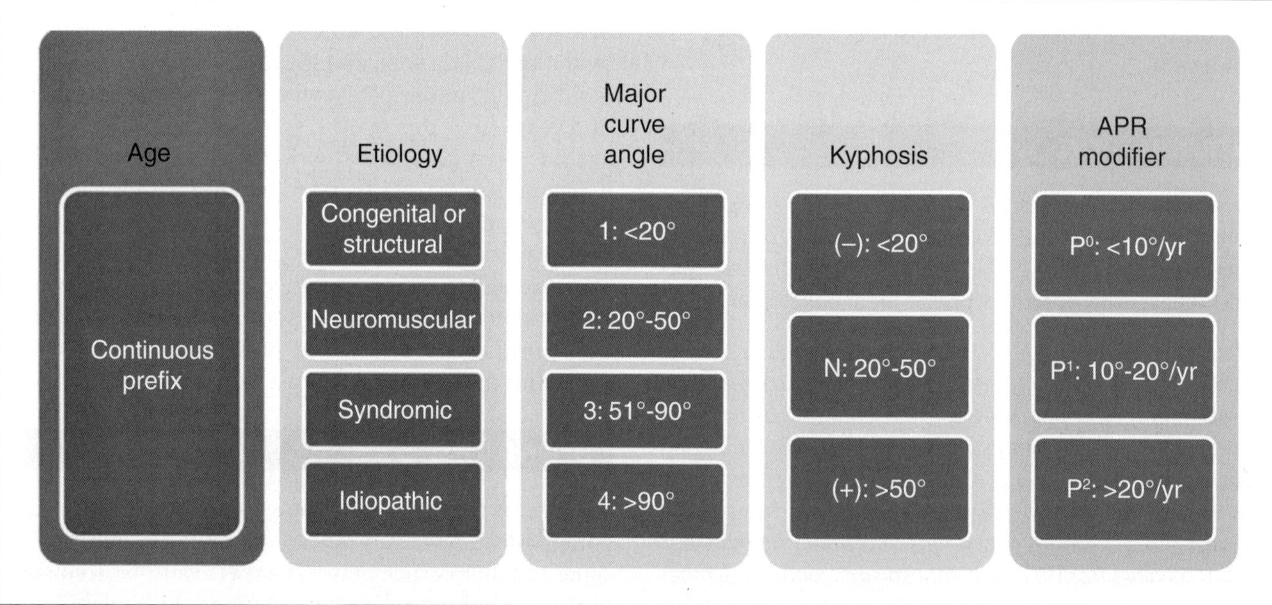

FIGURE 1 Illustration of the Classification of Early-Onset Scoliosis (C-EOS). This classification system consists of a continuous prefix (age), three core variables (etiology, major curve angle, and kyphosis), and an optional modifier (curve progression). APR = annual progression ratio, (−), N, and (+) = kyphosis variables, P = progression modifier. (Adapted with permission from Williams BA, Matsumoto H, McCalla DJ, et al: Development and initial validation of the Classification of Early-Onset Scoliosis (C-EOS). *J Bone Joint Surg Am* 2014;96[16]:1359-1367.)

between patients treated at different international centers. Combining patient-reported outcomes with radiographic and pulmonary functional data will likely aid in understanding the effects of treatment and observation on disease.

Management

The current management goals in EOS are to maximize thoracic volume and function, increase spine length, and maintain spine mobility throughout the child's growth while minimizing complications. Treatment decisions include both the type of treatment and the timing of intervention. Because the spinal deformity often includes a large portion of the spine, early definitive fusion is associated with poor outcomes.[11] Even in the absence of comorbid cardiac or pulmonary disease, patients with severe scoliosis who are younger than 5 years are at risk for long-term cardiopulmonary complications.[12,13]

Faced with a progressive deformity, a choice is often made between the effect of untreated progressive deformity versus the pulmonary growth restriction and loss of spinal height associated with spinal fusion. Less invasive options, such as bracing treatment or casting, may slow deformity progression and delay the need for surgery. Surgical intervention using growth-friendly instrumentation such as dual expandable growing rods, the vertical expandable prosthetic titanium rib (VEPTR; DePuy Synthes), growing rods such as MAGEC rods (Ellipse Technologies), tethers, or the SHILLA (Medtronic) growth guidance system can control a curve while preserving some growth of the spine and thoracic cavity. Earlier intervention may result in more complications and early spontaneous arthrodesis but may be required if the deformity is causing irreversible thoracic deformity and pulmonary compromise.[14,15] The development of the thorax should be the most heavily weighed factor in decision making. Although spinal imbalance and deformity can be improved at the end of growth, no such strategy exists to correct thoracic shape and dysfunction resulting from EOS.

EARLY-ONSET IDIOPATHIC SCOLIOSIS

Etiology

Because EOIS is less common than adolescent idiopathic scoliosis (AIS), it is important to rule out other causes of scoliosis such as neuromuscular or genetic conditions or an underlying spinal cord anomaly. By definition, EOIS has no clear underlying etiology. Intrauterine molding, a supine sleep position, and an undefined genetic contribution have all been postulated as causative factors. Previous terminology has divided the patient population into infantile (younger than 3 years) and juvenile (3 years to younger than 10 years) idiopathic scoliosis, but more current terminology combines these groups under the umbrella classification of EOIS, which includes all patients younger than 10 years.[1]

Natural History

Curves may resolve in many patients but may progress in some patients. A systematic review of the literature found that infantile scoliosis curves resolved in 573 patients, whereas the curves progressed in 333 patients.[16] Younger age and single curves have been postulated as predictive factors for progression, but the rib-vertebral angle difference (RVAD) is the most reliable indicator of curve progression[16,17] (**Figure 2**). When the RVAD is less than 20°, 83% of patients had resolution of the scoliosis. When the RVAD was greater than 20°, 84% of the patients had progressive curves. Subsequent studies have confirmed the usefulness of the RVAD in predicting curve progression in patients in this age group. The RVAD has traditionally been used for patients with infantile scoliosis and has not been applied to older patients with EOS (3 years to younger than 10 years).

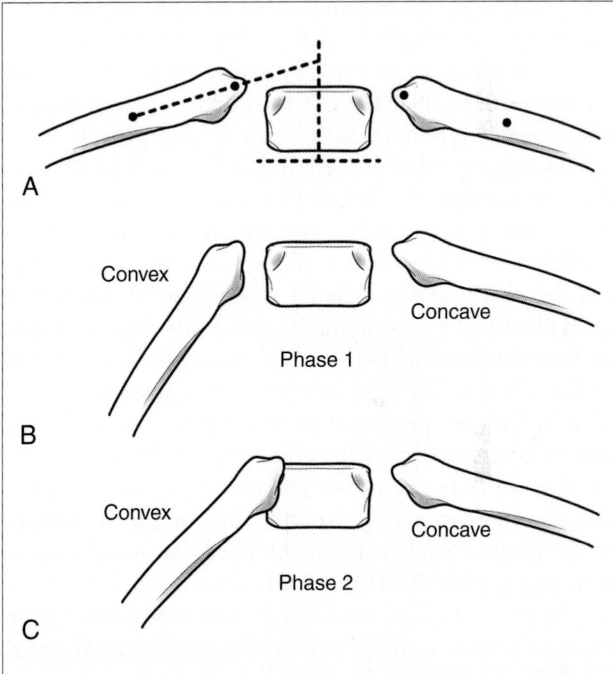

FIGURE 2 **A**, Illustration demonstrates the elements in the calculation of the rib-vertebral angle difference (RVAD). A line is drawn perpendicular to the end plate of the apical vertebra. A line is then drawn from the midpoint of the head of the rib to the midpoint of the neck of the rib on the convex side, and the created angle is calculated. The angle is calculated with the same method on the concave side. The difference between the two measurements is the RVAD. **B**, Illustration of the phase 1 relationship between the rib head and vertebra body demonstrating no overlap; an RVAD can be calculated. **C**, Illustration of the phase 2 relationship between the rib head and vertebra body with overlap of the rib on the vertebra, which is indicative of curve progression.

Clinical Evaluation

Patients with EOIS are more commonly males than females, especially patients younger than 3 years. Although left-sided curves are considered atypical in AIS, left-sided thoracic curves occur more frequently. Each patient with a spinal deformity should have a complete neurologic examination, including gait, patellar and Achilles reflexes, sensation, and abdominal reflexes. A skin examination should evaluate for cutaneous manifestations of a systemic condition or spinal dysraphism. Associated conditions include developmental dysplasia of the hip, inguinal hernia, and congenital heart disease.

Imaging

Standard radiographic examination includes full-length PA and lateral radiographs. Measurement of the Cobb angle and RVAD will help direct treatment decisions. The radiographic position should be considered when assessing curve progression. For example, a radiograph taken upright after the infant begins walking may cause a curve to appear larger than a previously obtained supine radiograph. Bending or traction radiographs are generally reserved for assessing flexibility and surgical planning. In patients with EOIS, MRI can be used to rule out associated neural axis abnormalities such as Chiari I malformation, syrinx, or tethered cord. In patients with EOIS who are younger than 3 years and have a curve greater than 20°, the rates of neural axis abnormality range from 13% to 22% despite normal neurologic examination findings and the absence of associated syndromes.[18,19] However, when identified, these anomalies frequently require neurosurgical intervention. Early recognition of these anomalies is clinically important, because they may cause irrevocable spine deformity progression. Recognition of tethering lesions is most accurately achieved by MRI, but spinal ultrasonography performed before 6 to 8 weeks of age will identify low conus, lipoma, and major anomalies of the filum while avoiding the need for anesthesia in very young patients. If there are neurologic abnormalities, deformed feet, urinary incontinence, or major spinal anomalies (such as diastematomyelia or congenital spinal dislocation), MRI is always indicated. In the setting of normal ultrasonography findings, an MRI should be pursued at a later date in a patient with a progressing curve.

Nonsurgical Management

In patients with a low RVAD, careful follow-up to assess for curve resolution is appropriate. In patients with an RVAD greater than 20°, there is a high likelihood of progression, and treatment should be considered. Options for nonsurgical management include casting, bracing treatment, or both.

In patients with a curve that is predicted to be progressive, bracing treatment or casting should be considered. Although bracing treatment has proved effective in a prospective randomized controlled trial of patients with AIS,[20] the efficacy of bracing treatment in younger patients is not supported by level I or level II evidence. However, other noninvasive treatments have recently gained popularity. Casting for EOS can be curative or, at a minimum, delay the need for surgical intervention.[21] In a study with minimum 5-year follow-up, 49% of children had improved scoliosis to less than 15° and 73% improved by at least 20°.[22] The rationale for cast treatment includes its ability to harness the rapid growth velocity that is common in young patients. It seems that patients with smaller Cobb angles who are treated at a younger age have a greater chance of a successful outcome.[21,23,24] The flexibility of the curve or the quality of the cast may also affect success rates. The goal of casting should be understood when initiating treatment. Although some patients (those with a smaller curve or younger age) treated with casting may be cured, there are many instances when a cure is not expected. However, casting can be used as a means to delay surgery in patients with larger curves so that surgical treatment can be initiated at an older age.[25] However, there are some concerns with this treatment strategy, given that young patients may require multiple anesthetics.

Surgical Management

Growth-friendly Instrumentation

There are multiple technologies used to treat patients with EOIS when nonsurgical management has been unsuccessful. All of these technologies attempt to maximize spinal and thoracic growth while controlling spinal deformity and minimizing complications. Because early spinal fusion has been associated with poor outcomes, growth-friendly strategies are currently accepted.

The traditional dual growing rod technique uses localized fusion with spine anchors at the top and the bottom of the curve and leaves the middle of the spine untouched to allow for serial distractions. Variations on this method include the use of rib anchors rather than spine anchors. The SHILLA system uses a strategy in which there is an apical fusion and correction at the area of deformity, with nonfusion/gliding implants proximally and distally that allow for guided growth through the normal spine segments.[26] The relative merit of this system is the avoidance of repetitive surgeries for routine surgical lengthening. New technologies that use a variety of convex tethers may provide another option for guided correction and growth.[27] Another new technology is a magnetically controlled growth rod (MCGR), which allows for magnetic lengthening through a device exterior to the skin.[28] It appears that at intermediate follow-up, MCGR has similar ability to lengthen the spine and control spinal curvature. Although anesthetic events are avoided with in office lengthening, complication rates are still high and unplanned return to the operating room is between 27% and 47%. Another technology, just recently approved by the FDA, anterior spinal growth tethering may also be an effective strategy[29] to stabilize/improve the curve in skeletally immature patients with significant growth remaining. Comparative[30,31] studies and long-term outcomes are lacking for these treatments to determine which strategy is best.

Outcomes and Complications

Except for young patients with EOIS who are cured with casting, a normal spine at the end of growth is achieved in only a few patients. After treatment with growth-friendly instrumentation, most patients require definitive fusion when they reach an appropriate age. In addition, junctional kyphosis is a frequently encountered complication. Junctional kyphosis is common in growth-friendly implants and is likely related to both the high underlying incidence of preoperative kyphosis and the mechanism by which the rods are lengthened, with posterior distraction promoting kyphosis.[32] Rod breakage or implant dislodgement is common and expected at some point during treatment.[33] Using a complication severity score has helped standardize the language used when assessing these complications.[34]

Although growth-friendly surgical treatment may lessen the deformity at final fusion, spontaneous fusion during the lengthening treatment and curve stiffness present challenging obstacles at the time of final fusion or may bring a premature end to growth-friendly treatment.[35] In addition, final fusion may not be the final procedure these children need, because many may require additional procedures related to complications after their final fusion procedure.[36]

The repetitive use of anesthetics often required along with the iatrogenic radiation exposure associated with treatment started at a young age may have detrimental effects on patient outcomes, such as psychologic disturbances and the role of radiation exposure in the development of secondary malignancies.[37,38] Also, early treatment may lead to a decrease in the effectiveness of repeated surgical lengthenings over time (the law of diminishing returns).[39] In the event of severe complications such as infection or spontaneous fusion, treatment may be ended before adequate space for lung development has been achieved.[40] The delicate balance between early intervention and curve control versus the complications associated with growth-friendly treatments is not yet established; however, it is hoped that data gathered from patient-reported outcome measures will help distinguish between treatment options. For example, the Early-Onset Scoliosis Questionnaire has begun to emerge as a tool to compare treatment modalities such as traditional growing rods versus MCGR.[41]

CONGENITAL SCOLIOSIS

Etiology

Similar to EOIS, congenital scoliosis has no clear etiology. Multiple environmental and genetic causes have been proposed but are unproved. Most cases are sporadic and have a low familial recurrence rate. Discovery of mutations in the genes of the notch family and their association with Alagille syndrome and spondylocostal dysostosis adds support to theories that genetic factors have a role in the etiology. The importance of *HOX* genes in the creation of the axial and appendicular skeleton offer further reasons to suspect a genetic etiology.[2]

Classification

Congenital spinal anomalies are classified as a failure of formation (**Figure 3**), a failure of segmentation (**Figure 4**), or a combination of both types.[42] In a failure of formation, the extent to which the vertebral body is not formed defines the deformity. A wedge vertebra has pedicles on both sides but asymmetric formation and growth of the vertebral body on one side, whereas a hemivertebra represents a complete unilateral failure of formation. Depending on the relationship to adjacent vertebrae and the number of disks present, the hemivertebrae can be defined as nonsegmented, partially segmented, or fully segmented. A hemimetameric shift describes a spine with balanced deformities and growth

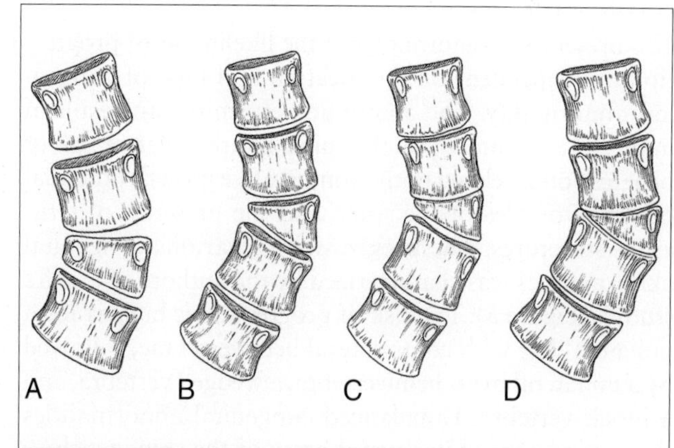

FIGURE 3 Illustration of formation defects. **A**, Wedge vertebra. **B**, Fully segmented hemivertebra. **C**, Partially segmented hemivertebra. **D**, Unsegmented hemivertebra. (Reproduced from Hedequist D, Emans J: Congenital scoliosis. *J Am Acad Orthop Surg* 2004;12[4]:266-275.)

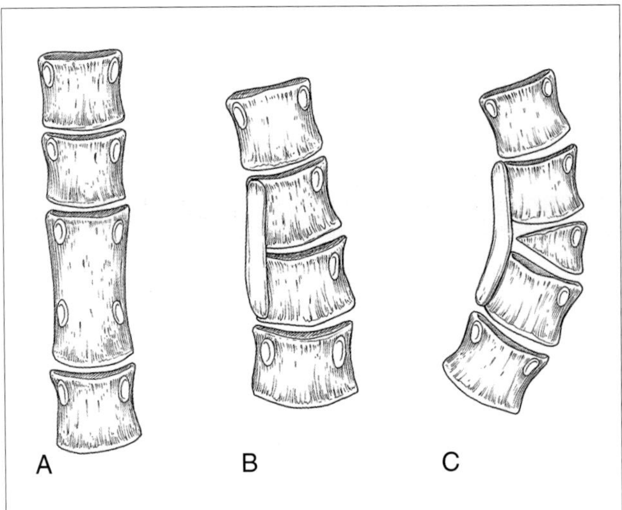

FIGURE 4 Illustrations of segmentation defects. **A**, Block vertebra. **B**, Unilateral segmentation (bar) defect. **C**, Unilateral bar with a contralateral hemivertebra. (Reproduced from Hedequist D, Emans J: Congenital scoliosis. *J Am Acad Orthop Surg* 2004;12[4]:266-275.)

potential on both sides of the spine, with similar hemivertebrae situated on opposite sides. With a failure of segmentation, adjacent vertebrae are inappropriately connected. In its most benign form, a block vertebra is symmetrically fused to an adjacent vertebra. On the severe end of the spectrum is a unilateral bar, in which on one side the vertebral bodies are fused, which allows for unchecked growth on the contralateral side. Fused ribs are commonly associated with congenital scoliosis. Many congenital spine deformities are more complex than can be described by this classification, with nonconcordance between anterior and posterior elements in the congenital spinal anomaly.

Natural History

The presence of deformity and the likelihood of progression are dependent on the location and type of congenital abnormality. The anatomic deformity can result in immediate asymmetry in the spine, but the relative risk of progression is related to the comparative growth potential of the two sides of the spine and the presence of tethering structures. The progression of various congenital abnormalities was characterized by the authors of a 1982 study[43] (**Figure 5**). The risk of progression is highest for a unilateral bar with contralateral hemivertebrae, followed by a unilateral bar, a hemivertebra, a wedged vertebra, and a block vertebra. Unbalanced congenital abnormalities that are present at junctional areas of the spine (such as cervicothoracic, thoracolumbar, and lumbosacral areas) are more likely to be clinically apparent. Progression typically occurs during rapid growth, either during the first 3 years of life or during the growth spurt in early adolescence.

Clinical Features

Patients with congenital scoliosis should be assessed with a full neurologic examination, including an evaluation of reflexes. Sagittal and coronal balance and rib cage deformity should be assessed. A thorough skin examination for evidence of spinal dysraphism as well as inspection for foot deformity or other neurologic dysfunction should be performed given the associated neural axis abnormalities. Exercise tolerance as well as inspiratory and expiratory capacity should be assessed because of the possible negative effect of chest wall and spinal deformity on pulmonary function. The presence of substantial rib fusions in the setting of congenital scoliosis may present as thoracic insufficiency syndrome.

As previously discussed, the formation of the spine occurs concurrently with other organ systems. Associated conditions include vertebral-anal-cardiac-tracheal-esophageal-renal-limb association, which is representative of the other organ systems commonly affected in patients with congenital scoliosis. Other musculoskeletal abnormalities include radial hypoplasia, hip dysplasia, and clubfoot and those seen in Klippel-Feil syndrome and Sprengel deformity. Congenital heart disease (such as a ventricular septal defect, an atrial septal defect, tetralogy of Fallot, or transposition of great vessels) is present in as many as 25% of patients with congenital scoliosis. A urologic or Müllerian duct abnormality (such as horseshoe kidney, renal aplasia, duplicate ureters, or hypospadias) is seen in up to 33% of patients.[2] Many of these associated conditions are readily apparent, but renal obstruction and unilateral hearing loss are easily missed unless screening is performed.

Imaging

Imaging begins with standard PA and lateral radiographs. In a nonambulatory patient, supine or sitting radiographs can be used. When a patient transitions to ambulatory status, any change in the deformity noted on radiographs must be interpreted in the context of the change in the radiographic position (eg, supine versus upright). Also, subtle changes may not be evident between radiographs, so comparing radiographs over time and to the earliest radiographs is useful in determining change over time. Measuring a Cobb angle may be more difficult in these patients and quantifying the amount of chest deformity is challenging. Similar landmarks should be used when comparing sequential radiographs. Even in the absence of neurologic abnormalities on examination, a screening MRI is generally recommended to rule out associated neural axial abnormalities, which are found in up to 35% of patients with congenital scoliosis.[2] However, anesthetic risks (including the unclear effects on the developing brain) associated with the patient's age should be weighed

Site of curvature	Type of congenital anomaly					
	Block vertebra	Wedged vertebra	Hemivertebra		Unilateral unsegmented bar	Unilateral unsegmented bar and contralateral hemivertebrae
			Single	Double		
Upper thoracic	<1°-1°	★ −2°	1°-2°	2°-2.5°	2°-4°	5°-6°
Lower thoracic	<1°-1°	2°-2°	2°-2.5°	2°-2.5°	5°-6.5°	6°-7°
Thoracolumbar	<1°-1°	1.5°-2°	2°-3.5°	5°-★	6°-9°	>10°-★
Lumbar	★	<1°-★	<1°-1°	★	>5°-★	★
Lumbosacral	★	★	<1°-1.5°	★	★	★

No treatment required — May require spinal fusion — Require spinal fusion

★ Too few or no curves

FIGURE 5 Illustration summarizing the natural history of congenital curves by the type of vertebral anomaly and curve location for a series of 251 patients. Median yearly deterioration is given for children younger than 10 years on the left and for children 10 years and older on the right of each cell. (Reproduced with permission from McMaster MJ, Ohtsuka K: The natural history of congenital scoliosis: A study of two hundred and fifty-one patients. *J Bone Joint Surg Am* 1982;64[8]:1128-1147.)

when determining the timing of radiologic studies. As previously mentioned, a spine ultrasonography can identify certain conditions and avoids the use of anesthesia in very young patients. However, immediate MRI is indicated depending on the presence of certain symptoms and/or the severity of the spinal anomaly. Substantial progression of curvature in a normally segmented spine requires MRI. CT should be used preoperatively to define the anatomy because posterior abnormalities may not correlate with findings on plain radiographs and there is frequent discordance of anterior and posterior anomalies.[44]

Nonsurgical Management

Observation is warranted for many congenital curves that have limited deformity or progression over time. Many congenital abnormalities may have relatively balanced growth and will not require treatment. Bracing treatment is generally viewed as ineffective treatment for congenital curves; however, it may be used for compensatory curves of a normally segmented spine. Casting or bracing treatment of congenital curves as a tactic to delay the need for surgery has been advocated; however, it is expected that this strategy is less successful in managing patients with congenital curves than those with normally segmented spines. In patients with associated chest wall and rib anomalies, casting and bracing treatment may have negative consequences, which are not well understood.

Surgical Management

As in patients with EOIS, the surgical management goals in patients with congenital deformity are to maximize spine and chest growth, control chest wall and spinal deformity, and minimize patient complications and distress. It is safe to use spinal instrumentation in these patients.[45] The use of preoperative traction can help with gradual, partial correction of severe deformity (with or without an anterior release).[46] Balancing early versus late intervention is challenging. It is known that early fusion leads to poor outcomes with regard to pulmonary function; therefore, other treatment strategies should be considered.[11] Because the types of deformity are broad, so are the possible treatment options.

If a small section of the spine is affected by a minimal deformity, an in situ fusion may prevent curve progression without detriment to the growing lungs. This is not a treatment option if the deformity is substantial enough that it requires more acute correction or if the deformity spans a large segment of spine, because in situ fusion would prevent adequate spinal growth. Hemiepiphysiodesis offers the potential for gradual deformity correction by slowing growth on the convex side and allowing the concave side to grow. Although historical results have been mixed, a 2015 literature has documented promising outcomes.[47]

If an isolated hemivertebra is causing coronal or sagittal imbalance, a hemivertebra excision offers an attractive surgical option. The most common hemivertebrae requiring this approach are fully segmented deformities at transition zones of the spine. When successful, spinal balance can be restored and the progression of adjacent compensatory curves can be prevented. Although historical reports include anterior and posterior resections, posterior-only approaches are currently advocated.[48]

In patients with adequate thoracic volume but an unacceptable coronal or sagittal deformity, an instrumented fusion with deformity correction is a reasonable option. If bending radiographs fail to demonstrate adequate flexibility for acceptable correction, treatment options include anterior and posterior approaches as well as posterior-based approaches such as pedicle subtraction osteotomies or vertebral column resection. The selected approach depends on the magnitude and location of the deformity.

Growth-friendly strategies are commonly used in the treatment of congenital scoliosis. Traditional growing rods are probably the most indicated instrumentation for patients with spinal deformity without substantial rib fusions or chest wall abnormality. If the chest wall is normal, spine-only fixation may be the better choice, as implants spanning or anchoring on the chest wall may lead to unwanted rib fusions and chest wall stiffness. Growing rods have been shown to increase spinal growth, control spinal curvature, and improve space available for lungs in patients with congenital scoliosis.[49] The use of VEPTR has been one of the most commonly adopted implant strategies for the management of congenital scoliosis (**Figure 6**). The ideal candidate for a VEPTR implant has progressive congenital spinal deformity, an associated hemithoracic constriction, and multiple fused ribs. In these patients, expansion thoracostomy and placement of a VEPTR expands the chest and controls deformity.[15,50] The VEPTR can be connected to the pelvis, spine, or ribs.

Less commonly, the SHILLA system has been used to correct the apical abnormality and allow guided growth cephalad and caudal to the deformity.[26]

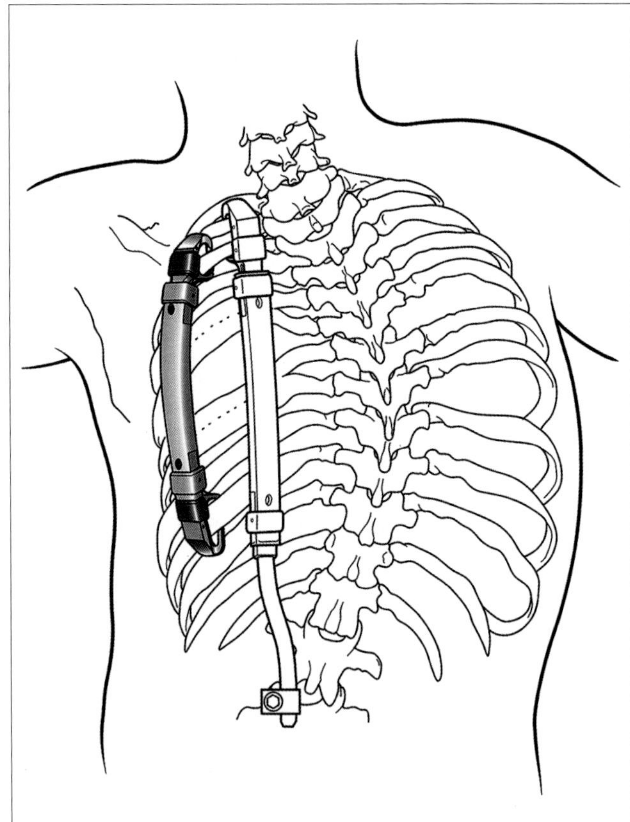

FIGURE 6 Schematic representation of vertical expandable prosthetic titanium rib devices used after an opening wedge thoracostomy in patients with congenital vertebral anomalies and fused ribs. A rib-rib device (shaded) or a hybrid rib prosthesis (unshaded) may be used to promote thoracic growth by lengthening the concave hemithorax. (Reproduced with permission from Campbell RM Jr, Smith MD, Hell-Vocke AK: Expansion thoracoplasty: The surgical technique of opening-wedge thoracostomy. Surgical technique. *J Bone Joint Surg Am* 2004;86[suppl 1]:51-64.)

Outcomes and Complications

Although chest wall expansion has been shown to increase the space available for lungs, a systematic review failed to demonstrate an improvement in pulmonary function.[51] Understanding the appropriate outcomes is challenging. Ultimately, improvement and maintenance of pulmonary function is the most important outcome. Because of substantial obstacles to obtaining meaningful pulmonary function tests in very young children, surrogate means such as radiographic measurements of spinal length and chest width are used to evaluate pulmonary function; however, it is unclear how well these measurements correlate with actual pulmonary function.[8] Better outcome measures are needed, specifically to understand the effects of treatment on pulmonary function. Patient-reported outcomes and cost-effectiveness studies will become increasingly important in evaluating treatment strategies.

Complications with the use of growth-friendly strategies for patients with scoliosis are common. Device migration, infection, rod breakage, and other complications have been reported with use of all growth-friendly strategies.[52,53] The C-EOS may be helpful in predicting complications such as anchor failure.[54] Complications may be more common in patients treated at a younger age, which is likely related to the severity of disease and the number of surgical treatments.[14] Junctional kyphosis is also an unsolved but common complication.[55]

SUMMARY

Both EOIS and congenital scoliosis present challenging clinical situations. Treatment goals common to patients with either diagnosis include maximizing spinal growth and pulmonary function while avoiding complications. Repetitive use of anesthetics and iatrogenic radiation exposure are problematic. Many treatments options are available, including a variety of growth-friendly implants.

Major challenges exist in understanding the disease and the effects of treatment on the disease. Junctional kyphosis, surgical site infection, and implant failure are common complications and areas of current research interest. Traditionally reported radiographic outcomes may not be good surrogates for actual patient outcomes or improvement in pulmonary function. Patient-reported outcomes require further study and correlation with traditionally collected radiographic outcomes.

KEY STUDY POINTS

- EOS is an all-encompassing term, and it is inclusive of all etiologies of scoliosis in patients younger than 10 years.
- Lung development in patients with a growing and changing thoracic cavity is uniquely important.
- Treatment goals and strategies in patients with EOS are directed at preserving the growth of the spine and thoracic cavity to maximize lung function.
- Less invasive treatment options, such as bracing treatment and casting, may slow deformity progression and delay the need for surgery.
- Surgical interventions using growth-friendly instrumentation, tethers, or a growth guidance system can control a curve while preserving growth of the spine and thoracic cavity.

ANNOTATED REFERENCES

1. Skaggs DL, Guillaume T, El Hawary L, et al: Early onset scoliosis consensus statement, SRS growing spine committee, 2015. *Spine Deform* 2015;3(2):107.
2. Hensinger RN: Congenital scoliosis: Etiology and associations. *Spine (Phila Pa 1976)* 2009;34(17):1745-1750.
3. Dimeglio A: Growth in pediatric orthopaedics. *J Pediatr Orthop* 2001;21(4):549-555.
4. Campbell RM Jr, Smith MD, Mayes TC, et al: The characteristics of thoracic insufficiency syndrome associated with fused ribs and congenital scoliosis. *J Bone Joint Surg Am* 2003;85(3):399-408.
5. Gillingham BL, Fan RA, Akbarnia BA: Early onset idiopathic scoliosis. *J Am Acad Orthop Surg* 2006;14(2):101-112.
6. Williams BA, Matsumoto H, McCalla DJ, et al: Development and initial validation of the Classification of Early-Onset Scoliosis (C-EOS). *J Bone Joint Surg Am* 2014;96(16):1359-1367.
7. Russo C, Trupia E, Campbell, et al, Children's Spine Study Group: The association between the Classification of Early-Onset Scoliosis and Smith complications after initiation of growth-friendly spine surgery: A preliminary study. *J Pediatr Orthop* 2019;39(10):e737-e741.

   The authors reviewed a multicenter registry and compared 245 Smith complications distributed among 116 patients. Using this terminology simplifies language to describe a complex pathology and complication scheme. Although there is an association of complication classification and complications, true risk stratification is not yet possible. Level of evidence: II.
8. Glotzbecker M, Johnston C, Miller P, et al: Is there a relationship between thoracic dimensions and pulmonary function in early-onset scoliosis? *Spine (Phila Pa 1976)* 2014;39(19):1590-1595.
9. Vitale MG, Corona J, Matsumoto H, et al: Development and initial validation of a disease specific outcome measure for early onset scoliosis. *Stud Health Technol Inform* 2010;158:172-176.
10. Corona J, Matsumoto H, Roye DP, Vitale MG: Measuring quality of life in children with early onset scoliosis: Development and initial validation of the early onset scoliosis questionnaire. *J Pediatr Orthop* 2011;31(2):180-185.
11. Karol LA, Johnston C, Mladenov K, Schochet P, Walters P, Browne RH: Pulmonary function following early thoracic fusion in non-neuromuscular scoliosis. *J Bone Joint Surg Am* 2008;90(6):1272-1281.
12. Pehrsson K, Larsson S, Oden A, Nachemson A: Long-term follow-up of patients with untreated scoliosis: A study of mortality, causes of death, and symptoms. *Spine (Phila Pa 1976)* 1992;17(9):1091-1096.
13. Branthwaite MA: Cardiorespiratory consequences of unfused idiopathic scoliosis. *Br J Dis Chest* 1986;80(4):360-369.
14. Upasani VV, Miller PE, Emans JB, et al, Children's Spine Study Group: VEPTR implantation after age 3 is associated with similar radiographic outcomes with fewer complications. *J Pediatr Orthop* 2016;36(3):219-225.

    VEPTR treatment resulted in similar deformity control and thoracic growth in patients younger than 3 years and in those 3 to 6 years of age. Lower complication rates were reported in the older age group. Level of evidence: III.
15. Campbell RM Jr, Smith MD, Mayes TC, et al: The effect of opening wedge thoracostomy on thoracic insufficiency syndrome associated with fused ribs and congenital scoliosis. *J Bone Joint Surg Am* 2004;86(8):1659-1674.

16. Fernandes P, Weinstein SL: Natural history of early onset scoliosis. *J Bone Joint Surg Am* 2007;89(suppl 1):21-33.

17. Mehta MH: The rib-vertebra angle in the early diagnosis between resolving and progressive infantile scoliosis. *J Bone Joint Surg Br* 1972;54(2):230-243.

18. Pahys JM, Samdani AF, Betz RR: Intraspinal anomalies in infantile idiopathic scoliosis: Prevalence and role of magnetic resonance imaging. *Spine (Phila Pa 1976)* 2009;34(12):E434-E438.

19. Gupta P, Lenke LG, Bridwell KH: Incidence of neural axis abnormalities in infantile and juvenile patients with spinal deformity: Is a magnetic resonance image screening necessary? *Spine (Phila Pa 1976)* 1998;23(2):206-210.

20. Dolan LA, Wright JG, Weinstein SL: Effects of bracing in adolescents with idiopathic scoliosis. *N Engl J Med* 2014;370(7):681.

21. Mehta MH: Growth as a corrective force in the early treatment of progressive infantile scoliosis. *J Bone Joint Surg Br* 2005;87(9):1237-1247.

22. Fedorak GT, D'Astous JL, Nielson AN: Minimum 5 year follow up of Mehta Casting to treat idiopathic early-onset scoliosis. *J Bone Joint Surg Am* 2019;101(17):1530-1538.

    The authors reviewed 54 children with early-onset scoliosis with minimum 5-year follow-up after treatment with Mehta Casting. In a recent study with minimum 5-year follow-up, 49% of children had improved scoliosis to less than 15° and 73% improved by at least 20°. The initial Cobb angle, first-cast Cobb angle, rib-vertebral angle difference, and traction Cobb angle were all predictive of sustained scoliosis of ≤15°. However, with continued growth, relapse of scoliosis was seen in three patients. Level of evidence: IV.

23. Iorio J, Orlando G, Diefenbach C, et al: Serial casting for infantile idiopathic scoliosis: Radiographic outcomes and factors associated with response to treatment. *J Pediatr Orthop* 2017;37(5):311-316.

    The authors report on 21 patients with an average age of 2.1 years who underwent serial casting for EOS. The patient's body mass index and age younger than 1.8 years at the initiation of casting were important predictors of success. Level of evidence: IV.

24. Gomez JA, Grzywna A, Miller PE, et al, Children's Spine Study Group, Growing Spine Study Group: Initial cast correction as a predictor of treatment outcome success for infantile idiopathic scoliosis. *J Pediatr Orthop* 2017;37(8):e625-e630.

    Sixty-eight patients were reviewed from a multicenter database. Infantile idiopathic scoliosis patients casted at an earlier age, with smaller major curves, and greater percent major curve correction in initial cast have the best prognosis. Level of evidence: III.

25. Waldron SR, Poe-Kochert C, Son-Hing JP, Thompson GH: Early onset scoliosis: The value of serial Risser casts. *J Pediatr Orthop* 2013;33(8):775-780.

26. McCarthy RE, McCullough FL: Shilla growth guidance for early-onset scoliosis: Results after a minimum of five years of follow-up. *J Bone Joint Surg Am* 2015;97(19):1578-1584.

27. Jain V, Lykissas M, Trobisch P, et al: Surgical aspects of spinal growth modulation in scoliosis correction. *Instr Course Lect* 2014;63:335-344.

28. Hickey BA, Towriss C, Baxter G, et al: Early experience of MAGEC magnetic growing rods in the treatment of early onset scoliosis. *Eur Spine J* 2014;23(suppl 1):S61-S65.

29. Newton PO, Kluck DG, Saito W: Anterior spinal growth tethering for skeletally immature patient with scoliosis: A retrospective review. *J Bone Joint Surg Am* 2018;100(19):1691-1697.

    Seventeen patients treated with anterior spinal growth tethering with a follow-up of 2 to 4 years were reviewed. Average curve correction was 51%, and 59% were viewed as clinically successful. Revision surgery was needed in seven patients. Level of evidence: IV.

30. Choi E, Yaszay B, Mundis G, et al: Implant complications after magnetically controlled growing rods for early onset scoliosis: A multicenter retrospective review. *J Pediatr Orthop* 2017;37(8):e588-e592.

    Fifty-four patients treated with MCGR were reviewed. Compared with traditional growing rods, MCGR has a lower infection rate but does not appear to prevent common implant-related complications. Level of evidence: IV.

31. Kwan KYH, Alanay A, Yazici M, et al: Unplanned reoperations in magnetically controlled growing rod surgery for early onset scoliosis with a minimum of two-year follow-up. *Spine (Phila Pa 1976)* 2017;42(24):E1410-E1414.

    Thirty patients with EOS underwent MCGR implantation at six institutions. Within the follow-up period (mean 37 months), 46.7% patients required an unplanned revision surgery. Level of evidence: IV.

32. Shah SA, Karatas AF, Dhawale AA, et al, Growing Spine Study Group: The effect of serial growing rod lengthening on the sagittal profile and pelvic parameters in early-onset scoliosis. *Spine (Phila Pa 1976)* 2014;39(22):E1311-E1317.

33. Yang JS, Sponseller PD, Thompson GH, et al, Growing Spine Study Group: Growing rod fractures: Risk factors and opportunities for prevention. *Spine (Phila Pa 1976)* 2011;36(20):1639-1644.

34. Michael N, Palmer C, Smith JT, et al: Complication severity score for growth-friendly surgery has strong interrater and intrarater agreement. *J Pediatr Orthop* 2018;38(4):e190-e193.

    Sixty-three cases were reviewed by 20 participants, and strong interrater and intrarater agreement for the published complications scheme was demonstrated. Level of evidence: I.

35. Flynn JM, Tomlinson LA, Pawelek J, et al, Growing Spine Study Group: Growing-rod graduates: Lessons learned from ninety-nine patients who completed lengthening. *J Bone Joint Surg Am* 2013;95(19):1745-1750.

36. Poe-Kochert C, Shannon C, Pawelek JB, et al: Final fusion after growing-rod treatment for early onset scoliosis: Is it really final? *J Bone Joint Surg Am* 2016;98(22):1913-1917.

    A hundred patients with multiple diagnoses with previous growing rod treatment were examined for complications after final fusion. Twenty of the patients (20%) had 30 complications requiring revision surgery (57 procedures). Level of evidence: IV.

37. Flynn JM, Matsumoto H, Torres F, Ramirez N, Vitale MG: Psychological dysfunction in children who require repetitive surgery for early onset scoliosis. *J Pediatr Orthop* 2012;32(6):594-599.

38. Khorsand D, Song KM, Swanson J, Alessio A, Redding G, Waldhausen J: Iatrogenic radiation exposure to patients with early onset spine and chest wall deformities. *Spine (Phila Pa 1976)* 2013;38(17):E1108-E1114.

 Children treated for thoracic insufficiency syndrome using a consistent protocol received iatrogenic radiation doses that were on average four times the estimated average US background radiation exposure of 3 mSv/yr. Radiation from CT accounted for 74% of the total dose. Level of evidence: III.

39. Sankar WN, Skaggs DL, Yazici M, et al: Lengthening of dual growing rods and the law of diminishing returns. *Spine (Phila Pa 1976)* 2011;36(10):806-809.

40. Kabirian N, Akbarnia BA, Pawelek JB, et al, Growing Spine Study Group: Deep surgical site infection following 2344 growing-rod procedures for early-onset scoliosis: Risk factors and clinical consequences. *J Bone Joint Surg Am* 2014;96(15):e128.

41. Doany ME, Olgun ZD, Kinikli GI: Health-related quality of life in early-onset scoliosis patients treated surgically: EOSQ scores in traditional growing rod versus magnetically controlled growing rods. *Spine (Phila Pa 1976)* 2018;43(2):148-153.

 Forty-four patients with EOS were enrolled. Scores of economic burden and overall satisfaction were superior in MCGR patients compared with those treated with traditional growing rods; however, this benefit was found to be less when controlled for duration of follow-up. Level of evidence: III.

42. Hedequist D, Emans J: Congenital scoliosis: A review and update. *J Pediatr Orthop* 2007;27(1):106-116.

43. McMaster MJ, Ohtsuka K: The natural history of congenital scoliosis: A study of two hundred and fifty-one patients. *J Bone Joint Surg Am* 1982;64(8):1128-1147.

44. Hedequist DJ, Emans JB: The correlation of preoperative three-dimensional computed tomography reconstructions with operative findings in congenital scoliosis. *Spine (Phila Pa 1976)* 2003;28(22):2531-2534, discussion 1.

45. Hedequist DJ, Hall JE, Emans JB: The safety and efficacy of spinal instrumentation in children with congenital spine deformities. *Spine (Phila Pa 1976)* 2004;29(18):2081-2086, discussion 2087.

46. Rinella A, Lenke L, Whitaker C, et al: Perioperative halo-gravity traction in the treatment of severe scoliosis and kyphosis. *Spine (Phila Pa 1976)* 2005;30(4):475-482.

47. Demirkiran G, Dede O, Ayvaz M, Bas CE, Alanay A, Yazici M: Convex instrumented hemiepiphysiodesis with concave distraction: A treatment option for long sweeping congenital curves. *J Pediatr Orthop* 2016;36(3):226-231.

 Convex instrumented hemiepiphysiodesis with concave distraction resulted in good curve correction while maintaining the growth of the thorax. The correction of the anomalous segment improved over time, proving the effectiveness of the hemiepiphysiodesis. Level of evidence: IV.

48. Hedequist D, Emans J, Proctor M: Three rod technique facilitates hemivertebra wedge excision in young children through a posterior only approach. *Spine (Phila Pa 1976)* 2009;34(6):E225-E229.

49. Elsebai HB, Yazici M, Thompson GH, et al: Safety and efficacy of growing rod technique for pediatric congenital spinal deformities. *J Pediatr Orthop* 2011;31(1):1-5.

50. Flynn JM, Emans JB, Smith JT, et al: VEPTR to treat nonsyndromic congenital scoliosis: A multicenter, mid-term follow-up study. *J Pediatr Orthop* 2013;33(7):679-684.

51. Sponseller PD, Yazici M, Demetracopoulos C, Emans JB: Evidence basis for management of spine and chest wall deformities in children. *Spine (Phila Pa 1976)* 2007;32(19 suppl):S81-S90.

52. Emans JB, Caubet JF, Ordonez CL, Lee EY, Ciarlo M: The treatment of spine and chest wall deformities with fused ribs by expansion thoracostomy and insertion of vertical expandable prosthetic titanium rib: Growth of thoracic spine and improvement of lung volumes. *Spine (Phila Pa 1976)* 2005;30(17 suppl):S58-S68.

53. Garg S, LaGreca J, St Hilaire T, et al: Wound complications of vertical expandable prosthetic titanium rib incisions. *Spine (Phila Pa 1976)* 2014;39(13):E777-E781.

54. Park HY, Matsumoto H, Feinberg N, et al: The Classification for Early-Onset Scoliosis (C-EOS) correlates with the speed of vertical expandable prosthetic titanium rib (VEPTR) proximal anchor failure. *J Pediatr Orthop* 2015;37(6):381-386.

 Survival analysis of C-EOS classes with more than three individuals, demonstrated that the C-EOS discriminates low-speed, medium-speed, and high-speed VEPTR anchor failure. This supports the validity of the C-EOS and its potential use in guiding decision making. Level of evidence: III.

55. El-Hawary R, Sturm P, Cahill P, et al: What is the risk of developing proximal junctional kyphosis during growth friendly treatments for early-onset scoliosis? *J Pediatr Orthop* 2015;37(2):86-91.

 The risk of developing proximal junctional kyphosis during distraction-based, growth-friendly management of EOS was 20% immediately after implantation and 28% at a minimum 2-year follow-up, with no difference observed between rib-based and spine-based treatment groups. Level of evidence: III.

CHAPTER 32

Adolescent Idiopathic Scoliosis

MATTHEW E. OETGEN, MD, MBA • BENJAMIN D. MARTIN, MD

ABSTRACT

Adolescent idiopathic scoliosis is a three-dimensional deformity of the spine affecting approximately 2% to 3% of children. Treatment goals are aimed at minimizing patient deformity and maximizing functional outcome throughout life. The risk of progression of scoliosis is affected by the magnitude of the deformity and growth potential, with younger children and larger deformities at higher risk of progression. Traditional treatment options include observation, brace treatment, and surgical intervention consisting of spinal fusion. Alternative treatments, such as scoliosis-specific physical therapy protocols and motion-preserving growth modulation surgery, are generating increasing interest from the public and the medical community. Although surgical techniques have evolved over time with more powerful correction ability, limited data exist regarding the changes in functional and patient-reported health-related outcomes associated with these changes in surgical technique.

Keywords: adolescent idiopathic scoliosis; nonsurgical treatment; spinal fusion

INTRODUCTION

Adolescent idiopathic scoliosis (AIS) is a three-dimensional deformity of the spine with a coronal curve magnitude of greater than 10°. Although the definition is based on the coronal plane, understanding the sagittal and axial planes is important.[1,2] In the sagittal plane, there is often a loss of kyphosis that produces a relative hypokyphotic sagittal alignment at the apex. In the axial plane, there is substantial deformity with maximal rotation of the apical vertebral body toward the coronal deformity. Taken together, these spinal malalignments produce the typical appearance of AIS.

CLASSIFICATION

The most basic classification system for AIS is a simple descriptive system indicating the location of the deformity (cervicothoracic, thoracic, thoracolumbar, or lumbar) and the magnitude of the deformity. A more structured classification system based on the radiographic description of the curve location introduced in 1983 by King and Moe[3] sought to determine when selective thoracic instrumentation was warranted by dividing curves into five types. However, because of some shortcomings in the King-Moe system, a more robust (and more complex) classification system was developed by Lenke and colleagues[4] in 1997. In an attempt to improve surgical planning, the Lenke system focuses mainly on surgical deformities.

The Lenke classification of AIS consists of six main categories defined by the location of the major spinal deformity (defined as the largest magnitude curve) and the location of any compensatory spinal deformities (defined as a curve with less than 25° of residual magnitude on bending radiographs).[4] In addition, the classification contains two modifiers: one for the lumbar curvature and one for the sagittal plane (**Figure 1**). This system allows for reproducible categorization of AIS and helps in surgical decision making.[5] The most common location of spinal deformity in patients with AIS is in the thoracic spine, with approximately 60% of deformities located in this region.[6]

Dr. Oetgen or an immediate family member serves as a board member, owner, officer, or committee member of the American Academy of Orthopaedic Surgeons, the Pediatric Orthopaedic Society of North America, and the Scoliosis Research Society. Dr. Martin or an immediate family member serves as a board member, owner, officer, or committee member of the Pediatric Orthopaedic Society of North America.

Curve Type	Proximal Thoracic	Main Thoracic	Thoracolumbar/Lumbar	Description
1	Nonstructural	Structural[a]	Nonstructural	Main thoracic (MT)
2	Structural†	Structural[a]	Nonstructural	Double thoracic (DT)
3	Nonstructural	Structural[a]	Structural[b]	Double major (DM)
4	Structural†	Structural[c]	Structural[c]	Triple major (TM)
5	Nonstructural	Nonstructural	Structural[a]	Thoracolumbar/lumbar (TL/L)
6	Nonstructural	Structural[b]	Structural[a]	Thoracolumbar/lumbar–main thoracic (TL/L-MT)

[a]Major curve: largest Cobb measurement, always structural; [b]Minor curve: remaining structural curves; [c]Type 4: MT or TL/L can be the major curve.

Structural Criteria
(Minor curves)

Proximal thoracic - Side-bending Cobb angle ≥25°
- T2-T5 kyphosis ≥+20°

Main thoracic - Side-bending Cobb angle ≥ 25°
- T10-L2 kyphosis ≥+20°

Thoracolumbar/lumbar - Side-bending Cobb angle ≥ 25°
- T10-L2 kyphosis ≥+20°

Location of Apex
(Scoliosis Research Society definition)

Curve	Apex
Thoracic	T2 to T11-12 disk
Thoracolumbar	T12-L1
Lumbar	L1-2 disk to L4

Modifiers

Lumbar Coronal Modifier	Center Sacral Vertical Line to Lumbar Apex
A	Between pedicles
B	Touches apical body(ies)
C	Completely medial

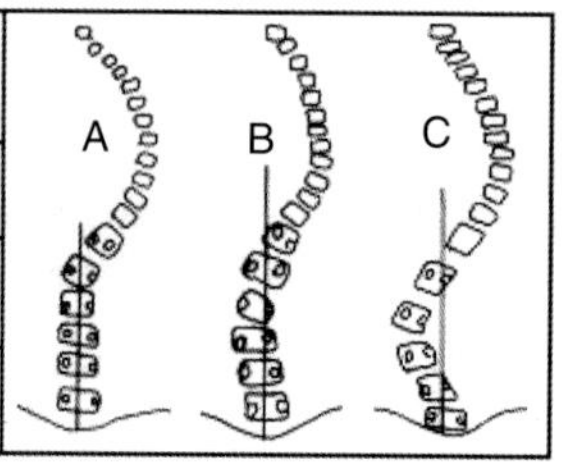

A B C

Thoracic Sagittal Profile (T5-T12)	
Modifier	Cobb Angle
– (hypo)	<10°
N (normal)	10°-40°
+ (hyper)	>40°

Curve type (1-6) + Lumbar coronal modifier (A, B, C) + Thoracic sagittal modifier (–, N, +) = Curve classification (eg, 1B+): _______

FIGURE 1 Charts show the Lenke classification system for adolescent idiopathic scoliosis. (Adapted with permission from Lenke LG, Betz RR, Harms J, et al: Adolescent idiopathic scoliosis: A new classification to determine the extent of spinal arthrodesis. *J Bone Joint Surg Am* 2001;83[8]:1169-1181. Copyright © The Journal of Bone and Joint Surgery, Incorporated.)

TREATMENT CONCEPTS

The treatment goals of AIS are the prevention of spinal deformity progression and the avoidance of physical impairment, pain, and disfigurement. The flexibility and movement of the spine should be maximized over time, and malalignment should be avoided because it can lead to future spondylotic degeneration. Traditionally, there are three mainstays of treatment of scoliosis depending on the age and skeletal maturity or growth potential of a patient. In patients with substantial remaining growth, observation of the spinal deformity is indicated when the deformity is less than 20°, a spinal orthotic is used to decrease the risk progression when the deformity is between 20° and 45°, and surgery is indicated for progressive deformities with magnitudes greater than 50°. Patients with little growth remaining or those who have reached skeletal maturity are typically not candidates for brace treatment, so observation and reassurance are indicated unless the deformity is greater than 50°, at which point surgical intervention should be considered. Although these are the traditional methods of treatment, this general algorithm has developed with a focus only on curve progression rather than understanding of the long-term repercussions and natural history of untreated scoliosis. As more focus is placed on objective measures of patient health as they relate to scoliosis (such as pulmonary function) and data regarding patient-reported outcomes become available, there will likely be important changes in these traditional treatment plans.

Alternative nonsurgical treatment modalities have been suggested to prevent scoliosis progression and, in some instances, to decrease the deformity; however, there is little evidence to support these treatments. While theoretically appealing after the clear demonstration that external brace applied forces can affect scoliosis's natural history, numerous physical therapy methods and protocols have been designed to prevent and reverse spinal deformity typically used in conjunction with brace treatment; however, limited data exist supporting these treatment modalities compared with the natural history.[7] There is a growing volume of reports in the physical therapy literature, focusing on small improvements in Cobb angles and quality of life scores.[8-10] Caution is indicated when assessing the role of physical therapy in the management of scoliosis, because a lack of evidence should not necessarily be taken to indicate a lack of effectiveness. Further investigations into the role of scoliosis-specific exercises are warranted and should include well-controlled, scientifically rigorous studies. Only when additional data are obtained can a clearer picture of the effectiveness and potential indications for this treatment be determined. The management of spinal deformity with chiropractic manipulation, electrical stimulation, and traction has been investigated, but there is no evidence to support the efficacy these methods.[11]

ETIOLOGY

A variety of possible pathogenetic factors have been suggested to explain AIS, including factors related to genetic susceptibility, biomechanics, and neurologic control of the body.[12] The underlying causes of AIS are being elucidated through experimental research. Population-based genetic studies comparing patients with idiopathic scoliosis with control subjects have identified DNA sequence variations that are associated with disease susceptibility. Such genome-wide association studies have effectively implicated several candidate genes and the biochemical functions of their encoded proteins in AIS. These genes include *CHL1*, *DSCAM*, and *CNTNAP2*, which participate in axon guidance;[13] *LBX1* and *PAX1*, which are important in muscle and spine pattern formation;[14-16] and *GPR126*, which is important in various processes such as myelination and disk chondrogenesis.[17] Importantly, *LBX1*, *PAX1*, and *GPR126* have been associated with AIS in both Asian and non-Hispanic White populations, and *PAX1* is specifically associated in females but not males, providing the first clue to the female prevalence of this disease. A 2015 gene-targeting study in which *GPR126* was specifically removed from chondrocytes produced an idiopathic scoliosis in a mice.[18] This is the first report of a genetically defined mouse model for AIS and opens the way for mechanistic studies to define its etiology. Although AIS is likely a multifactorial condition as opposed to being caused by a single gene,[19] continued genomic investigations of AIS using new and advanced techniques show promise for further understanding of this condition.

There appears to be evidence for inheritance of this disorder, with an increased prevalence in future generations, but the penetrance of scoliosis is variable. There is a relationship between AIS and sex, with an equal prevalence between males and females for small curves and an increasing prevalence of deformity in females as curve magnitude increases.

The prevalence of AIS has remained relatively constant over time, and it is present in approximately 2% of children aged 10 to 14 years. In this affected population, approximately 10% have progressive deformities of more than 20°, and 0.1% have deformities that progress to more than 50°.[20]

Progression of this disease is known to be affected by patient growth. In general, as the patient grows, there is a risk of spinal deformity progression, with the highest risk during the time of most rapid growth. Various clinical markers are used to assess growth and the risk of deformity progression. The Risser sign is a classic marker for skeletal maturity and is defined as the radiographic ossification of the iliac apophysis. This apophysis progressively ossifies from anterior to posterior and is graded from 0 (no ossification) to 5 (a fully fused apophysis), with interval measurements based on the progression of the appearance of the apophysis from anterior to posterior. The menarchal status in females is another marker used to indicate growth potential, although this has variable predictive ability compared with growth remaining. Menarche typically occurs following the peak height velocity, but the growth potential following the start of menarche is quite variable and ranges from 2.5 years to no growth remaining.

The peak height velocity, which is defined as the maximum change in skeletal growth of a child over time, also can be used to assess skeletal growth. The peak height velocity is reported to be approximately 8 cm per year for girls and 9.5 cm per year for boys. Although these markers are useful, many are not apparent until after the peak height velocity has occurred, which limits their usefulness during the time of maximal risk of deformity progression.[21] Evaluation of the skeletal maturation of the hand has been investigated and is suggested to be a better marker for growth velocity and the risk of scoliosis progression.[22]

NATURAL HISTORY

After an adolescent reaches skeletal maturity, the natural history of scoliosis appears to be dependent on the deformity magnitude. A long-term study at the University of Iowa reported little deformity progression over time if the curvature was less than 30° at skeletal maturity and a maximal risk of progression of deformity with curvatures greater than 50° at the time of skeletal maturity.[23] In 102 patients with an average follow-up of 40 years, the average progression of deformity over the follow-up period was 2.6° for thoracic curves of less than 30° at skeletal maturity, 10.2° for curves 30° to 50°, and 29.4° for curves 50° to

75°.[24] This pattern was also found in lumbar curves, with an average progression of 0°, 15.4°, and 18.5°, respectively.

Based on the University of Iowa data, recommendations for surgery have evolved, with a general indication for surgery being a deformity greater than 50° because of the risk of progressive deformity into adulthood. Radiographic outcomes for patients with curves between 30° and 50° at skeletal maturity are dependent on the location of the deformity, with lumbar curves being at increased risk for progression compared with thoracic curves.

Long-term data, published in 2003, have focused on both clinical and radiographic outcomes, suggesting the clinical effect of slowly progressing thoracic scoliosis continuing into adulthood may not be as important as originally suspected.[25] In addition, even moderate progression of smaller magnitude lumbar scoliosis into adulthood may be associated with more negative functional outcomes, such as increasing back pain, than previously thought. There may be unappreciated physiologic consequences of untreated thoracic scoliosis. A 2011 study reported that up to 19% of patients with AIS have moderately impaired pulmonary function (<65% predicted forced expiratory volume in 1 second) preoperatively, with a mean thoracic curve magnitude of 70°.[26] The authors concluded that, given the normally accepted age-related decline in pulmonary function, these patients are at substantial risk for serious pulmonary morbidity. Despite this conclusion, the 50-year long-term data comparing untreated patients with scoliosis with control subjects found no significant difference in reported shortness of breath with activity between groups.[25] However, higher rates of shortness of breath compared with control subjects was noted in patients with thoracic curves greater than 80°. Specific investigation comparing changes in pulmonary function in nonsurgically treated patients with those in surgically treated patients is needed.

Investigation of long-term functional outcomes (as defined by physiologic, psychological, and appearance-related patient-reported outcome measures) of various-sized AIS deformities at the time of skeletal maturity is needed to help redefine treatment algorithms during the adolescent period. In the absence of these data, current treatment algorithms are unfortunately based on the skeletal maturity of the patient, the magnitude of the deformity, and prognosis of curve progression rather than functional outcomes.

Given the lack of clear data regarding the long-term health risks of slowly progressive scoliosis through adulthood, it is worth reassessing the decision-making process. Although there is evidence that larger deformities will progress, an absolute correlation with decreased health is lacking. Other factors such as the risk of back pain, functional disability, and the disfiguring effects of spinal deformity must also factor into the decision for surgical correction; however, these factors may have different weights in different individuals. The decision to proceed with surgical correction of scoliosis should ultimately be made in a shared-decision process, with the physician providing the current knowledge of the long-term outcomes of both surgical intervention and observation and the patient and patient's family providing their preference for treatment.

DIAGNOSIS AND PRESENTATION

AIS is often identified by primary care physicians during a yearly well-child evaluation. The Adams forward bend test is the most common assessment test in this setting. The test is performed by having the patient bend forward at the waist until the back is horizontal to the ground. Spinal deformity is assessed by looking for asymmetry of the back, with an elevation of one side suggestive of the axial plane trunk deformity commonly seen in AIS (**Figure 2**). Use of a scoliometer adds a quantitative element to this examination, with varying suggestions regarding the threshold of rotational deformity that should trigger an orthopaedic referral. A threshold scoliometer value of 7° appears to be a suitable measurement to avoid missing deformities that could be braced and to limit unnecessary referrals.[27] Digital measurement of trunk rotation with a smartphone is possible using a scoliometer application and has been shown to be as accurate as classic scoliometer measurements.[28]

The cost versus benefit effectiveness of routine school-based scoliosis screening programs is controversial. Originally started as a program to detect spinal deformity associated with tuberculosis and polio, screening programs became increasingly recommended in the United States, with 21 states mandating screening and

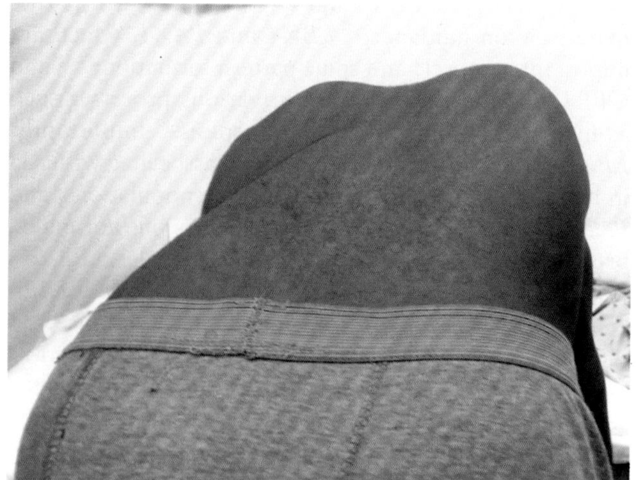

FIGURE 2 Clinical photograph of a patient with adolescent idiopathic scoliosis performing the Adam forward bend test. Note the rotational trunk deformity indicated by the asymmetry of the ribs, with the right rib cage being more prominent than the left.

an additional 12 recommending screening as of 2003. However, the U.S. Preventive Services Task Force[29] published a recommendation in 2004 against routine school-based scoliosis screening because of the ineffectiveness of these programs. Following that recommendation, several states reversed their recommendation for routine school-based screenings. Given the findings from a 2008 study on the effectiveness of bracing treatment for scoliosis to prevent progressive spinal deformity, renewed interest in screening for scoliosis has been demonstrated, and the Pediatric Orthopaedic Society of North America, the Scoliosis Research Society (SRS), and the American Academy of Pediatrics have declared joint support for these programs.[30] In 2018, the U.S. Preventive Services Task Force[31] again revised their recommendation in regard to screening for scoliosis in asymptomatic children, concluding there was insufficient evidence to assess the balance of benefits and harms in this patient population. They recommended clinicians use their own judgment in regard to patient screening until more evidence exists.

PHYSICAL EXAMINATION

Examination of a child with suspected idiopathic scoliosis is performed to define the appearance of the deformity and assess for signs of nonidiopathic scoliosis. Because AIS is a diagnosis of exclusion, other causes of spinal deformity must be ruled out through examination and imaging findings. The patient should be clothed in an examination gown to allow full assessment. Inspection of the skin is important to identify cutaneous stigmata of other diseases, specifically café au lait spots, sacral dimples, or hairy patches overlying the spine. Careful inspection of the entire patient, including the limbs, should be performed to look for subtle examination findings that may be associated with scoliosis-associated syndromes such as arachnodactyly and Marfan syndrome. With the patient standing, the shoulders, the pelvis, and trunk symmetry should be assessed and overall alignment documented. The Adams forward bend test is used to document axial plane trunk rotation, and gait assessment is important to document subtle neurologic deficits or muscle weakness. A full neurologic assessment of the upper and lower extremities is required, with documentation of the strength and sensation of all nerve root distributions as well as a complete reflex examination, including the presence of symmetric abdominal reflexes, which, if abnormal, can indicate associated intraspinal abnormalities.

IMAGING

Radiographic assessment of patients with suspected spinal deformity should start with PA and lateral radiographs performed on a full-length (36 × 14 inch) cassette in the weight-bearing position (**Figure 3**). Appropriate breast and gonadal shielding should be used to limit radiation exposure to these radiosensitive areas. Recent concerns regarding the cumulative effects of radiation exposure in immature patients and the future risk of malignancy has led to advances in lower dose imaging modalities. Digital radiography is the current standard in radiographic imaging because it leads to a substantial decrease in radiation exposure.[32] A recently introduced, novel imaging system using biplanar digital slot scanning substantially further decreases radiation exposure compared with traditional digital radiography, with no difference in image quality.[33] Nonradiation-based imaging systems such as surface imaging and ultrasonography have been assessed, but their use is limited.

MRI is used to assess the spinal cord for evidence of intraspinal abnormalities in patients with abnormal physical examination findings or, occasionally, for patients with substantial scoliosis-related pain. Routine evaluation of the spinal cord using MRI before surgical intervention in patients with normal physical examination or radiographic findings is a debated issue. Proponents of routine MRI point to the fact that the incidence of intraspinal abnormality in patients with suspected AIS can be up to 10%; however, other physicians argue that very few cases of intraspinal abnormality require neurosurgical intervention before spinal deformity correction, thus demonstrating the limited clinical effect of routine MRI evaluation.[34,35] Some findings, including limited axial

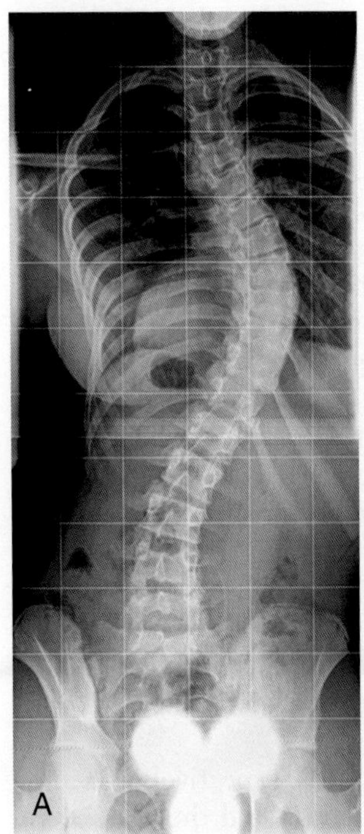

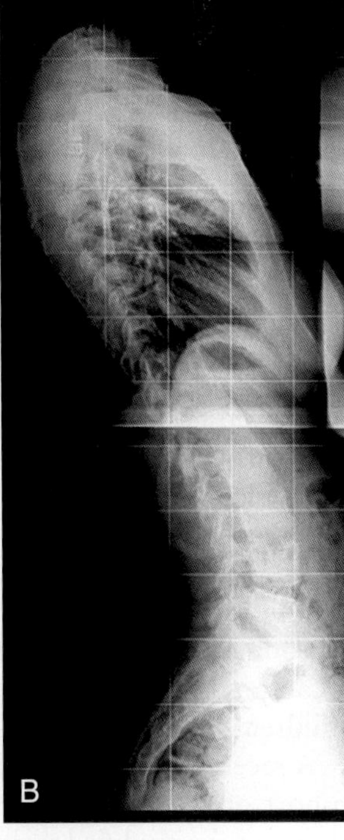

FIGURE 3 Appropriate full-length PA (**A**) and lateral (**B**) radiographs are used in the assessment of idiopathic scoliosis. A 55° right thoracic curve is shown.

plane rotation, abnormal reflexes on examination, lack of thoracic hypokyphosis, atypical curve direction (left thoracic or right thoracolumbar/lumbar), rapid deformity progression, and substantial back or radicular pain, warrant further investigation of the spine with MRI to assess for associated causative intraspinal abnormalities.

TREATMENT

Prediction

Treatment decisions for those with AIS are based mainly on the maturity of the patient and the size of the curve. Immature patients with substantial remaining growth have a higher risk of curve progression than more mature patients with the same size curve. Curve magnitude, in the context of maturity, is important in the decision-making process. Curve magnitudes greater than 20° have approximately a threefold increased risk of progression compared with curves less than 20° in patients with Risser grade 0, 1, or 2 skeletal maturity.[36]

Skeletal maturity has traditionally been judged by the ossification of the iliac apophysis, that is, the Risser sign, and the status of the triradiate cartilage. Although the Risser sign is simple and convenient, it is not sensitive at predicting peak height velocity. The Sanders staging system uses a hand radiograph and better predicts the behavior of idiopathic scoliosis.[22,37] Other radiographic assessments of skeletal growth and maturity have been introduced as well. The radiographic ossification of the olecranon progresses in a regular and predictable fashion during the period of peak height velocity and between the closure of the triradiate cartilage and development of the Risser sign. This elbow scoring system has been shown to correlate well with peak height velocity and allows radiographic assessment of skeletal maturity during this time frame.[38] More recently, growth velocity and skeletal maturity has been shown to be reliably measured by the proximal humeral ossification, offering another marker of skeletal maturity obviating the requirement a second radiograph.[39]

Several genetic markers of AIS have been identified. Currently, there is only one commercially available test available that advertises the ability to stratify the risk of progression.[40,41] Although promising in theory, clinical investigation of this test has been disappointing, as the results promoted by the developers were unable to be reproduced and there is little evidence to confirm that it can predict progressive curves in the at-risk cohort of children.[40,41]

A recent investigation, using a prospectively collected cohort of unbraced patients, evaluated the prognostic ability of the modified skeletal maturity system to predict deformity progression to ≥45° before skeletal maturity, an attempt to predict those patients at high risk for future surgery without treatment. A prognostic model, using the Sanders staging, Cobb angle, and curve pattern was developed, which reliably predicted the risk of curve progression with an associated online risk calculator developed based on this work.[42]

Observation

Observation is indicated for curves of less than 20° because of the relatively low risk of progression. Examination of skeletally immature children at 4- to 6-month intervals allows active treatment to be initiated when progression becomes clear. The exact definition of progression varies slightly among authors, but it is generally accepted that an increase greater than 5° is outside the range of interobserver and intraobserver measurement error. Despite this generally accepted value of progression, clinicians should be mindful of the long-term changes in scoliosis magnitude because single measurements have been shown to be variable. Diurnal variations in the Cobb angle have been shown to be up to 5°, so decisions regarding treatment based on curve progression should be made based on a broader deformity evaluation.[43]

Bracing Treatment

Bracing treatment is the mainstay of nonsurgical treatment of scoliosis for curves with an apex at T7 or below. The SRS criteria for bracing treatment are curves 25° to 45° in patients who are Risser grade 0, 1, or 2 and, if female, less than 1 year postmenarchal. In 2013, a randomized controlled study reported that bracing treatment was successful at avoiding progression past 50° in 72% of patients, compared with 48% of patients who were observed only.[44] The study was stopped early because of the clearly superior efficacy of bracing treatment compared with observation. The number of hours of brace wear is important to success, with those wearing the brace more than 12 hours per day having a greater than 80% chance of avoiding curve progression.[44,45] Treating approximately three patients with bracing treatment will avoid one surgical procedure,[44,46] assuming that the patients are compliant with bracing treatment protocols. Compliance is thought to be the main impediment to successful treatment, but because a large percentage of patients treated with observation alone do not progress to surgery, selection criteria clearly need to be refined. Most current studies use compliance monitors inside the brace to accurately measure time in the brace. These monitors are mainly used for research but are relatively inexpensive and are being adopted in clinical practices to monitor patient compliance.

A thoracolumbosacral orthosis is generally prescribed for treatment and is intended to be worn 18 to 20+ hours per day, given that the total number of hours influences success. A number of rigid braces are available, for example, Boston, Wilmington, Rigo Cheneau, but there is no convincing evidence that one is superior. There has been interest in using flexible bracing; however, a previous study showed the current flexible bracing model was inferior to rigid braces.[47]

The Charleston or Providence nighttime braces are bending braces that are used as an alternative to a full-time thoracolumbosacral orthosis. The goal of this type of nighttime brace is to create opposing forces about the apex of the curve and push it toward or past the midline. Although data exist demonstrating their effectiveness, current high-level studies comparing these two bracing treatment techniques are lacking.

After patients have adapted to their brace, a radiograph is taken with the patient in the brace to evaluate brace quality. Ideally, a thoracolumbosacral orthosis will reduce the curve approximately 50%, whereas a nighttime brace will achieve closer to 80% to 90% curve correction. Children are monitored every 6 months, usually with a radiograph taken when out of the brace, to evaluate for progression. Bracing treatment is discontinued at the conclusion of growth. Typically, for females, this is approximately 18 to 24 months after menarche, when the patient is at Risser grade 4, Sanders stage 7, or when growth has plateaued. Because males often continue to grow after Risser grade 4, height gain should be followed to determine when bracing treatment should be discontinued.[48] Recent evidence that calls into question the use of these growth markers to predicting which deformities are no longer at risk for progression has been published. In a study of 89 females with spinal deformities <50° and maturity of Sanders stage 7, 70% of these patients had further progression of the deformity up to 10° over 2 years of follow-up. Furthermore, 12% of these mature patients progressed to surgery in follow-up. The authors concluded those patients with a deformity >40° at Sanders stage 7 were at risk for further progression to surgery and should be followed beyond this marker of maturity.[49] Most physicians agree that bracing treatment has substantial effects on both the patient and his or her family; however, there are limited data evaluating the extent of the psychologic effect.[50]

Surgery

For adolescents presenting with curves greater than 50° or curves progressing past 45° in immature patients, traditionally, posterior spinal fusion is recommended. Curves of this magnitude tend to progress 1° per year even after skeletal maturity.[24] The primary goal of surgery is to prevent further progression by obtaining fusion while maintaining spinal balance in the coronal and sagittal planes. Secondary goals include decreasing the size of the curve and reducing the associated deformities such as trunk shift, waist asymmetry, shoulder height differences, and rotational prominences on the back. As few motion segments as necessary should be fused to achieve these goals. As discussed previously, this decision making is based primarily on the spinal deformity itself. The natural history studies have found limited evidence linking larger spinal deformity and poor functional outcomes, so the decision for surgical intervention should include discussion of the spinal deformity and long-term functional goals of the patient, and the final decision should be shared between patient and provider.

The Lenke classification provides guidance on the selection of fusion levels in the surgical management of AIS.[4] As opposed to the classic King-Moe classification, the Lenke classification includes curves with the major component in the thoracolumbar and lumbar spine and highlights the importance of the sagittal plane. The classification includes six curve types, three lumbar modifiers, and three sagittal modifiers, resulting in 42 different possible patterns. Supine bending radiographs are required to use the classification system to distinguish structural (curves that do not bend out to <25°) from nonstructural curves (curve that bend out to <25°). Despite the purpose of the Lenke classification in standardizing surgical planning, controversy still exists in which curves require fusion, the exact choice of fusion levels, and the appropriateness of fusing into the lower lumbar spine.

The most common curve patterns are Lenke types 1A and 1B. For these curves, the upper instrumented vertebra is typically the proximal end vertebra (often T4; **Figure 4**). The choice of the lowest instrumented vertebra is not as clear, but the lowest vertebra that is substantially touched by the center sacral vertical line is commonly the lowest instrumented vertebra. If the proximal thoracic curve is structural (Lenke type 2), the left shoulder is elevated, or there is kyphosis greater than 20° from T2 through T5, then T2 or T3 should be considered for the upper instrumented vertebra because this allows correction of the structural upper thoracic curve, which theoretically improves the ability to level the upper thoracic vertebrae with the goal of improving shoulder balance. Thoracolumbar and lumbar curves (Lenke type 5) are typically fused from the proximal end vertebra to the distal end vertebra.

Selective thoracic fusions are appealing for the preservation of lumbar motion. Having more available motion segments in the lumbar spine after fusion will allow for greater distribution of functional motion.[51] In addition, it seems intuitive that a curved, flexible spine offers a better long-term outcome than a straight, fused spine. However, there is no definitive connection between long fusions and symptomatic distal facet or disk degeneration. Historically, selective thoracic fusions were used for King-Moe type II curves in which the lumbar curve was considered compensatory. Lenke type 1B and 1C

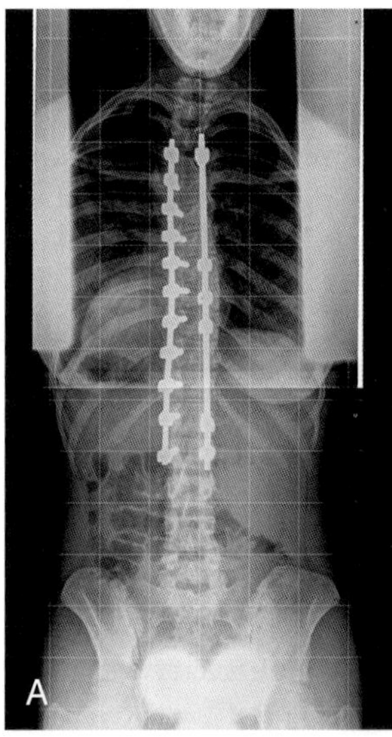

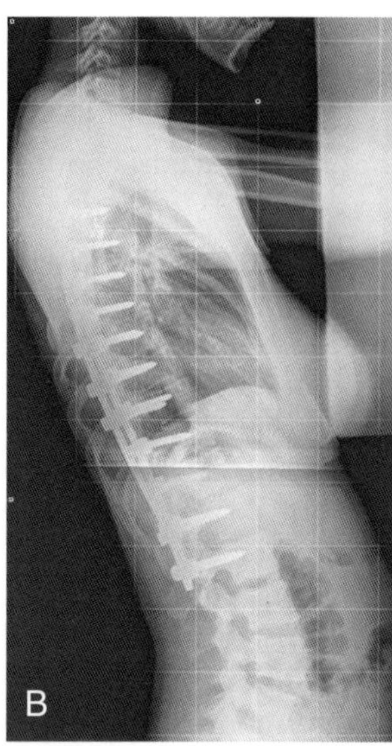

FIGURE 4 PA (**A**) and lateral (**B**) radiographs of the patient shown in **Figure 3** taken 2 years after a T4-L2 posterior spinal fusion for adolescent idiopathic scoliosis show correction of the deformity from 55° preoperatively to 14° postoperatively.

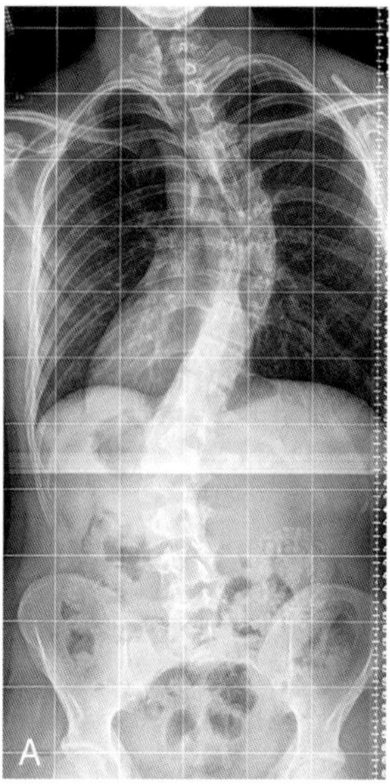

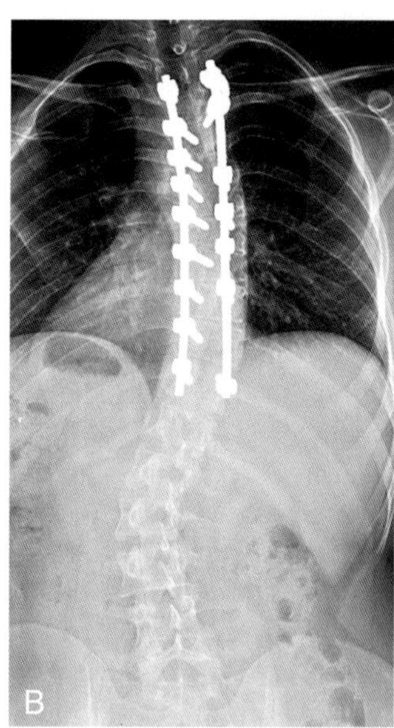

FIGURE 5 **A**, Preoperative radiograph of a patient with adolescent idiopathic scoliosis with a 55° right thoracic curve and a 45° left lumbar deformity. **B**, PA radiograph taken 3 years after a selective thoracic fusion. The postoperative radiograph shows correction of the right thoracic curve to 30° with spontaneous correction of the lumbar deformity to 26°.

patterns include these curve types. Spontaneous lumbar correction occurs with correction of the thoracic curve.[52] However, over time, the use of selective thoracic fusion has evolved to include Lenke type 3C curves.[53,54]

Commonly used criteria for selective fusion include a thoracic-to-lumbar curve magnitude ratio greater than 1.2, an apical vertebral translation ratio greater than 1.2, and a preoperative lumbar curve less than 45°[53] (**Figure 5**). In a 20-year follow-up study that included Lenke type 1B, 1C, and 3C curves, lumbar curve correction and overall balance were maintained over time; however, the patients had lower scores in self-image on the SRS-24 questionnaire compared with patients treated with fusions that included the lumbar spine.[55] Specifically, for Lenke type 3C patterns, patients with long fusions tend to have better balance and radiographic parameters than patients treated with selective fusions at 2-year follow-ups;[54] however, concerns remain about long-term function as patients age.

Most spinal fusions are now performed using a posterior approach. Historically, lumbar and thoracolumbar curves were approached anteriorly to decrease the number of levels needed to obtain correction. The use of pedicle screws that provide three-column fixation combined with wide posterior releases allows the posterior approach to provide similar radiographic outcomes as achieved with the anterior approach.[56,57]

Pedicle screws have become the standard implant for AIS correction because they provide more control of the vertebral body, allow for better three-dimensional correction, increase the strength of the construct, and avoid entry into the spinal canal. Although radiographic correction may be better than with hybrid constructs, no study has shown a difference in patient outcomes. Given that the costs of modern implants approaches 30% of the total cost for primary AIS surgical care,[58] there is interest in determining the clinical difference between implants with high-density and low-density constructs.[59,60] More research is needed to better understand the appropriate balance between cost, implant density, curve correction, and clinical outcomes.

An ideal treatment of AIS would provide curve correction without sacrificing motion. Anterior vertebral body tethering is a new technique that strives to achieve this goal.[61] To date, only small retrospective series have been published. Although the technique has shown the ability to alter the natural history of scoliosis and correct the deformity, it is not without complication and is not effective in all patients.[62,63] In a series of 17 patients, only 10 (59%) were considered clinically successful, with 41% requiring a revision surgery.[63] In August 2019, the FDA approved the first tethering system to treat idiopathic scoliosis ranging 30° to 65° in immature patients in whom bracing treatment had failed or who are intolerant to it. Currently, there is no consensus on the appropriate indication or physiologic timing for this intervention. More research is needed to better understand the long-term outcomes and potential complications of vertebral body tethering.

The perioperative care of patients undergoing spinal fusion has improved through the development of standardized care pathways. Decreasing variability of care in the preoperative, intraoperative, and postoperative periods has been consistently demonstrated to improve patient outcomes following posterior spinal fusion for idiopathic scoliosis. Multiple institutions have published results showing a significantly decreased length of stay, less use of opioid pain medications, improved pain control, and fewer blood transfusions with institution of a standardized care pathway.[64-66]

The overall complication rate for the surgical treatment of AIS is relatively low.[67] An infection within the first 3 months occurs in approximately 1% of patients and most commonly results from *Staphylococcus aureus*. Late infections may require hardware removal. The risk of spinal cord injury is less than 1%, but the risk is higher in revision settings and if osteotomies are performed.[67] Most spinal cord injuries are thought to be vascular in nature and result from the correction. Pseudarthrosis is uncommon in young, healthy patients undergoing spinal fusion.

OUTCOMES

Long-term studies investigating the natural history of AIS have demonstrated relatively few functional limitations in patients who were treated only with observation or bracing treatment.[68] In general, these studies have shown that spinal deformities tend to progress, but the risk of severe pulmonary or cardiac disease is limited; patients seem to lead functional lives without excessive pain; and social function is normal, with only self-image being consistently lower in patients with scoliosis compared with normal control subjects.[68-71] Although short-term studies have demonstrated improvements in patient-reported outcomes after surgery for AIS, midterm outcome investigations have shown that these results change over time.[72]

Questions remain regarding the incremental improvements in health-related quality of life with modern advancements in surgical techniques. Given the substantial increase in the cost associated with modern surgical interventions,[73] which are mainly associated with modern pedicle screw instrumentation, future studies are critically needed to determine the cost-benefit ratios of nonsurgical and surgical treatment options for AIS using patient-specific health-related outcome measures. The currently used scoliosis-specific patient-reported outcomes measure, the SRS-22, has been assessed and shows variable ability to discriminate between curve magnitudes. Although this tool has shown good discriminative validity between small nonsurgical curves and large preoperative curves, this was shown only in a few domains of the tool. In addition, few differences were noted within moderate-size curves.[74] This variable discriminative validity of the current scoliosis-specific patient-reported outcomes measure highlights the need for future improvements in the design of these outcome measures.

SUMMARY

AIS affects approximately 2% to 3% of patients between the ages of 10 and 14 years. Accurate diagnosis and prediction of the likelihood of deformity progression is important to determine optimal treatment strategies. Observation, scoliosis-specific exercises, brace treatment, and surgical intervention may be indicated based on the maturity of the patient and the magnitude of the deformity. Future investigations of patient outcomes after different treatments will be important in optimizing cost-effective treatments.

KEY STUDY POINTS

- AIS is a three-dimensional spinal deformity producing deviations in the coronal, sagittal, and axial planes, and it affects 2% to 3% of children.
- Treatment of AIS is based on the magnitude of the deformity and the skeletal maturity of the patient. In patients with substantial remaining growth, the basic treatment guidelines are observation for curves less than 20°, brace treatment for curves 20° to 45°, and spinal fusion for curves greater than 50°.
- Long-term studies for patients with untreated AIS have demonstrated relatively few functional differences compared with normal control subjects. Future investigations into the functional benefits of surgery for idiopathic scoliosis using detailed patient-reported health-related outcome tools will be important in optimizing treatment algorithms.

ANNOTATED REFERENCES

1. Labelle H, Aubin CE, Jackson R, Lenke L, Newton P, Parent S: Seeing the spine in 3D: How will it change what we do? *J Pediatr Orthop* 2011;31(1 suppl):S37-S45.
2. Newton PO, Fujimori T, Doan J, Reighard FG, Bastrom TP, Misaghi A: Defining the "three-dimensional sagittal plane" in thoracic adolescent idiopathic scoliosis. *J Bone Joint Surg Am* 2015;97(20):1694-1701.
3. King HA, Moe JH, Bradford DS, Winter RB: The selection of fusion levels in thoracic idiopathic scoliosis. *J Bone Joint Surg Am* 1983;65(9):1302-1313.
4. Lenke LG, Betz RR, Harms J, et al: Adolescent idiopathic scoliosis: A new classification to determine extent of spinal arthrodesis. *J Bone Joint Surg Am* 2001;83(8):1169-1181.
5. Richards BS, Sucato DJ, Konigsberg DE, Ouellet JA: Comparison of reliability between the Lenke and King classification systems for adolescent idiopathic scoliosis using radiographs that were not premeasured. *Spine (Phila Pa 1976)* 2003;28(11):1148-1156.

6. Lenke LG, Betz RR, Clements D, et al: Curve prevalence of a new classification of operative adolescent idiopathic scoliosis: Does classification correlate with treatment? *Spine (Phila Pa 1976)* 2002;27(6):604-611.

7. Romano M, Minozzi S, Bettany-Saltikov J, et al: Exercises for adolescent idiopathic scoliosis. *Cochrane Database Syst Rev* 2012;8:CD007837.

8. Burger M, Coetzee W, du Plessis LZ, et al: The effectiveness of Schroth exercises in adolescents with idiopathic scoliosis: A systematic review and meta-analysis. *S Afr J Physiother* 2019;75:904.

A meta-analysis of the impact of Schroth exercises shows limited statistical improvements in both Cobb angle and self-reported quality of life in patients who participated in this therapy. These improvements were quite modest, with questionable clinical significance despite statistical improvement. Additionally, this review is limited somewhat by the methodologic limitations. Level of evidence: II.

9. Day JM, Fletcher J, Coghlan M, Ravine T: Review of scoliosis-specific exercise methods used to correct adolescent idiopathic scoliosis. *Arch Physiother* 2019;9:8.

A literature review of studies investigated physiotherapy scoliosis-specific exercises to determine the effect of these exercises as a treatment method for scoliosis. This review found no evidence to suggest physiotherapy scoliosis-specific exercises are more effective at reducing Cobb angle compared with observation. Level of evidence: V.

10. Schreiber S, Parent EC, Hill DL, Hedden DM, Moreau MJ, Southon SC: Schroth physiotherapeutic scoliosis-specific exercises for adolescent idiopathic scoliosis: How many patients require treatment to prevent one deterioration? – Results from a randomized controlled trial – "SOSORT 2017 Award Winner". *Scoliosis Spinal Disord* 2017;12:26.

This is a randomized controlled trial of Schroth physical therapy for idiopathic scoliosis. This study showed a number needed to treat of 3.1 to decrease the risk of scoliosis progressing beyond 5°. Level of evidence: II.

11. Płaszewski M, Bettany-Saltikov J: Non-surgical interventions for adolescents with idiopathic scoliosis: An overview of systematic reviews. *PLoS One* 2014;9(10):e110254.

12. Dayer R, Haumont T, Belaieff W, Lascombes P: Idiopathic scoliosis: Etiological concepts and hypotheses. *J Child Orthop* 2013;7(1):11-16.

13. Sharma S, Gao X, Londono D, et al: Genome-wide association studies of adolescent idiopathic scoliosis suggest candidate susceptibility genes. *Hum Mol Genet* 2011;20(7):1456-1466.

14. Takahashi Y, Kou I, Takahashi A, et al: A genome-wide association study identifies common variants near LBX1 associated with adolescent idiopathic scoliosis. *Nat Genet* 2011;43(12):1237-1240.

15. Londono D, Kou I, Johnson TA, et al, TSRHC IS Clinical Group, International Consortium for Scoliosis Genetics, Japanese Scoliosis Clinical Research Group: A meta-analysis identifies adolescent idiopathic scoliosis association with LBX1 locus in multiple ethnic groups. *J Med Genet* 2014;51(6):401-406.

16. Sharma S, Londono D, Eckalbar WL, et al, TSRHC Scoliosis Clinical Group, Japan Scoliosis Clinical Research Group: A PAX1 enhancer locus is associated with susceptibility to idiopathic scoliosis in females. *Nat Commun* 2015;6:6452.

17. Kou I, Takahashi Y, Johnson TA, et al: Genetic variants in GPR126 are associated with adolescent idiopathic scoliosis. *Nat Genet* 2013;45(6):676-679.

18. Karner CM, Long F, Solnica-Krezel L, Monk KR, Gray RS: Gpr126/Adgrg6 deletion in cartilage models idiopathic scoliosis and pectus excavatum in mice. *Hum Mol Genet* 2015;24(15):4365-4373.

19. Gorman KF, Julien C, Moreau A: The genetic epidemiology of idiopathic scoliosis. *Eur Spine J* 2012;21(10):1905-1919.

20. Negrini S, Aulisa AG, Aulisa L, et al: 2011 SOSORT guidelines: Orthopaedic and rehabilitation treatment of idiopathic scoliosis during growth. *Scoliosis* 2012;7(1):3.

21. Busscher I, Kingma I, de Bruin R, Wapstra FH, Verkerke GJ, Veldhuizen AG: Predicting the peak growth velocity in the individual child: Validation of a new growth model. *Eur Spine J* 2012;21(1):71-76.

22. Sanders JO, Khoury JG, Kishan S, et al: Predicting scoliosis progression from skeletal maturity: A simplified classification during adolescence. *J Bone Joint Surg Am* 2008;90(3):540-553.

23. Weinstein SL, Zavala DC, Ponseti IV: Idiopathic scoliosis: Long-term follow-up and prognosis in untreated patients. *J Bone Joint Surg Am* 1981;63(5):702-712.

24. Weinstein SL, Ponseti IV: Curve progression in idiopathic scoliosis. *J Bone Joint Surg Am* 1983;65(4):447-455.

25. Weinstein SL, Dolan LA, Spratt KF, Peterson KK, Spoonamore MJ, Ponseti IV: Health and function of patients with untreated idiopathic scoliosis: A 50-year natural history study. *J Am Med Assoc* 2003;289(5):559-567.

26. Johnston CE, Richards BS, Sucato DJ, Bridwell KH, Lenke LG, Erickson M, Spinal Deformity Study Group: Correlation of preoperative deformity magnitude and pulmonary function tests in adolescent idiopathic scoliosis. *Spine (Phila Pa 1976)* 2011;36(14):1096-1102.

27. Korovessis PG, Stamatakis MV: Prediction of scoliotic Cobb angle with the use of the scoliometer. *Spine (Phila Pa 1976)* 1996;21(14):1661-1666.

28. Balg F, Juteau M, Theoret C, Svotelis A, Grenier G: Validity and reliability of the iPhone to measure rib hump in scoliosis. *J Pediatr Orthop* 2014;34(8):774-779.

29. U.S. Preventive Services Task Force: *Screening for Idiopathic Scoliosis in Adolescents: Recommendation Statement.* Rockville, MD, Agency for Healthcare Research and Quality, June 2004.

30. Richards BS, Vitale MG: Screening for idiopathic scoliosis in adolescents: An information statement. *J Bone Joint Surg Am* 2008;90(1):195-198.

31. US Preventive Services Task Force; Grossman DC, Curry SJ, Owens DK, et al: Screening for adolescent idiopathic scoliosis: US Preventive Services Task Force recommendation statement. *JAMA* 2018;319(2):165-172.

This was an update to the recommendations of the US Preventive Services Task Force (USPSTF) recommendation on screening for idiopathic scoliosis in asymptomatic adolescents from 2004. The task force found the evidence was insufficient to assess the balance of benefits and harms of screening for adolescent idiopathic scoliosis in children and adolescents aged 10 to 18 years.

32. Grieser T, Baldauf AQ, Ludwig K: Radiation dose reduction in scoliosis patients: Low-dose full-spine radiography with digital flat panel detector and image stitching system. *Rofo* 2011;183(7):645-649.
33. Ilharreborde B, Ferrero E, Alison M, Mazda K: EOS microdose protocol for the radiological follow-up of adolescent idiopathic scoliosis. *Eur Spine J* 2016;25(2):526-531.

    The authors present a prospective study of the EOS (EOS imaging) microdose protocol assessing dose exposure and image quality. A substantial decrease in patient radiation dose without image quality degradation was reported. Level of evidence: III.
34. Nakahara D, Yonezawa I, Kobanawa K, et al: Magnetic resonance imaging evaluation of patients with idiopathic scoliosis: A prospective study of four hundred seventy-two outpatients. *Spine (Phila Pa 1976)* 2011;36(7):E482-E485.
35. Richards BS, Sucato DJ, Johnston CE, et al, Spinal Deformity Study Group: Right thoracic curves in presumed adolescent idiopathic scoliosis: Which clinical and radiographic findings correlate with a preoperative abnormal magnetic resonance image? *Spine (Phila Pa 1976)* 2010;35(20):1855-1860.
36. Lonstein JE, Carlson JM: The prediction of curve progression in untreated idiopathic scoliosis during growth. *J Bone Joint Surg Am* 1984;66(7):1061-1071.
37. Minkara A, Bainton N, Tanaka M, et al: High risk of mismatch between Sanders and Risser staging in adolescent idiopathic scoliosis: Are we guiding treatment using the wrong classification? *J Pediatr Orthop* 2020;40(2):60-64.

    This radiographic evaluation study compared Risser grading with Sanders staging to assess skeletal maturity in patients with scoliosis. The authors found the Risser sign to underestimate skeletal maturity in 21.8% of patients and overestimate maturity in 3.6%. Risser grading appears to have limited sensitivity compared with Sanders staging in assessing skeletal growth remaining. Level of evidence: II.
38. Charles YP, Diméglio A, Canavese F, Daures JP: Skeletal age assessment from the olecranon for idiopathic scoliosis at Risser grade 0. *J Bone Joint Surg Am* 2007;89(12):2737-2744.
39. Li DT, Linderman GC, Cui JJ, et al: The proximal humeral ossification system improves assessment of maturity in patients with scoliosis. *J Bone Joint Surg Am* 2019;101(20):1868-1874.

    This study assesses the accuracy and predictive ability of a novel radiographic marker of skeletal growth and maturity using the ossification of the proximal humerus. Level of evidence: III.
40. Ogura Y, Takahashi Y, Kou I, et al: A replication study for association of 5 single nucleotide polymorphisms with curve progression of adolescent idiopathic scoliosis in Japanese patients. *Spine (Phila Pa 1976)* 2013;38(7):571-575.
41. Tang QL, Julien C, Eveleigh R, et al: A replication study for association of 53 single nucleotide polymorphisms in ScoliScore test with adolescent idiopathic scoliosis in French-Canadian population. *Spine (Phila Pa 1976)* 2015;40(8):537-543.
42. Dolan LA, Weinstein SL, Abel MF, et al: Bracing in Adolescent Idiopathic Scoliosis Trial (BrAIST): Development and validation of a prognostic model in untreated adolescent idiopathic scoliosis using the simplified skeletal maturity system. *Spine Deform* 2019;7(6):890-898.

    This study presents a reliable risk stratification system and online risk calculator using the Cobb angle, Sanders scoring, and curve pattern to predict the likelihood of a poor spinal deformity prognosis in untreated patients with AIS. Level of evidence: I.
43. Beauchamp M, Labelle H, Grimard G, Stanciu C, Poitras B, Dansereau J: Diurnal variation of Cobb angle measurement in adolescent idiopathic scoliosis. *Spine (Phila Pa 1976)* 1993;18(12):1581-1583.
44. Weinstein SL, Dolan LA, Wright JG, Dobbs MB: Effects of bracing in adolescents with idiopathic scoliosis. *N Engl J Med* 2013;369(16):1512-1521.
45. Katz DE, Herring JA, Browne RH, Kelly DM, Birch JG: Brace wear control of curve progression in adolescent idiopathic scoliosis. *J Bone Joint Surg Am* 2010;92(6):1343-1352.
46. Sanders JO, Newton PO, Browne RH, Katz DE, Birch JG, Herring JA: Bracing for idiopathic scoliosis: How many patients require treatment to prevent one surgery? *J Bone Joint Surg Am* 2014;96(8):649-653.
47. Guo J, Lam TP, Wong MS, et al: A prospective randomized controlled study on the treatment outcome of SpineCor brace versus rigid brace for adolescent idiopathic scoliosis with follow-up according to the SRS standardized criteria. *Eur Spine J* 2014;23(12):2650-2657.
48. Karol LA, Johnston CE II, Browne RH, Madison M: Progression of the curve in boys who have idiopathic scoliosis. *J Bone Joint Surg Am* 1993;75(12):1804-1810.
49. Grothaus O, Molina D, Jacobs C, Talwalkar V, Iwinski H, Muchow R: Is it growth or natural history? Increasing spinal deformity after Sanders stage 7 in females with AIS. *J Pediatr Orthop* 2020;40(3):e176-e181.

    This is a retrospective study of the progression of AIS in females with a Sanders 7 bone age after brace discontinuation. The authors found 70% of these patients had progressive deformities, with a deformity >40° at risk for progression to surgery. Level of evidence: III.
50. Negrini S, Minozzi S, Bettany-Saltikov J, et al: Braces for idiopathic scoliosis in adolescents. *Cochrane Database Syst Rev* 2015;6:CD006850.
51. Marks M, Newton PO, Petcharaporn M, et al: Postoperative segmental motion of the unfused spine distal to the fusion in 100 patients with adolescent idiopathic scoliosis. *Spine (Phila Pa 1976)* 2012;37(10):826-832.
52. Lenke LG, Betz RR, Bridwell KH, Harms J, Clements DH, Lowe TG: Spontaneous lumbar curve coronal correction after selective anterior or posterior thoracic fusion in adolescent idiopathic scoliosis. *Spine (Phila Pa 1976)* 1999;24(16):1663-1671.
53. Schulz J, Asghar J, Bastrom T, et al, Harms Study Group: Optimal radiographical criteria after selective thoracic fusion for patients with adolescent idiopathic scoliosis with a C lumbar modifier: Does adherence to current guidelines predict success? *Spine (Phila Pa 1976)* 2014;39(23):E1368-E1373.

54. Singla A, Bennett JT, Sponseller PD, et al: Results of selective thoracic versus nonselective fusion in Lenke type 3 curves. *Spine (Phila Pa 1976)* 2014;39(24):2034-2041.

55. Larson AN, Fletcher ND, Daniel C, Richards BS: Lumbar curve is stable after selective thoracic fusion for adolescent idiopathic scoliosis: A 20-year follow-up. *Spine (Phila Pa 1976)* 2012;37(10):833-839.

56. Geck MJ, Rinella A, Hawthorne D, et al: Comparison of surgical treatment in Lenke 5C adolescent idiopathic scoliosis: Anterior dual rod versus posterior pedicle fixation surgery. A comparison of two practices. *Spine (Phila Pa 1976)* 2009;34(18):1942-1951.

57. Shufflebarger HL, Geck MJ, Clark CE: The posterior approach for lumbar and thoracolumbar adolescent idiopathic scoliosis: Posterior shortening and pedicle screws. *Spine (Phila Pa 1976)* 2004;29(3):269-276.

58. Kamerlink JR, Quirno M, Auerbach JD, et al: Hospital cost analysis of adolescent idiopathic scoliosis correction surgery in 125 consecutive cases. *J Bone Joint Surg Am* 2010;92(5):1097-1104.

59. Bharucha NJ, Lonner BS, Auerbach JD, Kean KE, Trobisch PD: Low-density versus high-density thoracic pedicle screw constructs in adolescent idiopathic scoliosis: Do more screws lead to a better outcome? *Spine J* 2013;13(4):375-381.

60. Larson AN, Polly DW Jr, Diamond B, et al, Minimize Implants Maximize Outcomes Study Group: Does higher anchor density result in increased curve correction and improved clinical outcomes in adolescent idiopathic scoliosis? *Spine (Phila Pa 1976)* 2014;39(7):571-578.

61. Samdani AF, Ames RJ, Kimball JS, et al: Anterior vertebral body tethering for immature adolescent idiopathic scoliosis: One-year results on the first 32 patients. *Eur Spine J* 2015;24(7):1533-1539.

62. Samdani AF, Ames RJ, Kimball JS, et al: Anterior vertebral body tethering for idiopathic scoliosis: Two-year results. *Spine (Phila Pa 1976)* 2014;39(20):1688-1693.

63. Newton PO, Kluck DG, Saito W, Yaszay B, Bartley CE, Bastrom TP: Anterior spinal growth tethering for skeletally immature patients with scoliosis: A retrospective look two to four years postoperatively. *J Bone Joint Surg Am* 2018;100:1691-1697.

    This is a cohort study of 17 patients treated with anterior spinal growth tethering for idiopathic scoliosis. The cohort was found to have 51% deformity correction at a mean of 2.5 years' follow-up. Despite clinical success in 59% of patients, seven patients required revision surgery and three patients progressed to posterior spinal fusion. Level of evidence: IV.

64. Muhly WT, Sankar WN, Ryan K, et al: Rapid recovery pathway after spinal fusion for idiopathic scoliosis. *Pediatrics* 2016;137(4):e20151568.

    This is an assessment of a standardized recovery pathway for idiopathic scoliosis; this study showed this pathway led to a decrease in postoperative length of stay and daily pain scores. Level of evidence: III.

65. Fletcher ND, Andras LM, Lazarus DE, et al: Use of a novel pathway for early discharge was associated with a 48% shorter length of stay after posterior spinal fusion for adolescent idiopathic scoliosis. *J Pediatr Orthop* 2017;37:92-97.

    This is a comparative cohort study of the effectiveness of a standardized postoperative care pathway to facilitate early discharge following posterior spinal fusion for idiopathic scoliosis. The standardized care pathway led to a 48% shorter postoperative stay compared with no standardized postoperative pathway. Level of evidence: III.

66. Oetgen ME, Martin BD, Gordish-Dressman H, Cronin J, Pestieau SR: Effectiveness and sustainability of a standardized care pathway developed with use of lean process mapping for the treatment of patients undergoing posterior spinal fusion for adolescent idiopathic scoliosis. *J Bone Joint Surg Am* 2018;100:1864-1870.

    This study assessed the sustainability of a standardized postoperative care pathway for patients with idiopathic scoliosis. Implementation of this pathway demonstrated significant improvement in postoperative length of stay, improved pain scores, and lower postoperative opioid use. These clinical improvements were maintained over a 2.5-year period. Level of evidence: III.

67. Reames DL, Smith JS, Fu KM, et al, Scoliosis Research Society Morbidity and Mortality Committee: Complications in the surgical treatment of 19,360 cases of pediatric scoliosis: A review of the Scoliosis Research Society Morbidity and Mortality database. *Spine (Phila Pa 1976)* 2011;36(18):1484-1491.

68. Danielsson AJ, Hasserius R, Ohlin A, Nachemson AL: Health-related quality of life in untreated versus brace-treated patients with adolescent idiopathic scoliosis: A long-term follow-up. *Spine (Phila Pa 1976)* 2010;35(2):199-205.

69. Simony A, Hansen EJ, Carreon LY, Christensen SB, Andersen MO: Health-related quality-of-life in adolescent idiopathic scoliosis patients 25 years after treatment. *Scoliosis* 2015;10:22.

70. Rushton PR, Grevitt MP: Comparison of untreated adolescent idiopathic scoliosis with normal controls: A review and statistical analysis of the literature. *Spine (Phila Pa 1976)* 2013;38(9):778-785.

71. Danielsson AJ: Natural history of adolescent idiopathic scoliosis: A tool for guidance in decision of surgery of curves above 50°. *J Child Orthop* 2013;7(1):37-41.

72. Ghandehari H, Mahabadi MA, Mahdavi SM, Shahsavaripour A, Seyed Tari HV, Safdari F: Evaluation of patient outcome and satisfaction after surgical treatment of adolescent idiopathic scoliosis using Scoliosis Research Society-30. *Arch Bone Jt Surg* 2015;3(2):109-113.

73. Martin CT, Pugely AJ, Gao Y, et al: Increasing hospital charges for adolescent idiopathic scoliosis in the United States. *Spine (Phila Pa 1976)* 2014;39(20):1676-1682.

74. Berliner JL, Verma K, Lonner BS, Penn PU, Bharucha NJ: Discriminative validity of the Scoliosis Research Society 22 questionnaire among five curve-severity subgroups of adolescents with idiopathic scoliosis. *Spine J* 2013;13(2):127-133.

CHAPTER 33

Neuromuscular Spine Deformity

AMANDA T. WHITAKER, MD • PATRICK CURRAN, MD, MS • BRIAN D. SNYDER, MD, PhD

ABSTRACT

Spinal deformity (scoliosis and/or kyphosis) commonly affects children with neuromuscular maladies such as cerebral palsy, muscular dystrophy, spinal muscular atrophy, hereditary motor neuropathy (Charcot-Marie-Tooth disease), Rett syndrome, myelodysplasia, Friedreich ataxia, arthrogryposis, and spinal cord injury. The severity of the spinal deformity is often related to the extent of the neurologic impairment and the age of the child at presentation. Many comorbidities are associated with neuromuscular scoliosis, including hip instability, thoracic insufficiency, and cardiopulmonary compromise. Large curves in patients with the most involved and medically complicated disease are managed surgically, although risks are high and the perceived benefits may be limited. However, improvements in measuring outcomes and quality of life in patients with neuromuscular deformities may better demonstrate the benefits of surgical treatment.

Dr. Whitaker or an immediate family member serves as a paid consultant to or is an employee of Cartessa and serves as a board member, owner, officer, or committee member of the American Academy for Cerebral Palsy and Developmental Medicine and the Pediatric Orthopaedic Society of North America. Dr. Snyder or an immediate family member serves as an unpaid consultant to OrthoPediatrics and serves as a board member, owner, officer, or committee member of the American Academy of Orthopaedic Surgeons, the Orthopaedic Research Society, the Pediatric Orthopaedic Society of North America, and the Scoliosis Research Society. Neither Dr. Curran nor any immediate family member has received anything of value from or has stock or stock options held in a commercial company or institution related directly or indirectly to the subject of this chapter.

Keywords: kyphosis; neuromuscular; scoliosis; spinal deformity; spine

INTRODUCTION

Spinal deformity (scoliosis and/or kyphosis) commonly affects children afflicted with neuromuscular maladies such as cerebral palsy, muscular dystrophy, spinal muscular atrophy (SMA), hereditary motor neuropathy (Charcot-Marie-Tooth disease), Rett syndrome, myelodysplasia, Friedreich ataxia, arthrogryposis, and spinal cord injury (**Table 1**). The severity of the spinal deformity is often related to the extent of neurologic impairment and the age at which the child presents with disfigurement—more involved children frequently present with larger curves at a younger age; the likelihood of curve progression increases as a function of statural growth remaining.[1] Risk factors for developing neuromuscular spine deformity include truncal hypotonia, spasticity/dystonia, impaired sitting balance, and nonambulatory status. Large lumbar curves are associated with pelvic obliquity and hip instability; large thoracic curves are associated with thoracic insufficiency and cardiopulmonary compromise.[2,3] Unlike adolescent idiopathic scoliosis (AIS), in this population of children, nonsurgical interventions (bracing treatment, physical therapy, and/or wheelchair modification) have not been demonstrated to ameliorate curve progression over the long term.[4] Surgical interventions that stabilize or correct spinal deformity have been demonstrated to reduce curve magnitude, cause associated pelvic obliquity, and increase thoracic volume, which contribute to improved sitting posture, reduced dependence on external supports, and improved pulmonary function. However, the number and rate of complications associated with the surgical management of neuromuscular spine deformity are high, related to the frail health of these children who frequently suffer from complex medical comorbidities.[5] In this era of needing

TABLE 1

Incidence of Scoliosis in Neuromuscular Conditions

Diagnosis	Incidence (%)	Etiology	Presentation
Cerebral palsy	25-100	Brain injury	Spastic, dyskinetic, ataxic, and mixed variants that can affect all or part of the body, with varying severity of involvement present at or shortly after birth
Charcot-Marie-Tooth disease (hereditary motor and sensory neuropathy)	10-30	Genetic defect in axon or myelin composition (90% in *PMP22, MPZ, GJB1*, or *MFN2* gene)	Peripheral neuropathy with variable penetrance manifested by cavovarus feet, loss of intrinsic musculature, and loss of proprioception
Spina bifida	60-100	Folate deficiency	Neural tube defects ranging in level and severity of involvement present at birth
Rett syndrome	27-66	*MECP2* mutation	Regression of previously normal developmental milestones between 6 and 30 months of age
Spinal muscular atrophy	70-100	*SMN1* gene (survival motor neuron protein), SMN2 modifies severity	Death of anterior horn cells of the spinal cord causing progressive hypotonia and muscle weakness in early childhood
Friedreich ataxia	80	*FXN* gene (frataxin) trinucleotide repeats	Spinocerebellar disorder with onset of ataxia, weakness, stiffness, cardiomyopathy, diabetes, hearing loss, and impaired vision at puberty
Duchenne muscular dystrophy	60-90	*DMD* gene (dystrophin)	X-linked disorder appearing in early childhood with muscle weakness, pseudohypertrophy, and delayed milestones
Spinal cord injury	100	Trauma	Trauma to the spinal cord with neurologic injury

to establish the quality and value of our interventions, defining appropriate metrics to prove the success of managing neuromuscular scoliosis (NMS) is lacking. Patient-related outcome measures such as quality of life (QOL) are difficult to ascertain directly in this patient population who are limited by cognitive and physical impairments. The few prospective and retrospective studies that have evaluated QOL based on patient, parent, and caregiver surrogates demonstrate mixed results.[6-8] Assessment of the real cost of these treatments remains elusive.

PATIENT ASSESSMENT

The evaluation of a patient with NMS must consider the child's physiologic age, the magnitude and location of the spinal deformity, the underlying neuromuscular disease, associated medical comorbidities, and functional status. These findings will aid in the development of a rational treatment strategy based on the patient's prognosis, expected rate of curve progression, and exacerbation of musculoskeletal and medical ailments related to the scoliosis. Curve magnitudes <45° do not impair functional mobility, aggravate ischial decubiti, decrease oxygen saturation, or alter heart rate. Curve magnitudes >45° may compromise sitting posture that interferes with trunk balance and positioning.[3] Large (>70°) thoracic curves are often associated with rib cage distortion that contributes to thoracic insufficiency syndrome and restricted pulmonary function. Large thoracolumbar and lumbar curves are often associated with pelvic obliquity that contributes to hip instability and infrapelvic deformity from soft-tissue contractures. However, the causal relationship between hip and spine deformity has not been established. In nonambulatory children with unilateral hip instability, a compensatory lumbar curve may develop. As the lumbar curve and pelvic obliquity increase, the hip on the concave side becomes adducted and the hip on the convex side becomes abducted, creating a windswept posture. Increasing pelvic obliquity exacerbates the risk of hip subluxation and dislocation; however, posterolateral hip displacement may also be induced by flexion and adduction contractures about the hip rather than the scoliosis itself.[9]

The natural history of NMS varies significantly by underlying diagnosis[2,10-16] (**Table 1**). In children with cerebral palsy, the likelihood of developing scoliosis is not related to clinical subtype (spastic, athetoid, ataxic, and mixed).[10] The risk of development of spinal deformity in children with cerebral palsy is strongly related to the child's Gross Motor Function Classification Scale (GMFCS) level and age (ie, growth remaining) at presentation[10] (**Figure 1**). For children at GMFCS level I or II, the incidence of clinically significant scoliosis is low

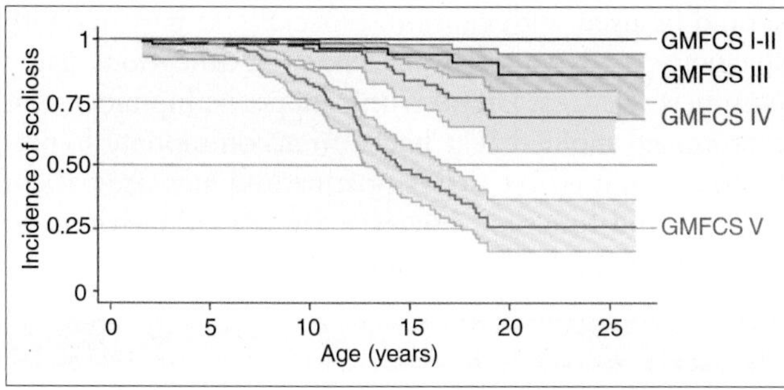

FIGURE 1 Graph showing incidence of scoliosis (Cobb angle ≥40°) diagnosed by Gross Motor Function Classification Scale (GMFCS) level and age.[10] (Reprinted from Hägglund G, Pettersson K, Czuba T, Persson-Bunke M, Rodby-Bousquet E: Incidence of scoliosis in cerebral palsy: A population-based study of 962 young individuals. *Acta Orthop.* 2018;89[4]: 443-447.)

and similar to that of the adolescent idiopathic population in typically developing children. In nonambulatory children with cerebral palsy (GMFCS levels IV and V), there is a significantly higher rate of early-onset and adolescent-onset NMS as well as progression past skeletal maturity[10] (**Figure 2**). Because of the high incidence and risk of progression of scoliosis in children with cerebral palsy, surveillance programs should be based on GMFCS level, start at a young age, and continue into adulthood.

In patients with hereditary motor and sensory neuropathies (eg, Charcot-Marie-Tooth disease), scoliosis typically becomes clinically apparent during pubertal growth. The curve may differ from AIS by atypical pattern (left thoracic) and progression despite bracing treatment.[11] In patients with spina bifida, the patient's age at diagnosis, clinical motor level of function, ambulatory status, and level of last intact laminar arch correlate with the development of scoliosis.[12] Most patients with spina bifida who do not develop scoliosis by the end of pubertal growth will not develop a curve later in life. Those who do develop scoliosis are at risk of rapid progression (2.5° to 6.2° per year) and may continue to progress after skeletal maturity.[13] In children with Rett syndrome, there is increased risk of developing severe scoliosis with increasing age, worse motor function (walking ability, voluntary use of hands), and worse severity of mutation type.[14,15] There is little known progression to severe scoliosis after maturity. Children with severe muscle weakness and truncal hypotonia as a consequence of muscle dystrophy, myopathy, or neuropathy (eg, type II spinal muscle atrophy is a prototype) develop early-onset scoliosis, pelvic obliquity, and hip instability by age 4 to 6 years. The scoliosis is rapidly progressive (8° per year) and severely compromises pulmonary function (relative vital capacity 54% predicted at age 4 to 6 years).[2,16] The rate of clinically significant and progressive scoliosis has significantly reduced with the introduction of glucocorticoid therapy for Duchenne muscular dystrophy (DMD).[17]

NONSURGICAL INTERVENTIONS

Braces, serial Risser or Mehta casts, and wheelchair modifications may be used to improve sitting posture, trunk balance, head control, and upper extremity function in patients with neuromuscular spinal deformity.[18] Although these interventions may slow the advancement of spinal deformity, they may not prevent progression. A 70% to

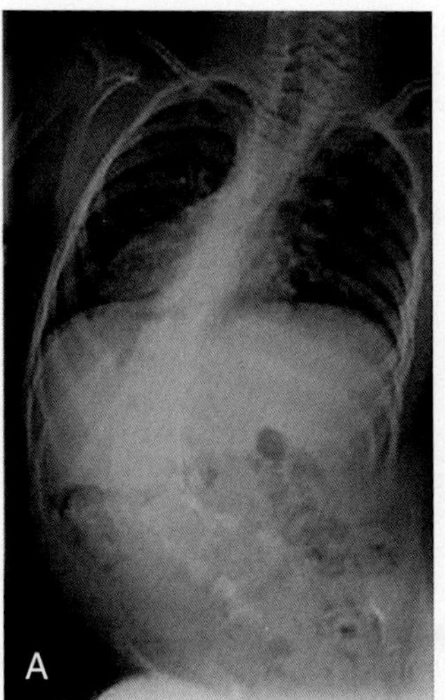

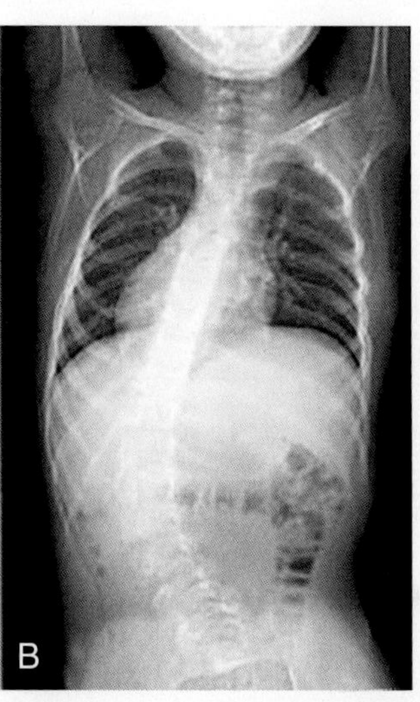

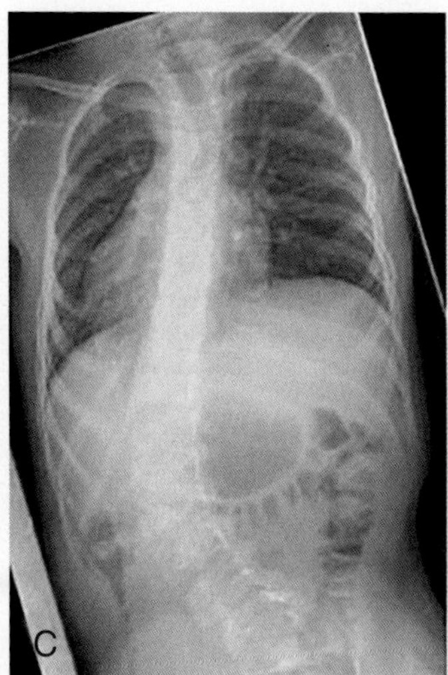

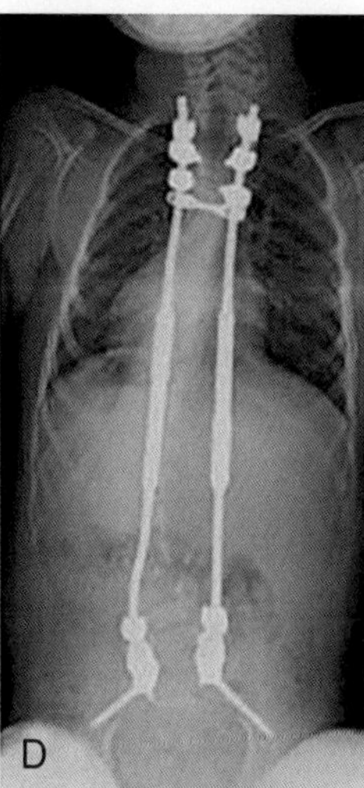

FIGURE 2 Radiographs from an 8-year-old boy with type II spinal muscular atrophy. **A**, Standard upright PA scoliosis radiograph shows a major curve measuring 82°. **B**, Supine traction PA scoliosis radiograph shows reduction in the major curve to 42°. **C**, Supine left bending (lumbar curve) PA scoliosis radiograph demonstrates approximately the same amount of correction (to 45°). **D**, PA upright radiograph after magnetic growing rod insertion shows that the major curve measures 41°, similar to the curve measurement in the traction radiograph.

80% failure rate has been reported with the use of a rigid thoracolumbosacral orthosis to correct NMS; this high failure rate may be attributable to incorrect implementation of the appliance and poor patient compliance.[4] A semirigid thoracolumbosacral orthosis with an anterior opening improves wear tolerance (10 to 12 hr/d) and sitting posture and makes breathing easier.[19] It is especially important that the brace include a large anterior window sufficient to accommodate the presence of a gastrostomy tube to allow for abdominal distension during feeding and to facilitate diaphragmatic breathing. Younger patients with smaller Cobb angles and long sweeping curves respond best to bracing treatment, which indicates that patient age, the extent of deformity, the number of vertebrae forming the scoliosis, and the flexibility of the curve correlate with the extent of in-brace curve correction.[20] Children with scoliosis as a consequence of spinal cord injury with curve magnitudes less than 40° may respond to bracing treatment; however, patients with curves greater than 40° have not demonstrated a consistent response to bracing treatment.[21] Although brace wear (>15 hr/d) and the extent of in-brace correction (50%) have been used as predictors of successful bracing treatment in patients with AIS, no such parameters have been shown to be predictive of effective bracing treatment in those with NMS. Serial Mehta or Risser casts have been used to control scoliosis progression in patients with early-onset scoliosis who have an underlying neuromuscular disease, but this approach should be used with caution, especially in patients with spasticity or dystonia. Wheelchair modifications using pummels, wedges, lateral trunk supports, hip blocks, or customized molded seat backs to accommodate hyperlordosis can improve sitting posture and increase patient comfort and function; however, these modifications do not treat the underlying spinal deformity.

SURGICAL INTERVENTION

Decision Making

If nonsurgical management is unsuccessful, surgical treatment is indicated for a severe (>50°), progressive, neuromuscular spinal deformity that is causing pain, interfering with sitting balance, contributing to ischial decubiti, inducing hip instability, or compromising cardiopulmonary function (**Figure 3**). The decision to surgically treat a patient with NMS requires consideration of many patient-related factors that influence the risks of surgery, the expected benefits from the intervention, the likelihood of success, and the potential for complications. The goals of surgery are to achieve solid arthrodesis to decrease progression of spinal deformity; relieve pain from costoiliac impingement syndrome; prevent decubiti by eliminating pelvic obliquity; improve sitting balance and wheelchair tolerance; enhance the ability for social interaction by aligning the head midline over level shoulders and pelvis; create a stable, balanced, upright torso to minimize use

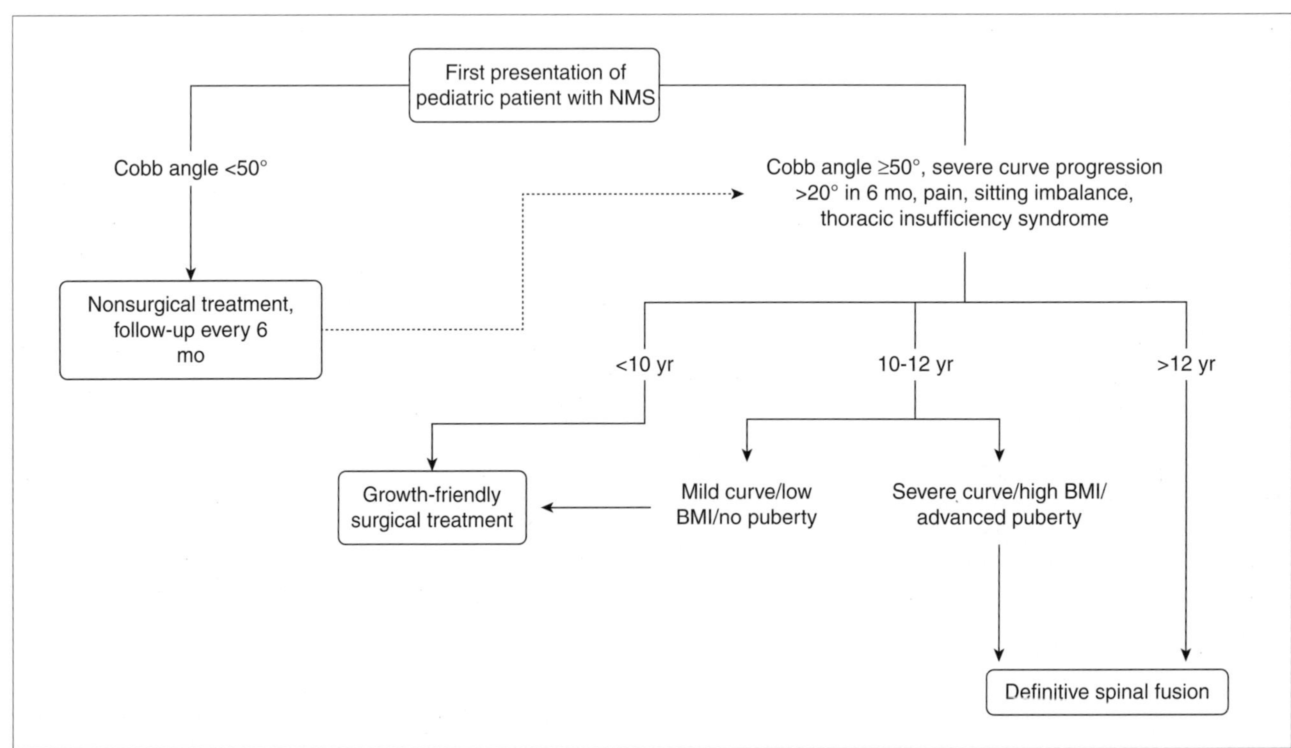

FIGURE 3 Clinical pathway for treatment of children presenting with neuromuscular scoliosis (NMS). BMI = body mass index.

of the upper limbs for auxiliary trunk support; facilitate daily care; decrease the need for assistance during activities of daily living; diminish thoracic distortion; and increase thoracic height to facilitate diaphragmatic excursion and pulmonary function.[22] Delayed intervention may allow further progression of disease resulting in increased complexity of surgery and rate of complications.[23] The benefits of surgery must outweigh the risks and improve on the natural history of the disease if the scoliosis remains untreated. To aid parents in deciding whether surgical treatment or palliative care is the appropriate choice for their child, a shared decision-making aid is available.[24] Caregivers should be provided with information about the risks and benefits of surgery and the expected issues that will likely be encountered during the perioperative and postoperative periods. Providers should be aware of caregiver perceptions about important information to convey to families considering spinal fusion surgery: it is important to simplify risks and benefits of surgery; delayed decision making may not benefit the child; anticipate anxiety and fear when making a decision about spinal fusion; understand that the child may experience a large amount of pain; anticipate a long recovery and healing process; and be engaged and advocate for the child throughout the spinal fusion process.[25]

Minimizing Adjustable Preoperative Risks

Children with NMS often have complex medical comorbidities that may increase perioperative risks, increase the need for prolonged admission to the intensive care unit, extend their hospitalization, and increase the probability of postoperative complications.[26] Common comorbidities include recurrent aspiration pneumonias from gastroesophageal reflux, the inability to manage oral secretions, respiratory failure from thoracic insufficiency syndrome, restrictive lung disease, cardiomyopathy, poor gastrointestinal function (reflux, constipation, malabsorption), malnutrition, seizures (in patients with cerebral palsy and Rett syndrome), coagulopathies (in patients with DMD and those taking antiseizure drugs), compromised immune function, anxiety, and osteopenia (disuse, vitamin D deficiency).[26] A careful evaluation by a multidisciplinary team of specialists and the institution of systematic protocols for anticipating and managing these comorbidities perioperatively may reduce perioperative risk and facilitate recovery.

Comprehensive pulmonary function tests are often difficult to perform in children with NMS because of their inability to cooperate. A 2011 study of 74 patients with NMS reported that postoperative pulmonary complications were probable in adolescents older than 16.5 years who have severe scoliosis (Cobb angle >69°) and a preoperative forced vital capacity of less than 39.5% of predicted value and a forced expiratory volume at 1 second of less than 40% of predicted value.[27] A forced expiratory volume at 1 second less than 40% of predicted value was prognostic for prolonged mechanical ventilation after surgery.[28] Of common medical comorbidities in children with NMS, chronic respiratory insufficiency has the highest contribution to increased length of stay and expenditures.[29] For patients with neurogenic scoliosis and compromised pulmonary function (forced vital capacity <30% to 40% of predicted value), pulmonary complications can be reduced by implementing pulmonary training before and after surgery.[30] This training can include noninvasive positive pressure ventilation to compensate for intrinsic respiratory muscle weakness and mechanical insufflation-exsufflation to augment mucous clearance.

Patients with Rett syndrome and scoliosis were found to have higher rates of postoperative complications compared with patients with cerebral palsy, with respiratory problems being the most severe complication.[31] In a retrospective case-control study, it was found that despite better preoperative motor function, shorter anesthesia, and shorter surgery durations, patients with Rett syndrome experienced more respiratory failure, prolonged positive pressure ventilation, and longer intensive care unit stays after posterior spinal fusion (PSF) than did children with cerebral palsy.[32] Tracheostomy before spinal surgery should be considered in patients with severe pulmonary insufficiency, poor pulmonary toilet, dependence on continuous positive airway pressure and bilevel positive airway pressure assistance, and a history of frequent intubation and/or prolonged extubation. Prophylactic tracheostomy expedites recovery of respiratory function, facilitates pulmonary toilet, and eliminates the need for urgent tracheostomy weeks after spinal surgery in a debilitated patient who has undergone multiple failed attempts at extubation.

Muscular dystrophies are often associated with cardiomyopathy and/or conduction abnormalities. An electrocardiogram and echocardiogram should be obtained preoperatively for these patients. A left ventricular ejection fraction less than 50% may be a relative contraindication to surgery. Consultation with a cardiologist to guide perioperative management is recommended. Transesophageal echocardiography and/or use of a Swan-Ganz catheter to monitor atrial filling pressures enables the intraoperative evaluation of cardiac function. Hypotensive anesthesia should be avoided. Fluid replacement with blood products and colloid (rather than crystalloid) helps to maximize the Starling curve.

Many children with NMS also have epilepsy. Some anticonvulsants adversely affect clotting (eg, valproic acid has a qualitative effect on platelet function that resolves over 4 to 6 weeks).[33] Postoperative ileus and delayed gastric motility can affect the serum concentration of anticonvulsants administered enterically, but several of these medications are unavailable for parenteral administration. Therefore, a neurologist should be consulted weeks before the surgery to adjust antiepileptic medications to avoid excess bleeding and decrease the risk of postoperative seizures. This should include a plan for bridging and to rescue antiseizure medications during the perioperative period. In addition, it is recommended that bleeding time be determined. Aspirin and NSAIDs should be avoided. If platelet function is abnormal, a hematology consultation is recommended in addition to having platelets and blood available for the procedure.[34] For children who use ventriculoperitoneal shunts, the functionality of the shunt should be assessed using appropriate imaging studies; preoperative clearance by a neurosurgeon should be obtained.

Osteopenia is common across the spectrum of neuromuscular disease because of poor nutrition, the long-term administration of anticonvulsant drugs, and the limited weight-bearing status of patients. Low bone mineral density decreases bone stiffness and strength and increases the risk of fragility fractures and the failure of bone anchor fixation. Proper diagnostic studies to determine the cause of osteopenia are required because osteoporosis (normal bone tissue mineralization but low bone mass) is managed differently than osteomalacia (low bone tissue mineralization). Dietary modifications to increase calcium and vitamin D intake in patients at risk for osteomalacia may be supplemented with diphosphonates to improve bone quality in patients with osteoporosis by decreasing osteoclastic bone resorption. The intravenous administration of zoledronic acid over a 2-year period has been shown to increase vertebral bone mineral density in children with cerebral palsy and Rett syndrome.[35] In anticipation of spinal fusion, a consultation with an endocrinologist can be considered so that a diphosphonate can be administered 9 to 12 months before surgery to allow for the maximization of bone anchor stability. Zoledronate administration in adults with osteoporosis undergoing lumbar spinal fusion decreased the time to fusion, increased the fusion rate, decreased the number of adjacent compression fractures, and improved clinical outcomes; no deleterious effects such as decreased fusion mass were reported.[36] Diphosphonate administration improves screw fixation in the spine and in osteoporotic bone.[37]

Higher infection rates have been reported in patients who have cerebral palsy and poor nutritional status (albumin <3.5 mg/dL and total lymphocyte count <1,500 cells/mm^3), who underwent surgery for scoliosis.[38] Discussion with a nutritionist and insertion of a nasogastric tube or gastrostomy tube to augment enteral feeding weeks before surgery should be considered. Gastrointestinal problems such as postoperative ileus, pancreatitis, gastroesophageal reflux, and constipation can complicate the postoperative course and lengthen the hospital stay. A bowel preparation (laxatives, enema) administered before surgery may improve gastrointestinal mobility, decrease constipation, and accelerate enteral feeding after surgery.

Urinary and bowel incontinence increase the risk of surgical site infections. The likelihood of a postoperative wound infection was increased in patients with myelomeningocele and a positive preoperative urine culture, thereby supporting the importance of prophylactic antibiotic treatment before surgery.[39] Quality and safety guidelines to mitigate the risk of surgical site infection in patients with neuromuscular spinal deformity undergoing spinal fusion endorse routine methicillin-resistant *Staphylococcus aureus* screening (nares, axilla, and groin), surgical site hair removal with clippers, the administration of gram-positive and gram-negative antibiotics within 1 hour of skin incision, and chlorhexidine skin preparation. This protocol has been found to significantly reduce the rate of deep infections in children with NMS undergoing PSF (8% to 1% of patients).[40]

Surgical Planning

The goal of spine surgery in patients with neuromuscular spinal deformity is to create a balanced spine, with the head centered over level shoulders and pelvis to improve sitting balance. In addition to frontal plane alignment, the sagittal spine contour should allow for sufficient thoracic kyphosis to lessen the likelihood of proximal junction kyphosis at the cervicothoracic junction and provide for sufficient lumbar lordosis to compensate for weak hip girdle muscles by aligning the trunk center of gravity at or slightly behind the hip joints. Careful preoperative planning that considers the age of the patient (spine and thoracic growth remaining), the flexibility of the spinal deformity, the causal pathophysiology, and associated intraspinal pathology (Chiari malformation, syrinx, or tethered cauda equina) will aid in the selection of growth-friendly spine implants versus definitive spinal fusion; the use of preoperative and/or intraoperative halo traction with or without femoral traction; and the choice of appropriate methods for intraoperative neuromonitoring, blood management, and spinal fixation.

Sitting (or standing) AP and lateral spine radiographs obtained on a single cassette that includes the head, neck, and pelvis will show the full scope of the spinal and trunk deformities requiring correction and will help identify the extent that associated hip pathology and/or pelvic obliquity and cervical spinal deformity (torticollis, laterocollis) are related to the overall deformity of the axial skeleton. Supine, push-pull longitudinal traction; right and left bending; and sagittal prone-supine bending (over a fulcrum) radiographs will demonstrate the flexibility of the spinal deformity (**Figures 2** and **4**). Syndromic patients (with storage diseases, Larsen syndrome, Down syndrome, Klippel-Feil syndrome, or arthrogryposis) should have static (AP, lateral, and open mouth) and dynamic (lateral

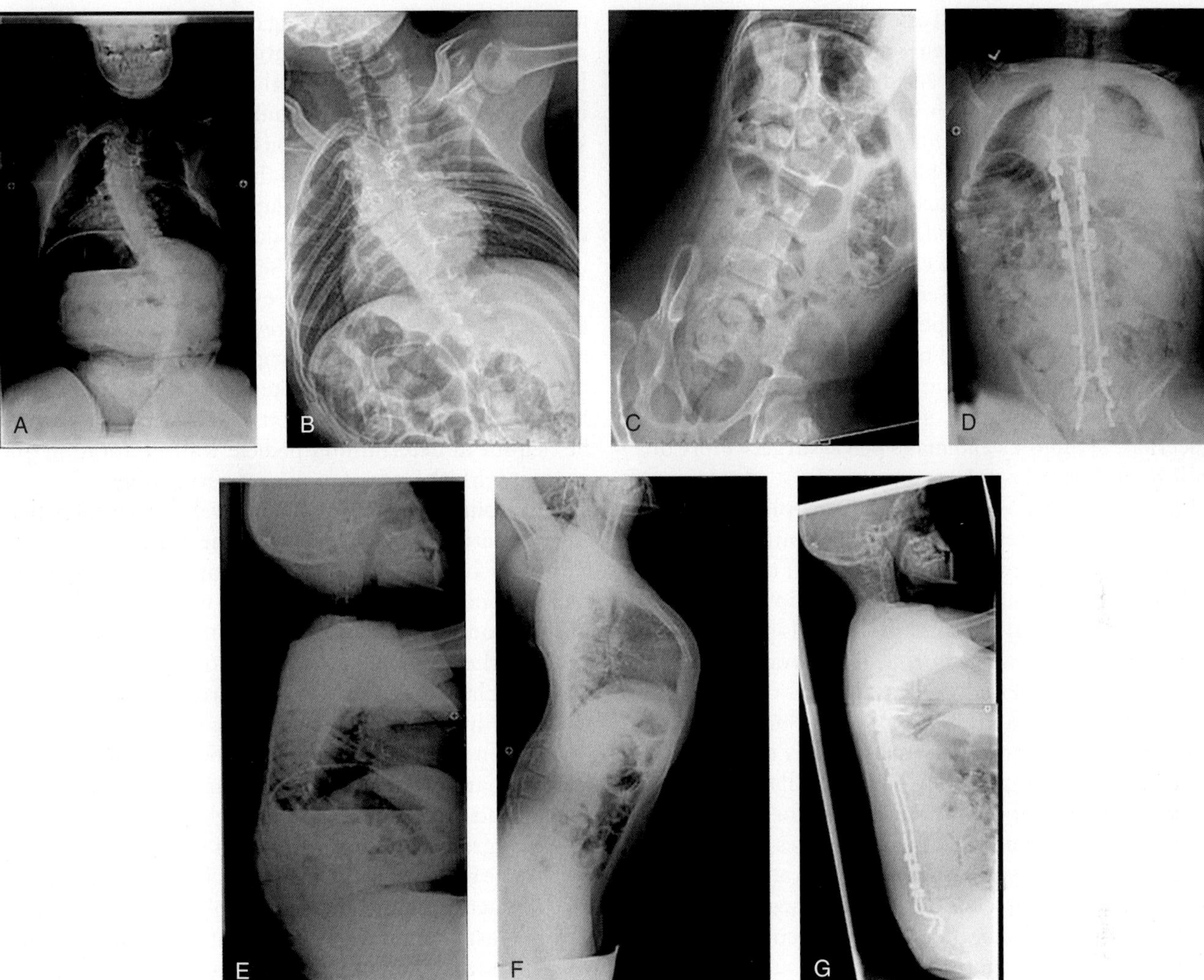

FIGURE 4 Radiographs from a 14-year-old boy with myelomeningocele. **A**, Sitting upright PA scoliosis radiograph shows a 57° main thoracic curve and a 44° lumbar curve. **B**, Supine left bending (thoracic curve) PA scoliosis radiograph shows main thoracic curve reduction to 11°, not including the congenital upper thoracic anomalies. **C**, Supine right bending (lumbar curve) PA scoliosis radiograph shows lumbar curve reduction to 3°. Sitting PA radiograph (**D**) and sitting lateral scoliosis radiograph (**E**) show 88° of lumbar kyphosis. **F**, Supine lateral radiograph taken with a bolster over the kyphosis shows residual kyphosis of 46°. **G**, Lateral radiograph after fusion and L1 vertebrectomy shows 18° of lumbar kyphosis.

Section 6: Spine

flexion-extension) views of the cervical spine to evaluate for associated axial and subaxial cervical spinal deformity that may contribute to occult mechanical instability and the risk of cervical spinal cord injury.

Serial transaxial CT of the entire spine and rib cage with two-dimensional and three-dimensional tomographic reconstructions is indicated to evaluate abnormal osseous anatomy related to congenital vertebral anomalies, neurofibromatosis, pathologic fractures, tumors, complex or unusual spinal deformity, and the morphology of the pedicles to accommodate pedicle screw anchors. MRI of the entire spine from the foramen magnum to the sacrum is required in rapidly progressing spinal deformities (>15° in a 1-year period), in myelomeningocele, in left thoracic curves or unusual patterns of spinal deformity, and in abnormally progressing foot deformity (equinovarus-cavovarus) to evaluate for Chiari malformation or intraspinal pathology.[41]

Hip dislocation and scoliosis are commonly seen together in children with neuromuscular diseases, and the more symptomatic one (hip or spine) should first be addressed with surgical intervention.[42] Because adequate hip range of motion is a prerequisite to facilitate sitting, transfers, toileting, and hygiene, intrapelvic and infrapelvic pathology (eg, windswept deformity) related to hip instability and/or contractures (psoas, adductors, tensor fascia lata, hamstrings) should be addressed before or coincident with spinal instrumentation. A fixed hip flexion contracture can increase lumbar lordosis, whereas a fixed proximal hamstring contracture can decrease lumbar lordosis, which will affect the sagittal alignment of a fused spine. In children with early-onset scoliosis, priority should first be given to treatment of the spine with growing rod insertion because of the risk of progression without intervention. In an adolescent patient with a level pelvis and flexible NMS (Cobb angle <60°), hip reconstruction before scoliosis surgery is acceptable in the case of painful, fixed, and/or nonmobile hips to reduce pain, improve daily care, and allow sitting after spine surgery. In an adolescent patient with larger stiff curves (≥60°) or increased pelvic obliquity (≥10°), spinal fusion should be addressed before hip surgery to reduce the risk of progression, improve sitting position, and level the pelvis, as fixation of the spine to the pelvis may exacerbate symptoms and make pelvic surgery more difficult to perform.

Preoperative halo-gravity traction applied full time for several weeks before spine instrumentation can be considered for the treatment of large, stiff curves (Cobb angle >60° on bending or traction radiographs). The child must have no cervical spine instability, and spasticity and/or seizures must be well controlled. The traction weight is increased incrementally to up to 50% of the child's body weight, with careful neurologic evaluation every 4 to 8 hours of the cranial nerves (especially the abducens nerve), cervical sympathetic chain (pupillary dilation), deviations in motor or sensory functions for dermatomes or myotomes C5-T1 and L1-S1, and changes in bowel and bladder function from baseline levels. Anterior release (open or thoracoscopic) of the anterior longitudinal ligament and intervertebral disk may be considered for excessive thoracic kyphosis (>65°) and/or a rigid scoliosis that failed to substantially improve with halo traction. Intraoperative halo-pelvic or halo-femoral traction in which the distal traction is applied to the concave side or the elevated hemipelvis facilitates deformity correction by viscoelastic creep that gradually stretches the soft-tissue connections. The total traction force (approximately 50% of body weight) is equally distributed between the halo and the lower extremity. In children with severe NMS, intraoperative halo-femoral traction is associated with reduced surgical time, greater correction of pelvic obliquity, less complications, and similar curve correction as combined anterior spinal fluid/PSF. This suggests that intraoperative traction may be a viable alternative to anterior release with posterior fusion in severe NMS.[43]

Neuromonitoring is recommended when correcting NMS because loss of residual bowel, bladder, motor, or sensory functions can substantially affect the patient's QOL. Most of these patients will be unable to cooperate with a wake-up test. In a patient who is incontinent and has spastic quadriplegia, a spinal cord injury may result in urinary and bowel retention that negatively alters daily care activities, with the need for catheterization and a bowel regimen requiring digital stimulation. Spinal somatosensory-evoked potentials (SSEPs) may be unreliable in NMS.[44] Transcranial motor-evoked potentials improve reliability when combined with SSEPs. In a study that included 39 patients with cerebral palsy, the responses to at least one modality could be monitored in 86% of the patients.[45] Stimulation to measure transcranial motor-evoked potentials does not elicit seizure activity or increase postoperative seizure activity. In patients with DMD or SMA, motor-evoked potentials may be absent but SSEPs are often present. Patients with hereditary sensory and motor neuropathy may exhibit abnormalities in both motor-evoked potentials and SSEPs. Electromyographic stimulation of each pedicle screw can be helpful in determining pedicle wall perforation and contact with the spinal cord or a nerve root.

Controlling for the number of levels fused and patient weight, patients with neuromuscular disease have a substantially higher amount of intraoperative blood loss during spinal fusion than patients with idiopathic scoliosis. Modifiable coagulopathies must be considered. Continual exudate of blood from osteoporotic bone is commonplace in children with neurogenic spinal deformity. An intraoperative coagulopathy often develops in children with DMD who have normal prothrombin time or partial thromboplastin time. Children taking valproic acid have qualitative platelet dysfunction. The overly aggressive administration of crystalloid solution to manage intraoperative blood loss further dilutes coagulation factors. Early judicious replacement with fresh frozen plasma and/or cryoprecipitate is required to prevent excessive exsanguination. Point-of-care devices and platelet mapping are used to determine coagulopathy and guide treatment, such as the use of fresh frozen plasma to treat hypofibrinogenemia (fibrinogen <1.5 g/L) and low factor XIII.[46] An arterial line facilitates continual monitoring of blood pressure with the goal of maintaining an intraoperative mean arterial pressure of 65 mm Hg. Insertion of a large-bore (≥18 gauge) central line or a peripherally inserted central catheter line with the tip at the superior vena cava allows for improved venous access for the administration of blood products and the intraoperative assessment of central venous pressure to evaluate hypovolemia.

The intraoperative administration of antifibrinolytic agents such as tranexamic acid and aminocaproic acid has been shown to substantially decrease intraoperative blood loss.[47] Tranexamic acid is given as a bolus (100 mg/kg before incision) and followed by an infusion (10 mg/kg per hour) until wound closure. Additional measures to decrease blood loss include dermal injection of 1:500,000 dilution of epinephrine along and deep to the skin incision; soft-tissue dissection with the electrocautery; tamponading bleeding by packing sponges along the lateral gutter deep to the paraspinal muscles (Hibb technique); packing decorticated bone and exposed dura with collagen sponges; injecting hemostatic matrix into pedicle tracks; using bipolar radiofrequency hemostatic sealer to coagulate bleeding muscle and bone; suctioning blood; and recycling via a cell salvage system.

Surgical Technique

Nonfusion Constructs

The previous paradigm of making a crooked spine straight by instrumenting multiple levels and fusing the spine early has been shown to inhibit lung growth, impair development, and decrease pulmonary function. For this reason, the goal of surgical treatment in the growing child with severe, progressive spinal deformity is to stabilize the spinal deformity while preserving the potential for longitudinal growth. These surgical techniques include distraction-based (vertical expandable prosthetic titanium ribs and growing rods), guided growth (Luque trolley and Shilla), compression-based (tether and staples), and early limited arthrodesis (**Figure 5**).

In distraction-based growing rod systems, two rods placed above the paravertebral muscles are fixed proximally to the spine or ribs and distally to the spine and/or pelvis using a variety of anchors, including sublaminar hooks, pedicle screws, rib cradles, and iliac crest S-hooks (**Figure 6**). Fusion is achieved cranially and caudally at bone anchor sites while the remaining spine is left free to allow correction and growth with lengthening. In traditional distraction-based growing rod systems, the device is lengthened surgically every 6 to 9 months to progressively correct scoliosis and maintain growth of the spine. In children with early-onset NMS, this technique has demonstrated medium-term and long-term success in increasing spinal length while improving or maintaining coronal plane deformity.[48] Patients are at risk of developing hyperkyphosis and should be monitored with serial radiographs. The frequency of sequential lengthening of the implants is controversial because more frequent lengthening increases infection risk but decreases stress on the implants.[49] Posteriorly placed, nonfusion systems have a 46% complication rate related to infection and wound dehiscence, which is exacerbated by multiple, open, manual lengthening procedures in addition to device failures.[50] More recently, dynamic growing rod implant systems such as MAGnetic Expansion Control (MAGEC, NuVasive) have gained popularity to allow control/correction and continued growth of early-onset scoliosis without the need for repeated open procedures to manually distract the rod. Sequential rod expansion is well tolerated by patients and can be performed without anesthesia in an office setting.

In guided growth techniques, the spinal deformity is corrected with two parallel rods affixed to the spine with either sublaminar wires or polyester bands (Luque trolley) or multiaxial nonlocking pedicle screws (Shilla growth guidance system, Medtronic). The rods act as rails for the wires or pedicle screws to slide along during normal vertebral growth. The Luque trolley technique has been used with sublaminar stainless steel wires and polyester bands that may be used in isolation or in hybrid pedicle screw systems. This technique has demonstrated success with correction of spinal deformity with variable success at maintaining longitudinal growth (35% to 88%

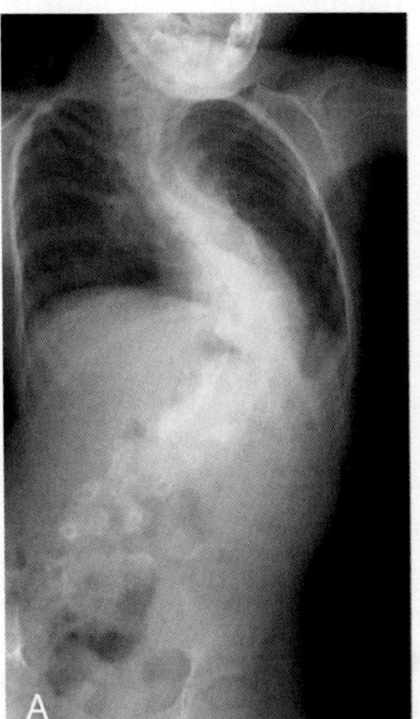

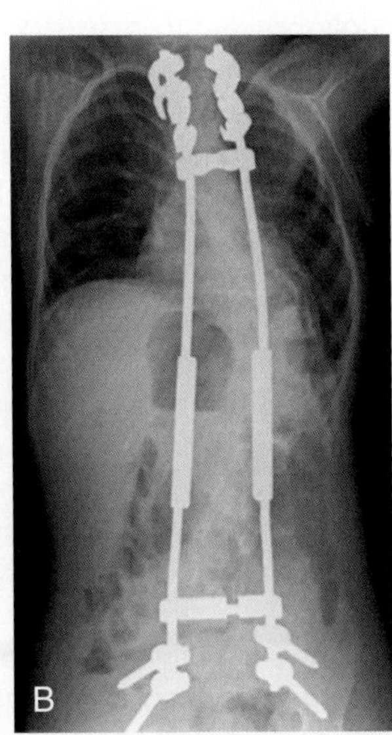

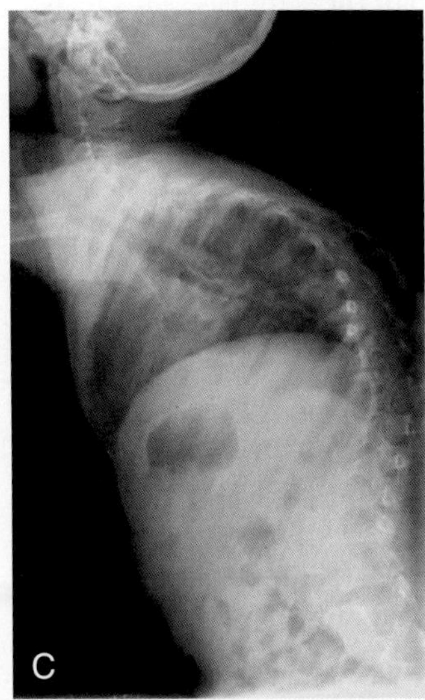

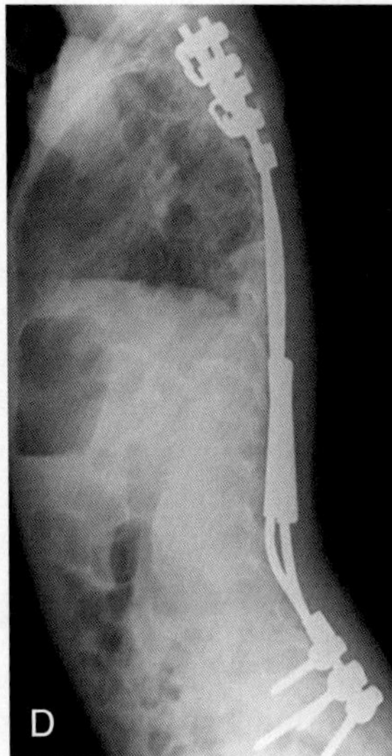

FIGURE 5 Radiographic images from a patient with neuromuscular scoliosis who was treated with growing rods, a hook-screw hybrid construct, and iliac screws. **A**, Preoperative PA scoliosis radiograph. **B**, Postoperative PA scoliosis radiograph shows the growing rod construct with hooks, cross-links, and iliac screws. **C**, Lateral preoperative scoliosis radiograph. **D**, Lateral postoperative scoliosis radiograph shows improvement in thoracic kyphosis and lumbar lordosis after treatment.

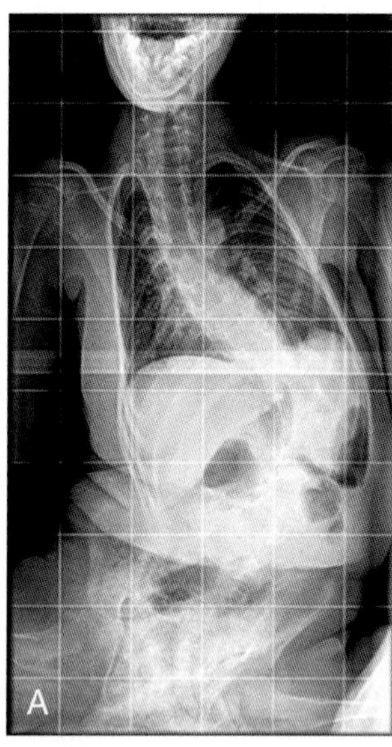

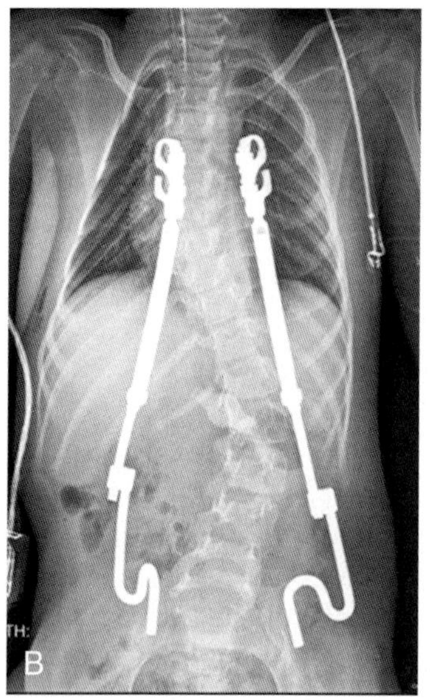

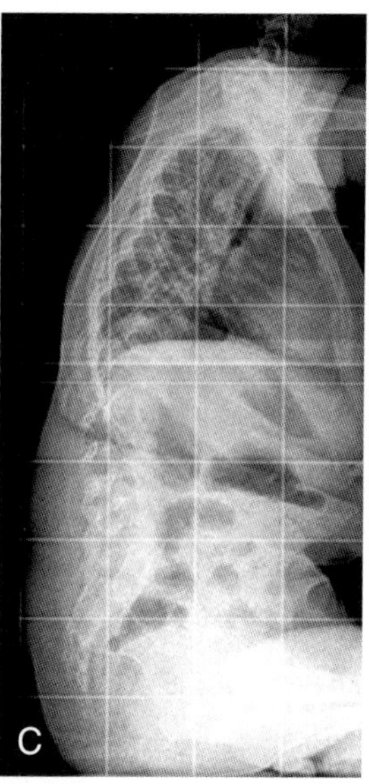

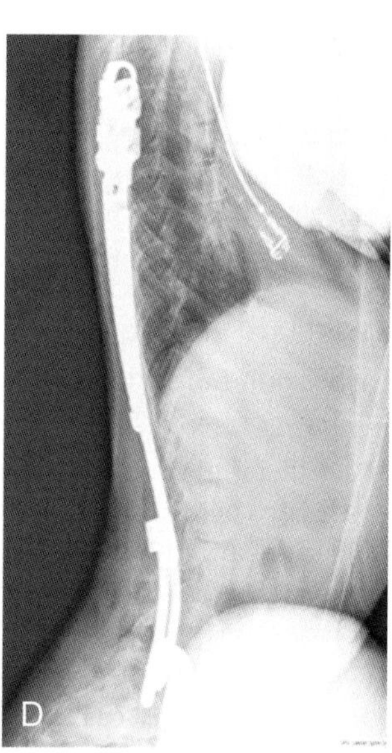

FIGURE 6 Radiographic images from a patient with neuromuscular scoliosis treated with the vertical expandable prosthetic titanium rib (VEPTR), growing rods, and S-rod pelvic fixation. Note that more than five proximal spine/rib anchors are required to provide sufficient mechanical stability and minimize the stress on each individual bone anchor. **A**, Preoperative PA scoliosis radiograph. **B**, Postoperative PA scoliosis radiograph shows the VEPTR proximally, S-rod pelvic fixation distally, and growing rods. **C**, Preoperative lateral scoliosis radiograph. **D**, Postoperative lateral scoliosis radiograph demonstrates improvement in lumbar lordosis.

of expected growth).[51] The complications include mechanical implant failure, metallosis at wire-rod interface, spontaneous fusion, and laminar fracture. This may be improved with the introduction of sublaminar polyester bands that allow for increased contact area between the sublaminar band, allowing higher corrective forces and reduced laminar fracture risk.[52] The Shilla growth guidance system (Medtronic) uses pedicle screws with locking set screws to fix the vertebrae at the apex of the deformity to dual rods that span the scoliosis. This technique achieves immediate deformity correction and local arthrodesis. Vertebrae proximal and distal to the apex of the deformity are captured using multiaxial pedicle screws with nonlocking, flanged set screws that slide along the rods. This approach seeks to allow guided longitudinal growth while maintaining alignment of the nonfused vertebrae. A 5-year, single-surgeon cohort demonstrated increased spinal growth by 15.8 mm/yr, increased space available for the lung by 29.1%, and a 73% complication rate.[53] More recently, a multicenter cohort has tempered enthusiasm for this technique with minimum 2-year follow-up, demonstrating spinal growth of only 4.2 mm/yr (36% predicted growth) with 75% of patients undergoing revision surgery for implant-related complications.[54]

These implants must serve multiple functions, including maintaining correction of the spinal deformity and modulating axial growth, without failing mechanically for an indeterminate number of years in a semimobile patient. Device fatigue fracture can be prevented by using the largest rod diameter possible. Minimizing the number of rod connectors helps prevent stress risers and crevice corrosion. The applied stress to each bone anchor is reduced by distributing the load among six bone anchors (three pairs of pedicle screws, sublaminar hooks, and/or rib cradles per rod) at the upper and lower end of each dual-rod construct, thus reducing the risk of anchor failure. Compared with single-rod constructs, dual-rod systems offer better structural stability and curve correction.[50]

Growing rod constructs may be lengthened through adolescence into maturity. To achieve the same gain in spine height over 2 years, lengthening a dual-rod system every 2 months decreases the resulting rod stress by 50% to 75% compared with lengthening every 6 months. This approach is now easily achievable using magnetic rod systems.[49] The magnetic systems may be lengthened by a distraction-to-stall and targeted distraction length technique with similar amount of achieved distraction. Early results with magnetic rods demonstrated improved scoliosis correction and higher forced vital capacity and forced expiratory volume at 1 second values.[55] In a systematic review of children with early-onset scoliosis, magnetically controlled growing rods improved coronal deformity (46% correction) while maintaining spinal growth (19.8 mm/yr) and have a complication rate of 44.5%. The most common implant-related complications include infection (5.5%), temporary loss of distraction (6.7%), implant failure (11.7%), rod breakage (10.6%), and anchor pullout (11.8%).[56] Overall rate of infection was lower in magnetically controlled growing rod than traditional growing rods (3.7% versus 11.1%).[57] With magnetically controlled growing rod, proximal spine anchors and greater anchor density (5+ anchors) impart superior deformity correction but does not significantly improve the risk of device complications.[58] At the conclusion of growth, patients with growth-friendly constructs may retain the implants with observational treatment or undergo definitive PSF. The criteria for conversion of growth-friendly constructs to PSF include unacceptable or progressive major curve deformity, sagittal malalignment, or complications with previous implants. However, growing rod removal without fusion should be avoided because of risk of progressive deformity. In a case-control series of 28 SMA patients with (n = 14) and without (n = 14) prior treatment with growing rod implants, curve angle before fusion, final scoliotic curve angle after fusion, and pelvic obliquity were significantly improved in the pretreated group.[59]

Fusion Constructs

A dual-rod construct fixed with multiple vertebral bone anchors spanning the entire spine deformity is essential to distribute corrective forces and moments in osteoporotic bone. Sagittal balance is as important as coronal plane correction to enable head control and sitting balance. Instrumentation should extend proximal to T4 to avoid upper thoracic junctional kyphosis. Sufficient lumbar lordosis (approximately 45°) is recommended to avoid pressure on the coccyx and ischium and transfer weight to the thighs while sitting. If the child is ambulatory, lumbosacral mobility should be preserved for walking and sitting; therefore, distal fixation proximal to L5 is indicated in an ambulatory patient whose spinal deformity is proximal to L5 and who has a level pelvis and stable hips. Fixation to L5 is indicated in a nonambulatory patient with a spinal deformity that extends to L5, a level pelvis (obliquity <15°), and stable hips. Fixation to the pelvis is indicated in a nonambulatory patient lacking independent trunk support, whose spinal deformity includes the pelvis or who has a collapsing curve so that the C7 plumb line projects lateral to the sacroiliac joint or who has hypolordosis (<15°), excessive pelvic obliquity (>15°), significant growth remaining, or a structural defect (deficient pars, absent L5 neural arch). Vertebral bone anchors include fixed-angle or variable-angle pedicle screws, sublaminar hooks, and sublaminar wires, cables, and bands. Pedicle screws provide rigid three-column fixation that enables improved deformity correction, potentially obviating the need for anterior procedures, which reduces blood loss and surgical time. Hybrid systems that combine pedicle screws, hooks, and/or sublaminar wires allow adequate curve correction and are less expensive than all-pedicle screw constructs but do not reduce surgical time or blood loss.[60]

Many techniques exist to achieve sacropelvic fixation[61] (**Figure 7**). A Galveston construct using dual-rod constructs or iliac screws extends distal lever arm fixation

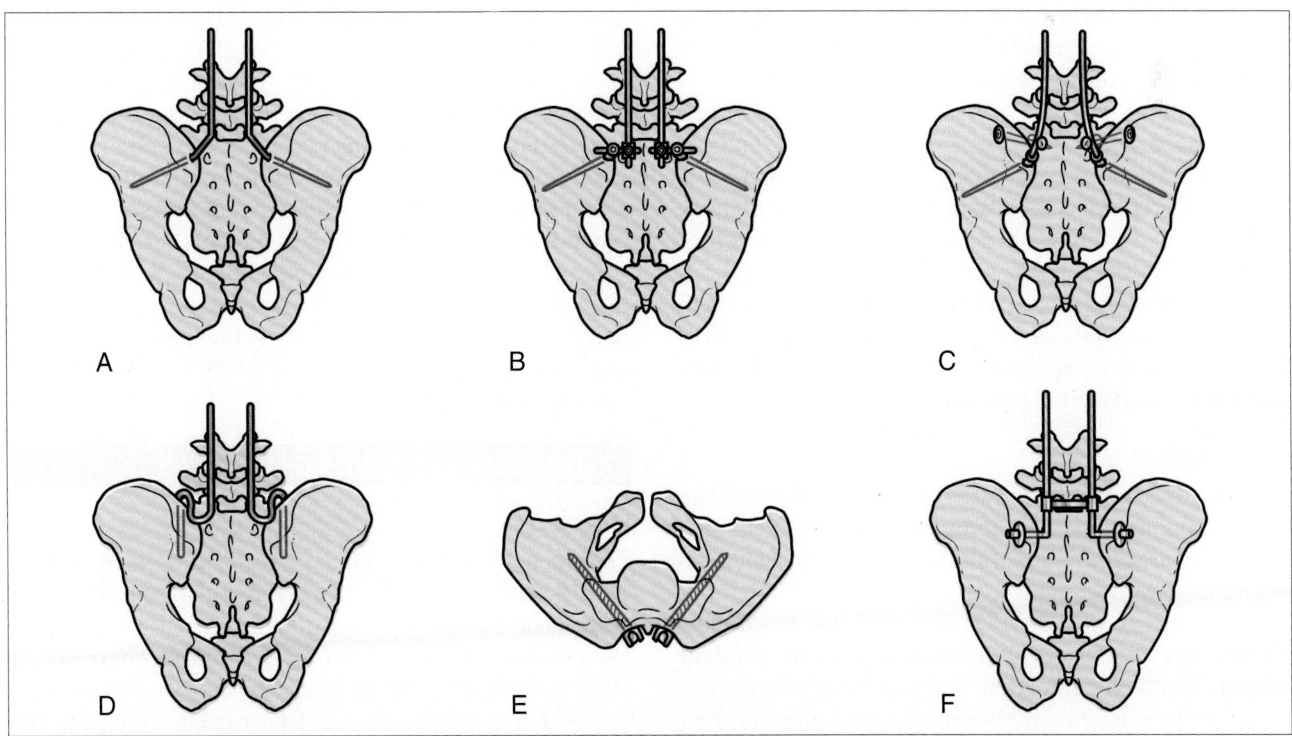

FIGURE 7 Illustrations of techniques to achieve sacropelvic fixation in patients with neuromuscular scoliosis. **A**, Galveston technique. **B**, Iliac screw technique. **C**, Technique using a maximum-width construct. **D**, S-rod (Dunn-McCarthy) technique. **E**, Technique using sacral alar iliac screws. **F**, Spinopelvic transiliac fixation technique.[61]

to better counteract the flexion moment created by the long spinal construct above. The authors of a 2015 study reported that at least six points of lumbar-sacral-pelvic fixation are required to achieve satisfactory stability.[62] Thirty-five percent of constructs with less than six bone anchors failed at 18 months, whereas constructs with at least six bone anchors remained intact at 28 months.

After release of the posterior interspinous ligaments (with or without the ligamentum flavum) and bilateral facetectomies, large rigid curves associated with excessive pelvic obliquity, thoracic kyphosis, or lumbar hyperlordosis may require Ponte or Smith Petersen osteotomies at multiple segments or pedicle subtraction or vertebral column resection at a specific level to sufficiently destabilize the spine to permit adequate realignment. In patients with myelodysplasia, pedicle subtraction vertebrectomy for collapsing C-shaped kyphosis or kyphectomy for rigid myelokyphosis (lumbar kyphosis and thoracic lordosis) may be necessary. Anterior ligamentous release with intervertebral disk resection and possible partial corpectomy may be indicated to improve the mobility of an inflexible hyperkyphotic spinal deformity or to facilitate arthrodesis in patients with neurofibromatosis or connective tissue disorders or those at risk for compromised bone healing. In skeletally immature patients, fusing the anterior spine prevents the crankshaft phenomenon. If both anterior and posterior procedures are required, controversy exists regarding staging of the procedures or completion of both in a single day with debates regarding degree of correction, morbidity, complication rate, length of stay, and associated costs.

The primary purpose of the procedure is to attain a stable, fused spine. After instrumentation, the lamina, facets, and transverse processes should be decorticated. Arthrodesis is induced by using local autologous bone graft obtained from resection of the facets, spinous processes, and lamina and is supplemented by autologous iliac crest or allogeneic cancellous bone graft. Excellent fusion rates are obtained using allogeneic bone graft.[63] The use of bone morphogenetic protein-2 is rarely indicated in primary spinal procedures.

Complications

Historically, complication rates vary from 44% to 80%, with pulmonary issues predominating (pneumonia, atelectasis, aspiration, pneumothorax).[5,64] Death has been reported in zero to 7% of cases. In a meta-analysis of 15,218 patients with NMS, the prevalence of complications was 22.7% for pulmonary, 12.5% for implant related, 10.9% for infection, 3.0% for neurologic, and 1.9% for pseudarthrosis.[65] In most neuromuscular diseases, spinal deformity is concomitant with intrinsic intercostal muscle weakness and restricted growth of the thoracic cavity, which compromise respiratory function by limiting excursion of the diaphragm and restricting inspiratory expansion of the rib cage. Aggressive postoperative pulmonary toilet including postural drainage and use of vibrating vest and cough assist to mobilize mucous plugs and continuous positive airway pressure/bilevel positive airway pressure to prevent atelectasis can ameliorate these problems. Increased infection risk has been related to inadequate prophylactic antibiotic dosing (timing, use of gram-positive and gram-negative coverage), length of construct, pelvic fixation, duration of hospitalization, and comorbidities.[66] A multifaceted approach may help reduce the incidence of surgical site infections, including preoperative assessment of patient nutrition and appropriate intervention, diligent use of preoperative skin cleansing, prophylactic use of perioperative antibiotics to cover methicillin-resistant *S aureus* and gram-negative bacteria, use of titanium instrumentation, meticulous handling of soft tissues, débridement of devitalized tissue, wound lavage with dilute povidone-iodine, instillation of vancomycin powder into the wound at closure, and careful postoperative wound care. Malnutrition, constipation, and ileus can be effectively managed by parenteral hyperalimentation until bowel motility returns and enteral feeds via nasogastric, gastric, or jejunum tube. Neuromonitoring can help anticipate neurologic injuries, and intraoperative CT transaxial imaging allows confirmation of proper placement of pedicle screws, decreasing likelihood of encroachment on neurologic or vascular structures. Device fatigue failure can be prevented by using the largest rod diameter possible. Implant failure is particularly associated with thoracic hyperkyphosis, which can be mitigated by anterior release, rigid, multilevel segment fixation using pedicle screws and/or sublaminar hook claw construct as well as in situ rod bending to accommodate kyphosis. In Friedreich ataxia, proximal junctional kyphosis occurred in patients fused to T4 but was prevented in patients fused above T4. In general, instrumentation to T2/3 and care to preserve the tension band created by the interspinous ligaments and facet joint capsule proximally help to mitigate the risk of proximal junctional kyphosis.

THE VALUE OF TREATING NMS

Outcomes

Treatment of NMS by spinal instrumentation and fusion is sufficiently successful in correcting spinal deformity and pelvic obliquity to create a balanced spine over a level pelvis.[67] However, spinal deformity progresses in 10% to 30% of patients after fusion.[68] Tools to assess the QOL of patients with NMS have been developed. The Caregiver Priorities and Child Health Index of Life with Disabilities (CPCHILD) questionnaire was specifically designed and validated to evaluate patients with cerebral palsy.[69] Measuring QOL after scoliosis surgery is difficult because many patients are incapable of independently responding to QOL questionnaires. The responses of caregivers to these surveys may reflect positive or negative bias. Caregivers report high satisfaction after spinal fusion for NMS, despite no change in pain, incidence of decubiti, function, or time required for daily care.[7,70] A prospective study of severely affected, nonambulatory children with cerebral palsy (GMFCS levels IV and V) and scoliosis demonstrated clinically significant improvements in the CPCHILD score 1 year after spinal surgery, but this regressed to baseline at 2 years reflecting that caregiver burden is little changed by spinal fusion.[7] A multicenter prospective study of nonambulatory children with cerebral palsy demonstrated 36.3% of patients had meaningful improvement in CPCHILD scores (≥10 point improvement) at 2-year postoperative follow-up. Patients who had meaningful improvement had significantly lower preoperative total CPCHILD scores (43.8 versus 55.2), suggesting more room for improvement with surgery.[8] Postoperative deep infection was associated with less improvement in CPCHILD total score. In a multicenter study of 69 patients with NMS undergoing spinal fusion, surgery demonstrated significant improvements in CPCHILD score, which was maintained at 5-year postoperative follow-up.[64] Overall, parents felt that their child's QOL, comfort, ease of care, and overall health improved a lot when surveyed after PSF. Although spinal fusion improved coronal alignment in patients with myelodysplasia, the rate of postoperative spine infections was high (32.4%), and the overall QOL in adulthood was unchanged compared with patients treated nonsurgically.[71] A cohort of 13 patients with DMD treated with spinal fusion demonstrated improved coronal alignment and improved comfort in life without bracing treatment, very good mental status, good sitting tolerance, and quality social integration as measured by a modified Scoliosis Research Society questionnaire.[72] A retrospective review of children with SMA found that definitive PSF was effective at controlling curve progression and pelvic obliquity without impairing space-available-for-lung ratio, trunk height, or pulmonary function at 10-year follow-up.[73]

Cost

Children with neuromuscular conditions incur high baseline medical expenditures. Compared with the treatment of AIS, the expenditure for health care and resource utilization is substantially higher for patients with neuromuscular spinal deformity.[26] Although PSF in children with neuromuscular conditions is marginally not cost effective, the cost effectiveness of fusion surgery depends on how children and their families perceive gains in QOL associated with fusion surgery.[74] The implant costs vary in spinal fusion but range from as low as $30 for Luque wire to greater than $500 for a pedicle screw. The length of hospitalization accounts for a large variability in costs.[75] Although hospital care accounts for most perioperative spending in children undergoing spinal fusion, multiple preoperative primary care visits in children with medical complexity have been shown to significantly lower hospital costs and reduce length of stay for spinal fusion surgery.[76] Often unaccounted for in real cost analyses is the time caregivers take off from work to care for their children in the hospital and after discharge. These analyses also fail to account for potential cost savings related to decreased emergency care visits and hospitalizations for pulmonary complications related to a severe spinal deformity.

Ethics

Managing NMS entails complex clinical decisions that account for medical indications, patient preferences, QOL, and contextual features.[77] A shared decision aid has been developed to properly educate caregivers and engage them in the decision-making process when choosing how to treat a neuromuscular patient with a spine deformity.[24] However, the inability to directly measure a patient's QOL obscures the true benefit of restoring an upright posture to a neuromuscular patient with a distorted spine.

SUMMARY

NMS associated with cerebral palsy, muscle dystrophies, and myelodysplasia typically presents as long, collapsing C-shaped curves associated with pelvic obliquity and kyphosis. The scope and magnitude of the deformity are inversely related to the patient's gross motor function and directly related to the severity of the disease or neurologic level (myelomeningocele or spinal cord injury). However, each disease entity presents different levels of patient functionality, different natural histories for curve progression, different surgical risk profiles, and inconsistent evidence for/against surgical treatment. In general, high rates of curve progression are associated with younger patients with more severe spinal deformities. Bracing treatment and other nonsurgical measures are ineffective in ameliorating curve progression over the long term but can be used to temporize until the child is sufficiently healthy and/or attains skeletally maturity to undergo definitive spine fusion. In young children with a rapidly progressive spine deformity unresponsive to bracing treatment, nonfusion, growth-friendly instrumentation systems have been shown to effectively correct the spinal deformity and improve thoracic volume. The assistance of a multidisciplinary team preoperatively can decrease modifiable risks related to cardiopulmonary, gastrointestinal, and neurologic comorbidities. Careful preoperative planning can decrease intraoperative complications and improve postoperative deformity correction. The goals of surgery are to establish a stable, balanced, painless spine fusion. The surgical approach and instrumentation must be individualized based on curve severity and stiffness, the extent of neurologic impairment, the patient's skeletal maturity, and baseline functional status. New outcome tools are being developed to assess patient and caregiver QOL and satisfaction. Increased quality, decreased cost, and shared decision making will increase the value of spinal fusion in NMS.

KEY STUDY POINTS

- Spinal deformity is proportional to the extent of neurologic disability.
- Nonsurgical management is palliative.
- Goals of surgery are to establish a stable, balanced, painless spine.
- The surgical approach and instrumentation must be individualized based on curve severity and stiffness, the extent of neurologic impairment, the patient's skeletal maturity, and baseline functional status.
- Preoperative medical comorbidities increase the risk of postoperative complications.
- A multidisciplinary team is required to anticipate and minimize complications.
- With appropriate anticipatory medical management and fourth-generation spinal instrumentation, prospective and retrospective outcome studies suggest improved long-term benefits are associated with spine fusion in life expectancy, lung function, sitting balance, and QOL.

ANNOTATED REFERENCES

1. Saito N, Ebara S, Ohotsuka K, Kumeta H, Takaoka K: Natural history of scoliosis in spastic cerebral palsy. *Lancet (London, England)* 1998;351(9117):1687-1692.
2. Granata C, Merlini L, Magni E, Marini ML, Stagni SB: Spinal muscular atrophy: Natural history and orthopaedic treatment of scoliosis. *Spine (Phila Pa 1976)* 1989;14(7):760-762.
3. Kalen V, Conklin MM, Sherman FC: Untreated scoliosis in severe cerebral palsy. *J Pediatr Orthop* 1992;12(3):337-340.
4. Olafsson Y, Saraste H, Al-Dabbagh Z: Brace treatment in neuromuscular spine deformity. *J Pediatr Orthop* 1999;19(3):376-379.
5. Benson ER, Thomson JD, Smith BG, Banta JV: Results and morbidity in a consecutive series of patients undergoing spinal fusion for neuromuscular scoliosis. *Spine (Phila Pa 1976)* 1998;23(21):2308-2317.
6. Suk KS, Baek JH, Park J-O, et al: Postoperative quality of life in patients with progressive neuromuscular scoliosis and their parents. *Spine J* 2015;15(3):446-453.
7. DiFazio RL, Miller PE, Vessey JA, Snyder BD: Health-related quality of life and care giver burden following spinal fusion in children with cerebral palsy. *Spine (Phila Pa 1976)* 2017;42(12):E733-E739.

   This prospective longitudinal cohort study of 26 patients with GMFCS IV-V cerebral palsy undergoing spine fusion found a significant increase in QOL by the CPCHILD at 1 year ($P = 0.005$), which regressed to baseline at 2 years ($P = 0.40$). Caregiver burden was not changed following spine fusion surgery as measured by the caregiver reported outcome measure at 1 year (0.09) and 2 years (0.72). Level of evidence: II.
8. Miller DJ, Flynn JM, Pasha S, et al: Improving health-related quality of life for patients with nonambulatory cerebral palsy: Who stands to gain from scoliosis surgery? *J Pediatr Orthop* 2020;40(3):E186-E192.

   This retrospective review of prospectively collected multicenter registry of nonambulatory children with cerebral palsy undergoing spinal fusion with minimum 2-year follow-up showed meaningful improvement of CPCHILD score in 36.3% of patients, with greatest improvement in those patients with lower preoperative scores. A lower score within the comfort, emotions, and behavior domain of the CPCHILD was predictive of meaningful improvement after surgery. Level of evidence: II.
9. Lonstein JE, Beck K: Hip dislocation and subluxation in cerebral palsy. *J Pediatr Orthop* 1986;6(5):521-526.
10. Hägglund G, Pettersson K, Czuba T, Persson-Bunke M, Rodby-Bousquet E: Incidence of scoliosis in cerebral palsy: A population-based study of 962 young individuals. *Acta Orthop* 2018;89(4):443-447.

    This prospective registry cohort of 1,025 children with cerebral palsy in Sweden reported that the prevalence and severity of scoliosis increased with the GMFCS level. Level of evidence: II.
11. Karol LA, Elerson E: Scoliosis in patients with Charcot-Marie-Tooth disease. *J Bone Joint Surg Am* 2007;89(7):1504-1510.
12. Trivedi J, Thomson JD, Slakey JB, Banta JV, Jones PW: Clinical and radiographic predictors of scoliosis in patients with myelomeningocele. *J Bone Joint Surg Am* 2002;84(8):1389-1394.
13. Eysel P, Hopf C, Schwarz M, Voth D: Development of scoliosis in myelomeningocele. Differences in the history caused by idiopathic pattern. *Neurosurg Rev* 1993;16(4):301-306.
14. Downs J, Torode I, Wong K, et al: The natural history of scoliosis in females with Rett syndrome. *Spine (Phila Pa 1976)* 2016;41(10):856-863.

    This retrospective review of Australian Rett Syndrome Database found median onset at 11 years, with earliest onset in p.Arg255 mutation subtype. Scoliosis was progressive in all mutation types except p.Arg306Cys mutation. Cobb angle and walking by age 10 years can predict patients who will develop severe scoliosis by age 16 years. Level of evidence: III.
15. Killian JT, Lane JB, Lee H-S, et al: Scoliosis in Rett syndrome: Progression, comorbidities, and predictors. *Pediatr Neurol* 2017;70:20-25.

This retrospective review of the Rett syndrome Natural History Study found severe scoliosis in 27% of 913 patients, of whom 113 developed severe scoliosis during follow-up assessments. Severe variant mutations of MECP2 showed higher proportions of scoliosis. Level of evidence: III.

16. Fujak A, Raab W, Schuh A, Richter S, Forst R, Forst J: Natural course of scoliosis in proximal spinal muscular atrophy type II and IIIa: Descriptive clinical study with retrospective data collection of 126 patients. *BMC Musculoskelet Disord* 2013;14:283.
17. Lebel DE, Corston JA, McAdam LC, Biggar WD, Alman BA: Glucocorticoid treatment for the prevention of scoliosis in children with Duchenne muscular dystrophy: Long-term follow-up. *J Bone Joint Surg Am* 2013;95(12): 1057-1061.
18. Pettersson K, Rodby-Bousquet E: Prevalence and goal attainment with spinal orthoses for children with cerebral palsy. *J Pediatr Rehabil Med* 2019;12(2):197-203.

    This is a cross-sectional analysis of the Swedish cerebral palsy registry assessing the frequency of brace use for NMS by age and GMFCS level, specifically assessing for achievement goals of brace treatment. Level of evidence: III.
19. Letts M, Rathbone D, Yamashita T, Nichol B, Keeler A: Soft Boston orthosis in management of neuromuscular scoliosis: A preliminary report. *J Pediatr Orthop* 1992;12(4):470-474.
20. Nakamura N, Uesugi M, Inaba Y, Machida J, Okuzumi S, Saito T: Use of dynamic spinal brace in the management of neuromuscular scoliosis: A preliminary report. *J Pediatr Orthop B* 2014;23(3):291-298.
21. Mehta S, Betz RR, Mulcahey MJ, McDonald C, Vogel LC, Anderson C: Effect of bracing on paralytic scoliosis secondary to spinal cord injury. *J Spinal Cord Med* 2004;27(suppl 1):S88-S92.
22. Adams AJ, Refakis CA, Flynn JM, et al: Surgeon and caregiver agreement on the goals and indications for scoliosis surgery in children with cerebral palsy. *Spine Deform* 2019;7(2): 304-311.

    This multicenter prospective survey of Harms Study Group to determine surgeon and caregiver agreement on goals and indications for scoliosis surgery in children with cerebral palsy found improved sitting, prevention of pulmonary compromise, pain improvement, and improved head control/position as most important factors. Level of evidence: II.
23. Hollenbeck SM, Yaszay B, Sponseller PD, et al: The pros and cons of operating early versus late in the progression of cerebral palsy scoliosis. *Spine Deform* 2019;7(3):489-493.

    This prospective multicenter case series to assess risks of surgery for NMS by curve severity demonstrated undergoing surgery after curve progressed greater than 90° increased the risk of infection, blood loss, and need for combined anterior and posterior procedure. Level of evidence: III.
24. Shirley E, Bejarano C, Clay C, Fuzzell L, Leonard S, Wysocki T: Helping families make difficult choices: Creation and implementation of a decision aid for neuromuscular scoliosis surgery. *J Pediatr Orthop* 2015;35(8):831-837.
25. Garrity B, Berry J, Crofton C, et al: Parent-to-parent advice on considering spinal fusion in children with neuromuscular scoliosis. *J Pediatr* 2019;213:149-154.

    The authors performed interviews of 18 families of children undergoing spinal fusion for NMS, identifying six common themes about decision making and preparation for spinal fusion surgery. Level of evidence: IV.
26. Murphy NA, Firth S, Jorgensen T, Young PC: Spinal surgery in children with idiopathic and neuromuscular scoliosis. What's the difference? *J Pediatr Orthop* 2006;26(2):216-220.
27. Kang G-R, Suh S-W, Lee I-O: Preoperative predictors of postoperative pulmonary complications in neuromuscular scoliosis. *J Orthop Sci* 2011;16(2):139-147.
28. Yuan N, Skaggs DL, Dorey F, Keens TG: Preoperative predictors of prolonged postoperative mechanical ventilation in children following scoliosis repair. *Pediatr Pulmonol* 2005;40(5):414-419.
29. Berry JG, Glotzbecker M, Rodean J, Leahy I, Hall M, Ferrari L: Comorbidities and complications of spinal fusion for scoliosis. *Pediatrics* 2017;139(3):e20162574.

    This retrospective analysis of 7,252 children of age 5 years and older with complex chronic condition demonstrated that chronic respiratory insufficiency was associated with increased length of stay and cost. Level of evidence: III.
30. Khirani S, Bersanini C, Aubertin G, Bachy M, Vialle R, Fauroux B: Non-invasive positive pressure ventilation to facilitate the post-operative respiratory outcome of spine surgery in neuromuscular children. *Eur Spine J* 2014;23(suppl 4):S406-S411.
31. Gabos PG, Inan M, Thacker M, Borkhu B: Spinal fusion for scoliosis in Rett syndrome with an emphasis on early postoperative complications. *Spine (Phila Pa 1976)* 2012;37(2):E90-E94.
32. Cohen JL, Klyce W, Kudchadkar SR, Kotian RN, Sponseller PD: Respiratory complications after posterior spinal fusion for neuromuscular scoliosis. *Spine (Phila Pa 1976)* 2019;44(19):1396-1402.

    This retrospective review of patients with NMS due to cerebral palsy (CP) or Rett syndrome (RS) who underwent spinal fusion found that despite better preoperative motor function (66% versus 96%), shorter anesthesia, and shorter surgery duration, patients with RS experienced more respiratory failure (43% versus 19%), prolonged positive pressure ventilation (67% versus 31%), and longer intensive care unit stay after PSF than children with CP. Level of evidence: IV.
33. Chambers HG, Weinstein CH, Mubarak SJ, Wenger DR, Silva PD: The effect of valproic acid on blood loss in patients with cerebral palsy. *J Pediatr Orthop* 1999;19(6):792-795.
34. Carney BT, Minter CL: Is operative blood loss associated with valproic acid? *J Pediatr Orthop* 2005;25(3):283-285.
35. Wiedemann A, Renard E, Hernandez M, et al: Annual injection of zoledronic acid improves bone status in children with cerebral palsy and Rett syndrome. *Calcif Tissue Int* 2019;104(4):355-363.

This study demonstrates the safety and efficacy of annual zolendronic acid infusion to improve bone status in children with cerebral palsy and Rett syndrome. Level of evidence: IV.

36. Chen F, Dai Z, Kang Y, Lv G, Keller ET, Jiang Y: Effects of zoledronic acid on bone fusion in osteoporotic patients after lumbar fusion. *Osteoporos Int* 2016;27(4):1469-1476.

    This randomized controlled trial reported on patients with osteoporosis who underwent single-level fusions for degenerative spondylolisthesis. Patients were assigned to zoledronic acid or saline infusions after spinal surgery. Those who received the zoledronic acid demonstrated more bridging bone ($P < 0.05$), no vertebral compression fractures ($P < 0.05$), and prevention of decline in bone mineral density compared with the control group. Level of evidence: I.

37. Moroni A, Faldini C, Hoang-Kim A, Pegreffi F, Giannini S: Alendronate improves screw fixation in osteoporotic bone. *J Bone Joint Surg Am* 2007;89(1):96-101.

38. Jevsevar DS, Karlin LI: The relationship between preoperative nutritional status and complications after an operation for scoliosis in patients who have cerebral palsy. *J Bone Joint Surg Am* 1993;75(6):880-884.

39. Hatlen T, Song K, Shurtleff D, Duguay S: Contributory factors to postoperative spinal fusion complications for children with myelomeningocele. *Spine (Phila Pa 1976)* 2010;35(13):1294-1299.

40. Glotzbecker M, Troy M, Miller P, et al: Implementing a multidisciplinary clinical pathway can reduce the deep surgical site infection rate after posterior spinal fusion in high-risk patients. *Spine Deform* 2019;7(1):33-39.

    This retrospective comparative study in children with NMS undergoing PSF before and after implementation of a high-risk protocol to reduce rate of deep infections demonstrated significantly reduced rate of deep infections in the postprotocol group (1%) compared with the preprotocol group (8%). Level of evidence: III.

41. Schwend RM, Hennrikus W, Hall JE, Emans JB: Childhood scoliosis: Clinical indications for magnetic resonance imaging. *J Bone Joint Surg Am* 1995;77(1):46-53.

42. Helenius IJ, Viehweger E, Castelein RM: Cerebral palsy with dislocated hip and scoliosis: What to deal with first? *J Child Orthop* 2020;14(1):24-29.

    This is a current expert opinion discussing treatment when hip dislocation and scoliosis occur in the same child. This suggests that when hip dislocation and scoliosis present at the same time, scoliosis-associated pelvic obliquity should be corrected before hip reconstruction. If the patient is not presenting with pelvic obliquity, the more symptomatic condition should be addressed first. Level of evidence: V.

43. Jackson TJ, Yaszay B, Pahys JM, et al: Intraoperative traction may be a viable alternative to anterior surgery in cerebral palsy scoliosis ≥100 degrees. *J Pediatr Orthop* 2018;38(5):e278-e284.

    This retrospective review of a prospective multicenter database on severe spinal deformity associated with cerebral palsy demonstrated that both intraoperative halo-femoral traction and anterior-posterior surgery aided in the correction of severe cerebral palsy scoliosis (>100°). Anterior surgery did not improve coronal alignment and was associated with increased surgical times, whereas traction was associated with greater correction of pelvic obliquity. Level of evidence: III.

44. Ashkenaze D, Mudiyam R, Boachie-Adjei O, Gilbert C: Efficacy of spinal cord monitoring in neuromuscular scoliosis. *Spine (Phila Pa 1976)* 1993;18(12):1627-1633.

45. DiCindio S, Theroux M, Shah S, et al: Multimodality monitoring of transcranial electric motor and somatosensory-evoked potentials during surgical correction of spinal deformity in patients with cerebral palsy and other neuromuscular disorders. *Spine (Phila Pa 1976)* 2003;28(16): 1851-1855.

46. Theusinger OM, Spahn DR: Perioperative blood conservation strategies for major spine surgery. *Best Pract Res Clin Anaesthesiol* 2016;30(1):41-52.

    This review article highlights the significance of Patient Blood Management with discussion of measures to reduce intraoperative blood loss including new surgical techniques; use of cell salvage where possible; bedside coagulation management with point-of-care devices; substitution of coagulation factors, antifibrinolytic agents, and desmopressin; induced hypotension; and avoidance of hypothermia. Level of evidence: V.

47. Dhawale AA, Shah SA, Sponseller PD, et al: Are antifibrinolytics helpful in decreasing blood loss and transfusions during spinal fusion surgery in children with cerebral palsy scoliosis? *Spine (Phila Pa 1976)* 2012;37(9):E549-E555.

48. ElBromboly Y, Hurry J, Padhye K, et al: Distraction-based surgeries increase spine length for patients with nonidiopathic early-onset scoliosis—5-year follow-up. *Spine Deform* 2019;7(5):822-828.

    This retrospective review of a multicenter prospectively collected database of children with nonidiopathic early-onset scoliosis found stable correction of coronal plane deformity and increased kyphosis with time. There was a mean increase in spine length by 8.2 cm. Level of evidence: III.

49. Agarwal A, Zakeri A, Agarwal AK, Jayaswal A, Goel VK: Distraction magnitude and frequency affects the outcome in juvenile idiopathic patients with growth rods: Finite element study using a representative scoliotic spine model. *Spine J* 2015;15(8):1848-1855.

50. Akbarnia BA, Breakwell LM, Marks DS, et al: Dual growing rod technique followed for three to eleven years until final fusion: The effect of frequency of lengthening. *Spine (Phila Pa 1976)* 2008;33(9):984-990.

51. Rosenfeld S, Schlechter J, Smith B: Achievement of guided growth in children with low-tone neuromuscular early-onset scoliosis using a segmental sublaminar instrumentation technique. *Spine Deform* 2018;6(5):607-613.

    This retrospective review of patients with low-tone early-onset neuromuscular scoliosis treated surgically with Luque trolley technique found that a this technique was safe and effective to allow guided growth while maintaining correction of their scoliosis. Level of evidence: IV.

52. Canavese F, Samba A: Sublaminar polyester bands for the correction of idiopathic and neuromuscular scoliosis. *Ann Transl Med* 2020;8(2):32.

This article discusses the utility of sublaminar bands to restore coronal and sagittal alignment. Level of evidence: V.

53. McCarthy RE, McCullough FL: Shilla growth guidance for early-onset scoliosis: Results after a minimum of five years of follow-up. *J Bone Joint Surg Am* 2015;97(19):1578-1584.

54. Nazareth A, Skaggs DL, Illingworth KD, et al: Growth guidance constructs with apical fusion and sliding pedicle screws (SHILLA) results in approximately 1/3rd of normal T1–S1 growth. *Spine Deform* 2020;8(3):531-535.

This retrospective review of patients with early-onset scoliosis undergoing treatment with Shilla technique demonstrated mean longitudinal growth of 4.2 mm per year. Level of evidence: IV.

55. Yoon WW, Sedra F, Shah S, Wallis C, Muntoni F, Noordeen H: Improvement of pulmonary function in children with early-onset scoliosis using magnetic growth rods. *Spine (Phila Pa 1976)* 2014;39(15):1196-1202.

56. Thakar C, Kieser DC, Mardare M, Haleem S, Fairbank J, Nnadi C: Systematic review of the complications associated with magnetically controlled growing rods for the treatment of early onset scoliosis. *Eur Spine J* 2018;27(9):2062-2071.

This is a systematic review of the literature to assess coronal correction, growth progression, and complications in children with early-onset scoliosis treated with magnetically controlled growing rods. The mean complication rate was 44.5%, with anchor pullout, implant failure, and rod breakage being most common. Level of evidence: II.

57. Choi E, Yaszay B, Mundis G, et al: Implant complications after magnetically controlled growing rods for early onset scoliosis: A multicenter retrospective review. *J Pediatr Orthop* 2017;37(8):e588-e592.

This multicenter retrospective review of magnetically controlled growing rod cases demonstrated 38.8% complication rate with broken rods, loss of lengthening, anchor failure, and infection. Level of evidence: IV.

58. Meza BC, Shah SA, Vitale MG, Sturm PF, Luhmann SJ, Anari JB: Proximal anchor fixation in magnetically controlled growing rods (MCGR): Preliminary 2-year results of the impact of anchor location and density. *Spine Deform* 2020;8(4):793-800.

This is a retrospective multicenter review of the effects of proximal anchor location and density on radiographic outcomes and complications in patients with early-onset scoliosis with minimum 2-year follow-up. This study showed that proximal spine anchors and greater anchor density impart superior deformity correction but do not significantly affect the risk of device complications. Level of evidence: III.

59. Hell AK, Braunschweig L, Tsaknakis K, et al: Children with spinal muscular atrophy with prior growth-friendly spinal implants have better results after definite spinal fusion in comparison to untreated patients. *Neurosurgery* 2020;87(5):910-917.

This retrospective review of 28 patients with SMA treated with (14) or without (14) prior growth-friendly implants before definitive spinal fusion found that prior growth-friendly implants were associated with better correction of curve and pelvic obliquity. Level of evidence: IV.

60. Mattila M, Jalanko T, Puisto V, Pajulo O, Helenius IJ: Hybrid versus total pedicle screw instrumentation in patients undergoing surgery for neuromuscular scoliosis: A comparative study with matched cohorts. *J Bone Joint Surg Br* 2012;94(10):1393-1398.

61. Dayer R, Ouellet JA, Saran N: Pelvic fixation for neuromuscular scoliosis deformity correction. *Curr Rev Musculoskelet Med* 2012;5(2):91-101.

62. Myung KS, Lee C, Skaggs DL: Early pelvic fixation failure in neuromuscular scoliosis. *J Pediatr Orthop* 2015;35(3):258-265.

63. Price CT, Connolly JF, Carantzas AC, Ilyas I: Comparison of bone grafts for posterior spinal fusion in adolescent idiopathic scoliosis. *Spine (Phila Pa 1976)* 2003;28(8):793-798.

64. Miyanji F, Nasto LA, Sponseller PD, et al: Assessing the risk-benefit ratio of scoliosis surgery in cerebral palsy: Surgery is worth it. *J Bone Joint Surg Am* 2018;100(7):556-563.

This prospective, multicenter study demonstrated that scoliosis surgery in patients with CP leads to significant improvements in health related quality of life which was maintained at 5 years postoperatively. Level of evidence: IV.

65. Sharma S, Wu C, Andersen T, Wang Y, Hansen ES, Bünger CE: Prevalence of complications in neuromuscular scoliosis surgery: A literature meta-analysis from the past 15 years. *Eur Spine J* 2013;22(6):1230-1249.

66. Ramo BA, Roberts DW, Tuason D, et al: Surgical site infections after posterior spinal fusion for neuromuscular scoliosis: A thirty-year experience at a single institution. *J Bone Joint Surg Am* 2014;96(24):2038-2048.

67. Larsson E-LC, Aaro SI, Normelli HCM, Oberg BE: Long-term follow-up of functioning after spinal surgery in patients with neuromuscular scoliosis. *Spine (Phila Pa 1976)* 2005;30(19):2145-2152.

68. Comstock CP, Leach J, Wenger DR: Scoliosis in total-body-involvement cerebral palsy. Analysis of surgical treatment and patient and caregiver satisfaction. *Spine (Phila Pa 1976)* 1998;23(12):1412-1424.

69. Narayanan UG, Fehlings D, Weir S, Knights S, Kiran S, Campbell K: Initial development and validation of the Caregiver Priorities and Child Health Index of Life with Disabilities (CPCHILD). *Dev Med Child Neurol* 2006;48(10):804-812.

70. Askin GN, Hallett R, Hare N, Webb JK: The outcome of scoliosis surgery in the severely physically handicapped child. An objective and subjective assessment. *Spine (Phila Pa 1976)* 1997;22(1):44-50.

71. Khoshbin A, Vivas L, Law PW, et al: The long-term outcome of patients treated operatively and non-operatively for scoliosis deformity secondary to spina bifida. *Bone Joint J* 2014;96-B(9):1244-1251.

Section 6: Spine

72. Nedelcu T, Georgescu I: Evaluation of the Unit Rod surgical instrumentation in Duchenne scoliosis. A retrospective study. *J Med Life* 2016;9(4):437-443.

This retrospective study of patients with NMS treated with Unit Rod fixation demonstrated good correction of deformity that was maintained at minimum 4 years follow-up. Level of evidence: IV.

73. Holt JB, Dolan LA, Weinstein SL: Outcomes of primary posterior spinal fusion for scoliosis in spinal muscular atrophy. *J Pediatr Orthop* 2017;37(8):e505-e511.

This retrospective review of 16 patients with SMA showed spinal fusion was effective at controlling curve progression and pelvic obliquity without impairing space-available-for-lung ratio, trunk height, or pulmonary function at 10-year follow-up. Level of evidence: IV.

74. Lin JL, Tawfik DS, Gupta R, Imrie M, Bendavid E, Owens DK: Health and economic outcomes of posterior spinal fusion for children with neuromuscular scoliosis. *Hosp Pediatr* 2020;10(3):257-265.

This cost-effectiveness analysis compares health and economic outcomes of spinal fusion to nonoperative treatment for children with NMS. They found that cost effectiveness is improved when NMS is the primary cause of debility. Level of evidence: IV.

75. Diefenbach C, Ialenti MN, Lonner BS, Kamerlink JR, Verma K, Errico TJ: Hospital cost analysis of neuromuscular scoliosis surgery. *Bull Hosp Jt Dis* 2013;71(4):272-277.

76. Berry JG, Glotzbecker M, Rodean J, et al: Perioperative spending on spinal fusion for scoliosis for children with medical complexity. *Pediatrics* 2017;140(4):e20171233.

In this retrospective review of 1,249 children aged 5 years and older with complex chronic conditions undergoing spinal fusion surgery, hospital care accounted for 78% of spending. Multiple preoperative primary care visits were associated with lower hospital costs and shorter length of stay. Level of evidence: IV.

77. Whitaker AT, Sharkey M, Diab M: Spinal fusion for scoliosis in patients with globally involved cerebral palsy: An ethical assessment. *J Bone Joint Surg Am* 2015;97(9):782-787.

CHAPTER 34

Kyphosis

MATTHEW E. OETGEN, MD, MBA

ABSTRACT

Kyphosis is a common deformity in children. Normally, sagittal alignment changes with age, with thoracic kyphosis decreasing and lumbar lordosis increasing, until normal adult spinal and sagittal pelvic alignment is achieved. Abnormal sagittal spinal alignment in pediatric patients can occur as the result of a variety of conditions, which are often associated with developmental structural abnormalities of the vertebral bodies. Regardless of the etiology, it is important to assess the neurologic status of patients with kyphosis because this spinal deformity is associated with the possibility of neurologic injury. Treatment depends on the age of the patient, the magnitude of the deformity, and the underlying etiology. Treatment options consist of observation, brace treatment, and spinal fusion. Long-term patient satisfaction and functional outcome may be improved with normal sagittal spinal alignment, which demonstrates the importance of treatment of pathologic kyphosis in this patient population.

Keywords: congenital kyphosis; kyphosis; sagittal spinal alignment; Scheuermann kyphosis

INTRODUCTION

The sagittal alignment of the skeletally mature spine is relatively well understood, with the normal values of cervical lordosis, thoracic kyphosis, lumbar lordosis, and pelvic parameters previously reported.[1] Despite this understanding of the adult spine, the normal development of spinal sagittal alignment throughout childhood and adolescence remains less clearly defined. It is particularly important to better define the effects of the many pediatric conditions that can result in pathologic sagittal spinal alignment and better monitor the growth of children with these conditions to assist in determining when intervention is needed.[2] A thorough understanding of the development of the sagittal plane may be important in optimizing long-term outcomes, because it will aid surgeons in determining when surgical interventions, such as contouring sagittal spinal alignment using modern segmental spinal instrumentation, are appropriate.

Despite its apparent importance, there is a relative paucity of information about the development of sagittal spinal alignment in children. An analysis of the normative sagittal spinal alignment of 121 children aged 3 to 15 years who were stratified into four age groups showed that the total global kyphosis measured from T1-T12 averaged 44.9° to 53.3° and was larger than adult normative values.[3] The total lumbar lordosis averaged −44.7° to −57.3° and was smaller than adult normative values. The average thoracic apex was the T7-T8 disk, and the lumbar apex was the L4 vertebra, which were both similar compared with these parameters in adults; however, there was an average of 3.6° of kyphosis across the thoracolumbar junction (T10-L2) in children. These findings suggest a more gradual transition from thoracic kyphosis to lumbar lordosis at the thoracolumbar junction, with greater kyphosis in this region in children compared with adults. This finding challenges the widely held belief that this area is essentially neutral in alignment. A change in alignment during growth also was found, with a notable decrease in global kyphosis and an increase in lumbar lordosis in children in the 10- to 12-year age group, with a later increase in kyphosis and decrease in lordosis in children in the 13- to 15-year age group. It was postulated that this change resulted from the adolescent growth

Dr. Oetgen or an immediate family member serves as a board member, owner, officer, or committee member of the American Academy of Orthopaedic Surgeons, the Pediatric Orthopaedic Society of North America, and the Scoliosis Research Society.

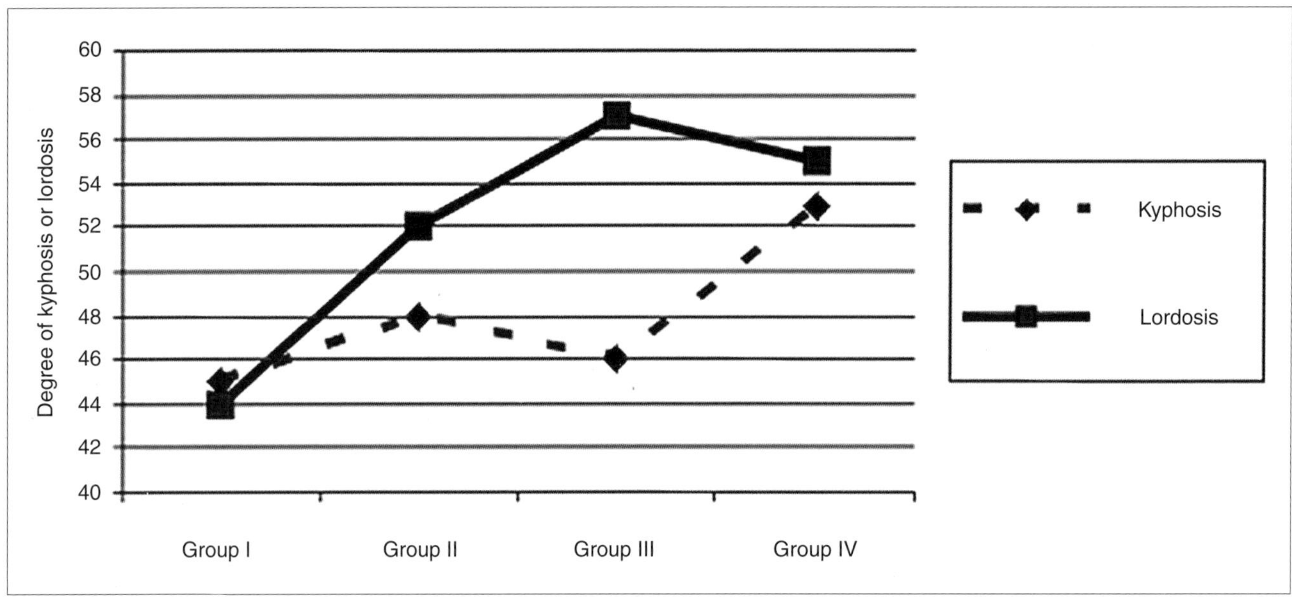

FIGURE 1 The line graph depicts the age-related changes in thoracic kyphosis and lumbar lordosis found in a study of radiographic sagittal spinal alignment in 151 normal children without musculoskeletal abnormalities. The children were divided into four groups based on age—group I: age 3-6 years; group II: age 7-9 years; group III: age 10-12 years; and group IV: age 13-15 years.

spurt with disproportionate anterior vertebral growth[3] (**Figure 1**); however, a 2016 study investigating the morphologic changes in the thoracic vertebral bodies with childhood development found no differences in vertebral body shape over time. These results suggest the overall changes in sagittal alignment in children are more likely related to maintenance of sagittal balance rather than changes in individual vertebral growth or shape.[4] A 2015 study reported that the normative sagittal spinal alignment of children in a sitting position showed less thoracic kyphosis and lumbar lordosis compared with normative standing sagittal alignment values.[5]

A better understanding of the relationship between the sagittal spinal alignment and sagittal pelvic alignment has emerged, with multiple investigations demonstrating that the interaction of these two areas leads to global sagittal balance (**Figure 2**). Although few data exist demonstrating normative sagittal pelvic values in children and the progressive changes that take place during development, these parameters in children were investigated in a 2004 study.[6] The authors found that the complex interaction between the sagittal spinal and pelvic parameters exists in children as it does in adults. In children, the pelvic incidence increases linearly from age 4 to 18 years; this was hypothesized to correlate with changing sagittal spinal alignment to maintain a constant sagittal balance.[6]

In general, it appears likely that global and segmental sagittal spinal alignment and sagittal pelvic alignment in a growing child is quite dynamic and should be carefully considered when planning a surgical intervention.

PHYSIOLOGIC CONSEQUENCES OF KYPHOSIS

Excessive thoracic kyphosis and abnormal global sagittal plane alignment has been shown to lead to a variety of physiologic effects, including the potential association with adolescent back pain, the risk of neurologic injury, and a decrease in self-reported patient satisfaction. In a cross-sectional study of Flemish adolescents, a correlation was found between poor sagittal standing posture and back and neck pain; however, this study used observational sagittal alignment of patients rather than radiographic parameters of spinal alignment.[7] A systematic review of patients with thoracic spine pain reported poor posture as a potential factor associated with pain, although the study authors found that there were many variables associated with spine pain in the pediatric population.[8]

Neurologic injury associated with excessive kyphosis in pediatric patients has been widely reported in the literature. In general, neurologic injury is suspected to occur as a result of excessive compression of the spinal cord when it is draped over a curve with a substantial kyphotic thoracic angle. Neurologic involvement has been most often reported in patients with congenital kyphotic deformities or those with rapidly progressing sharp kyphotic deformities such as those that occur in patients with neurofibromatosis type 1.[9] Patients with a substantial kyphotic deformity may be at greater risk for neurologic injury when undergoing lower limb surgery. A 2015 case report described the development of paraplegia in two children with skeletal dysplasia and

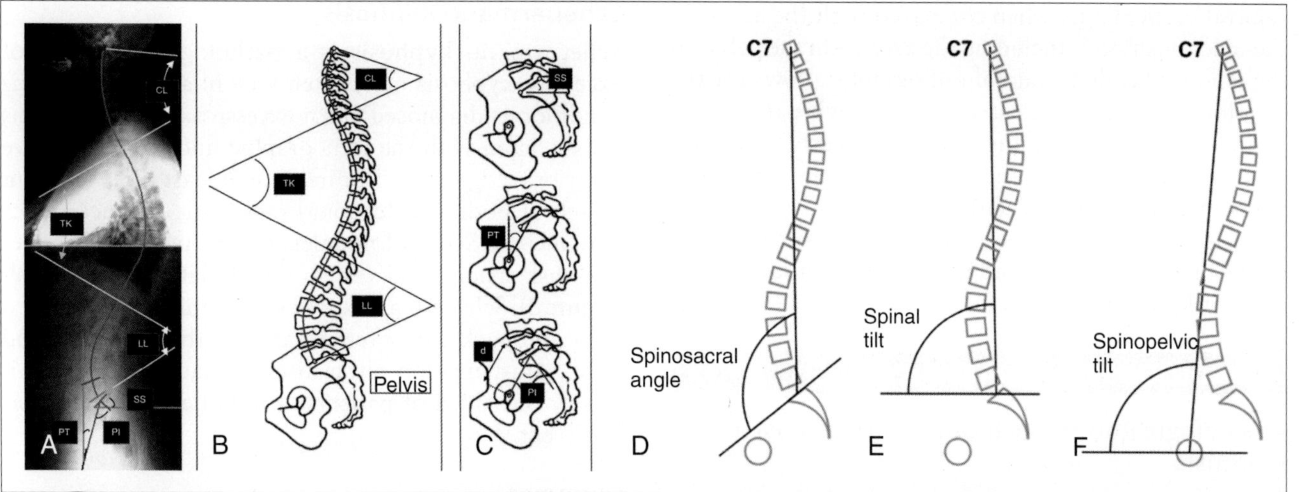

FIGURE 2 **A** through **C**, Techniques for measuring spinal sagittal plane alignment and pelvic parameters. **A**, Sagittal radiograph of the spine and pelvis show the simplified curve model of the spine and the shape and orientation parameters of the pelvis. **B**, Illustration of the spine with the shape parameters delineated. **C**, Illustration of the pelvis with its shape and orientation parameters delineated. The relationship of the pelvic parameters is PI = PT + SS. Illustration of techniques for measuring the global spinal sagittal alignment include measurement of the spinosacral angle (**D**), spinal tilt (**E**), and spinopelvic tilt (**F**). CL = cervical lordosis, d = distance from center of sacral plate to femoral head axis of rotation, LL = lumbar lordosis, PI = pelvic incidence, PT = pelvic tilt, SS = sacral slope, TK = thoracic kyphosis. (Panels **A** through **C** reproduced with permission from Berthonnaud E, Dimnet J, Roussouly P, Labelle H: Analysis of the sagittal balance of the spine and pelvis using shape and orientation parameters. *J Spinal Disord Tech* 2005;18:40-47 and panels **D** through **F** reprinted with permission from Springer Nature: *Eur Spine J*. Mac-Thiong JM, Labelle H, Roussouly P: Pediatric sagittal alignment. 2011;20[suppl 5]:586-590.)

associated thoracic kyphosis who were surgically treated for a lower limb deformity.[10] These outcomes highlight the need to take precautions to avoid iatrogenic spinal cord injury in patients with hyperkyphosis.

Patient-reported outcomes appear to be negatively associated with increased thoracic kyphosis. Evaluation of a prospectively collected spinal deformity database demonstrated worse self-reported values in all domains of the Scoliosis Research Society-22 questionnaire in patients with Scheuermann kyphosis compared with patients with scoliosis and normal control subjects. The self-image domain had the highest negative correlation with increasing kyphosis.[11] This negative correlation also was demonstrated in patients with thoracic hyperkyphosis (>45°) that was not associated with Scheuermann kyphosis.[12]

PATIENT PRESENTATION AND ASSESSMENT

The typical presentation of kyphosis varies based on the age of the patient and the location of the deformity. In infants and children who are not yet of walking age, excessive thoracic or thoracolumbar kyphosis is often appreciated as an obvious gibbus with inspection of the back. Commonly, this is a flexible deformity that is easily straightened with gentle three-point bending of the spine and is likely associated with relatively weak core strength in patients in this young age group. In older children of walking age, the presentation of kyphosis is dependent on the location of the deformity and the underlying etiology. Congenital kyphosis or kyphosis associated with underlying conditions that lead to structural abnormalities of the vertebral bodies often present as relatively short, sharp deformities of the spine. Overall sagittal spinal alignment is affected by the location of the kyphosis. Excessive thoracic kyphosis is often associated with increased lumbar lordosis, which is used as a compensatory mechanism to improve global alignment, whereas thoracolumbar kyphosis is associated with a compensatory thoracic lordosis or a mild crouching gait to compensate for global alignment.

Given the rare but reported occurrence of progressive myelopathy in pediatric patients with acute kyphosis often associated with congenital or syndromic conditions, a thorough neurologic assessment, including strength, sensation, and reflex testing, should be included in the evaluation of all patients presenting with kyphosis. Any evidence of abnormalities on examination should be further evaluated with MRI to assess for evidence of spinal cord compression or other neural axis anomalies.

Radiologic assessment of patients with kyphosis typically starts with upright, full-length radiographs of the spine. Positioning of the arms to move them out of the way of the spine when obtaining lateral radiographs has been shown to affect overall spinal alignment. Although a variety of techniques exist to limit this effect, it appears that passively supporting the arms in approximately 30° of forward flexion limits the amount of shifting of the sagittal vertical axis when compared with the arms-at-the-sides position.[13] Including the area from the pelvis to the femoral heads on lateral radiographs allows for the simultaneous measurement of sagittal pelvic parameters.

Cross-sectional imaging is useful in certain circumstances to further assess the spine. CT is helpful in defining bony anatomy, particularly for preoperative planning. MRI is useful in assessing intraspinal anomalies and the health of the spinal cord in patients with substantial angular kyphosis.

CONDITIONS OF PEDIATRIC KYPHOSIS

Physiologic Round-back Deformity or Postural Kyphosis

Postural kyphosis is a nonpathologic condition of excessive kyphotic alignment. It is often a relatively flexible deformity that can be passively corrected by active spinal extension by the patient. When viewed from the side, the patient often demonstrates a relatively gentle kyphotic alignment on forward bending as opposed to a sharp, angular kyphosis seen in other conditions. Other than the excessive kyphosis, radiographic findings are normal, with no evidence of abnormal development of the vertebral bodies. Treatment is directed at educating the patient and family about the condition and providing reassurance. Postural exercises consisting of paraspinal and core muscle strengthening to improve postural alignment are prescribed. Brace treatment or surgical intervention is rarely, if ever, indicated for postural kyphosis.

Scheuermann Kyphosis

Scheuermann kyphosis is a pathologic condition of excessive kyphosis most often seen in adolescents. This condition is diagnosed when excessive clinical kyphosis is associated with the radiographic finding of excessive anterior wedging of 5° or more of at least three adjacent vertebral bodies. Additional radiologic characteristics may include Schmorl nodules, narrowing of intervertebral disk spaces, and vertebral end plate irregularities[14] (**Figure 3**). Scheuermann kyphosis is commonly associated with dull back pain over the apex of the deformity and tight hamstrings on physical examination; in approximately one-third of patients, a mild degree of scoliosis is present.[15]

Outcomes

The natural history of both treated and untreated Scheuermann kyphosis is poorly documented in the medical literature. In a 1993 report on the long-term follow-up of 67 patients with Scheuermann kyphosis and an age-matched and sex-matched control group, it was found that patients in the Scheuermann group tended to have more back pain, jobs requiring lower activity levels, and less range of motion and strength of the trunk compared with the control group.[16] No differences in the groups were found regarding educational levels, the extent of pain interference with activities of daily living, self-consciousness, self-esteem, or social limitations. Some degree of restrictive pulmonary disease was seen in those individuals with greater than 100° of kyphosis. These

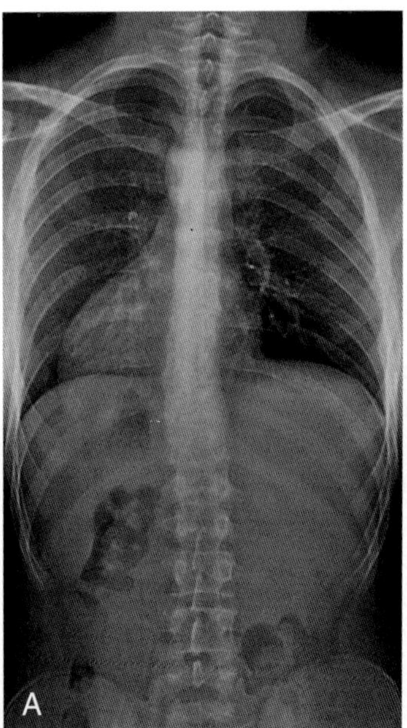

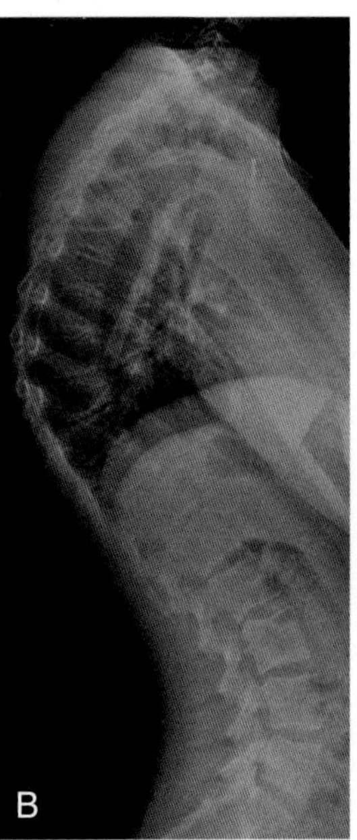

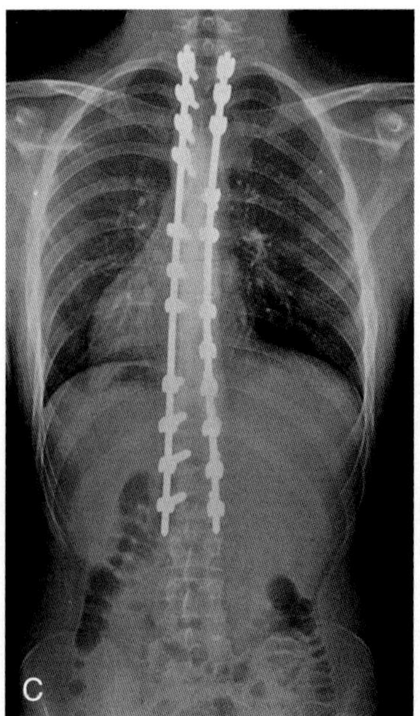

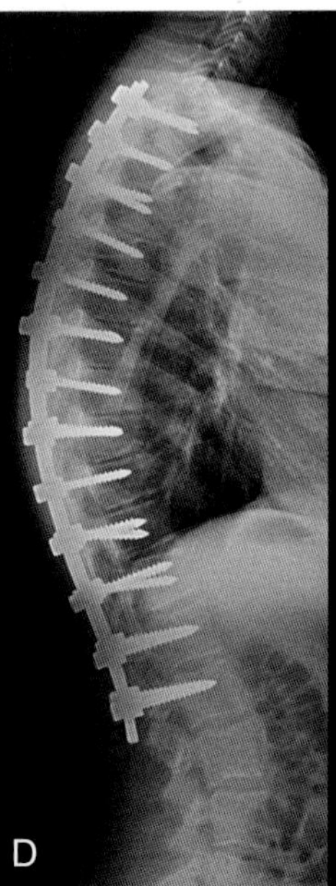

FIGURE 3 Preoperative PA (**A**) and lateral (**B**) radiographs of the spine of a 16-year-old boy with Scheuermann kyphosis measuring 93°. Postoperative AP (**C**) and lateral (**D**) radiographs after kyphosis correction using a segmental pedicle screw construct and multiple Ponte osteotomies.

long-term results are interesting in light of the lower levels of self-reported outcomes in patients with Scheuermann kyphosis compared with normal control subjects noted in a 2013 study.[11] The reasons for this discrepancy may be that outcomes of the cohort in the 1993 study were not generalizable; the natural history of patients in that study were not typical of patients with Scheuermann kyphosis; or differences exist between younger patients with Scheuermann kyphosis and older patients, with the inferior outcomes reported by younger patients improving over time. A 2012 report of long-term outcomes demonstrated increased odds for back pain and functional disability in patients with Scheuermann kyphosis; however, the amount of pain and disability was not related to the degree of kyphosis.[17] More recently a study of the functional impact of exercise tolerance in patients with Scheuermann kyphosis found patients with kyphosis had decreased maximum aerobic power compared with healthy controls, which inversely correlated with the magnitude of the kyphotic deformity.[18] Given these discrepancies in reported outcomes, additional and longer term follow-up studies are needed.

Treatment

Treatment options consist of observation, physical therapy, bracing treatment, and surgical intervention. Physical therapy, consisting of hamstring stretching and core and paraspinal muscle strengthening, has been shown to improve symptomatic pain but does not affect the degree of kyphosis.[19] Brace treatment of Scheuermann kyphosis has been demonstrated to be effective at improving the spinal deformity in patients with less rigid curves. Bracing treatment is considered for those with less severe deformity (<65°) who have at least 1 year of growth remaining. Despite the radiographic improvement seen with brace wear in this population, there is a high degree of deformity recurrence (up to 30% of patients) after bracing treatment is discontinued.[15]

Because of the relatively benign long-term results reported for patients with Scheuermann kyphosis, surgical intervention is controversial and there is little evidence-based material defining surgical indications. Relative surgical indications include progressive deformity greater than 70°, disabling back pain that is recalcitrant to nonsurgical treatment, and serious cosmetic concerns expressed by the patient.[15] Given the relatively low percentage of patients with uncontrolled deformity progression and severe back pain, cosmetic concerns of the patient are often the most influential consideration in surgical decision making.

The surgical treatment of Scheuermann kyphosis has changed over time. Currently, the most popular approach is a posterior spinal fusion with posterior column shortening osteotomies. Although a combined AP approach is effective, studies have demonstrated equivalent correction and decreased complications with the posterior-only approach.[20,21] A recent analysis of the trend of surgical intervention from 2003 to 2012 confirmed the increasing use of posterior-only surgery and the improved results from this approach, but found an associated increased length of fusion and use of osteotomies as well.[22] Although the current method of surgical management of this condition is generally considered safe, it has been shown to have a higher complication rate than management for adolescent idiopathic scoliosis. A 2013 comparison of patients treated for Scheuermann kyphosis and those treated for adolescent idiopathic scoliosis showed a higher rate of postoperative neurologic injury (2.1% versus 0.13%), instrumentation complications (3.1% versus 0.63%), and surgical site infection (10.3% versus 0.75%) in the patients with Scheuermann kyphosis than in those with idiopathic scoliosis, respectively.[11] Despite these results, surgical intervention of patients with Scheuermann kyphosis is associated with significantly greater improvements in patient-reported outcomes, especially in the self-image, mental health, and total score domains compared with patients with adolescent idiopathic scoliosis.[23] In addition, subtle preoperative neurologic abnormalities are present in up to 9% of patients with Scheuermann kyphosis, so careful preoperative assessment and judicious use of neurologic imaging is needed.[24] Two recent studies have investigated the utility of MRI scans for patients with Scheuermann kyphosis, both finding a relative high incidence of intraspinal pathology in this population. Despite this finding, the studies differed in the clinical impact of this information, with one study reporting no eventual change in surgical intervention,[25] and the other reporting a change in treatment plan of 4.7% due to the MRI findings.[26]

Congenital Kyphosis

Congenital kyphosis is a varied group of spinal deformities, with abnormal embryologic formation of the vertebral bodies being the common etiology. This group of deformities is broadly categorized into those with a failure of vertebral formation, a failure of vertebral segmentation, or a mix of these two conditions.[27] Congenital kyphosis should be distinguished from postural, early upper lumbar kyphosis seen in some children before walking age, which is likely associated with poor muscle tone of the trunk. Postural kyphosis is commonly seen without evidence of vertebral body abnormality (as opposed to congenital kyphosis or the vertebral body anterior-inferior beaking seen in patients with mucopolysaccharidoses) and will typically resolve with time and normal motor development. In addition, early infantile kyphosis resulting from mild anterior-superior upper lumbar body hypoplasia has been described and has been shown to resolve spontaneously with growth.[28]

The natural history of congenital kyphosis is variable and mainly influenced by the location and type of deformity and the number of vertebral levels involved. In general, progressive kyphotic deformity is typical, with progression seen most commonly during periods of rapid spinal growth. Little data exist regarding the effects of congenital kyphosis on patient-reported outcomes, but a recent analysis in Egypt showed health-related quality of life is significantly affected with much lower SRS-22 scores in patients with congenital kyphosis compared with healthy controls.[29]

A three-part classification system is used to describe congenital kyphosis based on the type of vertebral anomaly associated with the deformity[27,30] (**Figure 4**). Patients with kyphosis involving failures of vertebral body formation (type 1) typically have rapid progression during periods of growth and are at higher risk for neurologic deterioration because of the typically short, sharp deformity pattern (**Figure 5**). Type 2 deformities are associated with failures of vertebral body segmentation and often progress less rapidly and are rarely associated with progressive neurologic deterioration because the deformity is less sharply angulated. Mixed pattern deformities (type 3) and those associated with congenital vertebral dislocation have the most aggressive natural history, with deformity progression and neurologic deterioration almost assured without intervention.

Treatment of congenital kyphosis is dependent on patient age, neurologic status, and progression of the deformity. Management typically involves observation, with radiographic and neurologic examinations performed at regular intervals. Brace treatment has not been shown to be efficacious in this condition. Surgical intervention is required if deformity progression is noted or neurologic deterioration is found.

In patients with congenital kyphosis associated with failures of formation, posterior arthrodesis can lead to progressive correction of the deformity over time via anterior spinal column growth. This treatment is more successful in patients younger than 5 years and those with a deformity of less than 50°. Anterior and posterior arthrodesis is indicated in patients with progressive congenital kyphosis who are older than 5 years or have a curve magnitude greater than 50°. The anterior surgery can be performed through a separate anterior approach, via a costotransversectomy, or through an all-posterior approach, depending on the need for anterior decompression and the skill and comfort level of the treating surgeon.[31,32]

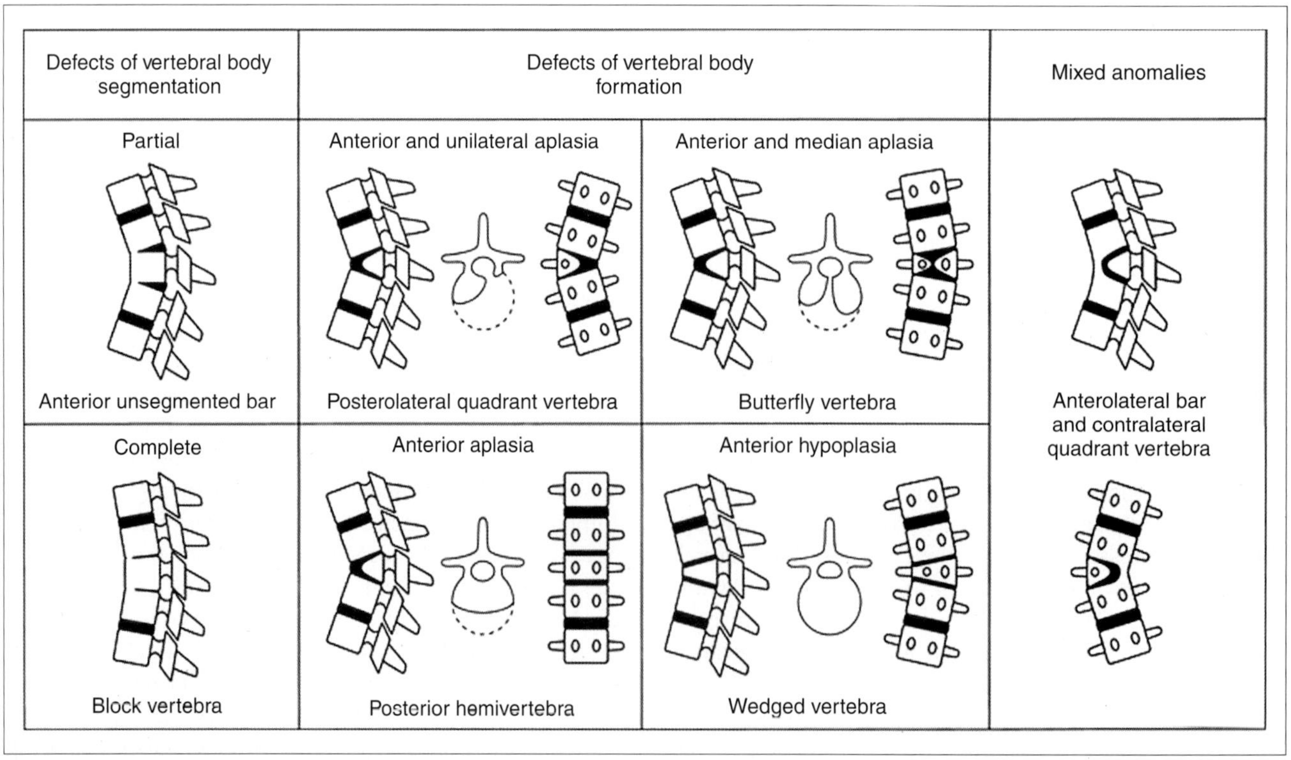

Defects of vertebral body segmentation	Defects of vertebral body formation		Mixed anomalies
Partial Anterior unsegmented bar	Anterior and unilateral aplasia Posterolateral quadrant vertebra	Anterior and median aplasia Butterfly vertebra	Anterolateral bar and contralateral quadrant vertebra
Complete Block vertebra	Anterior aplasia Posterior hemivertebra	Anterior hypoplasia Wedged vertebra	

FIGURE 4 Illustration of a three-part classification system used to describe congenital kyphosis based on the type of vertebral body anomaly associated with the deformity.

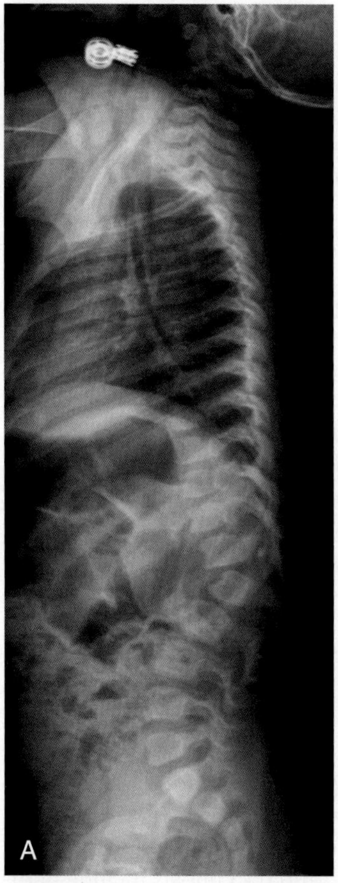

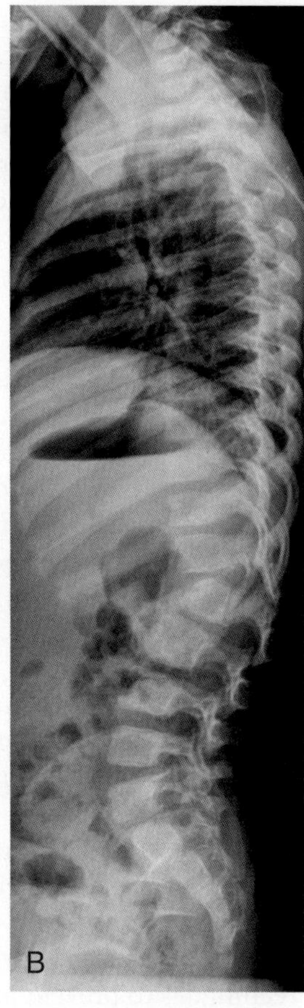

FIGURE 5 **A**, Sitting lateral radiograph of the spine of a 2-year-old boy with 32° of congenital thoracolumbar kyphosis resulting from a type 1 defect in the L1 vertebral body. **B**, Sitting lateral radiograph obtained at 3 years of age shows continued thoracolumbar kyphosis of 32° resulting from the failure of anterior vertebral body formation at L1.

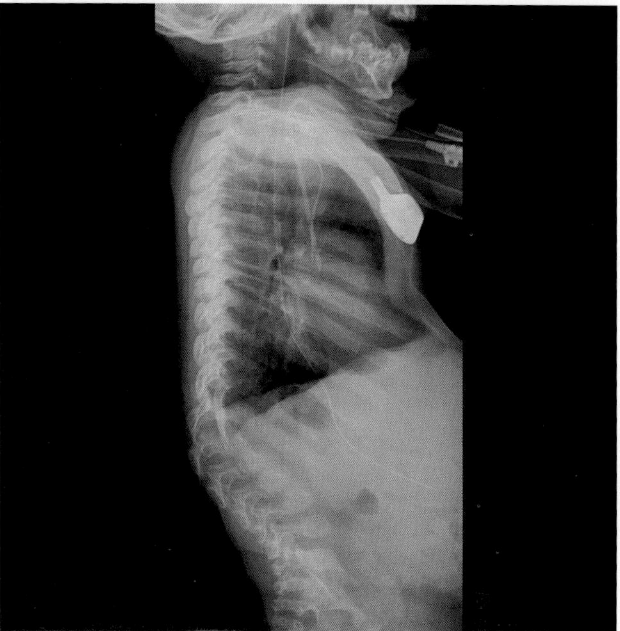

FIGURE 6 Lateral weight-bearing radiograph of a 2-year-old patient with type 1 mucopolysaccharidosis. The patient has 48° of kyphosis with an apex at L1. Note the anterior vertebral body beaking that is pathognomonic for this condition.

OTHER CONDITIONS ASSOCIATED WITH KYPHOSIS

Mucopolysaccharidosis

Mucopolysaccharidosis is a family of six genetic disorders defined by abnormal lysosomal storage caused by deficiency of enzymes required for degradation of intracellular glycosaminoglycans.[33] Although these conditions have a multitude of musculoskeletal manifestations, acute thoracolumbar kyphosis associated with abnormalities of vertebral development (inferior L1-L2 vertebral body beaking) is considered pathognomonic for this condition[33] (**Figure 6**). Although nonsurgical management can be considered as a method to delay definitive treatment in patients with deformity progression, long-term outcomes of brace or cast treatment of kyphosis associated with mucopolysaccharidosis are unproven. A recently published international consensus guideline on treatment of kyphosis in patients with mucopolysaccharidosis type 1 suggested the timing of surgery depends on the progression and flexibility of the deformity along with the presence of symptoms, growth potential, and comorbidities. Although no definitive treatment rules were suggested, this group recommended surgery be performed between the ages of 5 and 13 years if indicated.[34] Progressive deformity is definitively treated with circumferential spinal fusion to achieve maximal correction with the lowest risk of recurrent deformity.[35,36]

Achondroplasia

Achondroplasia is the most common skeletal dysplasia, with an incidence of approximately 1 in 30,000 live births each year.[37] The disorder is characterized by abnormal enchondral ossification of long bones caused by a mutation in the fibroblast growth factor receptor-3 gene (*FGFR3*). One of the most common skeletal manifestations of achondroplasia is the development of thoracolumbar kyphosis, with a reported prevalence of 87% in patients younger than 2 years, 39% in patients aged 2 to 5 years, and 11% in patients older than 5 years.[37] The most common clinical course is one of gradual improvement as the child matures and trunk and core strength increase with growth and progressing functional development (from sitting to standing to walking). Risk factors for

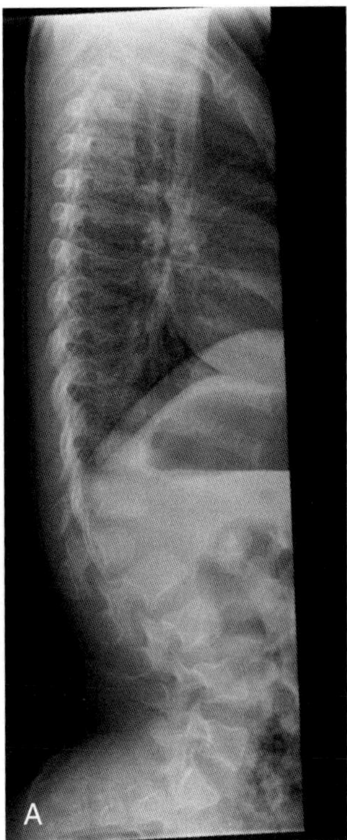

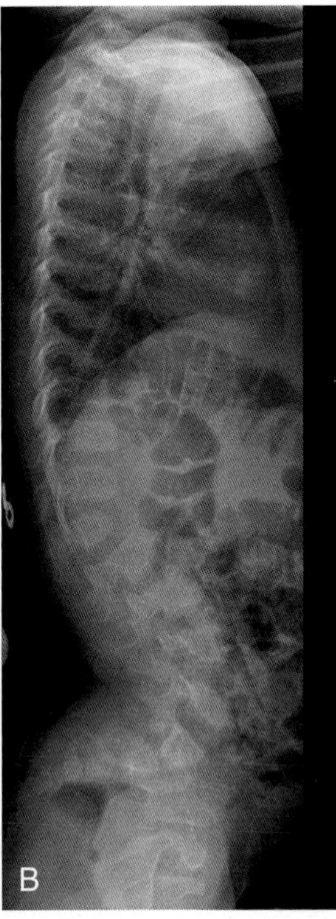

FIGURE 7 **A**, Weight-bearing lateral radiograph of a 2.5-year-old girl with achondroplasia shows a 44° thoracolumbar kyphosis with an apex at L1. **B**, Weight-bearing lateral radiograph shows some improvement of the kyphosis to 38° in a thoracolumbar orthosis.

progressive kyphosis have been reported with delayed motor development, initial kyphosis greater than 25°, and a greater percentage of apical vertebral wedging and translation.[38] In patients with persistent or progressive thoracolumbar kyphosis after walking age, a brace has been suggested to improve alignment and possibly help correct the deformity by allowing improved anterior vertebral body growth and development[39] (**Figure 7**). Although the natural history of thoracolumbar kyphosis in patients with achondroplasia has not been thoroughly documented, a recent study evaluated the likelihood of spontaneous resolution of this deformity and assessed factors associated with nonresolution of thoracolumbar kyphosis in this patient population. This study of 60 patients found 70% of patients had spontaneous deformity resolution over a 5.7-year follow-up, with 58% of patients resolving by 1 year after walking. Factors that were found to be associated with nonresolution of the deformity included apical vertebral translation, greater percentage of apical vertebral wedging, and developmental motor delay. Despite this information, the authors did not make any evidence-based recommendations in regard to the indications for surgical management of these nonresolving deformities.[40] Surgery has been proposed for patients with persistent or progressive deformity because of concerns about poor long-term function. In general, persistent thoracolumbar kyphosis greater than 50° after 5 years of age is considered an indication for corrective spinal fusion. A combined anterior-posterior approach and posterior-only fusion have both been shown to be effective methods of treatment.[37]

Iatrogenic Kyphosis

Proximal junctional kyphosis and distal junctional kyphosis are complications seen after spinal instrumentation in pediatric patients. Although no clear definition exists, this type of kyphosis is typically characterized by a progression of deformity of greater than 5° to 10° at the proximal or distal end of a fusion.[41] The difficulty in determining the existence of this complication is further accentuated by the difficulty in obtaining accurate radiographic measurements. Multiple studies have demonstrated a high degree of variability in measurements and poor interclass correlation between practitioners measuring proximal junction kyphosis in patients with adolescent idiopathic scoliosis or early-onset scoliosis.[42,43]

The prevalence of junctional kyphosis is varied and depends on the underlying spinal pathology, the underlying condition of the patient, the age of the patient, and the amount of postoperative deformity correction.[44] Techniques to prevent junctional kyphosis include planning deformity correction to achieve appropriate global sagittal balance, which may be predicted by baseline sagittal pelvic parameters; choosing appropriate proximal and distal end vertebrae in surgical planning; and using proper surgical techniques to minimize disruption of adjacent nonfused facet joint capsules and interspinous ligaments, which provide inherent junctional stability.[44-46]

SUMMARY

Patients with normal sagittal spinal alignment have been shown to have better long-term outcomes compared with patients with excessive spinal kyphosis. Increased back pain, poorer self-image, and possible neurologic deterioration over time can be seen with excessive kyphosis, which demonstrates the importance of diagnosis and proper treatment of this condition. A variety of underlying conditions are associated with kyphosis in the pediatric population, so a thorough evaluation and appropriate imaging are needed when this spinal deformity is encountered. Treatment aimed at correcting and maintaining sagittal alignment is important and should be undertaken within the context of the underlying condition of the individual patient.

KEY STUDY POINTS

- Normal pediatric sagittal spine alignment is dynamic and changes as children develop. Thoracic kyphosis decreases and lumbar lordosis increases until normal adult sagittal plane alignment is achieved. The pelvic incidence appears to increase during development to maintain overall global alignment based on changes in the spinal alignment.
- Abnormal sagittal plane alignment resulting from excessive thoracic kyphosis has been associated with increased back pain and possible delayed neurologic injury. Long-term patient-reported satisfaction and functional outcomes are better in those with normal sagittal spinal alignment compared with patients with abnormal sagittal alignment.
- Pathologic kyphosis is associated with a variety of pediatric conditions. The most common cause is Scheuermann kyphosis, which can be treated with observation, brace treatment, or surgery, depending on the magnitude of the deformity and skeletal maturity of the patient.
- Other conditions associated with abnormal kyphosis include congenital kyphosis, skeletal dysplasia, mucopolysaccharidosis, and iatrogenic junctional kyphosis after surgical intervention. A thorough patient and radiographic evaluation is needed when a diagnosis of kyphosis is made.

ANNOTATED REFERENCES

1. Vialle R, Levassor N, Rillardon L, Templier A, Skalli W, Guigui P: Radiographic analysis of the sagittal alignment and balance of the spine in asymptomatic subjects. *J Bone Joint Surg Am* 2005;87(2):260-267.
2. Mac-Thiong JM, Labelle H, Roussouly P: Pediatric sagittal alignment. *Eur Spine J* 2011;20(suppl 5):586-590.
3. Cil A, Yazici M, Uzumcugil A, et al: The evolution of sagittal segmental alignment of the spine during childhood. *Spine (Phila Pa 1976)* 2005;30(1):93-100.
4. Dede O, Büyükdogan K, Demirkıran HG, Akpınar E, Yazıcı M: The development of thoracic vertebral sagittal morphology during childhood. *Spine Deform* 2016;4(6):391-394.

   The authors present a cross-sectional radiographic study of children aged 3 to 16 years, assessing the relative anterior and posterior vertebral body height changes over time. They found the relative anterior to posterior height does not change as children age, suggesting sagittal alignment changes as associated to maintenance of balance rather than changes in shape of the vertebral body. Level of evidence: II.
5. Kamaci S, Yucekul A, Demirkiran G, Berktas M, Yazici M: The evolution of sagittal spinal alignment in sitting position during childhood. *Spine (Phila Pa 1976)* 2015;40(13):E787-E793.
6. Mac-Thiong JM, Berthonnaud E, Dimar JR II, Betz RR, Labelle H: Sagittal alignment of the spine and pelvis during growth. *Spine (Phila Pa 1976)* 2004;29(15):1642-1647.
7. Dolphens M, Cagnie B, Coorevits P, et al: Sagittal standing posture and its association with spinal pain: A school-based epidemiological study of 1196 Flemish adolescents before age at peak height velocity. *Spine* 2012;37(19):1657-1666.
8. Briggs AM, Smith AJ, Straker LM, Bragge P: Thoracic spine pain in the general population: Prevalence, incidence and associated factors in children, adolescents and adults. A systematic review. *BMC Musculoskelet Disord* 2009;10:77.
9. Zhang Z, Wang H, Liu C: Compressive myelopathy in severe angular kyphosis: A series of ten patients. *Eur Spine J* 2015;25(6):1897-1903.
10. Pruszczynski B, Mackenzie WG, Rogers K, White KK: Spinal cord injury after extremity surgery in children with thoracic kyphosis. *Clin Orthop Relat Res* 2015;473(10):3315-3320.
11. Lonner B, Yoo A, Terran JS, et al: Effect of spinal deformity on adolescent quality of life: Comparison of operative Scheuermann kyphosis, adolescent idiopathic scoliosis, and normal controls. *Spine (Phila Pa 1976)* 2013;38(12):1049-1055.
12. Petcharaporn M, Pawelek J, Bastrom T, Lonner B, Newton PO: The relationship between thoracic hyperkyphosis and the Scoliosis Research Society outcomes instrument. *Spine (Phila Pa 1976)* 2007;32(20):2226-2231.
13. Marks M, Stanford C, Newton P: Which lateral radiographic positioning technique provides the most reliable and functional representation of a patient's sagittal balance? *Spine (Phila Pa 1976)* 2009;34(9):949-954.
14. Tribus CB: Scheuermann's kyphosis in adolescents and adults: Diagnosis and management. *J Am Acad Orthop Surg* 1998;6(1):36-43.
15. Tsirikos AI, Jain AK: Scheuermann's kyphosis: Current controversies. *J Bone Joint Surg Br* 2011;93(7):857-864.
16. Murray PM, Weinstein SL, Spratt KF: The natural history and long-term follow-up of Scheuermann kyphosis. *J Bone Joint Surg Am* 1993;75(2):236-248.
17. Ristolainen L, Kettunen JA, Heliövaara M, Kujala UM, Heinonen A, Schlenzka D: Untreated Scheuermann's disease: A 37-year follow-up study. *Eur Spine J* 2012;21(5):819-824.
18. Lorente A, Barrios C, Lorente R, Tamariz R, Burgos J: Severe hyperkyphosis reduces the aerobic capacity and maximal exercise tolerance in patients with Scheuermann disease. *Spine J* 2019;19(2):330-338.

    A functional assessment of 41 adolescent patients with Scheuermann kyphosis compared with healthy controls demonstrated the kyphosis cohort had a decreased maximal aerobic power. An inverse relationship between kyphosis and maximal aerobic power was found with kyphosis >75° showing severe decrease in cardiovascular efficiency. Level of evidence: III.
19. Weiss HR, Dieckmann J, Gerner HJ: Effect of intensive rehabilitation on pain in patients with Scheuermann's disease. *Stud Health Technol Inform* 2002;88:254-257.

20. Etemadifar M, Ebrahimzadeh A, Hadi A, Feizi M: Comparison of Scheuermann's kyphosis correction by combined anterior-posterior fusion versus posterior-only procedure. *Eur Spine J* 2016;25(8):2580-2586.

21. Tsutsui S, Pawelek JB, Bastrom TP, Shah SA, Newton PO: Do discs "open" anteriorly with posterior-only correction of Scheuermann's kyphosis? *Spine (Phila Pa 1976)* 2011;36(16):E1086-E1092.

22. Horn SR, Poorman GW, Tishelman JC, et al: Trends in treatment of Scheuermann kyphosis: A study of 1,070 cases from 2003 to 2012. *Spine Deform* 2019;7(1):100-106.

This study is a retrospective review of the KID Inpatient database of adolescents treated for Scheuermann kyphosis between 2003 and 2012. Over that period, the authors found no changes in demographics or prevalence of surgery, but an increase in posterior-only surgery, length of fusions, use of osteotomies over time, and a decrease in the rate of complications associated with posterior-only surgery. Level of evidence: III.

23. Toombs C, Lonner B, Shah S, et al: Quality of life improvement following surgery in adolescent spinal deformity patients: A comparison between Scheuermann kyphosis and adolescent idiopathic scoliosis. *Spine Deform* 2018;6(6):676-683.

This study reports the comparison of self-reported health-related quality of life scores for 82 patients with Scheuermann kyphosis and 995 patients with adolescent idiopathic scoliosis, all surgically treated. Patients with Scheuermann kyphosis reported worse preoperative scores in self-image, mental health, and total score compared with patients with idiopathic scoliosis. At 2 years postoperatively, scores improved more in the Scheuermann group than the scoliosis group and achieved equivalence to those in patients with idiopathic scoliosis. Level of evidence: II.

24. Cho W, Lenke LG, Bridwell KH, et al: The prevalence of abnormal preoperative neurological examination in Scheuermann kyphosis: Correlation with X-ray, magnetic resonance imaging, and surgical outcome. *Spine (Phila Pa 1976)* 2014;39(21):1771-1776.

25. Demiroz S, Ketenci IE, Yanik HS, Bayram S, Ur K, Erdem S: Intraspinal anomalies in individuals with Scheuermann's kyphosis: Is the routine use of magnetic resonance imaging necessary for preoperative evaluation? *Asian Spine J* 2018;12(4):697-702.

This is a radiographic study of 120 patients undergoing spinal fusion for Scheuermann kyphosis. The authors found a 5.8% rate of intraspinal pathology (all syringomelia) with no patient requiring preoperative neurosurgical intervention. Level of evidence: IV.

26. Lonner BS, Toombs CS, Mechlin M, et al: MRI screening in operative Scheuermann kyphosis: Is it necessary? *Spine Deform* 2017;5(2):124-133.

This is a radiographic study of 86 patients undergoing spinal fusion for Scheuermann kyphosis. The authors found 4.7% of patients required a change in surgical plan based on the findings on the preoperative MRI. Given this, the authors recommended preoperative MRI screening for patients with Scheuermann kyphosis undergoing spinal fusion. Level of evidence: IV.

27. McMaster MJ, Singh H: Natural history of congenital kyphosis and kyphoscoliosis: A study of one hundred and twelve patients. *J Bone Joint Surg Am* 1999;81(10): 1367-1383.

28. Campos MA, Fernandes P, Dolan LA, Weinstein SL: Infantile thoracolumbar kyphosis secondary to lumbar hypoplasia. *J Bone Joint Surg Am* 2008;90(8):1726-1729.

29. Soliman HAG: Health-related quality of life of adolescents with severe untreated congenital kyphosis and kyphoscoliosis in a developing country. *Spine (Phila Pa 1976)* 2018;43(16):E942-E948.

This study reports the results of the Arabic version of the SRS-22 for a cross section of 134 patients with congenital kyphosis and congenital kyphoscoliosis compared with health controls. In general, patient reported health related quality of life was significantly decreased in patients with congenital kyphosis and congenital kyphoscoliosis compared to health controls. These results correlated with the amount of deformity, with lower scores reported as magnitude of kyphosis increased. Level of evidence: III.

30. Winter RB, Moe JH, Wang JF: Congenital kyphosis: Its natural history and treatment as observed in a study of one hundred and thirty patients. *J Bone Joint Surg Am* 1973;55(2):223-256.

31. Spiro AS, Rupprecht M, Stenger P, et al: Surgical treatment of severe congenital thoracolumbar kyphosis through a single posterior approach. *Bone Joint J* 2013;95-B(11): 1527-1532.

32. Zeng Y, Chen Z, Qi Q, et al: The posterior surgical correction of congenital kyphosis and kyphoscoliosis: 23 cases with minimum 2 years follow-up. *Eur Spine J* 2013;22(2): 372-378.

33. White KK, Sousa T: Mucopolysaccharide disorders in orthopaedic surgery. *J Am Acad Orthop Surg* 2013;21(1):12-22.

34. Kuiper GA, Langereis EJ, Breyer S, et al: Treatment of thoracolumbar kyphosis in patients with mucopolysaccharidosis type I: Results of an international consensus procedure. *Orphanet J Rare Dis* 2019;14(1):17.

This study includes the internationally developed consensus treatment guidelines for kyphosis in patients with mucopolysaccharidosis type I. Level of evidence: V.

35. Abelin Genevois K, Garin C, Solla F, Guffon N, Kohler R: Surgical management of thoracolumbar kyphosis in mucopolysaccharidosis type 1 in a reference center. *J Inherit Metab Dis* 2014;37(1):69-78.

36. Garrido E, Tomé-Bermejo F, Adams CI: Combined spinal arthrodesis with instrumentation for the management of progressive thoracolumbar kyphosis in children with mucopolysaccharidosis. *Eur Spine J* 2014;23(12):2751-2757.

37. Shirley ED, Ain MC: Achondroplasia: Manifestations and treatment. *J Am Acad Orthop Surg* 2009;17(4):231-241.

38. Borkhuu B, Nagaraju DK, Chan G, Holmes L Jr, Mackenzie WG: Factors related to progression of thoracolumbar kyphosis in children with achondroplasia: A retrospective cohort study of forty-eight children treated in a comprehensive orthopaedic center. *Spine (Phila Pa 1976)* 2009;34(16):1699-1705.

39. Pauli RM, Breed A, Horton VK, Glinski LP, Reiser CA: Prevention of fixed, angular kyphosis in achondroplasia. *J Pediatr Orthop* 1997;17(6):726-733.

40. Margalit A, McKean G, Lawing C, Galey S, Ain MC: Walking out of the curve: Thoracolumbar kyphosis in achondroplasia. *J Pediatr Orthop* 2018;38(10):491-497.

    This is a retrospective review of 60 patients with thoracolumbar kyphosis and achondroplasia. Of those patients presenting before walking age, 70% had spontaneous resolution of the kyphosis by 5.7 years of follow-up. Factors associated with persistence of kyphosis included apical vertebral translation, greater percentage of apical vertebral wedging, and developmental motor delay. Level of evidence: II.

41. Cho SK, Kim YJ, Lenke LG: Proximal junctional kyphosis following spinal deformity surgery in the pediatric patient. *J Am Acad Orthop Surg* 2015;23(7):408-414.

42. Barrett KK, Andras LM, Tolo VT, Choi PD, Skaggs DL: Measurement variability in the evaluation of the proximal junction in distraction-based growing rods patients. *J Pediatr Orthop* 2015;35(6):624-627.

43. Basques BA, Long WD III, Golinvaux NS, et al: Poor visualization limits diagnosis of proximal junctional kyphosis in adolescent idiopathic scoliosis. *Spine J* 2017;17(6):784-789.

    The authors reported a high degree of interobserver and intraobserver variability in radiographic measurements of proximal junctional kyphosis in patients with adolescent idiopathic scoliosis. Level of evidence: III.

44. Kim YJ, Lenke LG, Bridwell KH, et al: Proximal junctional kyphosis in adolescent idiopathic scoliosis after 3 different types of posterior segmental spinal instrumentation and fusions: Incidence and risk factor analysis of 410 cases. *Spine (Phila Pa 1976)* 2007;32(24):2731-2738.

45. Cho KJ, Lenke LG, Bridwell KH, Kamiya M, Sides B: Selection of the optimal distal fusion level in posterior instrumentation and fusion for thoracic hyperkyphosis: The sagittal stable vertebra concept. *Spine (Phila Pa 1976)* 2009;34(8):765-770.

46. Denis F, Sun EC, Winter RB: Incidence and risk factors for proximal and distal junctional kyphosis following surgical treatment for Scheuermann kyphosis: Minimum five-year follow-up. *Spine (Phila Pa 1976)* 2009;34(20):E729-E734.

CHAPTER 35

Pediatric Cervical Spine Disorders

FIROZ MIYANJI, MD, FRCSC

ABSTRACT

The diagnosis and management of pediatric cervical spine disorders pose many unique challenges for the treating physician. To optimize care for these children, it is critical to have a clear understanding of the variations in normal growth and development and the disparate presentations of the many disorders of the pediatric cervical spine from infancy through adolescence.

Keywords: cervical spine; dysplasia; subluxation; synchondrosis

INTRODUCTION

The unique growth and development of the pediatric cervical spine lends itself to a spectrum of disorders not commonly seen in the adult population. The spectrum of disease, patterns of injury, and any nontraumatic instability also may be different from infancy through childhood and into adolescence. Many congenital syndromes and skeletal dysplasias have pathognomonic involvement of the cervical spine, which is important for the pediatric orthopaedic surgeon to recognize. Understanding variations of normal in the developing cervical spine may aid in understanding the natural history of disease. Emphasis should be placed on important principles of the growing pediatric cervical spine, common osseoligamentous afflictions, challenges in diagnoses, and treatment options.

Dr. Miyanji or an immediate family member serves as a paid consultant to or is an employee of DePuy, a Johnson & Johnson Company, Orthopediatrics, and Zimmer and has received research or institutional support from DePuy, a Johnson & Johnson Company.

EMBRYOLOGY AND DEVELOPMENTAL ANATOMY

Embryologic formation of the spine (and the spinal cord) progresses in an organized manner beginning with the formation of the primitive streak, the notochord, somites, and sclerotomes. Initial spine development begins during the third week of gestation, with the axial skeleton arising from somites. Paired somites appear approximately on gestational day 20. They arise from the paraxial mesoderm in a cranial-to-caudal fashion at a rate of approximately three to four somites per day. Initially, 42 to 44 somite pairs flank the notochord, forming the base of the skull, and extend caudally. The basiocciput develops from somites 1 to 4, the atlantoaxial column from somites 5 to 7, and the subaxial spine from somites 7 to 12.

The somites then separate into sclerotomes, which ultimately form the bony spinal column. After sclerotome division is complete, the caudal half of the supra-adjacent sclerotome merges with the cranial half of the subadjacent sclerotome, forming the vertebra precursor. The division and subsequent re-fusion explains why eight cervical nerves but only seven cervical vertebrae are present. The cranial division of the first cervical sclerotome (the proatlas) contributes to form the base of the occiput and the tip of the odontoid process, whereas the caudal division of the first cervical sclerotome and the cranial division of the second cervical sclerotome forms the first cervical vertebra. The ventral sclerotome forms the vertebral body, and the dorsal sclerotome becomes the ventral arch (**Figure 1**).

Atlas

The first cervical vertebra has several morphologic characteristics that distinguish it from the other cervical vertebrae. It is incompletely ossified at birth and develops from three ossification centers. The two posterolateral ossification centers (which give rise to the lateral masses

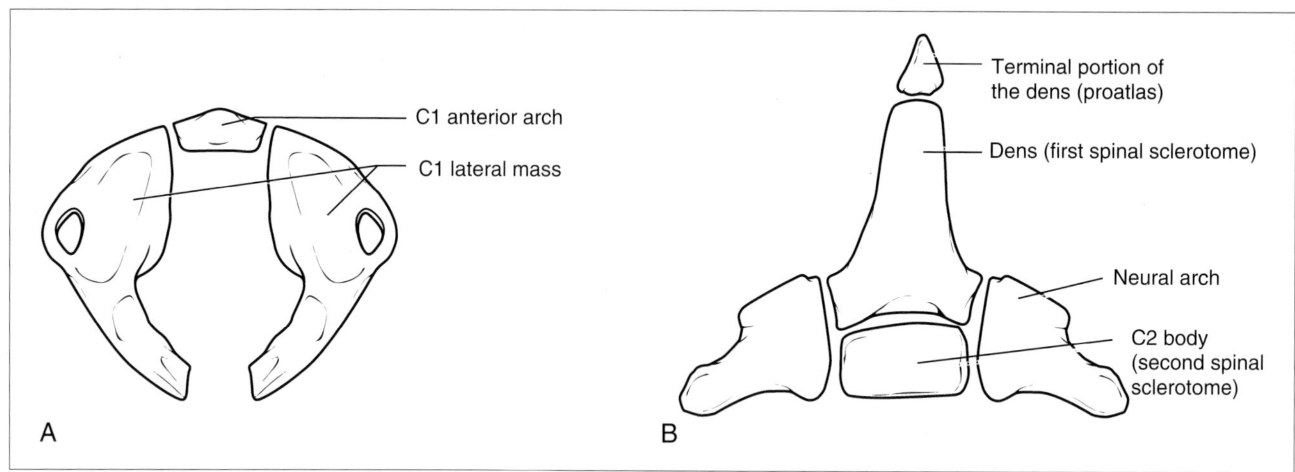

FIGURE 1 Schematic drawings of the developmental anatomy of C1 and C2. **A**, Cross-sectional view of C1. **B**, Anterior view of C2. (Adapted from Miyanji F: Cervical abnormalities, back pain, and the surgical treatment of spondylolysis and spondylolisthesis, in Song KM, ed: *Orthopaedic Knowledge Update®: Pediatrics*, ed 4. Rosemont, IL, American Academy of Orthopaedic Surgeons, 2011, pp 293-313.)

and the posterior arch) are present at birth, and the anterior ossification center (the anterior arch) appears between 6 months and 2 years of age. The age at which closure of the synchondroses occurs remains controversial. It was initially reported in 1937 that the posterior midline synchondrosis fuses by 3 to 5 years of age, whereas the two anterior synchondroses fuse by 7 to 9 years of age.[1] Later, it was reported the posterior synchondrosis closed by age 5 years, and the anterior synchondroses closed by age 6 years.[2] A 2011 study found that the median age of complete ossification of the anterior synchondroses was 8.5 years, with an interquartile range (IQR) of 5.5 to 13 years; however, approximately 45% of the patients showed incomplete ossification at age 10 years.[3] A 2013 quantitative, age-dependent, cross-sectional analysis of the closure of the C1 synchondroses noted complete closure of the posterior synchondrosis by 3 years of age in all but 1 of 54 patients (1.9%). Also in the series, closure of the anterior synchondroses was generally found after 3 years of age, and it was observed that the widths of the synchondroses decreased linearly with age as ossification progressed.[4] An analysis of 841 CT studies of the atlas also confirmed the universal features of the development of C1, notably the three ossification centers with two anterolateral synchondroses and one posterior midline synchondrosis.[2] The authors, however, noted an anterior midline synchondrosis in up to 20% of cases, highlighting the fact that the anterior arch may develop from a pair of symmetric ossification centers, not from a single anterior ossification center in some instances.[3]

In a retrospective review of CT scans of patients younger than 8 years, a group of authors found up to 21% with multiple anterior ossification centers, with incomplete ossification of the anterior arch in 46% of those aged 7 to 8 years.[5] The authors also noted incomplete ossification of the posterior synchondrosis in 16% of those older than 5 years, highlighting the variability present in C1 ossification patterns and the timing of synchondrosis fusion.

Axis

The axis is formed from five ossification centers: paired neural arch ossification centers (lateral masses), a basal central ossification center (body), a dentate center (dens), and an apical center (the odontoid tip). In fetal life, the dens arises from paired ossification centers that are symmetric about the sagittal midline plane. Although by birth these centers have usually fused and all that remains is a sagittally oriented cleft at the tip of the ossifying odontoid, some authors think that the fusion may occur within the first 3 months of life.[6] The C2 body appears by the fifth fetal month and is separated from the dens by the dentocentral synchondrosis, which fuses at 3 to 6 years of age. A 2011 CT study of 835 patients noted that the dentocentral synchondrosis closure occurred earlier than previously reported.[3] Most of the patients in the study with complete radiolucency of the dentocentral synchondrosis were younger than 3.3 years. The authors noted that beyond this age, sclerotic traces of the synchondrosis remained visible.

Historically, the ossiculum terminale at the tip of the dens has been reported to appear in children aged 5 to 8 years, with fusion to the dens between the ages of 10 and 13 years.[7] In 2011, however, researchers found that the ages of initial ossification and fusion are younger than what had been previously suggested,[3] with a median age at initial ossification of the apical center of 2.7 years

(IQR, 1.9 to 3.6 years). The oldest child in this study with no ossification in the apical center was 12.8 years. The authors found that the median age of incorporation of the apical center was 8.2 years (IQR, 7.1 to 9.9 years). The neural arch ossification centers appear bilaterally at fetal age 7 months and fuse posteriorly by age 3 years. The estimated median age of initial ossification of the neurocentral synchondroses was reported to be 3.8 years (IQR, 2.9 to 4.6 years).[3] It also is well recognized that the superior portion of the neurocentral synchondrosis (between the neural arches and the odontoid) closes later than the inferior portion (between the arches and the C2 body).

Lower Cervical Vertebrae

The lower cervical vertebrae are formed from two lateral ossification centers and a third one for the body. The neural arches appear by fetal age 7 to 9 weeks, and the body appears by fetal age 5 months. The neurocentral synchondroses separating the lateral masses from the body close between 3 and 6 years of age. The posterior synchondrosis usually unites by 2 to 4 years of age. The superior and inferior epiphyseal rings appear at puberty and unite with the body at about 25 years of age and are responsible for the vertical growth of the body.

IMAGING PARAMETERS AND EVALUATION

Numerous lines, angles, and measurements have been applied to diagnostic images to assess the craniocervical junction. As shown in **Figure 2**, the most widely used craniometric measurements include the McRae line, Chamberlain line, the Wackenheim clivus baseline, the Welcher basal angle, the Powers ratio, the anterior atlantodens interval (AADI), and the posterior atlantodens interval (PADI).

Although AP, lateral, and open-mouth odontoid plain radiographs are traditionally obtained to evaluate the cervical spine, the routine use of open-mouth odontoid radiographs in children remains questionable. In 2000, researchers reported on 51 children with cervical spine injuries and found that the open-mouth odontoid radiographs were not useful, especially for children younger than 9 years.[7]

The Chamberlain line is useful for identifying basilar invagination; however, as a normal variant, the dens may project a few millimeters (1 mm ± 3.6 to 6.6 mm) above the line.[8] If the opisthion is not clearly visualized in very young children, the McGregor line may be useful by connecting the posterior pole of the palate to the lowest point of the occipital squamosal surface. The Wackenheim

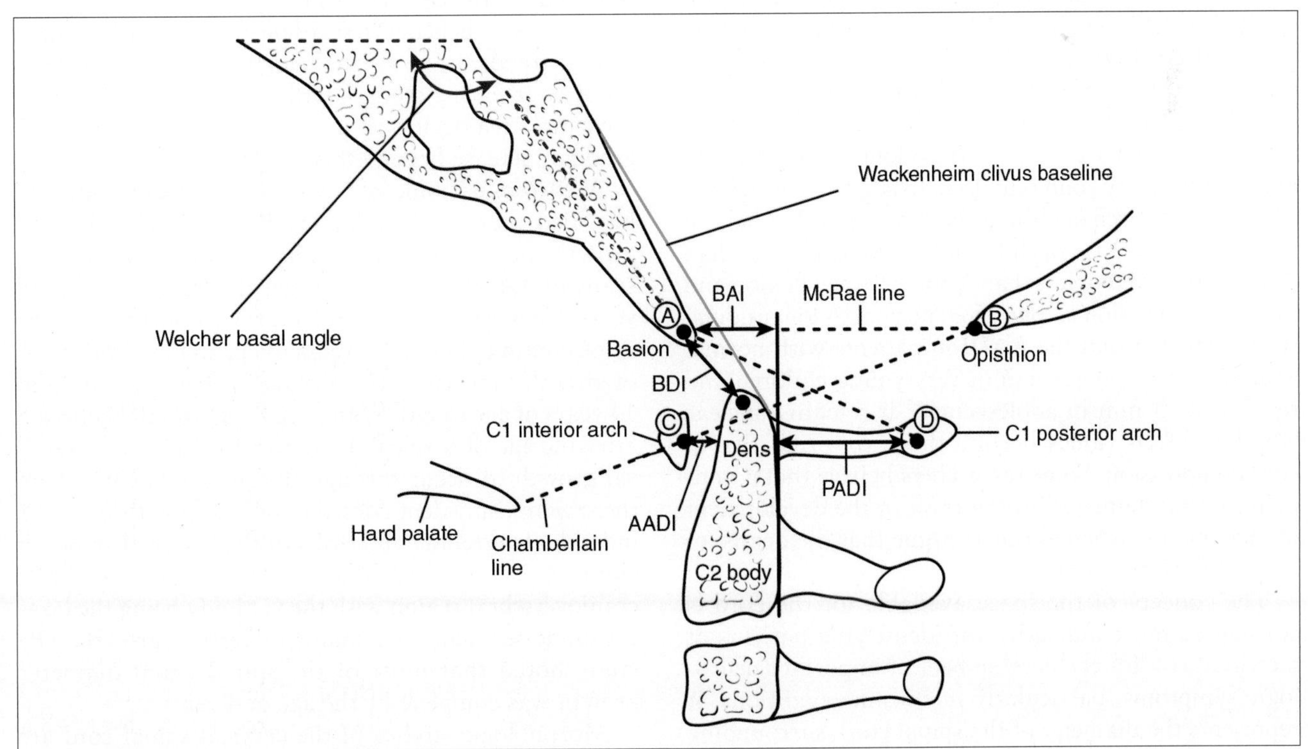

FIGURE 2 Schematic drawing of the upper cervical spine showing a lateral view of the common radiographic parameters. AADI = anterior atlantodens interval, BAI = basion-axial interval, BDI = basion-dens interval, PADI = posterior atlantodens interval, Powers ratio = AD/BC

clivus baseline can be used to identify basilar invagination, atlantoaxial dislocation, and atlanto-occipital dislocation. The angle formed by the Wackenheim clivus line with a line drawn along the posterior surface of the odontoid is called the craniovertebral angle and varies from 150° to 180° with flexion and extension, respectively.[8] The Welcher basal angle should always be less than 140°. Platybasia is associated with an increase in this angle.

Other useful parameters to assess atlanto-occipital instability include the Powers ratio, the basion-axial interval, the basion-dens interval, and the atlanto-occipital joint space (**Figure 2**). Although studies have reported the Powers ratio to be 33% to 60% sensitive, the basion-dens interval to be 50% sensitive, and the basion-axial interval to be close to 100% sensitive in children, these radiographic parameters have been difficult to assess because of the inherent challenges of visualizing the anatomic structures on plain radiographs in very young patients or those with anatomic abnormalities.[9] Studies have encouraged the use of CT scans in this setting and report improvements in sensitivity, specificity, and positive and negative predictive values in diagnosing atlanto-occipital instability compared with plain radiographs. In 2005, a basion-dens interval of greater than 10 mm on a CT scan was considered to be diagnostic of atlanto-occipital dissociation.[10]

The AADI has commonly been used to assess motion at C1-C2 and is emphasized as a marker for predicting potential cord compression at the atlantoaxial junction. In children younger than 8 years, it is agreed that an AADI of up to 5 mm is acceptable because of the increased cartilage content of the odontoid and the ring of the atlas in very young children. In addition, overriding of the anterior arch of the atlas on top of the odontoid can be seen in up to 20% of children.[11] In patients older than 8 years, an AADI of less than 3 mm between flexion and extension excursion is considered normal. A longitudinal study reported that the AADI in patients with normal anatomy averaged 1.9 mm in very young children and reached 2.45 mm in adolescents.[12] It remains unclear whether AADI values beyond these are predictive of cord compression. Some researchers believe that a minimal sagittal diameter is important in the development of myelopathy, whereas others argue that the degree of instability is more important.

The concept of the space available for the cord is considered most indicative for identifying patients at increased risk for the development of important neurologic symptoms, particularly in chronic conditions. It represents the diameter of the spinal cord, surrounding cerebrospinal fluid, and the dura mater at the level of C1 and was established with MRI. Conceptually, the space available for the cord is represented by the PADI, which can be measured on plain lateral radiographs. In adults, absolute stenosis is defined as a flexion PADI of less than 10 mm, whereas relative stenosis is considered to be between 10 and 13 mm. In children, however, the amount of narrowing of the canal diameter beyond which cord compression occurs is uncertain. In adults, cord compression has been reported when the canal diameter is less than 14 mm.

In children, cord compression may be inferred from the age-related diameter of the spinal canal. Morphologic investigations of the C1 vertebra in the growing spine, however, are limited. A prospective longitudinal study in 2001 attempted to provide more reliable reference values to objectively assess the developing cervical spine. The authors noted that cervical spine growth is most rapid in the first 3 years of life, by which time it has reached nearly 95% of its mature diameter. In males, the authors found the canal diameter of the upper cervical spine at C2 averaged 12.8 mm at 6 months of age, which increased to 16 mm in adolescence.[12] In a study using only lateral radiographs, the sagittal canal diameter at C1 in a developing spine was reported to increase from an average of 19.9 mm at age 3 to 6 years to 20.6 mm at the age of 7 to 10 years and 21.3 mm at the age of 11 to 14 years.[13] Another study described the average increase in the sagittal canal size at C1 from 3 to 18 years of age to be 1.8 mm in boys and 2.9 mm in girls.[14] In 2013, researchers reported on the developmental morphology of the C1 vertebra using helical CT scans on 54 children and noted similar trends in the sagittal canal dimensions as those reported in earlier studies, with substantial increases in the canal area occurring up to 6 years of age and more gradual increase beyond this age.[4]

A 2016 morphometric analysis of the pediatric spine has also increased understanding of cervical spine growth and development. The authors analyzed CT scans of 1,458 children between the ages of 1 and 18 years. They found that vertical growth of the pediatric spine continued up to 18 years of age in boys with 50% of growth occurring after the age of 9 years, and up to 14 years of age in girls with 33.2% of growth occurring after the age of 9 years. They also found 75% of vertical growth to occur through the subaxial spine where there were equivalent contributions of growth from the individual vertebrae and disks of the subaxial spine. In contrast, 25% of vertical growth occurred through the craniovertebral region with the C2 body being the largest single-segment contributor to vertical growth. The study noted that most of the spinal canal diameter growth was complete by the age of 4 years.[15]

Morphologic studies of the cervical spinal cord are very limited. A review of 110 normal myelograms in children (age range, 1 month to 15 years) found that the ratio of the cord to subarachnoid space was independent of age and sex, with very little variability at different vertebral levels.[16] The spinal canal was found to be narrowest at C4 followed by C5, whereas the spinal cord was largest at C4-C5.[17] The area and circularity of the cervical spinal cord were not significantly correlated with any parameter of the spinal canal, and the spinal cord showed less individual variation than the bony canal.

The canal dimensions determine, in part, the space available for the cord and the susceptibility to spinal cord injury. In a study of adults, a comparison of CT parameters of normal control subjects with those of patients who sustained spinal cord injury found no substantial differences between the groups with regard to the cross-sectional area of the spinal canal; however, the sagittal diameters of the spinal canal of the control group were significantly larger than those of the spinal cord injury group. The study authors concluded that it is not the total volume of space within the spinal canal, but rather the shape that is the critical factor.[18]

CT and MRI have obvious noted advantages when assessing the pathology of the upper cervical spine, especially given the inherent limitations of plain radiographs of visualizing many of the osseous landmarks of the craniocervical junction. These studies, however, provide static information; for patients with dynamic instability, flexion-extension radiographs are still warranted. Dynamic CT as well as MRI have been shown to be of value in patients with neurologic symptoms but equivocal plain radiographs. Despite the added potential value of CT compared with plain radiography in assessing the pediatric cervical spine, the associated radiation dose and estimated increased cancer risk are important considerations. In 2013, researchers evaluated seven US healthcare systems and noted a sharp increase in pediatric CT use, with a fourfold to ninefold increase in spinal CTs from 1996 to 2010.[19] The authors noted that the projected lifetime attributable risks of solid cancer were higher in younger patients, in girls, and for abdomen/pelvic and spinal CTs. The risk for leukemia was highest for head CT scans in children younger than 5 years.

CRANIOCERVICAL AND UPPER CERVICAL ABNORMALITIES

Atlantoaxial Rotatory Subluxation

Children with atlantoaxial rotatory subluxation (AARS) have a painful torticollis and limited neck motion. The head is rotated to one side and laterally flexed to the contralateral side. The associated muscle spasm is on the side of the long sternocleidomastoid muscle because the muscle is attempting to correct the deformity. This contrasts with congenital muscular torticollis, in which the muscle causes the deformity and is found to be tight on the opposite side of the deformity.

In normal rotation, C1 moves first; only after C1 rotates beyond 23° does C2 begin to rotate. As C2 begins to rotate, C1 continues to move at a greater rate, such that the angular relationship between C1 and C2 continues to increase. The ligaments between C1 and C2 become taut after C1 has rotated approximately 65° from midline, at which point C1 and C2 rotate together until maximum head turn is achieved. It is important to note that the difference in rates of motion between the axis and the atlas produce a natural subluxation of the atlantoaxial facets during normal rotation. In AARS, the subluxation of the C1-C2 facets is prevented from returning to normal.[20]

Of the numerous causes of AARS, trauma and infection (Grisel syndrome) are the most common. The authors of a 2017 study reported on a large, multicenter study of pediatric blunt-trauma cervical spine injuries. AARS accounted for 10% of all injuries, with falls being the most frequently reported mechanism.[21] The common denominator in AARS is a rotation of the atlantoaxial complex that is held in a fixed position and caused by either a muscle spasm or a mechanical block. Suspected pathophysiology after a retropharyngeal infection is thought to be involved because of a direct connection between the pharyngeal veins, the periodontal venous plexus, and the suboccipital epidural sinuses. This anatomic feature may facilitate the translocation of pharyngovertebral inflammatory products to the upper cervical spine, causing spastic contracture of the cervical muscles.[6] The presence of synovial folds in some atlantoaxial joints, which may be increased in children, has been reported. This abundance of soft-tissue structures adjacent to the mobile C1-C2 articulation may provide material that can become swollen or incarcerated during atlantoaxial motion, thus leading to AARS.

Although the classification by the authors of a 1977 study is most widely used,[22] several authors have proposed newer classification systems in an attempt to select the most appropriate treatment regimen. One group of authors established a classification system in 2005 by plotting C1-C2 motion curves generated from the dynamic CT scans of AARS patients.[23] In a subsequent study, these same authors found that patients in group 1 who had symptoms for more than 3 months' duration were more likely to have recurrent subluxation, undergo more prolonged treatment, and require more aggressive therapies.[24] A retrospective case study in 2012 used three-dimensional CT to classify AARS based on the lateral inclination of the atlas on the axis and the presence of C2 deformity. These authors described three types of AARS depending on the severity of the inclination, the degree of C2 deformity, and the duration of symptoms.[25]

Although, in the past, CT has been the most widely used imaging modality and is integral to several classification systems,[23,25] the value of diagnostic CT may be questioned because of more recent evidence. Because many patients with AARS do not have any intrinsic bony abnormality, and the subluxation noted on imaging is in the normal range, AARS is considered primarily a clinical diagnosis.[23,26] In 2002, researchers noted poor reliability and reproducibility of dynamic CT scanning and recommended against its routine use, especially in the acute setting.[27] Other authors found no important motion abnormalities on dynamic CT scanning and called into question its use in the acute setting.[26] In addition, all previous studies using CT scans for classification and treatment algorithms found that the more minor types of AARS were more likely to occur in patients with acute presentations.[24] These patients were more likely to have fewer observable abnormalities on CT and respond favorably to nonsurgical management. In chronic AARS, however, CT with three-dimensional reconstructions has a high accuracy of diagnosis and provides excellent anatomic detail of the abnormal C1-C2 relationship.

The treatment options for AARS continue to include cervical collars, halter or skeletal traction, halo immobilization, and surgery. Meaningful treatment conclusions, however, remain difficult to make given significant institutional and surgeon variation reported in the current literature.[21] The use of anti-inflammatory drugs and/or muscle relaxants also has shown benefit. The duration of symptoms before diagnosis remains the most important predictor of the type of treatment required.[23,24,28,29] Interestingly a 2017 multicenter effort noted that the time to presentation after injury was greater than 24 hours in 20% of children with AARS.[21] No formal definition exists of when AARS is considered acute, but most studies have reported on differences in the treatment required when AARS is diagnosed within 1 month from the onset of symptoms. Although earlier reports favor surgery for chronic AARS, a 2012 study reported treatment success by nonsurgical means in this setting with remodeling of the C2 facet deformity.[25] In a 2014 study, researchers reported successful outcomes at a mean follow-up of 10.3 months in 73% of the patients with chronic AARS who underwent reduction with traction and halo-thoracic vests.[30] A retrospective study also reported on favorable outcomes in their cohort where 75% of patients presented with chronic AARS. Nonsurgical management resulted in treatment success in 83% of their patients.[31] The duration of treatment, in particular the time in an orthosis, remains variable, with ranges of 1 week to 6 months.[23,26,32] One group of researchers recommended an MRI protocol to determine the length of time in an orthosis. These researchers recommended immobilization in a cervical orthosis until repeat MRI shows resolution of hyperintensity in the transverse and alar ligaments.[32] A C1-C2 fusion is usually required for recurrent cases or those in whom nonsurgical treatment is unsuccessful. Rates of eventual fusion vary for chronic cases from 30% to 100%[23,29] (**Figure 3**). Some authors have highlighted novel methods in obtaining a closed reduction in AARS with use of interventional MRI[33] or by a closed transoral approach.[34] Evidence to support these approaches, however, currently remains limited.

Os Odontoideum

Os odontoideum is the most common anomaly of the dens and is seen as an oval-shaped, well-corticated bony ossicle positioned cephalad to the body of the axis. The cause of os odontoideum remains the subject of debate, but three general etiologies have been proposed: The os odontoideum represents (1) a fracture nonunion of the dens, (2) damage to the epiphyseal plate occurring in the first year of life, or (3) a congenital malformation of the dens itself. The congenital hypothesis has been challenged because the neurocentral synchondrosis is located below the level of the superior articular facet, whereas the gap in os odontoideum is frequently located above the plane of the superior articular facet. The most widely accepted etiology was proposed by a group of authors in 1980; these authors suggested that a fracture of the dens occurs in early childhood, and the alar ligaments attached to the apex gradually distract the fragment away from the base.[35] Subsequent case reports and series on the topic have highlighted the history of remote trauma in most patients, which has made the traumatic theory the most widely accepted theory.

The position of the os odontoideum can be either orthotopic or dystopic and should be carefully distinguished, especially if surgical stabilization is warranted. Orthotopic os odontoideum refers to an ossicle in anatomic position that moves in unison with the anterior arch of C1 and can be reducible to be normally aligned with the dens. In dystopic os odontoideum, it is abnormally positioned near the base of the clivus, where it may fuse with the basion and move functionally as an extension of the clivus, thus increasing the risk of neurologic injury. In orthotopic os odontoideum with instability, a C1-C2 arthrodesis can be considered; however, a dystopic os odontoideum with instability may require an occiput to C2 fusion (**Figure 4**).

In addition to cervical myelopathy, intracranial manifestations of vertebrobasilar ischemia, cerebral infarction, brainstem damage, and vertigo have been reported in patients with unstable os odontoideum.

Surgical intervention is warranted in patients with neurologic involvement, documented instability, or persistent cervical spine or neck symptoms. Patients with other risk factors for instability (eg, Down syndrome and skeletal dysplasias) also should be considered for surgical stabilization.

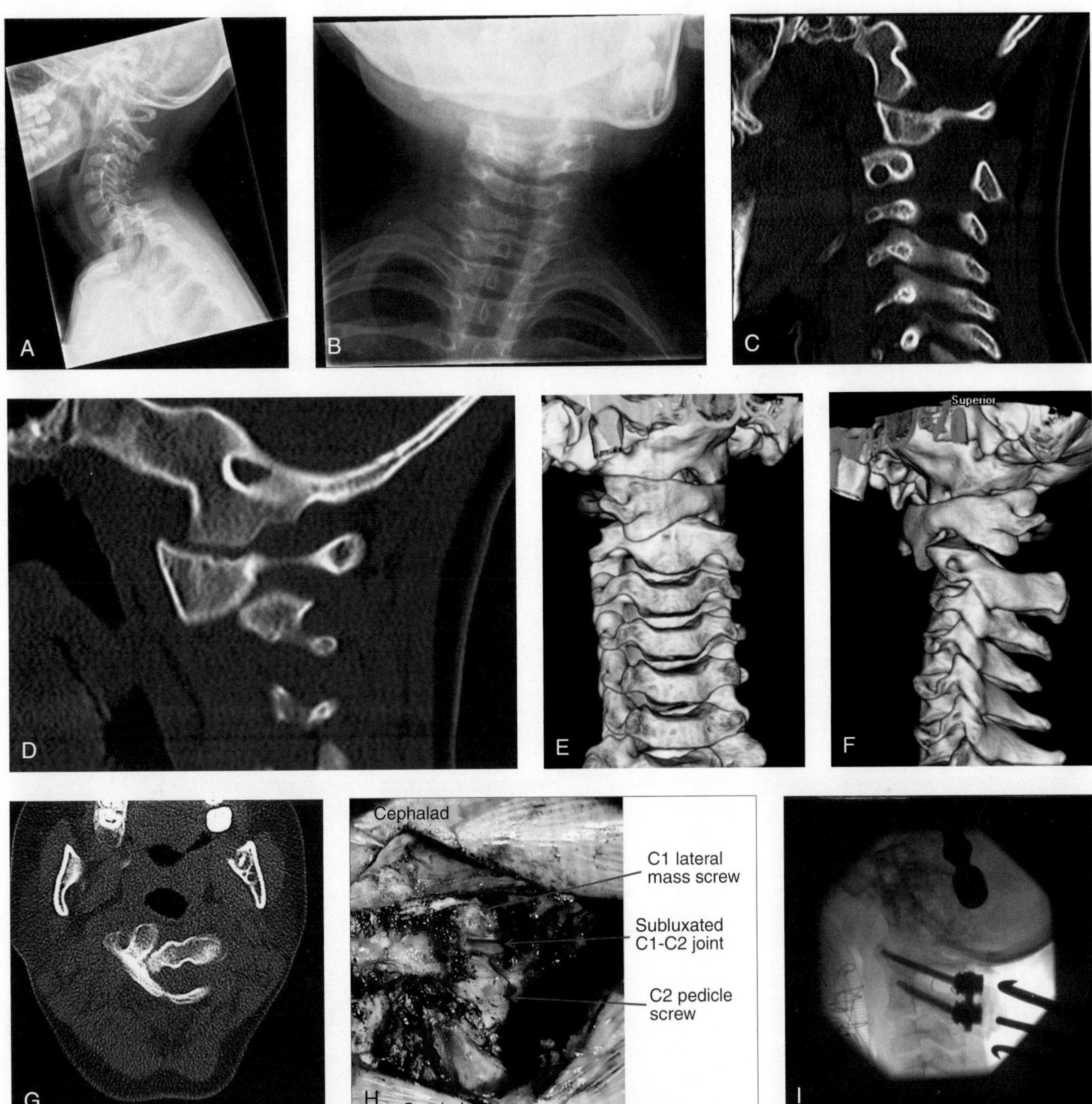

FIGURE 3 Images from a 9-year-old girl 6 months after torticollis secondary to Grisel syndrome. Lateral (**A**) and AP (**B**) radiographs show a decreased posterior atlantodens interval. **C**, Sagittal CT shows subluxated right C1-C2 joint. **D**, Sagittal CT shows subluxated left C1-C2 joint. AP (**E**) and lateral (**F**) three-dimensional CT reconstructions show gross subluxation of C1-C2. **G**, Axial CT shows gross subluxation of the C1-C2 facets. **H**, Intraoperative exposure of the right subluxated C1-C2 joint. **I**, Intraoperative lateral fluoroscopic image shows reduction and posterior segmental instrumented fusion of C1-C2.

The natural history and risks associated with untreated os odontoideum are unclear, so prophylactic arthrodesis remains controversial. With advances in surgical techniques, more recent literature supports a consideration for surgical stabilization for patients with incidental os odontoideum because of the potential for sudden death and substantial morbidity highlighted from earlier reports.[36-38] A 2010 study reported on 10 patients with incidental os odontoideum who sustained an acute cervical spinal cord injury after minor trauma and recommended prophylactic fusion in patients with asymptomatic os odontoideum.[38] The authors of a 2019

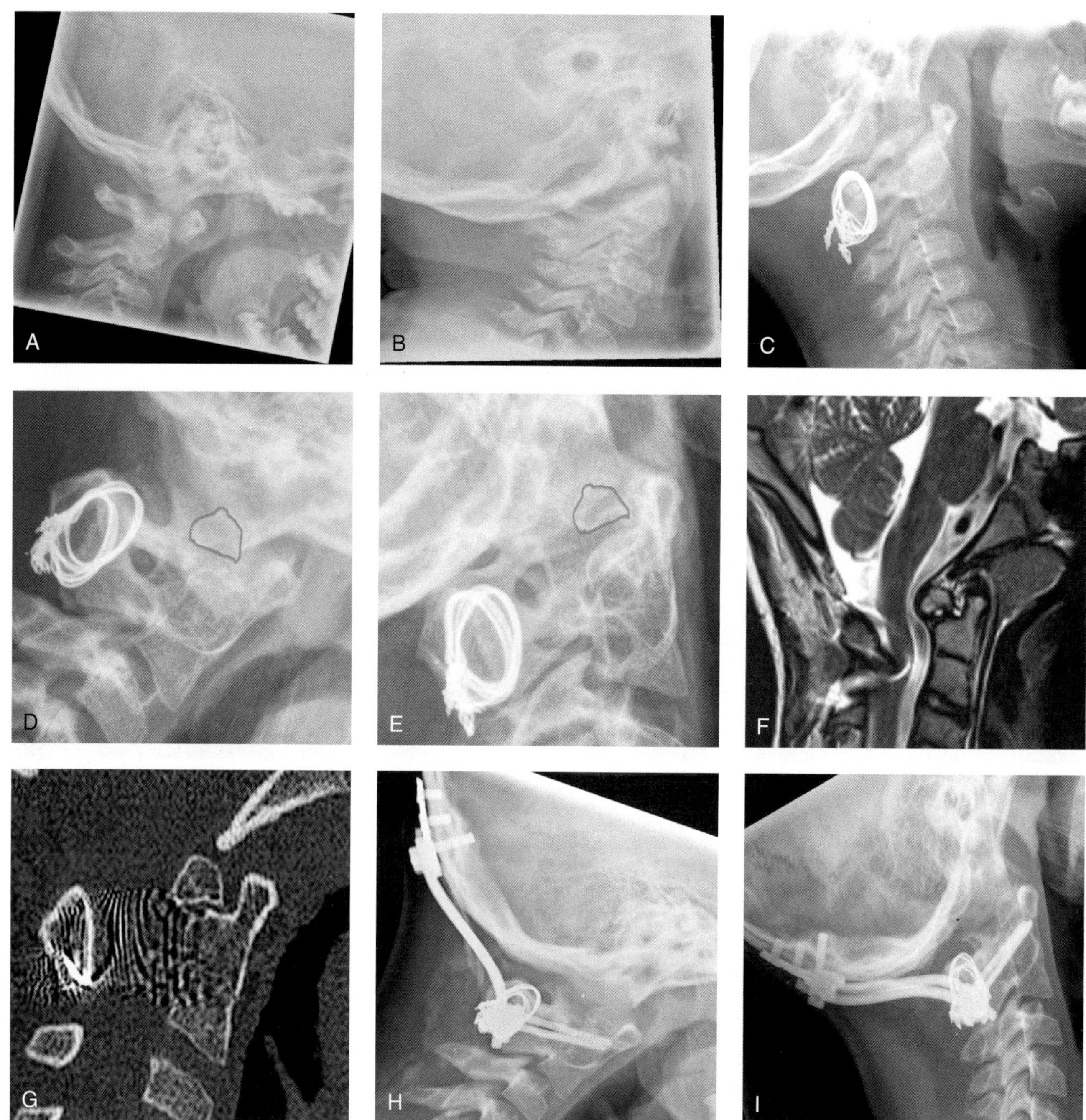

FIGURE 4 Images from an 8-year-old boy with os odontoideum diagnosed after a history of minor trauma. Lateral flexion (**A**) and lateral extension (**B**) cervical spine radiographs show unstable apparent orthotopic os odontoideum. **C**, Lateral cervical spine radiograph after the child was treated with C1-C2 fusion with a sublaminar wiring technique. Lateral flexion (**D**) and lateral extension (**E**) follow-up radiographs reveal os odontoideum behaving as the dystopic type. **F**, Sagittal midline magnetic resonance image shows anterior compression of the spinal cord caused by the dystopic os odontoideum. **G**, Sagittal midline CT image shows posterior displacement of dystopic os odontoideum causing canal compression. Lateral flexion (**H**) and lateral extension (**I**) radiographs after revision fusion to the occiput show the os odontoideum and C1 move as a unit with no further instability.

study, however, reported on 102 patients treated at 11 different centers over a 16-year period and highlighted good outcomes of nonsurgical management in 31 patients who had normal neurologic function and a stable atlantoaxial joint. Close surveillance of these patients was recommended as opposed to prophylactic fusion.[39] Although earlier studies advocate internal fixation using sublaminar wires, some authors caution against the use of posterior wiring techniques because the os odontoideum can be pulled back into the spinal canal.

Skeletal Dysplasias

Achondroplasia

Craniocervical manifestations in achondroplasia include foramen magnum stenosis and multisegmental spinal stenosis of the subaxial spine. Foramen magnum stenosis usually occurs within the first 2 years of life and is the direct result of defective enchondral bone growth and premature fusion of the two posterior basal synchondroses. The most common symptoms of this condition are excessive snoring and apnea; however, other signs and symptoms of chronic brainstem compression can manifest. These include lower cranial nerve dysfunction, hyperreflexia, hypotonia, weakness or paresis, clonus, swallowing difficulties, and developmental delay. Because foramen magnum stenosis can result in death, identification of the condition is critical. Polysomnography with or without other imaging studies may be used in making a diagnosis. Some authors recommend a screening MRI in all infants with achondroplasia to evaluate for foramen magnum stenosis.[40]

Decompression of the foramen magnum generally is required in patients who are symptomatic within the first 2 years of life; however, symptoms may develop in older children and require treatment at that time. A 2006 study reported on the outcomes after cervicomedullary decompression and noted that although improvement of respiratory symptoms occurred soon after surgery, several complications also were encountered. Cerebrospinal fluid leaks, recurrent stenosis requiring revision surgery, and infection were the reported complications in 16 of 43 patients.[41]

Cervical stenosis results from several factors. Endochondral ossification defects shorten vertebral bodies and pedicles. The pedicles are thickened with a decrease in the interpedicular distance. The soft-tissue elements also are affected with hyperplasia of the intervertebral disks and the ligamentum flavum. Previous reports have noted a 40% reduction in sagittal and coronal diameters because of these abnormalities. Stenosis typically becomes symptomatic in the third and fourth decades of life but also can be seen in skeletally immature patients. The incidence of symptomatic stenosis is reported to be 10% in 10-year-old children.[42] Cervical stenosis can occur in skeletally immature individuals, whereas lumbar spinal stenosis is more commonly problematic in adults. Multilevel laminectomy can be considered in symptomatic patients, but in skeletally immature patients, a concurrent fusion should be performed to avoid postlaminectomy kyphosis.

Morquio Syndrome

In Morquio syndrome, the degradation of keratan sulfate and chondroitin sulfate is defective. The upper cervical manifestations of this autosomal recessive disease virtually always include atlantoaxial instability from odontoid hypoplasia as well as the deposition of glycosaminoglycans posterior to the dens. The resultant cord compression causes substantial, progressive myelopathy in these patients. Timing of surgical intervention remains controversial. Prophylactic occipitocervical fusion has been advocated by some authors.[43,44] A recent long-term follow-up study (mean 7 years) reported on outcomes of 26 surgical patients with Morquio syndrome. The authors found that patients who were asymptomatic preoperatively remained clinically stable following cervical spine surgery. Those with preoperative myelopathy, however, did not improve and surgery failed to halt neurologic progression. Hence, surgical intervention before the development of neurologic symptoms has been recommended by the authors.[45] Similarly, the authors of a 2018 study recommend a close clinical and radiologic surveillance in this patient population for timely intervention, as in their series of 18 patients, neurologic improvement following surgery was limited when there was preexisting neurologic compromise. Because of the risk of acute neurologic deterioration, the authors support early surgery.[46] The anterior pannus at C1 typically resolves after posterior fusion, so anterior decompressive surgery usually is not warranted. Researchers in 2009 recommended that these patients should avoid contact sports and gymnastics and require cervical spine imaging before undergoing general anesthesia.[43]

Spondyloepiphyseal Dysplasia Congenita

Patients with spondyloepiphyseal dysplasia congenita (SEDC) are characterized by short-trunk disproportionate dwarfism. Atlantoaxial instability resulting from hypoplasia of the dens and/or lax ligaments can lead to myelopathy in up to 35% of patients. The sagittal atlas diameter also is reduced in most patients with SEDC, further compromising the spinal canal at C1. In a 2004 series, myelopathy developed in patients whose space available for the cord was less than 12 mm.[47] The authors also observed that a severe form of SEDC—with extreme short stature and coxa vara—was a risk factor for myelopathy. In their series, all patients with myelopathy were less than seven standard deviations below the mean. Spinal canal stenosis may not simply be addressed by reducing and stabilizing the atlantoaxial instability, and a concomitant C1 laminectomy may be required. The AADI in these patients increases with increasing age, so patients with SEDC should be followed into adulthood with regular cervical spine imaging.[48] The largest pediatric series of outcomes following cervical fusion in SEDC was reported by the authors of a 2017 study. They found 100% fusion rates and stable neurologic outcomes with instrumentation and iliac crest bone graft. The authors cautioned against noninstrumented in situ fusion because this was associated with a 60% pseudarthrosis rate requiring revision surgery.[49]

Syndrome-Related Abnormalities

Down Syndrome

Craniocervical instability has been reported in 8% to 63% of patients with Down syndrome, and atlantoaxial instability has been reported in 10% to 30% of these patients. Estimates of symptomatic disease, however, range from 1% to 2%. In addition to ligamentous laxity, patients with Down syndrome have a notably greater number of osseous anomalies of the upper cervical spine than do age-matched and sex-matched normal, healthy control subjects. Os odontoideum, persistent dentocentral synchondrosis of C2, spina bifida of C1, ossiculum terminale, and partial atlanto-occipital assimilation are the most frequently noted abnormalities. Patients with Down syndrome who have upper cervical instability are more likely to have bony anomalies than those without instability. Although no standard has been defined, occipitocervical subluxation of 7 to 10 mm is considered pathologic, and fusion is recommended. In 1996, some researchers noted difficulty with measuring occiput-C1 instability on plain radiographs and recommended confirmation with MRI;[50] other authors have suggested fusion for atlantoaxial instability in patients with an AADI greater than 10 mm or any symptomatic patients with cord changes on MRI.[51] Because of reported low interobserver and intraobserver reliability of the AADI, the authors of a 2014 study introduced the C1/C4 SAC ratio and the C1 inclination angle as a new radiologic parameter in assessing instability in patients with Down syndrome in an earlier study.[52] The authors have since demonstrated in a cohort of 272 children with Down syndrome normal values and those associated with a high risk of the development of neurologic symptoms. They found normal values of C1/C4 SAC ratio to be 1.2° and C1 inclination to be 15°. A C1/C4 SAC ratio of <0.8 was associated with the development of neurologic symptoms.[53] Most studies indicate that ligamentous instability at the occipitocervical or atlantoaxial joint is unlikely to progress to clinically relevant subluxation; however, those children with bony anomalies are at higher risk of progression and should be followed up closely.[54]

In 1983, the Special Olympics established radiographic screening guidelines,[55] which were endorsed in 1984 by the Committee on Sports Medicine of the American Academy of Pediatrics (AAP).[56] In 1995, the committee published a position paper questioning the value of lateral plain radiographs as a screening test in detecting patients with Down syndrome at risk for spinal cord injury and asserted that asymptomatic instability was not proven to be a risk factor for symptomatic instability.[57] Considerable debate exists regarding screening radiographs in the population with Down syndrome, and no consensus exists regarding the effectiveness of radiographs in preventing neurologic injury caused by upper cervical instability (**Figure 5**). The AAP published recommendations in 2001 and again in 2007 to screen all ambulatory children between the ages of 3 and 5 years, not just those participating in Special Olympics, using dynamic lateral cervical spine plain radiographs.[58,59] The need for subsequent serial radiographs in patients without instability on these index radiographs has not been agreed on, and it is important to note that instability may develop later in childhood in patients with Down syndrome despite normal screening radiographs at an early age (**Figure 5**). Therefore, more recently, the AAP changed its earlier 2001 and 2007 recommendations and now does not recommend routine radiologic evaluation of the cervical spine in asymptomatic patients. Pediatricians are advised by the AAP to rely on a careful history and physical examination to identify myelopathic signs and symptoms and to discuss with parents the importance of universal precautions for protection of the cervical spine during anesthetic, surgical, or radiographic procedures. Participation in certain sports, including football, soccer, and gymnastics, as well as trampoline use, is discouraged by the AAP because of the increased risk of spinal cord injury.[60]

Klippel-Feil Syndrome

Klippel-Feil syndrome occurs in a heterogeneous group of patients, all of whom have two or more fused cervical vertebrae. The classic triad of a low posterior hairline, short neck, and decreased range of motion of the cervical spine occurs in fewer than 50% of patients. Associated cervical conditions include occipitocervical synostosis, basilar impression, and odontoid anomalies. Noncervical-associated conditions include congenital scoliosis, Sprengel deformity, synkinesia, genitourinary abnormalities, sensorineural hearing loss, and cardiac disease. The authors of a 2018 study reported that the prevalence of Klippel-Feil syndrome was 0.58%, with most noted incidentally on imaging.[61] A 2011 study reported that the prevalence of cervical scoliosis in patients with Klippel-Feil syndrome was 53.3%, with the presence of congenitally fused patterns and associated vertebral malformations indicating the greatest risk for the development of cervical scoliosis.[62] Interestingly, cervical scoliosis was not associated with cervical spine-related symptoms in this series.

Three common patterns of cervical instability have been described: C2-C3 fusion with occipitocervical synostosis; extensive fusion over several cervical levels with abnormal occipitocervical junction; and two fused segments separated by an open joint space. Abnormal biomechanics may cause neurologic symptoms in the second or third decades of life resulting from either stenosis or arthritic changes of the unfused segments.[63,64] Surgical intervention is warranted in patients with progressive neurologic compromise.

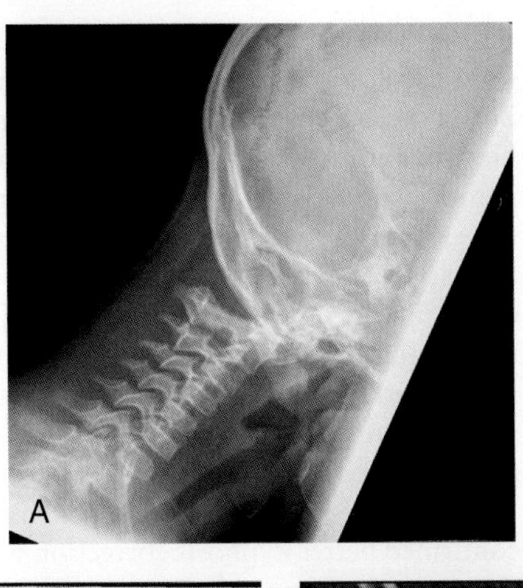

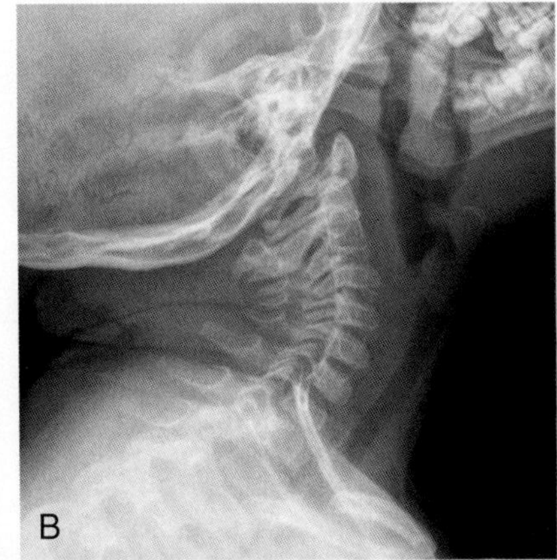

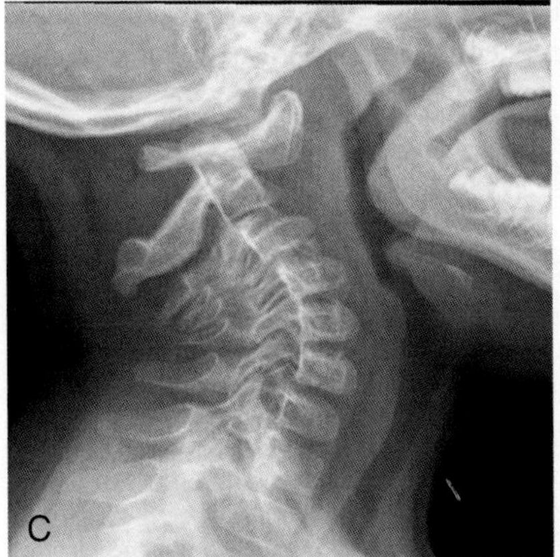

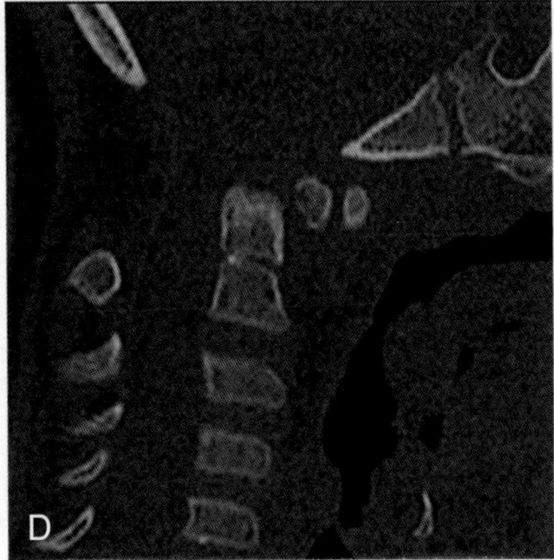

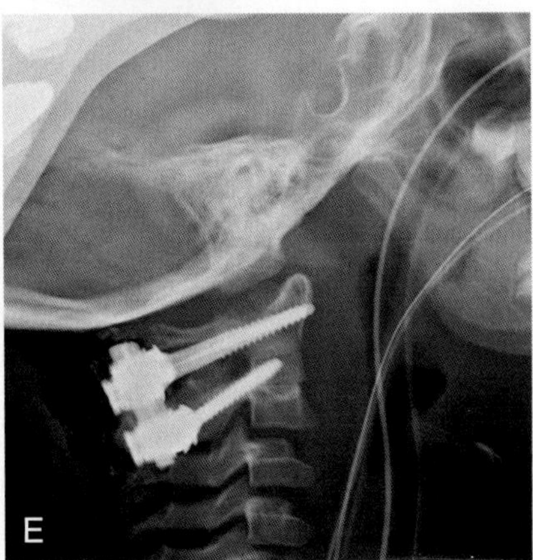

FIGURE 5 Images from a 9-year-old girl with Down syndrome. Screening lateral flexion (**A**) and extension (**B**) radiographs at age 5 years document no dynamic instability. **C**, Lateral radiograph obtained at age 9 years after the patient reported acute neck pain after going down a slide and dismounting uneventfully shows gross C1-C2 subluxation. **D**, Sagittal midline CT shows os odontoideum. **E**, Lateral radiograph after urgent C1-C2 reduction and arthrodesis.

Although patients may have a decreased range of motion of the cervical spine, most patients with stable fusion patterns are usually asymptomatic. Those in whom instability develops may have central or peripheral neurologic sequelae. Pathologic changes within the spinal cord, instability and hypermobility at the motion segment adjacent to the fused vertebrae, and basilar invagination are reported mechanisms of neurologic sequelae in this population. The authors of a 2017 study reported a relative risk of the development of degenerative cervical myelopathy in this patient population to be 3.3.[65] A recent analysis of a global Klippel-Feil syndrome patient-reported registry found brain fog and fatigue to be common complaints. In addition, nearly half of the patients reported problems with balance and 20% reported urinary incontinence. Most patients in this clinical study (>90%) had sought treatment, with 56% reporting having undergone an invasive procedure.[64] Interestingly, some researchers assessed atlantoaxial segmental motion in patients with Klippel-Feil syndrome and noted an increased AADI on flexion-extension radiographs, most notably in patients with occipitalization and a fused C2-C3 segment; however, this hypermobility was not associated with symptoms or neurologic signs.[63] Early recommendations of prophylactic stabilization of patients with Klippel-Feil syndrome with hypermobility have therefore been challenged, and more recent studies do not advocate this approach.[63,66]

SUBAXIAL ABNORMALITIES

Cervical Kyphosis

Larsen Syndrome

Larsen syndrome is rare genetic disorder that may have an autosomal dominant or autosomal recessive inheritance. It is a connective tissue disorder caused by mutations of filamin B, whose clinical presentation typically includes multiple joint dislocations, distinct facial anomalies, clubfoot, heart defects, cleft palate, and neonatal tracheomalacia.

C1-C2 instability, lysis of the C2 pedicles, and substantial progressive cervical kyphosis are the cervical manifestations of Larsen syndrome. The risk of cord compression leading to paralysis and death because of progressive cervical kyphosis and instability warrants close surveillance of these patients, with at least serial plain radiography supplemented with CT and MRI when required. Surgical intervention depends on the age of the patient, the severity of the kyphosis, and the severity of the syndrome. In very young children, anterior arthrodesis alone is not recommended because of its high risk for spinal cord injury and anterior growth arrest, thus eliminating the potential for kyphotic correction.[48] Posterior fusion alone in mild, flexible cases has been shown to produce good results. In patients with severe, rigid kyphosis with myelopathy, however, anterior decompression with circumferential fusion is warranted.[48,67]

Diastrophic Dysplasia

Diastrophic dysplasia is caused by mutations in the sulfate transporter gene, resulting in the production of abnormal cartilage that leads to many of the clinical manifestations associated with diastrophic dysplasia. Midcervical kyphosis with an apex at C3 or C4 present at birth typically occurs in up to one-third of this patient population. Kyphosis develops from ligamentous laxity and vertebral body wedging and hypoplasia. The natural history of cervical kyphosis in diastrophic dysplasia is favorable, with curves less than 60° typically resolving before the age of 6 years as the child holds up his or her head and strengthens the extensor muscles.[68] If the kyphosis exceeds 60° with an apical vertebra that is round or triangular and displaced posteriorly, then progression is likely.[68] Some authors advocate a Milwaukee brace in this setting to prevent progression; however, it remains unclear how effective nonsurgical treatment is in preventing the progression of kyphosis. Anterior decompression with posterior cervical arthrodesis has been shown to be the most effective method in preventing further progression and correcting the deformity.[48]

Neurofibromatosis

The most common cervical abnormality in patients with neurofibromatosis type 1 is kyphosis; this condition seldom requires surgery. Classic dystrophic changes of vertebral body scalloping, spinal canal widening, enlarged neural foramina, and defective pedicles may be present in cervical deformity. Severe progression of kyphosis and postoperative instability have been reported in 14% to 30% of patients after resection of intraspinal neurofibromas and spinal cord decompression[69,70] (**Figure 6**). Some authors advocate instrumented fusions as part of the decompressive laminectomy for patients with neurofibromatosis type 1 because of the frequency of severe postoperative kyphosis.[71] Hyperkyphosis that involves multiple vertebrae with dystrophic changes has been implicated as a predictor of curve progression.[72,73] In 2011, strong consideration of instrumented fusion has been recommended in the management of patients with neurofibromatosis type 1 who have cervical lesions, multiple levels of involvement, resection of lateral masses or facets, preexisting deformity, and involvement of either the occipitocervical or cervicothoracic junctions.[74] Despite the availability of more rigid modern instrumentation, many authors continue to favor preoperative traction with a combined circumferential fusion to optimize correction of the kyphosis and achieve a solid arthrodesis.[75] The authors of a 2016 retrospective multicenter review confirmed better kyphosis correction with combined anterior-posterior approaches compared with posterior fusion alone with no difference in fusion rates between the two.[76]

Cervical Spondylolysis

Cervical spondylolysis is a rare condition with approximately 100 cases reported in the literature, of which only 25% have been noted in the pediatric population.[77] A diagnosis is made incidentally on routine radiographs or after minor trauma (**Figure 7**). It is characterized by a disruption of the articular mass at the junction of the superior and inferior facet joints, and it has been reported at all levels except C1 but is most commonly reported at C6.[78] Controversy exists regarding the etiology of cervical spondylolysis, with some authors favoring a congenital cause and others reporting a traumatic etiology. Supporters for the traumatic theory base their argument on the fact that no cervical spondylolysis has been observed during autopsies of newborns, which implies that the disorder appears after birth. Repetitive trauma resulting in a stress fracture is now commonly accepted.[78] Rare reports of cord injury in cases of cervical spondylolysis have been noted. A 1999 study characterized cord compression in the presence of cervical spondylolysis.[79] Surgical management can be considered for pain, neurologic injury, instability on dynamic radiographs, or the presence of known risk factors for cervical spinal cord injury.[79] Optimal nonsurgical management in the absence of symptoms has yet to be fully defined.[77]

TRAUMA

Craniocervical and Upper Cervical Trauma

It is estimated that 1% of all pediatric injuries involve the cervical spine, with a male-to-female ratio of approximately 2:1.[80-83] The most common mechanism remains blunt trauma, with a fall from a height being the most common cause in patients younger than 8 years. Increased intrinsic elasticity with a large head-to-torso ratio results in a preponderance of upper cervical spine injuries in patients younger than 8 years.

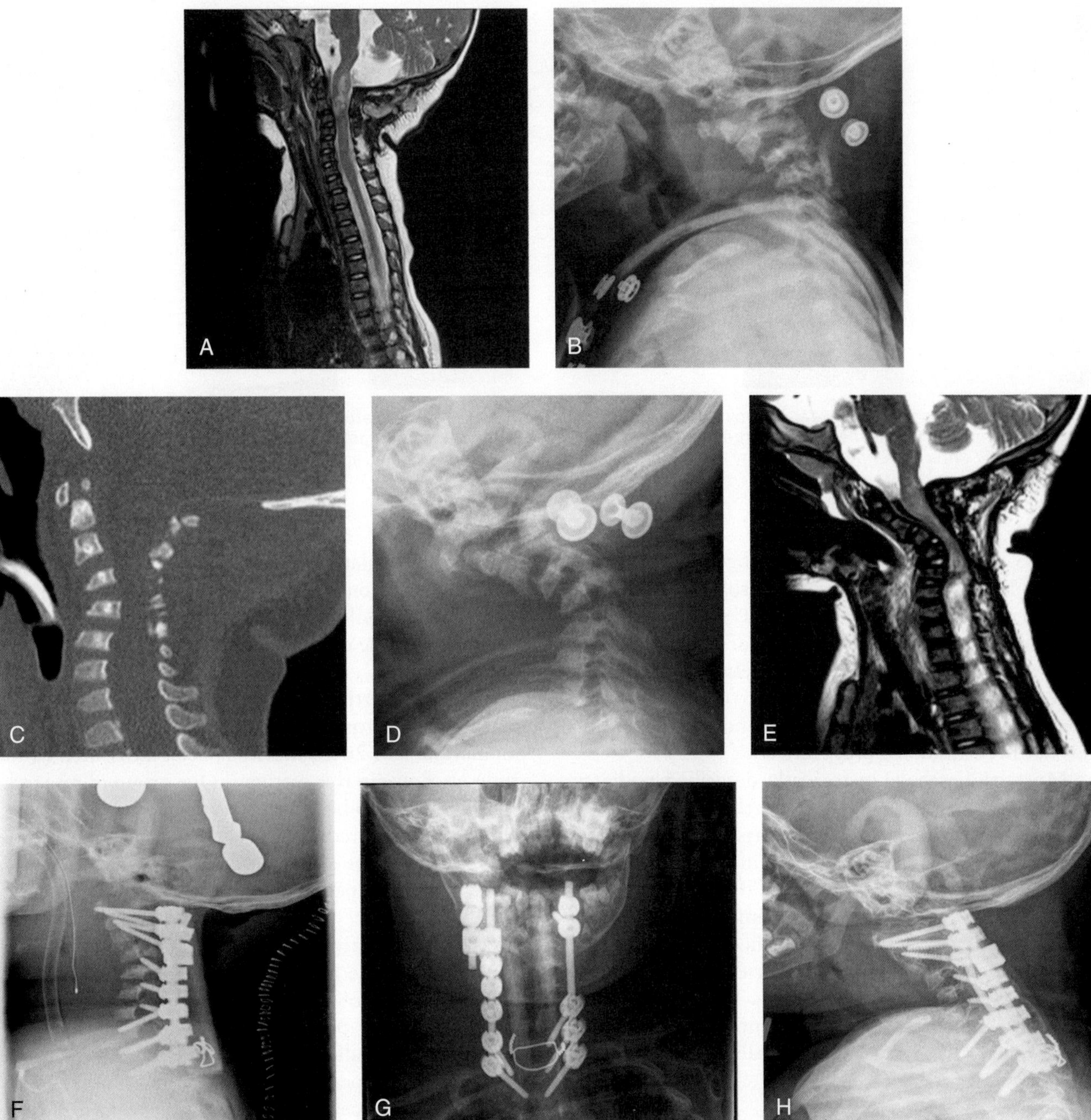

FIGURE 6 Images from a patient with neurofibromatosis type 1 at 3 months of age who underwent a C3-C5 laminectomy for debulking of an intraspinal tumor. Magnetic resonance image (**A**), lateral radiograph (**B**), and CT scan (**C**) at 10 months show postlaminectomy cervical kyphosis. Lateral cervical radiograph (**D**) and sagittal magnetic resonance image (**E**) show the rapid progression of cervical kyphosis despite attempts at bracing treatment with neurologic sequelae. **F**, Postoperative lateral cervical radiograph of the patient after undergoing C1-C7 posterior segmental instrumented fusion with tibial onlay allograft but no anterior procedure. AP (**G**) and lateral (**H**) radiographs show fusion with no recurrence of kyphosis at 4 years postoperatively.

Studies related to clinical decision making with regard to spinal imaging in pediatric cervical spine injuries are inconclusive. In adults, the National Emergency X-Radiography Utilization Study (NEXUS) criteria are well established. A 2001 study prospectively validated the NEXUS decision instrument in 3,065 pediatric patients and found a sensitivity of 100%, but the specificity was only 20%.[84] A major limitation of the NEXUS study was that only 2.8% of the included patients were younger than 2 years, which is the most crucial age group for the risk of ligamentous injury of the upper cervical spine. In 2008, two authors found a remarkably low sensitivity for the

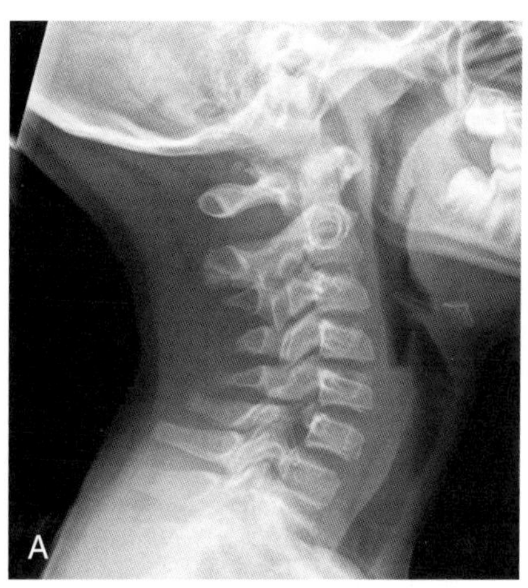

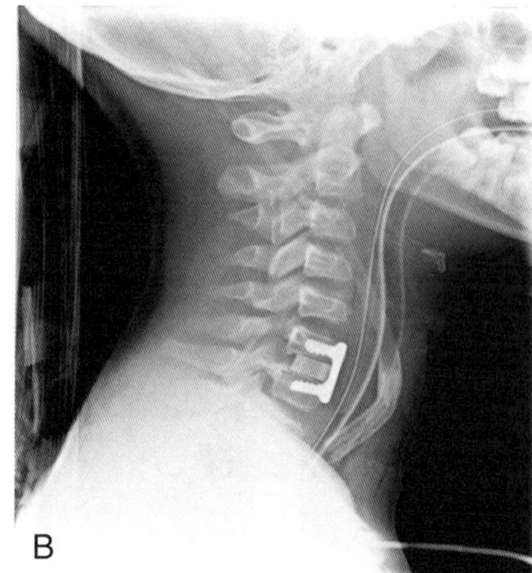

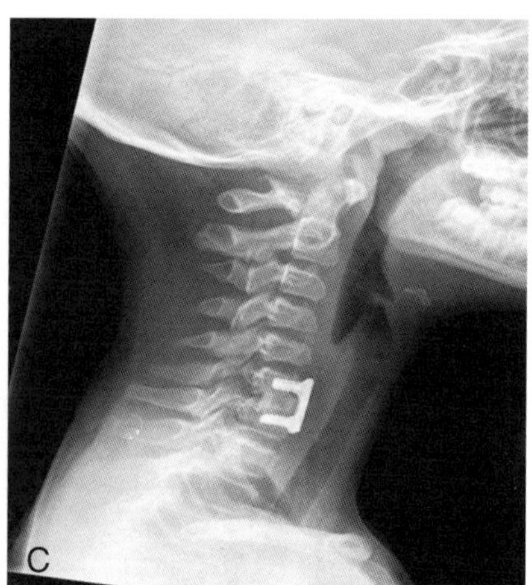

FIGURE 7 Images from an 8-year-old boy with a C6 pars defect and anterolisthesis after a minor fall. **A**, Lateral cervical spine radiograph shows C6 pars defect with anterolisthesis (C6 on C7). **B**, Immediate postoperative lateral cervical spine radiograph shows C6-C7 anterior cervical diskectomy and fusion. **C**, Lateral cervical spine radiograph at the 6-month follow-up shows graft incorporation.

NEXUS criteria among children younger than 9 years.[85] This finding led the Congress of Neurologic Surgeons to recommend application of the NEXUS decision instrument only in children older than 9 years.[86] The Pediatric Emergency Care Applied Research Network conducted a large, multicenter case-control study to define the clinical clearance criteria specific to children; however, this study has not been validated prospectively.[87]

Most studies have historically described pediatric spine trauma in patients younger than 8 years compared with patients older than 8 years. In 2014, a group of researchers assessed differences in the epidemiology and characteristics of spine trauma in patients younger than 4 years with those between 4 and 9 years of age.[82] Important differences were identified. Upper cervical spine injuries and ligamentous injuries were more common in patients younger than 4 years. The younger group also had a higher rate of nonaccidental trauma causing spinal injury (19%) and a substantially higher mortality rate (25%).

Subaxial Cervical Trauma

Injuries of the subaxial cervical spine mainly occur after high-energy trauma in older children and adolescents in whom the cervical spine has matured. After 8 years of age, the biomechanical properties of the cervical spine are more like those of adults, with injury patterns also similar to those in adults. The most common location of injury is between C5 and C7. The series reported in 2015 had similar findings with respect to mechanism of injury, mean age, level of injury, and associated injuries as earlier reports.[88] Because this injury occurs predominantly in older children, some advocate the NEXUS criteria for decision making.[89] It has been suggested that more than 7° of kyphotic angulation between adjacent vertebral bodies implies ligamentous instability. Translation of more than 3.5 mm also should raise suspicion of injury.[90]

Because of the diagnostic limitations of plain radiographs, CT has emerged as the imaging modality of choice in the setting of acute trauma. However, with increasing concerns of radiation exposure in the pediatric population,[19] in 2013, MRI has been advocated as the study of choice in this setting.[91] One group of researchers found MRI to be 100% sensitive and 97% specific, with a negative predictive value of 75% and a positive predictive value of 100%, in detecting osseous injuries in the setting of pediatric cervical trauma.[91] Another group of researchers used clinical decision analysis to determine the optimal cervical spine evaluation strategy, balancing the risk of missed cervical spine injury with the risk of radiation-induced malignancy. Using literature-derived probabilities and clinical clearance, screening plain radiographs were preferred over CT for the evaluation of pediatric patients with blunt trauma.[83]

Despite advances in modern instrumentation techniques for pediatric cervical spine injuries, most injuries can be managed with external immobilization. When surgery is warranted, consideration must be given to the small size and growth potential of the pediatric spine.

Athletic Injuries

Athletic activities are one of the leading causes of cervical spine injuries in the pediatric population, accounting for the second most common cause of spinal cord injury in people younger than 30 years.[92] In children aged 10 to 14 years, sports participation is the most common cause of cervical spine injuries.[93,94] Football and ice hockey account for most of these injuries, followed by rugby, wrestling, diving, skiing, snowboarding, cheerleading, and equestrian sports (**Figure 8**). The mechanism of injury can be sport related, but it is more commonly independent of the sport. Although the mechanics of a cervical spine injury in athletes have been extensively studied, the true mechanism of injury remains controversial. Injury patterns include cervical sprain or strain, stingers and burners, cord neurapraxia and transient quadriplegia, discoligamentous injury, and fractures with and without dislocation.

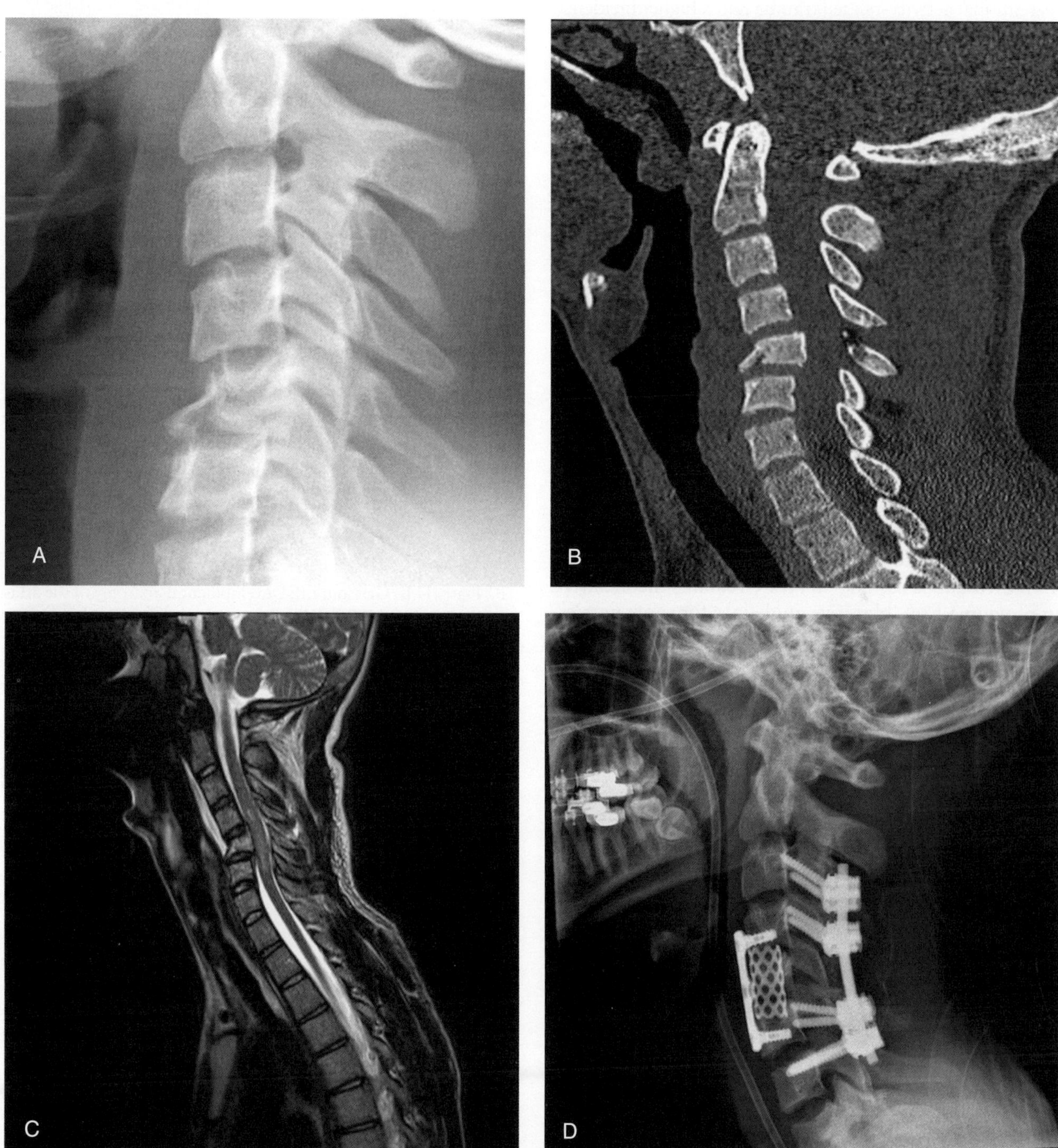

FIGURE 8 Images from a 14-year-old boy with a cervical unstable flexion-teardrop variant injury sustained after a snowboarding accident. Preoperative lateral radiograph (**A**) and CT scan (**B**) show the extent of the bony spinal column injury. **C**, Sagittal magnetic resonance image shows the spinal cord injury with cord edema and signal change. **D**, Lateral cervical spine radiograph after circumferential fusion.

The authors of a 2018 study attempted to highlight potential risk factors associated with cervical spine injuries in children due to sports and recreational activities by analyzing a multicenter retrospective case-control study through the Pediatric Emergency Care Applied Research Network. They found that children with sports-related and recreational activity-related trauma had a higher incidence of subaxial injuries and an increased odds of spinal cord injury without radiographic abnormality compared with cervical injuries from other mechanisms. Focal neurologic findings, neck pain, diving, or axial loading mechanism all increased the odds of a cervical spine injury in the setting of sports-related blunt trauma.[94]

The decision to allow an athlete to return to play after injury is complex and must be considered on an individual basis. Most published data offer expert opinion with limited objective data. In 1986, a point grading system was proposed to quantify a patient's clinical situation and offer an objective guideline for return to play.[95] In 2001, researchers attempted a questionnaire survey study to evaluate what factors, such as published guidelines, the type of sport of the patient, the physician's number of years in practice and subspecialty interests, and sport participation of the respondent, played a role in the return to play decision-making process.[96] The authors found that opinions vary regarding the decision to allow an athlete to return to play after a cervical spine injury. Most authors recommend that the decision be made on an individual basis. The literature remains inconclusive in providing firm, objective guidelines for sport participation after a cervical spine injury.

SUMMARY

Morphologic studies have advanced the understanding of the growth and development of the upper cervical spine in the pediatric population, highlighting important variability in ossification patterns and the timing of synchondrosis fusion. Although CT has been the imaging modality of choice to quantify osseous anomalies, recent concerns of radiation-induced malignancy are making MRI a more favorable choice. Screening radiographs in patients at high risk continue to be controversial because the association between instability and neurologic sequelae remains poorly understood. Historically, pediatric cervical trauma had a clear delineation between those younger than 8 years and those older than 8 years; more recent literature further characterizes important differences in patients younger than 4 years and those older than 4 years. Modern surgical stabilization techniques may provide outcomes that are more favorable in patients at high risk, with recent literature favoring surgical intervention, even in incidental findings of osseoligamentous instability in the pediatric cervical spine.

KEY STUDY POINTS

- The C1 posterior synchondrosis closure generally occurs by the age of 3 years, whereas the anterior C1 synchondrosis closure generally occurs at an older age.
- The duration of symptoms before the diagnosis of AARS is the most important predictor of the type of treatment required.
- The distinction between orthotopic and dystopic os odontoideum is critical in planning surgical stabilization.
- The AAP no longer recommends routine radiologic examinations in asymptomatic patients with Down syndrome to screen for upper cervical instability.
- The literature remains inconclusive in providing firm, objective guidelines for sport participation after a cervical spine injury.

ANNOTATED REFERENCES

1. Plaut HF: Fracture of the atlas or developmental abnormality. *Radiology* 1937;29(2):227-231.
2. Ogden JA: Radiology of postnatal skeletal development: XI. The first cervical vertebra. *Skeletal Radiol* 1984;12(1):12-20.
3. Piatt JH Jr, Grissom LE: Developmental anatomy of the atlas and axis in childhood by computed tomography. *J Neurosurg Pediatr* 2011;8(3):235-243.
4. Rao RD, Tang S, Lim C, Yoganandan N: Developmental morphology and ossification patterns of the C1 vertebra. *J Bone Joint Surg Am* 2013;95(17):e1241-e1247.
5. Junewick JJ, Chin MS, Meesa IR, Ghori S, Boynton SJ, Luttenton CR: Ossification patterns of the atlas vertebra. *AJR Am J Roentgenol* 2011;197(5):1229-1234.
6. Ghanem I, El Hage S, Rachkidi R, Kharrat K, Dagher F, Kreichati G: Pediatric cervical spine instability. *J Child Orthop* 2008;2(2):71-84.
7. Buhs C, Cullen M, Klein M, Farmer D: The pediatric trauma C-spine: Is the "odontoid" view necessary? *J Pediatr Surg* 2000;35(6):994-997.
8. Smoker WR: Craniovertebral junction: Normal anatomy, craniometry, and congenital anomalies. *Radiographics* 1994;14(2):255-277.
9. Harris JH Jr, Carson GC, Wagner LK, Kerr N: Radiologic diagnosis of traumatic occipitovertebral dissociation: 2. Comparison of three methods of detecting occipitovertebral relationships on lateral radiographs of supine subjects. *AJR Am J Roentgenol* 1994;162(4):887-892.
10. Dziurzynski K, Anderson PA, Bean DB, et al: A blinded assessment of radiographic criteria for atlanto-occipital dislocation. *Spine (Phila Pa 1976)* 2005;30(12):1427-1432.

11. Cattell HS, Filtzer DL: Pseudosubluxation and other normal variations in the cervical spine in children: A study of one hundred and sixty children. *J Bone Joint Surg Am* 1965;47(7):1295-1309.
12. Wang JC, Nuccion SL, Feighan JE, Cohen B, Dorey FJ, Scoles PV: Growth and development of the pediatric cervical spine documented radiographically. *J Bone Joint Surg Am* 2001;83(8):1212-1218.
13. Wills BP, Dormans JP: Nontraumatic upper cervical spine instability in children. *J Am Acad Orthop Surg* 2006;14(4):233-245.
14. Hinck VC, Hopkins CE, Savara BS: The size of the atlantal spinal canal: A sex difference. *Hum Biol* 1962;34:197-205.
15. Johnson KT, Al-Holou WN, Anderson RC, et al: Morphometric analysis of the developing pediatric cervical spine. *J Neurosurg Pediatr* 2016;18(3):377-389.

    CT scans of 1,458 children were analyzed, and the authors discuss the differences in growth of the cervical spine both in terms of location (subaxial versus craniocervical), sex, and age. This descriptive study also provides insight into the spinal canal diameter growth with age. Level of evidence: IV.
16. Boltshauser E, Hoare RD: Radiographic measurements of the normal spinal cord in childhood. *Neuroradiology* 1976;10(5):235-237.
17. Inoue H, Ohmori K, Takatsu T, Teramoto T, Ishida Y, Suzuki K: Morphological analysis of the cervical spinal canal, dural tube and spinal cord in normal individuals using CT myelography. *Neuroradiology* 1996;38(2):148-151.
18. Matsuura P, Waters RL, Adkins RH, Rothman S, Gurbani N, Sie I: Comparison of computerized tomography parameters of the cervical spine in normal control subjects and spinal cord-injured patients. *J Bone Joint Surg Am* 1989;71(2):183-188.
19. Miglioretti DL, Johnson E, Williams A, et al: The use of computed tomography in pediatrics and the associated radiation exposure and estimated cancer risk. *JAMA Pediatr* 2013;167(8):700-707.
20. Neal KM, Mohamed AS: Atlantoaxial rotatory subluxation in children. *J Am Acad Orthop Surg* 2015;23(6):382-392.
21. Powell EC, Leonard JR, Olsen CD, et al: Atlantoaxial rotatory subluxation in children. *Pediatr Emerg Care* 2017;33(2):86-91.

    This case-control study identified differences between AARS and other cervical spine injuries, noting that AARS often presents later with pain and torticollis and falls being the most common injury mechanism. The study also highlights variations in treatment across the 17 different hospitals where cases were identified. Level of evidence: III.
22. Fielding JW, Hawkins RJ: Atlanto-axial rotatory fixation. (Fixed rotatory subluxation of the atlanto-axial joint). *J Bone Joint Surg Am* 1977;59(1):37-44.
23. Pang D, Li V: Atlantoaxial rotatory fixation: Part 2. New diagnostic paradigm and a new classification based on motion analysis using computed tomographic imaging. *Neurosurgery* 2005;57(5):941-953.
24. Pang D, Li V: Atlantoaxial rotatory fixation: Part 3. A prospective study of the clinical manifestation, diagnosis, management, and outcome of children with atlantoaxial rotatory fixation. *Neurosurgery* 2005;57(5):954-972.
25. Ishii K, Toyama Y, Nakamura M, Chiba K, Matsumoto M: Management of chronic atlantoaxial rotatory fixation. *Spine (Phila Pa 1976)* 2012;37(5):E278-E285.
26. Hicazi A, Acaroglu E, Alanay A, Yazici M, Surat A: Atlantoaxial rotatory fixation–subluxation revisited: A computed tomographic analysis of acute torticollis in pediatric patients. *Spine (Phila Pa 1976)* 2002;27(24):2771-2775.
27. Alanay A, Hicazi A, Acaroglu E, et al: Reliability and necessity of dynamic computerized tomography in diagnosis of atlantoaxial rotatory subluxation. *J Pediatr Orthop* 2002;22(6):763-765.
28. Tauchi R, Imagama S, Ito Z, et al: Surgical treatment for chronic atlantoaxial rotatory fixation in children. *J Pediatr Orthop B* 2013;22(5):404-408.
29. Beier AD, Vachhrajani S, Bayerl SH, Aguilar CY, Lamberti-Pasculli M, Drake JM: Rotatory subluxation: Experience from the hospital for sick children. *J Neurosurg Pediatr* 2012;9(2):144-148.
30. Glotzbecker MP, Wasser AM, Hresko MT, Karlin LI, Emans JB, Hedequist DJ: Efficacy of nonfusion treatment for subacute and chronic atlanto-axial rotatory fixation in children. *J Pediatr Orthop* 2014;34(5):490-495.
31. Mifdud M, Abela M, Wilson NIL: The delayed presentation of atlantoaxial rotatory fixation in children: A review of the management. *Bone Joint J* 2016;98(5):715-720.

    The authors present a retrospective review of cases treated at their two institutions between 1988 and 2014 and found most of their cases (10 of 12) responsive to nonsurgical management and only two cases requiring fusion. Level of evidence: IV.
32. Landi A, Pietrantonio A, Marotta N, Mancarella C, Delfini R: Atlantoaxial rotatory dislocation (AARD) in pediatric age: MRI study on conservative treatment with Philadelphia collar. Experience of nine consecutive cases. *Eur Spine J* 2012;21(suppl 1):S94-S99.
33. Hannonen J, Perhomaa M, Salokorpi N, et al: Interventional magnetic resonance imaging as a diagnostic and therapeutic method in treating acute pediatric atlantoaxial rotatory subluxation. *Exp Ther Med* 2019;18(1):18-24.

    This is a single case report by authors to present a feasibility concept of utilizing interventional MRI to judge reduction of AARS after manual closed manipulation as opposed to dynamic CT. Level of evidence: V.
34. Jeszenszky D, Fekete T, Kleinstuck F, et al: Transoral closed reduction of fixed atlanto-axial rotatory-subluxation (AARS) in childhood and adolescence. *Clin Spine Surg* 2018;31(5):E252-E256.

    In this study, the authors describe their technique of closed reduction for AARS with no relevant patient outcomes. Level of evidence: V.
35. Fielding JW, Hensinger RN, Hawkins RJ: Os odontoideum. *J Bone Joint Surg Am* 1980;62(3):376-383.

Section 6: Spine

36. Klimo P Jr, Coon V, Brockmeyer D: Incidental os odontoideum: Current management strategies. *Neurosurg Focus* 2011;31(6):E10.

37. Arvin B, Fournier-Gosselin M-P, Fehlings MG: Os odontoideum: Etiology and surgical management. *Neurosurgery* 2010;66(3 suppl):22-31.

38. Zhang Z, Zhou Y, Wang J, et al: Acute traumatic cervical cord injury in patients with os odontoideum. *J Clin Neurosci* 2010;17(10):1289-1293.

39. Helenius IJ, Bauer JM, Verhofste B, et al: Os odontoideum in children: Treatment outcomes and neurological risk factors. *J Bone Joint Surg Am* 2019;101(19):1750-1760.

This study was a retrospective multicenter review that included 102 patients who were treated for os odontoideum. The authors note that the risk of the development of a neurologic deficit was strongly associated with instability and limited SAC and found fusion to resolve neurologic deficits in patients with symptomatic instability. Level of evidence: IV.

40. White KK, Bompadre V, Goldberg MJ, et al: Best practices in the evaluation and treatment of foramen magnum stenosis in achondroplasia during infancy. *Am J Med Genet A* 2016;170(1):42-51.

The authors present a consensus-based best-practice guideline with 22 recommendations for evaluating and treating foramen magnum stenosis in infants with achondroplasia. Level of evidence: V.

41. Bagley CA, Pindrik JA, Bookland MJ, Camara-Quintana JQ, Carson BS: Cervicomedullary decompression for foramen magnum stenosis in achondroplasia. *J Neurosurg* 2006;104(3 suppl):166-172.

42. Hunter AG, Bankier A, Rogers JG, Sillence D, Scott CI Jr: Medical complications of achondroplasia: A multicentre patient review. *J Med Genet* 1998;35(9):705-712.

43. White KK, Steinman S, Mubarak SJ: Cervical stenosis and spastic quadriparesis in Morquio disease (MPS IV): A case report with twenty-six-year follow-up. *J Bone Joint Surg Am* 2009;91(2):438-442.

44. Ransford AO, Crockard HA, Stevens JM, Modaghegh S: Occipito-atlanto-axial fusion in Morquio-Brailsford syndrome: A ten-year experience. *J Bone Joint Surg Br* 1996;78(2):307-313.

45. Broomfield A, Zuberi K, Mercer J, et al: Outcomes from 18 years of cervical spine surgery in MPS IVA: A single centre's experience. *Childs Nerv Syst* 2018;24:1705-1716.

This single-center long-term retrospective review of 26 surgical patients with Morquio syndrome found that delayed surgical treatment after patients developed neurologic deficits did not improve their myelopathic symptoms and so recommend early surgery to prevent neurologic symptoms from developing. Level of evidence: IV.

46. William N, Narducci A, Eastwood D, et al: An evidence-based approach to the management of children with Morquio A syndrome presenting with craniocervical pathology. *Spine* 2018;43(24):E1443-E1453.

This is an 18-patient case series that demonstrated poor neurologic improvement following surgery if neurologic symptoms were present preoperatively. Therefore, the authors support early surgery in patients with mucopolysaccharidosis. Level of evidence: IV.

47. Miyoshi K, Nakamura K, Haga N, Mikami Y: Surgical treatment for atlantoaxial subluxation with myelopathy in spondyloepiphyseal dysplasia congenita. *Spine (Phila Pa 1976)* 2004;29(21):E488-E491.

48. McKay SD, Al-Omari A, Tomlinson LA, Dormans JP: Review of cervical spine anomalies in genetic syndromes. *Spine (Phila Pa 1976)* 2012;37(5):E269-E277.

49. Serhan M, Abousamra O, Rogers K, et al: Upper cervical fusion in children with spondyloepiphyseal dysplasia congenita. *J Pediatr Orthop* 2017;37(7):466-472.

A retrospective analysis of 20 children with SEDC and cervical instability who underwent upper cervical fusion at an early age found a higher rate of pseudarthrosis in patients who had noninstrumented fusions. This series found instrumentation and iliac crest grafting resulted in a 100% fusion rate. Level of evidence: IV.

50. Karol LA, Sheffield EG, Crawford K, Moody MK, Browne RH: Reproducibility in the measurement of atlanto-occipital instability in children with Down syndrome. *Spine (Phila Pa 1976)* 1996;21(21):2463-2467, discussion 2468.

51. Pizzutillo PD, Herman MJ: Cervical spine issues in Down syndrome. *J Pediatr Orthop* 2005;25(2):253-259.

52. Nakamura N, Inaba Y, Oba M, et al: Novel 2 radiological measurements for atlantoaxial instability in children with Down syndrome. *Spine* 2014;39(26):E1566-E1574.

53. Nakamura N, Inaba Y, Aota Y, et al: New radiological parameters for the assessment of atlantoaxial instability in children with Down syndrome. *Bone Joint J* 2016;98-B(12):1704-1710.

The authors compared previously published radiographic parameters of C1/C4 SAC and C1 inclination angle to assess instability in patients with Down syndrome. They compared 272 patients with Down syndrome with 141 control patients and found normal values of C1/C4 SAC ratio to be 1.2° and C1 inclination to be 15°. A C1/C4 SAC ratio of <0.8 was associated with the development of neurologic symptoms. Level of evidence: III

54. Hankinson TC, Anderson RC: Craniovertebral junction abnormalities in Down syndrome. *Neurosurgery* 2010;66(3 suppl):32-38.

55. Participation by individuals with Down syndrome who suffer from the atlantoaxial dislocation condition. *Special Olympics Bulletin*, March 31, 1983.

56. American Academy of Pediatrics, Committee on Sports Medicine: Atlantoaxial instability in Down syndrome. *Pediatrics* 1984;74(1):152-154.

57. American Academy of Pediatrics, Committee on Sports Medicine and Fitness: Atlantoaxial instability in Down syndrome: Subject review. *Pediatrics* 1995;96(1 pt 1):151-154.

58. American Academy of Pediatrics, Committee on Genetics: Health supervision for children with Down syndrome. *Pediatrics* 2001;107(2):442-449.

59. Policy statement: AAP publications reaffirmed and retired. *Pediatrics* 2007;120(3):683-684.

60. Bull MJ, Committee on Genetics: Health supervision for children with Down syndrome. *Pediatrics* 2011;128(2):393-406.

61. Gruber J, Saleh A, Bakhsh W, Rubery PT, Mesfin A: The prevalence of Klippel-Feil syndrome: A computed tomography-based analysis of 2917 patients. *Spine Deform* 2018;6(4):448-453.

    This was a cross-sectional study in which the authors reviewed 2,917 CT scans obtained at a Level 1 emergency department. The prevalence of Klippel-Feil syndrome was found to be 0.0058% with C5-C6 and C2-C3 being the most commonly fused levels. Level of evidence: IV.

62. Samartzis D, Kalluri P, Herman J, Lubicky JP, Shen FH: Cervical scoliosis in the Klippel–Feil patient. *Spine (Phila Pa 1976)* 2011;36(23):E1501-E1508.

63. Shen FH, Samartzis D, Herman J, Lubicky JP: Radiographic assessment of segmental motion at the atlantoaxial junction in the Klippel-Feil patient. *Spine (Phila Pa 1976)* 2006;31(2):171-177.

64. Nouri A, Patel K, Evans H, et al: Demographics, presentation amd symptoms of patients with Klippel-Feil syndrome: Analysis of a global patient-reported registry. *Eur Spine J* 2019;28(10):2257-2265.

    The authors report the demographics, presentation, and symptoms of Klippel-Feil syndrome from data obtained through the CoRDS registry. They found associated comorbidities including Sprengel deformity to be more common in patients with multilevel cervical fusions. Brain fog, fatigue, balance issues, and urinary incontinence were common complaints in this patient population. Level of evidence: III.

65. Nouri A, Martin AR, Lange SF, Kotter MRN, Mikulis DJ, Fehlings MG: Congenital cervical fusion as a risk factor for development of cervical degenerative myelopathy. *World Neurosurg* 2017;100:531-539.

    A retrospective analysis of three prospective databases on degenerative cervical myelopathy aimed to determine the prevalence of Klippel-Feil syndrome and congenital cervical fusion in patients with degenerative myelopathy. The authors found the prevalence of Klippel-Feil syndrome higher in degenerative cervical myelopathy than the general population, suggesting a predisposition to cervical myelopathy in patients with KFS. Level of evidence: IV.

66. Nagashima H, Morio Y, Teshima R: No neurological involvement for more than 40 years in Klippel-Feil syndrome with severe hypermobility of the upper cervical spine. *Arch Orthop Trauma Surg* 2001;121(1-2):99-101.

67. Johnston CE II, Birch JG, Daniels JL: Cervical kyphosis in patients who have Larsen syndrome. *J Bone Joint Surg Am* 1996;78(4):538-545.

68. Remes V, Marttinen E, Poussa M, Kaitila I, Peltonen J: Cervical kyphosis in diastrophic dysplasia. *Spine (Phila Pa 1976)* 1999;24(19):1990-1995.

69. Isu T, Miyasaka K, Abe H, Ito T, Iwasaka Y, Tsuru M: Atlantoaxial dislocation associated with neurofibromatosis: Report of three cases. *J Neurosurg* 1983;58(3):451-453.

70. Yong-Hing K, Kalamchi A, MacEwen GD: Cervical spine abnormalities in neurofibromatosis. *J Bone Joint Surg Am* 1979;61(5):695-699.

71. Crawford AH: Pitfalls of spinal deformities associated with neurofibromatosis in children. *Clin Orthop Relat Res* 1989;245:29-42.

72. Funasaki H, Winter RB, Lonstein JB, Denis F: Pathophysiology of spinal deformities in neurofibromatosis: An analysis of seventy-one patients who had curves associated with dystrophic changes. *J Bone Joint Surg Am* 1994;76(5):692-700.

73. Wilde PH, Upadhyay SS, Leong JC: Deterioration of operative correction in dystrophic spinal neurofibromatosis. *Spine (Phila Pa 1976)* 1994;19(11):1264-1270.

74. Taleb FS, Guha A, Arnold PM, Fehlings MG, Massicotte EM: Surgical management of cervical spine manifestations of neurofibromatosis type 1: Long-term clinical and radiological follow-up in 22 cases. *J Neurosurg Spine* 2011;14(3):356-366.

75. Kawabata S, Watanabe K, Hosogane N, et al: Surgical correction of severe cervical kyphosis in patients with neurofibromatosis type 1. *J Neurosurg Spine* 2013;18(3):274-279.

76. Helenius IJ, Sponseller PD, Mackenzie W, et al: Outcomes of spinal fusion for cervical kyphosis in children with neurofibromatosis. *J Bone Joint Surg Am* 2016;98(21):e95.

    A retrospective multicenter review of cervical fusion in 22 patients with neurofibromatosis. The authors confirm better alignment and kyphosis correction with a combined anterior-posterior approach but no difference in fusion rates when compared with a posterior only approach. Level of evidence: IV.

77. Alton TB, Patel AM, Lee MJ, Chapman JR: Pediatric cervical spondylolysis and American football. *Spine J* 2014;14(6):e1-e5.

78. Ahn PG, Yoon DH, Shin HC, et al: Cervical spondylolysis: Three cases and a review of the current literature. *Spine (Phila Pa 1976)* 2010;35(3):E80-E83.

79. Fessy MH, Durand JM, Gunepin FX, Chavane H, Béjui JB, Bouchet A: An unusual anomaly: Cervical spondylolysis in an adult [French]. *Rev Chir Orthop Reparatrice Appar Mot* 1999;85(2):174-177.

80. Firth GB, Kingwell SP, Moroz PJ: Pediatric noncontiguous spinal injuries: The 15-year experience at a level 1 trauma center. *Spine (Phila Pa 1976)* 2012;37(10):E599-E608.

81. Schottler J, Vogel LC, Sturm P: Spinal cord injuries in young children: A review of children injured at 5 years of age and younger. *Dev Med Child Neurol* 2012;54(12):1138-1143.

82. Knox JB, Schneider JE, Cage JM, Wimberly RL, Riccio AI: Spine trauma in very young children: A retrospective study of 206 patients presenting to a level 1 pediatric trauma center. *J Pediatr Orthop* 2014,34(7):698-702.

83. Hannon M, Mannix R, Dorney K, Mooney D, Hennelly K: Pediatric cervical spine injury evaluation after blunt trauma: A clinical decision analysis. *Ann Emerg Med* 2015;65(3):239-247.

84. Viccellio P, Simon H, Pressman BD, et al, for the NEXUS Group: A prospective multicenter study of cervical spine injury in children. *Pediatrics* 2001;108(2):e20.

85. Garton HJ, Hammer MR: Detection of pediatric cervical spine injury. *Neurosurgery* 2008;62(3):700-708.

86. Hadley MN, Walters BC, Grabb PA, et al: Management of pediatric cervical spine and spinal cord injuries. *Neurosurgery* 2002;50(3 suppl):S85-S99.

87. Leonard JR, Jaffe DM, Kuppermann N, Olsen CS, Leonard JC, Pediatric Emergency Care Applied Research Network (PECARN) Cervical Spine Study Group: Cervical spine injury patterns in children. *Pediatrics* 2014;133(5):e1179-e1188.

88. Murphy RF, Davidson AR, Kelly DM, et al: Subaxial cervical spine injuries in children and adolescents. *J Pediatr Orthop* 2015;35(2):136-139.

89. Baumann F, Ernstberger T, Neumann C, et al: Pediatric cervical spine injuries: A rare but challenging entity. *J Spinal Disord Tech* 2015;28(7):E377-E384.

90. Mortazavi M, Gore PA, Chang S, Tubbs RS, Theodore N: Pediatric cervical spine injuries: A comprehensive review. *Childs Nerv Syst* 2011;27(5):705-717.

91. Henry M, Riesenburger RI, Kryzanski J, Jea A, Hwang SW: A retrospective comparison of CT and MRI in detecting pediatric cervical spine injury. *Childs Nerv Syst* 2013;29(8):1333-1338.

92. Bettencourt RB, Linder MM: Treatment of neck injuries. *Prim Care* 2013;40(2):259-269.

93. Benjamin HJ, Lessman DS: Sports-related cervical spine injuries. *Clin Pediatr Emerg Med* 2013;14(4):255-266.

94. Babcock L, Olsen CS, Jaffe DM, et al: Cervical spine injuries in children associated with sports and recreational activities. *Pediatr Emerg Care* 2018;34(10):677-686.

A retrospective case-control analysis of patients younger than 16 years who underwent cervical spine imaging following blunt trauma. The authors found that sport or recreational activity-related trauma had increased odds of cervical spine injury in children if they had focal neurologic findings (odds ratio 3.1), were injured diving (odds ratio 43.5), or sustained axial loading impacts (odds ratio 2.2). Football, diving, and bicycle crashes were leading activities associated with cervical spine injury. Level of evidence: III.

95. Watkins RG: Neck injuries in football players. *Clin Sports Med* 1986;5(2):215-246.

96. Morganti C, Sweeney CA, Albanese SA, Burak C, Hosea T, Connolly PJ: Return to play after cervical spine injury. *Spine (Phila Pa 1976)* 2001;26(10):1131-1136.

CHAPTER 36

Back Pain, Disk Disease, Spondylolysis, and Spondylolisthesis

A. NOELLE LARSON, MD

ABSTRACT

Back pain is a common problem in children. Because many conditions can cause back pain, it is important to use appropriate physical examination and imaging methods to rule out serious conditions, including those that are unique to children. Constant pain, night pain, abnormal findings on the physical examination, and progressive symptoms should prompt additional workup. Disk disease, spondylolysis, and spondylolisthesis are frequent causes of back pain in children. With the exception of high-grade spondylolisthesis, treatment for these conditions is typically driven by symptomatology. Most patients respond to physical therapy, rest, and/or bracing treatment. If nonsurgical measures are unsuccessful, surgical treatment may restore function.

Keywords: disk herniation; pars defect; pediatric back pain; spondylolisthesis; spondylolysis

INTRODUCTION

Historically, back pain in children was thought to indicate serious pathology and necessitated an extensive workup. However, back pain, particularly in adolescents, is quite common and has no identifiable underlying cause in up to 80% of patients. Intermittent back pain is experienced by one-third of adolescents.[1] An insurance registry evaluation of more than 200,000 adolescents with back pain reported that fewer than 20% had a specific associated diagnosis such as spondylolysis or disk disease given within 1 year.[2]

Conflicting evidence exists on whether back pain is more common in patients who are active and participate in sports and whether heavy schoolbags or backpacks contribute to pediatric back pain.[3-5] Idiopathic back pain has been associated with older age, increased body mass index, and parental smoking.[6,7] A patient with idiopathic back pain may have detectable differences in his or her spine. A study using upright MRIs to analyze the response to backpack loads showed increased compression of the L5-S1 disks with backpack wear in children with idiopathic back pain compared with normal control subjects.[8] Effective management of back pain in adolescents is essential because back pain in children is associated with back pain in adulthood.[9,10]

It is important to identify the structural causes of back pain; however, these causes are present in only 20% to 30% of patients. Many diagnoses involving back pain can be specific to the pediatric population, including tumor, infection, fracture, inflammatory arthritis, Scheuermann disease, spondylolysis, and spondylolisthesis. A diagnosis of idiopathic back pain can be made only after other important causes of back pain are ruled out by appropriate evaluations that are proportionate to the symptomatology.

PATIENT EVALUATION

A thorough patient history, a physical examination, and, in many cases, standing PA and lateral radiographs make up the initial evaluation.[11,12]

Dr. Larson or an immediate family member has received research or institutional support from Globus Medical, Medtronic, Orthopediatrics, and Zimmer and serves as a board member, owner, officer, or committee member of the Pediatric Orthopaedic Society of North America and the Scoliosis Research Society.

History

Patients should be asked about the duration, characteristics, and onset of their pain, as well as any aggravating or alleviating factors. Night pain, progressive pain, or constant pain may indicate tumor or infection. Pain from osteoid osteoma is classically relieved by NSAIDs. Pain that results in a loss of function or missed participation in sports is more concerning than activity-related back pain or mild symptoms at the end of the day. Extensive periods of missed school accompanied by chronic back pain may point to underlying psychosocial factors. Patients should be asked about constitutional symptoms, pertinent past medical history, and extracurricular activities that may put them at higher risk for spinal pathology. Patients who participate in hyperextension sports, such as gymnastics or diving, are at risk for spondylolysis. Weight lifting has been associated with lumbar Scheuermann disease and disk disease. A focused family history should be taken because disk disease may be a common condition in a patient's family. Careful questioning is needed regarding bowel and bladder function to elicit an accurate history because many patients and their families are reluctant to volunteer this information. Tobacco or e-cigarette use should also be verified.

Physical Examination

The physical examination should include inspection of the back for spinal deformity, including coronal balance and spinal asymmetry. The Adam forward bend test is used to assess for scoliosis and focal kyphosis. Pain or spasm from a tumor or structural cause can cause an atypical scoliosis, which resolves after treatment of the underlying problem. The skin should be examined for markings over the spine, such as a hairy patch or dimple, which may indicate spinal cord pathology. Findings such as multiple café au lait lesions or axillary freckling should prompt an evaluation for neurofibromatosis. Sagittal plane alignment, as well as spinal range of motion, should be noted. Restricted range of motion is concerning for an underlying pathologic process. Pain elicited from palpation or percussion also warrants evaluation. Excessive range of motion and generalized ligamentous laxity may be associated with idiopathic back pain. A complete neurologic examination is necessary, including motor strength, sensation, and reflexes. Gait should be assessed for asymmetry or limp. The feet should be examined for asymmetry or deformity, which could indicate a spinal cord tumor or a tethered cord.

Hip range of motion should be symmetric and pain free. Pain with provocative maneuvers, including pain with hip flexion and internal rotation or groin pain with resisted straight leg raises, may indicate hip pathology. Pain with the FABER (flexion, abduction, external rotation) maneuver or tenderness to palpation over the sacroiliac joints may indicate sacroiliac joint pathology, which may be attributable to degenerative causes, inflammatory arthritis, or infection (if unilateral). Hamstring tightness indicated by an increased popliteus angle is associated with spondylolysis, spondylolisthesis, kyphosis, and a tethered cord. Pain radiating below the knee with passive straight leg raises is indicative of nerve root tension. A positive, crossed straight leg raise is characterized by radicular pain in the opposite leg, which has even greater specificity. Radicular symptoms with palpation of the sciatic notch may indicate piriformis syndrome.

Imaging

Radiography is the first imaging study to be considered and should be obtained before CT or MRI. Imaging studies should be performed based on clinical judgment and may be ordered selectively. In the absence of red flags, such as abnormal neurologic examination or clinical and laboratory findings suggesting an infectious, traumatic, or neoplastic process, a period of observation or physical therapy is typically warranted before obtaining advanced imaging.[12] Full-length standing two-view spine radiographs may show a spondylolytic defect, spondylolisthesis, scoliosis, diskitis (disk space narrowing), congenital segmentation anomalies, limb-length discrepancy, Scheuermann disease, or a compression fracture. A lumbar spine lateral view or L5-S1 spot lateral view may better show spondylolisthesis or spondylolysis because of parallax on a standard full-length lateral view unless low-dose biplanar slot scanning technology is used, which provides a true lateral at every level. Oblique views and flexion-extension views are not typically indicated in the pediatric population, particularly for the initial evaluation, because of the high radiation dose, particularly for the oblique views, which transmit as much radiation as a focal lumbar CT scan.

A variety of advanced imaging modalities are effective for evaluating severe or atypical back pain or symptoms that have not responded to a period of nonsurgical management. Advanced imaging is not warranted for every pediatric patient with back pain and should be used selectively. MRI can be useful for detecting disk or spinal cord pathology, lumbar Scheuermann disease, fracture, tumor, infection, or spondylolysis.[13] Evidence of diskitis can sometimes be seen on plain radiographs, although MRI is more sensitive. The hallmark of infection is a T2 signal change crossing a disk space and involving two adjacent levels. Inflammation of the lumbar apophyseal joints and interspinous ligament seen on MRI may be found in patients with enthesitis-related arthritis.[14] MRI is costly, may not be readily available, and requires sedation in younger children; however, it provides excellent visualization of soft tissues and does not expose the patient to radiation. Bone scintigraphy can be used to evaluate for spondylolysis, infection, tumor, and an apophyseal ring fracture, but it exposes the patient to deep ionizing radiation. Scintigraphy will not show spinal cord pathology.[15] A bone scan is also helpful in localizing the anatomic area of pain in a patient who is nonverbal and has back pain or leg pain. A normal bone scan can provide peace of mind for patients with severe, persistent generalized back pain that has not improved with nonsurgical management and has no other obvious diagnoses; however, bone scans should be used sparingly because of the high radiation exposure.

Currently, CT provides the best three-dimensional visualization of bony structures. It is readily available at most centers, and images can be obtained quickly, so sedation in a younger child is less frequently needed. An apophyseal ring fracture may be better appreciated with CT than MRI. In addition, CT allows for careful evaluation of the pars anatomy for spondylolytic defects and is more sensitive than radiography. Based on the injury mechanism, emergent CT of the spine may be warranted in an obtunded trauma patient or a patient with a distracting injury. CT entails greater ionizing radiation, although this modality typically has a lower dose than a bone scan.[16] Specific CT protocols should be adjusted based on the body weight and age of the child to limit radiation exposure. A 2013 high-quality population-based study from Australia with a mean 10-year follow-up showed one additional cancer for every 1,800 pediatric CT scans performed.[17] Therefore, CT should be reserved for patients with clear indications. CT myelography involves injection of dye into the dural sac and can be used to evaluate compression of the neural elements in patients who are unable to undergo MRI because of incompatible medical devices such as specific cochlear implants. The choice of imaging study should be tailored to the individual patient and the suspected diagnosis.

Laboratory Investigation

Certain signs and symptoms of back pain should prompt additional evaluation. For patients with constant pain, night pain, radicular pain, or an abnormal neurologic examination, further evaluation is indicated. Idiopathic back pain is more frequently seen in adolescents, so additional evaluation in a younger child may be warranted. A laboratory workup is indicated for patients with a history of fevers, weight loss, or fatigue. This evaluation should include a complete blood count with differential, C-reactive protein level, and erythrocyte sedimentation rate. A peripheral smear to evaluate cell morphology may identify early cases of leukemia. Routine screening for rheumatoid factor, antinuclear antibodies, and HLA-B27 are low yield in the pediatric population and are not typically indicated unless other presenting features indicate a rheumatologic cause.

COMMON CATEGORIES OF BACK PAIN AND TREATMENT OPTIONS

Idiopathic Back Pain

If findings from the patient history, the physical examination, and radiography are all consistent with idiopathic back pain, a physical therapy program focused on core strengthening, hamstring stretches, and lumbar stabilization should be initiated. Treatment with physical therapy and strengthening exercises has been shown to improve idiopathic back pain in children.[18] Activity modification and a period of rest from sports may help relieve symptoms. Regular physical aerobic activity also may help improve back pain symptoms. In addition, smoking cessation and weight loss may be beneficial. The use of narcotic pain medications or muscle relaxants should be avoided. If the pain seems to warrant these types of prescriptions, further investigation is needed. Empiric spinal injections or oral corticosteroids are not warranted unless a discrete lesion is identified on imaging and other conservative measures have failed to improve symptoms.

Disk Disease

Degenerative disk disease may be seen in adolescents and can result in back pain and, occasionally, radicular symptoms. Asymptomatic degenerative disk disease has been seen on MRIs of 22% of children without back pain and herniated disks noted in up to 13% of pediatric athletes without back pain.[19,20] Imaging findings should be correlated with the physical examination findings. Degenerative disk disease may be familial in origin and has been associated with several genetic abnormalities. L4-L5 and L5-S1 are the most commonly affected levels.

Most patients younger than 21 years who have discogenic back pain can successfully be treated with nonsurgical measures,[21] including back and abdominal strengthening, weight loss, NSAIDs, activity restriction, low-impact aerobic conditioning, smoking cessation, and career counseling. Selective nerve root or epidural injections may be used as a second-line treatment and may achieve complete symptom relief.

Patients with disk herniation and congenital spinal stenosis (defined as less than 12 mm between the posterior wall of the vertebral body and the anterior margin of the lamina) may more frequently require surgical management.[21] Surgical management is indicated for cauda equina syndrome, neurologic deficit, or radicular symptoms refractory to 6 months of nonsurgical management (**Figure 1**). Although open diskectomy is the standard of care, successful microdiskectomy for symptomatic disk herniation in adolescents has been

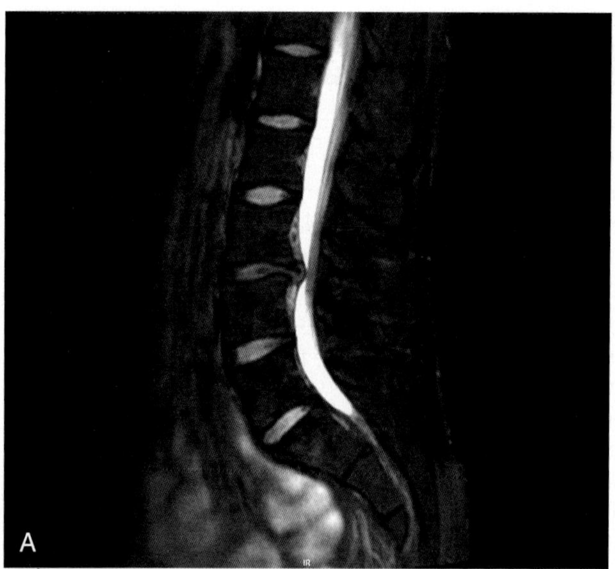

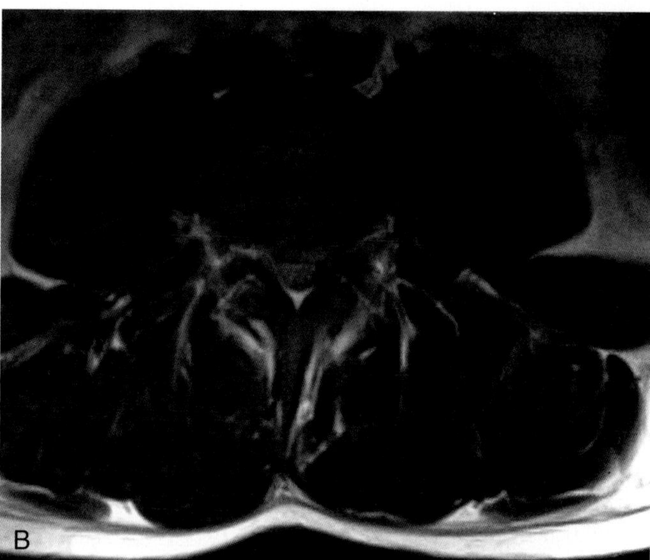

FIGURE 1 Magnetic resonance images from a 17-year-old boy who presented with bilateral radicular pain and a positive straight leg raise test. He had increased knee and ankle jerk reflexes on the right side. **A**, Sagittal T2 magnetic resonance image shows an L3 disk herniation. **B**, Axial T2 magnetic resonance image shows pressure on the nerve roots. The patient was subsequently treated with microdiskectomy after 6 months of nonsurgical treatment with physical therapy, rest, and epidural steroid injections proved unsuccessful.

reported.[22,23] CT may be used to rule out an accompanying apophyseal ring fracture. Fusion is not indicated for discogenic back pain in children.

Surgeons should be aware of posterior spinal cord infarct, which is a rare condition associated with participation in high-intensity sports and degenerative disk changes in children and is thought to be caused by a fibrocartilaginous embolus.[24] Patients have acute back pain and neurologic deficit after minor trauma or a high-intensity activity. A spinal cord infarct can be detected on MRI with diffusion-weighted imaging.

Apophyseal Ring Fracture

Apophyseal ring fractures (also known as limbus fractures) can occur in adolescents and young adults and have been reported in 28% to 38% of pediatric patients presenting with lumbar disk herniation.[25-27] Patients may have findings similar to a spondylolytic defect, with tight hamstrings, pain with hyperextension, possible radicular symptoms, a positive straight leg raise test, and/or neurologic findings.[25] The onset of symptoms may be insidious or acute after trauma. The lesion is best visualized on CT and may not be apparent on plain radiographs or MRI (**Figure 2**). On MRI, the disk herniation may be evident, but it can be difficult to appreciate the apophyseal fracture. Four types of apophyseal ring fractures have been described: (1) separation of the entire posterior vertebral margin; (2) an avulsion fracture, including a portion of the vertebral body; (3) a posterolateral fracture; and (4) a full-length fracture of the vertebral body between the end plates.

Compared with patients with disk herniation alone, patients with apophyseal ring fractures may be less likely to improve with nonsurgical treatment. Surgical treatment typically entails fragment excision, which is more complex than a simple diskectomy, requires wider exposure, and may require the use of a burr or an osteotome to remove the fragment. Patients with large apophyseal fragments treated nonsurgically are at risk for chronic back pain.[27] A 2012 study reported on 16 patients with apophyseal ring fractures treated nonsurgically and 8 patients treated surgically. At a mean follow-up of 13.8 years, no detectable difference in clinical outcomes occurred between the two groups.[28]

Lumbar Scheuermann Disease

Lumbar or atypical Scheuermann disease can be characterized on plain radiographs by Schmorl nodes, end plate irregularity, and loss of normal lumbar lordosis. MRI will show Schmorl nodes, degenerative disk disease, and narrowing of the disk space (**Figure 3**). The substantial kyphotic deformity and vertebral wedging seen in typical Scheuermann disease may not be present. Patients present with back pain and tend to be athletic male adolescents, sometimes with a history of weight lifting.[29,30] Treatment is nonsurgical. Interestingly, Schmorl nodes and end plate changes have been reported in up to 18% of the adult population

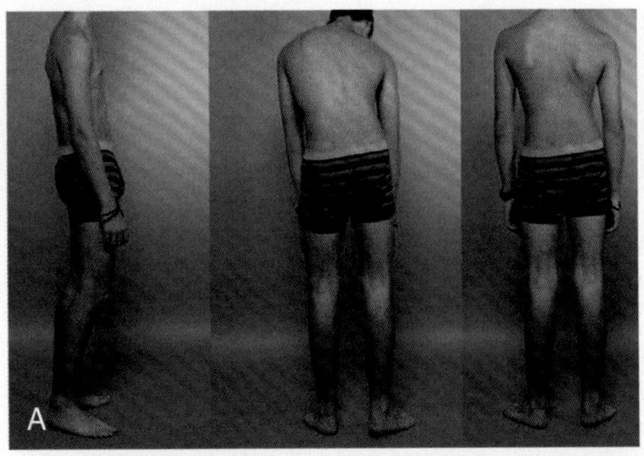
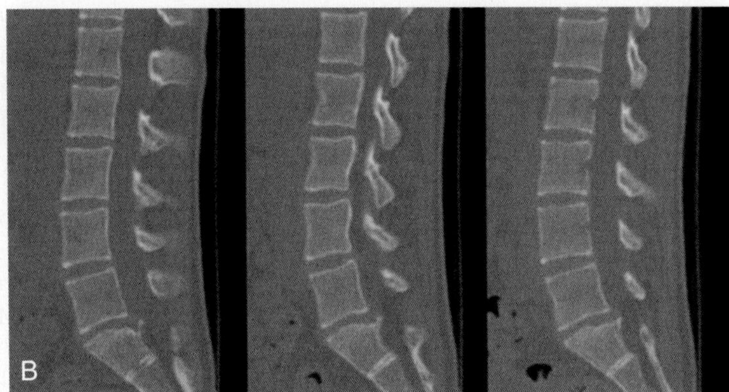
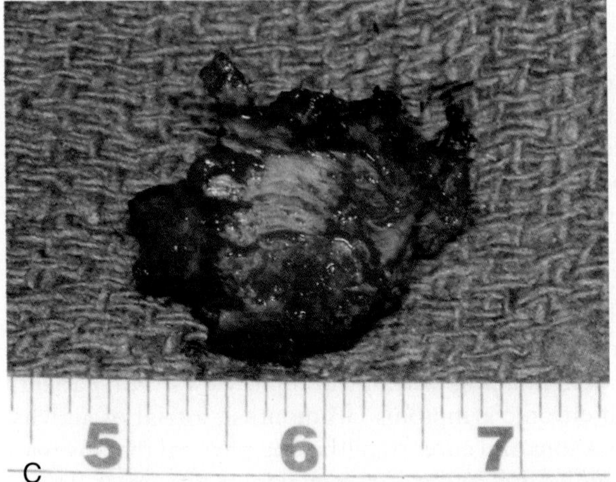
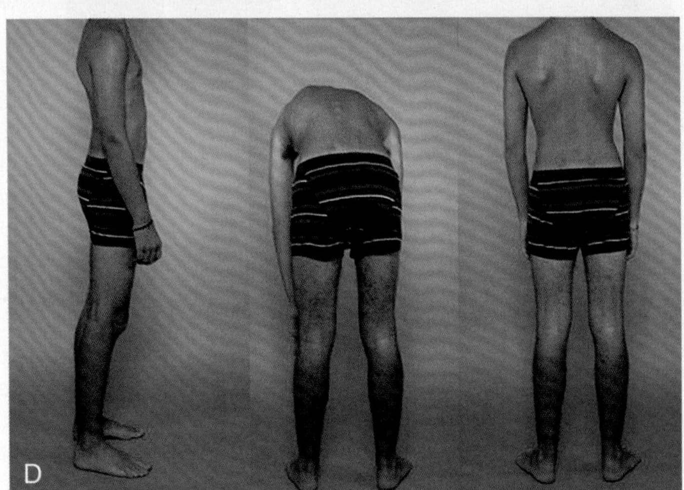

FIGURE 2 A 14-year-old boy presented with back pain, gait dysfunction, and bilateral radicular pain. **A**, Clinical photographs show atypical scoliosis, limited flexibility on forward bending (center panel), and loss of lumbar lordosis. **B**, Sagittal CT scans show an S1 apophyseal ring fracture associated with an L5-S1 disk herniation. **C**, Gross photograph of the resected lesion. **D**, Postoperative clinical photographs show resolution of scoliosis and improved forward bending (center panel).

and may be associated with chronic back pain.[31] Disk herniation in atypical Scheuermann disease can cause neurologic symptoms, but this is rare.[32]

Spondylolysis

Spondylolysis, a common cause of back pain in the pediatric population, is a defect of the lumbar pars interarticularis and can occur unilaterally or bilaterally. Patients may have acute or chronic low back pain in a bandlike fashion across the lumbar spine. Hyperextension characteristically worsens the pain. Occasionally, patients may have radicular pain and/or a positive straight leg raise test.

Two structured literature reviews summarize the current state of knowledge and imaging recommendations for pediatric spondylolysis.[33,34] It is an acquired condition and more common in athletes, particularly those who participate in sports requiring hyperextension, such as gymnastics. A unilateral defect can lead to a subsequent bilateral defect, which supports a mechanical etiology. L5 is the most commonly affected level. In the pediatric population, the prevalence of spondylolysis is 3% to 7%, although many individuals are asymptomatic.

Plain radiographs may show a defect up to 75% of the time, particularly when there is bilateral involvement.[16] Oblique radiographs do not add sensitivity or specificity in detecting spondylolysis and substantially increase radiation exposure.[35] Because limited CT through the pars interarticularis has a similar radiation dose as oblique lumbar spine radiographs and improved interrater reliability, oblique radiographs are not indicated in the pediatric population.[36] Standard CT also is an effective study and has a lower radiation dose than a bone scan (**Figure 4**). Increased lumbar lordosis and smaller vertebral cross-sectional area may be found in pediatric patients with spondylolysis.[37] Skeletal single photon emission computed tomography (SPECT) is very sensitive for acute or subacute spondylolysis with increased uptake over the pars interarticularis. This imaging study results in substantial radiation exposure, with organ radiation

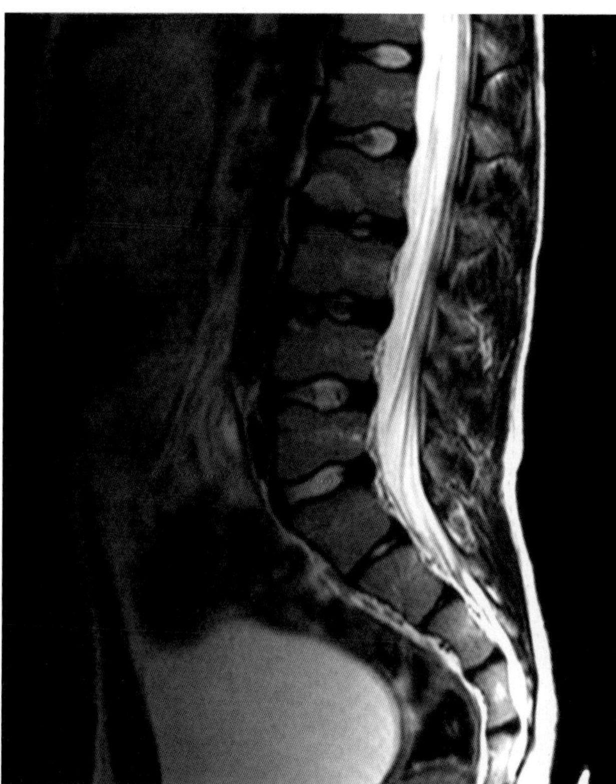

FIGURE 3 Sagittal magnetic resonance image of the spine of a 14-year-old boy who was active in multiple sports, including football, hockey, and snowmobiling, shows disk degeneration and Schmorl nodes.

doses up to 15 mSv, which is five times the annual background radiation and several times higher in radiation dose than a focal CT scan.[14,15,38] The incidence of cancer in individuals increases by 24% when these individuals had childhood exposure to a CT scan (mean estimated dose = 4.5 mSv) compared with those without childhood exposure to CT.[17] Because first-line management for most cases of spondylolysis is physical therapy, the benefits of this type of imaging should be carefully weighed.[37]

MRI also can be used to evaluate T2 signal change over the pars interarticularis or visualize a fracture, and MRI is more sensitive than plain radiography. It is worthwhile to contact a musculoskeletal radiologist to develop a specific MRI protocol to best visualize the pars. In general, the MRI must be obtained with thin section images (3 mm) with both T1 and T2 fat suppression sequences in the axial and sagittal planes at high resolution. T2 edema in the pars corresponds to a subacute process. Specific sequences have been described in the literature.[39,40] Similar to SPECT or bone scans, MRI may identify prelytic lesions that may not be evident on CT.[38-40]

The preferred initial evaluation for spondylolysis is standing AP and L5-S1 spot lateral or low-dose slot-scanner imaging without oblique views. For patients with chronic symptoms (>3 months), a trial of activity limitations and core strengthening physical therapy with scheduled follow-up is reasonable. Acute onset, severe

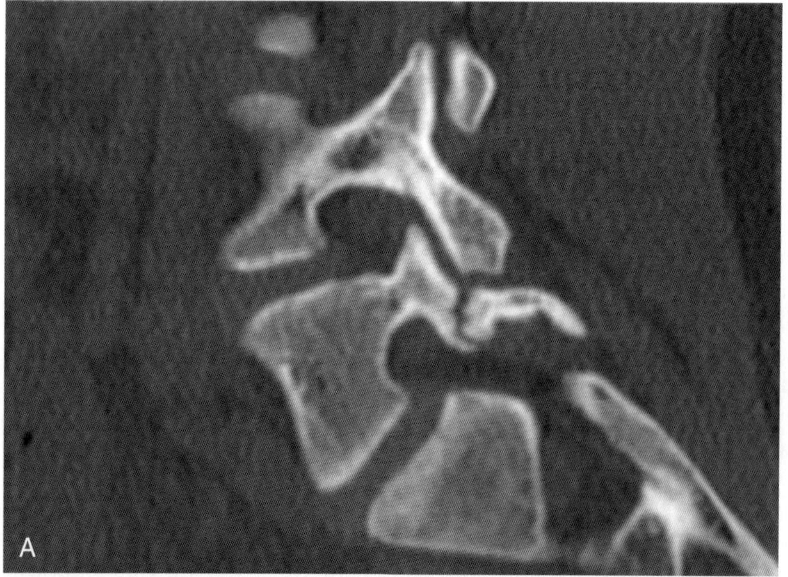

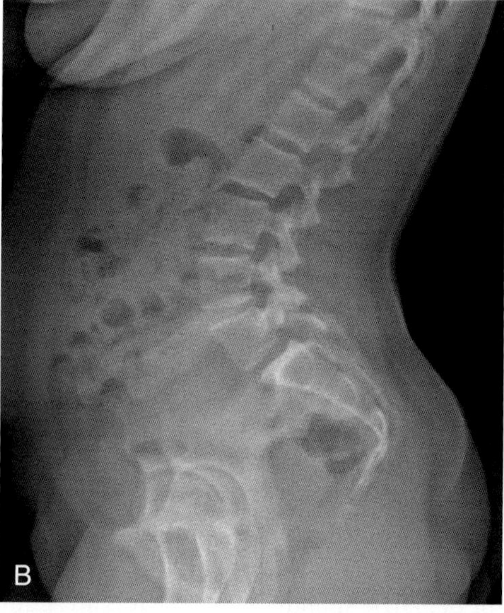

FIGURE 4 Images from a 13-year-old girl who presented with back pain. **A**, Sagittal CT scan shows a chronic-appearing L5 spondylolytic defect and increased sclerosis about the L4 pars interarticularis. After a period of rest followed by extensive core strengthening exercises, the patient successfully returned to all sports. **B**, Radiographic image obtained by biplane radiographic imaging (EOS imaging) taken at 2-year follow-up shows bilateral L5 pars defects and grade 1 spondylolisthesis; however, the patient was asymptomatic.

pain, radicular symptoms, or the need for immediate return to sporting activities should prompt axial imaging with either selective CT of L4-S1 or MRI depending on imaging capabilities. Ongoing controversy exists if CT, MRI, or SPECT is the best imaging study for the evaluation of spondylolysis.[34] Specialized protocols can be used to lower the radiation dose of CT scans or provide effective imaging of the pars on MRI.

Nonsurgical treatment with rest has been shown to result in a good or excellent outcome in more than 80% of pediatric athletes.[41] Nonsurgical treatment consists of 2 to 6 months of activity restriction; physical therapy, with core strengthening and hamstring stretches; and/or bracing treatment.[42] Cessation of sporting activities is more closely associated with a positive outcome than achieving bony union.[43] At mean 8-year follow-up, a 90% return to sports has been reported following diagnosis of spondylolysis, although 40% of patients still had back pain.[44] Rest, activity restrictions, and immobilization in a thoracolumbosacral orthosis can be used to achieve bony union in over 80% of early-stage lesions.[45] Healing is unlikely for patients with chronic-appearing unilateral lesions, bilateral disease, or spondylolisthesis. From 43% to 75% of patients with chronic bilateral pars defects will progress to low-grade spondylolisthesis.

Surgical treatment is indicated when 1 to 2 years of nonsurgical treatment is unsuccessful at achieving acceptable pain relief and the desired level of physical activity. Pars repair avoids fusion, and high success rates have been reported with methods such as intralaminar screw fixation or a pedicle screw/rod/laminar hook construct.[46,47] Higher success rates are reported in L4 than L5 spondylolytic defects. Spondylolisthesis is a contraindication to pars repair. L5-S1 fusion also predictably relieves symptoms but may contribute to adjacent-segment disease later in life.

Spondylolisthesis

Spondylolisthesis refers to the forward translation of a vertebral body with respect to the vertebra beneath it. Isthmic spondylolisthesis and dysplastic spondylolisthesis are the most common types in children (**Table 1**). MRIs of children who are asymptomatic have shown spondylolisthesis in 2.3% of patients. Grade 1 and 2 spondylolisthesis (zero to 50% slip) is managed symptomatically. Nonsurgical treatment includes physical therapy, bracing treatment, and activity modification. For a patient with persistent symptoms or neurologic deficit, in situ instrumented fusion is a treatment option. Six spinopelvic postures have been described for patients with spondylolisthesis, with types 1 through 3 slips being low grade and types 4 through 6 slips being high grade[48] (**Figure 5**). It is posited that increased pelvic incidence in a low-grade type 3 slip results in a higher risk of slip progression. Patients with types 3 and 4 slips have increased lumbar lordosis and are compensated in the sagittal plane. Types 5 and 6 slips are decompensated, and patients may have more symptoms and poorer patient-reported quality-of-life scores. If reduction is to be performed, types 5 and 6 slips may most benefit from correction of the slip angle. This classification has good reliability, but prospective long-term evidence to support these management recommendations is still needed.

Because of the high rate of progression and subsequent deformity, high-grade spondylolisthesis traditionally warrants surgical management, even in a patient who is asymptomatic. Although several studies reported

TABLE 1

The Wiltse-Newman Classification of Spondylolisthesis

Type	Description
Dysplastic Congenital Developmental	Increased risk of slippage and incompetent L5-S1 articulation. The pars may be intact but elongated or fractured. The sacrum may be domed. L5 spina bifida occulta may be present.
Isthmic Spondylolytic	Secondary to bilateral stress fractures of the pars. Posterior elements are still in place.
Degenerative	Secondary to degenerative changes in adulthood.
Posttraumatic	Acute fracture and slippage.
Pathologic	Attenuation of the pars from bone pathology (such as osteogenesis imperfecta or Ehlers-Danlos syndrome).

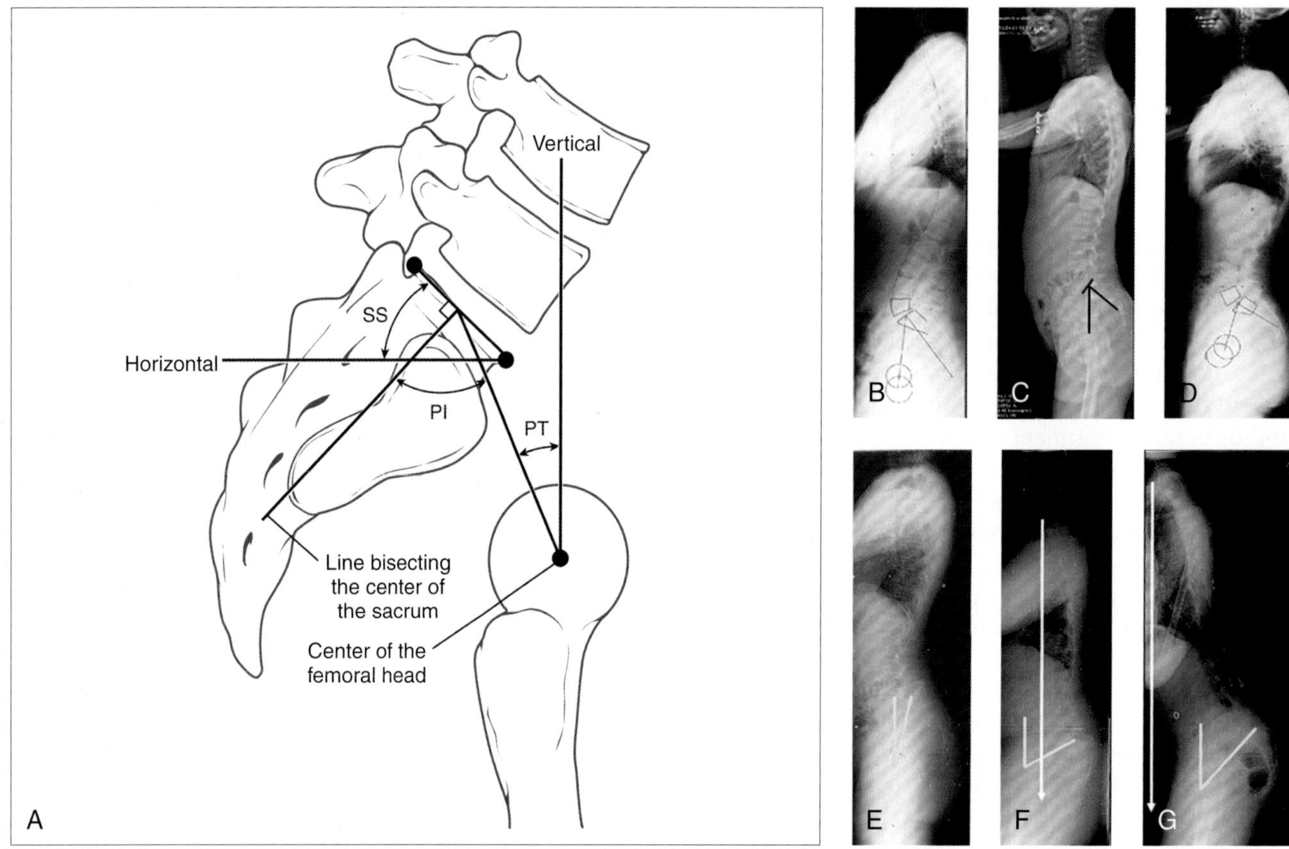

FIGURE 5 **A**, Schematic diagram shows a lateral view of the lumbosacral junction with standard parameters of pelvic morphology and spinopelvic balance in spondylolisthesis. In low-grade spondylolisthesis, the subtype depends on whether the pelvic incidence (PI) and the sacral slope (SS) are high or low. In high-grade spondylolisthesis, the subtype depends on whether the pelvic tilt (PT) and SS are high or low. **B** through **G**, Lateral radiographs demonstrate the six spinopelvic postures that have been described for patients with spondylolisthesis. **B**, Low-grade spondylolisthesis with low PI and low SS (nutcracker type). **C**, Low-grade spondylolisthesis with normal PI and SS. **D**, Low-grade spondylolisthesis with high PI and high SS (shear type). **E**, High-grade spondylolisthesis with a balanced pelvis, high SS, and low PT. **F**, High-grade spondylolisthesis with a retroverted pelvis, low SS, high PT, and a balanced spine. **G**, High-grade spondylolisthesis with an unbalanced spine. (Panel **B** through **G** reprinted with permission from Springer Nature: *Eur Spine J*. Labelle H, Mac-Thiong JM, Roussouly P: Spino-pelvic sagittal balance of spondylolisthesis: A review and classification. 20[suppl 5]:641-646. Copyright © 2011.)

successful nonsurgical management of even high-grade slips, the authors concluded that patients with symptoms benefit most from surgery.[49-51] An increased slip angle is associated with progression to surgical management. Decreased sacral slope is associated with more back pain.[52]

Most patients with high-grade spondylolisthesis have back pain and/or radicular symptoms and merit surgical management. A variety of surgical strategies exist. Historically, in situ fusion was performed and achieved with postoperative immobilization in a pantaloon spica cast or a thoracolumbosacral orthosis with a thigh extension. Circumferential in situ fusion can be achieved using the Bohlman technique to place a fibular strut through the sacrum and into L5 to augment a standard posterolateral fusion. In situ fusion can result in progression of the slippage over time and may necessitate later reduction, particularly for patients with a high slip angle (**Figure 6**). Combined anterior-posterior or all-posterior approaches can achieve reduction and circumferential fusion (**Figure 7**). The risk of neurologic deficit is substantially higher with reduction and can result in L5 nerve root irritation and foot drop. Performing a reduction to correct the slip angle is controversial because reduction is associated with a higher rate of neurologic compromise, although it is proposed to result in improved long-term durability compared with in situ fusion.

Bone morphogenetic protein is occasionally used in children for the surgical management of spondylolisthesis, although the indications and dosing are not clear and its use in children remains off-label.[53] Overall, there is an 11.5% rate of new neurologic defects after surgical

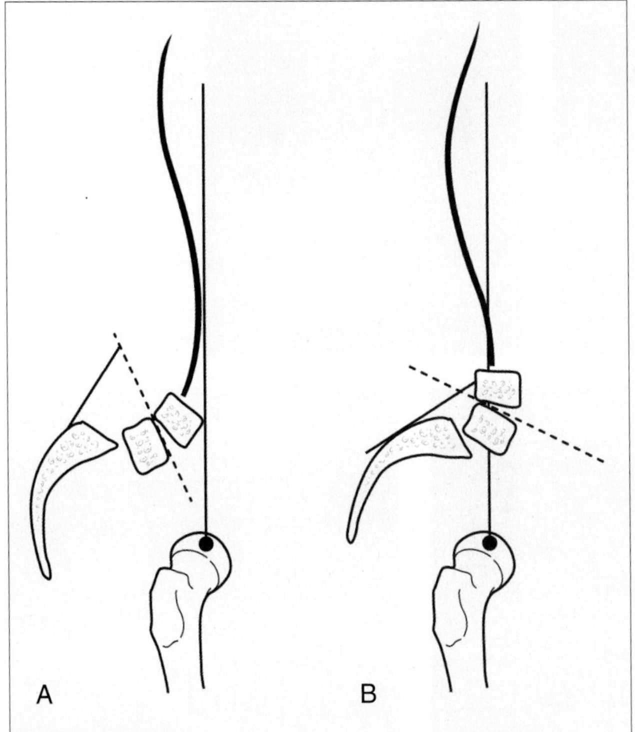

FIGURE 6 Illustrations of the slip angle, which can be used to describe the degree of spinal deformity. Surgical management of high-grade spondylolisthesis is focused on correcting the slip angle. **A**, Patients with a high slip angle, vertical sacrum, low sacral slope, and high pelvic tilt (a retroverted pelvis) may require correction of the deformity at the time of surgery. Patients with a retroverted pelvis may have a balanced spine or positive sagittal balance (as seen in **Figure 5**, **G**). **B**, Patients with a low slip angle may tolerate fusion in situ without reduction of the slip. These patients have neutral sagittal balance.

management of spondylolisthesis.[54] Patients with neurologic symptoms should undergo either direct posterior or indirect anterior decompression as part of the surgical management process.

OTHER CAUSES OF BACK PAIN IN CHILDREN

Transitional anomalies at the lumbosacral junction are common and, occasionally, may generate back pain known as Bertolotti syndrome. Evaluation may include plain radiographs and MRI to evaluate radicular symptoms, if present. Bone scans or SPECT can be used to detect symptomatic articulations. Treatment begins with nonsurgical management. The injection of corticosteroid and local anesthetic at the site of a symptomatic articulation can temporarily improve symptoms and help target surgical management if nonsurgical measures are unsuccessful. The role of surgical treatment is unclear and entails fusion or resection of the symptomatic articulation.[55]

Diskitis and vertebral osteomyelitis can occur in children who are prone to hematogenous infections because of low-flow blood vessels and anastomoses to the disk and vertebral end plates. Young children may have a limp or refuse to walk, whereas adolescents typically have back pain or abdominal pain.[56] An altered gait pattern in an adolescent may indicate pelvic pyomyositis or psoas abscess. The patient also may have a fever. Elevation may be seen in the white blood cell count, the platelet count, the C-reactive protein level, and/or the erythrocyte sedimentation rate. The evaluation should include blood cultures; however, they are rarely positive.[56,57] End plate changes and disk space narrowing may be seen on plain radiographs. MRI will show changes earlier in the disease course and can rule out a paravertebral abscess or an epidural abscess (**Figure 8**). Biopsy is not indicated unless empiric treatment with anti-inflammatory drugs, rest, and oral or intravenous antibiotics fails. Bracing treatment may be used for symptom management. Atypical organisms such as *Mycobacterium tuberculosis* should be suspected in multilevel disease, disease with an insidious onset, and in patients who are immunocompromised or have a history of exposure to such organisms. In a series of 103 pediatric patients presenting with a spinal infection, 77% were younger than 4 years, and methicillin-sensitive *Staphylococcus aureus* and *Kingella kingae* infections were the most frequently isolated pathogens.[57,58] Generally, patients can be treated nonsurgically.

Tumor is a rare cause of back pain in children. Radiographs may show a vertebra plana lesion, which can be caused by eosinophilic granuloma among other diagnoses (**Figure 9**). Osteoid osteoma and osteoblastoma classically affect the posterior vertebral elements. Of the total, 20% to 30% of patients with multiple hereditary exostosis may have a spinal osteochondroma, which can cause progressive pain and/or neurologic deficit.[59-61] Patients with neurofibromatosis frequently have dural ectasia and plexiform neurofibromas involving the spine, which can result in chronic back pain. These lesions typically are not amenable to resection. Aneurysmal bone cysts can be locally aggressive and result in spinal instability. Preoperative embolization may reduce perioperative blood loss.[62,63] Malignant lesions, such as osteosarcoma, chondrosarcoma, lymphoma, leukemia, Ewing sarcoma, and metastatic disease, are rare. Spinal cord tumors include astrocytoma, ependymoma, and chordoma. CT or open biopsy may be necessary for making a diagnosis. A multidisciplinary team should treat malignant tumors. The management of nonmalignant tumors depends on the type and location of the tumor, spinal stability, and symptomatology.

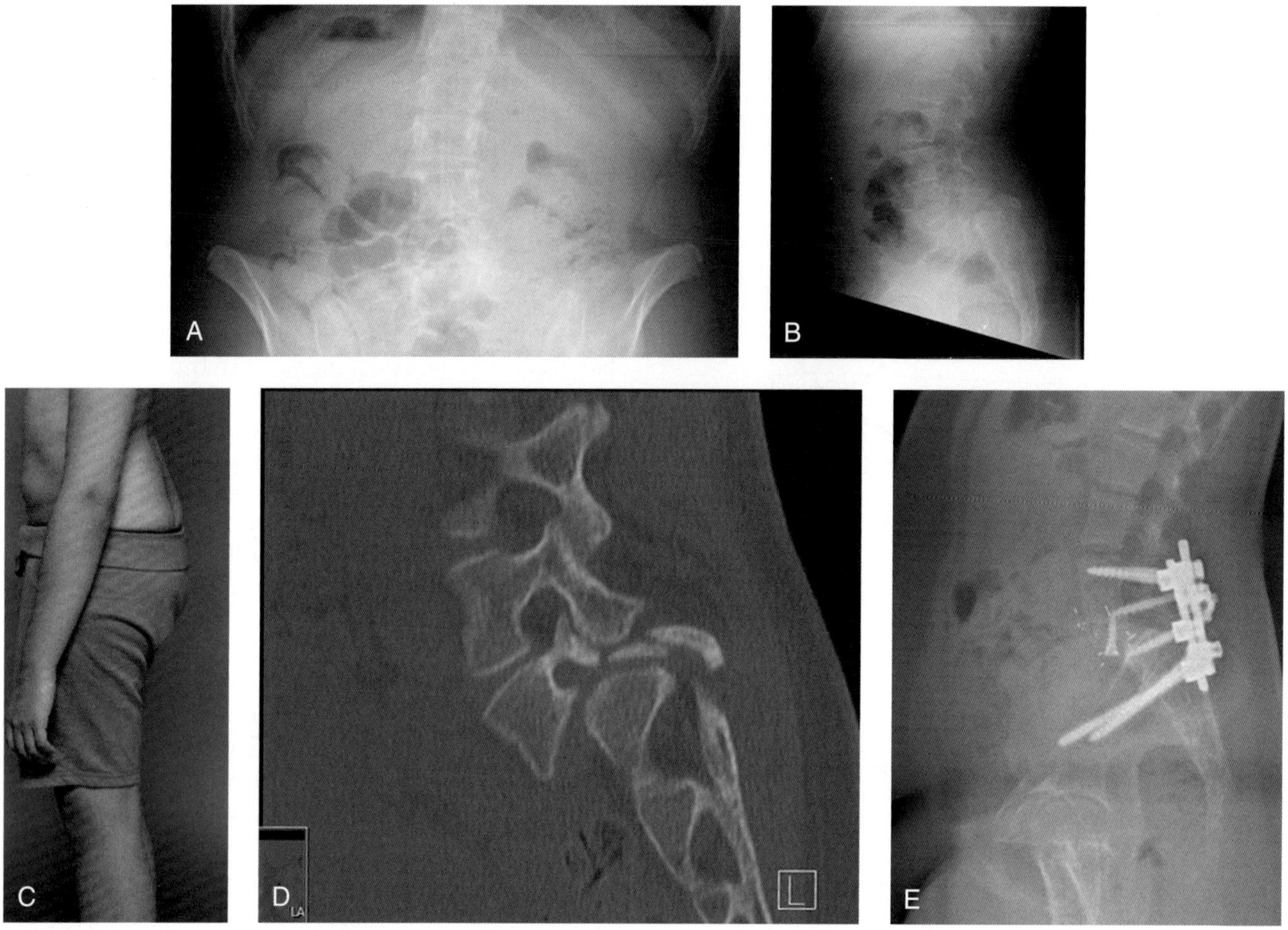

FIGURE 7 Images from a 13-year-old girl with back pain and deformity. **A**, PA standing radiograph shows apparent absence of the L5 vertebral body (the Napoleon hat sign). **B**, Lateral radiograph shows grade 4 spondylolisthesis and a retroverted pelvis. **C**, Clinical photograph shows a flattened sacrum. The L5 spinous process was not palpable. Lateral radiographs shows correction of the slip angle after anterior sacral dome osteotomy and fusion (**D**) and posterior instrumentation and fusion (**E**).

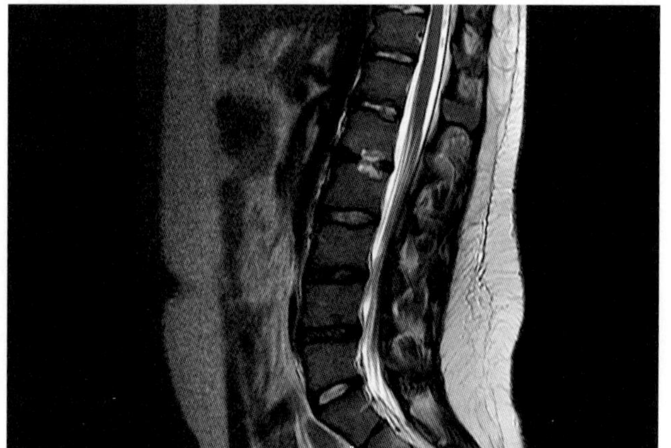

FIGURE 8 Magnetic resonance image from a 15-year-old boy who presented with a 5-week history of acute severe back pain and elevated C-reactive protein level and erythrocyte sedimentation rate. The image shows diskitis at L2-L3 and vertebral osteomyelitis at L2 and L3. Symptoms resolved with oral antibiotics and anti-inflammatory medications.

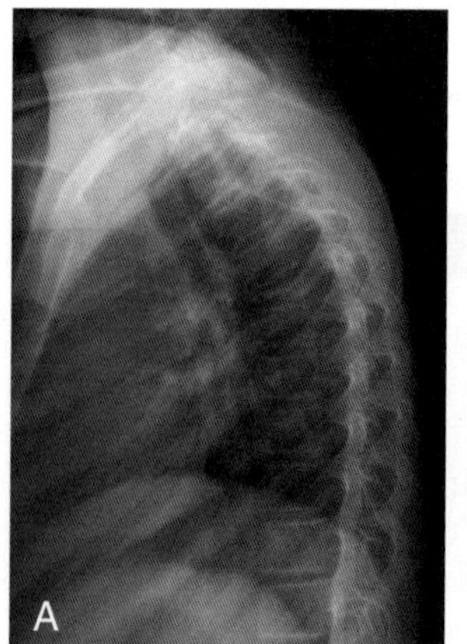

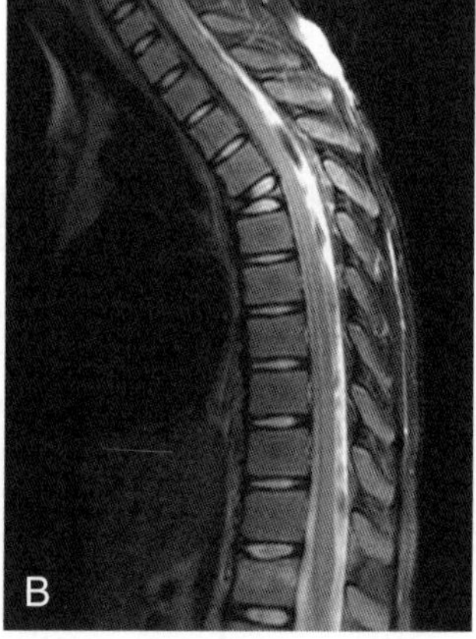

FIGURE 9 An 11-year-old girl had a 6-month history of severe back pain. **A**, Lateral radiograph shows vertebra plana secondary to eosinophilic granuloma. **B**, Sagittal magnetic resonance image shows vertebra plana. The patient should be monitored in the future for progressive kyphosis with serial radiographs, but her current spinal alignment is satisfactory.

SUMMARY

Pediatric orthopaedic surgeons will frequently need to evaluate and treat back pain in their patients. It is essential to be aware of the features for common back pain diagnoses specific to children. Although most adolescents and school-age children have idiopathic back pain, severe pain or symptoms that do not respond to nonsurgical management warrant additional workup. Disk disease and spondylolytic conditions may occur in children but rarely require surgical management. High-grade spondylolisthesis typically requires surgical management, and although the need for reduction is controversial, correction of the slip angle will likely improve the long-term durability of the surgery by improving sagittal plane correction.

KEY STUDY POINTS

- Patients younger than 18 years frequently have back pain, with 20% to 30% of patients having an underlying structural diagnosis.
- Further workup should be guided by the patient history and the findings of a careful neurologic examination and plain radiography. If the findings are benign, physical therapy and activity modification can be initiated without the need for advanced imaging.
- Symptoms from disk disease, spondylolysis, and low-grade spondylolisthesis are typically responsive to nonsurgical treatment. Surgery is indicated for patients with refractory symptoms.
- The management of high-grade spondylolisthesis is controversial, but surgery is typically recommended, particularly for patients who are symptomatic or those with documented progression.

ANNOTATED REFERENCES

1. Fabricant PD, Heath MR, Schachne JM, Doyle SM, Green DW, Widmann RF: The epidemiology of back pain in American children and adolescents. *Spine (Phila Pa 1976)* 2020;45(16):1135-1142.

   The authors of this cross-sectional survey evaluated patients between 10 and 18 years of age to determine prevalence of back pain in US adolescents. Level of evidence: IV.

2. Yang S, Werner BC, Singla A, Abel MF: Low back pain in adolescents: A 1-year analysis of eventual diagnoses. *J Pediatr Orthop* 2017;37(5):344-347.

   A review of the US National Insurance Registry between 2007 and 2010 identified 215,592 adolescents with back pain; less than 20% were given a secondary diagnosis within 1 year. Level of evidence: III.

3. Aartun E, Hartvigsen J, Boyle E, Hestbaek L: No associations between objectively measured physical activity and spinal pain in 11-15-year-old Danes. *Eur J Pain* 2016;20(3):447-457.

   Physical activity monitors revealed no association between physical activities and reported back pain in patients aged 11 to 15 years. Measurements were taken during a 2-year period. Level of evidence: III.

4. Sato T, Ito T, Hirano T, et al: Low back pain in childhood and adolescence: Assessment of sports activities. *Eur Spine J* 2011;20(1):94-99.

5. Yamato TP, Maher CG, Traeger AC, Wiliams CM, Kamper SJ: Do schoolbags cause back pain in children and adolescents? A systematic review. *Br J Sports Med* 2018;52(19):1241-1245.

   Evaluation of 69 studies showed no convincing evidence that backpacks or book bags were associated with back pain in children. Level of evidence: II.

6. Sano A, Hirano T, Watanabe K, Endo N, Ito T, Tanabe N: Body mass index is associated with low back pain in childhood and adolescence: A birth cohort study with a 6-year follow-up in Niigata city, Japan. *Eur Spine J* 2015;24(3):474-481.

7. Wirth B, Knecht C, Humphreys K: Spine day 2012: Spinal pain in Swiss school children. Epidemiology and risk factors. *BMC Pediatr* 2013;13:159.

8. Shymon SJ, Yaszay B, Dwek JR, Proudfoot JA, Donohue M, Hargens AR: Altered disc compression in children with idiopathic low back pain: An upright magnetic resonance imaging backpack study. *Spine (Phila Pa 1976)* 2014;39(3):243-248.

9. Brattberg G: Do pain problems in young school children persist into early adulthood? A 13-year follow-up. *Eur J Pain* 2004;8(3):187-199.

10. Harreby MS, Neergaard K, Hesselsøe G, Kjer J: Are low back pain and radiological changes during puberty risk factors for low back pain in adult age? A 25-year prospective cohort study of 640 school children [Danish]. *Ugeskr Laeger* 1997;159(2):171-174.

11. Expert Panel on Pediatric Imaging, Booth TN, Iyer RS, Falcone RA Jr, et al: ACR Appropriateness Criteria® back pain-child. *J Am Coll Radiol* 2017;14(5S):S13-S24.

    American College of Radiology Appropriateness Criteria are evidence-based guidelines for imaging of pediatric back pain developed by a multidisciplinary expert panel with extensive analysis of peer-reviewed journals and the application of RAND Corporation/University of California, Los Angeles Appropriateness Criteria. Level of evidence: IV.

12. Ramírez N, Olivella G, Valentín P, Feneque J, Lugo S, Iriarte I: Are constant pain, night pain, or abnormal neurological examination adequate predictors of the presence of a significant pathology associated with pediatric back pain? *J Pediatr Orthop* 2019;39(6):e478-e481.

    A total of 388 patients with unexplained back pain were included in this study. An underlying pathologic condition was identified in 56 of 132 of patients (42%) with constant pain, 61 of 162 (38%) with night pain, and 8 of 9 (89%) with abnormal neurologic examination. Level of evidence: III.

13. Ramirez N, Flynn JM, Hill BW, et al: Evaluation of a systematic approach to pediatric back pain: The utility of magnetic resonance imaging. *J Pediatr Orthop* 2015;35(1):28-32.

14. Vendhan K, Sen D, Fisher C, Ioannou Y, Hall-Craggs MA: Inflammatory changes of the lumbar spine in children and adolescents with enthesitis-related arthritis: Magnetic resonance imaging findings. *Arthritis Care Res (Hoboken)* 2014;66(1):40-46.

15. Alkhawaldeh K, Ghuweri AA, Kawar J, Jaafreh A: Back pain in children and diagnostic value of (99m)Tc MDP bone scintigraphy. *Acta Inform Med* 2014;22(5):297-301.

16. Miller R, Beck NA, Sampson NR, Zhu X, Flynn JM, Drummond D: Imaging modalities for low back pain in children: A review of spondylolysis and undiagnosed mechanical back pain. *J Pediatr Orthop* 2013;33(3):282-288.

17. Mathews JD, Forsythe AV, Brady Z, et al: Cancer risk in 680,000 people exposed to computed tomography scans in childhood or adolescence: Data linkage study of 11 million Australians. *Br Med J* 2013;346:f2360.

18. Michaleff ZA, Kamper SJ, Maher CG, Evans R, Broderick C, Henschke N: Low back pain in children and adolescents: A systematic review and meta-analysis evaluating the effectiveness of conservative interventions. *Eur Spine J* 2014;23(10):2046-2058.

19. van den Heuvel MM, Oei EHG, Bierma-Zeinstra SMA, van Middelkoop M. The prevalence of abnormalities in the pediatric spine on MRI: A systematic review and meta-analysis. *Spine (Phila Pa 1976)* 2020;45(18):E1185-E1196.

    This systematic review of pediatric MRIs showed that the pooled prevalence in nonathletes without low back pain, participants with low back pain, and athletes without low back pain was, respectively, 22%, 44%, and 22% for disk degeneration; 1%, 38%, and 13% for herniated disks; 5%, 22%, and 11% for end plate changes; and 0%, 30%, and 6% for pars fractures. Level of evidence: II.

20. Urrutia J, Zamora T, Prada C: The prevalence of degenerative or incidental findings in the lumbar spine of pediatric patients: A study using magnetic resonance imaging as a screening tool. *Eur Spine J* 2016;25(2):596-601.

    In this study of 103 patients with mean age of 6.6 years evaluated by MRI for abdominal and pelvic complaints, 10.7% had one Pfirrmann 2 disc and 1% had disc bulging. Level of evidence: IV.

21. Wiley MR, Hee Jo C, Khaleel MA, McIntosh AL: Size matters: Which adolescent patients are most likely to require surgical decompression for lumbar disk herniations? *J Pediatr Orthop* 2019;39(10):e791-e795.

    In pediatric patients with lumbar herniated nucleus pulposis, patients treated surgically had a smaller canal diameter (10 mm versus 14 mm) at L5 compared with those who were successfully treated nonsurgically. Level of evidence: III.

22. Thomas JG, Hwang SW, Whitehead WE, Curry DJ, Luerssen TG, Jea A: Minimally invasive lumbar microdiscectomy in pediatric patients: A series of 6 patients. *J Neurosurg Pediatr* 2011;7(6):616-619.

23. Çelik S, Göksu K, Çelik SE, Emir CB: Benign neurological recovery with low recurrence and low peridural fibrosis rate in pediatric disc herniations after lumbar microdiscectomy. *Pediatr Neurosurg* 2011;47(6):417-422.

24. Nagata K, Tanaka Y, Kanai H, Oshima Y: Acute complete paraplegia of 8-year-old girl caused by spinal cord infarction following minor trauma complicated with longitudinal signal change of spinal cord. *Eur Spine J* 2017;26(5):1432-1435.

    This case study reports on consecutive MRIs of a child with fibrocartilaginous embolism who developed complete paraplegia following minor trauma. Level of evidence: IV.

25. Bonic EE, Taylor JA, Knudsen JT: Posterior limbus fractures: Five case reports and a review of selected published cases. *J Manipulative Physiol Ther* 1998;21(4):281-287.

26. Singhal A, Mitra A, Cochrane D, Steinbok P: Ring apophysis fracture in pediatric lumbar disc herniation: A common entity. *Pediatr Neurosurg* 2013;49(1):16-20.

27. Chang CH, Lee ZL, Chen WJ, Tan CF, Chen LH: Clinical significance of ring apophysis fracture in adolescent lumbar disc herniation. *Spine (Phila Pa 1976)* 2008;33(16):1750-1754.

28. Higashino K, Sairyo K, Katoh S, Takao S, Kosaka H, Yasui N: Long-term outcomes of lumbar posterior apophyseal endplate lesions in children and adolescents. *J Bone Joint Surg Am* 2012;94(11):e74.

29. Greene TL, Hensinger RN, Hunter LY: Back pain and vertebral changes simulating Scheuermann's disease. *J Pediatr Orthop* 1985;5(1):1-7.

30. Blumenthal SL, Roach J, Herring JA: Lumbar Scheuermann's: A clinical series and classification. *Spine (Phila Pa 1976)* 1987;12(9):929-932.

31. Liu N, Guo X, Chen Z, et al: Radiological signs of Scheuermann disease and low back pain: Retrospective categorization of 188 hospital staff members with 6-year follow-up. *Spine (Phila Pa 1976)* 2014;39(20):1666-1675.

32. Song KS, Yang JJ: Acutely progressing paraplegia caused by traumatic disc herniation through posterior Schmorl's node opening into the spinal canal in lumbar Scheuermann's disease. *Spine (Phila Pa 1976)* 2011;36(24):E1588-E1591.

33. Crawford CH III, Ledonio CG, Bess RS, et al: Current evidence regarding the surgical and nonsurgical treatment of pediatric lumbar spondylolysis: A report from the Scoliosis Research Society Evidence-Based Medicine Committee. *Spine Deform* 2015;3(1):30-44.

34. Ledonio CG, Burton DC, Crawford CH III, et al: Current evidence regarding diagnostic imaging methods for pediatric lumbar spondylolysis: A report from the Scoliosis Research Society Evidence-Based Medicine Committee. *Spine Deform* 2017;5(2):97-101.

    A structured literature review evaluating imaging techniques for pediatric spondylolysis. Level of evidence: II.

35. Beck NA, Miller R, Baldwin K, et al: Do oblique views add value in the diagnosis of spondylolysis in adolescents? *J Bone Joint Surg Am* 2013;95(10):e65.

36. Fadell MF, Gralla J, Bercha I, et al: CT outperforms radiographs at a comparable radiation dose in the assessment for spondylolysis. *Pediatr Radiol* 2015;45(7):1026-1030.

37. Wren TAL, Ponrartana S, Aggabao PC, Poorghasamians E, Skaggs DL, Gilsanz V: Increased lumbar lordosis and smaller vertebral cross-sectional area are associated with spondylolysis. *Spine (Phila Pa 1976)* 2018;43(12):833-838.

    MRI morphology study of 35 adolescents with spondylolysis and 86 control subjects showed increased lumbar lordosis and decreased vertebral body cross-sectional area in children with spondylolysis. Level of evidence: IV.

38. Tofte JN, CarlLee TL, Holte AJ, Sitton SE, Weinstein SL: Imaging pediatric spondylolysis: A systematic review. *Spine (Phila Pa 1976)* 2017;42(10):777-782.

    On review of 10 articles, when compared with SPECT, the average sensitivity of CT was 85% and the sensitivity of MRI was 80% for detecting a pars lesion. Level of evidence: III.

39. Kobayashi A, Kobayashi T, Kato K, Higuchi H, Takagishi K: Diagnosis of radiographically occult lumbar spondylolysis in young athletes by magnetic resonance imaging. *Am J Sports Med* 2013;41(1):169-176.

40. Rush JK, Astur N, Scott S, Kelly DM, Sawyer JR, Warner WC Jr: Use of magnetic resonance imaging in the evaluation of spondylolysis. *J Pediatr Orthop* 2015;35(3): 271-275.

41. Álvarez-Díaz P, Alentorn-Geli E, Steinbacher G, Rius M, Pellisé F, Cugat R: Conservative treatment of lumbar spondylolysis in young soccer players. *Knee Surg Sports Traumatol Arthrosc* 2011;19(12):2111-2114.

42. Sairyo K, Sakai T, Amari R, Yasui N: Causes of radiculopathy in young athletes with spondylolysis. *Am J Sports Med* 2010;38(2):357-362.

43. El Rassi G, Takemitsu M, Glutting J, Shah SA: Effect of sports modification on clinical outcome in children and adolescent athletes with symptomatic lumbar spondylolysis. *Am J Phys Med Rehabil* 2013;92(12):1070-1074.

44. Sousa T, Skaggs DL, Chan P, et al: Benign natural history of spondylolysis in adolescence with midterm follow-up. *Spine Deform* 2017;5(2):134-138.

    Patients treated nonsurgically for spondylolysis were surveyed at a mean of 8 years following diagnosis regarding back pain and activity levels. Level of evidence: III.

45. Sakai T, Tezuka F, Yamashita K, et al: Conservative treatment for bony healing in pediatric lumbar spondylolysis. *Spine (Phila Pa 1976)* 2017;42(12):E716-E720.

    Bony healing was achieved in pediatric patients with early-stage spondolytic defects in the spine treated with bracing treatment, but recurrence rates were high. Level of evidence: III.

46. Menga EN, Kebaish KM, Jain A, Carrino JA, Sponseller PD: Clinical results and functional outcomes after direct intralaminar screw repair of spondylolysis. *Spine (Phila Pa 1976)* 2014;39(1):104-110.

47. Karatas AF, Dede O, Atanda AA, et al: Comparison of direct pars repair techniques of spondylolysis in pediatric and adolescent patients: Pars compression screw versus pedicle screw-rod-hook. *Clin Spine Surg* 2016;29(7):272-280.

    In this retrospective study, nine patients with spondylolysis who were treated with an intralaminar screw and seven patients treated with a pedicle screw, rod, and laminar hook construct had similar excellent results. Level of evidence: III.

48. Labelle H, Mac-Thiong JM, Roussouly P: Spino-pelvic sagittal balance of spondylolisthesis: A review and classification. *Eur Spine J* 2011;20(suppl 5):641-646.

49. Lundine KM, Lewis SJ, Al-Aubaidi Z, Alman B, Howard AW: Patient outcomes in the operative and nonoperative management of high-grade spondylolisthesis in children. *J Pediatr Orthop* 2014;34(5):483-489.

50. Harris IE, Weinstein SL: Long-term follow-up of patients with grade-III and IV spondylolisthesis: Treatment with and without posterior fusion. *J Bone Joint Surg Am* 1987;69(7):960-969.

51. Bourassa-Moreau É, Mac-Thiong JM, Joncas J, Parent S, Labelle H: Quality of life of patients with high-grade spondylolisthesis: Minimum 2-year follow-up after surgical and nonsurgical treatments. *Spine J* 2013;13(7):770-774.

52. Wang Z, Wang B, Yin B, Liu W, Yang F, Lv G: The relationship between spinopelvic parameters and clinical symptoms of severe isthmic spondylolisthesis: A prospective study of 64 patients. *Eur Spine J* 2014;23(3):560-568.

53. Nwachukwu BU, Schairer WW, Pan T, et al: Bone morphogenetic proteins in pediatric spinal arthrodesis: A statewide analysis of trends and outcome of utilization. *J Pediatr Orthop* 2017;37(6):e369-e374.

    This review of a statewide database from New York showed a peak of bone morphogenetic protein use in pediatric spine fusions around 2008, and no association between bone morphogenetic protein use and subsequent revision surgery was found. Level of evidence: III.

54. Kasliwal MK, Smith JS, Shaffrey CI, et al: Short-term complications associated with surgery for high-grade spondylolisthesis in adults and pediatric patients: A report from the scoliosis research society morbidity and mortality database. *Neurosurgery* 2012;71(1):109-116.

55. Li Y, Lubelski D, Abdullah KG, Mroz TE, Steinmetz MP: Minimally invasive tubular resection of the anomalous transverse process in patients with Bertolotti's syndrome: Presented at the 2013 Joint Spine Section Meeting. Clinical article. *J Neurosurg Spine* 2014;20(3):283-290.

56. Spencer SJ, Wilson NI: Childhood discitis in a regional children's hospital. *J Pediatr Orthop B* 2012;21(3):264-268.

57. Dayer R, Alzahrani MM, Saran N, et al: Spinal infections in children: A multicentre retrospective study. *Bone Joint J* 2018;100-B(4):542-548.

    In 103 pediatric patients with diskitis or other spinal infection, 8 had positive blood cultures, and of 20 who were biopsied 8 had isolated pathogens, most commonly methicillin-sensitive *S aureus* and *K kingae*. Level of evidence: IV.

58. Ceroni D, Belaieff W, Kanavaki A, et al: Possible association of *Kingella kingae* with infantile spondylodiscitis. *Pediatr Infect Dis J* 2013;32(11):1296-1298.

59. Roach JW, Klatt JW, Faulkner ND: Involvement of the spine in patients with multiple hereditary exostoses. *J Bone Joint Surg Am* 2009;91(8):1942-1948.

60. Ashraf A, Larson AN, Ferski G, Mielke CH, Wetjen NM, Guidera KJ: Spinal stenosis frequent in children with multiple hereditary exostoses. *J Child Orthop* 2013;7(3):183-194.

61. Jackson TJ, Shah AS, Arkader A: Is routine spine MRI necessary in skeletally immature patients with MHE? Identifying patients at risk for spinal osteochondromas. *J Pediatr Orthop* 2019;39(2):e147-e152.

Of 227 patients with multiple hereditary exostoses, 21 underwent advanced spinal imaging, of whom 8 had spinal lesions and 4 had intracanal lesions. Level of evidence: IV.

62. Zenonos G, Jamil O, Governale LS, Jernigan S, Hedequist D, Proctor MR: Surgical treatment for primary spinal aneurysmal bone cysts: Experience from Children's Hospital Boston. *J Neurosurg Pediatr* 2012;9(3):305-315.

63. Novais EN, Rose PS, Yaszemski MJ, Sim FH: Aneurysmal bone cyst of the cervical spine in children. *J Bone Joint Surg Am* 2011;93(16):1534-1543.

SECTION 7

Trauma

Section Editor:
Mark R. Sinclair, MD, FAAOS

CHAPTER 37

Principles of Pediatric Trauma Care

MAURICIO SILVA, MD • ANTHONY A. SCADUTO, MD

ABSTRACT

Fractures are common in children, with most caused by ground-level falls and sports activities. Certain fracture patterns, however, should raise concerns for an abusive etiology. For children with a fracture, younger age, black race, intracranial injury, a concomitant rib fracture, and burns are positive predictive factors of nonaccidental trauma. The anatomy and physiology of children influences the types of fractures seen as well as the treatment options. By considering the effect of age and fracture location on the capacity for remodeling, most fractures in children can be safely managed nonsurgically. Ketamine and intravenous sedation are commonly used during closed manipulation, but local and regional drugs can also provide effective analgesia in the pediatric population. Effective casting is less dependent on the casting material than the technique used. Careful cast application and removal reduces the risk of complications associated with immobilization, such as thermal injuries and pressure sores. Infections after an open fracture, compartment syndrome, and premature physeal arrest are some important complications of fractures in children. If intravenous antibiotics are administered soon after an open fracture, infections can be minimized. This should be coupled with irrigation and débridement within 24 hours of the injury in most cases. An increasing need for pain medication can be the only sign of an impending compartment syndrome in a child. Physeal fractures that have a high risk of growth arrest, such as those of the distal femur and tibia, require long-term surveillance to avoid angular deformities and limb-length discrepancies. The treatment of a traumatic growth arrest includes bar resection, epiphysiodesis, osteotomy, or limb lengthening or/shortening—depending on the extent of the arrest and the amount of growth remaining.

Keywords: compartment syndrome; fracture; management; physeal injury; polytrauma

Neither of the following authors nor any immediate family member has received anything of value from or has stock or stock options held in a commercial company or institution related directly or indirectly to the subject of this chapter: Dr. Silva and Dr. Scaduto.

INTRODUCTION

Each year, one out of every four children in the United States requires urgent medical care for accidental injury.[1] Roughly, this accounts for more than 9 million visits per year.[2] Although most of these injuries are sprains and contusions, nearly 50% of all boys and 25% of all girls sustain at least one fracture before reaching 16 years of age,[3] with the incidence of fractures peaking in children aged 10 to 14 years. Pediatric fractures managed in the emergency department most commonly involve the forearm, humerus, hand, or wrist[2,4] and most (94%) are managed on an outpatient basis.[4] The most common pediatric fractures requiring hospitalization are femur (20%) and humerus (18%) fractures.[5]

Although access to pediatric trauma care has diminished in many regions of the United States during the past decade,[6] orthopaedic surgeons continue to provide the bulk of fracture care to children. To optimize care, it is essential to understand the influence growth can have on both fracture healing and remodeling as well as recognize the complications unique to the growing skeleton.

MECHANISMS OF INJURY

The rate and pattern of musculoskeletal injuries vary by age. Children younger than 5 years most commonly sustain low-energy fractures at home, whereas recreational and playground injuries are more common in school-aged children. Children who are obese may have an increased risk for fractures caused by ground-level falls.[7] Sleep deprivation also increases injury rates among middle and high school athletes. One study found adolescents who slept less than 8 hours a day were 1.7 times more likely to have an injury than students who slept more than 8 hours.[8]

Children older than 10 years are physically larger, stronger, and practice longer than younger children, all of which may contribute to a greater risk for sports-related injuries. Single-sport specialization has become more common in youth athletics. Even while accounting for more hours of physical activity, sports specialization is independently associated with higher injury rates.[9,10]

In 2000, the Centers for Disease Control and Prevention reported the top eight sports-related activities associated with injuries in children aged 5 to 14 years: baseball, basketball, bicycling, football, playground equipment, roller sports, soccer, and trampolining. One national database study found that sports-specific injury rates had significantly improved over the past decade for many sports, including bicycling (38%), roller sports (20%), and trampolining (17%). In contrast, football injuries increased by 22% during the same period. Of concern to many is that football-related concussions have more than doubled in the past decade.[11]

High-energy Trauma

Severe and life-threatening musculoskeletal injuries in children are most commonly caused by falls from a height or motor vehicle accidents. Between 2007 and 2011, 2,238 pediatric traumatic amputations were reported in the national trauma databank. The most common injury mechanisms were being caught between two objects, machinery, powered lawn mowers, and motor vehicle collisions.[12] Motor vehicle collisions caused 8% of all amputations and were the leading cause of all amputations in adolescents. The increased use of child safety seats has reduced morbidity and mortality rates in children who are involved in motor vehicle crashes. Current safety guidelines include the recommended use of booster seats for children in the age range of 5 to 12 years.[13] Recent studies have shown that proper restraints in children involved in motor vehicle collisions are less common in children between the ages of 4 and 8 years, reinforcing the importance of proper use of child safety devices, including booster seats.[14,15] Most children with motor vehicle–related injuries are pedestrians who were struck by a vehicle. All-terrain vehicle (ATV)–related injuries disproportionally affect children. Although only 14% to 18% of ATV riders are children, they account for 37% to 57% of those injured in such vehicles.[16] Rollover is the most common mechanism of injury; however, children are substantially more likely than adults to be involved in collisions.[17,18] Snowmobile, ATVs, and dirt bike accidents involving children result in severe orthopaedic and associated injuries with distinct profiles. Snowmobile injuries are more likely to have a higher Injury Severity Score and higher incidence of axial fractures, lower extremity fractures, and abdominal and genitourinary injuries. ATV injuries are more likely to result in upper extremity fractures, open fractures, and head and thoracic injuries. Dirt bike injuries commonly include femur, clavicle, and thoracic fractures.[19]

Nonaccidental Trauma

Fractures are a common finding in children who have sustained nonaccidental trauma. The orthopaedic surgeon plays a critical role in recognizing and treating child abuse. It is estimated that between one-third and one-half of all children who are abused are seen by an orthopaedic surgeon.[20] The overall prevalence of nonaccidental trauma in children admitted to a hospital with a fracture has been reported to be 1.54%.[21] Certain fractures have a high likelihood of an abusive etiology, including posterior fractures of the ribs, metaphyseal corner fractures, long bone fractures in nonambulatory children, or multiple fractures in different stages of healing. A spiral fracture of the femur in a young child had been thought to be possibly indicative of nonaccidental trauma; however, several studies have shown that a transverse fracture pattern of the femoral shaft is more predictive of nonaccidental trauma.[20,22] For children with a fracture, younger age, black race, intracranial injury, a concomitant rib fracture, and burns are positive predictive factors of nonaccidental trauma.[21]

PEDIATRIC SKELETAL SYSTEM AND FRACTURE PATTERNS

Anatomy

Unlike adult bones, pediatric bones contain open epiphyseal plates and a thick periosteal layer. The presence of this thickened, highly osteogenic periosteum allows for faster fracture healing and the ability to remodel over time. With increasing age, the periosteum thins and its osteogenic capability decreases. Pediatric bones are less dense, are more porous, are penetrated by more vascular channels, and have a lower mineral content. Consequently, they have a lower modulus of elasticity and bending strength. The diaphysis, where the primary center of ossification is located during development, is highly vascular in a newborn. With age, vascularity decreases and the cortices thicken because of periosteum-induced bone formation. The metaphysis is wider than the diaphysis and has an increased amount of trabecular bone. After a fracture, much of the remodeling process happens in the metaphysis. The physis is composed of an expandable matrix that allows long bone growth through endochondral ossification. Most epiphyses are completely cartilaginous at birth. The epiphysis is rarely injured in its cartilaginous form. As the ossification of the epiphysis increases through the secondary center of ossification, so does the risk of injury.

Fracture Patterns

Pediatric bones are anatomically and mechanically different than adult bones. As such, many fracture patterns are unique to children. In general, pediatric fractures can be classified into five different types: plastic deformation, torus or buckle fractures, greenstick fractures, complete fractures, and physeal fractures. Plastic deformation is most commonly seen in the ulna and the fibula. Buckle fractures are mostly seen in the metaphyseal portion of long bones where porosity is greatest and the cortex is thin. Greenstick fractures demonstrate a characteristic failure of the tension cortex with a mirroring plastic deformity of the compression cortex. Complete fractures can be further subdivided into spiral, oblique, and transverse patterns. Comminution can occur but is less common than in adults. The thick periosteum tends to limit the amount of fracture displacement. An injury to the epiphysis frequently includes an associated injury to the epiphyseal plate. Conversely, not all epiphyseal plate injuries have an associated epiphyseal (or articular surface) injury. The physis and the epiphysis are firmly connected to the metaphysis by periosteum. In children, most joint capsules and ligaments originate and insert on the epiphysis of a long bone. It has been generally accepted that such capsules and ligaments are stronger than the bones in which they attach; therefore, an injury that results in ligament stretching would result in a fracture in a child. (In an adult, however, ligament stretching results in a ligament strain.) This concept has been challenged with advanced imaging studies in pediatric patients with suspected nondisplaced physeal fractures of the distal fibula, suggesting that ligament sprains are actually quite common in this clinical scenario.[23] Injuries that involve the epiphyseal plate usually occur through the hypertrophic zone, although variability of the fracture plane within the physis has been suggested.[24]

Classification

Traditionally, fractures that involve the epiphyseal plate in a child have been classified using the Salter-Harris system (**Figure 1**). In general, better prognosis is expected with lower energy injuries not involving the epiphysis (types I-II); the prognosis is poorer for those that involve the epiphysis (types III-IV) or are associated with high energy (type V). Anatomic reduction is usually necessary to minimize growth arrest with types III and IV fractures. Although it has generally been accepted that anatomic reduction is not necessary for types I and II fractures, this might not be generalized to all anatomic locations. The risk of growth arrest is less reliably predicted by the Salter-Harris fracture type if the fracture is through a nonplanar physis.[25,26] It has been suggested that, when treating Salter-Harris I and II fractures of the distal tibia, a residual physeal gap (>3 mm) may represent entrapped periosteum that could lead to a higher incidence of premature physeal closure if not removed surgically.[25] However, a 2013 study demonstrated that surgical management with removal of interposed tissue and stable anatomic reduction improved joint alignment but did not reduce the incidence of premature physeal closure.[27] Although less commonly used, a comprehensive classification of long bone fractures in children has also been described.[28] This comprehensive classification allows for a detailed description of fracture patterns associated with fractures of the upper and lower extremities.[29,30]

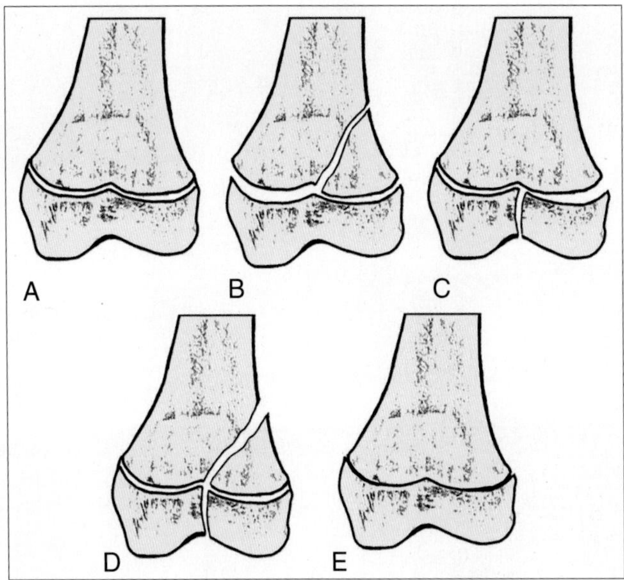

FIGURE 1 Illustration of the Salter-Harris classification for fractures. **A**, Type I. **B**, Type II. **C**, Type III. **D**, Type IV. **E**, Type V.

Healing and Remodeling

Fractures in children heal faster and more predictably than those in adults. Contributing factors include a thick and highly osteogenic periosteum, a more rapid initial inflammatory response because of higher bone vascularity (effectively shortening the early stages of fracture healing), and a lower likelihood of soft-tissue disruption. Pediatric bones have the ability to straighten residual deformities. The stresses and strains of the regular use of the bone (Wolff law), as well as reorientation of the

Section 7: Trauma

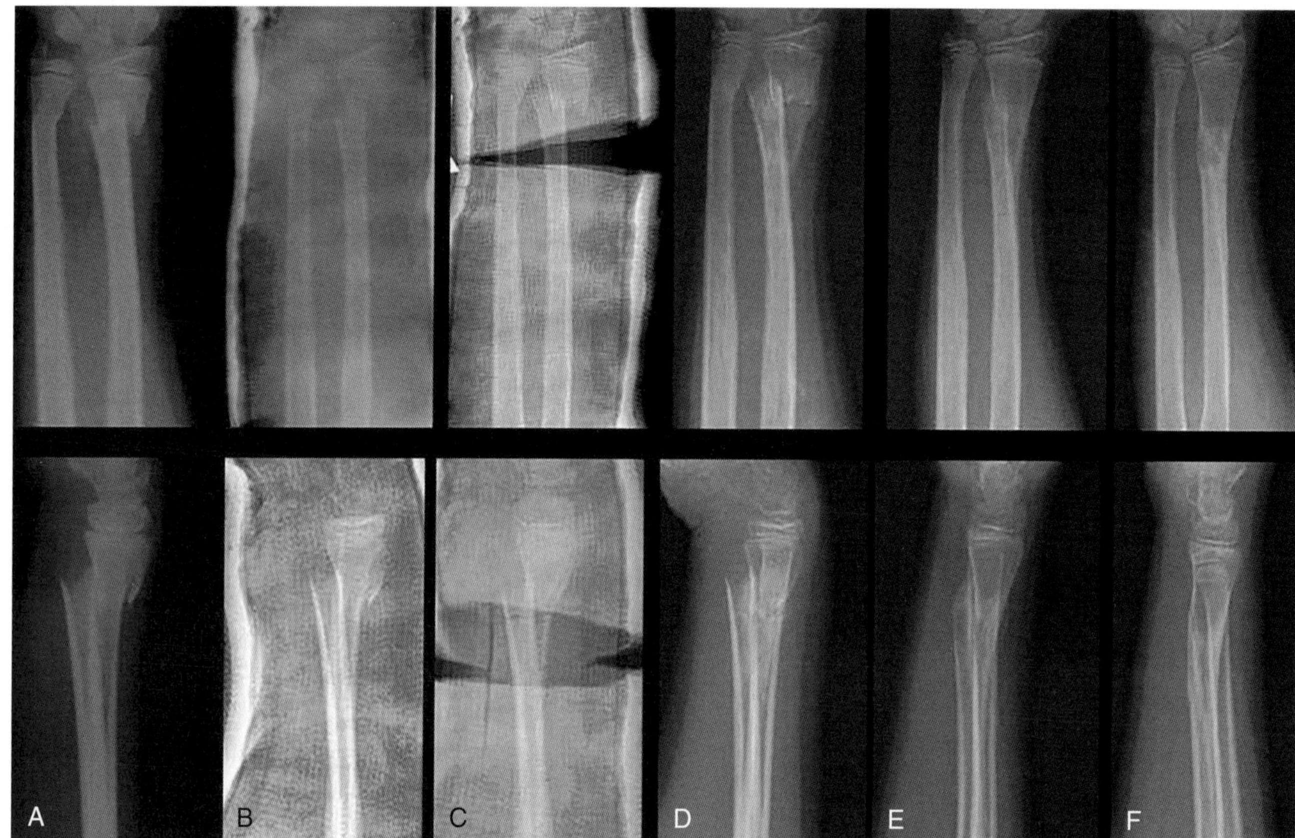

FIGURE 2 AP (top row) and lateral (bottom row) radiographs of remodeling after fracture of the distal radius and ulna. **A**, The initial injury. **B**, The fractures after reduction. **C**, The fractures after cast-wedging at 1 week after injury. The fractures 1 month (**D**), 3 months (**E**), and 8 months (**F**) after injury.

physis by asymmetric growth after a fracture (Hueter-Volkmann law), contribute to the remodeling capacity of pediatric fractures (**Figure 2**). The ranges of acceptable fracture reduction parameters are, therefore, broader than those for adults. In general, the ability to remodel varies based on the bone involved, the patient's skeletal maturity, the location of the fracture and its proximity to the physis, the contribution of the closest physis to the overall growth of the affected bone, and the plane of deformity.[31] A 10-year-old boy with a sagittal malunion of the metaphysis of the distal radius will have a greater potential for remodeling than a 12-year-old girl with a sagittal malunion of the proximal neck of the radius. In general, nonunion is uncommon in children. It appears that the risk of nonunion is highest with lateral condyle fractures of the humerus and open diaphyseal fractures of the tibia[32,33] (**Figure 3**).

FRACTURE MANAGEMENT

History and Physical Examination

A complete patient history and thorough physical examination are of primary importance when assessing a child with a possible fracture. It is crucial to determine the mechanism of injury. Although most fractures in children are isolated and the result of low-energy trauma, some are associated with high-energy mechanisms that can often involve multiple systems and result in life-threatening conditions. In such cases, a coordinated management of all injuries by members of the trauma team is critical to minimize morbidity and mortality. The presence of comorbidities should be considered. For instance, obese children have been shown to have a higher risk of loss of reduction after forearm fractures, more severe supracondylar fractures,[34] and more frequent complications with femur fractures.[35]

In the event of an isolated, low-energy injury, the affected extremity is inspected for the presence of deformity, swelling, ecchymosis, skin breakdown, and the possibility of exposed bone. All occluding dressings and splints should be removed to ensure a proper examination. Careful palpation of the entire affected extremity, with localization of the point of maximum tenderness, is helpful to determine the location of the possible fracture. Tenderness in more than one anatomic location should suggest the possibility of additional fractures.

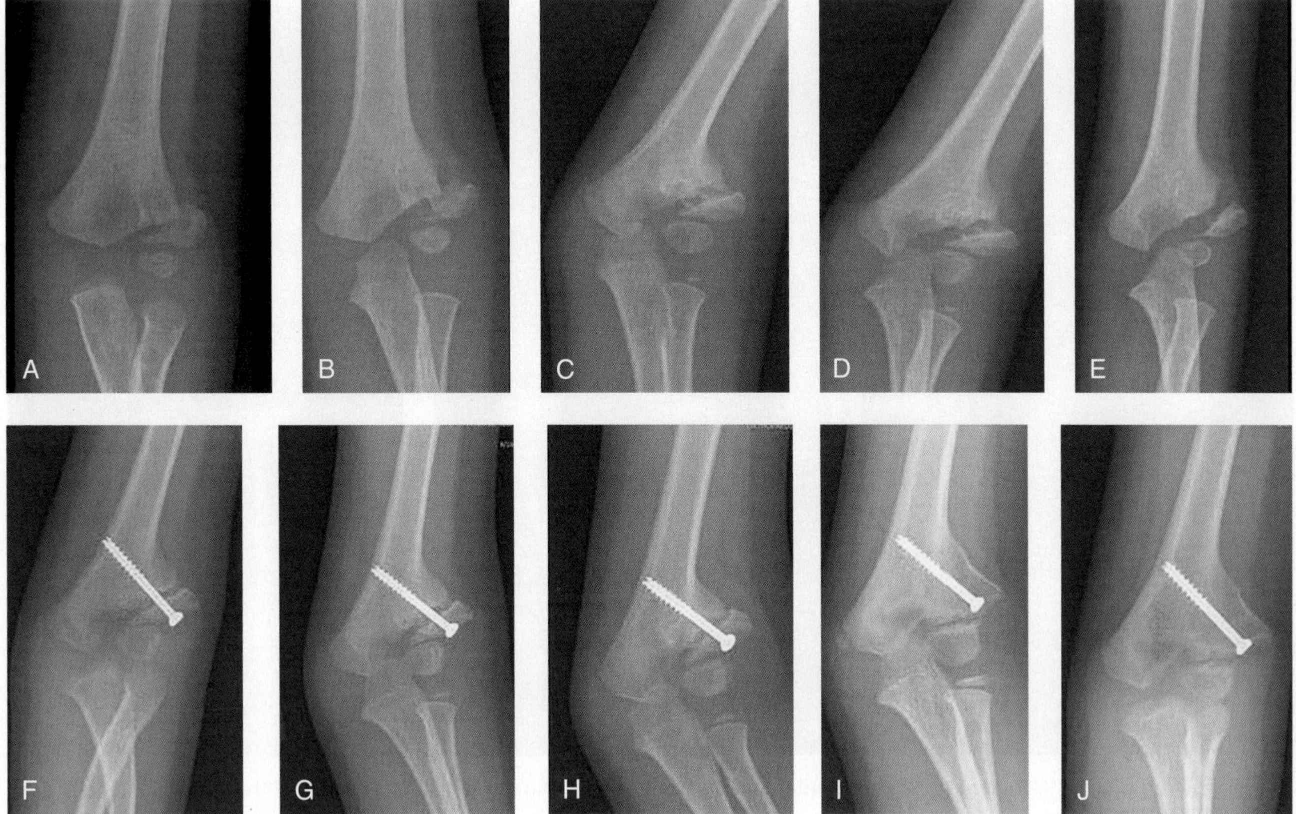

FIGURE 3 AP radiographs of fracture nonunion in a child, which is generally uncommon. The lateral condyle of the humerus is one of the few anatomic areas where nonunion can be observed. In this patient, a nonunion of the lateral condyle of the humerus was managed with percutaneous in situ screw fixation. **A**, The initial injury. The fracture at 2 months (**B**), 1 year (**C**), and 1.5 years (**D** and **E**) after injury. The fracture at 1 month (**F**), 2 months (**G**), 3 months (**H**), 1 year (**I**), and 2 years (**J**) after surgical fixation.

The compartments should be evaluated for the presence of excessive swelling and pain. A careful neurovascular examination should be performed, including motor and sensory examinations, the documentation of pulses, and assessment of capillary refill. After a focused examination of the affected extremity is performed, a rapid assessment of the remaining extremities should be completed to rule out the presence of additional injuries.

Imaging

Most fractures can be adequately evaluated with high-quality orthogonal radiographs of the affected area, including images of the joints above and below the suspected site of fracture. Oblique radiographs of the pediatric elbow and ankle are routinely obtained to facilitate the diagnosis of minimally displaced fractures (**Figure 4**). Special views could be helpful to determine displacement in specific anatomic areas. The routine use of comparison radiographs does not appear to increase diagnostic accuracy and is no longer favored. Although CT is useful for assessing pelvic, spinal, and intra-articular injuries, it is not routinely used for fracture assessment because it involves a large amount of ionizing radiation. Ultrasonography has been used to detect minimally displaced fractures of the upper extremity in children.[36,37]

Pain Control

Local and Regional Drugs

Effective and safe levels of analgesia and sedation are desirable to minimize pain and apprehension during the closed reduction and immobilization of fractures in children. Several local and regional techniques have been described and are used in the pediatric population, including hematoma blocks, intravenous regional blocks, and regional nerve blocks. Infiltration of the fracture hematoma has commonly been used to reduce distal forearm and ankle fractures in children. It has been suggested that in the setting of a pediatric distal forearm fracture, local anesthesia is less frequently used than sedation[38] and, as an adjunct to sedation, confers no additional benefits.[39] However, a 2015 report suggested that the use of a hematoma block in this setting provides similar clinical and radiographic outcomes (including pain

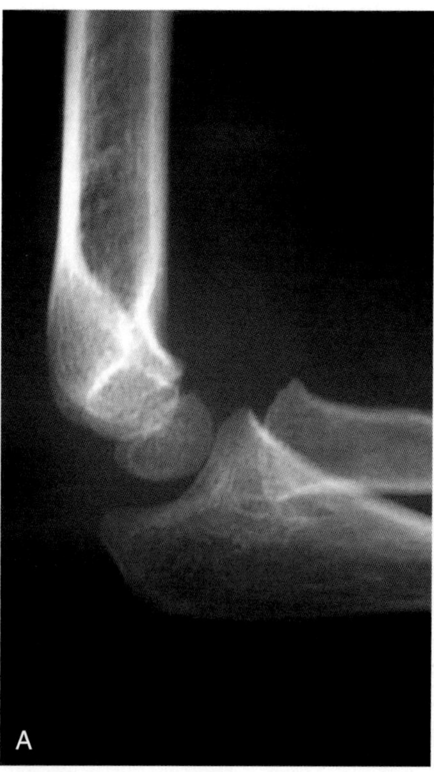

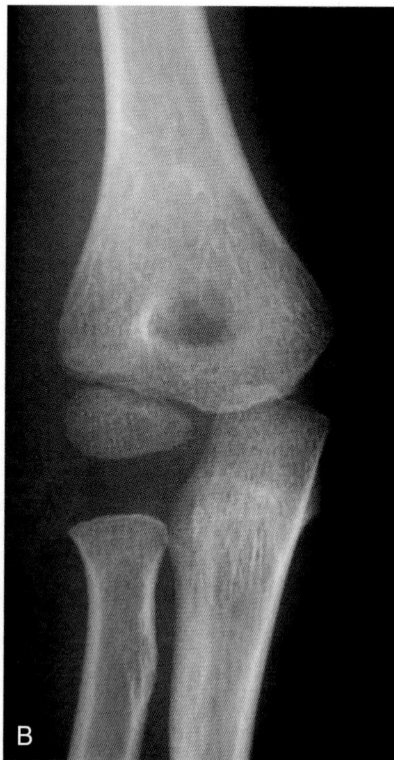

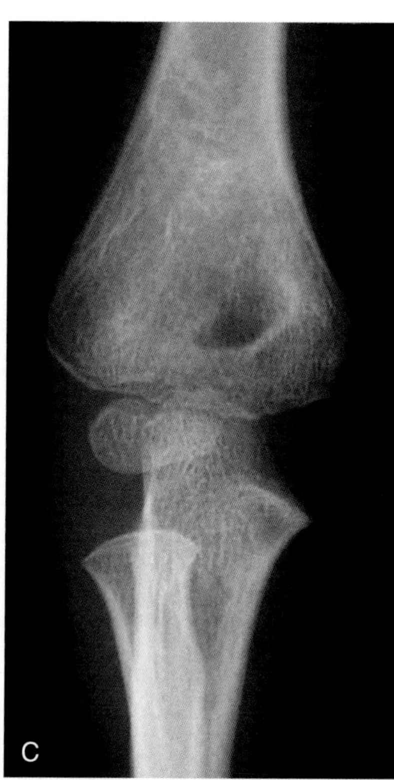

FIGURE 4 Lateral (**A**), AP (**B**), and internal oblique (**C**) radiographs of a minimally displaced fracture of the lateral condyle of the humerus in a child.

and patient satisfaction) as those obtained with sedation, while significantly reducing the patient's time in the emergency department and the use of resources.[40] Intravenous regional anesthesia has been shown to be safe and cost-effective when reducing pediatric fractures, providing satisfactory analgesia in more than 90% of patients.[41,42] Although regional nerve blocks (brachial plexus) are more commonly used in surgical settings, their use in the emergency department has proved safe for pediatric forearm fracture manipulation and results in procedural distress and pain levels comparable with those obtained with deep sedation.[43]

Conscious Sedation and Dissociative Anesthesia

Conscious sedation, a state of depressed consciousness in which the patient maintains a patent airway and protective reflexes, is commonly used to achieve fracture reduction in the pediatric population. Sedation can be obtained by using either inhalational (nitrous oxide) or parenteral (opiate analgesics and benzodiazepines) agents. Pain relief and a safe level of sedation are usually obtained with these techniques. A combination of inhalational agents and a hematoma block has also been described.[44]

Dissociative anesthesia, a cataleptic, trancelike state induced by pharmacologic agents capable of causing dissociation of the thalamoneocortical and limbic areas of the brain, can impede the perception of noxious stimuli and provides a combination of sedation, analgesia, and amnesia.[42,45] Dissociative anesthesia is commonly used for fracture reduction in pediatric patients in emergency settings.[45-47] Ketamine, a dissociative anesthetic, is commonly coupled with midazolam. When compared with other parenteral drug combinations, the ketamine-midazolam therapy demonstrates fewer respiratory events and less need for supplemental oxygen and airway maneuvers.[46,47] Specific protocols to ensure the safety of the sedation procedure should be adopted.[48] The availability of personnel with up-to-date training and skills and appropriate equipment for airway management is essential.

Perioperative Pain

The use of perioperative opioid medications has been commonplace in the management of pain associated with pediatric fractures.[49] Hydrocodone in combination with acetaminophen is the most prescribed drug in the United States.[49] The misuse of unused portions of opioid prescriptions has contributed to the ongoing opioid epidemic in the United States. Several strategies have been suggested to address the crisis, including physician-patient education, prescription monitoring and drug disposal programs, use of peripheral nerve blocks, and nonopioid analgesic alternatives.[49]

Preoperative education of patients should include specific instructions on the postoperative tapering of narcotics and when to be discontinued.[49] The potential for overprescription and opioid diversion was demonstrated in a prospective study involving pediatric supracondylar humerus fractures, in which patients used less than 25% of the prescribed opioid medication. The authors suggested that a prescription of seven opioid doses should be sufficient to effectively manage postoperative pain after these types of fractures.[50] The use of surgical site–specific peripheral regional anesthetic techniques as part of multimodal analgesia has been recommended for children undergoing extremity surgery.[51] Acetaminophen, alone or in combination with NSAIDs, has been recommended for the management of postoperative pain in children undergoing treatment for fractures.[51,52] Use of systemic NSAIDs perioperatively during the management of supracondylar humerus fractures has shown to effectively decrease postoperative pain, opioid usage, hospitalization costs, and length of stay.[53]

Splinting and Casting

Most pediatric fractures can be managed with immediate reduction and immobilization in a well-molded cast. Traditional splinting is usually preferred for patients if the injury is associated with severe swelling, in patients who are unable to communicate or insensate, or as a temporary measure in patients undergoing subsequent surgical treatment. It is generally accepted that a well-molded cast is more reliable than a traditional splint for maintaining fracture reduction. Removable splints have been shown to be advantageous for the management of some stable fractures.[54] Advocates of splint immobilization highlight the fact that splints can be taken off without exposing the child to the noise associated with a cast saw, a factor that has been identified as one of the most negative aspects of cast use from a child's perspective.[55-57]

No consensus is available on the optimal casting material for pediatric fractures. Plaster is more easily molded and is less expensive than fiberglass, but it is heavier and less resistant to water. Fiberglass is less malleable than plaster during the setting period and has a reduced capacity to create a good mold, but it is stronger, lighter, and water resistant.[58]

When applied by well-trained personnel, the use of casting is usually safe. However, it is critical to be aware of potential complications associated with casting, including stiffness, thermal injuries, localized pressure, and compartment syndrome.[59] The setting of plaster involves an exothermic reaction that generates heat. Care must be taken to avoid using a dip water temperature greater than 24°C (75°F), using excessively thick plaster, folding over the edges of splints (effectively increasing thickness), and placing the limb on a pillow during the curing process.[59,60] Although the risk of thermal injury is much lower with fiberglass, the risk of creating a constrictive bandage is greater. Proper application by stretching the material and allowing it to relax before rolling it on the affected extremity is critical to minimize this risk. In addition, overwrapping of plaster in fiberglass should be delayed until the plaster is fully cured and cooled. The application of padding, including self-adhesive foam padding, over pressure-sensitive areas can minimize pressure sores. For example, the addition of heel padding has proven to be effective in reducing the incidence of cast-related skin complications for patients receiving a lower extremity cast.[61]

The presence of increased pain and/or neurovascular change after cast application demands a careful evaluation and consideration of the possibility of compartment syndrome. Splitting or removing the cast might be necessary. Care must be taken to minimize the risk of cast saw cuts and burns. Sliding the oscillating saw along the cast should be avoided. The risk of burns and cuts can be reduced by applying appropriate padding during casting, properly training personnel in the use of cast saws, frequently changing the saw blade (dull blades generate more heat), and cooling the blade periodically during cast removal.[62] A recent study highlighted the effectiveness of simulation-based training for orthopaedic surgical residents in reducing cast saw injuries. The authors reported an 11-to-1 return of investment when considering the cost of medicolegal payments associated with cast burns.[63]

SPECIAL SITUATIONS

Polytrauma

Trauma is the leading cause of death in children aged 1 to 19 years in the United States.[64] Although extremity fractures are present in more than 60% of pediatric patients with polytrauma, approximately 80% of the deaths associated with high-energy trauma result from traumatic brain injury.[65] Compared with adult trauma centers, it has been reported that the treatment of a pediatric patient with multiple injuries at a pediatric trauma center results in 20% to 50% lower rate of mortality.[66,67] The initial care of the pediatric patients with polytrauma should include a rapid assessment of any respiratory or circulatory compromise, with prompt management of any deficiency in oxygenation, ventilation, or perfusion. Unlike adult trauma patients, multisystem failure in children often occurs during resuscitation, affecting all organs almost simultaneously. However, reported rates of acute lung injury are nearly six times lower in children.[68,69] The lower rate of systemic damage is probably the result of an imbalanced inflammatory response to trauma in children, with a strong response at the tissue level but a diminished one at the systemic level.[70] Best outcomes are achieved with aggressive treatment of all musculoskeletal injuries and careful surveillance to detect any missed injuries.

Emergency Orthopaedic Management

The orthopaedic surgeon plays a critical role in the treatment of a child with polytrauma. A careful evaluation to identify potentially limb-threatening or life-threatening injuries, including those to the spinal cord, the pelvic ring when associated with hemodynamic instability, fractures associated with vascular injury, and open fractures, is critical. When an injury to the cervical spine is suspected in a younger child, appropriate immobilization should be obtained using a backboard with an occipital recess. The use of a standard trauma backboard will result in an unsafe position because of neck flexion. Early stabilization with pelvic binders and external fixation may be beneficial in the presence of pelvic ring fractures associated with hemodynamic instability.[64] Temporary reduction and immobilization of pediatric fractures associated with vascular injury can facilitate definitive vascular reconstruction and improve the overall outcome. Provisional splinting of affected extremities will increase patient comfort and minimize further tissue damage. Skeletal traction pins, external fixators, or splinting can be considered for polytrauma patients if definitive treatment of femoral or unstable pelvic fractures is anticipated to be delayed by more than 24 hours.[64]

Timing of Orthopaedic Surgery in Polytrauma Patients

The timing of the treatment of patients with trauma has been the subject of extensive research. In general, complications are minimized when isolated fractures of the femur, pelvis, acetabulum, and spine are stabilized on an early basis.[71] However, in patients with multiple injuries, injuries to other body systems, and/or severe hemorrhage, additional factors should be taken into consideration. A major traumatic event results in a sustained response of the immune system, with an early hyperinflammatory stage. The early definitive management of all fractures in a patient with polytrauma, or early total care, is associated with substantial blood loss and hypothermia; as a result, an excessive inflammatory reaction (second hit) can be generated, potentially triggering a systemic inflammatory response syndrome, acute respiratory distress syndrome, and multiple organ failure.[72]

In an effort to minimize this phenomenon, the concept of damage control orthopaedics in the trauma setting emerged: it equates to performing only immediate lifesaving procedures aimed at stopping bleeding during the initial phase of care, achieving primary stabilization of major fractures by using external fixation.[72-74] The placement of external fixation in the acute period minimizes the risk of the second hit; definitive reconstruction occurs later, once the patient's physiologic parameters have improved.[72]

The preferential fixation of femoral fractures in the first 24 hours after injury, in contrast to other extremity fractures that could be splinted and fixed at a later date, has been described as early appropriate care.[75] Advocates of early appropriate care suggest that it represents a compromise between the earlier approach (wherein all fractures were treated immediately) and the staged treatment, as long as an aggressive approach to resuscitation is used. In general, severely injured patients benefit from damage control orthopaedics, including those with an Injury Severity Score greater than 40, multiple injuries combined with thoracic trauma (an Injury Severity Score greater than 20), multiple injuries combined with severe abdominal or pelvic injury and hemorrhagic shock, moderate or severe head trauma, radiographic evidence of a pulmonary contusion, bilateral femoral fractures, and those with body temperature less than 35°C.[74] Although not specifically studied in children, damage control orthopaedics can be considered in the setting of children with severe head injuries who have an intracranial pressure greater than 30 mm Hg, those who are unstable and not easily controlled medically, those with profound hypothermia on admission, and in those who are hypovolemic and hypotensive despite adequate ongoing resuscitation. Compared with adults, pediatric patients with polytrauma have a lower risk of sequential multiorgan failure in the first 48 hours after injury.[64] Early definitive orthopaedic stabilization after adequate resuscitation is critical to avoiding complications associated with prolonged immobilization.

Open Fractures

Although the principles of management of open fractures in children are similar to those in adults, the thicker and more active periosteum in children provides greater fracture stability. More rapid and reliable fracture healing also is usually achieved.

Open fractures typically result from high-energy or penetrating trauma. As with open fractures in adults, the Gustilo-Anderson system is used to classify open fractures in children. Open fractures represent approximately 2% of all pediatric fractures.[76,77] Careful evaluation of the patient in the emergency setting, after removing all dressings to allow for a complete skin assessment, is critical to diagnose smaller skin openings. The child's tetanus status should be confirmed. Little controversy exist with regard to the management of types II and III open fractures, including débridement of any devitalized tissue and abundant irrigation, in addition to the administration of intravenous antibiotics.[78] A first-generation cephalosporin is usually used in children with types II and III open fractures; an aminoglycoside and/or penicillin is added if the wound is severely contaminated or has been exposed to soil. The surgical management of type I open fractures has been questioned, with small studies suggesting that povidone-iodine and saline irrigation followed by closed reduction and cast immobilization in the emergency department (with either oral or intravenous antibiotics) have similar outcomes as those obtained with surgical treatment.[79-81] A recent, multicenter study on type I open forearm, wrist, and tibia fractures compared the outcome of 49 fractures managed with superficial wound débridement and antibiotics in the emergency department with that of 170 fractures managed with formal surgical débridement and antibiotics. The authors reported no significant differences in infection rates between the two treatment strategies.[82] Prospective, randomized controlled studies are required to validate these findings.[78]

Timing of Irrigation and Débridement

In an effort to minimize the risk of infection, emergent surgical treatment was traditionally recommended for all open fractures. This recommendation was challenged by a large study in which the outcome of 554 open fractures in children was analyzed. All patients received intravenous antibiotics at the time of admission to the emergency department, which were continued for 24 hours. Patients were retrospectively grouped based on whether they received surgical treatment before or after 6 hours from the time of injury. The infection rate was similar in both groups, regardless of the severity of the initial fracture.[83] Current recommendations suggest that emergent surgery is not required if intravenous antibiotics are administered soon after an injury.[78] Careful consideration of the vascular status of the limb and the severity of bone and soft-tissue injuries should help determine the need for immediate surgical treatment. All open fractures that require surgical treatment should receive it within 24 hours of the injury.

Surgical Considerations

The original wound should be extended as needed to gain adequate exposure to the bone ends. Muscle and other tissues should be inspected for signs of vitality. Any obviously devitalized tissue, including bone fragments completely stripped off the periosteum, and other debris should be removed. If the vitality of any tissue is in question, it is best to preserve it and reevaluate it under general anesthesia 48 hours later.

Obtaining cultures before and after débridement appears to be of limited or no value in the management of open fractures.[78] A 2015 study in the adult population suggests that the use of very low pressure irrigation (1 to 2 psi) is an acceptable, low-cost alternative for the irrigation of open fractures, with rates of revision surgery similar to those obtained with high (>20 psi) and low (5 to 10 psi) pressure.[84] Castile soap, as an additive in the irrigation fluid, has proved as effective as antibiotic (bacitracin) but with fewer wound healing problems.[85] However, castile soap appears to be associated with a higher revision surgery rate when compared with normal saline irrigation.[84]

Small, noncontaminated wounds can be closed over a drain. Negative pressure wound therapy with a vacuum-assisted closure system is helpful to reduce the need for free flaps and the risk of infection.[86,89] In general, stable fracture fixation is preferable to cast immobilization in patients with unstable fractures or a large soft-tissue injury. Sparse information is available regarding the length of antibiotic treatment after open fractures in children. In adults, the use of a first-generation cephalosporin for 24 to 48 hours after a type I open fracture and for 48 hours for types II and III open fractures has been recommended.[90]

Outcomes

Compared with adults who have open fractures, children have better outcomes and a lower overall rate of infection. The rate of infection in children with open fractures is approximately 3%,[83] with an increasing rate as fracture severity increases (8% for type III fractures).[83] Although unlikely, delayed union and nonunion can occur, especially after a type III open fracture of the tibial shaft in an adolescent.

Compartment Syndrome

Compartment syndrome can be caused by a variety of factors, including fractures, crush injuries, vascular problems, burns, infections, casting complications, and intravenous infiltrations.[91] Regardless of the etiology, compartment syndrome occurs when an increase in intracompartmental pressure causes a decrease of perfusion pressure, which leads to hypoxemia of the tissues within the compartment. With hypoxemia, oxidant stress is increased. Because insufficient adenosine triphosphate is present, cell membrane potential is lost and a resultant influx of chloride ions leads to cellular swelling and necrosis.[92]

Making a diagnosis of acute extremity compartment syndrome in a child can be challenging and is often delayed; the classic signs seen in adults are usually not helpful in children. The clinical diagnosis of acute extremity compartment syndrome in children should be based on the three As: anxiety, agitation, and increasing analgesic requirement.[92,93] Although the most common scenarios for an acute extremity compartment syndrome in a child include a tibial shaft fracture or a supracondylar humerus fracture, others include intravenous infiltrates, crush injuries, and thigh casts.[92]

For patients who are very young, are uncooperative, have altered mental status, or have unreliable or inconsistent clinical symptoms, the measurement of compartment pressures should be considered. The normal compartment pressures in children are higher than in adults. In one study comparing average pressures in the four lower leg compartments in healthy children and adults, the average pressure in the four compartments varied between 13.3 and 16.6 mm Hg in children and between 5.2 and 9.7 mm Hg in adults.[94] An absolute pressure greater than 30 mm Hg was thought to indicate impaired tissue perfusion and the need for emergency surgical fasciotomy; however, it is common practice now to use the differential pressure (Δp = diastolic blood pressure – intracompartmental pressure), with a proposed threshold of 30 mm Hg, as a more reliable indication.[92] Some pediatric providers recommend using the mean arterial pressure – intracompartmental pressure < 30 mm Hg because of the higher resting pressures in the pediatric and adolescent population.

Although time is of the essence in the diagnosis and management of acute compartment syndrome in both children and adults, there is some evidence that children may have more reserve in tolerating increased compartmental pressures or greater potential for recovery. In a study of 43 cases of acute compartment syndrome of the leg from two pediatric trauma centers, a 2011 study reported excellent functional outcomes in 41/43 patients. The average time from injury to fasciotomy was 20.5 hours (3.9 to 118 hours). The two patients who lost function had their fasciotomies performed more than 80 hours after injury.[95] Despite extended periods of time from injury to surgery in many cases, excellent outcomes were still observed in most patients.

There is no consensus in the literature regarding the best method for closure of fasciotomy wounds.[96] Negative pressure wound therapy with a vacuum-assisted closure system can be helpful. Repeat evaluation and débridement are often needed after 48 to 72 hours, when delayed primary closure is sometimes possible. Split-thickness skin grafts are infrequently needed. In certain cases, passive stretching exercises and splinting might be helpful to minimize contractures. Timely diagnosis and prompt management with an appropriate fasciotomy can result in recovery of function and favorable outcomes for children with acute compartment syndrome.

Growth Disturbance

The incidence of significant disturbance of normal growth after a physeal injury is relatively low (<10%). Factors than can determine the extent of the growth abnormality include the location and size of the physeal bar, the growth potential of the physis involved, and the age of the patient at the time of injury. Growth arrest can be complete or partial. With complete arrest, limb-length inequality may ensue. With a partial arrest, angular deformities or joint irregularities may be observed. The most common anatomic locations for growth arrest after a traumatic injury include the distal femur, the proximal tibia, and the distal tibia.[97,98]

Etiologies of Growth Arrest

In general, posttraumatic growth arrest usually is the result of partial or complete destruction of the physis at the time of injury, inadequate reduction of a physeal fracture, or tissue interposition at the fracture site.[97,98] A bridge of bone connecting the epiphysis and the metaphysis is responsible for the arrest in growth. Growth arrest can occur in the presence of an anatomic reduction.[97] Other causes of physeal bar formation include infection, tumors, irradiation, burns, vascular insufficiency, and metabolic disorders.[97] Crossing the physis with metal pins and drills, especially when threaded, and performing aggressive dissection of tissues, including the perichondrial ring, can also result in growth arrest.

Patterns of Bar Formation

Depending on the location of the bar within the physis, three common patterns are commonly seen: peripheral, central, or elongated (**Figure 5**). Peripheral bars are relatively common and can lead to angular deformities. Central bars are located away from the periphery and can tether growth, resulting in limb-length discrepancy or joint deformity. Elongated or linear bars run from one edge of the physis to the opposite one (usually anterior to posterior) and can result in a combination of angular and joint deformity.

Management

One of the earliest signs of growth arrest is the evidence of asymmetric growth recovery (Harris) lines. When growth is normal, growth recovery lines are parallel to the physis. With an arrest, the lines tend to converge toward the area of abnormal physis. Surveillance for growth arrest for 2 years is necessary after most physeal fractures. Particular attention should be paid to younger children with an injury known to have a high risk of growth disturbance, such as a distal femur fracture. Indistinct physeal margins and asymmetry or tilting at the joint are indirect radiologic signs that indicate the presence of a physeal bar.[99] Angular deformity and/or limb-length discrepancy are usually late radiographic manifestations. However, plain radiographs have limited ability to provide early identification and quantification of the extension of the physeal bar. Although CT scan has a better capacity to determine the size and location of physeal bars, it lacks the ability to detect early fibrous bars and is associated with high

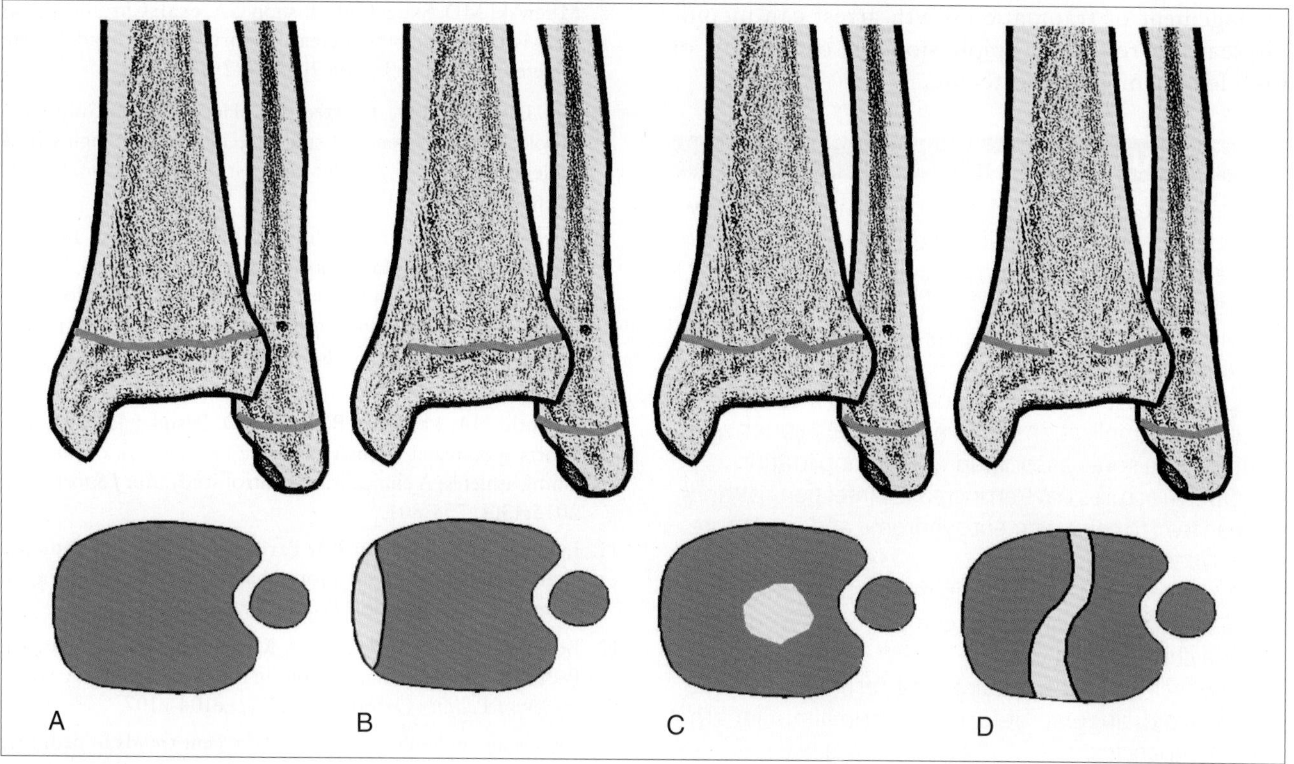

FIGURE 5 Illustrations of common patterns of bar formation. **A**, Normal physis. **B**, Peripheral bars are relatively common and can lead to angular deformities. **C**, Central bars are located away from the periphery and can tether growth. **D**, Elongated or linear bars run from one edge of the physis to the other and can result in a combination of angular and joint deformities.

levels of radiation.[99] MRI is now widely accepted as the method of choice to provide early and complete evaluation of physeal bars, particularly when the three-dimensional gradient-recalled echo sequence is used.[99]

The precise location and size of the bar should be determined when surgical management is planned. Several factors should be considered when planning surgical treatment after growth arrest, including the extent of the arrest, the anticipated discrepancy, and the age of the patient. In the presence of a complete arrest, contralateral epiphysiodesis is chosen if the anticipated discrepancy is less than 5 cm. If the anticipated discrepancy is greater than 5 cm, lengthening of the short limb is performed. Partial arrest can be managed by resecting the physeal bar, completing the arrest through an epiphysiodesis (if no angular deformities have been noted) or by a combination of epiphysiodesis and osteotomies and/or lengthening procedures if angular deformities and shortening is noted. Bar resection is indicated if the size if the bar represents less than 50% of the physis, the angular deformity is less than 20°, and at least 2 years of growth remains. Best results with resection are observed with physeal bars that are recognized early in younger children, are located centrally, and have a small size (less than 25% of the entire size of the physis).[100]

SUMMARY

Most fractures in children result from falls from low height or sports activities; however, certain fracture patterns should raise concern for an abusive etiology. The anatomy and physiology of children influences the types of fractures and treatment options. The age of the child and the location of the fracture affect the capacity for remodeling. Most fractures in children can be managed nonsurgically. Ketamine and intravenous sedation are commonly used during closed manipulation, but local and regional drugs can also provide effective analgesia. Careful cast application and removal reduce the risk of complications, such as thermal injuries and pressure sores associated with immobilization. Open fractures are violent injuries that not only have an increased infection risk but can also lead to compartment syndrome and premature physeal arrest. An increasing need for pain medication can be the only sign of an impending compartment syndrome in a child. Physeal fractures, particularly in the long bones of the lower extremities, require long-term surveillance to avoid angular deformities and limb-length discrepancies. Depending on the extent of the arrest and the amount of growth remaining, the management of traumatic growth arrest can include physeal bar resection, epiphysiodesis, osteotomy, or limb lengthening or shortening.

KEY STUDY POINTS

- Most fractures in children result from falls from low height or sports activities.
- Certain fracture patterns should raise concern for an abusive etiology.
- Most fractures in children can be managed nonsurgically.
- Careful cast application and removal reduce the risk of complications such as thermal injuries and pressure sores associated with immobilization.
- Open fractures have an increased infection risk and can lead to compartment syndrome and premature physeal arrest.
- An increasing need for pain medication can be the only sign of an impending compartment syndrome in a child.
- Physeal fractures require long term surveillance to avoid angular deformities and limb length discrepancies.

ANNOTATED REFERENCES

1. Danseco ER, Miller TR, Spicer RS: Incidence and costs of 1987-1994 childhood injuries: Demographic breakdowns. *Pediatrics* 2000;105(2):E27.
2. Wolfe JA, Wolfe H, Banaag A, Tintle S, Perez Koehlmoos T: Early pediatric fractures in a universally insured population within the United States. *BMC Pediatr* 2019;19(1):343.

   This epidemiologic report aimed to determine the prevalence and risk factors for fracture in a large cohort of pediatric patients younger than 5 years. Level of evidence: III.
3. Landin LA: Epidemiology of children's fractures. *J Pediatr Orthop B* 1997;6(2):79-83.
4. Naranje SM, Erali RA, Warner WC Jr, Sawyer JR, Kelly DM: Epidemiology of pediatric fractures presenting to emergency departments in the United States. *J Pediatr Orthop* 2016;36(4):e45-e48.

   Epidemiologic report aimed to identify the most frequent pediatric fractures in the United States using the 2010 National Electronic Injury Surveillance System (NEISS) database and 2010 US Census information. Level of evidence: III.
5. Nakaniida A, Sakuraba K, Hurwitz EL: Pediatric orthopaedic injuries requiring hospitalization: Epidemiology and economics. *J Orthop Trauma* 2014;28(3):167-172.
6. Iobst C, Arango D, Segal D, Skaggs DL: National access to care for children with fractures. *J Pediatr Orthop* 2013;33(6):587-591.
7. Manning RL, Teach SJ, Searcy K, et al: The association between weight status and pediatric forearm fractures resulting from ground-level falls. *Pediatr Emerg Care* 2015;31(12):835-838.
8. Milewski MD, Skaggs DL, Bishop GA, et al: Chronic lack of sleep is associated with increased sports injuries in adolescent athletes. *J Pediatr Orthop* 2014;34(2):129-133.
9. Bell DR, Post EG, Trigsted SM, Hetzel S, McGuine TA, Brooks MA: Prevalence of sport specialization in high school athletics: A 1-year observational study. *Am J Sports Med* 2016;44(6):1469-1474.

   Three hundred two high school athletes (aged 13 to 18) completed a sport specialization survey and an injury history survey. Highly specialized athletes were more likely to report a history of overuse knee or hip injuries, especially if participating in a single sport for more than 8 months per year. Level of evidence: III.
10. Jayanthi NA, LaBella CR, Fischer D, Pasulka J, Dugas LR: Sports-specialized intensive training and the risk of injury in young athletes: A clinical case-control study. *Am J Sports Med* 2015;43(4):794-801.
11. Lykissas MG, Eismann EA, Parikh SN: Trends in pediatric sports-related and recreation-related injuries in the United States in the last decade. *J Pediatr Orthop* 2013;33(8):803-810.
12. Borne A, Porter A, Recicar J, Maxson T, Montgomery C: Pediatric traumatic amputations in the United States: A 5-year review. *J Pediatr Orthop* 2017;37(2):e104-e107.

    This is an epidemiologic review of recent trends in pediatric traumatic amputations in the United States. Level of evidence: IV.
13. Mannix R, Fleegler E, Meehan WP III, et al: Booster seat laws and fatalities in children 4 to 7 years of age. *Pediatrics* 2012;130(6):996-1002.
14. Caskey S, Hammond J, Peck J, Sardelli M, Atkinson T: The effect of booster seat use on pediatric injuries in motor vehicle frontal crashes. *J Pediatr Orthop* 2018;38(7):e382-e386.

    This study highlights the efficacy of booster seats in preventing orthopaedic injury in children. Level of evidence: III.
15. Loftis CM, Sawyer JR, Eubanks JW III, Kelly DM: The impact of child safety restraint status and age in motor vehicle collisions in predicting type and severity of bone fractures and traumatic injuries. *J Pediatr Orthop* 2017;37(8):521-525.

    This study evaluates correlations between childhood injuries in motor vehicle collisions and their age and restraint status. Children between the ages of 4 and 8 years were commonly improperly restrained. The authors suggest that changes in regulations or automotive safety equipment might be required. Level of evidence: III.
16. Doud AN, Moro R, Wallace SG, et al: All-terrain vehicle injury in children and youth: Examining current knowledge and future needs. *J Emerg Med* 2017;53(2):222-231.

    The authors analyze data from 16 published reviews regarding epidemiology and risk factors among ATV-related injuries. They demonstrate that ATV-related injuries disproportionately affect children. Level of evidence: IV.
17. Su W, Hui T, Shaw K: All-terrain vehicle injury patterns: Are current regulations effective? *J Pediatr Surg* 2006;41(5):931-934.

18. Sawyer JR, Kelly DM, Kellum E, Warner WC Jr: Orthopaedic aspects of all-terrain vehicle-related injury. *J Am Acad Orthop Surg* 2011;19(4):219-225.
19. Shannon SF, Hernandez NM, Sems SA, Larson AN, Milbrandt TA: Pediatric orthopaedic trauma and associated injuries of snowmobile, ATV, and dirtbike accidents: A 19-year experience at a level 1 pediatric trauma center. *J Pediatr Orthop* 2018;38(8):403-409.

    The authors evaluate the type and severity of orthopaedic and associated injuries for snowmobile, ATV, and motorized dirt bike accidents in a pediatric patient population. Level of evidence: IV.
20. Sink EL, Hyman JE, Matheny T, Georgopoulos G, Kleinman P: Child abuse: The role of the orthopaedic surgeon in nonaccidental trauma. *Clin Orthop Relat Res* 2011;469(3):790-797.
21. Zhao C, Starke M, Tompson JD, Sabharwal S: Predictors for nonaccidental trauma in a child with a fracture–A national inpatient database study. *J Am Acad Orthop Surg* 2020;28(4):e164-e171.

    Using an inpatient database, the authors aimed to develop an evidence-based likelihood of nonaccidental trauma in a child presenting with a fracture. Level of evidence: III.
22. Leaman LA, Hennrikus WL, Bresnahan JJ: Identifying nonaccidental fractures in children aged <2 years. *J Child Orthop* 2016;10(4):335-341.

    The authors analyzed the data on 115 consecutive patients aged 2 years and younger, who presented with a fracture. They reported that age younger than 1 year, multiple fractures, corner fractures, transverse fractures, and covered by Medicaid were the most common factors associated with reporting of nonaccidental trauma. Level of evidence: III.
23. Boutis K, Narayanan UG, Dong FF, et al: Magnetic resonance imaging of clinically suspected Salter-Harris I fracture of the distal fibula. *Injury* 2010;41(8):852-856.
24. Wattenbarger JM, Gruber HE, Phieffer LS: Physeal fractures, part I: Histologic features of bone, cartilage, and bar formation in a small animal model. *J Pediatr Orthop* 2002;22(6):703-709.
25. Barmada A, Gaynor T, Mubarak SJ: Premature physeal closure following distal tibia physeal fractures: A new radiographic predictor. *J Pediatr Orthop* 2003;23(6):733-739.
26. Arkader A, Warner WC Jr, Horn BD, Shaw RN, Wells L: Predicting the outcome of physeal fractures of the distal femur. *J Pediatr Orthop* 2007;27(6):703-708.
27. Russo F, Moor MA, Mubarak SJ, Pennock AT: Salter-Harris II fractures of the distal tibia: Does surgical management reduce the risk of premature physeal closure? *J Pediatr Orthop* 2013;33(5):524-529.
28. Slongo T, Audige L, Lutz N, et al: Documentation of fracture severity with the AO classification of pediatric long-bone fractures. *Acta Orthop* 2007;78(2):247-253.
29. Joeris A, Lutz N, Blumenthal A, Slongo T, Audige L: The AO Pediatric Comprehensive Classification of Long Bone Fractures (PCCF). *Acta Orthop* 2017;88(2):123-128.

    This study is part of the validation process of the AO Pediatric Comprehensive Classification of Long Bone Fractures (AO PCCF) of the upper extremity. Level of evidence: IV.
30. Joeris A, Lutz N, Blumenthal A, Slongo T, Audige L: The AO Pediatric Comprehensive Classification of Long Bone Fractures (PCCF). *Acta Orthop* 2017;88(2):129-132.

    This study is part of the validation process of the AO Pediatric Comprehensive Classification of Long Bone Fractures (AO PCCF) of the lower extremity. Level of evidence: IV.
31. Wilkins KE: Principles of fracture remodeling in children. *Injury* 2005;36(suppl 1):A3-A11.
32. Herman MJ, Martinek MA, Abzug JM: Complications of tibial eminence and diaphyseal fractures in children: Prevention and treatment. *Instr Course Lect* 2015;64:471-482.
33. Tejwani N, Phillips D, Goldstein RY: Management of lateral humeral condylar fracture in children. *J Am Acad Orthop Surg* 2011;19(6):350-358.
34. Li NY, Bruce WJ, Joyce C, Decker NM, Cappello T: Obesity's influence on operative management of pediatric supracondylar humerus fractures. *J Pediatr Orthop* 2018;38(3):e118-e121.

    Using a national database, the authors aimed to determine if obese children with supracondylar humerus fractures are more likely to require open reduction and internal fixation than nonobese children. Level of evidence: IV.
35. Ashley P, Gilbert SR: Obesity in pediatric trauma. *Orthop Clin North Am* 2018;49(3):335-343.

    This study reviews the effect of obesity on the outcome of pediatric trauma. Level of evidence: V.
36. Supakul N, Hicks RA, Caltoum CB, Karmazyn B: Distal humeral epiphyseal separation in young children: An often-missed fracture-radiographic signs and ultrasound confirmatory diagnosis. *AJR Am J Roentgenol* 2015;204(2):W192-W198.
37. Neri E, Barbi E, Rabach I, et al: Diagnostic accuracy of ultrasonography for hand bony fractures in paediatric patients. *Arch Dis Child* 2014;99(12):1087-1090.
38. Constantine E, Steele DW, Eberson C, Boutis K, Amanullah S, Linakis JG: The use of local anesthetic techniques for closed forearm fracture reduction in children: A survey of academic pediatric emergency departments. *Pediatr Emerg Care* 2007;23(4):209-211.
39. Constantine E, Tsze DS, Machan JT, Eberson CP, Linakis JG, Steele DW: Evaluating the hematoma block as an adjunct to procedural sedation for closed reduction of distal forearm fractures. *Pediatr Emerg Care* 2014;30(7):474-478.
40. Bear DM, Friel NA, Lupo CL, Pitetti R, Ward WT: Hematoma block versus sedation for the reduction of distal radius fractures in children. *J Hand Surg Am* 2015;40(1):57-61.
41. Aarons CE, Fernandez MD, Willsey M, Peterson B, Key C, Fabregas J: Bier block regional anesthesia and casting for forearm fractures: Safety in the pediatric emergency department setting. *J Pediatr Orthop* 2014;34(1):45-49.

42. McCarty EC, Mencio GA, Green NE: Anesthesia and analgesia for the ambulatory management of fractures in children. *J Am Acad Orthop Surg* 1999;7(2):81-91.

43. Kriwanek KL, Wan J, Beaty JH, Pershad J: Axillary block for analgesia during manipulation of forearm fractures in the pediatric emergency department a prospective randomized comparative trial. *J Pediatr Orthop* 2006;26(6):737-740.

44. Luhmann JD, Schootman M, Luhmann SJ, Kennedy RM: A randomized comparison of nitrous oxide plus hematoma block versus ketamine plus midazolam for emergency department forearm fracture reduction in children. *Pediatrics* 2006;118(4):e1078-e1086.

45. McCarty EC, Mencio GA, Walker LA, Green NE: Ketamine sedation for the reduction of children's fractures in the emergency department. *J Bone Joint Surg Am* 2000;82-A(7):912-918.

46. Godambe SA, Elliot V, Matheny D, Pershad J: Comparison of propofol/fentanyl versus ketamine/midazolam for brief orthopedic procedural sedation in a pediatric emergency department. *Pediatrics* 2003;112(1):116-123.

47. Kennedy RM, Porter FL, Miller JP, Jaffe DM: Comparison of fentanyl/midazolam with ketamine/midazolam for pediatric orthopedic emergencies. *Pediatrics* 1998;102(4):956-963.

48. Cote CJ, Wilson S: Guidelines for monitoring and management of pediatric patients during and after sedation for diagnostic and therapeutic procedures: An update. *Pediatrics* 2006;118(6):2587-2602.

49. Raney EM, van Bosse HJP, Shea KG, Abzug JM, Schwend RM: Current state of the opioid epidemic as it pertains to pediatric orthopaedics from the Advocacy Committee of the Pediatric Orthopaedic Society of North America. *J Pediatr Orthop* 2018;38(5):e238-e244.

    The authors suggest that education of care providers, patients, and families; standardization of narcotic prescribing practices; and appropriate plans for disposal of unused narcotics are immediate concepts to consider in correcting the current opioid epidemic. Level of evidence: V.

50. Nelson SE, Adams AJ, Buczek MJ, Anthony CA, Shah AS: Postoperative pain and opioid use in children with supracondylar humeral fractures: Balancing analgesia and opioid stewardship. *J Bone Joint Surg Am* 2019;101(2):119-126.

    In this study, the authors aimed to characterize postoperative pain and opioid use after closed reduction and percutaneous pinning of a supracondylar humeral fractures. The authors report that pain levels and opioid usage decrease to a clinically unimportant level by postoperative day 3. The authors suggest that a prescription for seven opioid doses after discharge should allow adequate postoperative analgesia in most patients while improving narcotic stewardship. Level of evidence: IV.

51. Chou R, Gordon DB, de Leon-Casasola OA, et al: Management of postoperative pain: A clinical practice guideline from the American Pain Society, the American Society of Regional Anesthesia and Pain Medicine, and the American Society of Anesthesiologists' Committee on Regional Anesthesia, Executive Committee, and Administrative Council. *J Pain* 2016;17(2):131-157.

52. Swanson CE, Chang K, Schleyer E, Pizzutillo PD, Herman MJ: Postoperative pain control after supracondylar humerus fracture fixation. *J Pediatr Orthop* 2012;32(5):452-455.

53. Adams AJ, Buczek MJ, Flynn JM, Shah AS: Perioperative ketorolac for supracondylar humerus fracture in children decreases postoperative pain, opioid usage, hospitalization cost, and length-of-stay. *J Pediatr Orthop* 2019;39(6):e447-e451.

    The authors demonstrate that administration of ketorolac reduces postoperative pain and opioid use in children with displaced supracondylar humerus fractures undergoing closed reduction and percutaneous pinning. Level of evidence: III.

54. Boutis K, Willan A, Babyn P, Goeree R, Howard A: Cast versus splint in children with minimally angulated fractures of the distal radius: A randomized controlled trial. *Can Med Assoc J* 2010;182(14):1507-1512.

55. Carmichael KD, Westmoreland J: Effectiveness of ear protection in reducing anxiety during cast removal in children. *Am J Orthop (Belle Mead NJ)* 2005;34(1):43-46.

56. Katz K, Fogelman R, Attias J, Baron E, Soudry M: Anxiety reaction in children during removal of their plaster cast with a saw. *J Bone Joint Surg Br* 2001;83(3):388-390.

57. Liu RW, Mehta P, Fortuna S, et al: A randomized prospective study of music therapy for reducing anxiety during cast room procedures. *J Pediatr Orthop* 2007;27(7):831-833.

58. Inglis M, McClelland B, Sutherland LM, Cundy PJ: Synthetic versus plaster of Paris casts in the treatment of fractures of the forearm in children: A randomised trial of clinical outcomes and patient satisfaction. *Bone Joint J* 2013;95-B(9):1285-1289.

59. Halanski M, Noonan KJ: Cast and splint immobilization: Complications. *J Am Acad Orthop Surg* 2008;16(1):30-40.

60. Halanski MA, Halanski AD, Oza A, Vanderby R, Munoz A, Noonan KJ: Thermal injury with contemporary cast-application techniques and methods to circumvent morbidity. *J Bone Joint Surg Am* 2007;89(11):2369-2377.

61. Difazio RL, Harris M, Feldman L, Mahan ST: Reducing the incidence of cast-related skin complications in children treated with cast immobilization. *J Pediatr Orthop* 2017;37(8):526-531.

    This study suggests that incorporating padding to the heel of lower extremity cast is an effective intervention in decreasing the incidence of cast-related skin complications. Level of evidence: II.

62. Puddy AC, Sunkin JA, Aden JK, Walick KS, Hsu JR: Cast saw burns: Evaluation of simple techniques for reducing the risk of thermal injury. *J Pediatr Orthop* 2014;34(8):e63-e66.

63. Bae DS, Lynch H, Jamieson K, Yu-Moe CW, Roussin C: Improved safety and cost savings from reductions in cast-saw burns after simulation-based education for orthopaedic surgery residents. *J Bone Joint Surg Am* 2017;99(17):e94.

    This study highlights the effectiveness of simulation-based training for orthopaedic surgical residents in reducing cast saw injuries. Level of evidence: III.

64. Pandya NK, Upasani VV, Kulkarni VA: The pediatric polytrauma patient: Current concepts. *J Am Acad Orthop Surg* 2013;21(3):170-179.

65. Jawadi AH, Letts M: Injuries associated with fracture of the femur secondary to motor vehicle accidents in children. *Am J Orthop (Belle Mead NJ)* 2003;32(9):459-462.

66. Oyetunji TA, Haider AH, Downing SR, et al: Treatment outcomes of injured children at adult level 1 trauma centers: Are there benefits from added specialized care? *Am J Surg* 2011;201(4):445-449.

67. Myers SR, Branas CC, French B, Nance ML, Carr BG: A national analysis of pediatric trauma care utilization and outcomes in the United States. *Pediatr Emerg Care* 2019;35(1):1-7.

    The authors provide a description of the proportion of injured children treated at pediatric trauma centers in the United States. Level of evidence: III.

68. Zimmerman JJ, Akhtar SR, Caldwell E, Rubenfeld GD: Incidence and outcomes of pediatric acute lung injury. *Pediatrics* 2009;124(1):87-95.

69. Rubenfeld GD, Caldwell E, Peabody E, et al: Incidence and outcomes of acute lung injury. *N Engl J Med* 2005;353(16):1685-1693.

70. Wood JH, Partrick DA, Johnston RB Jr: The inflammatory response to injury in children. *Curr Opin Pediatr* 2010;22(3):315-320.

71. Vallier HA, Wang X, Moore TA, Wilber JH, Como JJ: Timing of orthopaedic surgery in multiple trauma patients: Development of a protocol for early appropriate care. *J Orthop Trauma* 2013;27(10):543-551.

72. Stinner DJ, Edwards D: Surgical management of musculoskeletal trauma. *Surg Clin North Am* 2017;97(5):1119-1131.

73. Lichte P, Kobbe P, Dombroski D, Pape HC: Damage control orthopedics: Current evidence. *Curr Opin Crit Care* 2012;18(6):647-650.

74. Pape HC, Tornetta P III, Tarkin I, Tzioupis C, Sabeson V, Olson SA: Timing of fracture fixation in multitrauma patients: The role of early total care and damage control surgery. *J Am Acad Orthop Surg* 2009;17(9):541-549.

75. Nahm NJ, Como JJ, Wilber JH, Vallier HA: Early appropriate care: Definitive stabilization of femoral fractures within 24 hours of injury is safe in most patients with multiple injuries. *J Trauma* 2011;71(1):175-185.

76. Cheng JC, Ng BK, Ying SY, Lam PK: A 10-year study of the changes in the pattern and treatment of 6,493 fractures. *J Pediatr Orthop* 1999;19(3):344-350.

77. Cheng JC, Shen WY: Limb fracture pattern in different pediatric age groups: A study of 3,350 children. *J Orthop Trauma* 1993;7(1):15-22.

78. Pace JL, Kocher MS, Skaggs DL: Evidence-based review: Management of open pediatric fractures. *J Pediatr Orthop* 2012;32(suppl 2):S123-S127.

79. Iobst CA, Spurdle C, Baitner AC, King WF, Tidwell M, Swirsky S: A protocol for the management of pediatric type I open fractures. *J Child Orthop* 2014;8(1):71-76.

80. Iobst CA, Tidwell MA, King WF: Nonoperative management of pediatric type I open fractures. *J Pediatr Orthop* 2005;25(4):513-517.

81. Doak J, Ferrick M: Nonoperative management of pediatric grade 1 open fractures with less than a 24-hour admission. *J Pediatr Orthop* 2009;29(1):49-51.

82. Godfrey J, Choi PD, Shabtai L, et al: Management of pediatric type I open fractures in the emergency department or operating room: A multicenter perspective. *J Pediatr Orthop* 2019;39(7):372-376.

    This study was aimed to compare the outcomes in type I open fractures managed nonsurgically with those in patients treated with surgical intervention. Level of evidence: III.

83. Skaggs DL, Friend L, Alman B, et al: The effect of surgical delay on acute infection following 554 open fractures in children. *J Bone Joint Surg Am* 2005;87(1):8-12.

84. Bhandari M, Jeray KJ, Petrisor BA, et al: A trial of wound irrigation in the initial management of open fracture wounds. *N Engl J Med* 2015;373(27):2629-2641.

85. Anglen JO: Comparison of soap and antibiotic solutions for irrigation of lower-limb open fracture wounds. A prospective, randomized study. *J Bone Joint Surg Am* 2005;87(7):1415-1422.

86. Dedmond BT, Kortesis B, Punger K, et al: Subatmospheric pressure dressings in the temporary treatment of soft tissue injuries associated with type III open tibial shaft fractures in children. *J Pediatr Orthop* 2006;26(6):728-732.

87. Shilt JS, Yoder JS, Manuck TA, Jacks L, Rushing J, Smith BP: Role of vacuum-assisted closure in the treatment of pediatric lawnmower injuries. *J Pediatr Orthop* 2004;24(5):482-487.

88. Mooney JF III, Argenta LC, Marks MW, Morykwas MJ, DeFranzo AJ: Treatment of soft tissue defects in pediatric patients using the V.A.C. system. *Clin Orthop Relat Res* 2000;376:26-31.

89. Halvorson J, Jinnah R, Kulp B, Frino J: Use of vacuum-assisted closure in pediatric open fractures with a focus on the rate of infection. *Orthopedics* 2011;34(7):e256-e260.

90. Hauser CJ, Adams CA Jr, Eachempati SR: Surgical Infection Society guideline: Prophylactic antibiotic use in open fractures. An evidence-based guideline. *Surg Infect (Larchmt)* 2006;7(4):379-405.

91. Kanj WW, Gunderson MA, Carrigan RB, Sankar WN: Acute compartment syndrome of the upper extremity in children: Diagnosis, management, and outcomes. *J Child Orthop* 2013;7(3):225-233.

92. von Keudell AG, Weaver MJ, Appleton PT, et al: Diagnosis and treatment of acute extremity compartment syndrome. *Lancet* 2015;386(10000):1299-1310.

93. Noonan KJ, McCarthy JJ: Compartment syndrome in the pediatric patient. *J Pediatr Orthop* 2010;30(2 suppl):96-101.

94. Staudt JM, Smeulders MJ, van der Horst CM: Normal compartment pressures of the lower leg in children. *J Bone Joint Surg Br* 2008;90(2):290-295.

95. Flynn JM, Bashyal RK, Yeger-McKeever M, Garner MR, Launay F, Sponseller PD: Acute traumatic compartment syndrome of the leg in children: Diagnosis and outcome. *J Bone Joint Surg Am* 2011;93(10):937-941.

96. Jauregui JJ, Yarmis SJ, Tsai J, Onuoha KO, Illical E, Paulino CB: Fasciotomy closure techniques: A meta-analysis. *J Orthop Surg* 2017;25:1-8.

97. Khoshhal KI, Kiefer GN: Physeal bridge resection. *J Am Acad Orthop Surg* 2005;13(1):47-58.

98. Wuerz TH, Gurd DP: Pediatric physeal ankle fracture. *J Am Acad Orthop Surg* 2013;21(4):234-244.

99. Wang DC, Deeney V, Roach JW, Shah AJ: Imaging of physeal bars in children. *Pediatr Radiol* 2015;45(9):1403-1412.

100. Yuan BJ, Stans AA, Larson DR, Peterson HA: Excision of physeal bars of the distal femur, proximal and distal tibia followed to maturity. *J Pediatr Orthop* 2019;39(6):e422-e429.

This study reported the results of physeal bar resection surgery in a group of patients followed up to skeletal maturity. Level of evidence: IV.

CHAPTER 38

High-Energy Injury and Polytrauma

NIRAV K. PANDYA, MD • KRISTIN S. LIVINGSTON, MD

ABSTRACT

Although most fractures in children are caused by low-energy falls and sports injuries, there are a small but significant subset of injuries in which a large amount of energy is transferred to the pediatric skeleton and soft tissues. Because of pediatric physiology, children typically experience better soft-tissue and bone healing and have better functional outcomes than adults with high-energy trauma, yet these injuries can still cause substantial morbidity at a young age with lifelong consequences. Although fundamental orthopaedic principles are followed in many cases, there are myriad ways in which pediatric injuries must be considered and managed differently than adult injuries. It is important to be knowledgeable on penetrating trauma, mangled extremities, extremity trauma with vascular injury, acute compartment syndrome, wound management, and polytrauma considerations in the pediatric patients with trauma.

Keywords: compartment syndrome; firearm; mangled extremity; open fracture; polytrauma; vascular injury

Dr. Pandya or an immediate family member serves as a paid consultant to or is an employee of OrthoPediatrics and serves as a board member, owner, officer, or committee member of the Pediatric Orthopaedic Society of North America. Neither Dr. Livingston nor any immediate family member has received anything of value from or has stock or stock options held in a commercial company or institution related directly or indirectly to the subject of this chapter.

INTRODUCTION

Because of changing patterns of activity and exposure, pediatric and adolescent patients are increasingly subject to high-energy injury. As a result, the orthopaedic clinician must be well versed in not only the management of these injuries but also the underlying physiology of the pediatric response to polytrauma. Adult principles of management are not always applicable in this setting, and significant morbidity and mortality can occur if appropriate care is not delivered. The areas to which special attention must be paid in children include polytrauma physiology, penetrating trauma (particularly gunshot wounds [GSWs]), the mangled extremity (particularly lawn mower injuries), extremity injuries requiring vascular repair, compartment syndrome, and traumatic wound management.

OVERVIEW OF THE PEDIATRIC PATIENT WITH POLYTRAUMA

The incidence of severe, multisystem trauma in the pediatric patients continues to increase and remains the leading cause of death in children aged between 1 to 19 years in the United States.[1] Use of all-terrain vehicles, dirt bikes, and snowmobiles in the pediatric population along with motor vehicle–related accidents can result in severe multisystem injury.[2] Although rarely the cause of mortality, orthopaedic injuries are frequently seen in this age group and can lead to morbidity if not appropriately addressed. Delayed diagnosis of orthopaedic injuries in the pediatric patients with trauma has been noted to be as high as 20%.[3,4] A retrospective analysis of 196 pediatric trauma patients with orthopaedic injury in 2017 found that lower Glasgow Coma Scale, higher Injury Severity Score (ISS), and greater hospital length of stay were associated with delays in diagnosis of orthopaedic injury.[4]

It is therefore essential for orthopaedic clinicians to be intimately involved in the care of these patients and also have an understanding of the unique physiology of pediatric patients in contrast to the adult patient population.

Initial Trauma Assessment

Pediatric Advanced Life Support and Advanced Trauma Life Support principles should guide the initial assessment in the trauma bay. Respiratory or circulatory compromise must be identified and managed to prevent acidosis, hypothermia, and coagulopathy. Large-bore intravenous access and/or intraosseous infusion distal to the tibial tuberosity can be used. Unlike adult patients, pediatric patients will not become hypotensive until 25% of the blood volume is lost, so heart rate should be used to assess for inadequate perfusion rather than blood pressure.

Radiographs of the chest, pelvis, and cervical spine along with CT scans of the chest, abdomen, and pelvis may be performed in a stepwise fashion to rapidly identify multisystem organ injury. Because of a difference in head-body ratios, pediatric patients should have cervical spine immobilization with a backboard with an occipital recess or a mattress pad to elevate the body.[5] Patients with extremity injuries should be splinted until surgical intervention can be undertaken. Open fractures should be managed with prompt antibiotics and tetanus prophylaxis until the patient is systemically stable to undergo intervention. When severe systemic injuries delay orthopaedic intervention, Buck traction can be used for unstable femoral or pelvic fractures for less than 24 hours. If traction is needed for longer periods, skeletal traction pins can be placed proximal to the distal femoral physis (**Figure 1**); proximal tibial pins should be avoided because of risk of damage to the tibial tubercle and subsequent recurvatum deformity.

Unlike the adult population, exsanguination from bleeding related to pelvic ring injury is rare.[6] Although morbidity and mortality from bleeding is less, mortality has not been shown to be different when these injuries occur.[6,7] This largely is because pediatric patients who sustain pelvic fractures are generally involved in high-energy trauma, and other associated visceral injuries are quite severe (leading to increased mortality). Thus, the clinician must thoroughly investigate for associated injuries in the presence of a pelvic fracture in this population. Albeit not the source of mortality, these fractures should be aggressively managed as long-term sequelae are common in untreated injuries.[8,9]

Pediatric Physiology

The pediatric and adult systemic responses to acute trauma vastly differ. Treatment of patients with polytrauma at pediatric trauma centers has been associated with improved outcomes.[10] This has been particularly true with the American College of Surgeons formal verification

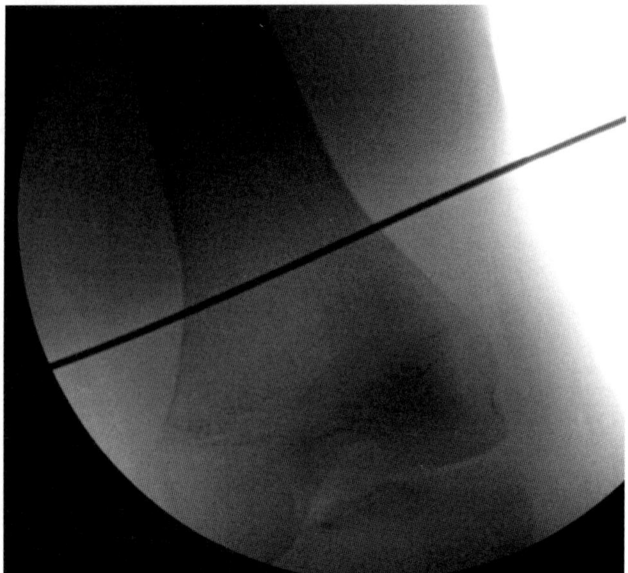

FIGURE 1 Intraoperative fluoroscopic image from a 14-year-old boy with head injury with a displaced femur fracture stabilized with skeletal traction proximal to the distal femoral physis before surgical fixation.

process for level I trauma centers.[11] It is important to note that as some older adolescents (aged 12 to 17 years) transition to more adult pattern injury and physiology, they may benefit from care at adult trauma centers, particularly when severe blunt polytrauma injury is present. A 2017 study retrospectively reviewed 1,606 patients (aged 12 to 17 years) from a Pennsylvania state database who had sustained severe polytrauma and found lower functional status at discharge and higher total complication rates when these adolescent patients were treated at pediatric trauma centers as opposed to adult centers.[12] In addition, careful resource allocation is critical in the transport of these patients. Although helicopter transport has been shown to improve the odds of survival of severely injured children, the benefit may only exist for patients with an ISS >15.[13,14] Overutilization of air transport for children with minor injuries, particularly those who are discharged within 24 hours, may burden the healthcare system.[14]

Understanding the differences in adult and pediatric physiology is critical in terms of understanding fracture management in this population[15] (**Table 1**). Adult physiology is characterized by an inflammatory cascade leading to endothelial permeability, interstitial edema, intravascular occlusion, microvascular ischemia, and eventual organ failure.[16,17] There is a robust *systemic* inflammatory response with organ failure occurring 48 hours after injury in a sequential fashion beginning with lungs.[18-21] In contrast in the pediatric population, multiorgan failure occurs early after the initial resuscitation process with simultaneous organ involvement with a robust

TABLE 1

Comparison of Adult and Pediatric Physiologic Response to Polytrauma

Factor	Adults	Children
Timing of organ failure	48-72 hr after injury	Immediately after injury
Organ failure sequence	Sequential	Simultaneous
Acute lung injury	High risk	Low risk
Systemic inflammatory response	Robust	Dampened
Local inflammatory response	Dampened	Robust
Death due to pelvic fracture	High risk	Low risk
Morbidity	Associated with pelvic fracture	Associated with organ injuries
Neurologic injury	Low recovery rate	High recovery rate

Reproduced with permission from Pandya NK, Upasani VV, Kulkarni VA: The pediatric polytrauma patient: Current concepts. *J Am Acad Orthop Surg* 2013;21(3):170-179.

local inflammatory response.[18-21] In addition, the rate of acute lung injury has been found to be six times lower in children than the adults.[22,23] Further understanding of cytokine levels such as interleukin 6 (which has been shown to correlate with injury severity in multiple injured pediatric patients) can help to guide management.[24]

Timing of Surgical Fixation

Because of the differences in adult and pediatric systemic responses to severe injury, timing of fracture fixation differs. Yet, there is limited high-quality prospective data regarding the timing of fracture fixation in the pediatric patient with polytrauma.[15] Definitive fracture stabilization in the adult population is many times delayed for 48 to 72 hours until resuscitation is complete, and the true extent of organ system failure is evident. Because the systemic inflammatory response occurs within the first 24 hours after injury in children, early fixation can be undertaken in the immature population. A 1987 study examined a series of 27 patients with polytrauma and found that early fracture fixation led to shorter hospital stay, intensive care unit time, and length of ventilatory support.[25] If fixation occurred after 72 hours, patients in this series sustained increased complications, particularly those with neural and thoracoabdominal injuries. In addition, patients with polytrauma older than 7 years and with ISS greater than 40 who were immobilized have been shown to have an increased risk of complications.[26]

As a result, prolonged immobilization should be avoided as aggressively as possible. Injuries that are typically managed nonsurgically when they are found in isolation (ie, humeral shaft, clavicle, proximal humerus) should have a much lower threshold for fixation to allow for progressive weight bearing and mobilization.[15] In addition, the utilization of internal fixation methods that allow immediate weight bearing with minimal blood loss (ie, rigid intramedullary nailing, flexible nailing) in long bone injuries should be encouraged. Although not as well studied as in adults, early mobilization may also prevent the risk of venous thromboembolism in older adolescent patients with risk factors such as presence of central venous catheter, infection, or family history.[27] A 2016 study also identified major vascular injury and orthopaedic surgery as predictors of pediatric venous thromboembolism in a cohort of pediatric patients with trauma.[28] This was further demonstrated by a 2013 review of 402,329 patients that found that injury severity was correlated with development of venous thromboembolism including requiring critical care, blood transfusion, central line placement, mechanical ventilation, and surgery; the most dramatic risk increase occurred when patients were aged 16 years or older.[29] It is also important to note that pulmonary embolism and even death can occur in this population.[27] Further study is necessary to develop clinical guidelines for treatment and prophylaxis in the severely injured population.

Nonorthopaedic Injury Including Neurologic Injury

The orthopaedic clinician must be versed in not only the overall systemic response to polytrauma in regard to surgical fixation but also the rates of nonmusculoskeletal injury. Because the pediatric pelvic ring is able to absorb more high-energy trauma without disruption (compared with the adult population), the force is transferred to other organ systems contained within the pelvis and thorax.[30,31] In addition, because of the smaller surface area of pediatric patient, there is a greater chance of simultaneous injury to multiple organs. As a result, injuries to genitourinary system (bladder/urethra), abdomen (spleen/intestine), or thorax (rib/pneumothorax) play a greater role in morbidity and/or mortality in the young population.[32] As a result, predictive calculations such as the unadjusted shock index (heart rate/systolic blood pressure) are accurate and specific markers of morbidity and mortality in the pediatric patients with polytrauma, predicting the need for blood transfusion, ventilation, interventional procedure, or intensive care unit stay.[33]

Neurologic injury (particularly head injury) remains the leading cause of long-term disability in this population.[34] However, neurologic recovery is quite high and noticeably higher than the adult population.[34,35] Therefore, aggressive management of orthopaedic injuries should be undertaken because what may seem to be severe, life-altering neurologic events in the adult population may be recoverable in the pediatric population. Management of musculoskeletal trauma should be designed under the assumption (in coordination with the neurosurgical team) that the patients will make substantial recovery from the injuries. Failure to do so may place a patient at a deficit after recovery because of nonsurgical management of extremity injuries (**Figure 2, A through D**).

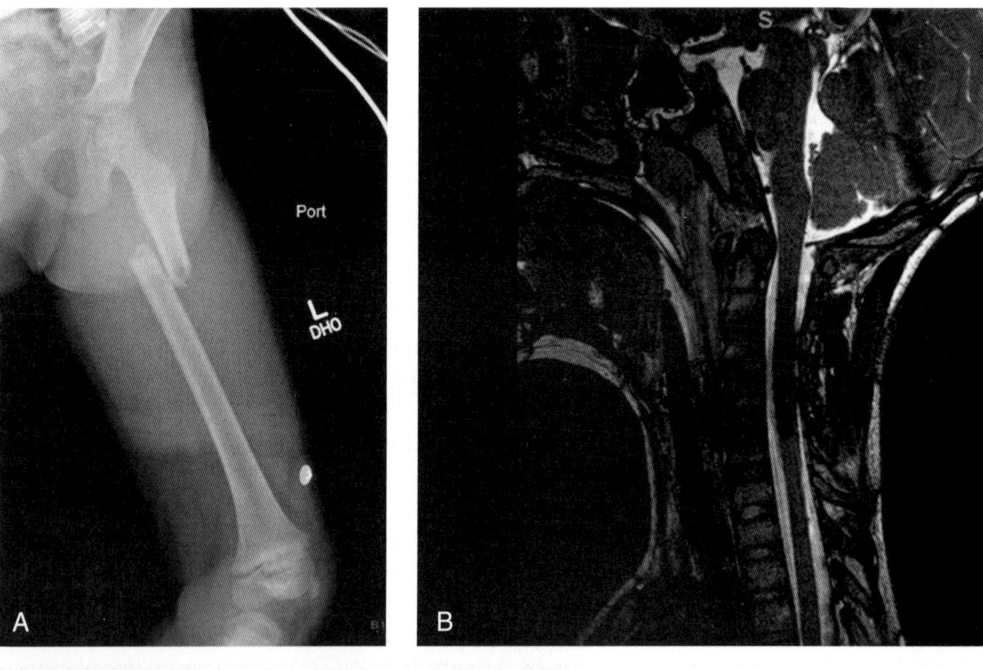

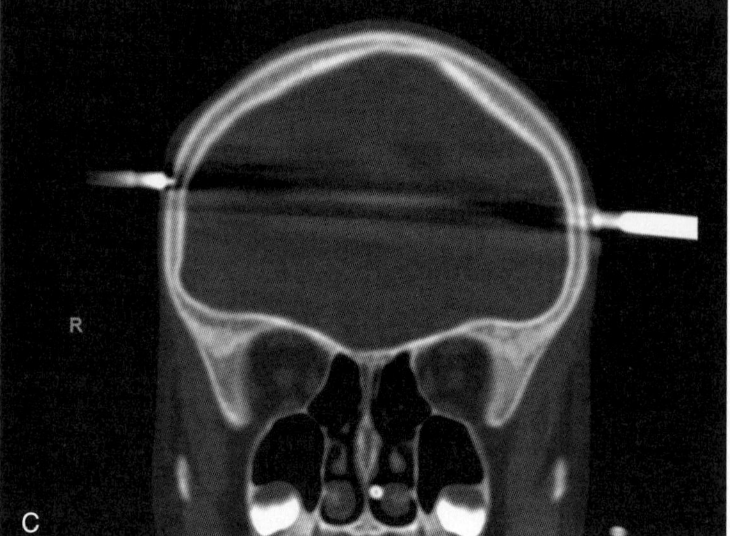

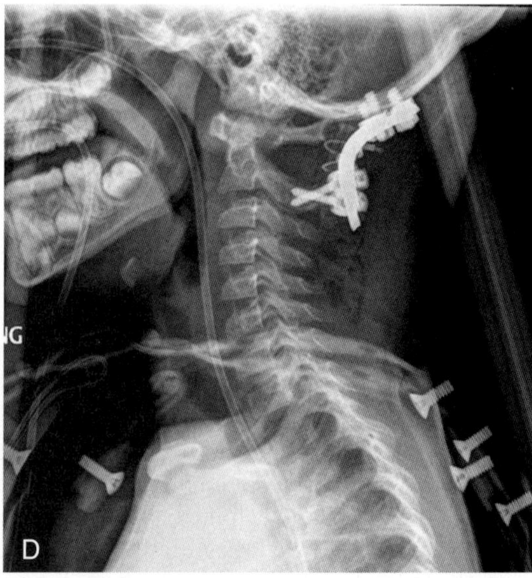

FIGURE 2 **A**, AP radiograph of the left femur from a 7-year-old boy ejected from a motor vehicle who sustained a displaced left femur fracture. **B**, Sagittal T2 magnetic resonance image demonstrating anterior translation of the skull relative to C1, which required delay of femur stabilization. **C**, Coronal CT image after halo placement by the neurosurgery team before flexible nail stabilization. **D**, After flexible nailing of the femur, the patient then underwent occiput to C2 fusion, shown in lateral c-spine radiograph.

Because of the risk of intramedullary fixation in the context of closed head injury (increased intracranial pressure), coordination of treatment with the neurosurgery team is essential during treatment of the patients with multiple injuries.[36]

PENETRATING TRAUMA

Epidemiology and Prevention

The effect of gun violence on the pediatric and adolescent population continues to escalate. Firearms are the third leading cause of death in children aged between 1 to 17 years.[37] A 2017 study reported that nearly 1,300 children die and 5,790 are treated per year in the emergency department for gun-related injury.[38] This increase in penetrating trauma also includes other mechanisms such as stabbings.[39] The burden of GSW-related violence is unequally distributed, with minorities, immigrants, lower socioeconomic status families, and males disproportionately affected. Complex social factors are inherently tied to this problem.[39-43] Trauma center prevention programs should be well versed in safe firearm storage education, which can effectively decrease intentional and unintentional gun injuries among youth.[44,45] Implementation of firearm safety laws, expansion of mental health services, and strong antiviolence messaging in the media are all mechanisms through which gun violence can be curbed in the pediatric and adolescent population.[46]

Initial Evaluation and Stabilization

Physiologic predictors of mortality for pediatric patients who sustain firearm injuries include low initial pH (≤7.15) or hematocrit (≤30), high ISS (>15), and head injury,[47] as well as self-inflicted injuries.[43] Although there exists a relative abundance of pediatric and general surgery literature in regard to the management of GSW injuries in this population, there is very limited orthopaedic literature. Orthopaedic clinicians must understand the management of these injuries because the penetrating trauma from firearms can affect the soft tissues and vital neurovascular structures in addition to the musculoskeletal injury. Because most cases of penetrating trauma will result in a trauma activation, initial treatment of patients with a penetrating injury should include a coordinated effort with the trauma service to ensure hemodynamic stability and assess for multisystem organ injury, particularly when multiple penetrating injuries are present.

It is essential for the orthopaedic clinician to understand the effect of the bullet on the surrounding soft tissue in addition to the fracture pattern. Handguns have a short barrel and can be characterized as creating low-energy tissue damage. In contrast, rifles fire bullets at much higher velocities creating high-energy soft-tissue damage.[48] Injuries caused by shotguns are unique in that they are directly related to the victim's proximity to the weapon at the time of discharge, with severe injuries occurring at close range. Although the injuries to the bone may appear innocuous in patients who are victims of high-energy gunshot injury, the surrounding soft tissues can be severely compromised requiring a much more aggressive treatment strategy.[49] In all penetrating trauma, careful attention should be paid to the distal neurovascular status of the affected extremity.

Most GSW-related fractures are closed but contaminated injuries. All patients should receive tetanus prophylaxis. Yet, there is no consensus in the literature for antibiotic prophylaxis for both low-energy and high-energy gunshot injuries. A 2013 study performed a systematic review of the role of antibiotics in the management of low-energy GSWs and found that prophylactic antibiotics did not significantly reduce the infection rate for fractures managed nonsurgically (1.7% with antibiotics versus 5.1% without). Duration of treatment also did not affect infection rate, and there was no difference between intravenous and oral antibiotics for nonsurgically managed fractures.[50] High-energy injuries (particularly with gross contamination, joint involvement, and open fractures) benefit from at least 24 to 48 hours of intravenous antibiotics[51] similar to Gustilo grade II and III injuries from blunt trauma.

Low-energy gunshots in which the bony injury can be managed in a closed fashion (using standard pediatric orthopaedic principles of acceptable reductions) can be irrigated at the bedside in the emergency department and immobilized. Typically, the wounds are left open to heal via secondary intention. High-energy injuries, however, require early aggressive débridement in the operating room to assess the extent of soft-tissue injury, remove devitalized tissue, and provisionally stabilize fractures with external fixation until the soft-tissue environment is free of infection and able to support definitive fixation[46,49] (**Figure 3**, **A** through **E**).

In the absence of indications to take the patient to the operating room for débridement and/or surgical stabilization, removal of retained bullets is not indicated unless there is joint retention, compression of neurovascular structures, or it is in a clinically symptomatic subcutaneous position (**Figure 4**). In general, the bullet creates tissue damage during its entry into the body. Once the bullet comes to rest, further injury to the body is minimized. A 2012 study examined 244 children who sustained GSWs, of which 107 had retained foreign bodies. Although 22% of these patients experienced complications (ie, infection, pain, inflammation, elevated lead levels) related to the retained foreign bodies (with 13% requiring removal), the authors concluded that prophylactic removal is not necessary as long as close follow-up is performed.[52]

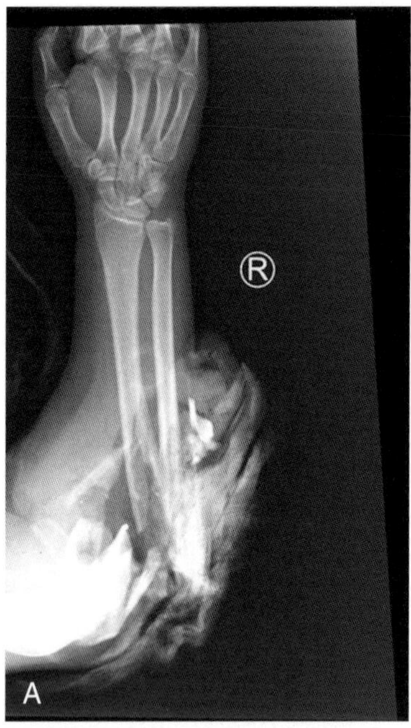

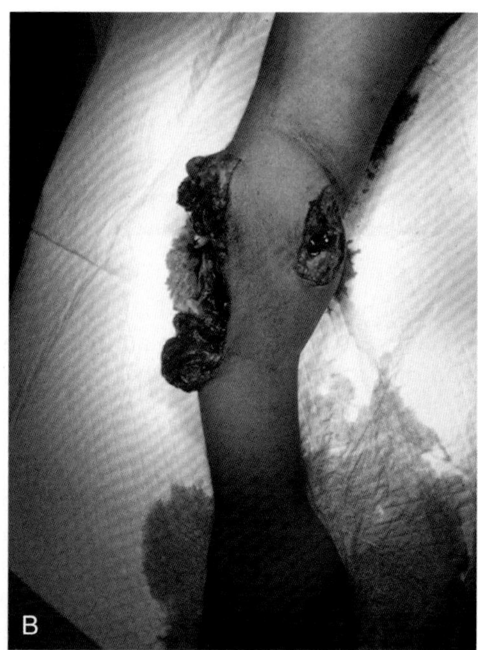

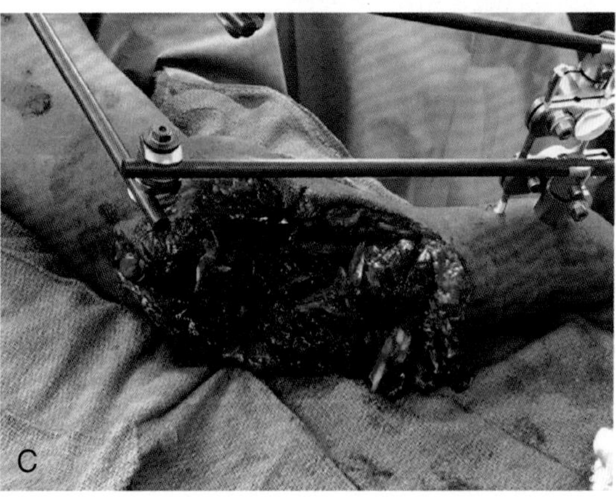

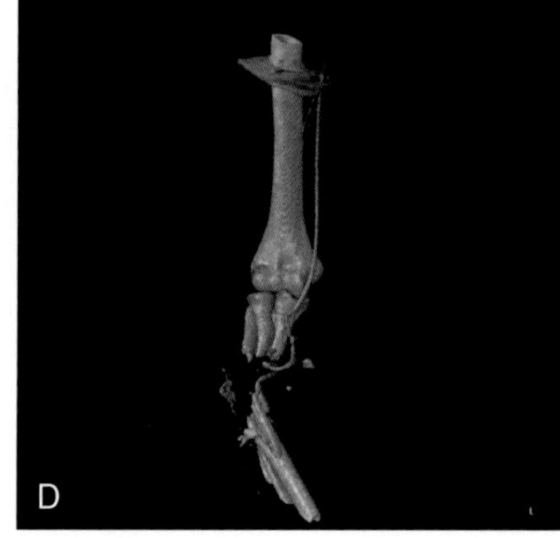

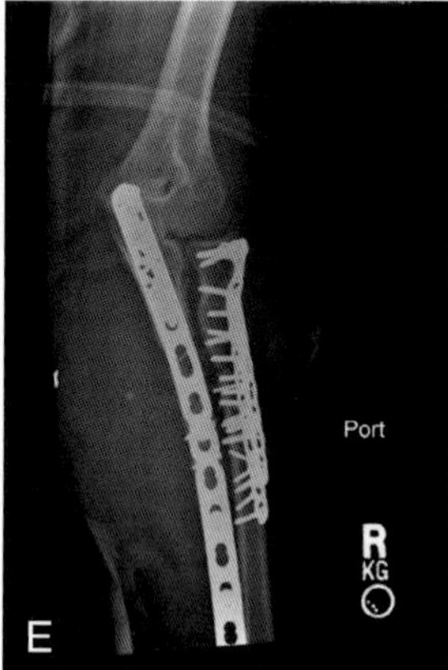

FIGURE 3 **A**, AP radiograph of the elbow from a 13-year-old girl who sustained a high-energy gunshot wound to the elbow. **B**, Intraoperative clinical photograph demonstrating entry and exit wound. **C**, Intraoperative clinical photograph after external fixation demonstrating extensive damage to the soft tissues about the elbow including muscle, tendon, nerve, and vascular injury on exploration of the wound. **D**, Reconstructed CT angiogram demonstrating intact vascular flow after radial artery repair with saphenous vein graft. **E**, AP radiograph of the elbow after definitive fixation and soft-tissue coverage.

Clinicians should educate parents and patients about the signs of lead toxicity including abdominal pain, constipation, nausea, vomiting, learning disability, growth disturbance, headache, appetite loss, memory loss, and/or irritability that may occur because of a retained bullet.

Surgical Management

General Principles

Extremity fracture can occur via direct contact of the bullet with the bone or secondary to energy transmission from the bullet to the bone when it passes through the surrounding soft tissue. The decision to proceed to the operating room should be based on both the soft-tissue injury and fracture stability. If the patient has a healthy soft-tissue envelope and a fracture that would not routinely require stabilization, then nonsurgical treatment can be performed.

Patients who have open injuries (both fracture and joints), unstable fracture patterns, bone loss, or severe soft-tissue injury should be taken to the operating room for treatment. Basic principles of trauma management are applicable; fractures should be provisionally stabilized via external fixation until the soft-tissue envelope can support internal fixation. Soft-tissue defects may require skin grafting, rotational flaps, or free flap coverage in conjunction with fracture stabilization. Extensive bone loss may need staged grafting procedures as well (**Figure 5**).

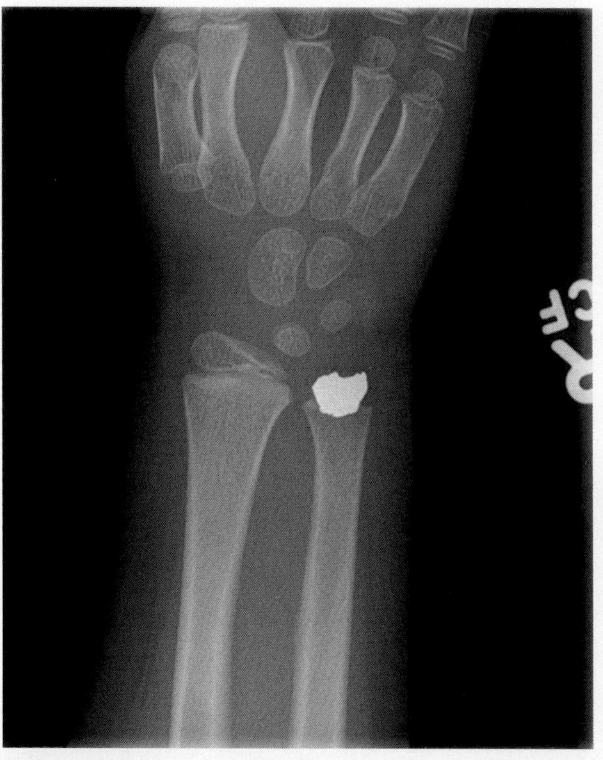

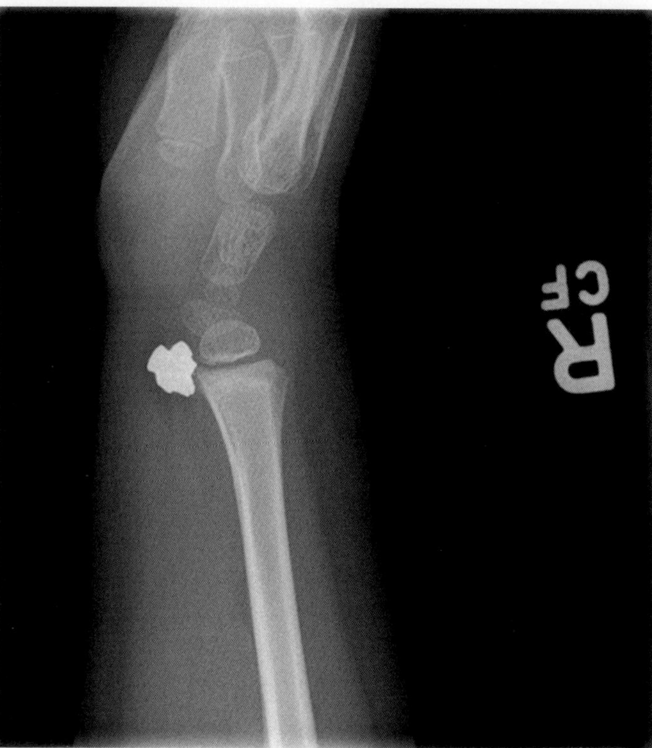

FIGURE 4 AP and lateral radiographs of the right wrist from a 5-year-old boy who sustained a gunshot wound to the wrist. The bullet came to rest on the ulnar nerve and was causing compression of the nerve but no transection.

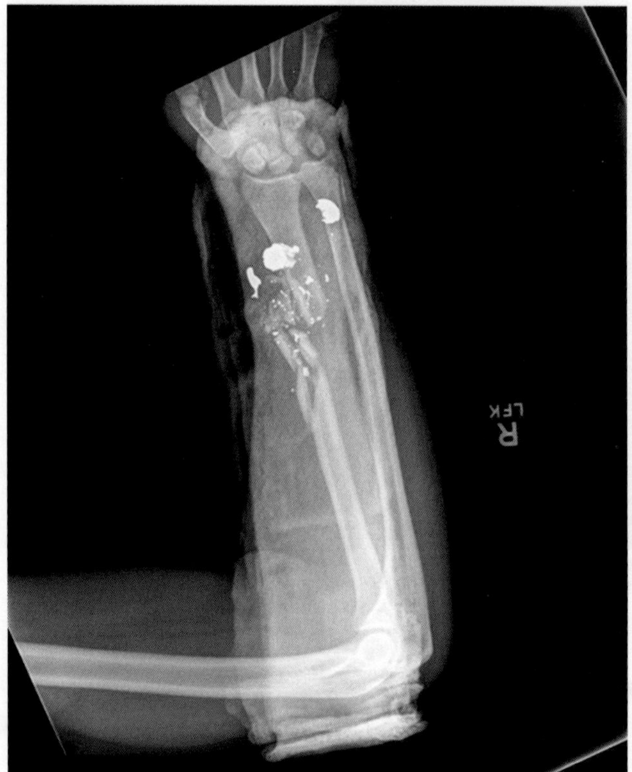

FIGURE 5 AP radiograph of the forearm from a 16-year--old boy who sustained a high-energy gunshot wound to the forearm with extensive bone loss that required eventual bone grafting.

Intra-articular Injuries

GSWs that violate the articular surface can be a devastating injury, particularly for young patients. These injuries require urgent irrigation and débridement via open or arthroscopic techniques with removal of retained bullet material. Joint penetration may not be immediately obvious, and radiographic findings such as air in the joint, hematoma in the joint, or articular fracture should raise suspicion for intra-articular bullet penetration (**Figure 6, A and B**).

The energy from the bullet can destroy a wide zone of articular cartilage. If present, large osteochondral fragments may need to be restored via fixation if possible. In addition, associated ligamentous injury may be present and may require staged reconstruction. Complete removal of foreign material from joints is necessary to decrease mechanical irritation. It is also necessary to limit the risk of lead toxicity and lead arthropathy in the future.[53] It has the added benefit of improving quality of advanced imaging if that will be required to assess for future reconstructive procedures.

Pelvis and Spine

Patients presenting with pelvic and spinal column injuries secondary to gunshot trauma require special consideration. Because of the proximity of the abdominal organs to the pelvis, a complete imaging workup should

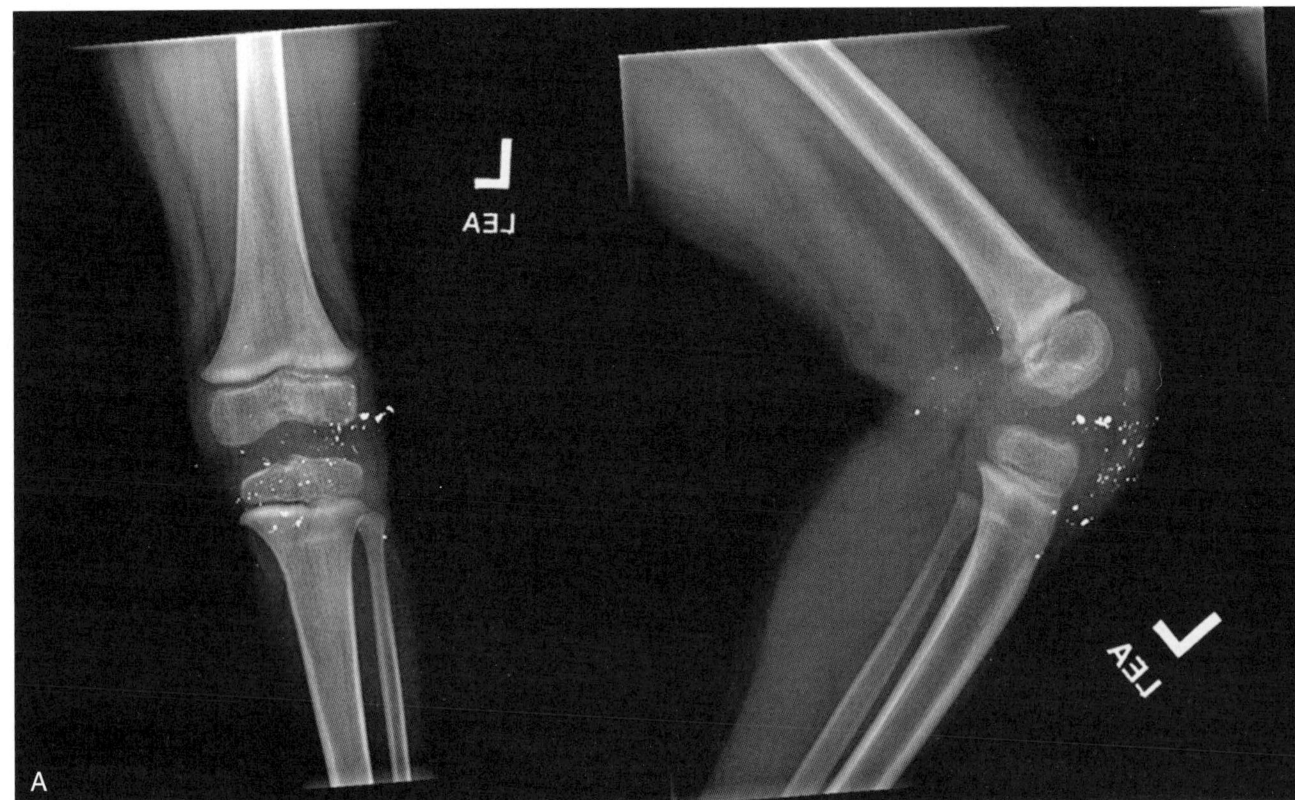

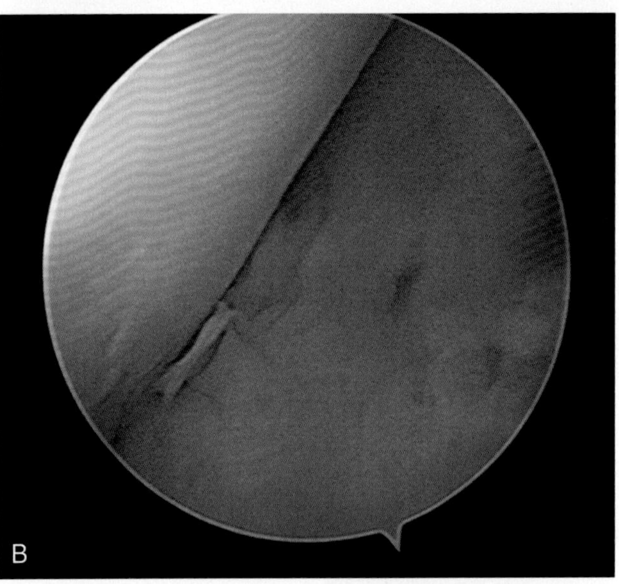

FIGURE 6 **A**, AP and lateral radiographs of the knee from a 3-year-old child who presented several months after being shot in the knee during an assault in other country with lead synovitis. **B**, Intraoperative arthroscopic image during synovectomy demonstrating lead fragments within the synovium.

be performed to ensure multisystem injury, and gastrointestinal tract perforation is not present. Extra-articular fractures do not necessitate débridement even in the case of bowel contamination.[54,55] As with appendicular injury, fractures that involve joints and/or retained bullet fragments in the joint should undergo débridement and stabilization. The infection rate is higher with concomitant bowel injury, and in this situation, treatment for 48 to 72 hours with broad-spectrum antibiotics is prudent.[56]

Management of spinal gunshot–induced injuries depends on several factors including neurologic function and any change in that function over time, spinal stability, the missile tract through the body, and concomitant injuries. Careful attention should be paid to cardiac, pulmonary, and abdominal injury (**Figure 7**). Sensory, motor, and reflex function of the cervical, thoracic, and lumbar regions should be tested and documented to pick up evolving neurologic function. As with pelvic injuries, routine débridement and bullet removal is not necessary even with transperitoneal contamination.[57,58] With concomitant bowel injury, treatment for 48 to 72 hours with broad-spectrum antibiotics is indicated.[59] Vertebral column instability that requires surgical intervention is rare. In a review of 60 adolescent patients with GSWs to the spine, no spinal instability was noted even in the presence of 34 patients with complete neurologic deficits.[60]

A progressive loss of neurologic function with radiographic evidence of neural compression is an indication for surgical intervention. Symptomatic dural tears as well as epidural hematomas or abscesses will also require surgical treatment. Retained bullet fragments in the disk space can result in lead toxicity and may need to be removed. However, surgery for stable, complete neurologic deficits has not been shown to improve sensory or motor recovery. Therefore, patients without clear indications for surgical intervention should be treated nonsurgically.[59]

Nerve Injury

Injuries to peripheral nerves can be frequently seen in the setting of gunshot injuries from both direct projectile transection and/or transmission of energy to the nerve from the surrounding tissue through which the bullet travels. A careful preoperative examination documenting neurologic function of both motor and sensory nerves is critical because the prognosis of peripheral nerve injuries is not as good as that seen with blunt trauma. If wound exploration is performed in the acute setting, the nerve should be assessed. A 2019 study outlined a suggested treatment algorithm for nerve injuries.[61] If a nerve palsy is found and there is a vascular injury or another indication for surgical intervention exists, acute exploration is warranted.[61] The nerve laceration rate with acute palsy is surprisingly low: 27% in a 2017 study.[62] Tendon lacerations and high-energy mechanism have also been cited as indications for nerve exploration.[63]

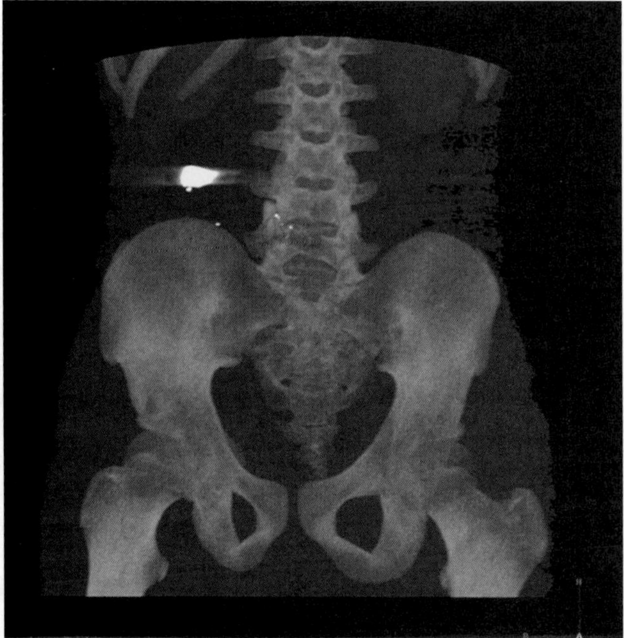

FIGURE 7 Reformatted coronal CT image from a 14-year-old patient demonstrating injury to the L5 pedicle after a gunshot wound to the spine.

If complete nerve transection is found, end-to-end repair can be attempted or the nerve ends can be tagged to prevent retraction and ease identification for later repair. Delayed repair of nerves may be preferable after acute exploration to allow the zone of injury to be better declared. Nerves found to be in continuity, or nerve palsies in which no surgical intervention is performed, can be observed for recovery for 3 months.[61] If incomplete recovery is present at 3 months, an electromyography should be considered to assess nerve function. Surgical exploration with external neurolysis, direct repair, or nerve grafting can be considered. It is important not to excessively delay intervention because muscles can sustain irreversible changes.

Physeal Injury

As with any fracture that involves a skeletally immature patient, physeal injury with subsequent risk of deformity and/or leg length discrepancy must be considered. It is important to note that premature physeal arrest can occur from either direct bullet injury to the physis or transmission of energy to the physis from a bullet that traverses the extraphyseal bone or surrounding soft tissue.[64] Follow-up radiographs of individuals who experience gunshot injury near the physis are indicated, and intervention should be taken based on patient age, skeletal maturity, and deformity (**Figure 8, A** through **D**).

Outcomes

There is limited literature examining orthopaedic injuries from GSWs in the pediatric population. A 2016 study examined 46 pediatric patients with orthopaedic firearm injuries at the trauma center over an 8-year period: 44 fractures and 6 traumatic arthrotomies. Eight patients sustained neurovascular injuries. Twenty-five patients had an orthopaedic procedure with five deep infections and four nonunions.[65] Mean hospital stay was 6.8 days. Another 2016 study examined 49 pediatric patients with 58 fractures over an 8-year period

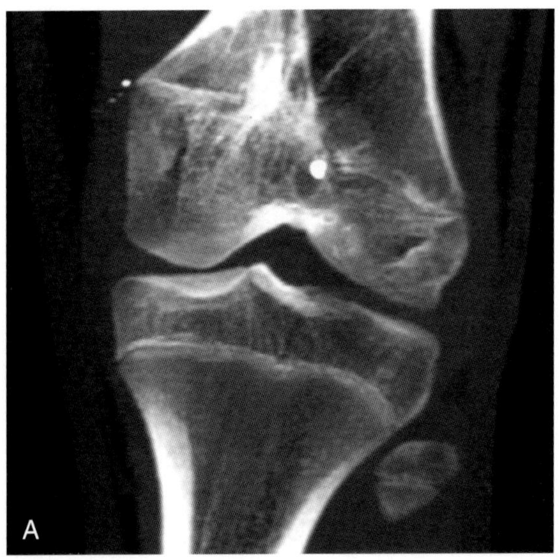
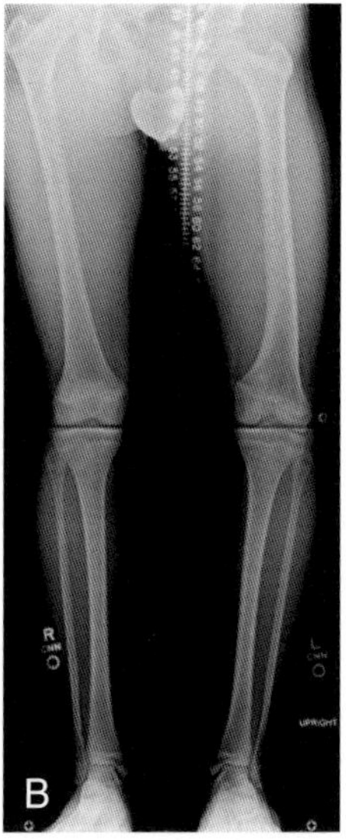
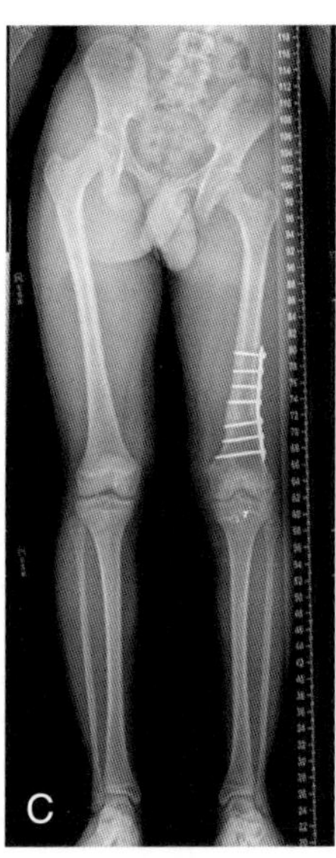
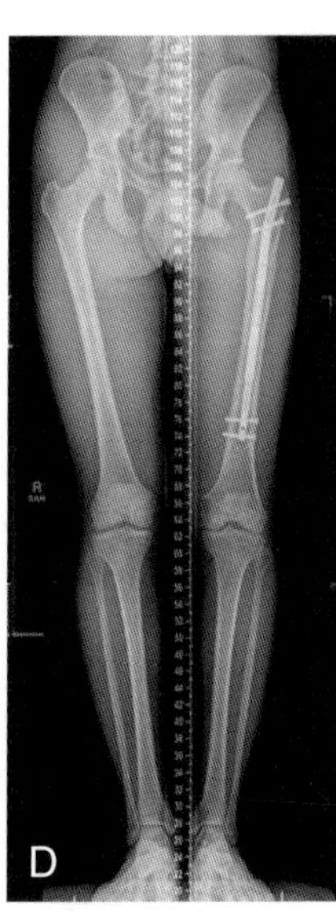

FIGURE 8 **A**, CT image from a 13-year-old boy who had been shot 10 years prior in the left knee with resultant physeal arrest. **B**, Bone length radiograph demonstrating subsequent leg length discrepancy and varus deformity. **C**, Bone length radiograph after osteotomy to correct varus alignment. **D**, Bone length radiograph after plate removal and lengthening to correct leg length discrepancy after angular correction.

at two level I pediatric trauma centers. The tibia and femur (19% each) were most commonly affected followed by foot and fibula. Nearly half of the patients had additional injuries including abdominal, genitourinary, and neurovascular injuries. Nearly three-fourths of the fractures were managed nonsurgically. Two patients developed infection, three patients developed compartment syndrome, and four patients required vascular injury repair.[66]

PEDIATRIC MANGLED EXTREMITY

Etiology

Most patients who present with mangled extremities are men aged 20 to 39 years,[67] although children of all ages may sustain these injuries, primarily from motor vehicle accidents (or pedestrian versus motor vehicle accident), lawn mowers, farm machinery, train, or all-terrain vehicle accidents.[68] These injuries are also seen in the setting of disasters such as earthquakes, blast injuries, or acts of terrorism.

Lawn Mower Injuries

Lawn mower injuries, affecting 17,000 children per year in the United States and costing $90 million per year,[69] have caught the attention of the media and national organizations such as the American Academy of Pediatrics and Pediatric Orthopaedic Society of North America.[70,71] These injuries are notable because they are highly preventable and have the potential to cause significant disability at a very young age (**Figure 9, A** through **D**). These injuries have a high amputation rate given the extreme amount of energy imparted by a lawn mower blade, which is equivalent to dropping a 211-lb object from a height of 100 feet.[69,72,73]

Despite various prevention strategies and educational outreach, there has not been a significant decrease in the incidence of these injuries over the past decade.[72] A study published in the *Journal of Bone & Joint Surgery* in 2018 described the patterns of lawn mower injury and found that these injuries tend to occur in warmer months with a bimodal age distribution with peaks at age 4 and 15 years and mainly in boys.[69] These injuries were most frequently from riding lawn mowers where children were bystanders, passengers, or operators.[72] Grandparent operators have been shown to be independently associated with a higher injury severity.[69]

The most frequent injuries tend to include the foot (84%), although upper extremity injuries occurred in 28%. Around 40% to 53% of pediatric victims of lawn mower injuries sustain traumatic amputation, and these lawn mower injuries account for 12% to 29% of all traumatic amputations in kids.[69,74] The youngest lawn mower victims tend to be the most severely injured with longer hospital stays and more frequent need for intensive care unit admission.[72,74] Additionally, children younger than 5 years have a six times higher rate of amputation compared with children aged 6 years or older.[75] Given these statistics, it is the recommendation of the American Academy of Pediatrics that children should be at least 12 years of age to operate a walk-behind power mower or hand mower and at least 16 years of age to operate a riding lawn mower and should never be passengers on ride-on mowers.[76]

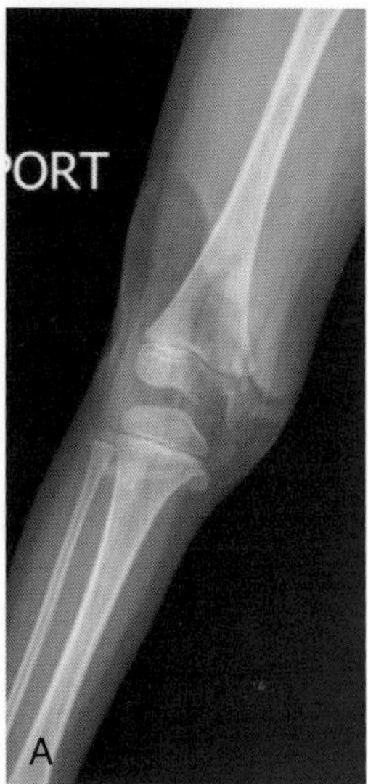

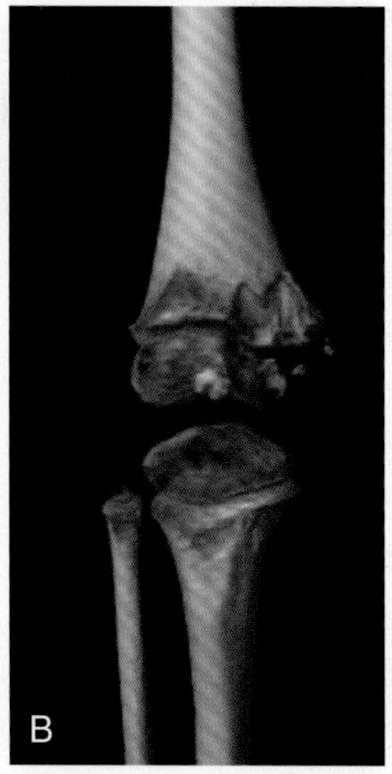

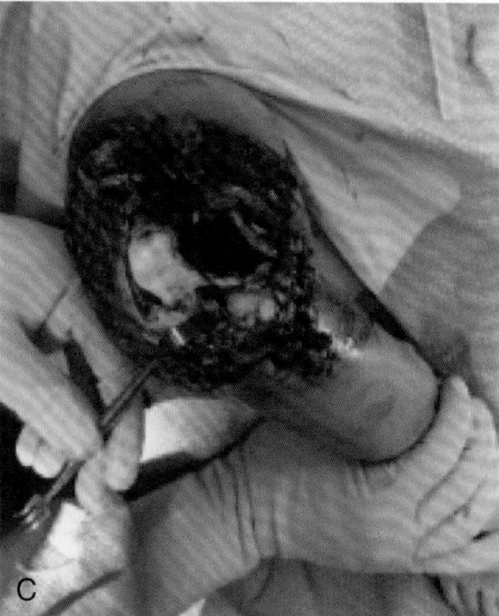

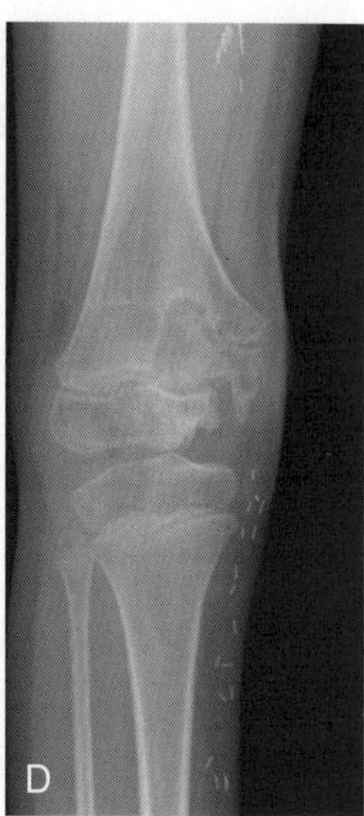

FIGURE 9 **A**, AP radiograph from 3-year-old girl injured by the blade of a lawn mower with fracture of medial femoral condyle. **B**, Three-dimensional CT reconstruction of knee demonstrating significant bone loss of medial femoral condyle, crossing physis. **C**, Intraoperative photograph demonstrating severe soft-tissue injury and bone loss of medial femoral condyle (Photograph courtesy of Dr. Coleen Sabatini). **D**, Follow-up radiograph showing joint deformity and irregular growth of the distal femur.

Treatment Decisions

In the setting of lawn mower injury or other severe extremity injury resulting in a mangled extremity in a child, the decision of limb salvage versus amputation can be extremely difficult. Luckily, in these situations, children tend to have superior outcomes compared with adults with lower rates of delayed union, nonunion, and osteomyelitis.[68,77-79] Despite the excellent healing abilities of children, the risks of indiscriminate attempts at limb salvage are documented in the literature, so the ability to make a well-informed decision for primary amputation versus limb salvage is paramount.

Different scoring systems have been developed in adults and extrapolated to children to help predict the need for amputation versus limb salvage. The Mangled Extremity Severity Score (MESS) is the most recognized score in orthopaedic literature and includes points for skeletal and soft-tissue injury, vascular status, blood pressure, and patient age, all taken together to assess the need for amputation versus possibility of salvage, with amputation predicted in scores ≥7[68] (**Table 2**).

MESS has been shown to have the ability to predict salvage versus amputation in children in several studies including a 2002 study that showed 93% accuracy of predicting limb salvage in pediatric patients.[68,80] A study in 2012 suggested a score over 6.5 was a good predictor of the need for amputation in children; however, this finding was questioned in a rebuttal that highlighted children's superior outcomes with nerve repair, higher likelihood of fracture union, lower wound infection rate, and superior neural plasticity.[81,82] Similarly, another study advocated to salvage limbs in children with MESS less than 10.[83] A study in 2017 evaluated a different scoring system, the Ganga Hospital Open Injury Severity Scoring system that includes assessment of skin loss, bone loss, musculotendinous, and nerve units as well as comorbidities (**Table 3**). In type IIIB open fractures of the tibia or femur in children with open physes, it was found that a Ganga Hospital Open Injury Severity Scoring of ≥17 had 75% sensitivity and 93.75% specificity for predicting amputation and was more accurate than MESS.[84]

Unfortunately, there is a lack of studies that look at functional outcomes of limb salvage versus amputation in severe lower extremity injuries in children. Regardless of which prediction algorithm is used, it is imperative that these decisions are made by experienced surgeons with multidisciplinary consultation. The prudent clinician will provide adequate documentation of the decision-making process because these decisions may be scrutinized after the fact.

VASCULAR TRAUMA

Evaluation

Traumatic vascular injury, albeit rare in children, can have serious clinical consequences. Hemorrhage in children with smaller total blood volumes can be rapidly lethal. Warm ischemia time is critical to irreversible tissue injury. Therefore, appropriate and efficient evaluation and management of vascular traumatic injuries is paramount. A coordinated response between pediatric trauma, vascular, and orthopaedic surgeons must occur. Careful and prompt diagnosis is key. A 2011 study divided signs of vascular injury into hard and soft signs.[85] Hard signs

TABLE 2

Mangled Extremity Severity Score

Variable	Points
Skeletal/soft-tissue injury	
Low-energy (stab, simple fracture, small-caliber gunshot wound)	1
Medium-energy (open or multiple fractures, dislocations, moderate crush injuries)	2
High-energy (close-range shotgun or high-velocity gunshot wound, crush injury)	3
Very high–energy (same as high-energy plus gross contamination, soft-tissue avulsion)	4
Limb ischemia	
Pulsatile limb without signs of ischemia	0[a]
Pulse reduced or absent but perfusion normal	1[a]
Pulseless, paresthesias, diminished capillary refill	2[a]
Cool, paralyzed, insensate, numb without capillary refill	3[a]
Shock	
Normotensive, blood pressure stable in the field and in operating room	0
Transient hypotension, blood pressure responsive to intravenous fluid	1
Persistent hypotension	2
Age (years)	
Younger than 30	0
30-50	1
Older than 50	2

[a]Points × 2 if ischemia time exceeds 6 hours.

Reproduced with permission from Johansen K, Daines M, Howey T, et al: Objective criteria accurately predict amputation following lower extremity trauma. *J Trauma* 1990;30[5]:568-573.

(ie, pulselessness, pallor, and pulsatile bleeding) require prompt intervention. Soft signs (ie, diminished pulses, history of bleeding in transit, and hematoma) need to be monitored and worked up as clinically indicated (**Table 4**).

Although guidelines for the management of the pulseless supracondylar humerus fracture exist,[86] the management of extremity vascular injury in the setting of other pediatric extremity trauma is less well defined. In the setting of penetrating trauma, a careful examination must be done to assess for compromised vascular flow. If soft signs of vascular injury are present, an ankle-brachial or arterial pressure index may be calculated, with a difference <0.9 indicating the need for further

TABLE 3

Ganga Hospital Open Injury Severity Scoring

Components	Score
Covering structures: skin and fascia	
Wounds without skin loss	
Not over the fracture	1
Exposing the fracture	2
Wounds with skin loss	
Not over the fracture	3
Exposing the fracture	4
Circumferential wound with skin loss	5
Skeletal structures: bone and joints	
Transverse/oblique fracture/butterfly fragment <50% circumference	1
Large butterfly fragment >50% circumference	2
Comminution/segmental fractures without bone loss	3
Bone loss <4 cm	4
Bone loss >4 cm	5
Functional tissues: musculotendinous and nerve units	
Partial injury to musculotendinous unit	1
Complete but repairable injury to musculotendinous units	2
Irreparable injury to musculotendinous units/partial loss of a compartment/complete injury to posterior tibial nerve	3
Loss of one compartment of musculotendinous units	4
Loss of two or more compartments/subtotal amputation	5
Comorbid conditions: add 2 points for each condition present	
• Injury—débridement interval >12 hr	2
• Sewage or organic contamination/farmyard injuries	2
• Age older than 65 yr	2
• Drug-dependent diabetes mellitus/cardiorespiratory diseases leading to increased anesthetic risk	2
• Polytrauma involving chest or abdomen with Injury Severity Score >25/fat embolism	2
• Hypotension with systolic blood pressure <90 mm Hg at presentation	2
• Another major injury to the same limb/compartment syndrome	2

Republished with permission of British Editorial Society of Bone & Joint Surgery from Rajasekaran S, Naresh Babu J, Dheenadhayalan J, et al: A score for predicting salvage and outcome in Gustilo type-IIIA and type-IIIB open tibial fractures. *J Bone Joint Surg Br* 2006;88-B[10]:1351-1360.

TABLE 4

Hard and Soft Signs of Vascular Injury Associated With Extremity Trauma

Hard signs
Pulselessness
Pallor
Paresthesia
Pain
Paralysis
Rapidly expanding hematoma
Massive bleeding
Palpable or audible bruit
Soft signs
History of bleeding in transit
Proximity-related injury
Neurologic finding from a nerve adjacent to a named artery
Hematoma over a named artery

Reproduced with permission from Halvorson JJ, Anz A, Langfitt M, et al: Vascular injury associated with extremity trauma: Initial diagnosis and management. *J Am Acad Orthop Surg* 2011;19(8):495-504.

vascular studies, such as a CT angiogram.[87] Similar to the adult population, the pediatric orthopaedic surgeon should perform timely reduction and stabilization of the fracture to allow for definitive vascular reconstruction and reduction of stress on the vascular repair. In addition, after fracture fixation, any change in postoperative vascular status should be meticulously evaluated (**Figure 10, A** and **B**). Documentation of vascular flow before leaving the operating room is paramount to ensure iatrogenic damage has not taken place.

Pelvic Fractures

Pelvic fractures require special consideration as bleeding can be life-threatening and/or limb threatening. The combination of vascular injury and pelvic trauma has a much higher incidence of mortality than extremity trauma–related vascular injury.[88] Stabilization of the unstable pelvic ring injury with a pelvic binder is key with arteriography/angiography and embolization used to control bleeding if needed, which has been shown to be safe in the pediatric population as well.[88-90]

Multiligament Knee Injury

Multiligament knee dislocations are at extremely high risk for concurrent vascular injury. The popliteus artery is most at risk. A 2014 systemic review of these injury patterns demonstrated an 18% incidence of vascular injury and 25% incidence of nerve injury.[91] Of note, 12% of patients with vascular injury had a resultant amputation. Because these injuries are associated with high-energy mechanisms, particularly in the pediatric population, a full trauma workup should be performed.

Indications for further vascular workup in the patient with a knee dislocation include asymmetry on pulse examination and abnormality of ankle-brachial indices.[92] Arteriography has been used historically, but CT angiogram has been increasingly used because it can be combined with CT of other extremities/systemic areas in the patient with multiple injuries. It has been shown to correlate with the results of intraoperative angiography.[93] Magnetic resonance angiography can be used as well and allows for ligamentous evaluation at the time of vascular assessment. In patients with documented injury, the knee should be reduced and stabilized with a joint-spanning external fixation device. Ligamentous reconstruction can be performed in a staged fashion, although limited literature exists in regard to timing and technique of multiligament knee fixation in the skeletally immature population.

Pediatric Acute Compartment Syndrome

Pediatric acute compartment syndrome (PACS) is a feared complication of high-energy extremity trauma and can lead to severe disability if not diagnosed expeditiously and managed appropriately. It must be noted that PACS, although similar to adult acute compartment syndrome in many ways including general pathophysiology, does have some unique qualities.

Epidemiology and Etiology

PACS most commonly occurs when a bicyclist or pedestrian is struck by a car resulting in a tibia fracture.[94,95] Open fractures carry a notably high risk of compartment syndrome because of the significant energy transfer, severe soft-tissue damage, and swelling but with only modest fascial decompression created by the open wound.[96] Although one must be vigilant in monitoring for PACS at any age with high-risk injury patterns (eg, high-energy tibia fractures that account for 40% of PACS), one must be particularly cognizant of this risk in adolescent population. Teenage boys are at highest risk of acute compartment syndrome of any demographic with ~23 of 100,000 average annual incidence.[97] A study from 2013 showed that the incidence of PACS after a tibia fracture was 11.6%, and this risk was 48% if the child was aged 14 years or older and involved in a motor vehicle crash.[98] This high risk in teenage boys is thought to be because of a rapidly growing muscle bulk with relatively inelastic fascia that may predispose to high compartment pressures. Additionally, resting compartment pressures in children have been shown to

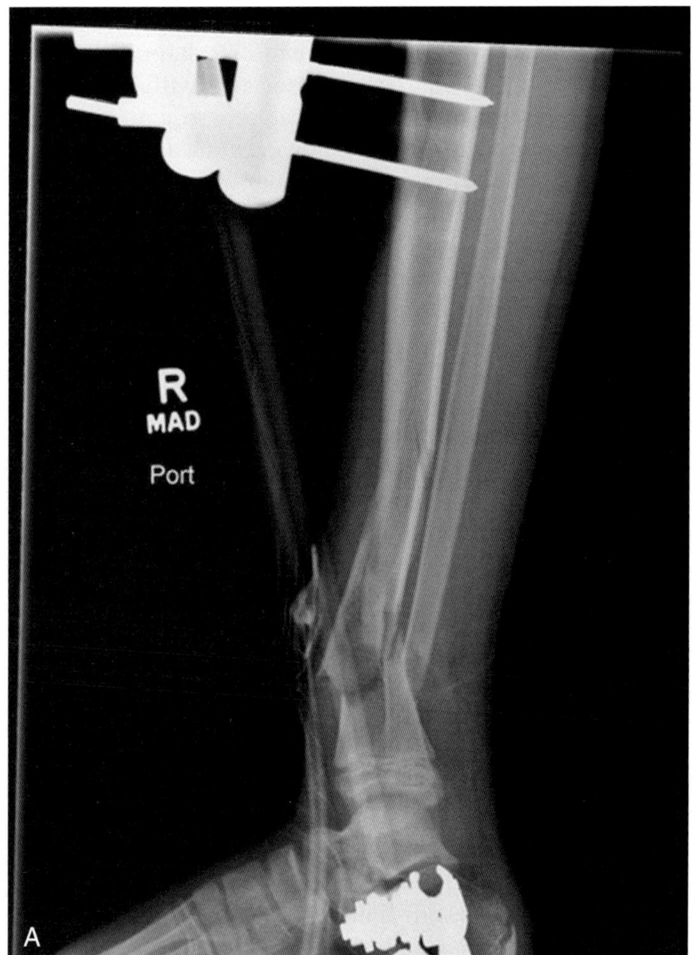

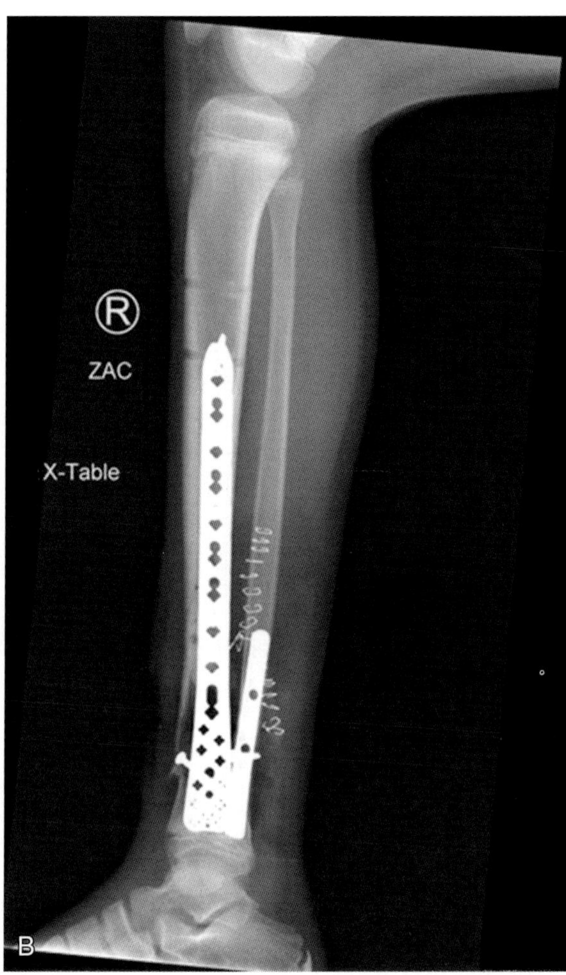

FIGURE 10 **A**, Lateral radiograph of the tibia from a 13-year-old boy with severe open grade IIIC tibia fracture from an all-terrain vehicle accident after initial external fixation in the operating room. **B**, Lateral radiograph after staged internal fixation. After fixation, the patient had an acute change in perfusion. Exploration demonstrated compression of the neurovascular bundle from the distal lag screw and bone spike that had to be revised with subsequent return of flow.

be slightly higher than in adults. One study from 2008 showed that children have resting pressures in the leg of 13.3 to 16.6 mm Hg compared with 5.2 to 9.7 mm Hg in adults.[99] Likewise, a 2016 study that compared normal with injured forearm pressures in children with forearm fractures requiring reduction reported that pressures in the noninjured forearm compartments averaged 9.66 mm Hg (superficial volar), 10.22 mm Hg (deep volar), and 12.9 mm Hg (dorsal), which are higher than reported adult pressures of 9.0 mm Hg.[100,101] Although the clinical significance of this elevated resting pressure is unclear, it has also been suggested that children may tolerate higher sustained pressures without developing muscle ischemia. In adult literature, many studies recommend an absolute pressure greater than 30 mm Hg as an indication for fasciotomy; however, the same forearm study showed that 15 patients had pressures greater than 30 mm Hg in the fractured forearm, 3 had pressures greater than 45 mm Hg, and only 1 of these patients had PACS.[101] A study from 1998 also showed that children tolerated pressures greater than 30 mm Hg without clinical sequelae as long as they were not within the delta-P of 30 mm Hg from mean arterial pressure.[102]

Diagnosis

Unfortunately in many cases it may be difficult or impossible to measure a compartment pressures at the bedside in a scared, awake child. This presents the conundrum that very young children, who are the hardest to diagnose, would be the best candidates for compartment pressure measurements, yet they are the least likely to tolerate the procedure. Pressure monitoring remains an important part in managing high-risk injuries in the obtunded or intubated trauma patient.

Although compartment pressures are used in most cases to diagnose PACS (48% to 77% of cases according to several pediatric case series[94,98,103-105]), one must not diminish the fundamental importance of a good clinical examination.

The 5 Ps (pain, paresthesias, paralysis, pallor, and pulselessness) are well-known diagnostic criteria in adults; however, this constellation of symptoms often represents a late compartment syndrome and is unreliable in children,[98,105,106] especially preverbal children who may not follow commands when scared or in pain or cannot give accurate answers about sensation and whose pain level may be difficult to judge. Even the hallmarks of pain out of proportion and pain with passive stretch may be difficult to interpret in an agitated and frightened child. Children may be more accurately diagnosed by the 3 As, namely increasing anxiety, agitation, and analgesia requirement.[107] A study in 2001 showed that an increasing need for analgesia preceded neurovascular changes by an average of 7 hours in children and is therefore a more reliable indicator of evolving PACS.[103] This difficulty in diagnosis often results in delay in diagnosis and prolonged time to surgery, which is a common theme in reported series of PACS.[94,95,98,104,105]

Treatment

When considering a diagnosis of PACS, one must ensure that patients are normotensive (hypotension is risk factor), traction is reduced, the ankle is allowed to plantarflex (in case of tibia fracture), circumferential dressings are loosened or bivalved, limb is not elevated, and supplemental oxygen is provided.[102,108,109] Once a diagnosis has been made or is strongly suspected, one must proceed with emergent fasciotomy. Decompression should be extensive and include all involved compartments. Frank necrotic tissue should be débrided, keeping in mind that, in kids, dusky muscle may have improved viability on subsequent washouts, and therefore débridement of muscle should be nonsurgical at first inspection.[96,105] Some authors emphasize the robust potential of nerve and muscle recovery after PACS, which suggests that thorough decompressive fasciotomy even in cases of significantly delayed diagnosis may be warranted.[94,98,110] Infection is rarely reported in series of PACS, and therefore concern for infection should not be used as a primary reason to avoid fasciotomy in cases of delay in diagnosis (as it may be in adults).[96] Open wounds may be managed with negative pressure dressings until definitive wound closure is possible. Delayed primary closure after fasciotomy is possible in most cases (75% to 88%) of PACS, although skin grafting or other forms of coverage may be needed in cases of greater soft-tissue compromise.[103,105,111,112]

Outcomes

Typically, it is unknown whether a late fasciotomy is late because of delay in diagnosis or just a longer time from injury to peak pressure. Fortunately, despite longer times from injury to surgery in children, the outcomes of PACS are generally good with robust nerve and muscle recovery and excellent functional outcomes in most series of PACS.[94,96,110] A 2011 study of 43 cases of PACS had nearly uniformly excellent outcomes (95% excellent). The only poor outcomes occurred in patients with fasciotomies after 80 hours from injury.[94] Another 2011 study evaluated outcomes in 24 children with fasciotomies on an average of 27 hours after admission with an overall complication rate of 4.2%.[111] Among another series of 32 children undergoing fasciotomy for PACS, the most common complication was concern about scar appearance (23%), whereas more serious complications occurred less frequently: neurapraxia (6.7%), stiffness (6.7%), swelling (3.3%), scar pain (3.3%), and weakness (3.3%).[112]

TRAUMATIC WOUND MANAGEMENT

There is a paucity of literature focused exclusively on high-energy open fractures and traumatic wounds in children. Open fractures occur in 0.7% to 2% of all pediatric fractures.[113-115] High-energy injuries are more likely to have associated open wounds. The mechanism of an open fracture in a child typically involves motor vehicle accident, bicycle versus motor vehicle accidents, or fall from height. The most common anatomic location of open fracture in a child is tibia/fibula followed by radius/ulna and then metacarpals.[116,117]

Classification

Similar to adults, the Gustilo-Anderson classification is used in children to describe severity of wounds associated with open fractures, despite some limitations in interobserver variability.[118,119] The grade is frequently assigned in the operating room once an assessment of the extent of the wound is possible and may change on serial débridement. Higher grades of injuries often portend a more complicated clinical course. Although grade I and II fractures may be successfully managed with primary or delayed primary closure and rarely experience infection, grade III fractures require longer time to wound closure, longer duration of antibiotics, higher rates of infection, longer stay in hospital, and longer time to union.[116] Grade of injury may also influence the timing and type of treatment, as discussed later.

Timing of Surgery

In general, surgical management of an open fracture should be conducted as quickly as is reasonable and possible, although enthusiasm for prior dogma of the 6-hour rule is waning. Some studies have shown that children with open fractures do not have higher infection rates when surgery is delayed for greater than 6 hours and even up to 24 hours as long as antibiotics are administered immediately on presentation.[117,120] Although most surgeons thought that it may be reasonable to wait over 6 hours for surgery for a grade I open fracture, very few agree with this stance in a grade III open fracture.[121]

Type I Poke Hole Open Fractures

Several studies have questioned the standard practice of formal wound débridement in the operating room for type I open poke hole fractures, particularly of the forearm and wrist and also of the tibia. Several studies have shown similar infection rates in children with type I open fractures treated with superficial wound irrigation and débridement in the emergency department compared with children treated with formal surgical irrigation and débridement.[122-124] A recent large multicenter study of 219 patients with type I open fractures showed a 2% infection rate (1 of 49 patients) in the nonsurgically treated group, which was not significantly different than the infection rate (0/170) in the group treated with formal surgical débridement.[125] Such patients receiving nonsurgical treatment may experience shorter hospital stays and reduced cost. Despite these studies and the fact this practice is becoming more mainstream, high-powered level I evidence is still lacking to establish nonsurgical treatment as the standard practice. Furthermore, there is no consensus as to antibiotic protocol (ie, route and duration) when managing open fractures surgically or surgically.

Surgical Techniques for Soft Tissues

On initial irrigation and débridement of soft-tissue wounds, one should thoroughly clean and inspect the bone and soft tissues and be conservative in the amount of tissue that is removed given children's remarkable healing potential. In young children, muscle of questionable viability should be left in place, as it may recover, and bone that has been stripped off the periosteum may be left in place to incorporate.[126] Periosteum should be meticulously maintained as this can reconstitute bone even when large sections of bone are lost in a child, particularly in upper extremity fractures.[127] On closure, one should ensure that nerves, vessels, tendons, articular cartilage, and bone are covered with local soft tissue or skin. Antibiotic bead placement, while commonly used in adults, sustains a paucity of literature support in children; however, the practice is supported in adults and may be considered on a case-by-case basis in children.[128] Choice of implants is also important when considering soft-tissue loss. Certain fracture patterns, especially distal tibia fractures in young children, may be amenable to K-wire fixation as an alternative to internal fixation when there is large soft-tissue injury to minimize risk of infection and further soft-tissue damage.[116]

Primary wound closure, if possible, is preferable as long as tissues are clean (without gross contamination), healthy, and viable, particularly in grade I and II open fractures where skin can be closed without tension. A 2020 study demonstrated that most grade II and even grade IIIA fractures in children can be safely treated with early primary wound closure, a conclusion which challenges the dogma that closure of more severe wounds should be delayed.[129] That said, one must always consider compartment pressures when making a decision to close the wound primarily at the first surgery.

If the traumatic wound is unable to be primarily closed, then different techniques such as rubber band lacing, saline-soaked sponges, or negative pressure therapy/vacuum-assisted closure (NPT/VAC) may be used to encourage wound closure over time or to prepare tissue for flap coverage.

Negative Pressure Therapy/Vacuum-Assisted Closure

NPT/VAC has many suspected and proven benefits for management of open wounds in orthopaedic trauma, including decreased extremity edema, increased local tissue perfusion, and stimulation of granulation tissue.[130] NPT/VAC has been shown to be safe and effective in children with traumatic wounds including type III open fractures[131,132] and may be particularly useful in children because it obviates the need for more frequent bedside dressing changes, which can be traumatic to a child. One study evaluating NPT/VAC in pediatric open fractures showed only a 5.4% wound infection rate,[132] although it may be higher in severe injuries, as suggested by a study of grade III open tibia fractures managed with NPT/VAC where 5 of 16 fractures were complicated by infection.[131] A 2005 retrospective study of children treated with NPT/VAC demonstrated that kids with traumatic soft-tissue wounds experienced wound healing in all cases at 10 days after initial surgery with a functional limb and acceptable cosmesis without the need for a skin graft.[133] NPT/VAC may decrease the need for complex soft-tissue reconstruction, as demonstrated by a study of type III open tibia fractures in children, which showed a 50% decrease in the need for free tissue transfer or pedicled muscle flap coverage with use of NPT/VAC compared with historical control subjects.[131] This study argued that use of NPT/VAC may be able to avoid the need for free tissue transfer or pedicled rotational flaps in these severe injuries.

Risk of Infection

Prompt administration of antibiotics in open fractures is often considered the most important factor in reducing infection.[134] Superficial and deep infections, for the most part, seem to occur to a lesser extent in children compared with adults with similar injuries.[116,134] Although adult rates of infections with open tibia fractures range from 1.3% to ~50% depending on Gustilo-Anderson grade, a study of more than 500 open pediatric fractures found the incidence of infection to be 2% in grade I and II injuries and 8% in grade III injuries.[117] Similarly, a 2017 study of 61 children with open tibia fractures demonstrated a 6.6% rate of superficial infection and 4.9% rate of deep infection, all of which occurred in grade III open fractures.[116] In addition to grade of open fracture, age of patient is also an important distinguishing factor, with children aged 12 years and older having a higher rate of infection compared with children younger than 12 years.[77]

Definitive Soft-Tissue Coverage

Pediatric physiology with higher soft-tissue elasticity and greater vascularity lends to a greater likelihood of closing traumatic wounds primarily without the need for skin grafting or flap coverage.[34,105] In more complex wounds, specifically grade IIIB and IIIC injuries, it may be helpful to involve plastic surgery early because synchronous bony stabilization and plastic surgical treatment is mostly favored to complete soft-tissue coverage either at the first surgery or within 48 to 72 hours, although evidence for this is for the most part extrapolated from adult literature.[116,135] In general, early soft-tissue coverage is preferred with orthopaedic and plastic surgery comanagement.

SUMMARY

Appropriate treatment of the pediatric patients with polytrauma is critical for clinicians who work in trauma centers. The physiology of the pediatric patient is different than that of the adult, leading to differences in both presentation of injury and management. Early definitive fixation in this population can lead to decreased complications because many patients with severe injury, particularly neurologic, will recover. Compartment syndrome should be high on the differential in adolescent patients who sustain high-energy lower extremity injuries with increasing analgesic requirements raising concern. Although polytrauma continues to rise, education around firearms and lawn mower safety can help to curb the increase in severe injury. Soft-tissue management is critical in these injuries. Although children and adolescents will heal traumatic wounds more reliably than the adult population, this fact should not lead to the undertreatment of severe soft-tissue lesions associated with GSWs, lawn mower injuries, and grade III open fractures.

KEY STUDY POINTS

- The pediatric systemic response to trauma is characterized by a robust local inflammatory response with simultaneous early organ failure unlike the adult population, which has a robust systemic inflammatory response with stepwise organ failure occurring after 48 hours.
- Early definitive fixation of the patient with multiple injuries should be performed to limit complications from immobilization and encourage early weight bearing.
- Firearm-related injuries continue to rise in the pediatric and adolescent population. The clinician should understand that the bullet can cause damage not only to the bone but also to the soft-tissue envelope because of the energy transmitted throughout the surrounding environment.
- PACS is common in adolescent boys, particularly with tibia fractures related to a motor vehicle accident. Compartment syndrome may present differently in children than in adults, and different signs and symptoms should be recognized.
- Pediatric lawn mower injuries impart severe physical trauma, especially in the youngest patients who have high rates of amputation. The American Academy of Pediatrics recommends that no child should be a passenger in a ride-on lawn mower.
- The soft tissues of pediatric patients in general are more resilient than adults, although the soft tissues still require meticulous care and planning for early soft-tissue coverage in severe traumatic wounds. Grade 1 open fractures may be managed nonsurgically, whereas grade II open fractures and even grade IIIA open fractures may be amenable to early primary wound closure.

ANNOTATED REFERENCES

1. Centers for Disease Control and Prevention: *National Center for Injury Prevention and Control (WISQARS)*. Available at: https://www.cdc.gov/injury/wisqars/index.html. 2017. Accessed September 26, 2019.

   The CDC's WISQARS is an online database that provides information on leading cause of death and injury by age group.

2. Shannon SF, Hernandez NM, Sems SA, Larson AN, Milbrandt TA: Pediatric orthopaedic trauma and associated injuries of snowmobile, ATV, and dirtbike accidents: A 19-year experience at a level 1 pediatric trauma center. *J Pediatr Orthop* 2018;38(8):403-409.

   This single-center retrospective review over a 19-year period of 758 patients with 441 fractures demonstrated that

Section 7: Trauma

snowmobile and all-terrain vehicle injuries had higher ISS scores than dirtbike patients. Level of evidence: III.

3. Perno JF, Schunk JE, Hansen KW, et al: Significant reduction in delayed diagnosis of injury with implementation of a pediatric trauma service. *Pediatr Emerg Care* 2005;21:367-371.

4. Podolnick JD, Donovan DS, Atanda AW Jr, et al: Incidence of delayed diagnosis of orthopaedic injury in pediatric trauma patients. *J Orthop Trauma* 2017;31(9):e281-e287.

   This single-center retrospective review of 196 patients found 18 patients with a delayed orthopaedic injury diagnosis. Lower Glasgow Coma Scale, higher ISS, and greater hospital length of stay were associated with delayed diagnosis. Level of evidence: IV.

5. Copley LA, Dormans JP: Cervical spine disorders in infants and children. *J Am Acad Orthop Surg* 1998;6(4):204-214.

6. Hermans E, Cornelisse ST, Biert J, Tan ECTH, Edwards MJR: Paediatric pelvic fractures: How do they differ from adults? *J Child Orthop* 2017;11(1):49-56.

   In this single-center retrospective study, 51 pediatric and 268 adult pelvic fractures were compared. Although mortality did not differ between groups, adults had significantly higher ISS and were more often hemodynamically unstable. Level of evidence: III.

7. Swaid F, Peleg K, Alfici R, et al: A comparison study of pelvic fractures and associated abdominal injuries between pediatric and adult blunt trauma patients. *J Pediatr Surg* 2017;52(3):386-389.

   This single-center retrospective review of 7621 patients with blunt trauma sustaining pelvic fractures found no difference in mortality although adults sustained significantly more severe fractures. Level of evidence: III.

8. Kruppa CG, Khoriaty JD, Sietsema DL, Dudda M, Schildhauer TA, Jones CB: Pediatric pelvic ring injuries: How benign are they? *Injury* 2016;47(10):2228-2234.

   The authors demonstrated that 33 pediatric pelvic fractures with radiographic deformity did not remodel with risk of low back and sacroiliac joint pain as well as leg length discrepancy. Level of evidence: IV.

9. Amorosa LF, Kloen P, Helfet DL: High-energy pediatric pelvic and acetabular fractures. *Orthop Clin North Am* 2014;45(4):483-500.

10. Oyetunji TA, Haider AH, Downing SR, et al: Treatment outcomes of injured children at adult level 1 trauma centers: Are there benefits from added specialized care? *Am J Surg* 2011;201(4):445-449.

11. Choi PM, Hong C, Woods S, Warner BW, Keller MS: Early impact of American College of Surgeons-verification at a level-1 pediatric trauma center. *J Pediatr Surg* 2016;51(6):1026-1029.

    This retrospective review of an experience at a trauma center before and after acute compartment syndrome verification demonstrated a reduction in pediatric intensive care unit admissions and morbidity from hospital-acquired conditions as well as readmission rates. Level of evidence: III.

12. Rogers AT, Gross BW, Cook AD, et al: Outcome differences in adolescent blunt severe polytrauma patients managed at pediatric versus adult trauma centers. *J Trauma Acute Care Surg* 2017;83(6):1082-1087.

    This retrospective review of 1,606 adolescent patients with trauma from a state-based database found that adolescents treated at adult trauma center had higher functional status at discharge and lower complications when treated at adult versus pediatric center. Level of evidence: III.

13. Brown JB, Leeper CM, Sperry JL, et al: Helicopters and injured kids: Improved survival with scene air medical transport in the pediatric trauma population. *J Trauma Acute Care Surg* 2016;80(5):702-710.

    This review of patients aged 15 years and younger undergoing scene transport from the National Trauma Data Bank over a 5-year period found 25,700 ground/helicopter pairs from 166,594 patients. Patients transported by helicopter had improved odds of survival compared with ground transport. Level of evidence: III.

14. Polites SF, Zielinski MD, Fahy AS, et al: Mortality following helicopter versus ground transport of injured children. *Injury* 2017;48(5):1000-1005.

    The authors of this 2017 study found from a 1-year study of the National Trauma Data Bank that only patients with an ISS >15 had a survival benefit when transported via helicopter. Level of evidence: III.

15. Pandya NK, Upasani VV, Kulkarni VA: The pediatric polytrauma patient: Current concepts. *J Am Acad Orthop Surg* 2013;21(3):170-179.

16. Rankin JA: Biological mediators of acute inflammation. *AACN Clin Issues* 2004;15(1):3-17.

17. Lee CC, Marill KA, Carter WA, Crupi RS: A current concept of trauma-induced multiorgan failure. *Ann Emerg Med* 2001;38(2):170-176.

18. Calkins CM, Bensard DD, Moore EE, et al: The injured child is resistant to multiple organ failure: A different inflammatory response? *J Trauma* 2002;53(6):1058-1063.

19. Proulx F, Gauthier M, Nadeau D, Lacroix J, Farrell CA: Timing and predictors of death in pediatric patients with multiple organ system failure. *Crit Care Med* 1994;22(6):1025-1031.

20. Tantaleán JA, León RJ, Santos AA, Sánchez E: Multiple organ dysfunction syndrome in children. *Pediatr Crit Care Med* 2003;4(2):181-185.

21. Goh A, Lum L: Sepsis, severe sepsis and septic shock in paediatric multiple organ dysfunction syndrome. *J Paediatr Child Health* 1999;35(5):488-492.

22. Zimmerman JJ, Akhtar SR, Caldwell E, Rubenfeld GD: Incidence and outcomes of pediatric acute lung injury. *Pediatrics* 2009;124(1):87-95.

23. Rubenfeld GD, Caldwell E, Peabody E, et al: Incidence and outcomes of acute lung injury. *N Engl J Med* 2005;353(16):1685-1693.

24. Andruszkow H, Fischer J, Sasse M, et al: Interleukin-6 as inflammatory marker referring to multiple organ dysfunction syndrome in severely injured children. *Scand J Trauma Resusc Emerg Med* 2014;22:16.

25. Loder RT: Pediatric polytrauma: Orthopaedic care and hospital course. *J Orthop Trauma* 1987;1(1):48-54.

26. Loder RT, Gullahorn LJ, Yian EH, Ferrick MR, Raskas DS, Greenfield ML: Factors predictive of immobilization complications in pediatric polytrauma. *J Orthop Trauma* 2001;15(5):338-341.

27. Kim SJ, Sabharwal S: Risk factors for venous thromboembolism in hospitalized children and adolescents: A systemic review and pooled analysis. *J Pediatr Orthop B* 2014;23(4):389-393.

28. Allen CJ, Murray CR, Meizoso JP et al: Risk factors for venous thromboembolism after pediatric trauma. *J Pediatr Surg* 2016;51(1):168-171.

    The authors examined 1934 consecutive pediatric admissions at a level I trauma center and found a 1.2% rate of venous thromboembolism with major vascular injury and orthopaedic surgery as predictors of the development of venous thromboembolism. Level of evidence: III.

29. Van Arendonk KJ, Schneider EB, Haider AH et al: Venous thromboembolism after trauma: When do children become adults? *JAMA Surg* 2013;148(12):1123-1130.

30. Stafford PW, Blinman TA, Nance ML: Practical points in evaluation and resuscitation of the injured child. *Surg Clin North Am* 2002;82(2):273-301.

31. Silber JS, Flynn JM, Koffler KM, Dormans JP, Drummond DS: Analysis of the cause, classification, and associated injuries of 166 consecutive pediatric pelvic fractures. *J Pediatr Orthop* 2001;21(4):446-450.

32. Schalamon J, Bismarck SV, Schober PH, Höllwarth ME: Multiple trauma in pediatric patients. *Pediatr Surg Int* 2003;19(6):417-423.

33. Strutt J, Flood A, Kharbanda AB: Shock index as a predictor of morbidity and mortality in pediatric trauma patients. *Pediatr Emerg Care* 2019;35(2):132-137.

    Using the National Trauma Data Bank, the authors compared the age-adjusted shock index with the unadjusted index and found that elevated shock index (heart rate/systolic blood pressure) was more accurate and specific predictor of complications than tachycardia or hypotension alone. Level of evidence: III.

34. Wang MY, Hoh DJ, Leary SP, Griffith P, McComb JG: High rates of neurological improvement following severe traumatic pediatric spinal cord injury. *Spine (Phila Pa 1976)* 2004;29(13):1493-1497.

35. Slovis JC, Gupta N, Li NY, Kernie SG, Miles DK: Assessment of recovery following pediatric traumatic brain injury. *Pediatr Crit Care Med* 2018;19(4):353-360.

    This retrospective review of a pediatric patients with traumatic brain injury over an 11-year period found that even with a poor neurologic status at discharge, many children with traumatic brain injury will significantly improve. Level of evidence: III.

36. Pandya NK, Edmonds EW: Immediate intramedullary flexible nailing of open pediatric tibial shaft fractures. *J Pediatr Orthop* 2012;32(8):770-776.

37. Centers for Disease Control and Prevention: *National Center for Injury Prevention and Control Web-Based Injury Statistics Query and Reporting System (WISQARS)*. 2005. Available at: www.cdc.gov/injury/wisqars. Accessed October 2, 2016.

38. Fowler KA, Dahlberg LL, Haileyesus T, Gutierrez C, Bacon S: Childhood firearm injuries in the United States. *Pediatrics* 2017;140(1):e20163486.

    This retrospective database review examined fatal firearm injuries from the National Electronic Injury Surveillance System from 2002 to 2014. Level of evidence: IV.

39. Schecter SC, Betts J, Schecter WP, Victorino GP: Pediatric penetrating trauma: The epidemic continues. *J Trauma Acute Care Surg* 2012;73(3):721-725.

40. Bachier-Rodriguez M, Freeman J, Feliz A: Firearm injuries in a pediatric population: African-American adolescents continue to carry the heavy burden. *Am J Surg* 2017;213(4):785-789.

    This retrospective case-control study reviewed 5 years of data and found that males older than 15 years and of African-American race were more likely to experience severe gun violence. Level of evidence: III.

41. Saunders NR, Lee H, Macpherson A, Guan J, Guttmann A: Risk of firearm injuries among children and youth of immigrant families. *CMAJ* 2017;189(12):E452-E458.

    This retrospective cohort study found that the risk of assault-related firearm injuries was higher among refugees and immigrants from Central America and Africa. Level of evidence: III.

42. Blumberg TJ, DeFrancesco CJ, Miller DJ, Pandya NK, Flynn JM, Baldwin KD: Firearm-associated fractures in children and adolescents: Trends in the United States 2003-2012. *J Pediatr Orthop* 2018;38(7):e387-e392.

    This retrospective cohort study analyzing the Kids' Inpatient Database from 2003 to 2012 found an increase in firearm-associated fractures during the study period, particularly among the younger than 4 years age group, males, and minorities. Level of evidence: III.

43. Monuteaux MC, Mannix R, Fleegler EW, Lee LK: Predictors and outcomes of pediatric firearm injuries treated in the emergency department: Differences by mechanism of intent. *Acad Emerg Med* 2016;23(7):790-795.

    The authors found in this retrospective study that multiple factors including race and lower socioeconomic status are tied to firearm injury. Level of evidence: IV.

44. Monuteaux MC, Azrael D, Miller M: Association of increased safe household firearm storage with firearm suicide and unintentional death among US youths. *JAMA Pediatr* 2019; 173(7):657-662.

    This modeling study demonstrated that even modest increased compliance with safe firearm storage recommendations would have a meaningful reduction in firearm-related injury. Level of evidence: III.

45. Hamilton EC, Miller CC III, Cox CS Jr, Lally KP, Austin MT: Variability of child access prevention laws and pediatric firearm injuries. *J Trauma Acute Care Surg* 2018;84(4):613-619.

The authors in this study analyzed the Healthcare Cost and Utilization Project Kids' Inpatient Database from 2006 to 2009 to determine that strong state-level child access prevention laws could significantly reduce pediatric firearm-related injuries. Level of evidence: III.

46. Carter CW, Sharkey MS, Fishman F: Firearm-related musculoskeletal injuries in children and adolescents. *J Am Acad Orthop Surg* 2017;25(3):169-178.

This review article examines the issues related to the public health issue of pediatric musculoskeletal injuries from firearms, and describes child specific factors for this mechanism of injury.

47. Feldman KA, Tashiro J, Allen CJ, et al: Predictors of mortality in pediatric urban firearm injuries. *Pediatr Surg Int* 2017;33(1):53-58.

This retrospective review at a single center over a 20-year period found that children admitted with initial pH ≤7.15 (odds ratio = 14.8), initial hematocrit ≤30 (odds ratio = 3.24), or ISS >15 (odds ratio = 1.08) had higher mortality rates ($P < 0.05$) from firearm injuries. Level of evidence: III.

48. Farjo L, Miclau T: Ballistics and mechanisms of tissue wounding. *Injury* 1997;28(S3):C12-C17.

49. Bartlett CS, Helfet DL, Hausman MR, Strauss E: Ballistics and gunshot wounds: Effects on musculoskeletal tissues. *J Am Acad Orthop Surg* 2000;8(1):21-36.

50. Papasoulis E, Patzakis MJ, Zalavras CG: Antibiotics in the treatment of low-velocity gunshot-induced fractures: A systematic literature review. *Clin Orthop Relat Res* 2013;471:3937-3944.

51. Simpson BM, Wilson RH, Grant RE: Antibiotic therapy in gunshot wound injuries. *Clin Orthop Relat Res* 2003;408:82-85.

52. Mazotas IG, Hamilton NA, McCubbins MA, Keller MS: The long-term outcome of retained foreign bodies in pediatric gunshot wounds. *J Trauma Nurs* 2012;19(4): 240-245.

53. Dougherty PJ, Vaidya R, Silverton CD, Bartlett CS III, Najibi S: Joint and long-bone gunshot injuries. *Instr Course Lect* 2010;59:465-479.

54. Rehman S, Slemenda C, Kestner C, Joglekar S: Management of gunshot pelvic fractures with bowel injury: Is fracture debridement necessary? *J Trauma* 2011;71(3):577-581.

55. Watters J, Anglen JO, Mullis BH: The role of débridement in low-velocity civilian gunshot injuries resulting in pelvis fractures: A retrospective review of acute infection and inpatient mortality. *J Orthop Trauma* 2011;25(3): 150-155.

56. Sathiyakumar V, Thakore RV, Stinner DJ, Obremskey WT, Ficke JR, Sethi MK: Gunshot-induced fractures of the extremities: A review of antibiotic and debridement practices. *Curr Rev Musculoskelet Med* 2015;8:276-289.

57. Lin SS, Vaccaro AR, Reisch S, Devine M, Cotler JM: Low-velocity gunshot wounds to the spine with an associated transperitoneal injury. *J Spinal Disord* 1995;8(2):136-144.

58. Heary RF, Vaccaro AR, Mesa JJ, Balderston RA: Thoracolumbar infections in penetrating injuries to the spine. *Orthop Clin North Am* 1996;27(1):69-81.

59. Jakoi A, Iorio J, Howell R, Zampini JM: Gunshot injuries of the spine. *Spine J* 2015;15:2077-2085.

60. Aryan HE, Amar AP, Ozgur BM, Levy ML: Gunshot wounds to the spine in adolescents. *Neurosurgery* 2005;57(4):748-752.

61. Omid R, Stone MA, Zalavras CG, Marecek GS: Gunshot wounds to the upper extremity. *J Am Acad Orthop Surg* 2019;27(7):e301-e310.

This review article provides evidence-based guidance on clinical management of upper extremity gunshot wounds including soft tissue, nerve, vascular, and bone injuries.

62. Pannell WC, Heckmann N, Alluri RK, et al: Predictors of nerve injury after gunshot wounds to the upper extremity. *Hand (NY)* 2017;12:501-506.

The authors in this retrospective case series of 41 patients with gunshot injuries with 59 nerve explorations found a higher frequency of fractures, retained fragments, vascular injury, and compartment syndrome in patients with nerve palsies. Patients with preoperative nerve palsies were significantly more likely to have nerve laceration found intraoperatively. Level of evidence: IV.

63. Stoebner AA, Sachanandani NS, Borschel GH: Upper and lower extremity nerve injuries in pediatric missile wounds: A selective approach to management. *Pediatr Surg Int* 2011;27:635-641.

64. Letts RM, Miller D: Gunshot wounds of the extremities in children. *J Trauma* 1976;16(10):807-811.

65. Perkins C, Scannell B, Brighton B, Seymour R, Vanderhave K: Orthopaedic firearm injuries in children and adolescents: An eight-year experience at a major urban trauma center. *Injury* 2016;47:173-177.

The authors found in this single-center retrospective review of 46 patients that gunshot-related fractures had higher than anticipated morbidity, including permanent neurologic deficits, infection (11%), and fracture nonunion (9%). Level of evidence: IV.

66. Naranje SM, Gilbert SR, Stewart MG, et al: Gunshot-associated fractures in children and adolescents treated at two level 1 pediatric trauma centers. *J Pediatr Orthop* 2016;36(1):1-5.

This retrospective review of 49 patients at two level I trauma centers over an 8-year period demonstrated that tibia and femur fractures were the most common sites of injury with nearly half of all patients having additional injuries including gastrointestinal/genitourinary and neurovascular injury. Level of evidence: IV.

67. Fodor L, Sobec R, Sita-Alb L, Fodor M, Ciuce C: Mangled lower extremity: Can we trust the amputation scores? *Int J Burns Trauma* 2012;2(1):51-58.

68. Fagelman MF, Epps HR, Rang M: Mangled extremity severity score in children. *J Pediatr Orthop* 2002;22(2):182-184.

69. Fletcher AN, Schwend RM, Solano M, Wester C, Jarka DE: Pediatric lawn-mower injuries presenting at a level-I trauma center, 1995 to 2015: A danger to our youngest children. *J Bone Joint Surg Am* 2018;100(20):1719-1727.

This retrospective review of pediatric lawn mower injuries presenting to a level-1 trauma center demonstrated that predictors of higher ISS with these injuries included young age (0 to 9 years), a riding lawn mower, a grandparent operator, and a nonmetro/rural location. Young children fared worse after such injuries. Level of evidence: IV.

70. Pediatric Orthopaedic Society of North America: *Lawnmower Safety*. OrthoKids. Available at: http://orthokidsorg/Safety/Lawnmower-Safety. Accessed October 13, 2019.

71. American Academy of Pediatrics: *Lawn Mower Safety Tips From the American Academy of Pediatrics*. 2018. Available at: https://healthychildren.org/English/safety-prevention/at-home/Pages/Lawnmower-Safety.aspx.

This public resource provides education on the dangers posed to children by lawn mowers and offers suggestions for lawn mower safety.

72. Branch LG, Crantford JC, Thompson JT, Tannan SC: Pediatric lower extremity lawn mower injuries and reconstruction: Retrospective 10-year review at a level 1 trauma center. *Ann Plast Surg* 2017;79(5):490-494.

This retrospective review underscored the danger of lawn mower injuries to children, with young patients aged 2 to 5 years suffering the most severe injuries, including a higher rate of amputation. Level of evidence: IV.

73. Park WH, DeMuth WE Jr: Wounding capacity of rotary lawn mowers. *J Trauma* 1975;15(1):36-38.

74. Garay M, Hennrikus WL, Hess J, Lehman EB, Armstrong DG: Lawnmowers versus children: The devastation continues. *Clin Orthop Relat Res* 2017;475(4):950-956.

This retrospective database study evaluated the incidence and characteristics of lawn mower-related injury in children. The authors concluded that young children had higher injury severity, and many of these injuries could be prevented with proper education. Level of evidence: IV.

75. Borne A, Porter A, Recicar J, Maxson T, Montgomery C: Pediatric traumatic amputations in the United States: A 5-year review. *J Pediatr Orthop* 2017;37(2):e104-e107.

This retrospective review analyzed the clinical characteristics of pediatric traumatic amputations. Young children more commonly suffered finger amputations while adolescents were more likely to sustained higher energy amputations. The authors highlight the importance of prevention strategies. Level of evidence: IV.

76. American Academy of Pediatrics, Committee on Injury and Poison Prevention: Lawn mower-related injuries to children. *Pediatrics* 2001;107:1480-1481.

77. Blasier RD, Barnes CL: Age as a prognostic factor in open tibial fractures in children. *Clin Orthop Relat Res* 1996;331:261-264.

78. Grimard G, Naudie D, Laberge LC, Hamdy RC: Open fractures of the tibia in children. *Clin Orthop Relat Res* 1996;332:62-70.

79. Kreder HJ, Armstrong P: A review of open tibia fractures in children. *J Pediatr Orthop* 1995;15(4):482-488.

80. Mommsen P, Zeckey C, Hildebrand F, et al: Traumatic extremity arterial injury in children: Epidemiology, diagnostics, treatment and prognostic value of mangled extremity severity score. *J Orthop Surg Res* 2010;5:25.

81. Behdad S, Rafiei MH, Taheri H, et al: Evaluation of Mangled Extremity Severity Score (MESS) as a predictor of lower limb amputation in children with trauma. *Eur J Pediatr Surg* 2012;22(6):465-469.

82. Stewart D, Coombs C, Graham H: Evaluation of mangled extremity severity score (MESS) as a predictor of lower limb amputation in children with trauma. *Eur J Pediatr Surg* 2013;23(4):333-334.

83. Lin CH, Wei FC, Levin LS, Su JI, Yeh WL: The functional outcome of lower-extremity fractures with vascular injury. *J Trauma* 1997;43(3):480-485.

84. Venkatadass K, Grandhi TSP, Rajasekaran S: Use of Ganga Hospital Open Injury Severity Scoring for determination of salvage versus amputation in open type IIIB injuries of lower limbs in children–An analysis of 52 type IIIB open fractures. *Injury* 2017;48(11):2509-2514.

This study demonstrates the utility of the Ganga Hospital Open Injury Severity Score (GHOISS) in predicting injury severity in type IIIB open fractures in children to assist with decision for amputation vs limb salvage. Level of evidence: IV.

85. Halvorson JJ, Anz A, Langfitt M, et al: Vascular injury associated with extremity trauma: Initial diagnosis and management. *J Am Acad Orthop Surg* 2011;19(8):495-504.

86. Mooney JF III, Hosseinzadeh P, Oetgen M, Cappello T: AAOS appropriate use criteria: Management of pediatric supracondylar humerus fractures with vascular injury. *J Am Acad Orthop Surg* 2016;24(2):e24-e28.

This AAOS appropriate use criteria provides guidance in management of pediatric supracondylar humerus fractures with associated vascular injuries.

87. Wang SK, Drucker NA, Raymond JL, et al: Long-term outcomes after pediatric peripheral revascularization secondary to trauma at an urban level 1 center. *J Vasc Surg* 2019;69:857-862.

This is a retrospective review of pediatric vascular injuries at a level I trauma center over 7 years. Twenty-three patients required arterial revascularization surgery. Bone fractures were associated with 39.1% of these injuries. Restoration of in-line flow was achieved by endovascular solution in one patient, and open surgery was required for the remainder. Direct repair was performed in 40.9% and arterial bypass in 59.1%. At last follow-up, all patients had patent vascular repairs, and all but one reported normal function of the affected limb. Level of evidence: IV.

88. Gilbert F, Schneemann C, Scholz CJ, et al: Clinical implications of fracture-associated vascular damage in extremity and pelvic trauma. *BMC Musculoskelet Disord* 2018;19(1):404.

In this single-center retrospective cohort study, 64 patients with fracture-associated vascular injuries were identified with 80% survival with pelvic injury and 97% survival in extremity injury. Level of evidence: III.

89. Vo NJ, Althoen M, Hippe DS, Prabhu SJ, Valji K, Padia SA: Pediatric abdominal and pelvic trauma: Safety and efficacy of arterial embolization. *J Vasc Interv Radiol* 2014;25(2):215-220.

90. Puapong D, Brown CV, Katz M, et al: Angiography and the pediatric trauma patient: A 10-year review *J Pediatr Surg* 2006;41(11):1859-1863.

91. Medina O, Arom GA, Yeranosian MG, Petrigliano FA, McAllister DR: Vascular and nerve injury after knee dislocation: A systematic review. *Clin Orthop Relat Res* 2014:472(9):2621-2629.

92. Mayer S, Albright JC, Stoneback JW: Pediatric knee dislocations and physeal fractures about the knee. *J Am Acad Orthop Surg* 2015;23(9):571-580.

93. Seamon MJ, Smoger D, Torres DM, et al: A prospective validation of a current practice: The detection of extremity vascular injury with CT angiography. *J Trauma* 2009;67(2):238-243.

94. Flynn JM, Bashyal RK, Yeger-McKeever M, Garner MR, Launay F, Sponseller PD: Acute traumatic compartment syndrome of the leg in children: Diagnosis and outcome. *J Bone Joint Surg Am* 2011;93(10):937-941.

95. Grottkau BE, Epps HR, Di Scala C: Compartment syndrome in children and adolescents. *J Pediatr Surg* 2005;40(4):678-682.

96. Gottlieb M, Adams S, Landas T: Current approach to the evaluation and management of acute compartment syndrome in pediatric patients. *Pediatr Emerg Care* 2019;35(6):432-437.

This review article offers evidence-based guidance for treating acute compartment syndrome in children.

97. McQueen MM, Gaston P, Court-Brown CM: Acute compartment syndrome. Who is at risk? *J Bone Joint Surg Br* 2000;82(2):200-203.

98. Shore BJ, Glotzbecker MP, Zurakowski D, Gelbard E, Hedequist DJ, Matheney TH: Acute compartment syndrome in children and teenagers with tibial shaft fractures: Incidence and multivariable risk factors. *J Orthop Trauma* 2013;27(11):616-621.

99. Staudt JM, Smeulders MJ, van der Horst CM: Normal compartment pressures of the lower leg in children. *J Bone Joint Surg Br* 2008;90(2):215-219.

100. Seiler JG III, Womack S, De L'Aune WR, Whitesides TE, Hutton WC: Intracompartmental pressure measurements in the normal forearm. *J Orthop Trauma* 1993;7(5):414-416.

101. Tharakan SJ, Subotic U, Kalisch M, Staubli G, Weber DM: Compartment pressures in children with normal and fractured forearms: A preliminary report. *J Pediatr Orthop* 2016;36(4):410-415.

The authors of this prospective comparative study showed that children have higher resting compartment pressure in the deep volar compartment of the forearm and may tolerate absolute pressures >30 mm Hg without clinical signs of ACS. Level of evidence: I.

102. Mars M, Hadley GP: Raised compartmental pressure in children: A basis for management. *Injury* 1998;29(3):183-185.

103. Bae DS, Kadiyala RK, Waters PM: Acute compartment syndrome in children: Contemporary diagnosis, treatment, and outcome. *J Pediatr Orthop* 2001;21(5):680-688.

104. Kanj WW, Gunderson MA, Carrigan RB, Sankar WN: Acute compartment syndrome of the upper extremity in children: Diagnosis, management, and outcomes. *J Child Orthop* 2013;7(3):225-233.

105. Livingston K, Glotzbecker M, Miller PE, Hresko MT, Hedequist D, Shore BJ: Pediatric nonfracture acute compartment syndrome: A review of 39 cases. *J Pediatr Orthop* 2016;36(7):685-690.

The authors of this retrospective review examined the clinical characteristics of the less common nonfracture acute compartment syndrome in children, and found a relatively high rate of delay in diagnosis, emphasizing the importance of clinical suspicion for NFACS in certain clinical scenarios. Level of evidence: IV.

106. Lee C, Lightdale-Miric N, Chang E, Kay R: Silent compartment syndrome in children: A report of five cases. *J Pediatr Orthop B* 2014;23(5):467-471.

107. Noonan K, McCarthy J: Compartment syndromes in the pediatric patient. *J Pediatr Orthop* 2010;30(2):S96-S101.

108. Roberts A, Shaw KA, Boomsma SE, Cameron CD: Effect of casting material on the cast pressure after sequential cast splitting. *J Pediatr Orthop* 2017;37(1):74-77.

This comparative study showed that type of padding influences the pressure inside a long arm cast. Cotton padding allowed for the greatest change in pressure and may best accommodate swelling. Level of evidence: I.

109. Weiner G, Styf J, Nakhostine M, Gershuni DH: Effect of ankle position and a plaster cast on intramuscular pressure in the human leg. *J Bone Joint Surg Am* 1994;76(10):1476-1481.

110. Livingston KS, Glotzbecker MP, Shore BJ: Pediatric acute compartment syndrome. *J Am Acad Orthop Surg* 2017;25(5):358-364.

This review articles examines the aspects of acute compartment syndrome that are unique to children, and emphasizes the special considerations in treating children with this condition.

111. Erdos J, Dlaska C, Szatmary P, Humenberger M, Vecsei V, Hajdu S: Acute compartment syndrome in children: A case series in 24 patients and review of the literature. *Int Orthop* 2011;35(4):569-575.

112. Shirley ED, Mai V, Neal KM, Kiebzak GM: Wound closure expectations after fasciotomy for paediatric compartment syndrome. *J Child Orthop* 2018;12(1):9-14.

This retrospective chart review showed that one in four pediatric patients requires skin grafting after fasciotomies. Concern with unpleasant scar is a frequent complication of upper extremity fasciotomies. Level of evidence: IV.

113. Cheng JC, Ng BK, Ying SY, Lam PK: A 10-year study of the changes in the pattern and treatment of 6,493 fractures. *J Pediatr Orthop* 1999;19(3):344-350.

114. Joeris A, Lutz N, Wicki B, Slongo T, Audige L: An epidemiological evaluation of pediatric long bone fractures – A retrospective cohort study of 2716 patients from two Swiss tertiary pediatric hospitals. *BMC Pediatr* 2014;14:314.

115. Rennie L, Court-Brown CM, Mok JY, Beattie TF: The epidemiology of fractures in children. *Injury* 2007;38(8):913-922.

116. Nandra RS, Wu F, Gaffey A, Bache CE: The management of open tibial fractures in children: A retrospective case series of eight years' experience of 61 cases at a paediatric specialist centre. *Bone Joint J* 2017;99-B(4):544-553.

    The authors of this retrospective review of tibia fractures in children showed longer time to union in older children, though high rate of union overall with better healing rates than adults. Level of evidence: IV.

117. Skaggs DL, Friend L, Alman B, et al: The effect of surgical delay on acute infection following 554 open fractures in children. *J Bone Joint Surg Am* 2005;87(1):8-12.

118. Brumback RJ, Jones AL: Interobserver agreement in the classification of open fractures of the tibia. The results of a survey of two hundred and forty-five orthopaedic surgeons. *J Bone Joint Surg Am* 1994;76(8):1162-1166.

119. Horn BD, Rettig ME: Interobserver reliability in the Gustilo and Anderson classification of open fractures. *J Orthop Trauma* 1993;7(4):357-360.

120. Skaggs DL, Kautz SM, Kay RM, Tolo VT: Effect of delay of surgical treatment on rate of infection in open fractures in children. *J Pediatr Orthop* 2000;20(1):19-22.

121. Lavelle WF, Uhl R, Krieves M, Drvaric DM: Management of open fractures in pediatric patients: Current teaching in Accreditation Council for Graduate Medical Education (ACGME) accredited residency programs. *J Pediatr Orthop B* 2008;17(1):1-6.

122. Bazzi AA, Brooks JT, Jain A, Ain MC, Tis JE, Sponseller PD: Is nonoperative treatment of pediatric type I open fractures safe and effective? *J Child Orthop* 2014;8(6):467-471.

123. Doak J, Ferrick M: Nonoperative management of pediatric grade 1 open fractures with less than a 24-hour admission. *J Pediatr Orthop* 2009;29(1):49-51.

124. Iobst CA, Tidwell MA, King WF: Nonoperative management of pediatric type I open fractures. *J Pediatr Orthop* 2005;25(4):513-517.

125. Godfrey J, Choi PD, Shabtai L, et al: Management of pediatric type I open fractures in the emergency department or operating room: A multicenter perspective. *J Pediatr Orthop* 2019;39(7):372-376.

    This multicenter retrospective review compared pediatric type I open forearm, wrist and tibia fractures treated either operatively or nonoperatively. The authors found no significant difference in infection or complication rates. Level of evidence: III.

126. Stewart DG Jr, Kay RM, Skaggs DL: Open fractures in children. Principles of evaluation and management. *J Bone Joint Surg Am* 2005;87(12):2784-2798.

127. Wimberly RL, Wilson PL, Ezaki M, Martin BD, Riccio AI: Segmental metadiaphyseal humeral bone loss in pediatric trauma patients: A case series. *J Pediatr Orthop* 2014;34(4):400-404.

128. Trionfo A, Cavanaugh PK, Herman MJ: Pediatric open fractures. *Orthop Clin North Am* 2016;47(3):565-578.

    This review article discusses the special consideration given to open fractures in children.

129. Wang KK, Rademacher ES, Miller PE, et al: Management of Gustilo-Anderson type II and IIIA open long bone fractures in children: Which wounds require a second washout? *J Pediatr Orthop* 2020;40(6):288-293.

    The authors at a level-1 pediatric trauma center evaluated outcomes of pediatric grade II and IIIA open fractures treated either with early primary versus delayed wound closure. They found that many of these fractures may be safely treated with early primary wound closure without need for additional washouts. Level of evidence: IV.

130. DeFranzo AJ, Argenta LC, Marks MW, et al: The use of vacuum-assisted closure therapy for the treatment of lower-extremity wounds with exposed bone. *Plast Reconstr Surg* 2001;108(5):1184-1191.

131. Dedmond BT, Kortesis B, Punger K, et al: Subatmospheric pressure dressings in the temporary treatment of soft tissue injuries associated with type III open tibial shaft fractures in children. *J Pediatr Orthop* 2006;26(6):728-732.

132. Halvorson J, Jinnah R, Kulp B, Frino J: Use of vacuum-assisted closure in pediatric open fractures with a focus on the rate of infection. *Orthopedics* 2011;34(7):e256-e260.

133. Caniano DA, Ruth B, Teich S: Wound management with vacuum-assisted closure: Experience in 51 pediatric patients. *J Pediatr Surg* 2005;40(1):128-132.

134. Patzakis MJ, Wilkins J: Factors influencing infection rate in open fracture wounds. *Clin Orthop Relat Res* 1989;243:36-40.

135. Laine JC, Cherkashin A, Samchukov M, Birch JG, Rathjen KE: The management of soft tissue and bone loss in type IIIB and IIIC pediatric open tibia fractures. *J Pediatr Orthop* 2016;36(5):453-458.

    The authors of this retrospective review propose an algorithm to guide management of pediatric type IIIB and IIIC tibia fractures. Level of evidence: IV.

CHAPTER 39

Child Abuse

BRIAN K. BRIGHTON, MD, MPH • BRIAN P. SCANNELL, MD

ABSTRACT

Fractures are one of the most common injuries found in children who have been physically abused. The evaluation of such children, the identification of any associated injuries, and the creation of a management plan require a multidisciplinary child maltreatment prevention team that includes communication and collaboration among pediatricians, orthopaedic surgeons, radiologists, nurses, and social workers.

Keywords: child abuse; fractures; nonaccidental trauma; physical abuse

INTRODUCTION

Child abuse remains a serious threat to the pediatric population. The incidence of nonaccidental trauma (NAT) in the pediatric population is high, with reports ranging from 0.47 per 100,000 to 2,000 per 100,000.[1,2] Musculoskeletal injuries are one of the most common manifestations of physical abuse in children. Soft-tissue injuries are the most common injury, followed by fractures.[3,4] Many orthopaedic surgeons feel unprepared to treat these patients, and they may benefit from improved education and training related to NAT.[5]

Dr. Brighton or an immediate family member serves as a board member, owner, officer, or committee member of the American College of Surgeons and the Pediatric Orthopaedic Society of North America. Neither Dr. Scannell nor any immediate family member has received anything of value from or has stock or stock options held in a commercial company or institution related directly or indirectly to the subject of this chapter.

BACKGROUND

Numerous early reports of violence or abuse toward children have been published. In 1946, an association was highlighted between multiple fractures and subdural hematomas in a case series of six infants.[6] Although indications existed that the injuries were traumatic in etiology, no direct link could made to child abuse. It was not until 1962 that the medical profession fully recognized the reality of child abuse—when researchers published a landmark article describing battered child syndrome.[7] The journal article described the clinical profile of a child who has been abused and when physicians should have high levels of suspicion for abuse. This article resulted in increased public awareness to the societal and emotional trauma of child abuse.

Within a few years of this landmark article, nearly all states mandated the reporting of suspected abuse. In addition, the Child Abuse Prevention and Treatment Act of 1974 provided assistance to states to develop child abuse and neglect prevention and identification programs. This act was amended in 2010, providing minimum standards to states for defining maltreatment; however, each state individually defines the parameters for the physical abuse of a child. The act defines child abuse as "any recent act or failure to act on the part of a parent or caretaker which results in death, serious physical or emotional harm, sexual abuse, or exploitation."[8]

RISK FACTORS FOR ABUSE

Several child, parent, and environmental risk factors can indicate child abuse (**Table 1**). Very young children appear to be at the greatest risk.[9] Nearly 80% of all fractures caused by child abuse occur in children younger than 18 months.[10] In 2009, researchers found that the mean age of children with orthopaedic injuries resulting from NAT was 11.8 months.[11] In addition, children with

TABLE 1

Child, Parental, and Environmental Risk Factors for Child Abuse

Child	Parental	Environment (Community and Society)
Emotional and/or behavioral difficulties	Low self-esteem	Social isolation
Chronic illness	Poor impulse control	Poverty
Physical disabilities	Substance and/or alcohol abuse	Unemployment
Developmental disabilities	Young maternal or paternal age	Low educational achievement
Premature birth	Parent abused as a child	Single parent
Unwanted child	Depression or other mental illness	Nonbiologically related male living in the home
Unplanned pregnancy	Poor knowledge of child development or unrealistic expectations for child	Family or intimate partner violence
	Negative perception of normal child behavior	

Reproduced with permission from Flaherty EG, Stirling J Jr: Clinical report: The pediatrician's role in child maltreatment prevention. *Pediatrics* 126(4):833-841. Copyright © 2010 by the AAP.

disabilities are three times more likely to be maltreated than children without disabilities.[12]

Parental and environmental factors also may make children more vulnerable to physical abuse. Factors such as low parental self-esteem, substance abuse, and alcohol abuse may decrease a parent's ability to cope with the stresses of parenting, which may then be a predisposing factor in abuse.[13,14] Parents who were abused or neglected as children are more likely to inflict abuse on their own children.[1,13] Socioeconomic status also appears to affect the incidence of abuse rates. Children from low socioeconomic households (annual income less than $15,000) are three times more likely to be abused.[15] Perpetrators of abuse often are known by the child and are more commonly male, with more than 50% of abusers being the child's father, the child's stepfather, or a male friend of the child's mother.[16] However, physical abuse can affect children of all ages, ethnicities, and socioeconomic groups.

PATIENT EVALUATION

History and Physical Examination

A detailed history and physical examination are of utmost importance in children when abuse is suspected. History taking may vary based on the age and communication level of the child. When children are of school age and able to communicate, they should be interviewed apart from their caregivers. Parents or caregivers should be asked to describe events surrounding the reported injury. If more than one caregiver is present, it can be helpful to interview each caregiver separately.

The history should include details of the event, the developmental history of the child, and the family's social history to determine who lives in the house and who was present at the time of the injury.[17] A thorough family history is important to identify any bleeding, bone, and metabolic or genetic disorders.

Numerous key findings from the history should raise concern for abuse, including the following: (1) explicit denial of trauma in a child with obvious injury; (2) no explanation or only a vague explanation given for a substantial injury; (3) unexplained or notable delay in seeking medical care; (4) an injury explanation that is inconsistent with the child's physical and/or developmental capabilities; (5) an injury explanation that is inconsistent with the pattern, age, or severity of the injury; and (6) markedly different explanations for the injury between caregivers or the child and the caregiver.[17,18]

Each child requires a comprehensive head-to-toe physical examination, and it is of utmost importance that this examination be performed with the child undressed. The examination should include a thorough musculoskeletal and age-appropriate neurologic examination. In general, young children should be examined for signs of neglect, including malnutrition, dental issues, or neglected wound and/or skin issues, such as diaper dermatitis.[17] The head, eyes, ears, nose, and throat should be assessed, including the anterior fontanelle in infants; a detailed ophthalmology examination if abuse is suspected and an evaluation for dental trauma and/or caries should be performed.

The skin examination may reveal bruises, lacerations, burns, or other injuries, and these should be documented in size, shape, and location.[17] Soft-tissue injuries are found in a high percentage (92%) of suspected child abuse cases.[4] Suspicion should be high for abuse for any soft-tissue injury in a child who is younger than 9 months or if multiple soft-tissue injuries are present in children ranging from 10 months to 2 years of age.[10] Certain sites of soft-tissue injury are more commonly associated with abuse, such as the face, back, buttocks, perineum, and genitalia; other locations, such as the anterior aspect of the lower leg, are more common with accidental injury.[19,20]

Imaging

In children undergoing an evaluation for both accidental and nonaccidental trauma, dedicated radiographs of the injured limb or joint should be obtained. In children younger than 2 years and select patients up to 5 years of age with injuries that are suspicious for physical abuse, a skeletal survey should be performed. A skeletal survey based on the parameters of the American College of Radiology and the Society for Pediatric Radiology includes images of the appendicular and axial skeleton[21] (**Table 2**). Using highly detailed skeletal surveys, additional unsuspected fractures may be present up to 20% of the time in cases of suspected abuse.[22] Repeating a skeletal survey 2 to 3 weeks after the initial evaluation of a child who has been abused improves the diagnostic accuracy of identifying skeletal injuries, including rib fractures and classic metaphyseal lesions.[23]

TABLE 2

Complete Skeletal Survey

Appendicular Skeleton	Imaging View
Humeri	AP
Forearms	AP
Hands	PA
Femurs	AP
Lower legs	AP
Feet	AP
Axial Skeleton	**Imaging View**
Thorax	AP, lateral, right and left obliques, including ribs and thoracic and upper lumbar spine
Pelvis	AP, including midlumbar spine
Lumbosacral spine	Lateral
Cervical spine	Lateral
Skull	Frontal and lateral

To document the level of suspicion for abuse in the presence of multiple fractures, surgeons must have a keen understanding of fracture healing in children. Typically, the resolution of soft-tissue swelling occurs in 4 to 10 days, and new periosteal reaction can be seen on radiographs in 10 to 14 days.[24]

In children with suspected head injuries and in infants younger than 1 year, CT is recommended to evaluate for a subdural hemorrhage or a brain injury. Brain MRI has become more frequently used for the diagnosis and prognostication of abusive head trauma.[25] In a recent study from two level 1 trauma centers, intracranial injuries were commonly seen in abused children, and fatalities from abuse accounted for a large proportion of trauma mortality in children younger than 5 years.[26] Clinical signs of spinal cord injury may be masked by respiratory depression and impaired consciousness associated with the head injury.[27] Children who have abusive head trauma and are undergoing a brain MRI also should be considered for an MRI of the spine to assess for occult spinal cord injury, ligamentous disruption, or intrathecal blood.[28-30] In addition, spinal MRI may help differentiate between a traumatic and a nontraumatic intracranial subdural hemorrhage.[28] A chest CT can be used to identify rib fractures.[18] Bone scans may be used to detect rib fractures or other fractures when a skeletal survey is negative but when a high index of suspicion for abuse is present.[31,32] Whole-body MRI also may have a limited role in the evaluation of the child who is physically abused.[33]

COMMON FRACTURES

Fractures in children commonly occur as the result of accidental trauma. However, in young children and infants with skeletal trauma, the timely recognition of injuries associated with abuse can protect victims from further abuse.[34] In children with skeletal injuries, physical abuse should be included in the diagnosis if certain injury patterns are present. Several factors to consider are the patient age and history, the mechanism of injury, the fracture location and pattern, and associated injuries. It is important to correlate fracture findings with the history and physical examination because certain fractures should provoke a suspicion for abuse (**Table 3**). Although no absolutes exist, a high index of suspicion is appropriate in children who have a history of trauma that does not support the associated injury or certain fractures of the femur or tibia in children who are nonambulatory. If the presentation is delayed or multiple fractures in various states of healing are present, the concern for abuse increases. In addition, unusual fractures in infants and

TABLE 3

Specificity of Radiographic and Injury Findings

Specificity	Injury
High	Classic metaphyseal lesions Rib fractures, especially posterior Scapular process fractures Spinous process fractures Sternal fractures
Moderate	Multiple fractures, especially bilateral Fractures of different ages Epiphyseal separations Vertebral body fractures and subluxations Digital fractures Complex skull fractures Pelvic fractures
Low	Subperiosteal new bone formation Clavicular fractures Long-bone shaft fractures Linear skull fractures

Adapted with permission of Cambridge University Press through PLSclear. Kleinman PK, Rosenberg AE, Tsai A: Skeletal trauma: General considerations, in Kleinman PK, ed: *Diagnostic Imaging of Child Abuse*, ed 3. New York, NY, Cambridge University Press, 2015, pp 23-52.

toddlers, such as rib fractures, sternal fractures, vertebral fractures, and classic metaphyseal lesions (metaphyseal corner fractures), without a history of trauma or known metabolic bone disorder should alert the physician to the high likelihood of abuse.[17] In a systematic review of the literature in 2008, researchers found that fractures resulting from abuse were most commonly found in infants younger than 1 year and toddlers (aged 1 to 3 years) and were located throughout the skeletal system.[35] Although any skeletal injury can be associated with physical abuse, rib fractures had the highest probability for abuse, followed by humeral, femoral, and skull fractures for a particular developmental stage.[35] A recent study using a large national inpatient database developed a predictive tool to help identify children presenting with a fracture and possible NAT. The authors found that risk factors such as younger age, black race, intracranial injury, concomitant rib fractures, and burns were positive predictors for NAT in children presenting with a fracture.[36]

Femoral Fractures

Fractures of the femur occur in association with both accidental and nonaccidental trauma. In general, a child younger than 18 months with a femoral fracture has a 1:3 to 1:4 chance of having been the victim of physical abuse. Femoral fractures in NAT occur more commonly in children who are nonambulatory.[35,37] In a single institution study in 2011, researchers found that among children with femoral fractures, evidence (physical and/or radiographic) of a prior injury and being younger than 18 months were risk factors for abuse.[38]

Diaphyseal fractures of the femur can be nondisplaced, transverse, spiral, oblique, or comminuted, but no single fracture pattern is pathognomonic for abuse.[39] Using a fracture ratio, which is calculated by measuring the length of the fracture and dividing it by the diameter of the bone, researchers found that patients with NAT had femoral fractures with lower mean anterior-posterior fracture ratios (ie, the fractures were more transverse).[40] As recommended in the American Academy of Orthopaedic Surgeons Clinical Practice Guideline on the management of pediatric diaphyseal femur fractures, children younger than 3 years with a femoral fracture should be evaluated for the possibility of physical abuse.[41,42]

Humeral Fractures

In approximately 50% of children younger than 3 years who have a humeral fracture, the fracture is associated with physical abuse.[31] Fractures of the humeral shaft are more common in abuse, whereas supracondylar humerus fractures are more commonly seen with accidental trauma; however, supracondylar humerus and transphyseal distal humerus fractures can also occur in abuse situations.[43-45] In a single institution study in 2010, researchers found that a history suspicious for abuse, evidence (physical and/or radiographic) of a prior injury, and being younger than 18 months were the strongest predictors of child abuse in children with humeral fractures.[46]

Classic Metaphyseal Lesions

Classic metaphyseal lesions, also called corner fractures or bucket-handle fractures, were initially described by John Caffey but later explained in great detail by pediatric radiologist Paul Kleinman in his radiologic-histopathologic study in 1996.[6,23,47] These fractures carry a high specificity for abuse. The injury pattern is a trans-metaphyseal fracture through the primary spongiosa and often is the result of a violent shake of the limbs or the trunk.[31] The resulting fractured disk of bone and calcified cartilage then appears as a corner fracture or a bucket-handle fracture based on the projection of the radiograph[48] (**Figures 1** and **2**).

DIFFERENTIAL DIAGNOSIS

In children with unexplained fractures, physical abuse remains a probable differential diagnosis; however, alternative diagnoses need to be considered. Osteogenesis

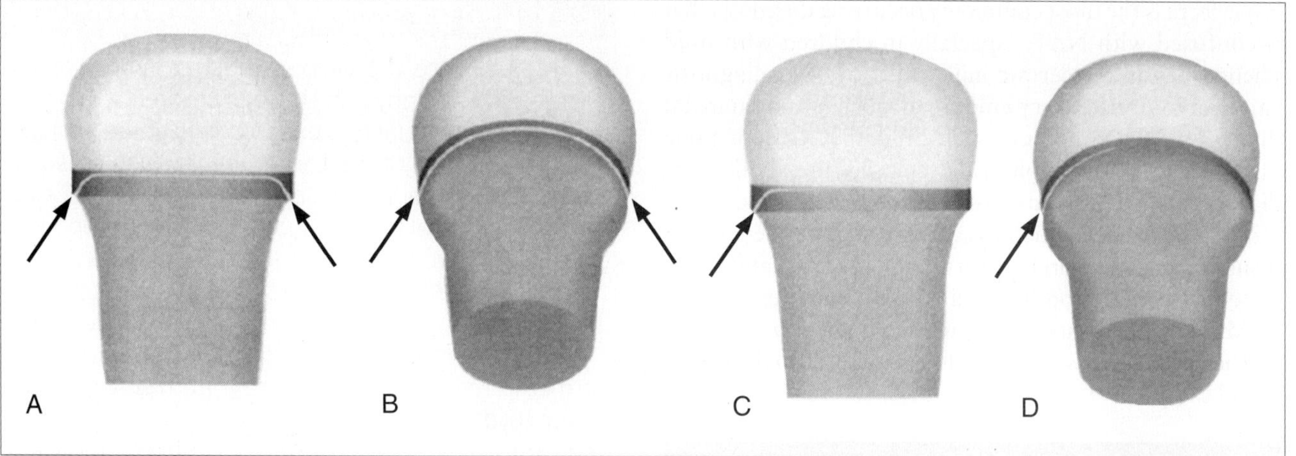

FIGURE 1 Diagrammatic representation of the relationship of the subperiosteal bone collar to a metaphyseal lesion. **A**, A tangential view of the metaphyseal margin shows a fracture line (arrows) that extends adjacent to the chondro-osseous junction centrally. Peripherally, the fracture line veers away from the epiphyseal plate to undermine a larger peripheral fragment incorporating the subperiosteal bone collar. **B**, When the fracture line (arrows) is projected obliquely, the thicker peripheral fragment, including the subperiosteal bone collar, is projected as a curvilinear fragment or a bucket-handle lesion. **C**, When the fracture line (arrow) is incomplete (it extends across only a portion of the metaphysis), the appearance suggests a focal, triangular-shaped peripheral fragment encompassing the subperiosteal bone collar. **D**, When the fracture line (arrow) is tipped obliquely, the peripheral margin of the fragment is projected as a curvilinear density. (Reproduced with permission from Kleinman PK, Marks SC Jr: Relationship of the subperiosteal bone collar to metaphyseal lesions in abused infants. *J Bone Joint Surg Am* 1995;77[10]:1471-1476.)

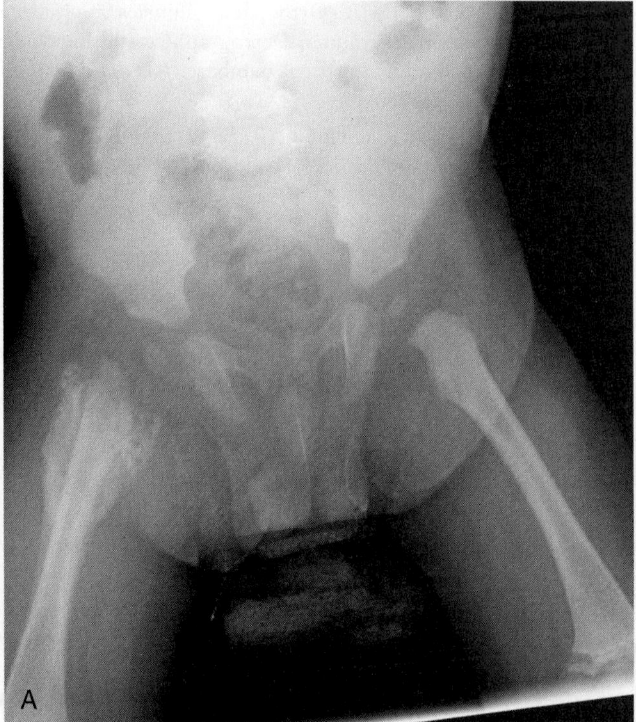

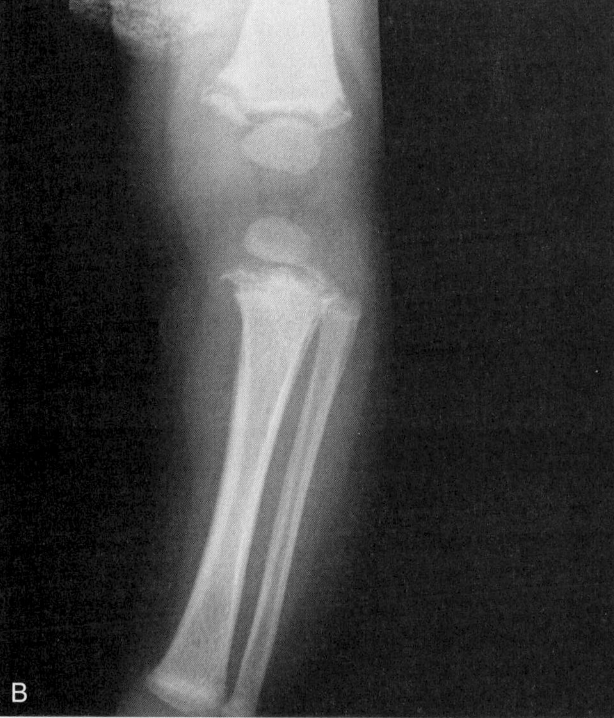

FIGURE 2 Radiographs from a 6-month-old infant with multiple fractures caused by nonaccidental trauma. AP radiographs show a right proximal femoral fracture (**A**) and left distal femoral and proximal tibial classic metaphyseal lesions (**B**). (Courtesy of Brian K. Brighton, MD, MPH, Charlotte, NC.)

imperfecta is the most commonly occurring diagnosis that is confused with NAT, especially in children with mild phenotypes and uncertain injury histories. Misdiagnosis can lead to unnecessary emotional, social, and financial distress for the families of such children.[49] Genetic bone disorders such as metaphyseal dysplasias, metabolic bone diseases such as vitamin D–deficient rickets, vitamin or mineral deficiencies such as scurvy or copper deficiency, disuse osteopenia, prematurity, osteomyelitis, and other systemic medical conditions also have been reported in children being evaluated for suspected abuse and can be further evaluated with laboratory or DNA analysis of a blood sample.[18,50]

MANAGEMENT OF ABUSE

After a diagnosis of physical abuse has been made or if abuse is suspected, the orthopaedic surgeon must not only be involved with the management of the child's injuries but also engage in ongoing evaluations with the multidisciplinary child maltreatment team.[51] Many children's hospitals and trauma centers caring for children suspected of NAT have developed multidisciplinary teams, including child abuse pediatricians, social work, and child protective services, to coordinate the screening, evaluation, and treatment of patients.[52]

Orthopaedic management of many injuries associated with abuse is nonsurgical and includes splints or casts. Displaced fractures, such as displaced femoral fractures, may require closed reduction and casting.

Suspected cases of child abuse must be reported to the appropriate state or local child protective service agencies. The diagnosis of abuse often carries substantial social and legal implications in addition to the medical issues. Initiating a report of abuse must be nonjudgmental and presented as the standard of care. Clear and detailed documentation of the injuries and management within the medical record is extremely important in the event the surgeon is asked to participate in later legal proceedings.[53]

SUMMARY

Orthopaedic surgeons play a critical role in the evaluation, treatment, and coordination of care of a child who is the victim of child abuse and suspected NAT. The physician must evaluate and treat the child's injuries in the context of the history and mechanism of injury and obtain additional imaging studies (such as a skeletal survey) if indicated. In addition, if abuse is suspected, involvement of a multidisciplinary child maltreatment prevention team is necessary.

KEY STUDY POINTS

- Fractures are the second most common injury related to the physical abuse of children.
- Numerous risk factors exist for child abuse, including young age of the child, parental factors (such a single marital status and poor coping skills), and environmental factors (such as low socioeconomic status). However, physical abuse can affect children of all ages, ethnicities, and socioeconomic groups.
- Although any skeletal injury can be associated with physical abuse, certain fractures, such as rib and metaphyseal corner fractures, are highly specific for child abuse.
- Suspicion for physical abuse mandates physician reporting to the appropriate services and should initiate a multidisciplinary approach to the treatment of these patients.

ANNOTATED REFERENCES

1. Altemeier WA III, O'Connor S, Vietze PM, Sandler HM, Sherrod KB: Antecedents of child abuse. *J Pediatr* 1982;100(5):823-829.
2. Sibert JR, Payne EH, Kemp AM, et al: The incidence of severe physical child abuse in Wales. *Child Abuse Negl* 2002;26(3):267-276.
3. Loder RT, Feinberg JR: Orthopaedic injuries in children with nonaccidental trauma: Demographics and incidence from the 2000 kids' inpatient database. *J Pediatr Orthop* 2007;27(4):421-426.
4. McMahon P, Grossman W, Gaffney M, Stanitski C: Soft-tissue injury as an indication of child abuse. *J Bone Joint Surg Am* 1995;77(8):1179-1183.
5. Tenenbaum S, Thein R, Herman A, et al: Pediatric nonaccidental injury: Are orthopedic surgeons vigilant enough? *J Pediatr Orthop* 2013;33(2):145-151.
6. Caffey J: Multiple fractures in the long bones of infants suffering from chronic subdural hematoma. *Am J Roentgenol Radium Ther* 1946;56(2):163-173.
7. Kempe CH, Silverman FN, Steele BF, Droegemueller W, Silver HK: The battered-child syndrome. *J Am Med Assoc* 1962;181(1):17-24.
8. The Child Abuse Prevention and Treatment Act (CAPTA). Available at: https://www.acf.hhs.gov/sites/default/files/cb/capta.pdf. Accessed September 1, 2020.
9. Wu SS, Ma CX, Carter RL, et al: Risk factors for infant maltreatment: A population-based study. *Child Abuse Negl* 2004;28(12):1253-1264.
10. Coffey C, Haley K, Hayes J, Groner JI: The risk of child abuse in infants and toddlers with lower extremity injuries. *J Pediatr Surg* 2005;40(1):120-123.

11. Pandya NK, Baldwin K, Wolfgruber H, Christian CW, Drummond DS, Hosalkar HS: Child abuse and orthopaedic injury patterns: Analysis at a level I pediatric trauma center. *J Pediatr Orthop* 2009;29(6):618-625.

12. Sullivan PM, Knutson JF: Maltreatment and disabilities: A population-based epidemiological study. *Child Abuse Negl* 2000;24(10):1257-1273.

13. Oates RK, Davis AA, Ryan MG: Predictive factors for child abuse. *Aust Paediatr J* 1980;16(4):239-243.

14. Kelleher K, Chaffin M, Hollenberg J, Fischer E: Alcohol and drug disorders among physically abusive and neglectful parents in a community-based sample. *Am J Public Health* 1994;84(10):1586-1590.

15. Sedlak AJ, Mettenburg J, Basena M, et al: *Fourth National Incidence Study of Child Abuse and Neglect (NIS-4): Report to Congress*. Washington, DC, US Department of Health and Human Services, Administration for Children and Families, 2010.

16. Starling SP, Sirotnak AP, Heisler KW, Barnes-Eley ML: Inflicted skeletal trauma: The relationship of perpetrators to their victims. *Child Abuse Negl* 2007;31(9):993-999.

17. Christian CW, Committee on Child Abuse and Neglect, American Academy of Pediatrics: The evaluation of suspected child physical abuse. *Pediatrics* 2015;135(5):e1337-e1354.

18. Flaherty EG, Perez-Rossello JM, Levine MA, et al: Evaluating children with fractures for child physical abuse. *Pediatrics* 2014;133(2):e477-e489.

19. Kemp AM, Maguire SA, Nuttall D, Collins P, Dunstan F: Bruising in children who are assessed for suspected physical abuse. *Arch Dis Child* 2014;99(2):108-113.

20. Fassier A, Gaucherand P, Kohler R: Fractures in children younger than 18 months. *Orthop Traumatol Surg Res* 2013;99(suppl 1):S160-S170.

21. American College of Radiology: *ACR Appropriateness Criteria. Suspected Physical Abuse–Child.* Available at: https://acsearch.acr.org/docs/69443/narrative. Accessed September 1, 2020.

22. Barber I, Perez-Rossello JM, Wilson CR, Kleinman PK: The yield of high-detail radiographic skeletal surveys in suspected infant abuse. *Pediatr Radiol* 2015;45(1):69-80.

23. Kleinman PK, Nimkin K, Spevak MR, et al: Follow-up skeletal surveys in suspected child abuse. *AJR Am J Roentgenol* 1996;167(4):893-896.

24. Dwek JR: The radiographic approach to child abuse. *Clin Orthop Relat Res* 2011;469(3):776-789.

25. Shaahinfar A, Whitelaw KD, Mansour KM: Update on abusive head trauma. *Curr Opin Pediatr* 2015;27(3):308-314.

26. Yu YR, DeMello AS, Greeley CS, Cox CS, Naik-Mathuria BJ, Wesson DE: Injury patterns of child abuse: Experience of two level 1 pediatric trauma centers. *J Pediatr Surg* 2018;53(5):1028-1032.

    Intracranial injuries occurring commonly in child abuse are associated with an increased risk of death. In this retrospective review of two level 1 pediatric trauma centers, the authors report that of the 4,623 trauma admissions in children younger than 5 years, 557 (12%) were due to NAT. Nearly half (43) of the 93 overall trauma fatalities were due to NAT. Head injuries were the most common injuries sustained (60%) and led to the greatest increased risk of death (risk ratio: 5.1, 95% confidence interval: 2.0 to 12.7). Level of evidence: II.

27. Kemp AM, Joshi AH, Mann M, et al: What are the clinical and radiological characteristics of spinal injuries from physical abuse: A systematic review. *Arch Dis Child* 2010;95(5):355-360.

28. Kadom N, Khademian Z, Vezina G, Shalaby-Rana E, Rice A, Hinds T: Usefulness of MRI detection of cervical spine and brain injuries in the evaluation of abusive head trauma. *Pediatr Radiol* 2014;44(7):839-848.

29. Choudhary AK, Bradford RK, Dias MS, Moore GJ, Boal DK: Spinal subdural hemorrhage in abusive head trauma: A retrospective study. *Radiology* 2012;262(1):216-223.

30. Knox J, Schneider J, Wimberly RL, Riccio AI: Characteristics of spinal injuries secondary to nonaccidental trauma. *J Pediatr Orthop* 2014;34(4):376-381.

31. Sink EL, Hyman JE, Matheny T, Georgopoulos G, Kleinman P: Child abuse: The role of the orthopaedic surgeon in nonaccidental trauma. *Clin Orthop Relat Res* 2011;469(3):790-797.

32. Bainbridge JK, Huey BM, Harrison SK: Should bone scintigraphy be used as a routine adjunct to skeletal survey in the imaging of non-accidental injury? A 10 year review of reports in a single centre. *Clin Radiol* 2015;70(8):e83-e89.

33. Perez-Rossello JM, Connolly SA, Newton AW, Zou KH, Kleinman PK: Whole-body MRI in suspected infant abuse. *AJR Am J Roentgenol* 2010;195(3):744-750.

34. Ravichandiran N, Schuh S, Bejuk M, et al: Delayed identification of pediatric abuse-related fractures. *Pediatrics* 2010;125(1):60-66.

35. Kemp AM, Dunstan F, Harrison S, et al: Patterns of skeletal fractures in child abuse: Systematic review. *Br Med J* 2008;337:a1518.

36. Zhao C, Starke M, Tompson JD, Sabharwal S: Predictors for nonaccidental trauma in a child with a fracture—A national inpatient database study. *J Am Acad Orthop Surg* 2020;28(4):e164-e171.

    Using data from the 2012 Kids' Inpatient Database, the authors developed a predictive model to determine the likelihood of NAT in a hospitalized child presenting with a fracture. Younger age, race, intracranial injury, concomitant rib fractures, and burns were all found to be positive predictors of NAT in children who present with fractures. Level of evidence: II.

37. Schwend RM, Werth C, Johnston A: Femur shaft fractures in toddlers and young children: Rarely from child abuse. *J Pediatr Orthop* 2000;20(4):475-481.

38. Baldwin K, Pandya NK, Wolfgruber H, Drummond DS, Hosalkar HS: Femur fractures in the pediatric population: Abuse or accidental trauma? *Clin Orthop Relat Res* 2011;469(3):798-804.

39. Scherl SA, Miller L, Lively N, Russinoff S, Sullivan CM, Tornetta P III: Accidental and nonaccidental femur fractures in children. *Clin Orthop Relat Res* 2000;376:96-105.

40. Murphy R, Kelly DM, Moisan A, et al: Transverse fractures of the femoral shaft are a better predictor of nonaccidental trauma in young children than spiral fractures are. *J Bone Joint Surg Am* 2015;97(2):106-111.

41. Kocher MS, Sink EL, Blasier RD, et al, American Academy of Orthopaedic Surgeons: American Academy of Orthopaedic Surgeons clinical practice guideline on treatment of pediatric diaphyseal femur fracture. *J Bone Joint Surg Am* 2010;92(8):1790-1792.

42. Blatz AM, Gillespie CW, Katcher A, Matthews A, Oetgen ME: Factors associated with nonaccidental trauma evaluation among patients below 36 months old presenting with femur fractures at a level-1 pediatric trauma center. *J Pediatr Orthop* 2019;39(4):175-180.

In this single-institution study, the authors found poor utilization of NAT evaluation for patients younger than 36 months presenting with femur fracture despite recent clinical practice guidelines. There are several recommendations presented to increase the screening and identification of NAT in patients admitted with femur fractures. Level of evidence: III.

43. Gilbert SR, Conklin MJ: Presentation of distal humerus physeal separation. *Pediatr Emerg Care* 2007;23(11):816-819.

44. Strait RT, Siegel RM, Shapiro RA: Humeral fractures without obvious etiologies in children less than 3 years of age: When is it abuse? *Pediatrics* 1995;96(4 pt 1):667-671.

45. Shaw BA, Murphy KM, Shaw A, Oppenheim WL, Myracle MR: Humerus shaft fractures in young children: Accident or abuse? *J Pediatr Orthop* 1997;17(3):293-297.

46. Pandya NK, Baldwin KD, Wolfgruber H, Drummond DS, Hosalkar HS: Humerus fractures in the pediatric population: An algorithm to identify abuse. *J Pediatr Orthop B* 2010;19(6):535-541.

47. Caffey J: Some traumatic lesions in growing bones other than fractures and dislocations: Clinical and radiological features. The Mackenzie Davidson Memorial Lecture. *Br J Radiol* 1957;30(353):225-238.

48. Kleinman PK, Marks SC Jr: Relationship of the subperiosteal bone collar to metaphyseal lesions in abused infants. *J Bone Joint Surg Am* 1995;77(10):1471-1476.

49. Singh-Kocher M, Dichtel L: Osteogenesis imperfecta misdiagnosed as child abuse. *J Pediatr Orthop B* 2011;20(6):440-443.

50. Pandya NK, Baldwin K, Kamath AF, Wenger DR, Hosalkar HS: Unexplained fractures: Child abuse or bone disease? A systematic review. *Clin Orthop Relat Res* 2011;469(3):805-812.

51. Ranade SC, Allen AK, Deutsch SA: The role of the orthopaedic surgeon in the identification and management of nonaccidental trauma. *J Am Acad Orthop Surg* 2020;28(2):53-65.

This is a review article detailing the role of the orthopaedic surgeon in the initial recognition, diagnosis, and management of NAT in children. Outlined are the important elements of the history and physical examination as well as recommendations for appropriate imaging studies in the suspected NAT workup. Level of evidence: V.

52. ACS Trauma Quality Programs: *Best Practice Guidelines for Trauma Center Recognition of Child Abuse, Elder Abuse, and Intimate Partner Violence.* 2019. Available at: https://www.facs.org/-/media/files/quality-programs/trauma/tqip/abuse_guidelines.ashx. Accessed September 1, 2020.

The American College of Surgeons and Trauma Quality Improvement Program best practice guidelines provide recommendations for hospitals to coordinate the screening, evaluation, and treatment of patients with suspected child physical abuse. Trauma centers are encouraged to admit suspected child abuse patients to a surgical trauma service because of the potential for polytrauma and to participate in a multidisciplinary team, including child abuse pediatricians, social work, and child protective services. Level of evidence: V.

53. Sullivan CM: Child abuse and the legal system: The orthopaedic surgeon's role in diagnosis. *Clin Orthop Relat Res* 2011;469(3):768-775.

CHAPTER 40

Pediatric Clavicle, Shoulder, and Humerus Trauma

JESSICA D. BURNS, MD, MPH • DAVID E. LAZARUS, MD • ERIC W. EDMONDS, MD, FAOA

ABSTRACT

Pediatric clavicle, shoulder, and humerus trauma is common, and management often differs from how adults are treated. Familiarity with specific injuries and a review of updates in the literature within the past 5 years pertaining to injuries about the clavicle, shoulder, and humerus will aid orthopaedic surgeons in caring for young patients with these types of traumatic injuries.

Keywords: clavicle dislocation; clavicle fracture; humerus fracture; shoulder trauma

INTRODUCTION

Traumatic injuries to the upper extremity are common and represent about one-third of pediatric musculoskeletal complaints that seek management. Specifically, injures to the clavicle, shoulder, and humerus represent about 11% of all musculoskeletal pediatric physician visits and 36% of upper extremity complaints.[1] These injuries can be managed with both surgical and nonsurgical modalities. When deciding on treatment, it is critical to understand the injury to avoid complications, such as deformity, physeal injury, and motion restriction.[2] Understanding the pathophysiology, associated conditions, appropriate workup, treatment options, and prognosis is critical for optimal outcome.

Dr. Edmonds or an immediate family member is a member of a speakers' bureau or has made paid presentations on behalf of Arthrex, Inc. and serves as a board member, owner, officer, or committee member of the American Academy of Orthopaedic Surgeons and the Pediatric Orthopaedic Society of North America. Neither of the following authors nor any immediate family member has received anything of value from or has stock or stock options held in a commercial company or institution related directly or indirectly to the subject of this chapter: Dr. Burns and Dr. Lazarus.

SHOULDER

Sternoclavicular Dislocations

Injuries to the sternoclavicular joint (SCJ) are rare, representing <1% of fractures, and include sternoclavicular dislocations or medial clavicular physeal fractures. The medial clavicular epiphysis does not ossify until age 18 years, making a true sternoclavicular dislocation difficult to radiographically differentiate from a medial physeal fracture in both children and adolescents, although the treatment is similar for both injury patterns.[3,4] Serendipity radiographs (40° of cephalic tilt) or CT scans can help delineate the position of the medial clavicle (**Figure 1**). CT is recommended to assess the presence of concomitant mediastinal compression in posteriorly directed injuries. Direct impact to the clavicle, or impact to the lateral shoulder, is the usual mechanism that can disrupt the robust posterior ligamentous support about the joint. The medial clavicular physis fuses around age 25 years, putting adolescents and young adults at risk for physeal fractures. An estimated 71% of SCJ injuries occur during sporting activity.[5] The sternocleidomastoid and sternohyoid muscles provide posterior dynamic support, whereas the clavicular head of the pectoralis major provides dynamic anterior stability.[3] Posterior injuries can have associated fractures of the ribs, scapula, spine, and extremities, but more importantly, can have life-threatening injuries to mediastinal structures, including tracheal compression (15%), esophageal compression (23%), compression or injury to the brachiocephalic or subclavian vein (14%), or brachial plexus or other neural injury (2%).[3,5]

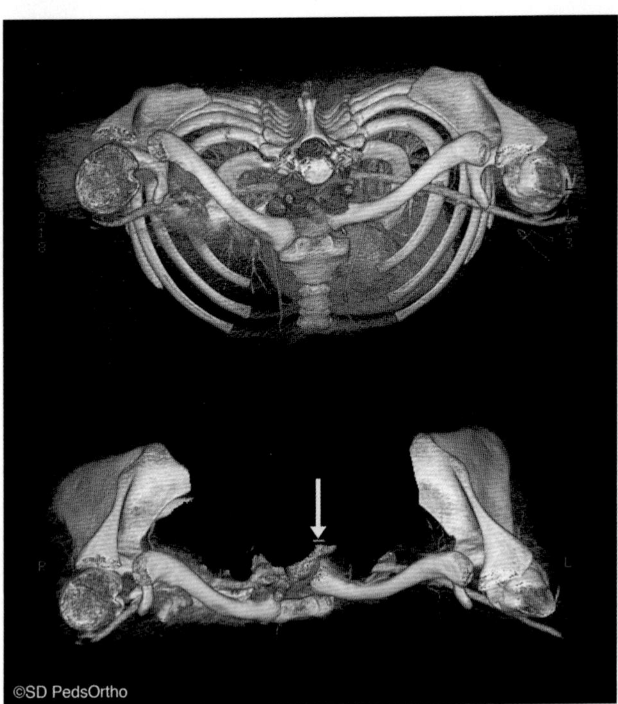

FIGURE 1 Three-dimensional CT reconstruction of a 15-year-old girl involved in a motor vehicle accident who presented complaining of left shoulder pain. Plain radiographs suggested a sternoclavicular injury that was confirmed on CT. Three-dimensional reconstructions (above) with ribs and vascular structures removed (below) identify a posterior dislocation (indicated by arrow). (Copyright James Bomar, San Diego Pediatric Orthopedics, San Diego, CA.)

Treatment includes closed reduction and open reduction with or without internal fixation. Closed reduction should be attempted if the patient presents within 48 hours of the injury, which is successful 30% to 50% of the time. A bolster is placed between the scapulae with lateral traction on the ipsilateral shoulder in abduction and extension. Alternatively, the arm can be adducted with posterior pressure applied to both shoulders.[5] Open reduction reduces recurrence and can allow earlier motion.[3,5] The patient is placed supine or in beach-chair position. A transverse incision is made directly over the SCJ, sparing supraclavicular sensory nerves during dissection. The platysma is divided in a single layer, with release of the sternocleidomastoid and pectoralis major as needed. The periosteum should be incised and the joint reduced with a towel clamp, shoehorn technique, or other methods. Methods for fixation of the fracture or joint include cannulated screws, anterior plating, cerclage with wire or sternal cable, direct repair of the costoclavicular and sternoclavicular ligaments, suture anchor fixation, figure-of-8 semitendinosus reconstruction, costoclavicular tenodesis using the subclavius, sternoclavicular tenodesis using sternal head of the sternocleidomastoid, and resection of the medial clavicle.[5] Kirschner wires (K-wires), Steinmann pins, or Hagie pins are no longer used because of the risk of intrathoracic migration. Outcomes are generally good with both closed and open reduction methods, resulting in more than 90% of patients achieving full pain-free range of motion. There are reports of late sequelae of chronic instability of the SCJ, undiagnosed mediastinal injury, and device complications.[3-5]

Clavicle Fractures

Pediatric clavicle fractures are common, representing 8% to 15% of all pediatric fractures. The spectrum of clavicle fractures ranges from birth-related injury to injuries in adolescents and young adults. Approximately 76% to 85% of fractures are in the middle third. The mechanism is usually a fall onto an outstretched arm, a direct fall on or blow to the lateral shoulder, or a direct blow to the clavicle itself, often related to a sports injury.[6-10] Traditional treatment for pediatric clavicle fractures has been nonsurgical, with the clavicle showing great potential for remodeling and union. The clavicle reaches 80% of its length at age 9 in girls and 12 in boys, growing at a rate of 2.6 mm and 5.4 mm per year in girls and boys, respectively.[6] Literature in the past 15 years has shown that surgical management of displaced midshaft clavicle fractures in adults can decrease the rate of symptomatic nonunion and malunion and decrease the time to return to functional activity, leading to controversy regarding appropriate management of displaced midshaft clavicle fractures in adolescents.[9-11]

The clavicle is the most commonly fractured bone during delivery of the neonate occurring in 0.035% to 3.2% of live births. Risk factors include high birth weight (>4,000 g), shoulder dystocia, and increased maternal age. Other risk factors depend on the region of the world, but can also include instrumentation at delivery, breech position, and length of delivery.[12,13] Cesarean section reduces the risk for clavicle fracture, but still occurs in 0.05% of live births via cesarean section with high birth weight and increased maternal age as the primary risk factors.[14] These injuries can be missed with up to 20% identified after discharge from the hospital.[13] These fractures are managed with immobilization for pain control by Velpeau splinting, using an ace bandage, or pinning the sleeve of the affected arm to the shirt body.[12,13] Pseudarthrosis of the clavicle should be considered in a nontender presumed clavicle fracture if the radiographic appearance does not suggest an acute fracture with sclerotic bone ends and no callus formation on follow-up imaging. This diagnosis is most commonly seen in the diaphysis of the right clavicle.[15]

Nonsurgical management with a sling, sling and swathe, or figure-of-8 brace is the standard of treatment for midshaft clavicle fractures in children. Indications for surgical management are open or impending open fractures, floating shoulder injuries with a completely displaced clavicle, and associated neurovascular injuries. Relative indications include polytrauma patients and completely displaced midshaft clavicles with >2 cm of shortening. These indications and relative indications are controversial among different authors.[6-8,10] There is trend for orthopaedic surgeons to manage displaced clavicle fractures surgically,[16] likely based on the adult orthopaedic literature. Half of the members of the Pediatric Orthopaedic Society of North America who responded to a survey reported that the adult literature influenced their decision making in choosing surgical management.[6]

The meta-analysis by the authors of a 2012 study of randomized controlled trials comparing surgical and nonsurgical management of displaced clavicle fractures in adults demonstrated earlier return to function, with 80% of surgically treated patients participating in moderate activity at 60 days, compared with 55% in the nonsurgical group. Patients treated with surgery had decreased rates of symptomatic nonunion and malunion, with a number needed to treat of 4.6.[11] Rates of symptomatic nonunion and malunion are significantly lower in the adolescent population. The largest series of pediatric clavicle nonunions showed that 4.6% of 545 diaphyseal clavicle fractures required surgical treatment for nonunion.[17] The primary risk factor for nonunion development was refracture. Nonunions managed with open reduction and internal fixation had a high rate of union.[17] Malunion can occur with fractures displaced >2 cm, but only 10% to 20% of these are symptomatic.[9,18]

Options for surgical treatment include open reduction with plate and screws, isolated screw fixation, and intramedullary implants. There is a variable rate of implant removal with reports from <10% to 88%. Over 75% of patients are satisfied with the cosmetic appearance of their clavicle treated nonsurgically, whereas patients can be dissatisfied with surgical scar in up to 20% of cases. There can be high rates of implant complications with intramedullary fixation, which can be converted to plate construct, which is why many authors prefer plate construct when surgical management is chosen.[8] Superior plating has been shown to have twice the load to failure in bending in an adult cadaver biomechanical study,[19] whereas anterior-inferior plating has limited evidence to suggest that there is a reduced rate of implant removal.[20]

Nonsurgical treatment for pediatric clavicle fractures remains the mainstay of treatment with surgical treatment in open and impending open fractures, floating shoulders, and neurovascular compromise. There is consideration for surgical management of midshaft clavicle fractures displaced >2 cm.

Shoulder Dislocations

The physis is a weak spot in the shoulder, thus making pediatric shoulder dislocations less common; however, pediatric shoulder dislocations do occur and can be recognized with proper imaging. Twenty percent of all shoulder dislocations occur in patients younger than 20 years and are more common in adolescents who participate in competitive contact sports, with most of the dislocations being anterior or anterior-inferior. A prospective study demonstrated that the incidence is much higher in males (86.5%) than in females (13.5%).[21]

Radiographs are used for diagnosis and reduction confirmation. The AP, scapular Y, and axillary views are critical for evaluating the shoulder. Secondary to pain and the occasional difficulty of an adequate axillary view, a Velpeau radiograph can be taken with minimal shoulder manipulation to confirm proper reduction (**Figure 2**). To evaluate for any bony lesions, the Westpoint view allows glenoid examination, and the Stryker notch view helps identify a Hill-Sachs lesion. An MRI or a magnetic resonance arthrogram is recommended for dislocations in younger patients to identify soft-tissue injuries that might make the shoulder prone to recurrent dislocations.

The natural history of shoulder dislocations has been well studied. The reported risk for recurrence in this younger cohort appears to be quite variable, yet previous studies have consistently demonstrated that young patients with shoulder dislocations have a higher rate of recurrence. Of 133 patients aged 13 to 18 years, the recurrence rate was 76.7%. In an evaluation of the survival of the shoulder reduction, 59% of reductions were intact at 1 year, but only 38% were without recurrence at 2 years, with decreasing numbers on the curve with time from the index event.[21] An epidemiologic study of

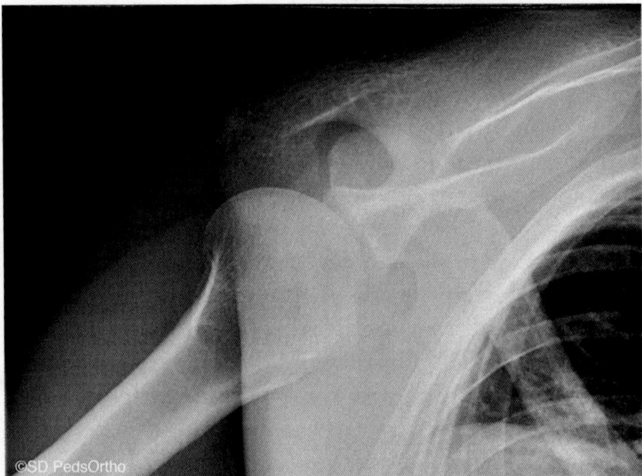

FIGURE 2 Lateral Velpeau radiographic view confirms a reduced glenohumeral joint. (Copyright James Bomar, San Diego Pediatric Orthopedics, San Diego, CA.)

Section 7: Trauma

shoulder dislocations in Canada in patients aged 10 to 16 years reported an overall recurrence rate of 38.2% at a mean of 10 months after the initial injury, although the authors of the study noted that the recurrence rate was lower in patients aged 10 to 13 years than in patients aged 14 to 16 years.[22]

After closed reduction, it is important to document a neurovascular examination. The axillary nerve is the most commonly injured neurovascular structure. Even if MRI shows structural pathology, nonsurgical treatment often is still recommended for the first traumatic shoulder dislocation, with a short period of sling immobilization followed by physical therapy. If a recurrent dislocation occurs, then the recommendations universally shift to surgical treatment, particularly if a large Hill-Sachs lesion, a Bankart tear, or a labral tear is present. The purpose of surgery is to prevent recurrence.

Arthroscopy is a good option if available and can be successful in managing a traumatic shoulder dislocation in an adolescent with a minimal risk of complications.[23,24] At 27-month follow-up, the overall return to sports was 87% after arthroscopic labral repair for anterior instability and 69% for achieving a preinjury level of performance.[25] However, despite the ability to return to full activities, adolescents treated with either an arthroscopic or an open Bankart repair for instability had a 5-year shoulder survival rate of 49%.[26] Moreover, adolescent patients who later had revision surgery after failure of the primary repair demonstrated a rate of 33% repeat failure after the revision surgery.[27] This is clearly an age cohort and pathology that requires further investigation to optimize treatment outcomes.

Scapula Fractures and Scapulothoracic Dissociation

Scapula fractures are relatively rare in the pediatric population and often secondary to high-energy trauma. Most scapula fractures in the literature are in the adult population. In these patients with shoulder girdle pain, swelling, or tenderness, it is important to rule out fractures about the scapula. When identified, it is important to ensure no other injuries of the thoracic cavity and its organs are present. A recent article looking at high-energy scapula fractures in the pediatric population found a higher rate of intracranial hemorrhage, skull fractures, thoracic injuries, upper extremity fractures, and spine fractures when compared against control patients without scapula fractures from motor vehicle accidents.[28] Scapula fractures in young children may also be associated with nonaccidental trauma, so it is important be diligent to rule this out as an etiology.[29]

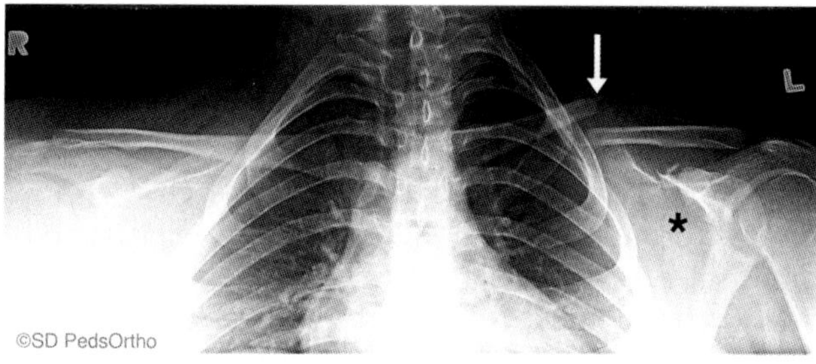

FIGURE 3 Radiograph of a 15-year-old girl involved in a motor vehicle accident who presented complaining of left and right shoulder pain. Plain radiographs demonstrate a left clavicle fracture (indicated by arrow), but there is also a left scapula body fracture (indicated by asterisk). (Copyright James Bomar, San Diego Pediatric Orthopedics, San Diego, CA.)

A full neurovascular examination should be performed and any other injuries managed. Dedicated scapula radiographs including an AP, scapular Y, and axillary lateral should be performed (**Figure 3**). CT scans can help further examine the fracture pattern and the involvement of the glenoid. The large majority can be treated with closed management of a sling and pain control, followed by early range of motion (**Figure 4**). Intra-articular involvement of the glenoid or severe displacement of the fracture may require surgery.[30]

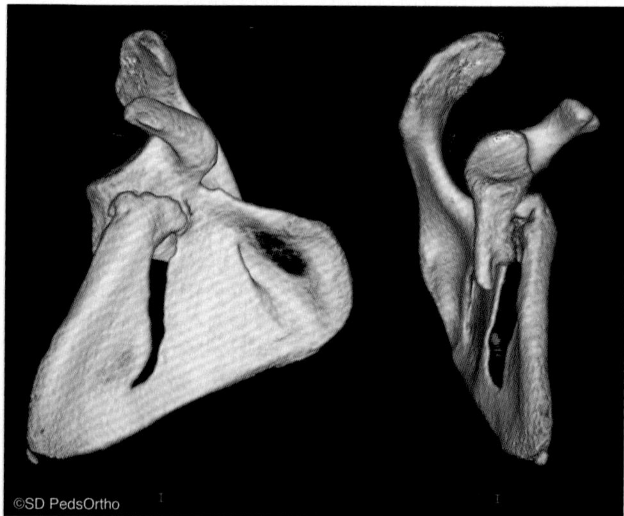

FIGURE 4 Three-dimensional CT reconstruction of the same teenager from **Figure 3**, who was treated nonsurgically for both the clavicle and scapula body fracture, 3 months after injury. On left-side image, there is delayed union of the body, but callus formation at the spine and base of acromion. On the right-side image, there is fusion of the fracture to the glenoid neck but no involvement of the glenoid itself. Full function and range of motion was restored to her shoulder. (Copyright James Bomar, San Diego Pediatric Orthopedics, San Diego, CA.)

Scapulothoracic dissociation is rare with only one case series of three patients in the pediatric literature. The condition involves a spectrum of skeletal, muscular, vascular, and neurologic injury resulting from traumatic disruption of the relationship of the scapula and upper extremity with the thorax. It occurs as a result of a high-energy distraction force applied to the upper extremity. Patients will usually exhibit noticeable asymmetric swelling of the injured shoulder compared with the contralateral side. Radiographs may show lateral displacement of the scapula relative to the spinous processes compared with the contralateral side (increased scapular index). Initial treatment depends on the vascular status of the extremity. Skeletal stabilization procedures include plate fixation of an associated clavicle fracture. The extensive disruption of the surrounding soft tissues necessitates repair with at least one point of fixation of the extremity to the axial skeleton. The extent of neurologic injury dictates clinical outcome. Initial conservative management is appropriate as the prognosis is guarded when severe brachial plexus injury has occurred.[31,32]

HUMERUS

Proximal Humerus and Humeral Shaft Fractures

Similar to clavicle fractures, proximal humerus fractures in children can range from birth trauma in the newborn to nonaccidental trauma in children and sports injuries in adolescents. As with suspected clavicle injuries, surgeons must always be aware of differential diagnoses, including infection and tumor. Proximal humerus fractures occur through the physis or the metaphysis. Younger children tend to fracture through the metaphysis and adolescents fracture through the physis. Because the proximal humeral physis contributes approximately 80% of the bone growth, the remodeling potential for fractures is excellent.[33,34] Generally accepted amounts of displacement depend on the location of the fracture. Fractures in newborns usually occur from a rotation or hyperextension of the extremity during birth. These fractures are treated with immobilization for pain control with a simple Velpeau splint or ace wrap to secure the arm to the torso for 3 to 4 weeks.[34,35]

In older children, a careful history can help narrow the differential diagnosis. Without a significant history of trauma, pathologic fracture through a unicameral bone cyst (UBC), osteomyelitis, and septic arthritis should be considered. Radiographs of the shoulder with an axillary view is critical to assess the glenohumeral relationship because these can be injured concurrently.[34,35] The Neer-Horowitz classification is commonly used for pediatric proximal humerus fractures. The capsule on the medial side attaches beyond the physis onto the metaphysis, which may lead to a Salter-Harris type II fracture pattern, which is often seen with the medial metaphysis still attached to the proximal piece.[36] Neer-Horowitz type I and II fractures can almost universally be managed nonsurgically, unless an open fracture or a neurovascular injury is present. Patient age and growth remaining are important factors. In those with substantial growth remaining, larger deformities will have time for remodeling. The management of displaced fractures in older children and adolescents should be individualized, including surgical considerations. Neer-Horowitz type III and IV fractures are commonly considered surgical fractures in children older than 10 years because displacement will have less remodeling potential in this age group. A 2015 study comparing nonsurgical to surgical management of Neer-Horowitz type III and IV fractures in patients who are skeletally mature demonstrated no differences in complications, rate of return to full activity, or functional outcome. There was a trend, however, for less desirable outcomes in children older than 12 years who were treated nonsurgically.[35]

Surgical treatment includes closed or open reduction with stabilization of the fracture with K-wires, cannulated screws, intramedullary nails, or plates and screws. Open reduction is typically reserved for intra-articular fractures or those with neurovascular compromise, which are rare. K-wires are relatively easy to use when closed reduction is amenable, but care must be taken to avoid branches of the axillary nerve. K-wires may extend from the skin or be buried, although the complication rate of leaving them exposed is approximately 55%, whereas the treatment expense substantially increases when a second surgical procedure is required to remove buried pins.[37] Intramedullary nails can be used with a lower complication rate and achieve outcomes similar to those with percutaneous fixation but may involve a longer surgery time as well as a second surgical procedure for implant removal.[38]

Critical evaluation of the radiographic findings is important. Proximal humerus fractures often are associated with a pathologic lesion, most commonly UBC. Risks of fracture through a UBC include involvement of 85% of the bone or a cyst wall less than 0.5 mm. In a study of 68 humeral UBCs, 94% exhibited a fracture.[39] Overall, the goal is healing of the fracture followed by management of the cyst, as appropriate. Complications from proximal humerus fractures can include brachial plexus injury in younger children, varus malunion, and growth disturbance. Deformity is generally well tolerated as is upper extremity limb-length discrepancy[34,35] (**Figure 5**).

Humeral shaft fractures represent about 5% of all pediatric fractures and are most commonly managed nonsurgically with minimal complications.[40] Open fractures

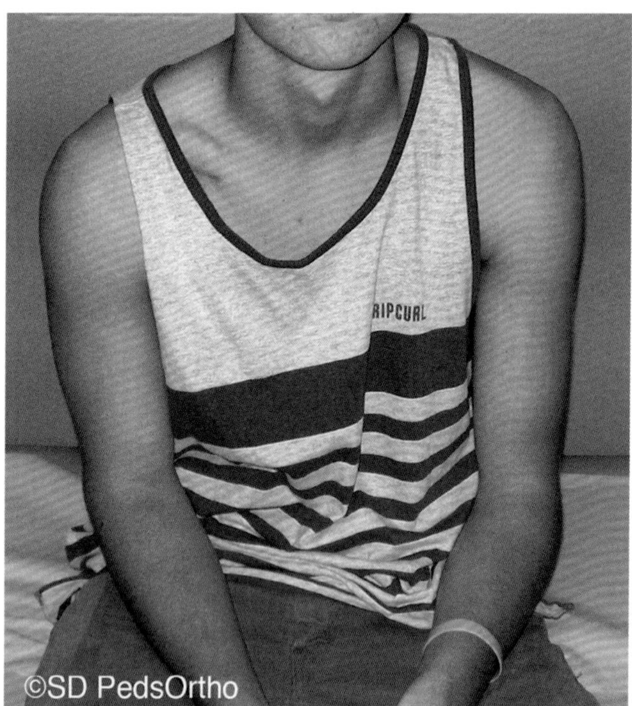

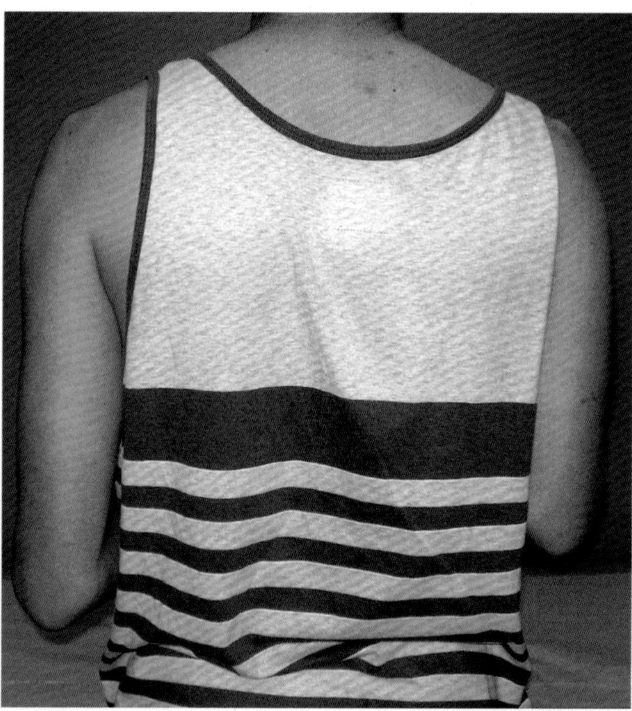

FIGURE 5 Clinical photographs of a 16-year-old boy, 6 years from a proximal humerus fracture, who presented for orthopaedic clearance for lacrosse participation. Clinical image of his front side demonstrates apparent equality of this arm length. The clinical image from behind demonstrates the 5 cm deficit in length of the right humerus. (Copyright James Bomar, San Diego Pediatric Orthopedics, San Diego, CA.)

will typically require surgical management. Surgical stabilization of the humerus is indicated with coexistent vascular injury as can be seen in cases of penetrating trauma. Relative surgical indications include improved mobilization of the polytrauma patient, bilateral injuries, floating elbow injuries, and failure of closed management. Surgical treatment in this age group can include external fixation, flexible intramedullary nails, and plate and screw constructs. In comparative studies of surgical and nonsurgical management, surgical management results in improved radiographic outcomes and faster return to mobilization.[41] Complications of humeral shaft fractures include radial nerve palsy, delayed and nonunion, and refracture. Radial nerve palsies are less common in pediatric fractures than adults. A course of initial observation for associated nerve palsies is supported.[34,42]

SUMMARY

Fractures and dislocations of the upper extremity must receive a correct diagnosis and optimal treatment to prevent complications. A thorough physical examination and appropriate imaging studies are important in determining proper management. Controversy exists in determining proper surgical indications in children and adolescents given the growth rate and healing potential of the skeletal structures around the shoulder.

KEY STUDY POINTS

- Posterior SCJ dislocations are difficult to discern from medial physeal fractures in adolescents, but both have good outcomes with open reduction and internal fixation.
- The management of clavicle fractures remains controversial in pediatric and adolescent cohorts; recent literature suggests that children and adolescents have less symptomatic nonunion and malunion than adults.
- Shoulder instability during adolescence can be managed surgically, as in adult patients; however, the outcomes are potentially worse with higher rates of recurrence.
- Scapula fractures usually occur in the setting of high-energy trauma. These fractures are rarely managed surgically in children, but care should be taken to ensure that scapular kinematics are maintained.
- Proximal humerus fractures have great remodeling potential, and patients can tolerate some deformity secondary to the motion at the shoulder.
- Radial nerve palsies associated with humerus shaft fractures are less common in the pediatric age group than in adults. Full recovery frequently occurs in the setting of blunt trauma, and a course of observation in this age group is supported.

ANNOTATED REFERENCES

1. Department of Research & Scientific Affairs, American Academy of Orthopaedic Surgeons: *Physician Visits for Musculoskeletal Symptoms and Complaints*. Available at: http://www.aaos.org/research/stats/patientstats.asp. Updated November 2013. Accessed August 27, 2019.
2. Dashe J, Roocroft JH, Bastrom TP, Edmonds EW: Spectrum of shoulder injuries in skeletally immature patients. *Orthop Clin North Am* 2013;44(4):541-551.
3. Chaudhry S: Pediatric posterior sternoclavicular joint injuries. *J Am Acad Orthop Surg* 2015;23(8):468-475.
4. Lee JT, Nasreddine AY, Black EM, Bae DS, Kocher MS: Posterior sternoclavicular joint injuries in skeletally immature patients. *J Pediatr Orthop* 2014;34(4):369-375.
5. Tepolt F, Carry PM, Heyn PC, Miller NH: Posterior sternoclavicular joint injuries in the adolescent population: A meta-analysis. *Am J Sports Med* 2014;42(10):2517-2524.
6. Assafiri I, Sraj S: Adolescent displaced midshaft clavicle fracture. *J Hand Surg Am* 2015;40(1):145-147.
7. Song MH, Yun YH, Kang K, Hyun MJ, Choi S: Nonoperative versus operative treatment for displaced midshaft clavicle fractures in adolescents: A comparative study. *J Pediatr Orthop B* 2019;28(1):45-50.

   This is a study of 41 patients comparing nonsurgical and surgical treatment for midshaft clavicle fractures. Time to union, subjective scores, shoulder abduction strength, and time to return to activity were compared, showing no differences between the two groups, with the exception that the surgical group regained motion and shoulder abduction strength more quickly. Level of evidence: III.
8. Scott ML, Baldwin KD, Mistovich RJ: Operative versus nonoperative treatment of pediatric and adolescent clavicle fractures: A systematic review and critical analysis. *JBJS Rev* 2019;7(3):e5.

   A review of 19 studies showed good outcomes for both surgical and nonsurgical management of displaced midshaft clavicle fractures. Surgical management was associated with higher rate of complications, including implant removal. There is conflicting evidence regarding both cosmesis and functional status of the patient between the two management strategies. Level of evidence: IV.
9. Schulz J, Moor M, Roocroft J, Bastrom TP, Pennock AT: Functional and radiographic outcomes of nonoperative treatment of displaced adolescent clavicle fractures. *J Bone Joint Surg Am* 2013;95(13):1159-1165.
10. McIntosh AL: Surgical treatment of adolescent clavicle fractures: Results and complications. *J Pediatr Orthop* 2016;36(suppl 1):S41-S43.

    This is a review of literature describing surgical indications for displaced midshaft clavicle fractures and the associated complications associated with symptomatic hardware. Level of evidence: IV.
11. McKee RC, Whelan DB, Schemitsch EH, McKee MD: Operative versus nonoperative care of displaced midshaft clavicular fractures: A meta-analysis of randomized clinical trials. *J Bone Joint Surg Am* 2012;94(8):675-684.
12. Ozdener T, Engin-Ustun Y, Aktulay A, et al: Clavicular fracture: Its prevalence and predisposing factors in term uncomplicated pregnancy. *Eur Rev Med Pharmacol Sci* 2013;17(9):1269-1272.
13. Ahn ES, Jung MS, Lee YK, Ko SY, Shin SM, Hahn MH: Neonatal clavicular fracture: Recent 10 year study. *Pediatr Int* 2015;57(1):60-63.
14. Choi HA, Lee YK, Ko SY, Shin SM: Neonatal clavicle fracture in cesarean delivery: Incidence and risk factors. *J Matern Fetal Neonatal Med* 2017;30(14):1689-1692.

    This is a retrospective review of more than 36,000 cesarean deliveries identifying 19 cases of clavicle fractures with maternal age and high birth weight as risk factors. Level of evidence: IV.
15. Brevaut-Malaty V, Guillaume JM: Neonatal diagnosis of congenital pseudarthrosis of the clavicle. *Pediatr Radiol* 2009;39(12):1376.
16. Suppan CA, Bae DS, Donohue KS, Miller PE, Kocher MS, Heyworth BE: Trends in the volume of operative treatment of midshaft clavicle fractures in children and adolescents: A retrospective, 12-year, single-institution analysis. *J Pediatr Orthop B* 2016;25(4):305-309.

    This retrospective review quantified the number of clavicle fractures and treatment trends over time. There was an increase in the number of clavicle fractures managed from 1999 to 2011 and an increase in the percentage managed surgically from 5% to 26%. Level of evidence: IV.
17. Pennock AT, Edmonds EW, Bae DS, et al: Adolescent clavicle nonunions: Potential risk factors and surgical management. *J Shoulder Elbow Surg* 2018;27(1):29-35.

    A multicenter review of 25 cases of nonunion in pediatric clavicle fractures showed high rates of union with surgical treatment and that refracture is a risk for nonunion. Displacement at the time of injury did not correlate with nonunion. Level of evidence: IV.
18. Bae DS, Shah AS, Kalish LA, Kwon JY, Waters PM: Shoulder motion, strength, and functional outcomes in children with established malunion of the clavicle. *J Pediatr Orthop* 2013;33(5):544-550.
19. Kontautas E, Gerulis V, Varzaityte L, Ambrozalitis KV, Burkauskiene A: Osteosynthesis of the clavicle after osteotomy in brachial plexus surgery: A biomechanical cadaver study. *Medicina (Kaunas)* 2015;51(2):112-116.
20. Serrano R, Borade A, Mir H, et al: Anterior-inferior plating results in fewer secondary interventions compared to superior plating for acute displaced midshaft clavicle fractures. *J Orthop Trauma* 2017;31(9):468-471.

    A retrospective comparative study of two level 1 regional trauma centers with 510 surgically managed midshaft clavicle fractures shows implant removal rate of 5.9% in anterior-inferior plating and 22.3% in superior plating. Level of evidence: III.
21. Roberts SB, Beattie N, McNiven ND, Robinson CM: The natural history of primary anterior dislocation of the glenohumeral joint in adolescence. *Bone Joint J* 2015;97-B(4):520-526.
22. Leroux T, Ogilvie-Harris D, Veillette C, et al: The epidemiology of primary anterior shoulder dislocations in patients aged 10 to 16 years. *Am J Sports Med* 2015;43(9):2111-2117.

23. Kraus R, Pavlidis T, Heiss C, Kilian O, Schnettler R: Arthroscopic treatment of post-traumatic shoulder instability in children and adolescents. *Knee Surg Sports Traumatol Arthrosc* 2010;18(12):1738-1741.

24. Edmonds EW, Lewallen LW, Murphy M, Dahm D, McIntosh AL: Peri-operative complications in pediatric and adolescent shoulder arthroscopy. *J Child Orthop* 2014;8(4):341-344.

25. Ozturk BY, Maak TG, Fabricant P, et al: Return to sports after arthroscopic anterior stabilization in patients aged younger than 25 years. *Arthroscopy* 2013;29(12):1922-1931.

26. Shymon SJ, Roocroft J, Edmonds EW: Traumatic anterior instability of the pediatric shoulder: A comparison of arthroscopic and open Bankart repairs. *J Pediatr Orthop* 2015;35(1):1-6.

27. Blackman AJ, Krych AJ, Kuzma SA, Chow RM, Camp C, Dahm DL: Results of revision anterior shoulder stabilization surgery in adolescent athletes. *Arthroscopy* 2014;30(11):1400-1405.

28. Shannon SF, Hernandez NM, Sems SA, Larson AN, Milbrandt TA: High-energy pediatric scapula fractures and their associated injuries. *J Pediatr Orthop* 2019;39(7):377-381.

    This is a series of high-energy fractures of the scapula and their injuries when compared with a control series of patients. Level of evidence: III.

29. Jayakumar P, Barry M, Ramachandran M: Orthopaedic aspects of paediatric non-accidental trauma. *J Bone Joint Surg Br* 2010;92-B(2):189-195.

30. Kannan S, Singh HP, Pandey R: A systematic review of management of clavicle fractures. *Acta Orthop Belg* 2018;84(4):497-508.

    This is a review of the management of fractures surrounding the shoulder girdle. Level of evidence: IV.

31. Lovejoy J, Ganey TM, Ogden JA: Scapulothoracic dissociation secondary to major shoulder trauma. *J Pediatr Orthop B* 2009;18(3):131-134.

32. Choo AM, Schottel PC, Burgess AR: Scapulothoracic dissociation: Evaluation and management. *J Am Acad Orthop Surg* 2017;25(5):339-347.

    A review article regarding the scapulothoracic dissociation that discusses outcomes and management strategies. Evidence of brachial plexus injury being significantly associated with worse prognosis. Level of evidence: IV.

33. Beaty JH, Kasser JR: *Rockwood and Wilkins' Fractures in Children*, ed 5. Philadelphia, PA, Lippincott Williams & Wilkins, 2001, pp 741-806.

34. Shrader MW: Proximal humerus and humeral shaft fractures in children. *Hand Clin* 2007;23(4):432-435.

35. Chaus GW, Carry PM, Pishkenari AK, Hadley-Miller N: Operative versus nonoperative treatment of displaced proximal humeral physeal fractures: A matched cohort. *J Pediatr Orthop* 2015;35(3):234-239.

36. Lefevre Y, Jouneau P, Angelliaume A, Bouty A, Dobremez E: Proximal humerus fractures in children and adolescents. *Orthop Traumatol Surg Res* 2014;100(1 suppl):S149-S156.

37. Shore BJ, Hedequist DJ, Miller PE, Waters PM, Bae DS: Surgical management for displaced pediatric proximal humeral fractures: A cost analysis. *J Child Orthop* 2015;9(1):55-64.

38. Hutchinson PH, Bae DS, Waters PM: Intramedullary nailing versus percutaneous pin fixation of pediatric proximal humerus fractures: A comparison of complications and early radiographic results. *J Pediatr Orthop* 2011;31(6):617-622.

39. Kadhim M, Sethi S, Thacker MM: Unicameral bone cysts in the humerus: Treatment outcomes. *J Pediatr Orthop* 2016;36(4):392-399.

    This is a treatment review of humeral UBCs. Level of evidence: III.

40. Caviglia H Garrido CP, Palazzi FF, Meana NV: Pediatric fractures of the humerus. *Clin Orthop Relat Res* 2005;432:49-56.

41. Canavese F, Marengo L, Mattia C, et al: Outcome of conservative versus surgical treatment of humeral shaft fracture in children and adolescents: Comparison between nonoperative treatment (Desault's bandage), external fixation and elastic stable intramedullary nailing. *J Pediatr Orthop* 2017;37(3):e156-e163.

    This is a 1-year follow-up study of 36 patients with humeral shaft fractures treated in three different ways reporting superior radiographic and return to function in surgically managed fractures. Level of evidence: III.

42. O'Shaughnessy MA, Parry JA, Liu H, Stans AA, Larson AN, Milbrandt TA: Management of paediatric humeral shaft fractures and associated nerve palsy. *J Child Orthop* 2019;13:508-515.

    Over a 20-year period, 80 humeral shaft fractures in the pediatric age group were reviewed. Nonsurgical management was successful in most patients. Surgical stabilization, when rarely indicated, had a low complication rate and improved radiographic alignment. All nerve injuries (6% incidence) fully recovered without surgical intervention. Level of evidence: IV.

CHAPTER 41

Elbow Trauma

MEGAN E. JOHNSON, MD

ABSTRACT

Fractures and injuries about the elbow are extremely common in the pediatric population. The unossified anatomy of the distal humerus in young children can make interpretation of injury radiographs challenging. A number of complications can occur with management. It is therefore important for orthopaedic surgeons to be able to recognize common patterns of pediatric elbow injury and be familiar with treatment principles.

Keywords: elbow dislocation; lateral condyle fracture; medial epicondyle avulsions; olecranon fracture; radial neck fracture; supracondylar humerus fracture

INTRODUCTION

Fractures and injuries about the elbow are very common in young children. As in other aspects of pediatric trauma, many elbow injuries can be managed nonsurgically or with minimally invasive techniques, such as closed reduction and percutaneous pinning. Displaced fractures may cause injury to neurovascular structures that are in close proximity. Other complications include residual deformity, loss of elbow motion, growth irregularities, and osteonecrosis. Because of the notable prevalence of pediatric elbow injuries, orthopaedic surgeons should be well versed in the diagnosis and management.

Neither Dr. Johnson nor any immediate family member has received anything of value from or has stock or stock options held in a commercial company or institution related directly or indirectly to the subject of this chapter.

SUPRACONDYLAR HUMERUS FRACTURES

Supracondylar humerus fractures are the most common type of elbow fracture in children. Although the mean age of injury is 5.5 years, most fractures (53.6%) occur in children aged 3 to 6 years.[1] Most of these fractures are sustained in the child's nondominant arm, and a near-equal incidence is seen between males and females.[2,3] A fall from a height less than 10 feet is the most common mechanism,[4] with extension-type injuries occurring >95% of the time.[5] The medial and lateral columns of the distal humerus are connected by a 1-mm-thick wafer of bone centrally, which separates the coronoid fossa anteriorly from the olecranon fossa posteriorly. Because children reflexively outstretch the arm to break the fall, the olecranon is driven into the thin fossa and fractures can occur.[6]

Clinical Presentation and Evaluation

On presentation, there is usually pain and fusiform swelling about the elbow. With increasing degrees of displacement, greater amounts of deformity will be seen. Open fractures are uncommon, occurring in approximately 1% of displaced fractures,[1] with the proximal fragment typically tearing through the skin anteriorly. The extent of soft-tissue injury, as measured by swelling, ecchymosis, puckering, and tenting, is correlated with the presence of neurovascular injury.[7] The overall incidence of nerve injury with displaced supracondylar humerus fractures is ~11%.[8] The anterior interosseous nerve, a motor branch of the median nerve, is the most commonly injured. This is distinguished from a more proximal median nerve palsy by intact sensation on the volar side of the radial digits and thumb. Radial nerve palsies are a close second in incidence. The ulnar nerve is rarely injured in extension supracondylar fractures but is the most common nerve injured in the rarer flexion-type fractures.[8] Because of pain, anxiety, language barriers, or poor cooperation, a thorough neurologic assessment in this age group can be difficult. The best assessment possible should be documented.

Accurate determination of the vascular status of the involved limb is essential during the assessment of displaced fractures. Presence or absence of a palpable radial pulse should be documented. Capillary refill of the fingertips should be assessed. If there is concern about the vascular status of the hand, Doppler imaging can be used to assess the radial artery flow and the signal compared with the contralateral side. As abundant collateral flow to the forearm and hand originates proximal to the site of fracture, clinical evaluation can yield a well-perfused hand without a palpable radial pulse. This normal color, pulseless hand can be a confusing clinical situation to manage.[9,10] A supracondylar fracture with poor distal circulation (the pale, pulseless hand) constitutes a surgical emergency, and fracture reduction with percutaneous pin fixation should proceed without delay.[11]

The distal extremity should be evaluated for an ipsilateral concomitant fracture. A concomitant fracture can be seen in 5% to 16% of patients with supracondylar fracture, with the most common additional fracture being the ipsilateral distal radius and/or ulna.[4,12] The presence of an ipsilateral forearm fracture with a surgical supracondylar humerus fracture is associated with a higher incidence of nerve palsy compared with isolated surgical supracondylar humerus fractures.[12] The use of an electronic assessment pro forma, or checklist, has been shown to improve on the preoperative clinical evaluation of pediatric patients with supracondylar fractures.[13]

Radiographic Evaluation

The patient in the emergency department with a suspected elbow fracture should have an AP and lateral radiograph centered on the elbow. When no fracture is visible, the presence of a posterior fat pad sign on the lateral view should be assessed. This radiographic finding is highly suggestive of an occult elbow fracture.[14] Ultrasonographic examination can improve diagnostic accuracy in cases of elbow injury without obvious radiographic abnormality.[15] The anterior humeral line is a radiographic marker drawn along the anterior humeral cortex and extended to the capitellum on the lateral radiograph. This line intersects the middle third of the capitellum ossification center in most children older than 4 years.[16] It may intersect more anteriorly in children younger than 4 years. Posterior displacement of extension-type fractures is present if the anterior humeral line does not intersect the capitellar ossification center. The presence of medial or lateral angulation or rotational malalignment on the AP view, in addition to the amount and direction of coronal displacement, can affect surgical decision making.[17,18]

Radiographic Classification

The Gartland classification is used to describe extension-type supracondylar humerus fractures. It is based on the position of the distal fragment in the sagittal plane. Type I fractures are nondisplaced, type II fractures demonstrate anterior angulation with posterior displacement of the distal fragment with an intact posterior humeral cortical hinge, and type III fractures are completely displaced.[19] The Gartland classification was modified by separating type II fractures into two specific subtypes based on coronal or rotational displacement. Type IIA fractures in this modified Gartland classification are fractures that are extended in the sagittal plane but have no rotational or coronal plane malalignment, whereas type IIB fractures demonstrate rotational and/or coronal plane malalignment.[18] The authors of a 2006 study described an additional subgroup of supracondylar fractures with multidirectional instability and labeled these type IV injuries.[20] These are frequently identified, and occasionally created, at the time of surgical reduction and pinning. Some radiographic findings that can help identify type IV fractures preoperatively have been identified.[21]

Management

Management of extension-type supracondylar humerus fractures is based on the Gartland classification. Type I fractures are managed nonsurgically with cast immobilization. Type IIA fractures can be managed with closed reduction and cast immobilization, whereas type IIB fractures are more typically managed with closed reduction and percutaneous pinning.[22] If a type II fracture is managed with closed reduction and casting, it must be followed closely to avoid loss of reduction because swelling decreases and the cast becomes less snug. Type III and IV fractures require closed or open reduction and pin fixation to obtain the best clinical result. Open reduction is indicated when an acceptable closed reduction cannot be obtained. Because entrapped soft-tissue structures are the most common cause of failed closed reduction, the open approach is usually determined by the position of the proximal metaphyseal fragment.[23] Obesity and posterolateral displacement have also been shown to be specific risk factors for conversion to open reduction.[24,25] Numerous studies have shown that management of most displaced supracondylar fractures can safely be delayed to the following morning and do not require emergent management.[26-29] Supracondylar fractures requiring emergent management are those that are open, have an abnormal vascular examination, or are at risk of compartment syndrome.[5] Children who may not be reliably examined and fractures causing tenting of the skin may also need more emergent management.

When managing supracondylar fractures with percutaneous pinning, the most stable pin configuration is crossed medial and lateral pins.[30,31] The use of all-lateral entry pins avoids the risk of iatrogenic ulnar nerve injury with medial pin placement. For more stable fractures, two lateral pins with sufficient pin spread at the fracture site provide adequate stabilization.[32,33] Less stable fracture patterns necessitate placement of a third lateral pin or a medial pin.[34] A recent study demonstrated the utility of intraoperative internal rotation stress testing in determining the need for additional pin fixation in type III supracondylar humerus fractures.[35]

Postoperatively, the extremity is immobilized in a cast, split cast, or splint depending on the degree of soft-tissue swelling. Because these metaphyseal fractures in young children heal quickly, most fractures are managed with immobilization for 3 to 4 weeks. If pins were used, they may be removed in the clinic at that time, and early motion is established. Many surgeons obtain postoperative radiographs in the early phase of postoperative treatment,[36,37] but a number of studies have questioned the clinical necessity of this practice.[18,19]

Outcomes and Complications

Recent data regarding patient-reported outcomes for supracondylar humerus fractures suggest that most patients have excellent outcomes, regardless of fracture type or direction of displacement.[38] Most nerve injuries associated with supracondylar humerus fractures recover within 6 months without further intervention. Isolated radial nerve injury or multiple nerve injuries are associated with prolonged recovery.[39]

Displaced supracondylar humerus fractures with an absent pulse, regardless of the vascularity of the hand, should undergo closed reduction and percutaneous pin fixation on an urgent-emergent basis. If the pulse returns, the arm should be immobilized and observed to ensure that the neurovascular status remains stable. Exploration of the brachial artery is not necessarily required, where the radial pulse does not return postreduction but the limb remains well perfused.[10] Exploration of the brachial artery should be performed if the vascular examination remains equivocal or the extremity is dysvascular.[11] An absent palpable radial pulse with a concomitant anterior interosseous nerve/median nerve palsy was thought to be an absolute indication for emergent brachial artery exploration,[40] although a recently published multicenter retrospective study of 71 such patients has called for this indication to be more relative.[26]

Compartment syndrome associated with supracondylar humerus fractures was a significant concern when displaced (type III/IV) fractures were managed with hyperflexion and casting.[41] The practice of percutaneous pinning and immobilization in less flexion has decreased the incidence of this feared complication, but not to zero.[42] Subgroups of patients have been identified as being at increased risk. A displaced supracondylar fracture with a displaced forearm fracture (floating elbow) has been associated with forearm compartment syndrome,[43] in addition to increased risk of neurologic injury.[12] In a large National Trauma Data Bank review, children with neurovascular injury, and in particular a vascular injury, were the subgroup most at risk for development of a compartment syndrome complication.[42]

Flexion

Flexion-type supracondylar humerus fractures are uncommon and occur as the result of a flexion force being placed on the distal fragment. These fractures tend to occur in older children (mean age of 7.5 years versus 5.8 years for extension-type fractures).[44] Although there is no difference in the incidence of neurovascular injury, ulnar nerve injuries were more common in flexion-type fractures than extension-type fractures (19% versus 3%).[44] A 2010 study found a 17% rate of nerve injury in flexion-type fractures, of which 91% involved the ulnar nerve.[8] The need for open reduction is more common with flexion-type supracondylar fractures.[45] When open reduction is necessary, a medial approach should be used so that exploration of the ulnar nerve can be performed to ensure that it is not trapped in the fracture site.[23] Flexion-type fractures are often more unstable than extension-type fractures, and the use of a transolecranon pin may be helpful to add stability to unstable fractures once reduction of the fracture in the sagittal plane is achieved. Malalignment in the coronal plane can then be corrected, and traditional laterally based pins can be placed, followed by removal of the transolecranon pin[46] (**Figure 1**).

Transphyseal

Transphyseal supracondylar humerus fractures represent fracture-separations of the distal humerus and typically occur in children younger than 3 years. Mechanisms of injury include birth trauma, fall on an outstretched hand with the elbow in extension, and nonaccidental trauma. In a study of 16 children with this fracture, child abuse was either proven or suspected in 6 children.[47] If there is concern for nonaccidental trauma, a skeletal survey should be performed and the child abuse team/social services consulted.[48]

These fractures are classified according to the age of the child and presence or absence of the capitellar ossification center.[47] Before the appearance of the capitellar ossification center, the key to diagnosis of transphyseal fractures is recognizing that the forearm is not aligned with the humeral shaft. These injuries can be mistaken for elbow dislocations. Elbow dislocations are exceedingly rare in this age group and are usually displaced posterolaterally, whereas transphyseal fractures are almost always displaced posteromedially. If the capitellar ossification center is present, it will be aligned with the radius, and both the radius and capitellum will be displaced in the same direction, usually posteromedially.[48] Because

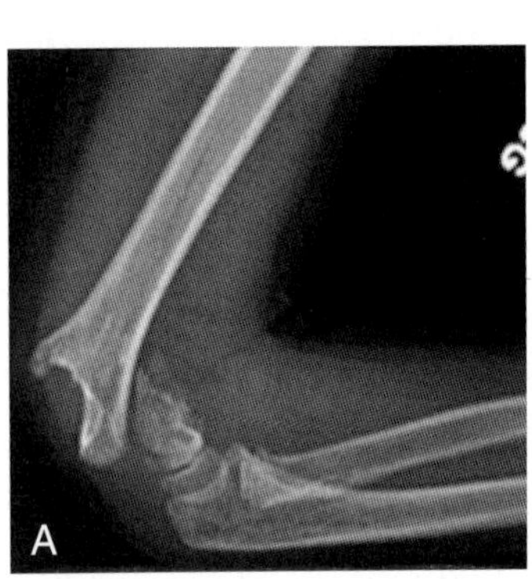

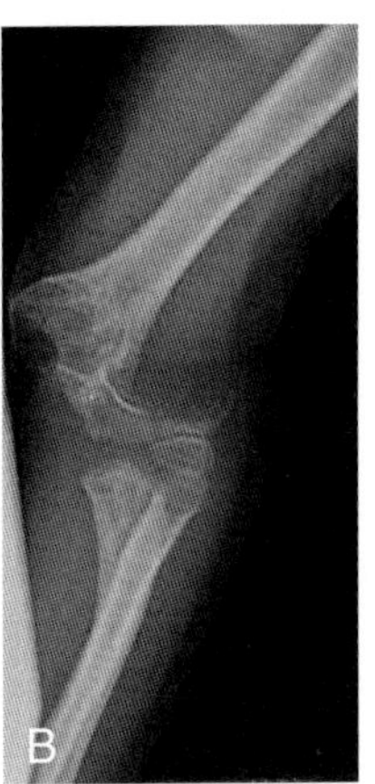

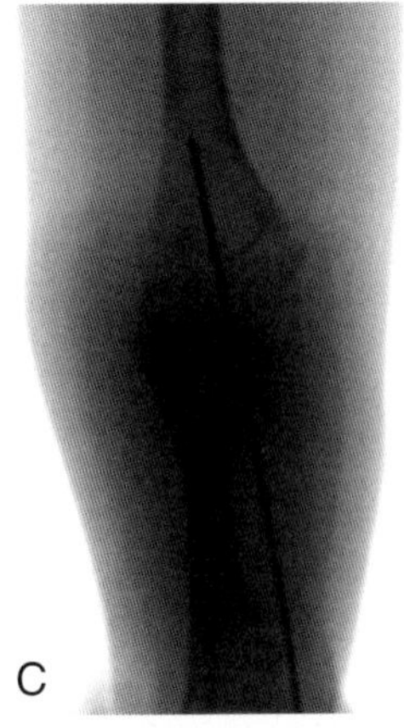

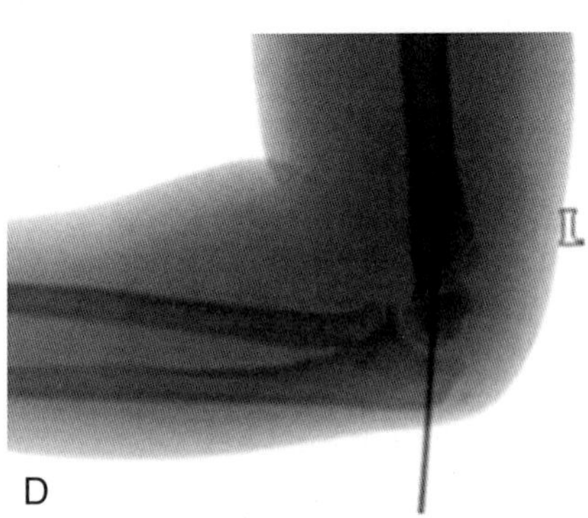

FIGURE 1 Transolecranon pin fixation for flexion-type supracondylar humerus fracture. **A**, Preoperative lateral radiograph of a flexion-type supracondylar humerus fracture. **B**, Preoperative AP radiograph of a flexion-type supracondylar humerus fracture. **C**, Intraoperative AP fluoroscopic image showing a transolecranon pin placed centrally up the humeral canal. **D**, Lateral intraoperative fluoroscopic image showing transolecranon pin holding sagittal alignment. (Reproduced with permission from Green BM, Stone JD, Bruce RW, Fletcher ND: The use of a transolecranon pin in the treatment of pediatric flexion-type supracondylar humerus fractures. *J Pediatr Orthop* 2017;37[6]:e347-e352.)

of the rarity and the irregular ossification in this area, the diagnosis of a transphyseal fracture may be missed by radiologists in >50% of cases.[49] Ultrasonography can be used to aid in the diagnosis of this injury. MRI can be diagnostic but not ideal because of the requirement of sedation or anesthesia in this young age group. Arthrography can be used at the time of treatment if necessary to determine the type of injury present and guide reduction and fixation.[48]

Closed reduction and percutaneous pin fixation is the recommended management for displaced transphyseal fractures because of the high incidence of cubitus varus after closed reduction alone. If diagnosis has been delayed, transphyseal fractures can be managed by in situ casting/splinting, especially if there is already evidence of healing on radiographs. The approach to closed reduction and pin fixation is the same as that used for supracondylar humerus fractures. It may be difficult to determine the adequacy of reduction if the capitellum has not yet started to ossify. The use of medial and lateral humeral lines drawn parallel to the medial and lateral humeral diaphysis can help determine if the alignment is adequate after closed reduction. Successful reduction is achieved when the ulnar axis falls within the boundaries of the medial and lateral humeral lines[50] (**Figure 2**). Using this method, cubitus varus developed in only 1 of 13 patients, compared with the 25% to 71% incidence reported in the literature. Transphyseal fractures caused by birth trauma can be managed closed with immobilization, even if displaced, because of the tremendous remodeling potential of the newborn.

T-condylar

T-condylar humerus fractures are characterized by a central intercondylar split with extension of the proximal fracture line through the medial and lateral columns of the distal humerus. This fracture is caused by high-energy mechanisms and typically occurs in older children and adolescents.[51] One should have a high index of suspicion for this pattern of injury in a child older than 9 or 10 years presenting with a supracondylar humerus fracture after a significant trauma. When concern for a T-condylar–type fracture is present, CT scan can help confirm the diagnosis and is also helpful to characterize the intra-articular and extra-articular components of the fracture.

The intra-articular portion of the fracture must be fixed anatomically to restore the joint surface of the distal humerus. Fractures that are minimally displaced can be managed with closed reduction and percutaneous fixation with Kirschner wires (K-wires) or cannulated screws depending on the age of the child.[52,53] If the articular surface cannot be restored through closed reduction, open reduction and internal fixation must be performed. Surgical approach can be performed through a triceps-splitting, paratricipital, or posteromedial (Bryan-Morrey) approach. In older children with closed physes, an olecranon osteotomy can be performed to visualize the articular surface of the distal humerus. A recent systematic review found the highest outcome scores with the triceps-splitting approach, as well as the best range of motion in follow-up.[54] When the articular surface of the distal humerus required direct visualization for fracture reduction, the Bryan-Morrey approach led to similar outcomes as the olecranon osteotomy, but with fewer approach-related complications.[54]

Bicolumnar or delta configurations provide the most stable fixation for T-condylar fractures. In the delta configuration, an interfragmentary screw or transverse K-wire is placed from lateral to medial parallel to the

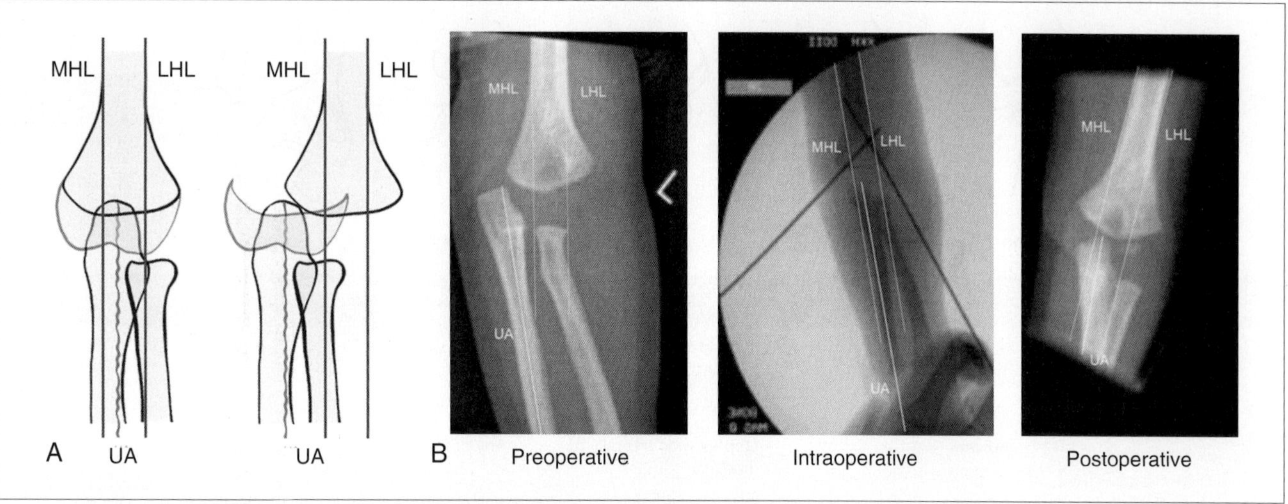

FIGURE 2 Medial and lateral humeral lines for evaluation of distal humerus physeal separations. **A**, Illustration showing the ulnar axis (UA), medial humeral line (MHL), and lateral humeral line (LHL) in a normal elbow on the left and distal humerus physeal separation on the left. **B**, Preoperative, intraoperative, and postoperative radiographs showing use of the MHL and LHL to judge reduction of distal humerus physeal separation. (Reproduced with permission from Chou ACC, Wong HYK, Kumar S, et al: Using the medial and lateral humeral lines as an adjunct to intraoperative elbow arthrography to guide intraoperative reduction and fixation of distal humerus physeal separations reduces the incidence of postoperative cubitus varus. *J Pediatr Orthop* 2018;38[5]:e262-e266.)

articular surface of the distal humerus to fix the intra-articular component of the fracture. Screws or K-wires are then placed up the medial and lateral columns of the distal humerus to complete the delta configuration. In older patients with closed physes, an intercondylar screw is placed followed by medial and posterolateral plates to provide bicolumnar fixation. This construct provides rigid fixation to allow for early motion to avoid joint stiffness.

LATERAL CONDYLE FRACTURES

Lateral condyle fractures are the second most common elbow fracture in children. They occur in a similar age demographic as supracondylar humerus fractures. These fractures also often occur with a fall on an outstretched arm, but with different coronal plane and rotational forces resulting in the difference in fracture pattern.[55] The fracture occurs through the lateral metaphysis of the distal humerus, across the physis, and into the epiphysis, often extending into the joint. Once the fracture extends into the joint, the fracture becomes notably less stable and frequently requires more aggressive management. Although they rarely have the neurovascular issues that supracondylar fractures have, they are known for a host of joint-related complications that can have a significant effect on long-term function.

Clinical Presentation and Evaluation

Patients will present with elbow pain usually associated with a fall and will typically demonstrate swelling of the elbow laterally. The amount of swelling is often indicative of the significance of the articular injury.[56] Neurovascular compromise is uncommon, but this should still be assessed and documented.

Radiographic Evaluation

An AP and lateral radiograph centered on the elbow may identify the fracture, but addition of an internal oblique view, which orients the radiograph beam with the typical fracture plane, can assist in diagnosis and classification.[57,58] The degree of displacement of the lateral condyle fragment will often dictate treatment. Because of the cartilaginous epiphysis in the young patients, plain radiographs cannot directly evaluate articular displacement. Ultrasonography, CT, MRI, and arthrography all have been used to assess and characterize fracture pattern, displacement, and stability.[59-62]

Radiographic Classification

As the amount of radiographic displacement correlates with fracture stability and articular congruency, classification schemes that prescribe treatment revolve around the displacement of the lateral condyle fragment from the remaining intact distal humerus on plain radiographs. Among numerous proposed classification systems, the Song classification appears most comprehensive without being too complex to be clinically useful (**Figure 3**). Good interobserver and intraobserver reliability has been documented with this system, which then reliably guides the clinician in prescribing appropriate treatment to obtain the best clinical result.[63] In this classification, these fractures are described in stages, with Song stage

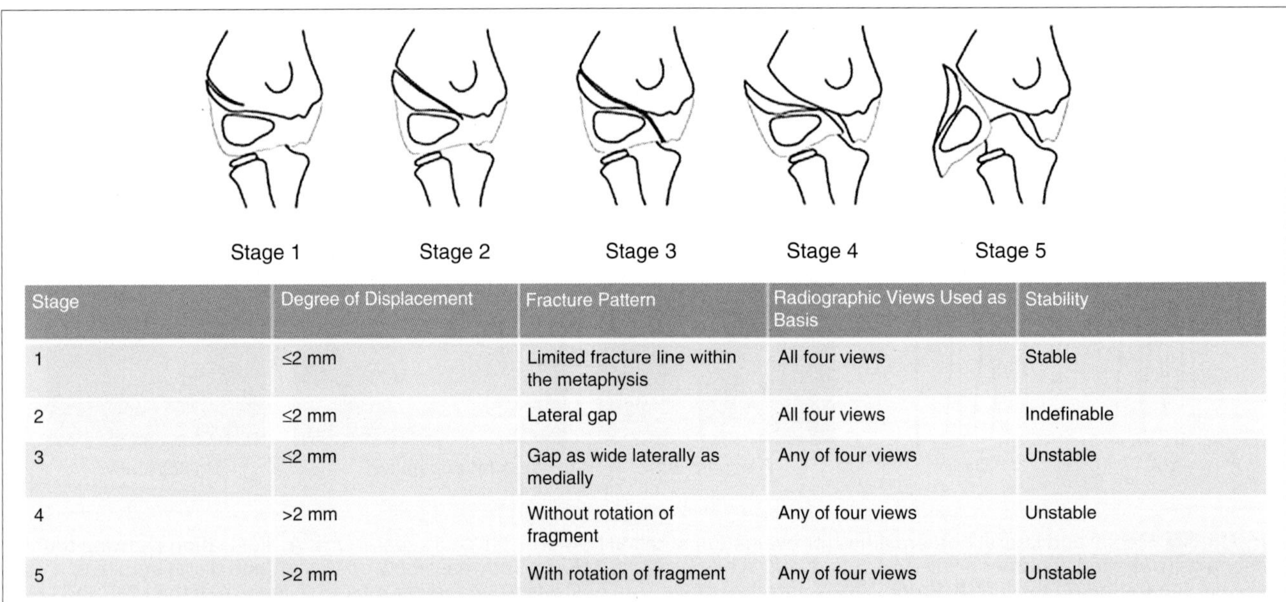

Stage	Degree of Displacement	Fracture Pattern	Radiographic Views Used as Basis	Stability
1	≤2 mm	Limited fracture line within the metaphysis	All four views	Stable
2	≤2 mm	Lateral gap	All four views	Indefinable
3	≤2 mm	Gap as wide laterally as medially	Any of four views	Unstable
4	>2 mm	Without rotation of fragment	Any of four views	Unstable
5	>2 mm	With rotation of fragment	Any of four views	Unstable

FIGURE 3 Illustration showing Song classification of lateral condyle fractures. (Reproduced with permission from Song KS, Kang CH, Min BW, et al: Closed reduction and internal fixation of displaced unstable lateral condyle fractures of the humerus in children. *J Bone Joint Surg Am* 2008;90[12]:2673-2681.)

1 being a nondisplaced metaphyseal fracture not extending into the epiphysis and Song stage 5 being a widely displaced and rotated fracture of the lateral condyle. In between these extremes, there is Song stage 2, which is a fracture into the epiphysis but not into the joint, Song stage 3, which is into the joint and hence unstable, but without rotational displacement, and Song stage 4, into the joint, with greater articular displacement but without the rotational displacement of stage 5.[64,65]

Management

The importance of all classification systems used in the management of lateral condyle fractures is to recognize fractures that, when managed closed, are likely to displace further in a cast and potentially go on to intra-articular malunion or nonunion with progressive deformity.[66] These complications are best avoided by decisive early management of fractures that require surgical stabilization.[67]

Using the Song classification, stage 1 and stage 2 fractures can be managed closed in a long arm cast with the forearm in supination and the wrist in extension. Any patient treated nonsurgically should be followed up closely (weekly) with radiographs (including the internal oblique) to confirm that no further displacement is occurring.[68] The risk of subsequent displacement in minimally displaced (<2 mm) fractures initially managed with immobilization is approximately 15% to 18%, with fracture displacement typically occurring within the first week following injury.[69,70] Cast immobilization is required for 3 to 6 weeks.

For Song stage 2 fractures for which nonsurgical management fails, and Song stage 3 fractures, in situ fixation or closed reduction and percutaneous pinning is recommended to prevent further displacement. This treatment avoids some of the complications seen with open reduction techniques.[71,72] An arthrogram can be performed after closed reduction to evaluate the quality of the articular reduction. The technique for closed reduction and percutaneous fixation of more displaced fractures has been described.[64] Arthroscopically assisted reduction techniques with percutaneous pinning have also been described.[73,74]

For Song stage 4 and 5 fractures not amenable to closed reduction techniques, an open reduction is performed (**Figure 4**). Although a Kocher approach is typically described, the approach into the joint is often done by the injury itself in more displaced fractures. Although visualization of the articular surface is essential, care is taken to avoid posterior dissection so as not to devascularize the lateral condyle fragment.[75] Following anatomic reduction, percutaneous pinning outside the surgical incision is the most common form of fixation. Two to three K-wires in a parallel or divergent pattern will provide adequate fixation as long as the distal pin engages the bone and is not solely engaged in the cartilaginous epiphysis.[75] Pins are typically removed at 4 weeks, but immobilization is carried out for an additional 2 weeks to ensure complete healing. Burying the pins is also an option.[76]

Screw fixation of lateral condyle fractures is an alternative to stabilization with K-wires. There is a slightly

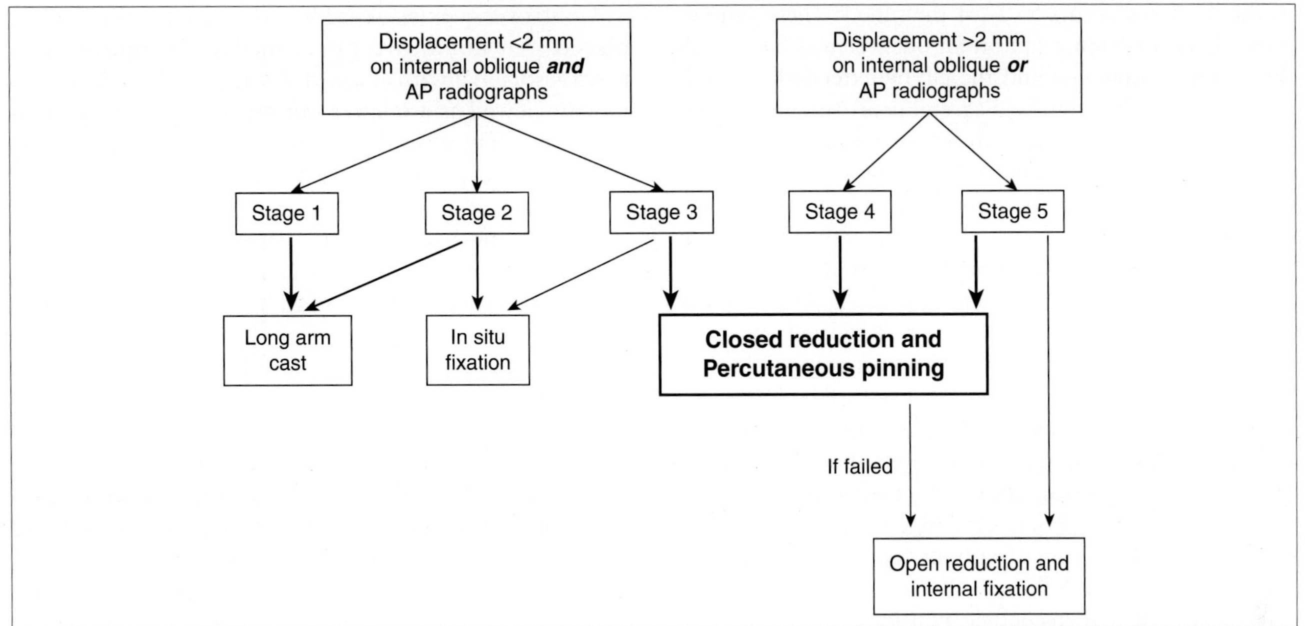

FIGURE 4 Treatment algorithm for lateral condyle fractures based on fracture displacement. (Reproduced with permission from Song KS, Kang CH, Min BW, et al: Closed reduction and internal fixation of displaced unstable lateral condyle fractures of the humerus in children. *J Bone Joint Surg Am* 2008;90[12]:2673-2681.)

higher rate of nonunion with K-wire fixation when compared with screws, but no difference in Baumann angle, carrying angle, or rate of complications.[77] Screw fixation is associated with shorter duration of immobilization, quicker time to union, and increased range of motion at follow-up but does require a secondary procedure for hardware removal.[78] Closed reduction with percutaneous cannulated screw fixation is associated with infection rates lower than those for traditional pin fixation.[79]

Patients may arrive to the treating surgeon on a delayed basis. A comparison of lateral condyle fractures managed within 7 days from injury versus those managed between 7 and 14 days after injury showed similar range of motion, a low and similar rate of complications, and comparable rates of satisfactory outcomes.[80] Fractures that present more than 14 days after injury are best managed between 3 and 4 weeks after injury, with outcomes only becoming slightly worse with increased duration from injury and degree of displacement.[81] A high rate of union (20 of 22 patients) and satisfactory elbow function can be achieved even in patients who undergo fixation more than 4 weeks after injury.[82]

Outcomes and Complications

The Song classification is successful in guiding the clinician to successful treatment and avoiding notable complications that can be seen with these fractures.[63] Delayed union (failure of the fracture to heal by 8 weeks) and nonunion (failure of the fracture to heal by 12 weeks) can occur.[65] Nonunion is most common in patients who are treated nonsurgically.[83] For surgically managed fractures, risk factors for delayed healing include the amount of residual displacement after reduction and the difficulty of obtaining reduction intraoperatively.[84] Nonunions have also been found to be associated with initial displacement at presentation and can be successfully managed with in situ screw fixation.[85] Surgical débridement of the fibrous nonunion, bone grafting, and internal fixation has also been described. Aggressive attempts at reduction of the lateral condyle in this situation should be avoided, however, to limit risk of osteonecrosis.[65]

Lateral condylar overgrowth (lateral spur) is the most common complication seen, occurring in up to 73% of fractures.[86] Cubitus varus can be seen in approximately 40% of cases.[87] Both of these issues are rarely symptomatic. Cubitus valgus is less common and can be seen because of nonunion or premature consolidation of the lateral condylar physis. In cases of progressive cubitus valgus, delayed (tardy) ulnar nerve palsy can occur and can be managed with ulnar nerve transposition.[88]

ELBOW DISLOCATIONS

Elbow dislocations are the most common traumatic joint dislocation during childhood.[89] These injuries occur in an older age group than do supracondylar and lateral condyle fractures, with a mean age of 11.3 years. Males are more likely to sustain this injury by a ratio of approximately 2:1.[90] Although the elbow can dislocate in any direction, dislocation of the radius and ulna posteriorly in relation to the humerus occurs 95% of the time.[90] These injuries typically occur from a fall on an outstretched hand with the forearm supinated and the elbow extended. As with any pediatric elbow injury, a careful neurovascular assessment must be performed both before and after reduction given the proximity of the brachial artery and peripheral nerves. Nerve palsy has been reported in 17% of pediatric traumatic elbow dislocations, with 83% of those involving the ulnar nerve.[91] Most traumatic elbow dislocations in children are accompanied by a fracture.[92] Closed reduction is typically successful in managing posterior elbow dislocations and should be performed as soon as possible after presentation. After reduction, stability of the elbow and concentricity of the reduction must be confirmed clinically and radiographically. Stable reductions should be immobilized for 1 to 2 weeks, followed by early mobilization to avoid joint stiffness. Long-term functional outcomes for simple elbow dislocations (without concomitant fracture) are routinely excellent.[93]

Although medial epicondyle avulsion is the most common associated fracture,[92] fractures of the radial neck, coronoid process, trochlea, and lateral condyle can be seen as well. Patients with multiple associated fractures tend to have a worse functional outcome.[91] Entrapment of the medial epicondyle after reduction should be suspected if the elbow is unstable or if the reduction does not appear concentric radiographically (**Figure 5**). An incarcerated medial epicondyle fracture is an absolute indication for surgical treatment. Ulnar nerve symptoms are more common with entrapped medical epicondyle fractures. It is hypothesized to be related to a higher energy mechanism of injury and not the entrapment itself. Most injuries are neuropraxias and resolve over time without specific treatment.[94]

Controversy exists regarding the management of displaced (but nonincarcerated) medial epicondyle fractures associated with elbow dislocation. This situation is mostly viewed as a relative indication for surgical management.[95] There are higher rates of medial epicondyle avulsion fracture nonunion when associated with an elbow dislocation, and loss of range of elbow motion is more frequent. Because of this, surgeons tend to be more aggressive with surgical management in this population. However, despite deficits on radiographic and physical examination, minimal functional disability in patients after nonsurgical management of elbow dislocations with medial epicondyle avulsion is reported.[96]

Although most patients have excellent outcomes from this injury, patients who require surgical management and have prolonged postdislocation immobilization have a higher incidence of loss of range of motion and residual discomfort.[91] Recurrent dislocation is rare in children but may be caused by capsuloligamentous laxity or osseocartilaginous depressions in the capitellum and radial head.[97-100] Posterolateral rotatory instability may develop because of laxity of the ulnar band of the radial collateral ligament.[101] Chronic instability of the elbow was identified in 5 of 145 patients (3.4%) with traumatic elbow dislocation reported in a 2017 study, with 4 of 5 patients undergoing instability reconstruction.[91]

MEDIAL EPICONDYLE AVULSION FRACTURES

Medial epicondyle fractures most commonly occur in children aged 10 to 14 years.[102] Most are avulsion-type fractures caused by the pull of the flexor-pronator muscle group during a fall on an outstretched hand with

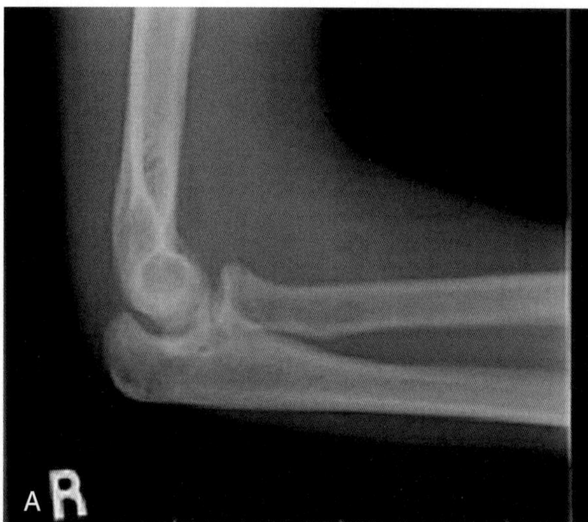

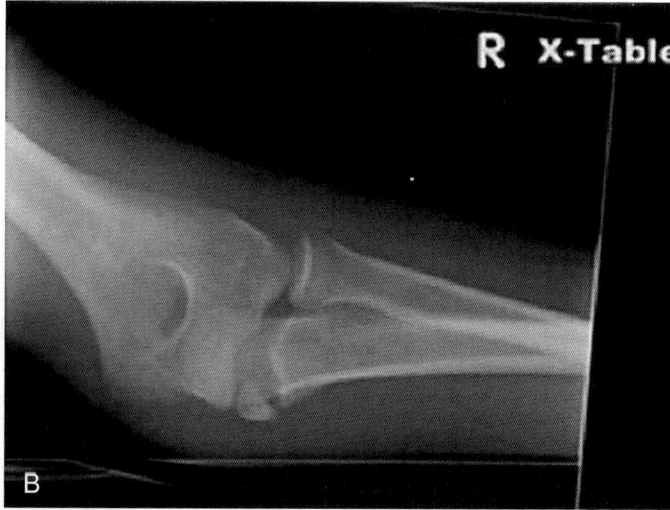

FIGURE 5 Lateral (**A**) and AP (**B**) elbow radiographs showing an incarcerated medial epicondyle after reduction of elbow dislocation. (Reproduced with permission from Vuillermin C, Donohue KS, Miller P, et al: Incarcerated medial epicondyle fractures with elbow dislocation: Risk factors associated with morbidity. *J Pediatr Orthop* 2019;39[9]:e647-e651.)

the elbow extended and forearm supinated. Although these injuries represent up to 20% of all pediatric elbow injuries, the optimal management remains unclear.[103] As with most pediatric fractures, with increasing amounts of fracture displacement, increasing rates of surgical treatment have been recommended.[95,104] The best technique for measurement of the true amount of fracture displacement has been controversial. Fractures considered to be nondisplaced or minimally displaced based on AP and lateral radiographs may actually be displaced as much as 1 cm based on CT.[105] AP radiographs overstate medial displacement, and anterior displacement is not accurately measured on lateral radiographs. Based on cadaver studies, 45° internal oblique radiographs are reliable in measuring the true amount of displacement of these fractures with high interobserver and intraobserver agreement.[106] The distal humeral axial view has been proposed as a better measurement of true displacement without the need for a CT scan.[107] This view is obtained by having the patient rest the elbow on the examination table with the humerus at a 45° angle from the vertical and the radiograph tube above the shoulder at a 25° angle from the long axis of the humerus. Using this technique, the mean error in measurement was 1.5 mm for fractures displaced less than 10 and 0.8 mm in fractures displaced more than 10 mm.[107] Other studies support the improved accuracy of the distal humeral axial view at detecting displacement of medial epicondyle fractures.[108]

Minimally displaced fractures (<5 mm) will often heal adequately with nonsurgical management. With increasing amounts of displacement, the rate of medial epicondyle fracture nonunion increases with nonsurgical management.[109] Because this is mostly an athletic injury, the demand for complete recovery and return to full function is high. Anatomic reduction and compression fixation with a screw has been shown to result in fracture union reliably.[110] Surgical techniques to make this procedure easier have been described.[111,112] Use of a washer does not increase fracture union rate over using a screw alone but has been found to increase the likelihood of a second surgery for removal of prominent hardware.[113] Fixation can be achieved by K-wires in younger children, where continued growth is a concern. Suture anchors can be used when the fragment is small or comminuted and obviate the need for later hardware removal.[114]

Although the rate of nonunion is higher in patients treated nonsurgically, there is debate about whether this is functionally or clinically significant.[56] Surgically and nonsurgically managed fractures with moderate displacement have a similar time to full range of motion with equal rates of complications. Surgically managed fractures did require return to operating room for hardware removal in 18% of patients.[57] Based on this, nonsurgical management seems to be a good option for low-energy injuries with minimal displacement in low-demand patients, whereas open reduction and internal fixation may be best for higher energy injuries with more displacement, especially in patients with high-level participation in sports.[115]

NURSEMAID ELBOW (ANNULAR LIGAMENT DISPLACEMENT)

This injury is caused by subluxation of the radial head with displacement of the annular ligament. It frequently occurs in children aged 6 months to 5 years.[116] It is typically caused by longitudinal traction placed on a forearm that is pronated. The annular ligament slips over the cartilaginous proximal radial epiphysis, causing the injury. This can be seen on ultrasonographic examination, and actual tearing of the annular ligament has been identified in 22% of cases.[117] Children with this injury present with the arm held in a partially extended and pronated position at the elbow. Classically, the reduction is achieved by supination and elbow flexion with pressure placed over the radial head. A palpable or audible click may be felt/heard followed by relatively rapid resolution of symptoms. The child will often go back to using the arm shortly after reduction. Successful treatment is confirmed by full elbow flexion and extension with normal forearm pronation and supination. Hyperpronation of the forearm has been proposed as an alternative reduction method and may produce better results with less pain.[118] Younger children are at increased risk of recurrent subluxation because of ligamentous laxity and pliability of the annular ligament.[119,120] Because the recurrence rate is reported to be from 27% to 45%, counseling the parents about pulling the young child's arm and demonstrating reduction maneuvers to parents at the first presentation may avoid repeat trips to the emergency department.[121]

OLECRANON FRACTURES

Olecranon fractures are relatively uncommon in children and are the result of a fall on an outstretched hand with a variable degree of elbow extension and forearm rotation. They can also occur from a direct blow to the proximal ulna. Olecranon fractures are not uncommon in patients with osteogenesis imperfecta.[122] In a series of 358 patients with osteogenesis imperfecta, 8.1% had an olecranon fracture at a mean age of 11.9 years. Of those patients, 41.4% fractured the contralateral side at an average of 5 months after the first fracture.[123]

Nondisplaced fractures can be managed with cast immobilization as long as the articular surface is anatomic. Displaced fractures require surgical management to restore the joint surface and maintain proper elbow mechanics. Most olecranon fractures in children and adolescents are transverse and can be fixed using a tension band technique using either wire or suture depending on the age of the patient.[124] Comminuted fractures are best managed with open reduction and internal fixation using plates and screws. In most cases, hardware will need to be removed because of prominence once the fracture is healed.

RADIAL NECK FRACTURES

Radial neck fractures are more common in children than radial head fracture. Associated injuries occur in 30% to 50% and are more likely in younger children. Olecranon fractures are the most commonly associated injury, followed by elbow dislocation and medial epicondyle fracture.[125,126] The mechanism of injury is a valgus force with a fall on an extended elbow. Radial neck fractures are classified based on the amount of displacement. Although the diagnosis can usually be made on AP and lateral radiographic views of the elbow, a Greenspan view of the radiocapitellar joint can aid in diagnosis.[66] The presence of a fat pad sign, suggestive of an occult fracture, often represents a nondisplaced fracture of the radial neck. In 16% of children younger than 5 years, the radiocapitellar line may not intersect the capitellum, especially in the AP view.[67] A new radiographic parameter, the lateral humeral line, has been proposed as a better measure of radiocapitellar alignment. The lateral humeral line is drawn parallel to the long axis of the humerus at the lateral-most extent of the ossified distal humerus and should lie lateral to the radial neck when extended distally on an AP view of the elbow[127] (**Figure 6**).

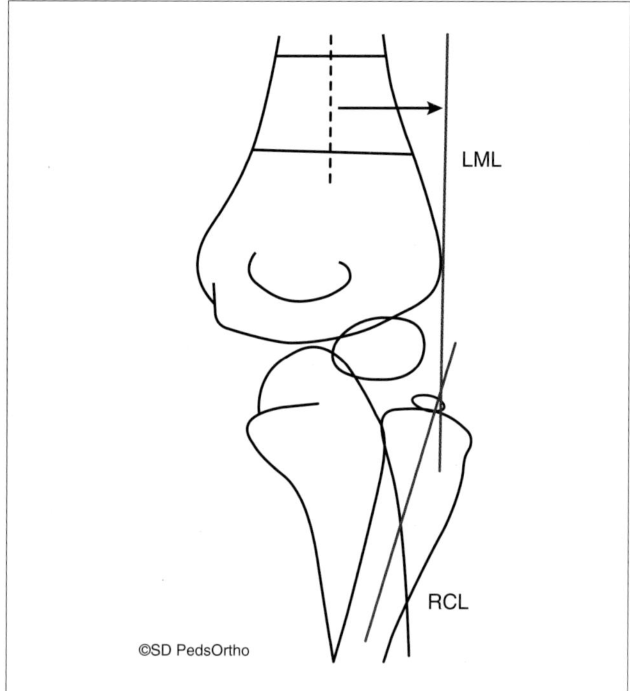

FIGURE 6 Illustration of lateral humeral line (LHL) shown in a laterally displaced radial head dislocation. The LHL is obtained by finding the long axis of the humeral shaft. This line is then translated to the most lateral extent of ossified distal humerus. The radiocapitellar line (RCL) is also marked. (Reproduced with permission from Souder C, Roocroft JH, Edmonds EW: Significance of the lateral humeral line for evaluating radiocapitellar alignment in children. *J Pediatr Orthop* 2017;37[3]:e150-e155.)

The amount of displacement of radial neck fractures requiring reduction is somewhat controversial, but most agree that in children 10 years and older, up to 30° of angulation is acceptable. Up to 45° of angulation may be accepted in younger children with greater remodeling potential.[128] Cast immobilization should be relatively brief (2 to 3 weeks) to avoid stiffness. Shorter immobilization times have been associated with improved outcomes for radial neck fractures.[129] Fractures with angulation more than 30° to 45° and/or translation greater than 3 to 4 mm should undergo reduction.

Several techniques have been described in the literature to achieve closed reduction. If reduction cannot be achieved via closed means, percutaneous reduction can be achieved by using a K-wire or Steinmann pin to lever the radial neck onto the shaft. The Wallace technique can be used when there is medial translation of the radial shaft. In this technique, a periosteal elevator is inserted medial to the radial shaft at the level of the biceps tuberosity. Lateral force is applied to the shaft, whereas pressure is placed on the radial head to reduce the fragment.[130] With any percutaneous technique, care must be taken to avoid injury to the posterior interosseous nerve. This is best avoided by pronating the forearm and using a more posterior approach. The Metaizeau technique involves retrograde insertion of an elastic titanium nail or K-wire from the distal radius into the intramedullary canal and across the fracture site to capture, reduce, and stabilize the radial head.[131] A similar technique involves use of a transphyseal K-wire inserted percutaneously into the distal radius and into the intramedullary canal to capture the radial head once the fracture has been reduced.[132] The advantage of this technique is that the K-wire can be removed in the office after the fracture has healed. Use of an elastic titanium nail, however, requires subsequent removal in the operating room. Excellent results can be achieved with both techniques.[133] For very young children in whom the radial head is not fully ossified, arthrography can be used to assess reduction.

Open reduction should be avoided if possible because of risk of stiffness and osteonecrosis of the radial head; however, if the fracture cannot be reduced by closed methods, open reduction is indicated. If the fracture is stable after open reduction, internal fixation is not necessarily required. If the fracture is not stable, percutaneous pin or flexible intramedullary nail fixation can be performed. Transcapitellar pins should be avoided because of the potential of breakage within the joint.[134]

Good or excellent outcomes can be achieved in most fractures, especially when treatment involves immobilization without the need for reduction. Worse outcomes are associated with greater initial displacement, associated injuries, age older than 10 years, articular involvement, need for open reduction, and inadequate fixation.[126,135] Elbow stiffness is a common complication after radial neck fracture and is associated with worse outcomes. Injury severity, associated fracture, multiple attempts at closed reduction, and open reduction all are correlated with increased joint stiffness.[136-138] Other complications include osteonecrosis, radial head overgrowth, and premature physeal closure. Nonunion is relatively uncommon.[126]

SUMMARY

Thorough physical examination is important because of the increased risk of neurovascular injury associated with certain fractures. Understanding the radiographic anatomy of the pediatric elbow, especially in young children who lack full ossification of numerous growth centers, is key to recognizing common injury patterns. Excellent outcomes can be achieved in most pediatric elbow fractures with appropriate management.

KEY STUDY POINTS

- Thorough preoperative clinical examination of the patient with a displaced supracondylar humerus fracture is critical, documenting preoperative neurologic and vascular status and looking for concomitant ipsilateral fractures.
- Clinical awareness of the transphyseal distal humerus fracture in infants and toddlers is important. The radiographic dissociation of the radius and ulna from the humerus and the posteromedial displacement is key to early diagnosis and appropriate treatment.
- Early decisive recognition and classification of lateral condyle fractures can lead to timely, appropriate treatment, avoiding difficult-to-manage complications such as nonunion and intra-articular malunion.
- There is an increased trend toward surgical fixation of pediatric medial epicondyle fractures despite documentation that nonsurgically managed fractures have similar outcomes. Fracture displacement and associated elbow dislocation are two factors associated with an increased likelihood of surgical treatment.
- Olecranon fractures are common in pediatric patients with osteogenesis imperfecta.

ANNOTATED REFERENCES

1. Holt JB, Glass NA, Shah AS: Understanding the epidemiology of pediatric supracondylar humeral fractures in the United States: Identifying opportunities for intervention. *J Pediatr Orthop* 2018;38:e245-e251.

   The Nationwide Emergency Department Sample database was queried for all children who presented with supracondylar humerus fractures from 2006 to 2011. There was no significant difference in fracture rate by sex. Mean age was 5.5 + 3.1 years, with 53.6% of fractures occurring in children aged 3 to 6 years. Open injuries accounted for 1% of fractures. These patients were older (mean 9.1 + 4.4 years) and predominantly male. Level of evidence: IV.

2. Farnsworth CL, Silva PD, Mubarak SJ: Etiology of supracondylar humerus fractures. *J Pediatr Orthop* 1998;18:38-42.

3. Cheng JC, Lam TP, Maffulli N: Epidemiological features of supracondylar fractures of the humerus in Chinese children. *J Pediatr Orthop B* 2001;10:63-67.

4. Pilla NI, Rinaldi J, Hatch M, Hennrikus W: Epidemiological analysis of displaced supracondylar humerus fractures. *Cureus* 2020;12(4):e7734.

   Seventy-five patients with displaced supracondylar humerus fractures were reviewed and compared with a sample from the literature. All 75 patients were injured in falls. This was similar to the 86% falls as mechanism of injury reported in the literature. The patients were older (average 6 years), but patients with displaced injuries requiring surgery skew older than studies of all supracondylar fractures (surgical and nonsurgical). Of the 75 patients, 12 patients (16%) had ipsilateral distal radius and/or ulna injuries. Nine percent presented with nerve injuries and 12% with skin puckering, similar to what was reported in the reviewed literature. Level of evidence: IV.

5. Abzug JM, Herman MJ: Management of supracondylar humerus fractures in children: Current concepts. *J Am Acad Orthop Surg* 2012;20:69-77.

6. Mencio GA: Fractures and dislocations about the elbow, in Mencio GA, Swiontkowski MF, eds: *Green's Skeletal Trauma in Children*, ed 5. Philadelphia, PA, Elsevier-Saunders, 2015, pp 182-245.

7. Ho CA, Podeszwa DA, Riccio AI, Wimberly RL, Ramo BA: Soft tissue injury severity is associated with neurovascular injury in pediatric supracondylar humerus fractures. *J Pediatr Orthop* 2018;38(9):443-449.

   This is a prospective study of 748 patients treated surgically for displaced supracondylar humerus fractures. Patients with severe swelling, tenting, puckering, ecchymoses, and open fractures were associated with the presence of either a nonpalpable pulse or neurologic injury. The overall incidence of nonpalpable pulse and neurologic injury in the study group was 7.8% and 14%, respectively. Level of evidence: II.

8. Babal J, Mehlman C, Klein G: Nerve injuries associated with pediatric supracondylar humeral fractures. A meta-analysis. *J Pediatr Orthop* 2010;30(3):253-263.

9. Shah AS, Waters PM, Bae DS: Treatment of the "pink pulseless hand" in pediatric supracondylar humerus fractures. *J Hand Surg* 2013;38:1399-1403.

10. Scannell BP, Jackson B III, Bray C, Roush TS, Brighton BK, Frick SL: The perfused, pulseless supracondylar humeral fracture: Intermediate term follow up of vascular status and function. *J Bone Joint Surg Am* 2013;95:1913-1919.

11. Badkoobehi H, Choi PD, Bae D, Skaggs DL: Management of the pulseless pediatric supracondylar humerus fracture. *J Bone Joint Surg Am* 2015;97:937-943.

12. Muchow RD, Riccio AI, Garg S, Ho CA, Wimberly RL: Neurological and vascular injury associated with supracondylar humerus fractures and ipsilateral forearm fractures in children. *J Pediatr Orthop* 2015;35:121-125.

13. Mayne AI, Perry D, Stables G, Dhotare S, Bruce CE: Documentation of neurovascular status in supracondylar fractures and the development of an assessment proforma. *Emerg Med J* 2013;30:480-482.

14. Skaggs DL, Mirzayan R: The posterior fat pad sign in association with occult fracture of the elbow in children. *J Bone Joint Surg Am* 1999;81:1429-1433.

15. Marcell V, Papp S, Kassai T, Bodzay T, Gáti N, Pintér S: Standardized sonographic examination of pediatric elbow injuries is an effective screening method and improves diagnostic efficiency. *Injury* 2020;S0020-1383(20):30133-30139.

A total of 365 children aged 1 to 14 years with suspected closed elbow injury underwent a standard five-point sonographic examination after clinical examination but before radiography. Ultrasonographic examination was very sensitive and specific regarding identification of an elbow injury by detecting a sonographic lipohemarthrosis. This was more sensitive than a posterior fat pad sign radiographically. Ultrasonography was not as effective at detecting the exact nature of the fracture, so patients with positive ultrasonographic findings still benefited from standard elbow radiograph. Level of evidence: IV.

16. Herman MJ, Boardman MJ, Hoover JR, Chafetz RS: Relationship of the anterior humeral line to the capitellar ossific nucleus: Variability with age. *J Bone Joint Surg Am* 2009;91:2188-2193.

17. Lim KBL, Lim CT, Tawng DK: Supracondylar humerus fractures in children: Beware the medial spike. *Bone Joint J* 2013;95-B:1290-1294.

18. Wilkins KE, Beaty JH, Chambers HG, et al: Fractures and dislocations of the elbow region, in Rookwood CA, Wilkens KE, Beaty J, eds: *Fractures in Children*. Philadelphia, PA, Lippincott Williams & Wilkins, 1996, vol 4, pp 653-904.

19. Gartland JJ: Management of supracondylar fractures of the humerus in children. *Surg Gynecol Obstet* 1959;109:145-154.

20. Leitch KK, Kay RM, Femino JD, Tolo VT, Storer SK, Skaggs DL: Treatment of multidirectionally unstable supracondylar humeral fractures in children: A modified Gartland type-IV fracture. *J Bone Joint Surg Am* 2006;88:980-985.

21. Mitchell SL, Sullivan BT, Ho CA, Abzug JM, Raad M, Sponseller PD: Pediatric Gartland type IV supracondylar humeral fractures have substantial overlap with flexion type fractures. *J Bone Joint Surg Am* 2019;101:1351-1356.

Thirty-nine type IV fractures were compared with a cohort of type III fractures. There were no preoperative clinical factors that were different between the two groups. There were five preoperative radiographic parameters associated with increased odds of having a type IV fracture. They were flexion angulation, valgus angulation, lateral translation, osseous apposition between the two fragments (as opposed to complete displacement), and propagation of the fracture line toward the diaphysis. Level of evidence: IV.

22. Silva M, Ebramzadeh E: Is the "appropriate use criteria" for type II supracondylar humerus fractures really appropriate? *J Pediatr Orthop* 2019;39(7):e563-e564.

A total of 1,120 type II supracondylar humerus fractures were reviewed. Both surgically and nonsurgically treated patients were compared. At final outcome, there was no difference between the groups. Patients with isolated extension deformity and no coronal or axial plane malalignment were more likely to be successfully treated without surgical intervention. Level of evidence: III.

23. Wingfield JJ, Ho CA, Abzug JM, Ritzman TF, Brighton BK: Open reduction techniques for supracondylar humerus fractures in children. *J Am Acad Orthop Surg* 2015;23:e72-e80.

24. Li NY, Bruce WJ, Joyce C, Decker NM, Cappello T: Obesity's influence on operative management of pediatric supracondylar humerus fractures. *J Pediatr Orthop* 2018;38(3):e118-e121.

In this database study, 31,905 patients with supracondylar humerus fractures were reviewed. Children with obesity aged between 8 and 12 years were four times more likely to require open reduction and internal fixation. Level of evidence: IV.

25. Novais EN, Carry PM, Mark BJ, De S, Miller NH: Posterolaterally displaced and flexion-type supracondylar fractures are associated with a higher risk of open reduction. *J Pediatr Orthop B* 2016;25(5):406-411.

This is a retrospective review of patients with supracondylar humerus fractures to determine the risk factors for open reduction. Flexion-type and posterolaterally displaced extension-type fractures were more likely to require open reduction. Level of evidence: IV.

26. Harris LR, Arkader A, Broom A, et al: Pulseless supracondylar humerus fracture with anterior interosseous nerve or median nerve injury-an absolute indication for open reduction? *J Pediatr Orthop* 2019;39(1):e1-e7.

This is a multicenter retrospective review of patients with type III/IV supracondylar humerus fractures presenting with absent distal palpable pulses and anterior interosseous nerve or median nerve injury. Of a total of 71 patients, 52 patients (73%) underwent closed reduction, and 50 of 52 patients (96%) did not need additional surgery. Of the 19 patients (27%) having open reduction, 11 (58%) required a procedure on the brachial artery (repair or detethering). Of 71 patients, 6 patients (8%) developed compartment syndrome. Compartment syndrome was associated with poor perfusion status at the time of presentation and delayed time from injury to surgery. Of 61 patients, 59 patients (97%) seen at 3-month follow-up had complete resolution of nerve palsy. Level of evidence: IV.

27. Mehlman CT, Strub WM, Roy DR, Wall EJ, Crawford AH: The effect of surgical timing on the perioperative complications of treatment of supracondylar humerus fractures in children. *J Bone Joint Surg Am* 2001;83:323-327.
28. Gupta N, Kay RM, Leitch K, Femino JD, Tolo VT, Skaggs DL: Effect of surgical delay on perioperative complications and need for open reduction in supracondylar humerus fractures in children. *J Pediatr Orthop* 2004;24:245-248.
29. Bales JG, Spencer HT, Wong MA, Fong YJ, Zionts LE, Silva M: The effect of surgical delay on the outcome of pediatric supracondylar humeral fractures. *J Pediatr Orthop* 2010;30:785-791.
30. Skaggs D, Hale J, Bassett J, Kaminsky C, Kay V: Operative treatment of supracondylar fractures of the humerus in children. The consequences of pin placement. *J Bone Joint Surg Am* 2001;83(5):735-740.
31. Herzenberg J, Koreska J, Carroll N, Rang M: Biomechanical testing of pin fixation techniques for pediatric supracondylar humerus fractures. *Orthop Trans* 1988;12(12):678-679.
32. Lee SS, Mahar AT, Miesen D, et al: Displaced pediatric supracondylar humerus fractures: Biomechanical analysis of percutaneous pinning techniques. *J Pediatr Orthop* 2002;22(4):440-443.
33. Bloom T, Robertson C, Mahar A, Newton P: Biomechanical analysis of supracondylar humerus fracture pinning for slightly malreduced fractures. *J Pediatr Orthop* 2008;28:766-772.
34. Jaeblon T, Anthony S, Ogden A, Andary JJ: Pediatric supracondylar fractures: Variation in fracture patterns and the biomechanical effects of pin configuration. *J Pediatr Orthop* 2016;36(8):787-792.

    This is a biomechanical study of pin configuration for supracondylar humerus fractures. Two lateral pins were found to be stiffer than three lateral pins and cross pins for sagittal oblique fractures. Two and three lateral pins were found to be stiffer than cross pins for low transverse fractures, and three lateral pins are preferred for high transverse fractures. For all fracture configurations, lateral pins were stiffer than cross pins. Level of evidence: V.
35. Bauer JM, Stutz CM, Schoenecker JG, Lovejoy SA, Mencio GA, Martus JE: Internal rotation stress testing improves radiographic outcomes of type 3 supracondylar humerus fractures. *J Pediatr Orthop* 2019;39(1):8-13.

    Intraoperative internal rotation stress test was utilized in a prospective cohort of patients with displaced supracondylar humerus fractures requiring fixation to determine the need for additional fixation with a medial column pin. Use of the internal rotation stress test resulted in improved final radiographic rotational alignment with no postoperative nerve injuries. Level of evidence: III.
36. Karalius VP, Stanfield J, Ashley P, et al: The utility of routine postoperative radiographs after pinning of pediatric supracondylar humerus fractures. *J Pediatr Orthop* 2017;37(5):e309-e312.

    This is a retrospective case series of patients with displaced supracondylar humerus fractures. The authors found that initial postoperative radiographs changed treatment in 1.6% of patients, whereas postoperative radiographs at 3 weeks led to changes in treatment in none of the patients. Based on this, it was recommended against obtaining radiographs at 3 weeks unless clinically warranted. Level of evidence: IV.
37. Mansor Y, Givon A, Sherr-Lurie N, Seltser A, Schindler A, Givon U: Is a radiograph needed one week after internal fixation of a supracondylar humeral fracture? *J Pediatr Orthop B* 2019;28(6):536-541.

    This is a retrospective review of patients who underwent surgical management of displaced supracondylar humerus fractures to determine the need for early follow-up radiographs. About 3.8% of patients had loss of reduction; however, there was evidence of inadequate fixation on intraoperative radiographs. Therefore, the authors conclude that early radiographs are not necessary for follow-up when adequate fixation is obtained intraoperatively. Level of evidence: IV.
38. Ernat J, Ho C, Wimberly RL, Jo C, Riccio AI: Fracture classification does not predict functional outcomes in supracondylar humerus fractures: A prospective study. *J Pediatr Orthop* 2017;37(4):e233-e237.

    The authors prospectively evaluated patients with supracondylar humerus fractures to evaluate fracture classification and functional outcomes using the Pediatric Outcomes Data Collection Instrument global functional scale score and Quick Disabilities of the Arm, Shoulder and Hand (QuickDASH) scores. All children had excellent functional outcomes with no difference in scores based on Gartland classification or direction of displacement. Level of evidence: II.
39. Shore BJ, Gillespie BT, Miller PE, Bae DS, Waters PM: Recovery of motor nerve injuries associated with displaced, extension-type pediatric supracondylar humerus fractures. *J Pediatr Orthop* 2019;39(9):e652-e656.

    This is a retrospective review of 244 nerve injuries associated with supracondylar humerus fractures. Sixty-two percent of injuries were associated with median nerve with an average recovery time of 2.3 months. Eighty-nine percent of patients overall experienced a nerve injury. Sixty percent had nerve recovery by 3 months, and 92% had complete nerve recovery. Radial nerve injuries took longer to recover. Level of evidence: IV.
40. Mangat KS, Martin AG, Bache CE: The 'pulseless pink' hand after supracondylar fracture of the humerus in children: The predictive value of nerve palsy. *J Bone Joint Surg Br* 2009;91:1521-1525.
41. Mubarak SJ, Carroll NC: Volkmann's contracture in children: Aetiology and prevention. *J Bone Joint Surg Br* 1979;61-B:285-293.
42. Robertson AK, Snow E, Browne TS, Brownell S, Inneh I, Hill JF: Who gets compartment syndrome?: A retrospective analysis of the national and local incidence of compartment syndrome in patients with supracondylar humerus fractures. *J Pediatr Orthop* 2018;38(5):e252-e256.

This is a retrospective review of patients with supracondylar humerus fractures to determine risk factors for compartment syndrome. The overall rate of compartment syndrome was 2 to 4 of 1,000 patients. Older age, male gender, floating elbow injury, and neurovascular injury were all found to be risk factors for compartment syndrome. Level of evidence: IV.

43. Blakemore LC, Cooperman DR, Thompson GH, et al: Compartment syndrome in ipsilateral humerus and forearm fractures in children. *Clin Orthop Relat Res* 2000;376:32-38.

44. Mahan S, May C, Kocher M: Operative management of displaced flexion supracondylar humerus fractures in children. *J Pediatr Orthop* 2007;27(5):551-556.

45. Flynn K, Shah A, Brusalis CM, Leddy K, Flynn JM: Flexion-type supracondylar humerus fractures: Ulnar nerve injury increases risk of open reduction. *J Bone Joint Surg Am* 2017;99:1485-1487.

A total of 2,783 consecutive pediatric supracondylar fractures were reviewed. Ninety-five (3.4%) were flexion-type injuries. Ten of 95 fractures (10.5%) had ulnar nerve injuries. Three of 95 fractures (3.2%) were open. Of the closed fractures, 21 of 82 fractures required open reduction (compared with 1.9% of the extension-type fractures). Open reduction was performed in 6 of 10 fractures (60%) with an associated ulnar nerve injury, as opposed to 15 of 82 fractures (18.3%) without an ulnar nerve injury. Level of evidence: III.

46. Green BM, Stone JD, Bruce RW Jr, Fletcher ND: The use of a transolecranon pin in the treatment of pediatric flexion-type supracondylar humerus fractures. *J Pediatr Orthop* 2017;37(6):e347-e352.

The authors propose a novel technique for reduction of unstable flexion-type supracondylar humerus fractures. The technique involves the placement of a temporary transolecranon pin to stabilize the fracture in the sagittal plane to allow for coronal and axial plane adjustments to be made and for lateral pins to be placed. Level of evidence: IV.

47. DeLee JC, Wilkins KE, Rogers KF, et al: Fracture-separation of the distal humeral epiphysis. *J Bone Joint Surg Am* 1980;62(1):46-51.

48. Abzug JM, Ho CA, Ritzman TF, Brighton BK: Transphyseal fracture of the distal humerus. *J Am Acad Orthop Surg* 2016;24(2):e39-e44.

This is a review article on transphyseal distal humerus fractures involving diagnosis, treatment, complications, and outcomes. Level of evidence: V.

49. Supakul N, Hicks RA, Caltoum CB, Karmazyn B: Distal humeral epiphyseal separation in young children: An often-missed fracture-radiographic signs and ultrasound confirmatory diagnosis. *AJR Am J Roentgenol* 2015;204(2):W192-W198.

50. Chou ACC, Wong HYK, Kumar S, Mahadev A: Using the medial and lateral humeral lines as an adjunct to intraoperative elbow arthrography to guide intraoperative reduction and fixation of distal humerus physeal separations reduces the incidence of postoperative cubitus varus. *J Pediatr Orthop* 2018;38(5):e262-e266.

The authors analyzed a novel method for determination of quality of reduction for distal humerus transphyseal fractures using the ulnar axis and medial and lateral humeral lines. Thirteen patients were included in the study. No patients experienced a complication. There was a low incidence of both angular deformity and cubitus varus at final follow-up. Level of evidence: IV.

51. Popkin CA, Rosenwasser KA, Ellis HB Jr: Pediatric and adolescent T-type distal humerus fractures. *J Am Acad Orthop Surg Glob Res Rev* 2017;1(8):e040.

This is a review article on pediatric T-type distal humerus fractures. Level of evidence: V.

52. Kanellopoulos A, Yiannakopoulos C: Closed reduction and percutaneous stabilization of pediatric T-condylar fractures of the humerus. *J Pediatr Orthop* 2004;24:13-16.

53. Ruiz A, Kealey W, Cowie H: Percutaneous pin fixation of intercondylar fractures in young children. *J Pediatr Orthop B* 2001;10:211-213.

54. Anari JB, Neuwirth AL, Carducci NM, Donegan DJ, Baldwin KD: Pediatric T-condylar humerus fractures: A systematic review. *J Pediatr Orthop* 2017;37(1):36-40.

This is a systematic review of pediatric T-condylar humerus fractures. Less invasive surgical approaches, such as the triceps-splitting approach, are preferred. If articular reduction is required, the Bryan-Morrey approach offers similar results to an olecranon osteotomy, but with fewer complications. In general, younger children can be treated with less invasive methods. Level of evidence: IV.

55. Jakob R, Fowles JV, Rang M, Kassab MT: Observations concerning fractures of the lateral humeral condyle in children. *J Bone Joint Surg Br* 1975;57:430-436.

56. Lee WC, Zainul-Abidin S, Kwan YH, Lam KY, Mahadev A: Prophylactic fixation or surveillance: Predicting subsequent displacement of lateral condyle of humerus fractures based on soft tissue swelling. *J Shoulder Elbow Surg* 2019;28:310-316.

Initial elbow radiographs of 87 minimally displaced lateral condyle fractures that subsequently displaced and 87 fractures with no subsequent displacement were compared. Lateral elbow swelling was quantitatively described using the lateral elbow swelling-humeral shaft diameter (LES-H) ratio. The LES-H ratio was significantly larger in the subsequent displacement group. An LES-H ratio of >1.90 was used as a threshold value to predict subsequent displacement. Level of evidence: III.

57. Bland DC, Pennock AT, Upasani VV, Edmonds EW: Measurement reliability in pediatric lateral condyle fractures of the humerus. *J Pediatr Orthop* 2018;38(8):e429-e433.

A radiographic review of lateral condyle fractures was performed. The authors found the internal oblique view to be the most reliable view measuring displacement. Level of evidence: III.

58. Song KS, Kang CH, Min BW, Bae KC, Cho CH: Internal oblique radiographs for diagnosis of non-displaced or minimally displaced lateral condylar fractures of the humerus in children. *J Bone Joint Surg Am* 2007;89:58-63.

59. Chapman V, Grottkau B, Albright M, Salamipour H, Jaramillo D: Multidetector computed tomography of pediatric lateral condylar fractures. *J Comput Assist Tomogr* 2005;29(6):842-846.

60. Horn B, Herman M, Crisci K, Pizzitullo P, MacEwen G: Fractures of the lateral humeral condyle: Role of the cartilage hinge in fracture stability. *J Pediatr Orthop* 2002;22(1):8-11.

61. Kamegaya M, Shinohara Y, Kurokawa M, Ogata S: Assessment of stability in children's minimally displaced lateral condyle fracture by magnetic resonance imaging. *J Pediatr Orthop* 1999;19(5):570-572.

62. Vocke-Hell A, Schmid A: Sonographic differentiation of stable and unstable lateral condyle fractures of the humerus in children. *J Pediatr Orthop B* 2001;10(2):138-141.

63. Ramo BA, Funk SS, Eliott ME, Jo CH: The Song classification is reliable and guides prognosis and treatment for pediatric lateral condyle fractures: An independent validation study with treatment algorithm. *J Pediatr Orthop* 2020;40:e203-e209.

    A total of 736 patients with lateral condyle fractures were identified. Sixty patients were selected to evaluate the interobserver and intraobserver reliability of the Song classification system. The Song classification was seen to have high interobserver and intraobserver reliability. The Song classification was then used to evaluate the clinical outcomes of the 736 fractures. The classification algorithm better distinguished fractures at risk for failure of nonsurgical treatment and guided management to improve treatment outcomes. Level of evidence: IV.

64. Song K, Kang C, Byung W, Bae K, Cho C, Lee J: Closed reduction and internal fixation of displaced unstable lateral condylar fractures of the humerus in children. *J Bone Joint Surg Am* 2008;90(12):2673-2681.

65. Flynn JC: Nonunion of slightly displaced fractures of the lateral humeral condyle in children: An update. *J Pediatr Orthop* 1989;9:691-696.

66. Greenspan A, Norman A: The radial head, capitellum view: Useful technique in elbow trauma. *AJR Am J Roentgenol* 1982;138:1186-1188.

67. Ramirez RN, Ryan DD, Williams J, et al: A line drawn along the radial shaft misses the capitellum in 16% of radiographs of normal elbows. *J Pediatr Orthop* 2014;34(8):763-767.

68. Song KS, Waters PM: Lateral condylar humerus fractures: Which ones should we fix? *J Pediatr Orthop* 2012;32:S5-S9.

69. Greenhill DA, Funk S, Elliott M, Jo CH, Ramo BA: Minimally displaced humeral lateral condyle fractures: Immobilize or operate when stability is unclear? *J Pediatr Orthop* 2019;39(5):e349-e354.

    The authors performed a retrospective review of Song type 2 lateral condyle fractures. Of those fractures managed closed with casting, only 18% were found to displace in the cast. Meaningful displacements occurred before 14 days. The conclusion of the study was that most Song type 2 lateral condyle fractures (82%) can be managed successfully with cast immobilization with the addition of only one extra clinic visit and radiography. Level of evidence: III.

70. Knapik DM, Gilmore A, Liu R: Conservative management of minimally displaced (<2 mm) fractures of the lateral humeral condyle in pediatric patients: A systematic review. *J Pediatr Orthop* 2017;37:e83-e87.

    A systematic literature review was performed to evaluate the fate of minimally displaced (<2 mm) lateral condyle fractures. The authors identified that the risk of subsequent displacement in these fractures managed nonsurgically was 14.9%. Fracture displacement, when it did happen, typically occurred in the first week post injury. Malunion, nonunion, and loss of elbow motion were the most commonly identified complications following subsequent displacement. Level of evidence: II.

71. Pennock AT, Salgueiro L, Upasani VV, Bastrom TP, Newton PO, Yaszay B: Closed reduction and percutaneous pinning versus open reduction and internal fixation for type II lateral condyle humerus fractures in children displaced >2 mm. *J Pediatr Orthop* 2016;36(8):780-786.

    This is a retrospective review of 74 children with lateral condyle fractures with >2 mm of displacement and no articular incongruity managed surgically with either open reduction and internal fixation or closed reduction and percutaneous pinning. All patients had good outcomes regardless of the type of treatment. Closed reduction and percutaneous pinning was associated with shorter surgical times and a 13% complication rate versus 25% in the group treated with open reduction and internal fixation. Level of evidence: III.

72. Shabtai L, Lightdale-Miric N, Rounds A, Arkader A, Pace JL: Incidence, risk factors and outcomes of avascular necrosis occurring after humeral lateral condyle fractures. *J Pediatr Orthop B* 2020;29:145-148.

    A total of 500 patients with lateral condyle fractures were evaluated for osteonecrosis. The incidence of osteonecrosis was 1.4%. All cases of osteonecrosis were associated with displaced fractures managed with open reduction. Without residual deformity and bony reconstitution, good clinical outcomes can be expected in cases of osteonecrosis. Level of evidence: IV.

73. Hausman MR, Qureshi S, Goldstein R, et al: Arthroscopically-assisted treatment of pediatric lateral humeral condyle fractures. *J Pediatr Orthop* 2007;27:739-742.

74. Perez Carro L, Golano P, Vega J: Arthroscopic-assisted reduction and percutaneous external fixation of lateral condyle fractures of the humerus. *Arthroscopy* 2007;23:1131-1134.

75. Tejwani N, Phillips D, Goldstein RY: Management of lateral humeral condylar fractures in children. *J Am Acad Orthop Surg* 2011;19:350-358.

76. Chan LW, Siow HM: Exposed versus buried wires for fixation of lateral humeral condyle fractures in children: A comparison of safety and efficacy. *J Child Orthop* 2011;5:329-333.

77. Ganeshalingam R, Donnan A, Evans O, Hoq M, Camp M, Donnan L: Lateral condylar fractures of the humerus in children: Does the type of fixation matter? *Bone Joint J* 2018;100-B(3):387-395.

This study reviewed 336 children treated with either K-wire fixation or screw fixation for displaced lateral condyle fractures. A higher rate of nonunion was found in the K-wire group, but otherwise, there were no differences between the two types of fixation. Level of evidence: III.

78. Gilbert SR, MacLennan PA, Schlitz RS, Estes AR: Screw versus pin fixation with open reduction of pediatric lateral condyle fractures. *J Pediatr Orthop B* 2016;25(2):148-152.

The authors retrospectively compared 84 patients with lateral condyle fractures treated with open reduction and internal fixation with K-wires or screws. Patients treated with screw fixation had a shorter duration of immobilization and better range of motion at follow-up with fewer nonunions and faster time to union; however, these patients did require a secondary procedure for hardware removal. Level of evidence: III.

79. Stein BE, Ramji AF, Hassanzadeh H, Wohlgemut JM, Ain MC, Sponseller PD: Cannulated lag screw fixation of displaced lateral humeral condyle fractures is associated with lower rates of open reduction and infection than pin fixation. *J Pediatr Orthop* 2017;37(1):7-13.

This is a review of 48 patients with displaced lateral condyle fractures treated surgically with either screw or pin fixation. More patients underwent closed reduction in the screw group with a significantly lower infection rate and earlier mobilization than traditional pin fixation. Level of evidence: III.

80. Silva M, Paredes A, Sadlik G: Outcomes of ORIF >7 days after injury in displaced pediatric lateral condyle fractures. *J Pediatr Orthop* 2017;37(4):234-238.

The authors completed a comparative study of displaced lateral condyle fractures managed within the first 7 days after injury versus fractures managed between 7 and 14 days. All fractures were managed with open reduction and internal fixation. All fractures showed similar range of motion at follow-up with a low and similar rate of complications and comparable rates of satisfactory outcomes. Level of evidence: II.

81. Saraf S, Khare G: Late presentation of fractures of the lateral condyle of the humerus in children. *Indian J Orthop* 2011;45(1):39-44.

82. Agarwal A, Qureshi N, Gupta N, et al: Management of neglected lateral condyle fractures of humerus in children: A retrospective study. *Indian J Orthop* 2012;46(6):698-704.

83. Launay F, Leet AI, Jacopin S, Jouve JL, Bollini G, Sponseller PD: Lateral humeral condyle fractures in children: A comparison of two approaches to treatment. *J Pediatr Orthop* 2004;24:385-391.

84. Salgueiro L, Roocroft JH, Bastrom TP, et al: Rate and risk factors for delayed healing following surgical treatment of lateral condyle humerus fractures in children. *J Pediatr Orthop* 2017;37(1):1-6.

This is a retrospective case series looking at surgically managed lateral condyle fractures. Thirty-three patients with delayed union (16%) were identified, seven of whom required additional surgery to achieve healing. Risk factors for delayed healing were residual displacement >1 mm after reduction and the difficulty of obtaining reduction, as measured by fluoroscopic time. For each 1 second increase in fluoroscopic time, there is a 3% increase in the risk of delayed healing. Level of evidence: IV.

85. Pace JL, Arkader A, Sousa T, Broom AM, Shabtai L: Incidence, risk factors, and definition for nonunion in pediatric lateral condyle fractures. *J Pediatr Orthop* 2018;38(5):e257-e261.

A total of 530 patients with lateral condyle fractures were retrospectively reviewed. The rate of nonunion was found to be 1.4%. The biggest risk factor for nonunion was fracture displacement. Level of evidence: IV.

86. Pribaz J, Bernthal N, Wont T, Silva M: Lateral spurring (overgrowth) after pediatric lateral condyle fractures. *J Pediatr Orthop* 2012;32:456-460.

87. So YC, Fang D, Leong JCY, Bong SC: Varus deformity following lateral humeral condylar fractures in children. *J Pediatr Orthop* 1985;5:569-572.

88. Shaerf DA, Vanhegan IS, Dattani R: Diagnosis, management and complications of distal humerus lateral condyle fractures in children. *Shoulder Elbow* 2018;10:114-120.

The authors present a review of lateral condyle fracture management in children, including a thorough discussion of complications seen with this fracture and the management of such complications. Level of evidence: V.

89. Stans AA, Lawrence JTR: Dislocations of the elbow, medial epicondylar humerus fractures, in Flynn JM, Skaggs DL, Waters PM, eds: *Rockwood and Wilkins' Fractures in Children*, ed 8. Philadelphia, PA, Wolters Kluwer Health, 2015, pp 625-698.

90. Hyvonen H, Korhonen L, Hannonen J, Serlo W, Sinikumpu JJ: Recent trends in children's elbow dislocation with or without a concomitant fracture. *BMC Musculoskelet Disord* 2019;20:294.

A population-based study was performed to evaluate the annual incidence and patient characteristics of children sustaining elbow dislocations. About 104 patients were identified with a mean age of 11.3 years. The average incidence was 6 per 100,000 in children and showed little variations during the study period of 1996 to 2014. Trampoline usage was the most common mechanism of injury in this population from Finland. Level of evidence: IV.

91. Murphy RF, Vuillermin C, Naqvi M, Miller PE, Bae DS, Shore BJ: Early outcomes of pediatric elbow dislocation-risk factors associated with morbidity. *J Pediatr Orthop* 2017;37(7):440-446.

The authors performed a retrospective review of pediatric elbow dislocations. Ninety percent of cases experience excellent outcomes. Risk factors associated with less than excellent outcomes were the presence of multiple associated fractures, surgical intervention, and prolonged immobilization. Level of evidence: IV.

92. Rasool MN: Dislocations of the elbow in children. *J Bone Joint Surg Br* 2004;86:1050-1058.

93. Nussberger G, Schadelin S, Mayr J, Studer D, Zimmerman P: Treatment strategy and long term functional outcome of traumatic elbow dislocation in childhood: A single center study. *J Child Orthop* 2018;12:129-135.

The authors studied 37 patients with traumatic elbow dislocations. The mean age was 10.2 years. Twenty-one patients (56.8%) underwent nonsurgical treatment and 16 patients (43.2%) underwent surgical treatment. A number of functional outcome and patient-reported outcome scores were used to calculate the overall posttreatment status. No significant differences regarding long-term functional outcomes were identified between the surgical and nonsurgical cohorts. The authors concluded that functional outcome after traumatic elbow dislocation in children was excellent, and unless a clear surgical indication was present, a nonsurgical approach should be followed. Level of evidence: III.

94. Vuillermin C, Donohue KS, Miller P, Bauer AS, Kramer DE, Yen YM: Incarcerated medial epicondyle fractures with elbow dislocation: Risk factors associated with morbidity. *J Pediatr Orthop* 2019;39(9):e647-e651.

The authors reviewed 32 patients who underwent surgical treatment for incarcerated medial epicondyle fractures. Fourteen patients had preoperative ulnar nerve symptoms, of which five were resolved with surgery. All but three patients had good to excellent outcomes. There was no correlation between complications and longer duration between initial presentation and surgery. Level of evidence: IV.

95. Hughes M, Dua K, O'Hara NN, et al: Variation among pediatric orthopaedic surgeons when treating medial epicondyle fractures. *J Pediatr Orthop* 2019;39(8):e592-e596.

The authors conducted a discrete choice experiment to determine which patient and injury attributes include the management of medial epicondyle fractures by pediatric orthopaedic surgeons. Substantial variations among surgeons regarding treatment were found. Degree of fracture displacement and associated elbow dislocation were the two factors that most heavily influenced surgeons to manage a medial epicondyle fracture surgically. Level of evidence: V.

96. Knapik DM, Fausett CL, Gilmore A, Liu RW: Outcomes of nonoperative pediatric medial humeral epicondyle fractures with and without associated elbow dislocation. *J Pediatr Orthop* 2017;37(4):e224-e228.

This is a systematic review of the literature evaluating nonsurgical outcomes for isolated medial epicondyle fractures and fracture-dislocations. Seven studies with 81 patients were identified. The authors found nonsurgical management of isolated medial epicondyle fractures with or without elbow dislocation to be successful with few long-term complications leading to functional disability. The authors did, however, find increased rates of nonunion, elbow stiffness, and joint laxity in patients with fracture-dislocation. The long-term functional consequences of this are not known. Level of evidence: II.

97. Osborne G, Cotterill P: Recurrent dislocation of the elbow. *J Bone Joint Surg Br* 1966;48(2):340-346.

98. Hassman G, Brunn F, Neer C: Recurrent dislocation of the elbow. *J Bone Joint Surg Am* 1975;57(8):1080-1084.

99. Symeonides P, Paschaloglu C, Stavrou Z, et al: Recurrent dislocation of the elbow. Report of three cases. *J Bone Joint Surg Am* 1975;57:1084-1086.

100. Trias A, Comeau Y: Recurrent dislocation of the elbow in children. *Clin Orthop Relat Res* 1974;100:74-77.

101. O'Driscoll SW, Spinner RJ, Mckee MD, et al: Tardy posterolateral rotatory instability of the elbow due to cubitus varus. *J Bone Joint Surg Am* 2001;83-A(9):1358-1369.

102. Gottschalk H, Eisner E, Hosalkar H: Medial epicondyle fractures in the pediatric population. *J Am Acad Orthop Surg* 2012;20(4):223-232.

103. Beck JJ, Bowen RE, Silva M: What's new in pediatric medial epicondyle fractures? *J Pediatr Orthop* 2018;38:e202-e206.

Medial epicondyle avulsions frequently occur in young athletes, and the goal of rapid return to full function has resulted in an abundance of recent literature on imaging modalities, treatment techniques, outcomes, and complications. The authors reviewed 30 new articles on this topic published between 2005 and 2016. Despite this new information, clear treatment algorithms still do not exist for this injury, and care frequently needs to be individualized for the patient and family to provide the optimum treatment plan. Level of evidence: V.

104. Masquijo JJ, Ferreyra A, Torres-Gomez A, Allende V: Medial epicondyle fractures: Current practices and preferences between SLAOTI members. *J Pediatr Orthop* 2020;40:267-270.

A web-based survey containing 19 questions regarding decision making for treatment of patients with medial epicondyle fractures was conducted by the active members of Sociedad Latinoamericana de Ortopedia y Traumatologia. Of the 354 completed questionnaires, 193 were returned (54% response). There were significant differences in opinion regarding optimal management. Most respondents considered >5 mm of displacement as the differentiation between nonsurgical and surgical management. Level of evidence: V.

105. Edmonds E: How displaced are "nondisplaced" fractures of the medial humeral epicondyle in children? Results of a three-dimensional computed tomography analysis. *J Bone Joint Surg Am* 2010;92(17):2785-2791.

106. Gottschalk H, Bastrom T, Edmonds E: Reliability of internal oblique elbow radiographs for measuring displacement of medial epicondyle humerus fractures: A cadaveric study. *J Pediatr Orthop* 2013;33(1):26-31.

107. Souder CD, Farnsworth CL, McNeil NP, Bomar JD, Edmonds EW: The distal humerus axial view: Assessment of displacement in medial epicondyle fractures. *J Pediatr Orthop* 2015;35(5):449-454.

108. Cao J, Smetana BS, Carry P, Peck KM, Merrell GA: A pediatric medial epicondyle fracture cadaveric study comparing standard AP radiographic view with the distal humerus axial view. *J Pediatr Orthop* 2019;39(3):e205-e209.

This is a two-part study involving identification of the anatomic orientation of the medial epicondyle physis in children based on CT and MRI and comparison of the accuracy of determining fracture displacement between axial and standard AP radiographs based on a cadaver model of medial epicondyle fracture. The medial epicondyle was found to be a posterior structure angled distally and posteriorly. When displacement was >5 mm, the distal humerus axial view was more accurate than the AP view at determining actual fracture displacement. Level of evidence: IV.

109. Pezzutti D, Lin JS, Singh S, Rowan M, Samora JB: Pediatric medial epicondyle fracture management: A systematic review. *J Pediatr Orthop* 2020;40(8):e697-e702.

A systematic review of the literature was performed looking at optimum management of medial epicondyle avulsions. Thirty-seven studies with 1,022 patients were reviewed. Surgical management was associated with a higher union rate than nonsurgical management (96% versus 28%). The most common complication was slight losses of elbow extension and flexion. Both surgical and nonsurgical management result in good outcomes. Level of evidence: IV.

110. Kamath AF, Baldwin K, Horneff J: Operative versus nonoperative management of pediatric medial epicondyle fractures: A systematic review. *J Child Orthop* 2009;3(5):345-357.

111. Kamath AF, Cody SR, Hosalkar HS: Open reduction of medial epicondyle fractures: Operative tips for technical ease. *J Child Orthop* 2009;3:331-336.

112. Glotzbecker MP, Shore B, Matheney T, Gold M, Hedequist D: Alternative technique for open reduction and fixation of displaced medial epicondyle fractures. *J Child Orthop* 2012;6:105-109.

113. Pace GI, Hennrikus WL: Fixation of displaced medial epicondyle fractures in adolescents. *J Pediatr Orthop* 2017;37(2):e80-e82.

The authors reviewed 17 fracture-dislocations of the medial epicondyle in children treated with screw fixation. The patients treated with a screw only versus patients treated with a screw and a washer were compared. No cases of fragmentation or penetration of the epicondyle was found when a washer was not used. The use of a washer increased the likelihood of a second procedure for hardware removal. Level of evidence: IV.

114. Rigal J, Thelen T, Angelliaume A, Pontailler JR, Lefevre Y: A new procedure for fractures of the medial epicondyle in children: Mitek® bone suture anchor. *Orthop Traumatol Surg Res* 2016;102(1):117-120.

This is a retrospective case series of patients treated with a new bone suture anchor technique for management of displaced medial epicondyle fractures. All patients achieved bony union with full range of motion at follow-up. No patients required removal of hardware. Level of evidence: IV.

115. Axibal DP, Carry P, Skelton A, Mayer SW: No difference in return to sport and other outcomes between operative and nonoperative treatment of medial epicondyle fractures in pediatric upper-extremity athletes. *Clin J Sport Med* 2020;30(6):e214-e218.

This is a comparison study of a matched cohort of 22 surgically versus 22 nonsurgically managed displaced medial epicondyle fractures. The authors found no difference in outcomes, including range of motion and complications between the two groups. Level of evidence: III.

116. Diab HS, Hamed MM, Allam Y: Obscure pathology of pulled elbow: Dynamic high resolution ultrasound-assisted classification. *J Child Orthop* 2010;4:539-543.

117. Browner EA: Nursemaid's elbow. *Pediatr Rev* 2013;34:366-367.

118. Bexkens R, Washburn FJ, Eygendaal D, van den Bekerom MP, Oh LS: Effectiveness of reduction maneuvers in the treatment of nursemaid's elbow: A systematic review and meta-analysis. *Am J Emerg Med* 2017;35(1):159-163.

This is a systematic review of the literature to identify randomized controlled trials comparing supination-flexion and hyperpronation reduction maneuvers for the management of nursemaid elbow. Seven trials with 350 patients were identified. Hyperpronation was found to be more effective than supination-flexion with a better success rate and less pain. Level of evidence: II.

119. Taha A: The treatment of pulled elbow: A prospective randomized study. *Arch Orthop Trauma Surg* 2000;120:336-337.

120. Teach S, Schutzman S: Prospective study of recurrent radial head subluxation. *Arch Pediatr Adoles Med* 1986;150:164-166.

121. Kimura M, Takentani T, Kurozawa Y: Parental questionnaire study showed annular ligament displacement was common in three year old children and almost half had reoccurring episodes. *Acta Paediatr* 2018;107:1983-1985.

A population-based study was performed to identify the incidence and recurrence of nursemaid elbow, also known as annular ligament displacement (ALD). A questionnaire was sent to 1098 families before the child's 3-year-old routine health check and 784 were completed (71.4% response rate). Sixty-one (7.8%) had a history of ALD. Mean and median age of first ALD occurrence was 25 months. Twenty-eight children (46%) had more than one episode. Because of the relatively high rate of recurrence, the authors thought that reduction techniques should be taught to the parents at the initial ALD presentation to avoid repeated emergency department visits for this condition. Level of evidence: IV.

122. Peddada KV, Sullivan BT, Margalit A, Sponseller PD: Fracture patterns differ between osteogenesis imperfecta and routine pediatric fractures. *J Pediatr Orthop* 2018;38(4):e20 7-e212.

This is a retrospective review of 29,101 pediatric patients with fractures. Patients with osteogenesis imperfecta were identified and compared with a control group without osteogenesis imperfecta. Transverse and diaphyseal humerus and olecranon fractures were the mostly likely fractures to indicate osteogenesis imperfecta. Level of evidence: III.

123. Tayne S, Smith PA: Olecranon fractures in pediatric patients with osteogenesis imperfecta. *J Pediatr Orthop* 2019;39(7):e558-e562.

The authors reviewed 358 patients with osteogenesis imperfecta and found the incidence of olecranon fracture to be 8.1%, most often occurring in patients with type I osteogenesis imperfecta. Of the total, 41.4% of patients were found to develop bilateral fractures, with a mean time to second fracture of 5 months. Level of evidence: IV.

124. Gortzak Y, Mercado E, Atar D, et al: Pediatric olecranon fractures: Open reduction and internal fixation with removable Kirschner wires and absorbable sutures. *J Pediatr Orthop* 2006;26(1):39-42.

125. Degnan AJ, Ho-Fung VM, Nguyen JC, Barrera CA, Lawrence JTR, Kaplan SL: Proximal radius fractures in children: Evaluation of associated elbow fractures. *Pediatr Radiol* 2019;49(9):1177-1184.

This is a retrospective review of 494 children with proximal radius fractures to evaluate associated injuries. Thirty-nine percent of patients had additional fractures, the most common being the olecranon (22%). Joint effusion and severity of displacement of the radial neck fracture were predictors of additional injuries. Level of evidence: IV.

126. Nicholson LT, Skaggs DL: Proximal radius fractures in children. *J Am Acad Orthop Surg* 2019;27(19):e876-e886.

This is a review article discussing proximal radius fractures in children. Level of evidence: V.

127. Souder CD, Roocroft JH, Edmonds EW: Significance of the lateral humeral line for evaluating radiocapitellar alignment in children. *J Pediatr Orthop* 2017;37(3):e150-e155.

This is a radiographic evaluation of 37 children to determine the position of the radiocapitellar joint in the coronal plane as well as the relationship of the lateral humeral line to the lateral cortex of the radial neck. The lateral humeral line was consistently found to lay lateral to the radial neck in normal elbows and can be used as an adjunct in evaluating the radiocapitellar joint on AP imaging. Level of evidence: III.

128. Gibly RF, Garg S, Mehlman CT: The community orthopaedic surgeon taking trauma call: Radial neck fracture pearls and pitfalls. *J Orthop Trauma* 2019;33(suppl 8):S17-S21.

This is a review article discussing management of pediatric radial neck fractures. Level of evidence: V.

129. Badoi A, Frech-Dorfler M, Hacker FM, Mayr J: Influence of immobilization time on functional outcome in radial neck fractures in children. *Eur J Pediatr Surg* 2016;26(6):514-518.

This is a case series looking at children with displaced radial neck fractures treated during two different periods. Primary outcome was achievement of full range of motion at final follow-up. Patients with longer duration of immobilization and worse fracture displacement were noted to have worse range of motion. Level of evidence: IV.

130. Kocialkowski A, Wallace WA: Closed percutaneous K-wire stabilization for displaced fractures of the surgical neck of the humerus. *Injury* 1990;21(4):209-212.

131. Metaizeau JP, Lascombe P, Lamelle JL, et al: Reduction and fixation of displaced radial neck fractures by closed intramedullary pinning. *J Pediatr Orthop* 1993;13(3):355-360.

132. Massetti D, Marinelli M, Facco G, et al: Percutaneous K-wire leverage reduction and retrograde transphyseal K-wire fixation of angulated radial neck fractures in children. *Eur J Orthop Surg Traumatol* 2020;30(5):931-937.

This is a retrospective review of 20 children with displaced radial neck fracture who underwent percutaneous K-wire leverage reduction and retrograde transphyseal K-wire fixation. Seventy-five percent of patients had excellent outcomes. No patient developed complications. Level of evidence: IV.

133. Qiao F, Jiang F: Closed reduction of severely displaced radial neck fractures in children. *BMC Musculoskelet Disord* 2019;20(1):567.

The authors reviewed 26 patients with displaced radial neck fractures who underwent percutaneous K-wire leverage and radial intramedullary pinning. All patients achieved bony union and had good to excellent function outcomes based on Mayo Elbow Performance Score. There were no complications recorded. Level of evidence: IV.

134. Newman JH: Displaced radial neck fractures in children. *Injury* 1977;9(2):114-121.

135. De Mattos CB, Ramski DE, Kushare IV, Angsanuntsukh C, Flynn JM: Radial neck fractures in children and adolescents: An examination of operative and nonoperative treatment and outcomes. *J Pediatr Orthop* 2016;36(1):6-12.

This is a retrospective review of 193 children with radial neck fractures treated both surgically and nonsurgically. Outcomes were evaluated based on range of motion at final follow-up. Older children were more likely to have more severely displaced fracture and had a greater risk of poor outcome. More complications were found with surgical treatment. Level of evidence: III.

136. Shabtai L, Arkader A: Percutaneous reduction of displaced radial neck fractures achieves better results compared with fractures treated by open reduction. *J Pediatr Orthop* 2016;36(suppl 1):S63-S66.

This is a review of surgical techniques for displaced radial neck fractures and presentation of the authors' evidence-based treatment algorithm. The conclusion is that most displaced fractures can be managed with closed reduction or percutaneous techniques and that open reduction should be reserved as a last resort in which all closed reduction techniques fail. Level of evidence: V.

137. Kaiser M, Eberl R, Castellani C, Kraus T, Till H, Singer G: Judet type-IV radial neck fractures in children: Comparison of the outcome of fractures with and without bony contact. *Acta Orthop* 2016;87(5):529-532.

This is a study comparing severely displaced radial neck fractures with and without bony contact. Patients who had fractures without bony contact were more likely to have additional injuries and to require open reduction. The patients were also more likely to have a poor outcome, irrespective of whether or not the fractures were managed with closed versus open reduction. The authors concluded that worse outcomes were associated with injury severity and not whether open reduction was required. Level of evidence: III.

138. Gutierrez-de la Iglesia D, Perez-Lopez LM, Cabrera-Gonzalez M, Knorr-Gimenez J: Surgical techniques for displaced radial neck fractures: Predictive factors of functional results. *J Pediatr Orthop* 2017;37(3):159-165.

This is a retrospective review of 51 children with displaced radial neck fractures comparing functional outcomes using the Mayo Elbow Performance Score (MEPS) for three different surgical techniques (closed reduction and casting, closed reduction and Metaizeau nail, and open reduction with intramedullary nailing). The authors found no difference in MEPS between the three surgical techniques, but did find an association between initial fracture displacement and final MEPS. Level of evidence: III.

CHAPTER 42

Fractures of the Forearm, Wrist, and Hand

JOSHUA M. ABZUG, MD • THERESA O. WYRICK, MD

ABSTRACT

Pediatric forearm, wrist, and hand fractures are the most common fractures in children. Most of these fractures can be successfully managed with immobilization alone. If required, closed reduction maneuvers and casting with proper techniques can result in excellent outcomes for patients with these fractures. When surgery is necessary, successful outcomes can be expected along with low complication rates.

Keywords: distal radius fracture; forearm fracture; pediatric; phalangeal neck; scaphoid fracture

INTRODUCTION

Forearm, wrist, and hand fractures are very common in the pediatric population. A study of the National Electronic Injury Surveillance System database assessed the epidemiology of pediatric fractures presenting to emergency departments in the United States and found that forearm fractures were the most common (17.8% of all fractures), followed by finger and wrist fractures.[1] Recently published information regarding the epidemiology, treatment, and outcomes of these fractures in children and adolescents is focused.

It is important to note that the reduction of displaced fractures in these anatomic locations was thought to involve less radiation when a mini C-arm was used; however, it has been shown that radiation exposure during pediatric upper extremity fracture reduction was greater with the use of a mini C-arm than with the use of conventional radiography.[2] Less experienced orthopaedic residents had higher levels of radiation exposure than those with more experience. The authors of that study recommended that formalized training and education be provided to residents about the use of a mini C-arm in fracture reduction.[2]

Furthermore, it is imperative that care providers in emergency departments and urgent care centers use proper splinting techniques when initially stabilizing these fractures to prevent complications from occurring, as a recent study found that 93% of splints are placed improperly. Therefore, orthopaedic providers must assess the splint at the initial outpatient visit to ensure adequacy if the splint is not being removed. Emergency department and urgent care center providers would benefit from education from local orthopaedic providers regarding optimal splint placement.[3]

FRACTURES OF THE FOREARM SHAFT

Pediatric forearm fractures of the radius and ulna are classified by location, displacement, and fracture and deformity characteristics. The peak incidence of these fractures occurs between 12 and 14 years of age, and they usually result from a fall onto an outstretched hand.[4] In pediatric patients, most of these fractures can be managed nonsurgically with excellent outcomes, which is not the case in adult patients. The rapid healing and remodeling potential of children allow for a less than perfect reduction of these fractures in young patients.[5]

The determination of an acceptable reduction depends on many factors, but it is largely influenced by the remodeling potential of the individual patient. Because most of the longitudinal growth of the forearm bones comes from the distal physes of the radius (75%) and ulna (81%),

Dr. Abzug or an immediate family member serves as a paid consultant to or is an employee of Axogen. Neither Dr. Wyrick nor any immediate family member has received anything of value from or has stock or stock options held in a commercial company or institution related directly or indirectly to the subject of this chapter.

distal forearm fractures have more remodeling potential than more proximal forearm fractures. A recent article used the Friberg equation to predict pediatric distal radius forearm fracture remodeling and found it to be reliable. Therefore, the Friberg equation ($V_t = V_0[e^{(-\beta t)}]$) can be used to improve clinical decision making and reduce unnecessary reduction procedures.[6] However, inadequate reduction or insufficient remodeling will result in malunion and contribute to loss of forearm rotation.[5] Remodeling of fractures of the forearm diaphysis cannot be expected in children who are within 1 to 2 years of skeletal maturity; therefore, these children should be treated in the same manner as adults, with anatomic reduction and internal fixation.[7]

Plastic deformations, incomplete fractures (greenstick fractures), and complete fractures of the forearm are observed variations. Forearm fractures with an apex volar deformity occur when the outstretched arm is in supination during a fall. Conversely, a fall onto an outstretched pronated arm results in apex dorsal angulation of the fracture. The closed reduction maneuver for a greenstick fracture includes rotation of the forearm in the opposite direction of that of the injuring force. In complete forearm fractures, a more complex maneuver may be needed to achieve adequate reduction.[5]

Current recommendations regarding what constitutes an acceptable deformity are based on the proximity of the fracture to the physis and the age of the patient. In children younger than 8 years, remodeling of up to 20° of angulation in diaphyseal fractures can be expected, whereas no more than 10° of diaphyseal angulation remodeling can be expected in children older than 10 years. Up to 1 cm of shortening is acceptable. Complete translation can remodel well in fractures located in the middle and distal forearm shaft in younger children, although translation in the radioulnar plane is less well tolerated and can lead to radioulnar impingement.[4] Malrotation of less than 45° is generally acceptable because functional motion is usually possible; however, remodeling will not occur. Bayonet apposition is acceptable in most instances except when the interosseous space is substantially narrowed because this leads to loss of motion secondary to radioulnar impingement with forearm rotation.[5,8]

Most pediatric forearm fractures can be managed with either immobilization alone or with closed reduction to achieve acceptable alignment, which is then followed by casting or sugar-tong splint placement.[9] Closed reduction is typically performed in the emergency department with the patient under conscious sedation or in the operating room. Most often, fluoroscopy is used in the reduction process; however, a 2016 study found that ultrasonography can be used as well.[10] Formal postreduction radiography is not necessary following a reduction with fluoroscopy as it increases cost, radiation exposure, and time in the emergency department without a change in management.[11] However, close follow-up is warranted in patients with displaced or angulated forearm fractures, potentially unstable fractures, and reduced fractures. In those who have undergone fracture reduction, periodic radiographs should be obtained during the first 3 weeks after the injury to monitor for any loss of reduction. In patients with a greenstick fracture, however, a less stringent follow-up protocol may be indicated. A 2016 study reported that only two office visits and a total of three sets of radiographs will provide adequate monitoring because only 1 of 109 study patients with greenstick fractures over a 10-year period required rereduction.[12] In contrast, loss of reduction occurs in 5% to 25% of patients with unstable forearm fractures of both bones. A substantial amount of literature has been published on preventing loss of reduction.[4] Most recently it has been shown that fractures that take 35 minutes or longer to reduce, a complete fracture of the radius, and fractures with more than 50% translation in either plane are at highest risk for loss of reduction.[13] Determination of the optimal type and position of immobilization (above-elbow or below-elbow) and analyses of all of the factors contributing to loss of reduction are ongoing.

Malunion of forearm fractures results in loss of range of motion in as many as 60% of children but may not result in functional limitations. The risk of loss of range of motion is increased in older children and adolescents with fracture malunion because there is less remodeling potential; therefore, the need for surgical fixation of displaced forearm fractures is greater in these patients. To determine predictors of loss of reduction, one study evaluated 282 patients with complete both-bone forearm shaft fractures who were treated nonsurgically.[8] Loss of reduction that exceeded acceptable angulation criteria was found in 144 of the patients, with most of the reduction loss occurring in the first and second weeks after the initial closed reduction procedure. Risk factors for loss of reduction were patient age of 10 years or older, fracture of the proximal radius, and initial angulation of the ulna fracture of less than 15°. Another study in a similar patient cohort identified initial fracture displacement greater than 50% and an inability to achieve an anatomic initial reduction as major risk factors for redisplacement.[14]

Distal forearm fractures of both the radius and ulna and isolated distal radius fractures can be successfully managed with a properly placed and molded below-elbow cast or splint. However, most displaced midshaft and proximal forearm fractures are better and more safely managed with an above-elbow cast. Careful attention to the casting technique is critical. The cast should be more narrow in the dorsal-ventral plane than in the

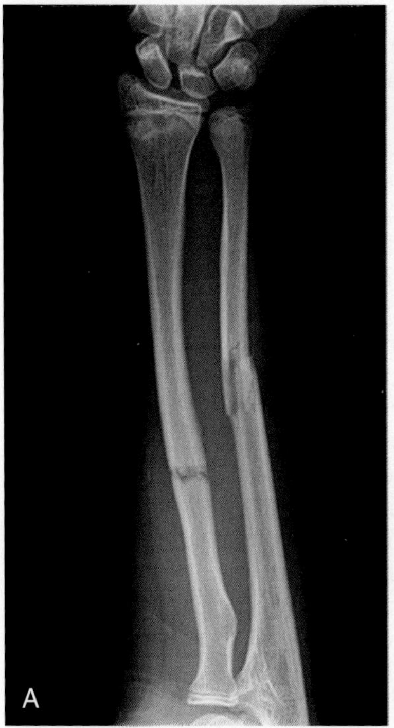

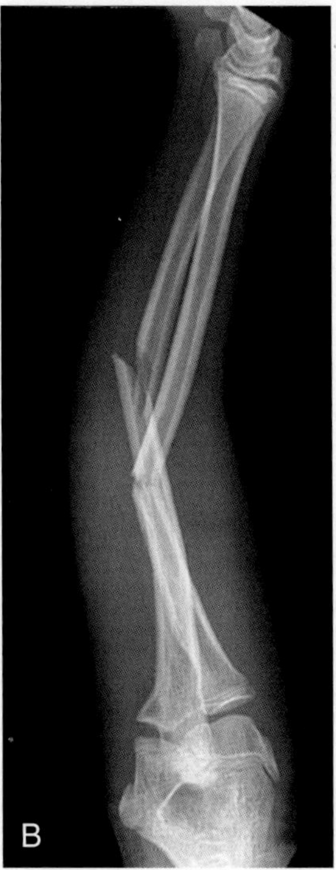

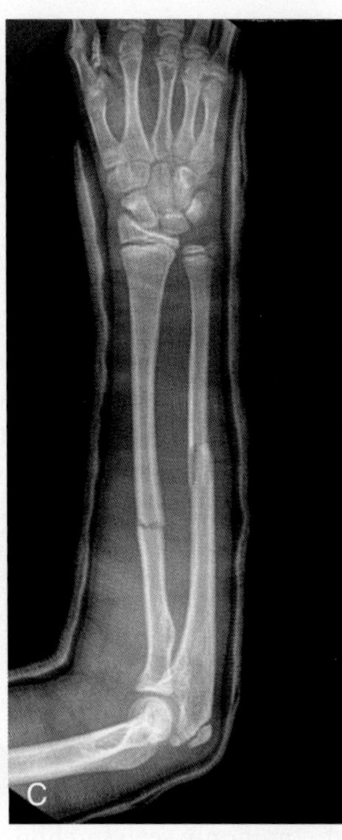

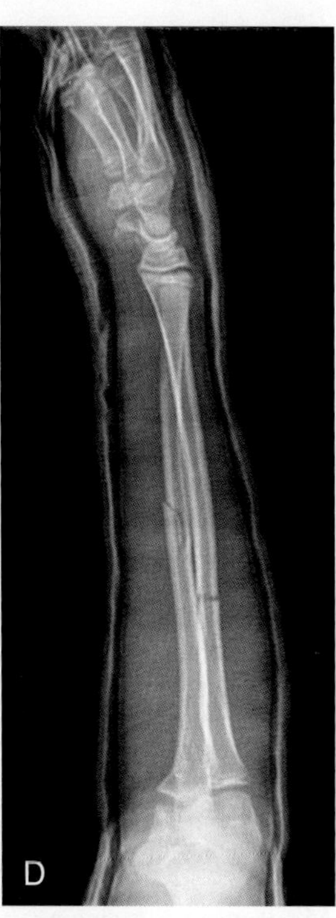

FIGURE 1 AP (**A**) and lateral radiographs (**B**) of the forearm of a 12-year-old girl who fell off a trampoline sustaining a both-bone forearm fracture. AP (**C**) and lateral (**D**) radiographs of the forearm after closed reduction and the application of a long arm cast. Note that the cast applied is wider in the radioulnar plane compared with dorsal-ventral plane, indicating a low cast index. (Courtesy of Joshua M. Abzug, MD.)

radioulnar plane by a radiographic ratio of 0.7 (cast-index) while producing an adequate three-point mold around the fracture site (three-point index)[15] (**Figure 1**). In the case that a long arm cast is necessary because of the proximal nature of the fracture, careful attention to a cast that does not migrate distally as swelling subsides is critical to prevent late apex ulnar angulation. Attention to creating 90° of flexion at the elbow and a straight ulnar border of the cast can help prevent this late angulation.

With the increase in obesity seen in the pediatric population, this comorbidity may be an additional risk factor contributing to the failure of nonsurgical management of forearm fractures. In a study of 157 pediatric patients with distal forearm fractures initially treated nonsurgically, 42% of the children were overweight and 29% of children met the criteria for obesity (body mass index >95th percentile).[16] The children who were obese more often required a closed reduction in the operating room after initial closed treatment compared with children of normal weight. Children who were obese were significantly ($P = 0.005$) less likely to have an initial anatomic reduction in the emergency department and also had a significantly ($P = 0.004$) greater number of visits with radiographic follow-up than children who were not obese. Obesity is an important risk factor for failure of nonsurgical management of forearm fractures in the pediatric population.

If nonsurgical treatment is unsuccessful, surgery is warranted. Surgical intervention is also warranted in patients with open fractures, fractures with severe soft-tissue injury, displaced floating elbow injuries, irreducible fractures, and unstable fractures. A relative indication for surgery is a refracture of a previously nonsurgically managed forearm fracture. Older studies suggested a refracture rate of 5%; however, a more recent large series reported a rate of 1.4%, with refractures most commonly occurring in the middle third of the forearm (72%) followed by the proximal third (24%).[17] Fractures with residual angulation of 15° or more refractured earlier than those with less angulation. Surgical treatment options include intramedullary fixation with Kirschner wires, Steinmann pins, elastic nails, or Rush rods; external fixation; and plate-and-screw fixation. Single-bone fixation is an option in some instances.[4]

Although most patients have excellent outcomes after surgical intervention, complications are relatively common, with reported complication rates of 14% to 21% for elastic nailing.[18,19] One study evaluating risk factors for tendon complications after intramedullary nailing of pediatric forearm fractures reported that 3 of 17 patients (18%) sustained extensor pollicis longus tendon ruptures.[20] No risk factors were identified, except all of the elastic nails had been placed using a dorsal approach to the radius, which suggested attritional tendon rupture secondary to implant prominence. Care should absolutely be taken to avoid tendon irritation in the presence of a dorsal entry elastic nail because of this potential complication, and it should be recognized and treated in a timely fashion. Treatment consists of extensor indicis proprius (EIP) to extensor pollicis longus (EPL) tendon transfer, EPL repair, or EPL reconstruction using a palmaris longus graft.[21]

A recent meta-analysis assessed the complication rates using a lateral approach compared with a dorsal approach during the insertion of a radius intramedullary nail. The overall major complication rate was 5.6% when using a lateral approach, whereas a major complication rate of 8.9% was found when using a dorsal approach. The lateral approach led to a permanent dorsal radial sensory nerve palsy in 0.3% of patients and a transient palsy in 2.9% of patients. The overall rate of EPL tendon rupture was 2.6% from the five articles included in the meta-analysis.[22]

MONTEGGIA FRACTURE-DISLOCATIONS

Monteggia injuries are most commonly seen in children between the ages of 6 and 10 years and are usually the result of a fall onto an outstretched arm. Although closed reduction and cast immobilization often provides sufficient treatment, close follow-up is warranted, with weekly radiographs for the first 3 weeks after injury to monitor for loss of fracture and radiocapitellar joint reduction. An algorithm to direct treatment strategies in patients with pediatric Monteggia fractures was described in 1998[23] and was expanded to a larger population of pediatric patients in 2015.[24] Using this algorithm, successful management of Monteggia fractures without subsequent loss of reduction of either the ulna or radiocapitellar joint at follow-up was reported.[23,24]

The treatment algorithm is directed by the ulna fracture pattern. In patients with plastic deformation or a greenstick fracture of the ulna, closed reduction with cast immobilization is recommended. For a complete fracture of the ulna that is length-stable (transverse or short oblique), intramedullary pin fixation of the ulna is recommended (**Figure 2**). In a complete fracture of the ulna that is length unstable (long oblique or comminuted), open reduction with plate fixation is recommended. Complete fractures of the ulna, regardless of the fracture pattern, are at risk of failure in the form of loss of reduction of the ulna fracture and subsequent radial head subluxation or dislocation if surgical stabilization of the ulnar fracture is not undertaken initially.[23,24] It is rare for soft-tissue interposition to prevent reduction of the radial head dislocation after anatomic reduction of an ulnar shaft fracture. However, open reduction of the radiocapitellar joint is indicated in the setting of an irreducible radial head dislocation.

Complications associated with Monteggia fracture-dislocations in the pediatric population include loss of reduction; persistent pain; decreased motion; nonunion; compartment syndrome; and nerve palsies, which are usually transient. Loss of reduction can usually be prevented by treating complete fractures of the ulna with surgical stabilization, regardless of the amount of

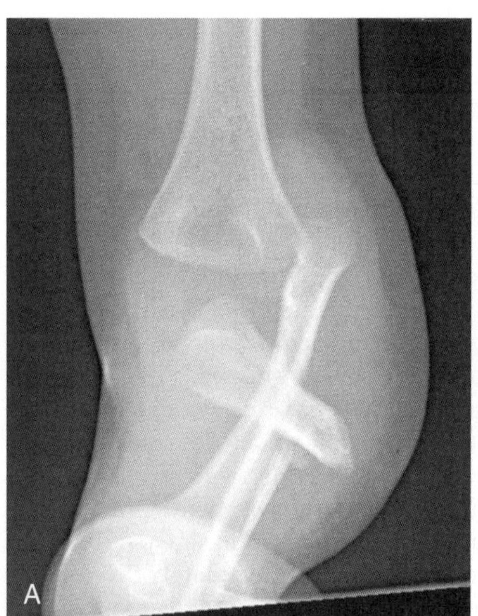

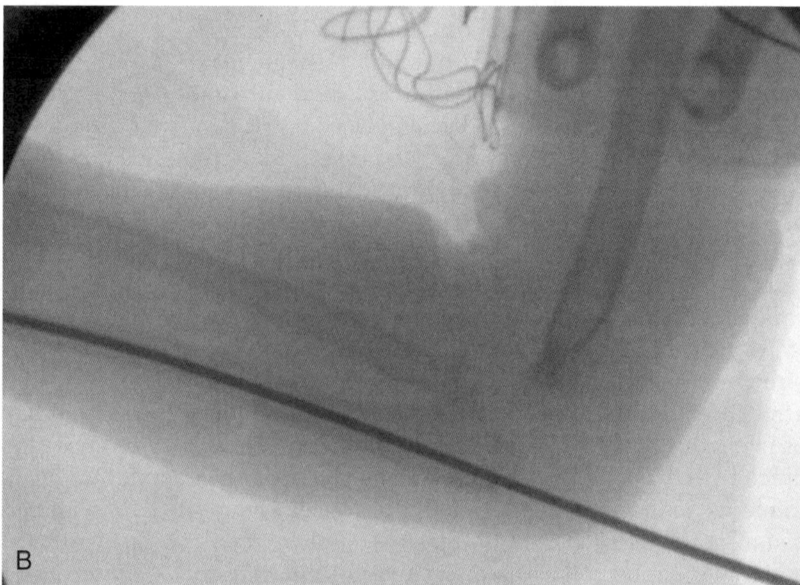

FIGURE 2 **A**, AP radiograph of the elbow of an 8-year-old girl with a Monteggia fracture-dislocation sustained in a fall from a bicycle. **B**, Intraoperative fluoroscopic lateral view of the elbow shows the reduction of the Monteggia fracture-dislocation and stabilization of the short oblique ulna fracture using intramedullary fixation. (Courtesy of Theresa O. Wyrick, MD.)

displacement. Close radiographic follow-up of patients with complete ulna fractures treated with closed reduction and cast immobilization is recommended, with early surgical intervention, including ulnar stabilization, if loss of anatomic radiocapitellar alignment is observed.[23,24]

Chronic Monteggia fracture-dislocations are occasionally seen in children and may result from a failure to recognize the initial radial head dislocation or subsequent loss of reduction during treatment. Initially, children often adapt well to a dislocated radial head, which usually causes little pain or functional deficit. However, over time, the radiocapitellar dislocation can cause valgus elbow instability, cubitus valgus, loss of motion, and pain.

Multiple techniques for corrective osteotomy of the ulna with subsequent closed or open reduction of the radiocapitellar joint have been described in the literature; results of these techniques have varied.[23] Soft-tissue reconstruction of the annular ligament also has been described using various methods. The age of the patient, the existing deformity of the radial head, and the length of time since the injury are all considerations when determining whether surgical management of a chronic Monteggia fracture-dislocation will be beneficial. Preferably, surgical management of this lesion should be undertaken within 1 year of the original injury for the best outcome. If little potential for remodeling exists and the radial head is radiographically deformed, the results of surgical treatment are less predictable.[23] No consensus exists on whether soft-tissue reconstruction of the annular ligament is warranted. In pediatric patients, overcorrection of an ulnar shaft deformity should be undertaken because of the extensive remodeling that occurs at the fracture site after the original injury. Fixation has been performed with various methods, including plate fixation, uniplane external fixation, intramedullary wire fixation, and ringed fixators; results have varied. Clearly, it is best to prevent the need for delayed treatment of this injury by pursuing diligent radiographic follow-up of the patient in the acute setting.

GALEAZZI FRACTURE-DISLOCATIONS

A fracture of the shaft of the radius with an associated dislocation of the distal radioulnar joint is known as a Galeazzi fracture. This type of fracture was first described in 1934 by Riccardo Galeazzi of Milan.[25] It has also been called a reverse Monteggia fracture or a fracture of necessity. Galeazzi fractures are typically the result of a fall onto an outstretched arm. Good results are seen with nonsurgical treatment in children and adolescents after closed reduction and cast immobilization. In adults, open rigid internal fixation is necessary for the management of a Galeazzi fracture.[26]

The incidence of this relatively uncommon fracture-dislocation in children is reported to be between 0.3% and 2.8%, and it most commonly occurs in children between the ages of 9 and 13 years. A Galeazzi fracture must be considered with any isolated fracture of the radius and is more common in radius fractures at the junction of the middle and distal thirds of the diaphysis. Usually, the distal ulna is dislocated dorsally. Examination of the distal radioulnar joint should be performed after closed reduction of the radial shaft fracture to assess for instability when an anatomic reduction of the radius is achieved. If the radius or distal radioulnar joint is irreducible, soft-tissue interposition is likely, and an open approach to either the radius fracture, the distal radioulnar joint, or both is necessary to obtain an adequate reduction. Immobilization above the elbow is recommended after an anatomic reduction is achieved. Close follow-up is warranted to evaluate for loss of reduction of the radius and subsequent subluxation or dislocation at the distal radioulnar joint. If closed reduction of the radius fracture and/or the distal radioulnar joint is not successful, then an open reduction of the fracture and/or the distal radioulnar joint is indicated. Periodic radiographic assessments are recommended over the first 3 weeks after reduction to monitor for possible redisplacement. Fortunately, long-term instability of the distal radioulnar joint is not typical in pediatric patients with this injury pattern.[27]

DISTAL BOTH-BONE FOREARM FRACTURES AND DISTAL RADIUS FRACTURES

Distal radius fractures are common in the pediatric population and include metaphyseal and physeal injuries. Most wrist fractures result from a fall onto an outstretched hand. A study evaluating the epidemiology of pediatric wrist fractures found that the mean age of patients was 10.9 years, with approximately two-thirds of the fractures occurring in boys.[28] The top five activities associated with these fractures were bicycling, football, playground activities, basketball, and soccer. Subgroup classifications showed that in patients from birth to 12 months of age, wrist fractures were most commonly associated with beds, whereas in children aged 13 to 36 months, the fractures were most commonly associated with stairs, and in children aged 11 to 17 years, wrist fractures were associated with playing football.[28]

An increase in the incidence of pediatric distal radius fractures may also be associated with patient factors such as bone density, increased body mass index, participation in more intense or higher risk activities, and younger ages of participation in these activities. Multiple treatment options exist and many factors must be considered, including physeal involvement, articular displacement, remodeling potential, the risk of growth arrest, patient factors, and family expectations.[29] However, it is important to note that there is substantial variation among pediatric orthopaedic surgeons regarding the diagnosis and management of pediatric distal radius fractures.[30]

A metaphyseal torus fracture of the distal radius is an incomplete or buckle fracture sustained as the result of an axial compression injury. Torus fractures do not require rigid immobilization or extended clinical follow-up and are expected to heal uneventfully within 3 weeks of injury. A removable splint provides sufficient immobilization. Splint removal at home 3 weeks after injury is acceptable and actually preferred by most families.[29,31] Similarly, minimally displaced and angulated metaphyseal fractures of the distal radius will typically remodel because of continued skeletal growth and the close proximity to the distal radial physis. Generally accepted radiographic parameters for this fracture pattern include 20° to 30° of sagittal plane angulation because sufficient remodeling will be possible.

Displaced fractures needing reduction require more discussion and consideration in decision making. An initial closed reduction is recommended for displaced fractures that are not expected to sufficiently remodel based on established parameters. Factors to consider include patient age, skeletal immaturity, remaining growth, fracture pattern, and the presence of associated injuries. Closed reduction is most commonly performed with the patient sedated; however, this can lead to long times in the emergency department and high costs. One study comparing reductions performed under sedation versus reductions performed with only hematoma blocks found that there were no important differences in radiographic alignment, patient satisfaction, and pain control.[32] However, the use of a hematoma block alone substantially reduced the time spent in the emergency department (average, 2.2 fewer hours) as well as the resources required to perform the reduction.[32]

Displaced intra-articular fractures are rare in skeletally immature patients. Because these fractures will not remodel, surgical treatment is recommended. Other indications for surgical treatment include open fractures, displaced floating elbow injuries, irreducible fractures, and the skeletally maturing adolescent with limited remodeling potential. Additionally, volar Barton fractures can be managed successfully using a buttress plate.[33]

At the initial closed reduction procedure, either a cast or a splint can be used and both short-arm and long-arm immobilization are acceptable. Patients and families generally prefer short-arm immobilization. Careful attention to immobilization technique, whether a splint or cast is used, is important to prevent loss of reduction. It is essential to use a high-quality mold, as measured by the cast index and three-point index. Close radiographic follow-up is recommended, with weekly radiographic studies for the first 2 to 3 weeks after the reduction.[29]

Physeal arrest is a known sequela of distal radius fractures, with reported rates between 1% and 7%. Because of the increased risk of posttraumatic physeal arrest in the distal radius following late manipulations of displaced physeal fractures in pediatric patients, it is recommended that manipulations not be performed more than 10 days after the initial injury.[34] Because treatment of a subsequent malunion may be required if sufficient remodeling does not occur, the family should be informed of this possibility.

Multiple studies have shown that there is a substantial risk of pin site complications with the acute use of pin stabilization of displaced distal radius fractures to prevent loss of reduction. Outcomes in patients treated with reduction and pinning compared with those treated with reduction and cast immobilization are equivalent. Therefore, pinning of all displaced distal radius fractures is not indicated.[29]

Substantial treatment variability exists among practitioners managing distal radius fractures in the pediatric population.[30,35] A study of hand, pediatric, and general orthopaedic surgeons reported that hand surgeons and general orthopaedic surgeons were 2.9 and 1.6 times more likely, respectively, than pediatric orthopaedic surgeons to treat the same distal radius fracture surgically. In addition, orthopaedic surgeons in private practice were 1.5 times more likely to recommend surgery than surgeons with academic affiliations. This variation in treatment choices indicates that surgeons managing distal radius fractures in the pediatric population have varying criteria for acceptable alignment. Further investigation of the optimal treatment of these fractures is warranted.[35]

SCAPHOID FRACTURES

Scaphoid fractures are relatively uncommon in children and adolescents; however, the incidence has increased as older children and adolescents are engaging in more intense sports participation and extreme sports.[36-38] Scaphoid fractures most commonly result from injuries sustained during participation in sports such as football, basketball, snowboarding, and skateboarding.[39]

Historically, scaphoid fractures were thought to more commonly involve the distal pole; however, recent studies have questioned the accuracy of this assumption. A retrospective analysis of 351 fractures seen over a 15-year period found that 71% of fractures occurred at the scaphoid waist, 23% at the distal pole, and 6% at the proximal pole.[39] In contrast, a smaller study that assessed 56 confirmed scaphoid fractures found that the most common fracture location was the distal pole (80%).[36] Both studies demonstrated that scaphoid fractures are more common in males. High-energy mechanisms, closed physes, and a high body mass index are associated with fractures of the scaphoid waist or proximal pole.[39]

Patients with a potential scaphoid fracture should be assessed with a thorough physical examination; the presence of tenderness to palpation in the snuffbox should be noted. Plain radiographs, including PA, lateral, and scaphoid views, are the mainstay of diagnostic imaging; however, ultrasonography can also identify an acute scaphoid fracture, even if it is not visualized on plain radiographs.[40] An MRI can be helpful in diagnosing an occult scaphoid fracture in the setting of normal plain radiographs. A CT scan can be helpful in determining the amount of displacement at the fracture site in subtle fractures in which the decision as to whether to proceed with nonsurgical or surgical treatment is unclear based on plain radiographs. It is important to assess for associated injuries, which can be present in up to 10% of scaphoid fractures, including distal radius fractures, transscaphoid perilunate dislocations, ulnar styloid fractures, capitate fractures, and bilateral scaphoid fractures.[39]

Cast immobilization is the mainstay of management of pediatric and adolescent scaphoid fractures with healing present in more than 90% of acute fractures.[39] Lower union rates are more likely in more proximal fractures, displaced fractures, and late-presenting fractures. In younger children who present acutely, union may occur as early as 4 to 6 weeks after injury, whereas longer times to union are more likely in older children and adolescents, older fractures, displaced fractures, more proximal fractures, and fractures in patients with osteonecrosis.[39] A CT scan is the most accurate and reliable way to assess for scaphoid fracture union. If a fracture does not unite with immobilization alone or in the case of displaced fractures or fractures with delayed presentation in which surgical treatment is indicated, surgical fixation is still likely to be successful. One study reported a 96.5% union rate seen in pediatric patients who underwent surgical fixation of scaphoid fractures for a variety of reasons.[39]

Surgical fixation is warranted for acute displaced fractures (>1 mm), open fractures, and fractures with associated injuries such as transscaphoid perilunate fracture dislocations and displaced distal radius fractures requiring surgical treatment. Greater times to union after surgical intervention are associated with open physes, fracture displacement, more proximal fractures, the type of screw used for fixation, and bone grafting at the time of surgery.[39]

Complications after nonsurgical and surgical management of pediatric and adolescent scaphoid fractures are relatively rare. However, late presentation of chronic fractures with nonunion is more common in this population. In one study, the use of immobilization only achieved union in 18 of 90 patients (20%) with chronic fractures.[39] Successful management of scaphoid nonunions occurs in 95% of patients.[41,42] A recent meta-analysis found a 95.6% union rate occurred when no bone graft was used, and a 94.7% union rate was present when bone graft was used. Avoidance of bone graft may avoid pain associated with obtaining the graft, decrease surgical time, and potentially have less complications.[42] These findings suggest that chronic scaphoid nonunions are optimally treated with surgical intervention.

HAND FRACTURES

Pediatric hand fractures are extremely common, with finger fractures representing the second most common pediatric fracture seen in emergency departments in the United States.[1] Most of these fractures can be managed nonsurgically with splint or cast immobilization followed by early active range of motion. Some fractures, including displaced fractures with malrotation or angulation, open fractures, displaced phalangeal neck fractures, and Seymour fractures, are best managed surgically[43-45] (**Figure 3**). The outcomes after surgical management of displaced pediatric proximal phalanx fractures are typically excellent, with no pain, full function, and perfect esthetics. However, 5% of patients have complications, including infection, pin site complications, and malunions. Approximately 30% of patients have stiffness and ultimately require a course of therapy to regain motion.[43]

Pediatric phalangeal neck or subchondral fractures deserve special mention because these fractures are often displaced and relatively unstable and require surgical treatment. One can optimally assess these fractures by understanding the ossification of the phalangeal condyles. As a child's age increases above 9 years, the volar phalangeal line will intersect the middle third of the phalangeal condyles, analogous to the anterior humeral line intersecting the capitellum. In children younger than 8 years, the volar phalangeal line commonly intersects the anterior third of the phalangeal condyles because of their eccentric ossification.[46]

A stepwise algorithm has been recommended to successfully manage pediatric phalangeal neck fractures.[45] The algorithm begins with an attempt at closed reduction. If this is successful, percutaneous pinning is performed. If closed reduction is not successful, a percutaneous reduction is recommended using a temporary intrafocal pin as a joystick for reduction and osteoclasis as needed. If these maneuvers fail, then open reduction with percutaneous pinning should be performed. Using this algorithm, the authors of a 2014 study reported that 80% of the fractures were treated with closed reduction and percutaneous pinning, and the remaining 20% were treated with percutaneous reduction and percutaneous pinning. In all of the fractures that were treated more

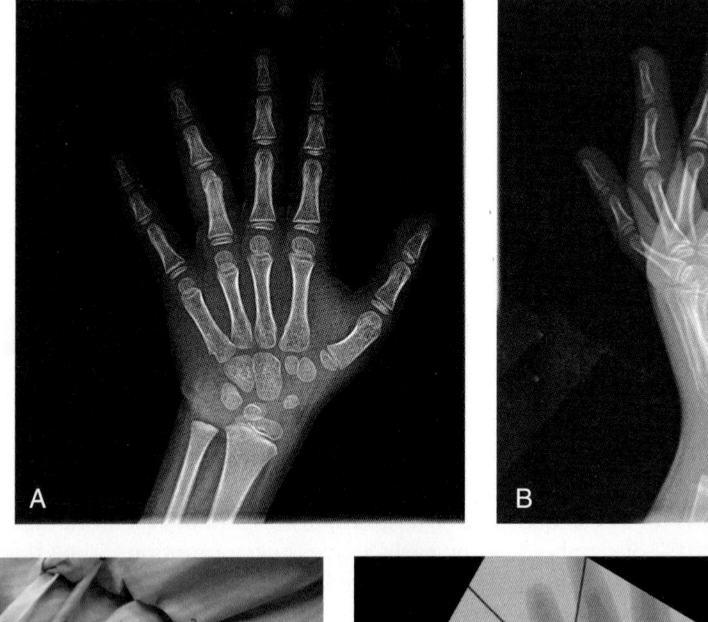

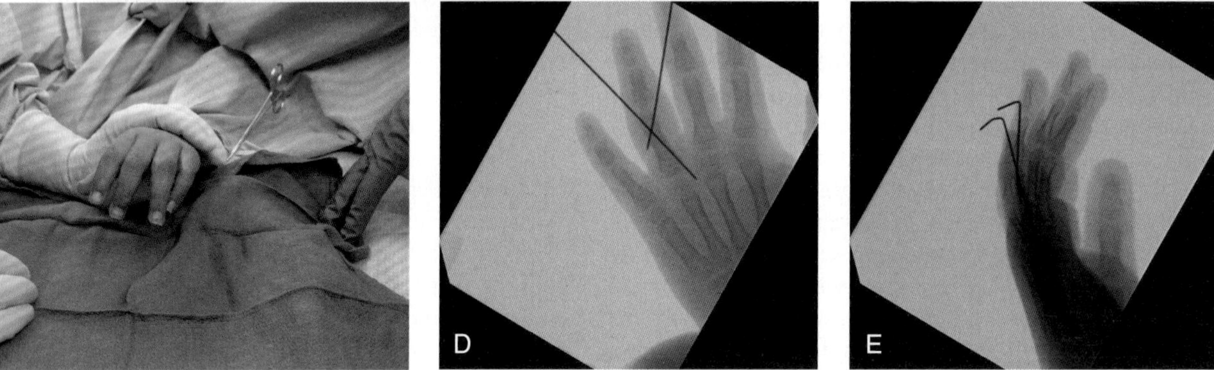

FIGURE 3 PA (**A**) and lateral (**B**) radiographs of a proximal phalanx phalangeal neck/subchondral fracture of the left ring finger of a 5-year-old boy sustained after his finger was caught in a door. Note the relatively benign appearance of the fracture. **C**, Intraoperative photograph shows the substantial deviation caused by the fracture. Intraoperative PA (**D**) and lateral (**E**) fluoroscopic images after closed reduction and percutaneous pinning of the fracture. (Courtesy of Joshua M. Abzug, MD.)

than 2 weeks after injury, percutaneous reduction and percutaneous pinning were required. Good or excellent outcomes were reported in 90% of the patients. Among those with fair or poor outcomes, four patients had complications, which included two patients with a flexion contracture, one patient with nonunion after a pin tract infection, and one patient with osteonecrosis after a crush injury.[45] A 2015 study that evaluated complications after surgical treatment of displaced proximal phalanx fractures reported that subcondylar fractures were associated with a greater likelihood of stiffness, angular deformity, and worse aesthetic outcomes.[43] In addition, a study assessing the sequelae of pediatric phalangeal fractures found that subcondylar fractures were associated with decreased range of motion, malunion, and osteonecrosis.[47]

Mallet fractures are avulsion fractures that occur at the insertion of the extensor tendon, which is on the epiphysis of a skeletally immature individual. Most of these fractures can be managed with splint immobilization with or without an overlying cast. Surgical intervention for pediatric and adolescent mallet fractures is typically reserved for those patients who have subluxation of the distal interphalangeal joint and/or large (>50%) bony fragments. One study compared percutaneous reduction and pin fixation in acute and chronic pediatric mallet fractures and noted that overall the outcomes were excellent in 84% of patients. The results were somewhat less optimal in patients who had chronic fractures, with 77% of patients having an excellent outcome and 23% having a good outcome. However, there were no reports of pain in any patients, and all patients were able to return to full activity.[48]

Seymour fractures were originally described in 1966 as juxta-epiphyseal fractures of the terminal phalanx in a child or adolescent.[49] The proximity of the fracture to the nail bed will result in a nail bed injury and an open fracture if the fracture is displaced. The lacerated germinal matrix will frequently become entrapped in the fracture site, preventing a complete reduction.[44,50] Timely recognition and appropriate management of Seymour fractures is crucial to obtain the best results and avoid complications. Appropriate treatment for these displaced fractures includes nail plate removal, irrigation and débridement, fracture reduction, and antibiotic administration. These injuries should be ideally treated within 24 hours of the time of injury.[51,52] Delayed or incomplete treatment will yield a higher acute and chronic infection rate.

SUMMARY

Pediatric forearm, wrist, and hand trauma is extremely common. Most fractures can be managed nonsurgically with immobilization. When fracture alignment is unacceptable, closed reduction and casting performed using appropriate technique can achieve successful outcomes. Surgical intervention, when needed, typically achieves excellent outcomes with a low complication rate.

KEY STUDY POINTS

- The casting technique plays an important role in the successful closed management of pediatric forearm fractures.
- Early recognition and treatment of Monteggia fracture-dislocations yields excellent outcomes, whereas a missed diagnosis may lead to permanent pain, instability, and decreased range of motion.
- Acute scaphoid fractures in children and adolescents can be successfully treated with immobilization alone in 90% of patients.
- Pediatric phalangeal neck and subchondral fractures are best managed surgically; however, even with optimal treatment, these fractures are more likely to have a poor outcome compared with other pediatric phalangeal fractures.

ANNOTATED REFERENCES

1. Naranje SM, Erali RA, Warner WC Jr, Sawyer JR, Kelly DM: Epidemiology of pediatric fractures presenting to emergency departments in the United States. *J Pediatr Orthop* 2016;36(4):e45-e48.

   This study is a National Electronic Injury Surveillance System database study that identified the annual occurrence of fractures in 2010. The annual occurrence rate for the pediatric population was 9.47 per 1000 children. Forearm fractures were the most common followed by finger and wrist fractures being second and third, respectively. Children between 10 and 14 years of age had the highest risk of having fractures. Level of evidence: III.

2. Sumko MJ, Hennrikus W, Slough J, et al: Measurement of radiation exposure when using the mini C-arm to reduce pediatric upper extremity fractures. *J Pediatr Orthop* 2016;36(2):122-125.

   This prospective study assessed the total amount of radiation exposure when performing a pediatric forearm fracture reduction. Eighty-six patients were included in the study. The authors noted that the amount of radiation exposure was affected by the resident using the mini C-arm and the fracture pattern. The amount of radiation from the mini C-arm exceeded the amount of radiation from conventional radiographs. Furthermore, PGY2 residents had a higher amount of radiation exposure per reduction compared with PGY3 residents. Level of evidence: III.

3. Abzug JM, Shwartz BS, Johnson AJ: Assessment of splints applied for pediatric fractures in an emergency department/urgent care environment. *J Pediatr Orthop* 2019;39(2):76-84.

   An evaluation of the adequacy of all splints applied in the emergency department/urgent care environment as well as the prevalence and type of complications that occurred with inadequate splints was performed. In the evaluation of 275 patients who presented to the pediatric orthopaedic clinic after being splinted at an outside emergency department or urgent care center, 93% (256/275) were found to have improperly placed splints. Level of evidence: II.

4. Bae DS: Pediatric distal radius and forearm fractures. *J Hand Surg Am* 2008;33(10):1911-1923.

5. Noonan KJ, Price CT: Forearm and distal radius fractures in children. *J Am Acad Orthop Surg* 1998;6(3):146-156.

6. Pearce SS, Honeycutt MW, Cutchen WA, Tillman MD, Nimityongskul P: Friberg equation to predict pediatric distal forearm fracture remodeling. *J Pediatr Orthop* 2019;39(6):e441-e446.

   The Friberg equation, $V_t = V_0[e^{(-\beta t)}]$ was found to accurately predict remodeling of distal radius forearm fractures. The mean predicted angles were similar to the measured angles present in the radioulnar plane and the measured angles were only 2° greater than the measured angles found in the dorsovolar plane. This equation can reliably be used to limit unnecessary reduction procedures. Level of evidence: II.

7. Zlotolow DA: Pediatric forearm fractures: Spotting and managing the bad actors. *J Hand Surg Am* 2012;37(2):363-366, quiz 366.

8. Bowman EN, Mehlman CT, Lindsell CJ, Tamai J: Nonoperative treatment of both-bone forearm shaft fractures in children: Predictors of early radiographic failure. *J Pediatr Orthop* 2011;31(1):23-32.

9. Dittmer AJ, Molina D IV, Jacobs CA, Walker J, Muchow RD: Pediatric forearm fractures are effectively immobilized with a sugar-tong splint following closed reduction. *J Pediatr Orthop* 2019;39(4):e245-e247.

   This study assessed the utilization of a sugar-tong splint after patients underwent a closed reduction of their forearm fractures by an orthopaedic surgery resident (either PGY2 or PGY3). The study found that, of the 168 patients, 38% (64/168) of those who underwent closed reduction demonstrated radiographic loss of reduction with 90% of the lost reductions occurring within the first 2 weeks after the reduction. The study also determined that using a sugar-tong splint had a rate of lost reduction similar to that reported for casting of fractures. The authors concluded that sugar-tong splinting was an effective method of immobilization for pediatric forearm fractures (distal, midshaft, and proximal). Level of evidence: IV.

10. Wellsh BM, Kuzma JM: Ultrasound-guided pediatric forearm fracture reductions in a resource-limited ED. *Am J Emerg Med* 2016;34(1):40-44.

    This prospective nonrandomized study evaluated 47 consecutive patients with pediatric forearm fractures using ultrasound to assess the adequacy of the reduction. The authors reported that 94% of patients were able to undergo a successful reduction. Based on these data, the authors were able to conclude that the use of ultrasound-guided closed reduction procedures for pediatric forearm fractures is safe and efficacious. Level of evidence: III.

11. Goodman AD, Zonfrillo MR, Chiou D, Eberson CP, Cruz AI Jr: The cost and utility of postreduction radiographs after closed reduction of pediatric wrist and forearm fractures. *J Pediatr Orthop* 2019;39(1):e8-e11.

    This study evaluated the cost and utility of postreduction radiographs after closed reduction of pediatric wrist and forearm fractures. Of the 119 patients in the study, none of the patients required rereduction following the formal postreduction radiograph. The study found that, although radiographs are needed to assess the adequacy of a reduction, formal postreduction radiographs did not change the management of a fracture and consumed 7.3% of the encounter time and cost. Therefore, the fluoroscopic images obtained during the reduction should be noted to be adequate in most circumstances, and formal plain radiographs should not be obtained in the immediate postreduction period. Level of evidence: IV.

12. Ting BL, Kalish LA, Waters PM, Bae DS: Reducing cost and radiation exposure during the treatment of pediatric greenstick fractures of the forearm. *J Pediatr Orthop* 2016;36(8):816-820.

    This study was a retrospective analysis of children treated with closed reduction and cast immobilization for greenstick fractures. The authors identified 109 patients, of which 94% maintained acceptable radiographic alignment. Only one patient underwent a rereduction. The authors also noted that if clinical follow-up was limited to visits and three sets of radiographs total, there would be an approximately 15% reduction in the total fracture care cost and an approximately 40% reduction in radiation exposure. Level of evidence: IV.

13. Kutsikovich JI, Hopkins CM, Cannon EW III, et al: Factors that predict instability in pediatric diaphyseal both-bone forearm fractures. *J Pediatr Orthop B* 2018;27(4):304-308.

    This study evaluated what variables (time course, demographic, and radiographic data) predicted loss of reduction and need for further intervention in pediatric diaphyseal both-bone forearm fractures. Of the 174 patients, 19 required a repeat procedure. The study found that lengthy reduction times (>35 minutes), degree of translation (>50% in any plane), and increasing age (>9 years) were all predictive factors for a repeat intervention after a closed reduction. Level of evidence: IV.

14. McQuinn AG, Jaarsma RL: Risk factors for redisplacement of pediatric distal forearm and distal radius fractures. *J Pediatr Orthop* 2012;32(7):687-692.

15. Schreck MJ, Hammert WC: Comparison of above- and below-elbow casting for pediatric distal metaphyseal forearm fractures. *J Hand Surg Am* 2014;39(2):347-349.

16. Auer RT, Mazzone P, Robinson L, Nyland J, Chan G: Childhood obesity increases the risk of failure in the treatment of distal forearm fractures. *J Pediatr Orthop* 2016;36(8):e86-e88.

    This retrospective study assessed 157 patients with consecutive distal radius fractures following a closed reduction in the emergency department or operating room. The study noted that obese children needed more visits requiring radiographs and were less likely to have an initial perfect reduction in the emergency room. The authors concluded that obesity results in higher rates of malreduction and subsequent manipulations. Level of evidence: III.

17. Tisosky AJ, Werger MM, McPartland TG, Bowe JA: The factors influencing refracture of pediatric forearms. *J Pediatr Orthop* 2015;35(7):677-681.

18. Flynn JM, Jones KJ, Garner MR, Goebel J: Eleven years experience in the operative management of pediatric forearm fractures. *J Pediatr Orthop* 2010;30(4):313-319.

19. Martus JE, Preston RK, Schoenecker JG, Lovejoy SA, Green NE, Mencio GA: Complications and outcomes of diaphyseal forearm fracture intramedullary nailing: A comparison of pediatric and adolescent age groups. *J Pediatr Orthop* 2013;33(6):598-607.

20. Lee AK, Beck JD, Mirenda WM, Klena JC: Incidence and risk factors for extensor pollicis longus rupture in elastic stable intramedullary nailing of pediatric forearm shaft fractures. *J Pediatr Orthop* 2016;36(8):810-815.

    This retrospective review identified patients who sustained an extensor pollicis longus rupture after fixation of a pediatric radial shaft fracture using an intramedullary nail. In this series, 3 patients of 17 in the cohort (18%) sustained EPL ruptures. No risk factors were identified. Level of evidence: IV.

21. Murphy HA, Jain VV, Parikh SN, Wall EJ, Cornwall R, Mehlman CT: Extensor tendon injury associated with dorsal entry flexible nailing of radial shaft fractures in children: A report of 5 new cases and review of the literature. *J Pediatr Orthop* 2019;39(4):163-168.

    The study evaluated the risks of EPL tendon injury following elastic stable intramedullary nailing of the radius when using the dorsal entry approach. For those with EPL tendon rupture or EPL tendon injury, treatment with EIP to EPL tendon transfer, tendon release/lysis of adhesions, EPL repair, or EPL graft reconstruction using the palmaris longus tendon resulted in near-anatomic extension at the thumb interphalangeal joint, no pain, and no further complications at the 12-month follow-up visit. The study suggests that a lateral approach be used to avoid EPL tendon injury as well as using a suggested technique involving K-wires for intramedullary fixation. Level of evidence: III.

22. Nøgaard SL, Riber SS, Danielsson FB, Pedersen NW, Viberg B: Surgical approach for elastic stable intramedullary nail in pediatric radius shaft fractures: A systematic review. *J Pediatr Orthop B* 2018;27(4):309-314.

This systematic review looked at the risks, complications, and outcomes associated with a dorsal versus lateral approach when placing an elastic stable intramedullary nail in pediatric radial shaft fractures. The review found that the dorsal approach had a major complication rate of 8.9%, with EPL tendon rupture being most prominent. The lateral approach was associated with risk to the superficial branch of the radial nerve and had a 5.6% major complication rate. The review suggests that with a large enough incision, the superficial branch of the radial nerve can be identified and protected during nail insertion from the lateral approach without the risk of EPL injury found when using the dorsal approach. Level of evidence: III.

23. Ring D, Jupiter JB, Waters PM: Monteggia fractures in children and adults. *J Am Acad Orthop Surg* 1998;6(4):215-224.

24. Ramski DE, Hennrikus WP, Bae DS, et al: Pediatric Monteggia fractures: A multicenter examination of treatment strategy and early clinical and radiographic results. *J Pediatr Orthop* 2015;35(2):115-120.

25. Sebastin SJ, Chung KC: A historical report on Riccardo Galeazzi and the management of Galeazzi fractures. *J Hand Surg Am* 2010;35(11):1870-1877.

26. Rettig ME, Raskin KB: Galeazzi fracture-dislocation: A new treatment-oriented classification. *J Hand Surg Am* 2001;26(2):228-235.

27. Eberl R, Singer G, Schalamon J, Petnehazy T, Hoellwarth ME: Galeazzi lesions in children and adolescents: Treatment and outcome. *Clin Orthop Relat Res* 2008;466(7):1705-1709.

28. Shah NS, Buzas D, Zinberg EM: Epidemiologic dynamics contributing to pediatric wrist fractures in the United States. *Hand (NY)* 2015;10(2):266-271.

29. Bae DS, Howard AW: Distal radius fractures: What is the evidence? *J Pediatr Orthop* 2012;32(2 suppl 2):S128-S130.

30. Dua K, Stein MK, O'Hara NN, et al: Variation among pediatric orthopaedic surgeons when diagnosing and treating pediatric and adolescent distal radius fractures. *J Pediatr Orthop* 2019;39(6):306-313.

This study evaluated diagnoses and treatment of distal radius fractures in the pediatric and adolescent populations. The study found that the greatest level of agreement was when diagnosing fractures. Most providers chose either long-arm splinting or short-arm casting as the form of immobilization, but there was poor agreement in the duration of immobilization. The study demonstrates that classification schemes (Salter-Harris classification, torus/buckle fractures, greenstick fracture, and extraphyseal fractures) used in the description of distal radius fractures in the pediatric and adolescent populations are subjective during radiographic interpretation. A more standardized management plan for pediatric distal radius fractures could lead to reduced patient morbidity, less radiation exposure, and lower patient healthcare costs. Level of evidence: II.

31. Kuba MHM, Izuka BH: One brace: One visit. Treatment of pediatric distal radius buckle fractures with a removable wrist brace and no follow-up visit. *J Pediatr Orthop* 2018;38(6):e338-e342.

The study evaluated the use of a removable brace and no follow-up visit or imaging when managing pediatric distal radius buckle fractures. The study of 41 wrists in 40 patients found that there were no complications noted in the 5- to 10-month period between the initial treatment and the second follow-up phone survey. This treatment approach allows for decreased patient radiation exposure from routine follow-up radiographs, lowers the out-of-pocket cost for families and the overall cost of health care for society, and allows for greater access to care for other patients in need of care because there is no need for a follow-up appointment from the distal radius buckle fracture patients. Level of evidence: IV.

32. Bear DM, Friel NA, Lupo CL, Pitetti R, Ward WT: Hematoma block versus sedation for the reduction of distal radius fractures in children. *J Hand Surg Am* 2015;40(1):57-61.

33. Cha SM, Shin HD: Buttress plating for volar Barton fractures in children: Salter-Harris II distal radius fractures in sagittal plane. *J Pediatr Orthop B* 2019;28(1):73-78.

This study evaluated the use of buttress plating in volar Barton fractures in the pediatric population. The study retrospectively evaluated 13 patients and found that the only statistically significant difference was in the flexion-extension movement arc during the range of motion assessment. Overall, the study found that buttress plating can be a useful treatment for volar Barton type injuries involving the physis in the pediatric population. Level of evidence: IV.

34. Abzug JM, Little K, Kozin SH: Physeal arrest of the distal radius. *J Am Acad Orthop Surg* 2014;22(6):381-389.

35. Bernthal NM, Mitchell S, Bales JG, Benhaim P, Silva M: Variation in practice habits in the treatment of pediatric distal radius fractures. *J Pediatr Orthop B* 2015;24(5):400-407.

36. Ahmed I, Ashton F, Tay WK, Porter D: The pediatric fracture of the scaphoid in patients aged 13 years and under: An epidemiological study. *J Pediatr Orthop* 2014;34(2):150-154.

37. Hayes JR, Groner JI: The increasing incidence of snowboard-related trauma. *J Pediatr Surg* 2008;43(5):928-930.

38. Larson AN, Stans AA, Shaughnessy WJ, Dekutoski MB, Quinn MJ, McIntosh AL: Motocross morbidity: Economic cost and injury distribution in children. *J Pediatr Orthop* 2009;29(8):847-850.

39. Gholson JJ, Bae DS, Zurakowski D, Waters PM: Scaphoid fractures in children and adolescents: Contemporary injury patterns and factors influencing time to union. *J Bone Joint Surg Am* 2011;93(13):1210-1219.

40. Tessaro MO, McGovern TR, Dickman E, Haines LE: Point-of-care ultrasound detection of acute scaphoid fracture. *Pediatr Emerg Care* 2015;31(3):222-224.

41. Masquijo JJ, Willis BR: Scaphoid nonunions in children and adolescents: Surgical treatment with bone grafting and internal fixation. *J Pediatr Orthop* 2010;30(2):119-124.

42. Jaurengui JJ, Seger EW, Hesham K, Walker SE, Abraham R, Abzug JM: Operative management for pediatric and adolescent scaphoid nonunions: A meta-analysis. *J Pediatr Orthop* 2019;39(2):e130-e133.

This meta-analysis evaluated surgical management for scaphoid nonunions in the pediatric and adolescent populations. It was found that only a small subset of scaphoid fractures develop a nonunion and that fractures of the proximal and distal poles as well as displaced fractures have a greater risk of nonunion. More than 4 weeks between the initial injury and immobilization was associated with a higher risk of nonunion. Overall, it was found that the various surgical techniques published resulted in excellent outcomes. However, the use of bone graft did not appear to be necessary and may lead to increased complications, longer surgical times, and pain at the donor site. Level of evidence: III.

43. Boyer JS, London DA, Stepan JG, Goldfarb CA: Pediatric proximal phalanx fractures: Outcomes and complications after the surgical treatment of displaced fractures. *J Pediatr Orthop* 2015;35(3):219-223.

44. Abzug JM, Kozin SH: Seymour fractures. *J Hand Surg Am* 2013;38(11):2267-2270, quiz 2270.

45. Matzon JL, Cornwall R: A stepwise algorithm for surgical treatment of type II displaced pediatric phalangeal neck fractures. *J Hand Surg Am* 2014;39(3):467-473.

46. Dua K, O'Hara NN, Shusterman I, Abzug JM: Ossification of the proximal and middle phalangeal condyles: Radiographic aid in phalangeal neck fracture reduction. *J Pediatr Orthop* 2019;39(3):e222-e226.

This study evaluated if radiographic landmarks can be used as reference tools for assessing phalangeal neck fracture alignment. The volar phalangeal line (VPL) can be used to evaluate the alignment following proximal and middle phalangeal neck fractures. It was found that the VPL and knowledge of ossification of the phalangeal condyles can help longitudinally monitor remodeling. The VPL should intersect the middle third of the phalangeal condyles above 9 years of age and commonly intersects the anterior third of the phalangeal condyles below 8 years of age. Level of evidence: III.

47. Huelsemann W, Singer G, Mann M, Winkler FJ, Habenicht R: Analysis of sequelae after pediatric phalangeal fractures. *Eur J Pediatr Surg* 2016;26(2):164-171.

This retrospective review assessed the complications associated with pediatric phalangeal fractures. Forty patients were identified to have complications following a phalangeal fracture. Thirteen of the 40 patients had complications following fractures involving the joint or surrounding bony structures. Ten patients had complications after sustaining a transcondylar or subcondylar fracture. Another 10 patients had complications because of extensive soft-tissue damage. The authors concluded that most sequelae of phalangeal fractures are consequences of the fracture itself as opposed to the treatment. Level of evidence: IV.

48. Reddy M, Ho CA: Comparison of percutaneous reduction and pin fixation in acute and chronic pediatric mallet fractures. *J Pediatr Orthop* 2019;39(3):146-152.

This study evaluated the use of percutaneous reduction and pin fixation to treat acute and chronic mallet fractures. Between the acute and chronic groups, the main differences were found in the time to surgical intervention, the initial articular gap, and the final articular gap. In each of these variables, the chronic mallet fracture group was found to have higher values. There was a clinically noticeable dorsal bump present in 18% of the acute group and 15% of the chronic group, but otherwise there were minimal complications reported. At the final follow-up, there were no reports of pain and all patients had returned to full activity. The study found that both the radiographic and clinical results of the percutaneous technique had better results in the pediatric population compared with the results published on surgical intervention for adult mallet fractures. Level of evidence: II.

49. Seymour N: Juxta-epiphyseal fracture of the terminal phalanx of the finger. *J Bone Joint Surg Br* 1966;48:347-349.

50. Banerjee A: Irreducible distal phalangeal epiphyseal injuries. *J Hand Surg Br* 1992;17:337-338.

51. Reyes BA, Ho CA: The high risk of infection with delayed treatment of open Seymour fractures: Salter-Harris I/II or juxta-epiphyseal fractures of the distal phalanx with associated nailbed laceration. *J Pediatr Orthop* 2017;37:247-253.

A total of 34 patients with 35 Seymour fractures were retrospectively studied: 31% received acute, appropriate treatment, and their infection rate was zero; 37% received acute, partial treatment, and their infection rate was 15%; 31% received delayed treatment, and their infection rate was 45%. The authors concluded that timing and quality of initial treatment significantly influences infection rates. Level of evidence: III.

52. Lin JS, Popp JE, Samora JB: Treatment of acute Seymour fractures. *J Pediatr Orthop* 2019;39:e23-e27.

A total of 65 Seymour fractures were retrospectively studied. Fifty-eight (89%) were initially managed in the emergency department (ED) with nail plate removal, irrigation and débridement, fracture reduction, and splinting under digital block. Seven cases were initially managed in the operating room (OR) with K-wire fixation. Of 58 cases managed in the ED 4 required a secondary procedure in the OR. Although 17% of these cases needed surgical intervention, most were managed in the ED setting successfully. Level of evidence: IV.

CHAPTER 43

Pelvis, Hip, and Femur Trauma

CAROLINE M. TOUGAS, MD • PABLO MARRERO BARRERA, MD
ANNA D. VERGUN, MD, FAAOS • JOSÉ A. HERRERA-SOTO, MD

ABSTRACT

Pelvis fractures are rare in younger patients but more common in adolescents. The mode of injury in older adolescents is similar to that of adults, and the management is similar. Hip fractures require urgent management and are at risk to develop osteonecrosis. The management of femur fractures depends on many factors including the age and weight of the patient, the fracture pattern, and the patient's level of skeletal maturity.

Keywords: apophysis; femur; fracture; hip; pelvis; trauma

Dr. Vergun or an immediate family member serves as a board member, owner, officer, or committee member of the Association of Children's Prosthetic and Orthotic Clinics. Dr. Herrera-Soto or an immediate family member has received royalties from Biomet; is a member of a speakers' bureau or has made paid presentations on behalf of Biomet and Biomet Spine; serves as a paid consultant to or is an employee of Biomet and Biomet Spine; and serves as a board member, owner, officer, or committee member of the Pediatric Orthopaedic Society of North America. Neither of the following authors nor any immediate family member has received anything of value from or has stock or stock options held in a commercial company or institution related directly or indirectly to the subject of this chapter: Dr. Tougas and Dr. Barrera.

INTRODUCTION

Fractures of the pelvis and acetabulum are infrequent but potentially debilitating injuries in children. Injuries that disrupt the pelvic ring are typically the result of high-energy trauma and can be associated with substantial morbidity and mortality. A comprehensive multidisciplinary approach to managing the concomitant injuries in these patients is warranted. A lack of pelvic remodeling can result in long-term sequelae such as leg-length discrepancy, scoliosis, gait abnormalities, sitting imbalance, chronic pain, and disability.

Acetabular fractures occur infrequently in skeletally immature patients but can be complicated by growth arrest of the triradiate cartilage (TRC) with development of posttraumatic dysplasia and/or arthritis. Hip dislocations generally occur because of sports injuries or motor vehicle accidents in adolescents and can be associated with acetabular fractures. Younger children can sustain hip dislocations after relatively minor trauma due to periarticular laxity. Urgent and gentle reduction is recommended to minimize the risk of iatrogenic epiphysiolysis and posttraumatic osteonecrosis.

Femoral neck fractures are relatively uncommon but are associated with a high complication rate. Femoral shaft fractures are the most common musculoskeletal injury resulting in hospital admission in the United States. The treatment is most frequently determined by the patient's age, weight, fracture pattern, and skeletal maturity.

This chapter is adapted from Hale G, Collins C, Herrera-Soto J: Pelvis, hip, femur, and knee, in Martus JE, ed: *Orthopaedic Knowledge Update®: Pediatrics*, ed 5. Rosemont, IL, American Academy of Orthopaedic Surgeons, 2016, pp 485-496.

PELVIC RING INJURIES

Pediatric Considerations

Relative pelvic skeletal maturity is best determined by fusion of the TRC as seen on radiographs.[1,2] Patency of the TRC can affect pelvic injury patterns and associated injuries.[1-5] Several key anatomic and physiologic differences exist between the mature and immature pelvis. The pediatric pelvis is more resistant to fracture than the adult pelvis because of its cartilaginous nature and greater capacity for energy absorption. Given the same mechanism of injury, it is estimated that an adult is two to seven times more likely to sustain a pelvic fracture than a child.[6,7] Furthermore, the plasticity and flexibility of the pediatric pelvis may allow for single disruptions of the pelvic ring, in contrast to the double-break phenomenon seen in adults. The relative ligamentous strength and joint elasticity in children render osseous structures (iliac wing or pubic rami), in general, more vulnerable to failure than ligamentous structures (pubic symphysis or sacroiliac joints).[1,6] Fracture displacement in children is also limited by their thick surrounding periosteum; this may explain the higher incidence of isolated pelvic fractures and lower incidence of unstable ring injuries in the skeletally immature.[2,4,5,8]

Although epiphyseal plates and apophyses provide additional flexibility to the pelvis, they are also vulnerable to injury. A 2017 study described differences in anterior ring failure patterns between skeletally immature and mature patients, most notably with regard to the presence of apophyseal avulsions in the skeletally immature.[9] A unique mechanism of posterior ring disruption in children has also been described, wherein sacroiliac joint failure occurred through the iliac wing apophysis rather than the posterior sacroiliac ligaments.[9,10] The presence of continuing growth and the associated vascularity that accompanies it permits healing and remodeling of these injuries. However, the degree of remodeling that occurs in the pelvis appears limited, and injury to the epiphyseal plates and apophyses can result in growth arrest and deformity.[9-11]

Because of its inherent resistance to injury, a great amount of force is required to disrupt the pediatric pelvic ring. The vast majority of these injuries are the result of high-energy trauma, particularly motor vehicle–related mechanisms.[4,12] Furthermore, young children are more often struck by motor vehicles, as opposed to adolescents and adults who are more likely to be motor vehicle occupants or operators.[2,5,13] Falls from a height are another common mechanism in children. These varying mechanisms of injury contribute to the difference in fracture patterns seen between the mature and immature pelvis.

Epidemiology

Pelvic ring injuries (PRIs) are rare in children, accounting for 1.6% to 7.0% of pediatric injuries.[14-16] When considering trauma-related admissions, the incidence of PRI increases toward 15%.[12] Regardless, the incidence of PRI in children is much lower than that in adults. A 2015 study reviewed the National Trauma Data Bank and calculated an incidence of four to five cases of PRI per 10,000 trauma admissions in the pediatric population. In contrast, the incidence in adults was 26 cases of PRI per 10,000 admissions.[17] Many recent studies have analyzed the epidemiology, demographics, and clinical characteristics of children with PRI.[2,4,5,8,12,17-21] Because of the heterogeneity of the methodologies and results, as well as the relative rarity of these injuries, it is difficult to summate their findings. It is possible to conclude that pelvic ring disruptions in children, which may appear less severe radiographically, are markers of high-energy injury, requiring the clinician to thoroughly investigate for associated injuries. Case in point: when compared with pediatric trauma patients without PRI, children with PRI have higher mortality rates, greater injury severity scores, longer intensive care unit stays, and greater transfusion requirements.[3]

Associated Injuries

Rates of associated injuries with PRI can exceed 80%.[2,15,22] Patients with PRI had on average 5.2 additional injuries involving multiple organ systems in one study,[23] and 50% of patients sustained injuries to two or more separate organ systems in another.[4] PRIs are considered complex when associated with open fractures and/or additional injury to the pelvic vessels and organs[18]—particularly the rectum, bladder, and urethra. Hematuria is common after pelvic trauma in children, and genitourinary injuries are reported in up to 12% of pediatric patients.[4,19,24]

Additional musculoskeletal injuries occur frequently in children with PRI. Most frequently seen are fractures of the femur, tibia, ankle, and clavicle. An important distinction must be made between acetabular fractures and PRI as they are often grouped together in studies because of their rarity. Although a PRI associated with an acetabular fracture designates a more severe injury, they are best thought of by clinicians and researchers as clinically separate entities.[25,26]

Despite their high rates of associated injuries at presentation, children are generally less likely than adults to suffer from subsequent major complications such as thromboembolism, acute respiratory distress syndrome, persistent neurologic deficit, and multiorgan failure.[6,17,18]

Mortality

Mortality rates of pediatric patients with PRI over the last decade range between 3% and 12%.[20,22] As with most aspects of pediatric trauma, head injury is the most commonly cited cause of death, followed by visceral injury and multiorgan failure.[2,5,18,19] Although lower overall mortality rates have previously been shown in children,[6] other studies have found mortality rates similar to those in adults.[4,7,8,18] In a review of the National Trauma Data Bank, a 2015 study subdivided the pediatric population into children and adolescents. In doing so, it demonstrated increased odds of death in children (younger than 13 years), but decreased odds of death in adolescents (aged 13 to 17 years), when compared with adults (older than 18 years). It concluded that comparing the entire pediatric population to adults may be inadequate as children and adolescents appear to have different outcomes after PRI.[17] A 2018 study, in a comparison of cohorts from 2006 to 2017 versus 1986 to 1996, found that despite the most recent cohort of patients having more unstable pelvic fracture patterns, they had lower mortality, suggesting both an increase in the rate of high-energy pediatric trauma as well as improved trauma care.[8]

Life-threatening bleeding and hemodynamic instability from lacerations of the venous and/or arterial plexus can occur in both adults and children. A 2017 study found that although children had a lower rate of hemodynamic instability on presentation compared with adults, both groups had similar transfusion requirements.[4] The decreased hemorrhage associated with the pelvic fracture itself in children may be due to differences in fracture pattern and a more effective hemostatic response.[5,6,14,26]

Classification

Several classification systems exist to guide the treatment of PRI, but none fully addresses the anatomic and pathologic variations that occur in the pediatric pelvis. After closure of the TRC, adult classification systems can be used more readily. Of these, the Tile (1996) classification is often used in children as it simplifies PRI into stable (type A), rotationally unstable (type B), and rotationally and vertically unstable (type C) patterns.[27]

The most commonly used classification system in the pediatric literature is that described by the authors of a 1985 study.[28] In their original description, pelvic injuries are classified as isolated avulsion fractures (type I), iliac wing fractures (type II), stable ring injuries (type III), or unstable (type IV) ring injuries. Modifications were then made to include CT data differentiating type III injuries into stable disruptions (with less than 2 mm of displacement) of the anterior ring alone (type IIIA) and stable disruptions of both the anterior and posterior pelvic ring (type IIIB).[3] Type I injuries are generally isolated sport-related injuries in adolescents. In the context of high-energy trauma, avulsions of the pubic symphysis and iliac crest apophyses have been described.[10,29] Type II injuries may occur more frequently in the skeletally immature, when bony failure is likely to occur before ligamentous failure.[1] Type IIIA injuries occur equally between skeletally mature and immature patients, whereas type IIIB and IV injuries occur more commonly in mature patients. When compared with type IIIA, type IIIB injuries were associated with greater transfusion and intensive care unit requirements, longer hospital stays, higher mortality, and more associated injuries.[3,19] Although type IIIB injuries clinically resemble type IV injuries, they are typically mechanically stable and can be adequately treated without surgery in most patients. The modified Torode classification is predictive of significant morbidity and mortality in the setting of polytrauma.[3,28]

Diagnosis

Trauma patients should be carefully examined for pelvic instability. Pelvic stress examinations have been shown to be sensitive and specific for pelvic fracture in children, albeit limited by altered levels of consciousness and distracting injuries.[30] Often, PRIs are diagnosed via an AP pelvic radiograph obtained in the emergency department (**Figure 1, A**). Additional radiographs that may then help delineate the injury include pelvic inlet (45° cranial) and outlet (60° caudal) views. CT scans are especially useful for evaluation of the posterior ring and may identify injuries otherwise missed on radiographs, particularly those associated with acetabular fractures and iliac crest apophyseal avulsions[5,9,15,28] (**Figure 1, B**). When reviewing pediatric pelvic imaging, it is important to understand the effect that variations in age have on the interpretation of both radiographs[31] and CT scans.[32] The ambiguity of diagnosis of pathologic diastasis can lead to the undertreatment or overtreatment of children with pelvic trauma and the potential for poor outcomes or unnecessary procedures. A 2017 study established normative values from CT and, in doing so, demonstrated an age-dependent decrease in width of the pubic symphysis and sacroiliac joints, but a relatively stable width of the TRC limbs until closure.[33] Similarly, a 2016 study established age-related and gender-related measurements of sacroiliac joint width, showing distinct changes with growth. It suggested values falling outside of the 97th percentile should strongly be considered for sacroiliac injury.[34]

In an effort to reduce radiation exposure to as low as reasonably achievable, there is debate regarding the necessity of pelvic radiographs and CT scans in the pediatric trauma patient. Some authors recommend low-dose abdominopelvic CT scans as a first-line

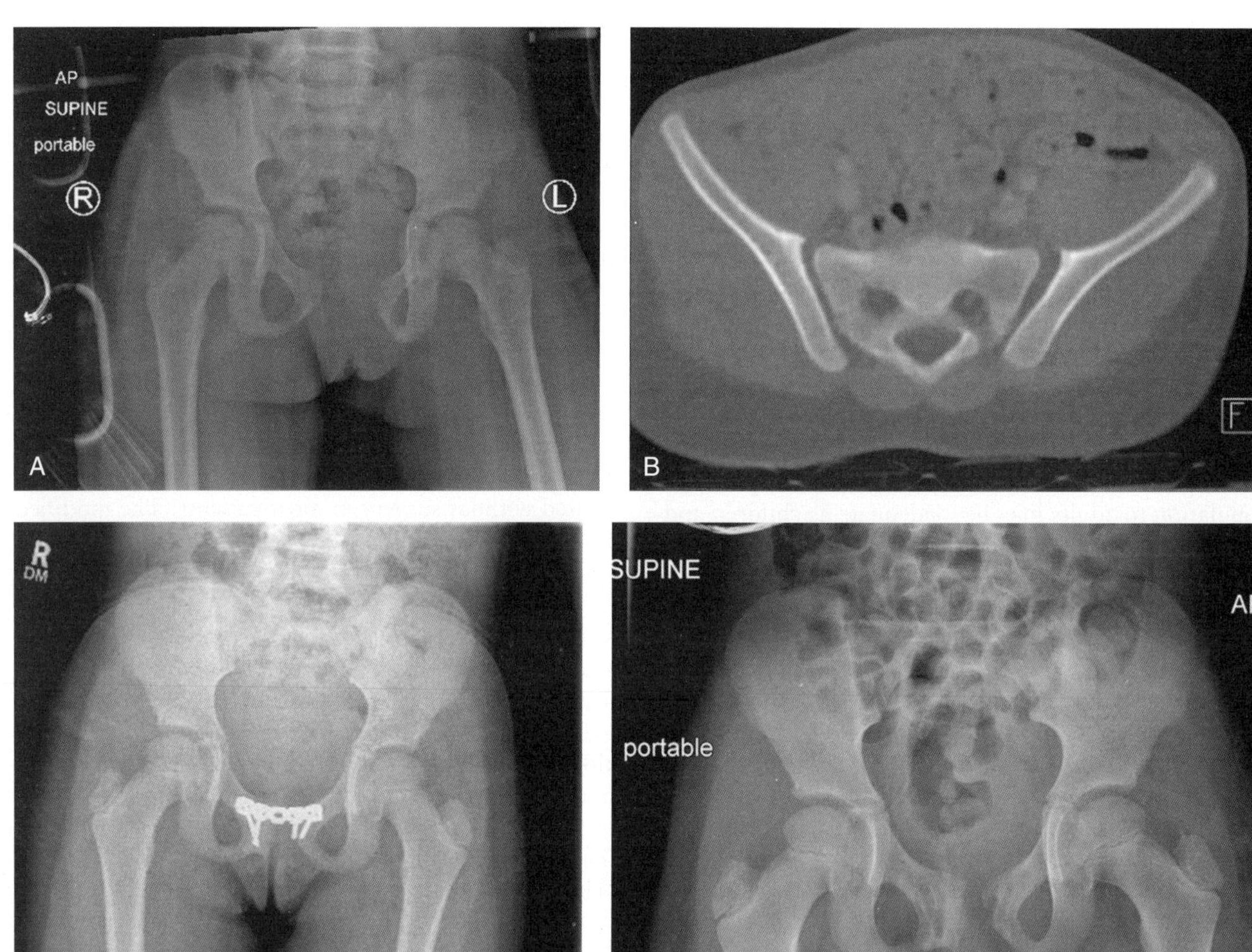

FIGURE 1 **A**, AP radiograph from a 7.5-year-old girl involved in a motor vehicle accident. **B**, Axial CT scan demonstrating concomitant posterior ring injury. **C**, AP radiograph after open reduction and internal fixation of the symphysis pubis. **D**, AP radiograph 9 months after removal of INFIX.

imaging modality for blunt trauma in lieu of radiographs,[35] whereas others recommend only selective use of CT scans with a greater emphasis on physical examination and radiographs.[4,36] However, in the pediatric population specifically, certain pelvic injuries, such as Torode and Zieg IIIB fractures, crescent fractures, and iliac apophyseal avulsions, that may not be discernible on plain radiographs have been associated with poorer clinical outcomes and may necessitate a change in management.[3,29,37]

MRI has a limited yet evolving diagnostic role in the acute management of PRI. Potential indications include evaluation of unossified portions of the pelvis in young children, assessment of posterior ligamentous structures, and/or iliac apophyseal disruptions, which may help guide surgical management.[29] Further study is required to better define the role of MRI in pediatric PRI.

Initial Management

Management of polytrauma in pediatric patients requires a multidisciplinary approach using validated protocols to optimize outcomes. Pediatric Advanced Life Support and Advanced Trauma Life Support principles should guide the initial assessment and management of these injuries. In cases of suspected PRI, the patient should be assessed for pelvic ring stability, soft-tissue injuries of the trunk and thigh, and neurovascular injury of the lower extremities. Associated rectal, vaginal, or urogenital injuries should be assessed. Complex and open fractures are associated with greater morbidity and mortality and may require multidisciplinary interventions such as orthopaedic débridement and stabilization, diverting colostomy, genitourinary repair, or specialized catheterization.[37] Generally, children require emergency surgery at similar rates as in adults.[4,18]

Initial orthopaedic management hinges on the hemodynamic stability of the patient and the mechanical stability of the pelvis. Hemodynamically unstable patients with an unstable PRI should receive fluid resuscitation in line with massive transfusion protocols. This must be coupled with manual reduction of the pelvic volume to tamponade bleeding. The initial step in achieving this is application of a pelvic binder. Limb traction can be applied for additional reduction and stabilization of vertically displaced injuries. Failure to reduce the pelvic ring using these methods may warrant emergent external fixation or internal fixation in select cases.[38] Principles of damage-control orthopaedics should be adhered to during this acute phase of management. Angiographic embolization and/or pelvic packing should be considered only after mechanical stabilization if hemodynamic stability is not achieved. A 2013 study found that mortality rates were higher in adult patients who underwent pelvic packing or angiographic embolization before external fixation of the pelvis.[39] Angiographic embolization is rarely required in children but is safe and effective if performed within 60 minutes of presentation.[26,40,41]

Definitive Management

Definitive orthopaedic treatment can be considered once hemodynamic stability has been achieved. The next consideration in management is reestablishing stability and symmetry of the pelvic ring. Most authors recommend surgical fixation of unstable PRI in children.[9,10,42-44] In addition to restoration of mechanical stability, treatment goals include prevention of deformity, limb-length inequality, and posterior arch malunion.[45] Other accepted indications for definitive fixation of the pelvic ring include complex injuries, optimization of mobility, and improved care of the polytraumatized patient.[12,18,21]

Instability can be determined clinically or radiographically; however, static imaging may not adequately identify dynamic or occult instability.[46] The pelvic stress examination under anesthesia (EUA) is an important diagnostic tool in adults, with rates of occult instability found in 30% to 50% of seemingly stable fracture patterns on static imaging.[47] Conversely, the EUA can accurately predict stable fractures amenable to unrestricted weight bearing.[2] Most pediatric PRIs are stable without significant displacement and can be managed nonsurgically with early mobilization and progressive weight bearing as tolerated with appropriate analgesia. Short-term casting for comfort or compliance with activity restrictions can be considered in younger children. Skeletally mature patients experience higher rates of unstable injuries, and surgical fixation is more frequently necessary than in skeletally immature patients.[3-5,12,18]

Surgical approaches and techniques depend on many factors, including injury pattern, patient comorbidities, and surgeon preference/experience.[45] The principles of management of PRI are well established in adults. Similar treatment goals are appropriate for pediatric patients with appropriate modifications and/or limitations to account for skeletal immaturity. Reduction and fixation can often be achieved by closed or percutaneous methods. Inability to obtain an acceptable closed reduction will require an open approach (**Figure 1, C**). The immature pelvis may be too small for standard-sized pelvic reduction clamps, and the cartilaginous nature of the immature pelvis may not tolerate the forces these clamps transmit. Consideration should be given to hardware removal in 6 to 12 months after fixation in skeletally immature patients to prevent bony overgrowth, growth disturbance, and iatrogenic deformities (**Figure 1, D**).

Posterior Ring

Percutaneous fixation of the posterior ring is the mainstay of treatment in the adult population and, with modifications for size, can be safely used in pediatric patients as well. A 2018 study performed percutaneous posterior pelvic fixation with sacroiliac screws in 56 patients with less than 50 mL of blood loss in all cases and no cases of iatrogenic nerve or visceral injury.[42] Three patients (ages 7, 9, and 10 years) required an open reduction of the sacroiliac joint, and planned hardware removal was performed 7 to 19 months postoperatively in three patients. Other authors have described inserting sacroiliac screws through plates to prevent screw head penetration into the soft iliac wing of skeletally immature patients.[9] Concern has also been raised regarding the safety of percutaneous sacroiliac fixation in younger children because of the relatively small size and dysmorphism of the immature sacrum.[37,48] A 2016 study studied the CT scans of children aged 2 to 16 years and found that in the first sacral segment, nearly all had radiographically safe pathways available for iliosacral style screws, whereas only half had safe pathways for transsacral style screws.[49] Contrary to the authors of a 2004 study,[48] the authors of a 2018 study[42] recommend against intraoperative CT scans to minimize ionizing radiation exposure. This recommendation should be tempered by surgeon experience. Careful preoperative CT evaluation of available osseous pathways and intraoperative fluoroscopy are sufficient to safely perform this technique in patients as young as 20 months.[50] A 2017 study described difficulties while placing retrograde posterior iliac (aka lateral column [LC] screws) in two of five patients in their series, mostly because of the small size and cartilaginous nature of the posterior crescent fracture in children. Accordingly, it recommended against this technique in the skeletally immature.[9]

Anterior Ring

Fixation options for the anterior ring include external fixation, plate osteosynthesis, and percutaneous screws. In a 2018 study, 24 patients underwent percutaneous superior pubic rami screw placement with minimal reported complications.[42] Of note, only 15% of patients in this series had open TRC epiphyseal plates, the patency of which should be respected when considering anterior ring fixation options. A 2017 study described supra-acetabular external fixation with pins placed at the level of the anterior inferior iliac spine to address anterior ring injuries in 21 patients, of which 50% had open TRC epiphyseal plates. It demonstrated that external fixation is a safe and reliable option with minimal complications in the growing pelvis.[9] A supra-acetabular pin on a hand chuck can also be used as a reduction tool for displaced posterior pelvic injuries.

Apophyseal Injuries

Isolated pelvic apophyseal avulsion injuries do not result in instability of the pelvic ring, and the vast majority can be managed nonsurgically. The pelvic apophyses most commonly injured are the anterior inferior iliac spine, ischial tuberosity, and anterior superior iliac spine. A 2017 literature review and meta-analysis of isolated pelvic apophyseal avulsions found that adolescents treated surgically had better overall outcomes, especially in patients who had >15 mm of displacement (50% versus 84%, $P = 0.003$). With similar overall complication rates (17% versus 19%), surgical consideration is recommended for patients with Torode and Zieg type I injuries displaced greater than 15 mm or with high functional demands.[51] A 2017 study of 29 surgically treated pediatric patients with PRI found iliac and pubic symphyseal apophyseal avulsions in nine and six children, respectively. Fixation of these unstable injuries by direct repair or indirect reduction with external fixation is recommended to decrease the risk of growth disturbance and pelvic asymmetry. In the context of unstable ring injuries with posterior disruption, this study highlighted that the iliac apophysis actually kept its normal anatomic relation to the axial skeleton and should be used as a landmark for reduction of the displaced bony pelvis.[9]

Outcomes

Children with multiple injuries treated at pediatric trauma centers have shown lower mortality and improved outcomes compared with those treated at nonpediatric centers.[52,53] These findings clearly demonstrate the importance of pediatric specialization and volume of care for improved outcomes after pediatric trauma.[14] Because of the rarity of pediatric PRI and the relative difficulty in obtaining adequate follow-up to assess outcomes, few studies have considered the long-term functional outcomes of children after PRI.[54] Good short-term functional outcomes have been reported, especially in younger children.[55,56] Overall, children have been found to have significantly better outcome scores than adults.[18]

Associated injuries account for a significant portion of the disability that occurs in children after PRI, particularly those that include other orthopaedic injuries, head injuries, genitourinary injuries, and psychiatric illnesses.[24] Nonetheless, unstable or displaced ring injuries can also cause significant morbidity and impairment in isolation. This is especially true for severely displaced or vertically unstable fractures.[55] Historically, the remodeling potential of pediatric extremity fractures had been extrapolated to the pelvis. However, many authors have demonstrated that unsatisfactory pelvic asymmetry will not remodel,[54] leading to permanent deformity and significant long-term sequelae.[10,37] Residual pelvic asymmetry of 1.1 cm or greater has been associated with scoliosis, chronic pain, gait disturbances, and sitting imbalance.[37,44,57] Additionally, pain and poor functional outcome was correlated with residual deformity of >5 to 10 mm of the posterior pelvic ring.[2,58] Other potential long-term complications include permanent neurologic deficit, delayed union and nonunion, sacroiliac joint subluxation or ankylosis, persistent pubic symphysis diastasis, and hemipelvic undergrowth.[9,10,13,28]

ACETABULAR FRACTURES

General

Acetabular fractures are uncommon injuries in childhood, accounting for less than 1% of all pediatric fractures.[6,15] Registry data suggest that acetabular fractures occur in up to 20% of pediatric bony pelvic trauma cases.[8,15,18] Acetabular fractures are more common in the skeletally mature, again best distinguished by the closure of the TRC.[1,6,18,59]

Acetabular development is a complex process that involves the simultaneous interaction of multiple intrinsic and extrinsic factors. The TRC, a Y-shaped physis interposed between the ilium, ischium, and pubis, closes at a skeletal age of approximately 12 years in girls and 14 years in boys.[34,60] Children with an open TRC are less likely to sustain acetabular fractures than those whose TRC has closed.[1,5,6,44] A 2017 study reported that 20% of PRIs had concomitant acetabular fractures in children with an open TRC, as compared with 35% with a closed TRC.[5] A 2002 study reported an even greater discrepancy with rates of 6% and 44%, respectively.[1] The elasticity and flexibility of the pediatric pelvis allows for greater resistance to fracture and displacement, and when a fracture does occur, fracture patterns are frequently different. Typically in the skeletally immature, more simple and/or elemental fracture patterns are seen,[61,62] whereas the majority of adult acetabular fractures involve complex associated patterns, frequently involving both columns.[63] The most common patterns of isolated acetabular fractures seen in the pediatric age group are posterior wall, posterior column, and transverse fracture types[2,6,8,15,59,64,65] (**Figure 2, A**). A 2018 study compared isolated and PRI-associated acetabular fractures in 32 children with a mean age of 12.8 years. They found that 84% of PRI-associated acetabular fractures were anterior column fractures.[2] A 2017 study similarly found that 87.5% of all acetabular fractures in their series were an extension of a high pubic root fracture into the anterior column. The mean age in their series was 8.3 years, suggesting a predisposition to such injury in the immature pelvis.[5] Injury to the TRC itself is thought to be rare, although it has been reported in 15% to 20% of children with bony pelvic trauma.[11,64]

Most of these fractures are caused by high-energy mechanisms such as traffic accidents and falls from height. Lower energy sport-related hip dislocations are another common cause of acetabular fractures in younger patients.[65] Generally, acetabular fractures do not carry the potential for life-threatening bleeding but can be associated with PRIs and other nonorthopaedic-related trauma.[26]

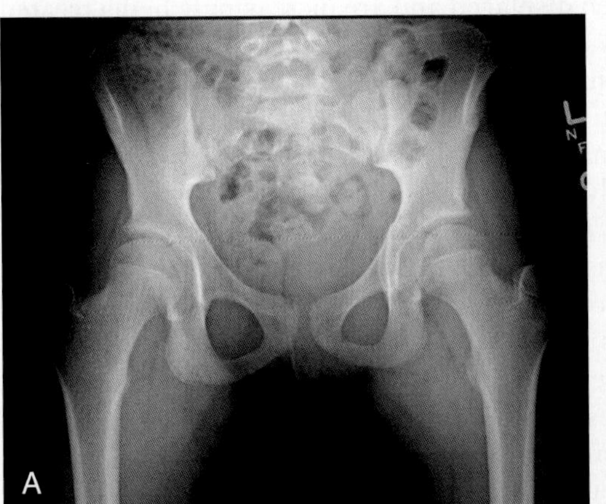

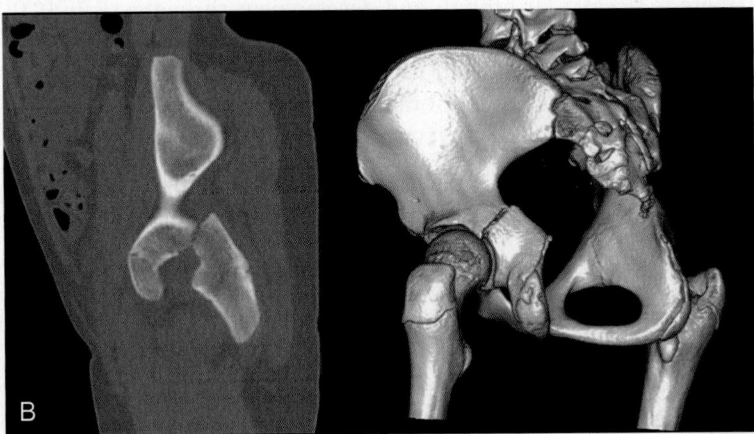

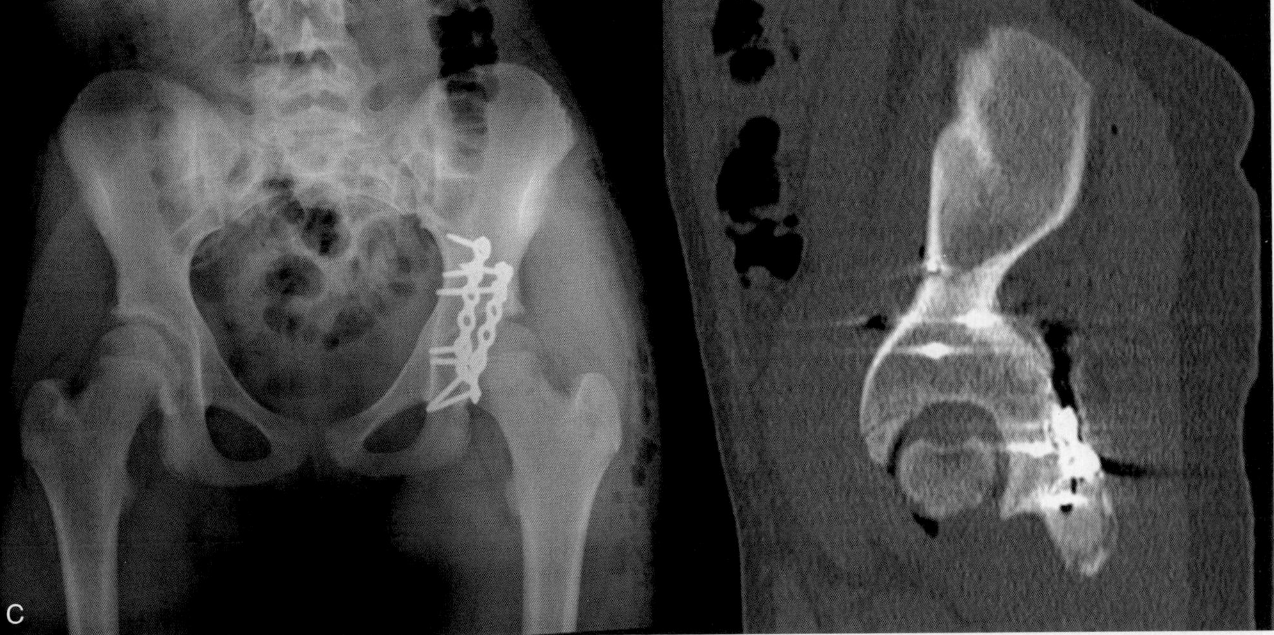

FIGURE 2 **A**, AP radiograph from a 12-year-old girl with left hip pain and a fracture through the closing triradiate cartilage after landing awkwardly while jumping. **B**, Sagittal and three-dimensional CT scans demonstrating a posterior column and wall fractures. Note the intra-articular displacement. **C**, AP radiograph and sagittal CT scan demonstrating anatomic fixation of the fractures.

Section 7: Trauma

Imaging

Acetabular fractures in children are not that easily identified on plain radiographs. A 2013 study found that 25% of acetabular fractures compared with 92% of PRIs were detected on AP pelvis radiograph. Patients younger than 12 years seem to be at particular risk.[21,66] Even CT can miss nonossified, cartilaginous portions of the acetabulum (**Figure 2, B**). In young patients with posterior wall fractures or fractures extending into the TRC, MRI is frequently required to evaluate the extent of the injury. Imaging in this area is made increasingly complicated by the presence of secondary ossification centers that develop in early adolescence while the TRC is still open.[67] These superior, anterior, and posterior ossification centers appear between 10 and 12 years of age and further contribute to acetabular growth and development through adolescence.[67,68] The posterior ossification center fuses just before TRC closure and needs to be differentiated from a traumatic posterior labral injury, frequently seen radiographically as a fleck sign on postreduction CT scans after hip dislocation.[69] Although CT is an excellent imaging modality for the skeletally mature pelvis, MRI should be considered to evaluate the acetabulum before TRC closure.[70]

Classification

After TRC closure, acetabular fractures in adolescents generally follow adult fracture patterns as described by the author of a 1980 study.[62] Before TRC closure, children can sustain fracture patterns not easily described using the Letournel classification. Classification systems established by the author of a 1976 study[61] and/or the author of a 1982 study[11] can be used in this age group. The Watts[61] classification is based on hip stability and includes four types: type A, small fracture fragment associated with hip dislocation; type B, stable linear fractures in association with pelvic fractures; type C, linear fractures associated with hip joint instability; and type D, fractures secondary to central fracture-dislocations of the hip. The Bucholz classification is centered more on the TRC and is based on the type of force and resulting Salter-Harris injury type: shearing type, which involves epiphysiolysis with or without bony extension (Salter-Harris type I or II), and crushing type, which results in an impaction injury to the epiphyseal plate (Salter-Harris type V).[11]

Treatment and Outcomes

Although the treatment of acetabular fractures in adults has been widely reported, limited data exist in the pediatric literature. Previous reports suggest nonsurgical management yields reasonable results in appropriately selected patients.[21] Acetabular fractures associated with PRI tend to be less displaced than those occurring in isolation and can be frequently treated nonoperatively.[2] In cases of minimally displaced but unstable fractures, consideration can be given to percutaneous column fixation to promote early mobilization.

Surgical management for acetabular fractures is indicated for articular displacement and joint instability. In adults, stress EUA has become the benchmark for assessing the stability of posterior wall fractures that are frequently seen with posterior hip dislocations, as other radiographic parameters have been shown to be unreliable.[71] This technique can be used in adolescents as well to determine if surgical stabilization is required. Acetabular fractures in adults with articular displacement, with few exceptions, are treated surgically. Isolated acetabular fractures in adolescents are more often displaced and are increasingly being treated surgically as well.[2,64] A 2015 study described experience with the surgical management of 37/38 acetabular fractures seen in patients aged 11 to 18 years.[65] It reported minor complications attributed to the surgical exposure that resolved spontaneously (ie, meralgia paresthetica, abductor weakness) and a 20% rate of revision surgery for removal of hardware or excision of heterotopic ossification. Because of the strong relation between anatomic reduction and clinical outcomes, emphasis should be placed on sound exposure and reduction techniques for these injuries when surgical treatment is undertaken[72] (**Figure 2, C**).

Acetabular injuries in younger children are sparsely reported in the literature and can present additional challenges, especially when the TRC is involved. Consideration must be given to surgical fixation that spares the epiphyseal plate whenever possible, such as temporary Kirschner wires, suture anchors, or interfragmentary lag screws.[69,73] Nonetheless, these modifications in technique should not compromise reduction or joint stability. Hardware removal is generally recommended 6 to 12 months after surgical fixation to prevent growth arrest and/or bony overgrowth. Additional surgical challenges in young children can include smaller anatomy, early callous formation, interposed periosteum, bony plastic deformation, and nonossified fragments. These challenges, as well as the previously overestimated remodeling potential of the pediatric pelvis,[37] likely contributed to most of the previously reported cases and series of acetabular fractures being treated nonsurgically.[15,44] Although the surgical management of acetabular fractures in younger patients has been desc ribed,[18,59,64] there is a lack of outcome studies to clearly evaluate the effectiveness of surgical versus conservative management in this age group.

Growth arrest and the development of posttraumatic dysplasia is a rare but potentially debilitating complication after injury to the TRC. In addition to direct injury, arrest of TRC can occur because of ossification of adjacent hematoma, perichondrium stripping, and callous formation and disruption of its blood supply.[11,74,75] Posttraumatic dysplasia presents as progressive medial wall thickening, shallowing of the acetabulum, and lateralization of femoral head with relatively normal proximal femoral anatomy. Routine surveillance radiographs until skeletal maturity are recommended to detect and monitor early signs of growth arrest as deformity may not be evident until ossification of the acetabulum in adolescence.[11] Similarly, patients may not complain of symptoms until decades after injury.[75] Patient age and severity of the injury are the most important factors in the development of posttraumatic deformity. The greatest risk of clinically significant growth disturbance occurs in children younger than 10 years.[11] Bucholz shearing-type injuries typically have a favorable prognosis, whereas impaction-type injuries experience high rates of growth arrest.[11,75] Although surgery is generally recommended for displaced fractures, it is unknown whether surgical management of these injuries alters their outcome as studies to date are limited to small case series. Reconstructive osteotomies, arthrodesis, and arthroplasty have successfully addressed established posttraumatic dysplasia.[75] More recently, a 2013 study reported successful early resection of a partial physeal bar of the TRC with methylmethacrylate and/or fat interposition in three patients.[76] Although they were successful in restoring growth, recurrence and/or residual dysplasia developed in all patients. The potential benefits of triradiate bar resection must be weighed against the risks of this invasive procedure with questionable efficacy, especially in light of other reliable reconstructive options in adolescence and adulthood.

TRAUMATIC HIP DISLOCATIONS

General

Traumatic hip dislocation is an uncommon but potentially devastating injury in children because of the associated risk of osteonecrosis. The magnitude of force required to produce such an injury decreases with decreasing age because of the relative periarticular laxity and pliability in young children.[77,78] Relatively minor trauma can cause a hip dislocation in children younger than 10 years.[79] In adolescents, these injuries are often related to traumatic sports injuries, falls from a height, or motor vehicle accidents.[70,78,80,81] Most pediatric traumatic hip dislocations are posterior in direction; anterior and inferior dislocations are rarely reported.[78,82] Abnormal hip morphology may be a predisposing factor to traumatic hip dislocation, with relative femoral and acetabular retroversion as the greatest influences on the mechanics of dislocation.[80,83]

Imaging and Initial Reduction

Patients will typically present with notable pain after a traumatic injury, a fixed deformity about the hip, and an AP radiograph showing an obvious dislocation. Sciatic and gluteal nerve palsies have also been reported to correlate with the force of injury, occurring in approximately 5% of patients. This should be evaluated when possible before reduction. Urgent closed reduction of these injuries under conscious sedation or general anesthesia is indicated to diminish the risk of osteonecrosis.[82,84] Traumatic and iatrogenic epiphysiolysis of the proximal femur has been reported in adolescents,[85,86] likely because of the mechanical susceptibility of the mature physis and/or the shear forces across the physis involved with higher energy mechanisms.[87,88] Even with adequate muscle relaxation, iatrogenic epiphysiolysis has been reported.[89] Therefore, it is generally recommended that adolescent patients be reduced in the operating room with muscle relaxation under fluoroscopy to prevent iatrogenic injury from a traumatic reduction and allow for provisional stabilization of suspected physeal injury if identified before reduction attempt. Hip stability after reduction should also be assessed while the patient is still sedated.

Postreduction Imaging and Definitive Management

Postreduction radiographs must be scrutinized as nonconcentric reduction has been reported in 20% to 50% of cases[78,82,90] (**Figure 3, A**). Although up to 6 mm of joint asymmetry has been shown because of hematoma or joint laxity, any concern for joint asymmetry or incongruity should be evaluated with cross-sectional imaging.[77,82,91] MRI has been shown to be superior to CT scan for detection of cartilaginous and soft-tissue structural pathologies after traumatic posterior hip dislocation without the additional ionizing radiation exposure.[70,92] Incomplete ossification of the posterior wall can lead to underestimated or missed posterior wall fractures in younger patients.[68,92-94] Deceivingly small posterior wall injuries identified on radiographs or CT may result in significant posterior instability, especially in children with an open TRC[66] (**Figure 3, B**). A 2020 study proposed a standard MRI protocol that allows for adequate detection of structural pathologies in the skeletally immature patient with traumatic hip injuries while minimizing scan time and variability. It recommended MRI as the standard diagnostic imaging modality after closed reduction of traumatic hip dislocations in children.[70]

Surgery is indicated for patients with a nonconcentric reduction or hip instability after reduction. The classically recommended surgical approach to the dislocated hip is from the direction of dislocation[77] (**Figure 3, C**). However, surgical hip dislocation (SHD) and hip arthroscopy have been shown to be safe and effective in children

Section 7: Trauma

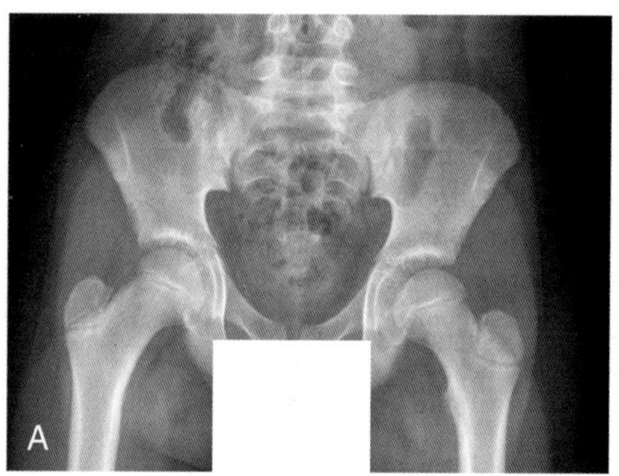

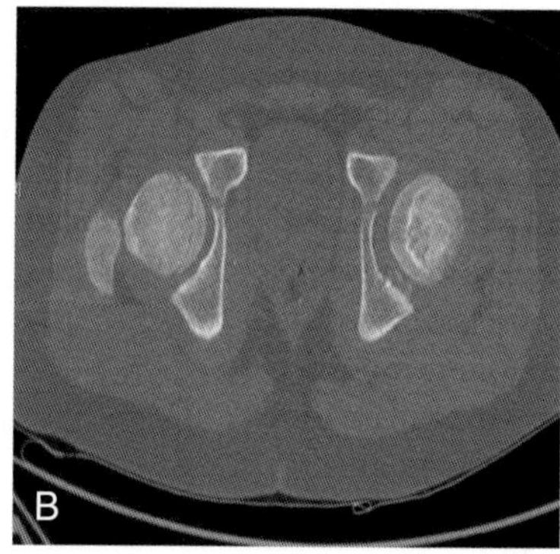

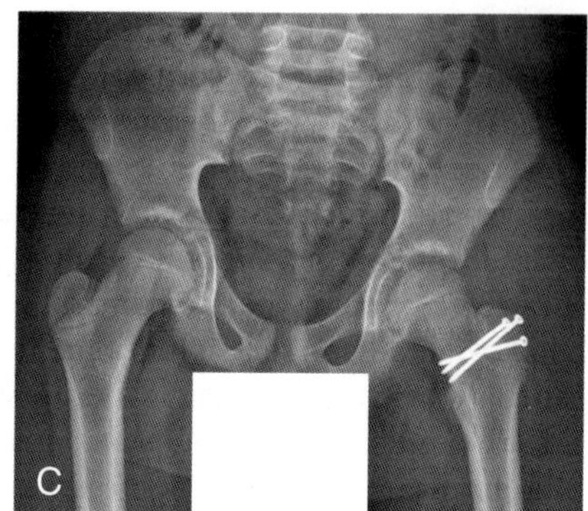

FIGURE 3 **A**, AP radiograph from a 13-year-old boy who got tackled while playing football with immediate left hip pain. Note the widening in the medial joint space when compared with the right side. **B**, Axial scan reveals joint asymmetry and posterior bony interposition. **C**, AP radiograph 6 weeks post surgery demonstrating symmetric joint space. Patient was ambulatory and pain free.

as well.[80,81,90] SHD has the advantage of direct access to periarticular hip pathology, whereas arthroscopy is less invasive. A 2016 study described three patients in whom osteochondroplasty was performed to correct their femoroacetabular impingement deformity during SHD given the potential role of femoroacetabular impingement in hip instability.[90] Reported impediments to a stable and/or concentric reduction include muscle interposition, capsule and/or labrum entrapment, acetabular fractures, and osteochondral fragment incarceration.[78,92,95] A 2018 study reported that 83% of posterior wall fractures associated with a traumatic posterior hip dislocation required surgical treatment after closed reduction because of interposed soft-tissue or osteochondral fragments.[96] Avulsion of the posterior labrum is commonly observed intraoperatively during open reductions of posterior hip dislocations.[90,92] In light of the published importance of the acetabular labrum on hip biomechanics and the association of labral tears with early degenerative hip disease in adults,[97] some authors have recommended surgical fixation for all patients with evidence of labral pathology on imaging.[69,90] However, the necessity of surgical fixation for these labral injuries in children has not yet been proven. A 2018 case report described a 5-year-old girl with MRI evidence of spontaneous healing of a large posterior labral avulsion 2 months after injury.[98] Additionally, a 2017 study reported satisfactory results after arthroscopic reduction without fixation of an interposed labral complex in seven pediatric patients with an average 10 months of follow-up.[81]

Complications/Outcomes

To prevent redislocation in children younger than 10 years, postreduction spica casting or abduction splinting is recommended for 4 to 6 weeks, whereas older children with stable and concentric reductions can be treated with protected weight bearing for 6 to 12 weeks.[77] A 2013 study reported recurrent dislocation in two of three young patients treated with a brief period of skin traction, compared with zero of 10 patients treated in postreduction spica casts.[79] Timely recognition and treatment of a hip dislocation is crucial, as delays greater than 6 hours have been associated with significantly increase rates of osteonecrosis.[78,82] Even with prompt treatment, osteonecrosis has been reported in 3% to 15% of patients after traumatic hip dislocation.[77] Postreduction nuclear scintigraphy or MRI does not appear to reliably predict the later development of osteonecrosis.[82,95] Asymptomatic coxa magna develops in approximately 20% of patients and has been associated with younger age at time of injury.[95]

A hip dislocation may go unrecognized in the pediatric patient with distracting injuries or spontaneous but incomplete reduction.[91] When children lack timely access to appropriate orthopaedic care, it has been shown that neglected traumatic hip dislocations are associated with high rates of osteonecrosis, early degenerative arthritis, and poor functional outcomes, even after successful delayed reduction of the hip.[99] In cases of delayed treatment, reduction of the femoral head within the acetabulum is recommended to equalize limb lengths, restore the stimulus for hip development, and facilitate future hip reconstruction as indicated.[91,99,100] A 2013 study demonstrated successful delayed reduction of hip dislocations by heavy traction alone up to 3 weeks after injury.[79] However, other authors have shown variable success with this technique and required open reductions with or without osteotomies in most cases of neglected hip dislocations.[99]

PEDIATRIC FEMORAL NECK FRACTURES

Pediatric femoral neck fractures are uncommon injuries but are associated with a high complication rate including osteonecrosis, malunion, nonunion, coxa vara, and proximal femoral growth abnormalities.[101] The high complication rate is related to the intra-articular nature of the majority of these fractures affecting healing, the biomechanics of the femoral neck, and the precarious vascular anatomy of the pediatric proximal femoral epiphysis.[102,103] Timely anatomic reduction and stable internal fixation are the two aspects of management that are under the control of the treating orthopaedic surgeon and are the best tools to limiting complications in the treatment of pediatric femoral neck fractures. Although these fractures can occur with awkward falls and sports injuries, they are also seen in the setting of high-energy trauma, carrying with that the risk of concomitant musculoskeletal and other related injuries. Pathologic fractures are also known to occur in the femoral neck, and this should always be kept in mind when evaluating the radiographs of these injuries.[104]

The most common classification system for femoral neck fractures in children is the Delbet system,[105] which is based on the location in the femoral neck of the fracture (**Table 1**). The Delbet system has been shown to have prognostic value for the risk of posttraumatic osteonecrosis,[106-108] as well as assisting with surgical fixation decision making.

Delbet I: Transepiphyseal Fractures

A Delbet type I fracture is the least common, accounting for <10% of all pediatric femoral neck fractures, but they carry the worst prognosis for developing osteonecrosis.[106,109,110] These fractures result from a traumatic separation of the femoral head from the femoral neck through the subcapital physis. These traumatic transphyseal separations are further classified into type IA, without femoral head dislocation, and type IB, with femoral head dislocation. The rate of osteonecrosis is worse with type IB injuries compared with type IA, with the largest series demonstrating an osteonecrosis rate of 75%.[111]

The rare nondisplaced type I fracture in a child younger than 4 years can be treated with a hip spica cast. Otherwise, the treatment of a type I femoral neck fracture starts with an attempt at closed reduction in the operating room with adequate muscle relaxation. The reduction technique was initially described by the author of a 2002 study, flexing the affected leg to 45° with slight abduction and then extending the hip with internal rotation as traction is being applied.[112] If closed reduction is unsuccessful, an open reduction is indicated, usually through a direct anterior (Smith Petersen) approach. In a type IB, a posterior approach may be necessary if the dislocation is posterior. Fixation usually involves transphyseal pins or screws depending on age. The use of a postoperative spica cast depends on patient age, quality of fixation, and anticipated compliance with postoperative weight-bearing and activity restrictions.[113,114]

TABLE 1

Delbet Classification of Pediatric Hip Fractures

Type	Description
I	Transepiphyseal fracture, with or without dislocation of the femoral head from the acetabulum
II	Transcervical fracture
III	Cervicotrochanteric fracture
IV	Intertrochanteric fracture

Delbet II and III: Transcervical and Cervicotrochanteric Fractures

Delbet type II and type III fractures are the most common. A 2013 review reported of 876 pediatric femoral neck fractures: 410 (46.8%) were Delbet type II and 307 (35.0%) were Delbet type III. In the same study, the type II fractures had a 27% incidence of osteonecrosis and the type III fractures 20%.[109] A nondisplaced type II or III fracture in a child younger than 5 years can be treated with spica casting and careful follow-up.[113] Percutaneous fixation should be considered in addition to cast immobilization as these fractures are prone to secondary displacement and varus angulation in cast.[115]

Most type II and III fractures are displaced, however, and require a near anatomic reduction (either closed or open) and internal fixation.[1] Acceptable reduction in a type II fracture consists of <5° of angulation and <2 mm of cortical translation. Acceptable reduction in a type III fracture consists of <10° of angulation.[116] If acceptable closed reduction cannot be obtained, then an open reduction through an anterior or anterolateral approach should be performed. A combination of these two approaches has been described for young adults and can be considered.[117] Smooth Kirschner wires can be used in patients younger than 4 years, and physeal sparring cannulated screws in the 4- to 9-year age group, with strong consideration to postoperative casting. In those older than 10 years, transphyseal screw fixation can be considered, as stable fracture fixation should not be compromised to spare the physis.[116]

Delbet IV: Intertrochanteric Fractures

Intertrochanteric fractures (Delbet type IV) account for approximately 15% of femoral neck fractures in children and have the lowest incidence of osteonecrosis (5%).[106] In children younger than 8 years, these fractures can be treated with closed reduction followed by hip spica casting. Because of remodeling, <10° of varus is considered acceptable.[106] Open reduction through a standard lateral approach and internal fixation with a pediatric hip screw, side plate, and derotation screw is a standard approach for older children and those that have failed a more conservative approach, although other pediatric proximal femoral implants can be used. In most type IV fractures, screw fixation can stop short of the physis. With a good reduction and stable fixation, weight bearing can be permitted as tolerated with type IV fractures.[111]

Pediatric Femoral Neck Fracture Complications

Osteonecrosis of the femoral head is the most common complication resulting from a pediatric femoral neck fracture.[106-118] As there is no curative treatment available for osteonecrosis once it has developed after a femoral neck fracture, the surgeon's treatment is best focused on its prevention. The risk of a patient developing osteonecrosis is directly related to the fracture pattern (Delbet classification) and the patient's age at the time of the injury, with older children having a higher risk.[106] These are nonmodifiable risk factors. Several other factors may contribute to the development of osteonecrosis. Initial fracture displacement, timing of reduction and treatment, open versus closed reduction, and decompression of the hip capsule releasing the tamponade effect on the epiphyseal circulation have been shown in a number of studies to have some contributing effect.[113,114,118-121] Other than initial displacement, these factors are modifiable by the treating orthopaedic surgeon.

Fracture displacement is associated with higher energy injuries, and displaced fractures typically have a higher rate of osteonecrosis.[106,110,122] Despite this, not all displaced femoral neck fractures develop osteonecrosis and some nondisplaced fractures do.[110] Timely reduction (<24 hours from time of injury) is thought to lessen osteonecrosis risk,[109] but this concept has not always been shown consistently to be predictive of lower osteonecrosis rates.[110,120,122] Decompression of the hip hemarthrosis with a hip capsulotomy or aspiration makes sense to do in the setting of closed reduction[123,124] but may not have a direct impact on lowering the rate of osteonecrosis.[109,110] Because timely reduction and hip joint decompression are aspects under the surgeon's control, many pursue a "cannot hurt, might help avoid osteonecrosis" approach.

Other complications associated with pediatric hip fractures include nonunion (10.8%), coxa vara (18.5%), and proximal femoral growth irregularity (21.8%).[109] Delbet II fractures have the highest rate of nonunion.[109] Factors affecting nonunion rates are quality of reduction, verticality of the femoral neck fracture angle (Pauwel angle), and stability of fixation.[111] Posttraumatic coxa vara may develop following loss of reduction, development of osteonecrosis, nonunion, greater trochanteric overgrowth, or premature physeal closure. It was more commonly seen with closed treatment without fixation of femoral neck fractures, and the use of fixation has decreased this complication.[125] Premature physeal closure/growth irregularity may occur from the traumatic injury or from implants crossing the physis. Based on the age of the patient, this can lead to leg length discrepancy, angular deformity of the hip, and/or greater trochanteric overgrowth.[101] Case reports and a small case series have suggested that delayed slipped capital femoral epiphysis is another potential complication that can occur after surgical fixation of a femoral neck fracture when the implants stop short of the physis.[126]

FEMUR SHAFT FRACTURES

The treatment of pediatric diaphyseal femur fractures (PDFFs) is a mainstay of pediatric orthopaedic trauma practice. These fractures are the most common pediatric orthopaedic injury resulting in hospital admission in the United States.[125] Given their frequency, the American Academy of Orthopaedic Surgeons (AAOS) created evidence-based guidelines for treatment of PDFFs. These were first published in 2009,[127] and an update was published in 2015.[128,129] These recommendations, however, lacked comprehensive guidance for many common clinical scenarios, and recent studies have shown that these guidelines are not routinely followed as the standard of care for PDFFs.[130,131]

When evaluating a patient with a PDFF, the orthopaedic surgeon aspires to provide the treatment with the optimal outcome that places the minimum burden on the patient and family.[132] This decision is made by considering the patient's age, weight, fracture pattern, and stage of skeletal maturation. This decision can be influenced by the patient's overall medical condition and specific resources available to the surgeon.

Treatment Options by Age

During the first 6 months of life, most femoral shaft fractures can be safely treated in a Pavlik harness.[133] Although this brace is designed for the treatment of hip dysplasia in this age group, it also positions the limb in the ideal position for femoral shaft fracture alignment as well as routine infant care. Because the brace is not rigid, infants may experience more discomfort until initial fracture callous develops. The trade-off for this is a significant decrease in the skin complications associated with having young patients in a spica cast.[133,134] Although fractures may heal with some angulation, a 2013 study reported excellent clinical outcomes at an average follow-up of 5 years post injury.[135] (Note: all femur fractures in children younger than 36 months should be assessed for possible nonaccidental trauma.[136]

Children aged 6 to 60 months (fifth birthday) are most frequently treated with reduction of their fracture as necessary and application of a hip spica cast. Incomplete and nondisplaced fractures can be treated in a walking spica cast.[137] Complete fractures with displacement or shortening are more commonly treated in a standard hip spica cast. A single or double leg spica cast may be used, although the single leg variety may place less stress on the family regarding care and transportation issues.[138] This is most often done with the child under anesthesia in the operating room, although this may be performed in the emergency department setting at substantially lower cost.[139,140] A degree of malunion will occur with this treatment, but the routine amount of shortening, rotation, and coronal and sagittal plane angulation seen with spica casting will regularly remodel to the point of clinical irrelevance.[141] Careful molding of the cast and placing the initial reduction in mild valgus and recurvatum can limit the degree of malunion.[142] Despite this, some authors propose elastic nailing in this age group. The authors noted similar healing times, with earlier return to independent ambulation and full activities in the elastic nailing group.[143]

In the 5-year-old to 11-year-old age group, the size of the children, the rate of malunion, and the time in cast required to heal start to make spica casting a less attractive option for treatment. Titanium elastic nails (TENs) has become the standard treatment in this age group. The nails are sized to fit the patient, are inserted via a retrograde physeal-sparing technique, and allow early mobilization without external stabilization.[144] Attention to specific technical points, such as >80% canal fill at the isthmus,[145] leaving <2.5 cm of the nail out of the entry point,[146] and diverging the position of the tips in the sagittal plane,[147] helped avoid some issues with malunion. With increased experience, however, it became evident that some subgroups in this age demographic had a higher complication rate with TENs. Specifically, older patients (older than 10 years),[146,148] heavier patients (greater than 50 kg),[149] and length-unstable fracture patterns (Orthopaedic Trauma Association A2, B, and C patterns)[150] were identified as having a higher complication rate, requiring modifications of the standard technique. The use of stiffer stainless steel nails,[151-153] Enders nails with a distal locking screw,[154] and stacked nails (more than two)[155,156] has expanded the ability to use flexible nailing technique in older and heavier patients. In unstable fracture patterns, submuscular plating has been described as another option to treat the patient with PDFF at risk of malunion with TENs management.[157,158] This technique can also be used to treat proximal or distal third femur fractures in this age demographic.[159] Submuscular plating technique, however, carries with it its own set of complications.[160,161]

Lateral trochanteric entry antegrade rigid locked nails have gained favor in such circumstances, particularly in patients older than 8 years with an intramedullary canal of ample size[162] (**Figure 4**). The safe lower age limit of rigid intramedullary nailing is unclear. This is not a physeal sparing technique, with trochanteric entry nails traversing the greater trochanteric epiphyseal plate. A 2014 study of 241 patients with 246 fractures identified postoperative changes in the articulotrochanteric distance in 15.1% of patients, but no patient had clinical symptoms associated with this.[163] A piriformis fossa entry

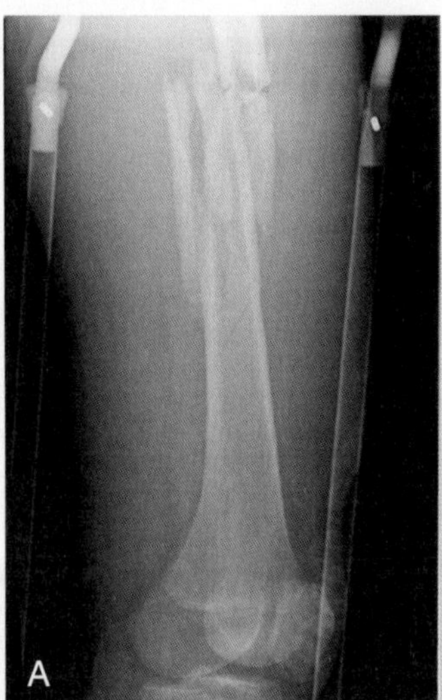

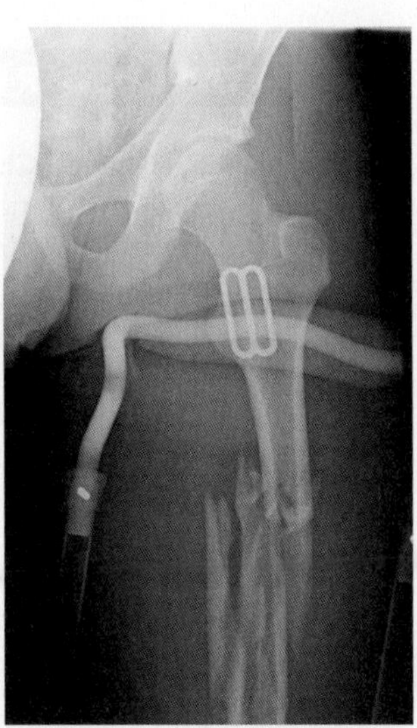
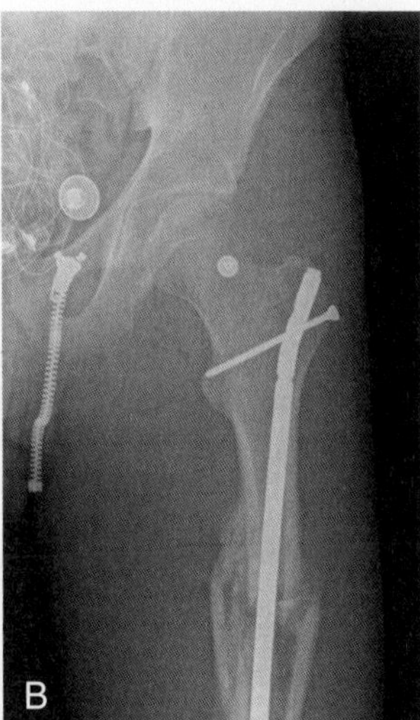

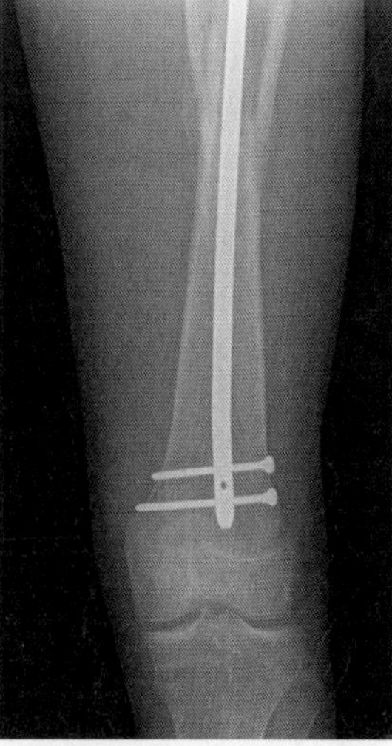

FIGURE 4 **A**, AP radiographs of the left femur of a 14-year-old boy involved in a motor vehicle accident. He underwent intramedullary fixation. Attention was given to the limb length because of the comminution as well as rotation. **B**, AP radiographs 6 weeks post surgery shows abundant callus formation. The patient had started full weight bearing the week before without any pain.

point cannot be used in the skeletally immature because of the risk of injury to the proximal femoral circulation and subsequent osteonecrosis. The incidence of osteonecrosis with trochanteric entry is substantially lower, but not zero,[164] and the surgeon must have an excellent understanding of the safe window through which trochanteric entry may be performed.[165,166] Locked rigid nailing is the treatment of choice in adults with femoral shaft fractures, and in patients 12 years of age and older, trochanteric entry antegrade rigid nailing becomes the preferred treatment as well.[128]

Subtrochanteric Femur Fractures

Subtrochanteric femoral fractures are more challenging to manage because of the opposing forces displacing the fracture fragments and the problems this causes with reduction and fixation. Although these fractures are relatively rare in children,[167] this makes their management all the more challenging for the treating surgeon. Because of the changing body dimensions of growing children, these fractures have been defined as occurring within 10% of the total femoral length (as measured from the top of the femoral head to the bottom of the medial femoral condyle) below the lesser trochanter.[168] With some modifications, these fractures can be managed within the age-specific and weight-specific guidelines outlined earlier. At a younger age, spica cast management is effective as these fractures will remodel notably. In the school-aged patient of appropriate size, flexible nailing can be considered if the standard technique is modified.[168,169] As the patients get older and heavier, plating or nailing has been advocated.[170-172]

SUMMARY

Fractures of the pelvis and acetabulum are rare in children. Pelvic ring injuries are typically secondary to high-energy trauma. The management of pelvis injuries should be multidisciplinary to manage the associated injuries in these patients that carry a substantial morbidity and mortality.

The presence of the TRC influences the fracture patterns of acetabular fractures. Fracture patterns before TRC closure are different than the more adult patterns of injury seen after TRC closure. Hip dislocations generally occur after high-energy trauma in adolescents. However, younger children can sustain hip dislocations after relatively minor trauma. Urgent and gentle reduction is recommended to minimize the risk of posttraumatic osteonecrosis and the potential of epiphysiolysis. Careful examination and imaging post reduction is necessary to confirm concentric reduction and joint stability.

Femoral neck fractures are associated with an inherent high complication rate. Femoral shaft fractures are the most common musculoskeletal injury requiring a hospital admission. The patient's age, weight, fracture pattern, and skeletal maturity status determine the treatment of femoral shaft fractures.

KEY STUDY POINTS

- Pelvic fractures in skeletally immature patients are a marker of high-energy injury, and evaluation for concomitant injuries, both musculoskeletal and other, is prudent.
- Pelvis fractures in pediatric patients are associated with less life-threatening hemorrhage than is seen in adults.
- MRI should be strongly considered when evaluating the acetabulum after hip dislocation in the skeletally immature. Large cartilaginous fragments and labral injuries can be easily underestimated by a plain radiograph and CT.
- Care must be taken when reducing hip dislocations in skeletally immature adolescents to avoid epiphysiolysis of the femoral head and subsequent osteonecrosis.
- The Delbet classification is the most reliable prognostic indicator of osteonecrosis risk in pediatric femoral neck fractures.
- Femur fractures are managed based on the age and weight of the patient, fracture type, and the patient's skeletal maturity. Undertreatment and overtreatment of these fractures can be avoided by respecting these treatment parameters.

ANNOTATED REFERENCES

1. Silber JS, Flynn JM: Changing patterns of pediatric fractures with skeletal maturation: Implications for classification and management. *J Pediatr Orthop* 2002;22:22-26.
2. Kruppa CG, Khoriaty JD, Sietsema DL, Dudda M, Schildhauer TA, Jones CB: Does skeletal maturity affect pediatric pelvic injury patterns, associated injuries and treatment intervention? *Injury* 2018;49(8):1562-1567.

   This is a retrospective review of pediatric patients with PRI. Skeletally mature children are more likely to sustain more complex injury patterns with a higher rate of surgical treatment. They also have a higher rate of associated injuries and higher injury severity score than immature patients. Level of evidence: III.
3. Shore BJ, Palmer CS, Bevin C, Johnson MB, Torode IP: Pediatric pelvic fracture: A modification of a preexisting classification. *J Pediatr Orthop* 2012;32(2):162-168.

4. Hermans E, Cornelisse ST, Biert J, Tan ECTH, Edwards MJR: Paediatric pelvic fracture: How do they differ from adults? *J Child Orthop* 2017;11:49-56.

   This is a retrospective chart review of 51 children and 368 adults with PRI demonstrating differences in their presentation, associated injuries, and treatment. Children had similar mortality rates to adults, and mortality was often due to concomitant injuries rather than exsanguination from a PRI. Adults had higher injury severity score and more severe PRI and were more often hemodynamically unstable. Level of evidence: III.

5. Shaath MK, Koury KL, Gibson PD, et al: Analysis of pelvic fracture pattern and overall orthopaedic injury burden in children sustaining pelvic fractures based on skeletal maturity. *J Child Orthop* 2017;11:195-200.

   This is a retrospective review comparing 178 pediatric patients with PRI and TRC-open versus TRC-closed. Patients with TRC-open were more likely to sustain rami fractures and stable PRI, whereas patients with TRC-closed were more likely to sustain acetabular fractures, hip dislocations, and unstable PRI. Additionally, patients with TRC-closed were more likely to be treated surgically for their pelvic injury. Level of evidence: III.

6. Ismail N, Bellemare JF, Mollit DL, DiScala C, Koeppel B, Tepas JJ: Death from pelvic fracture: Children are different. *J Pediatr Surg* 1996;31(1):82-85.

7. Demetriades D, Karaiskakis M, Velmahos GC, Alo K, Murray J, Chan L: Pelvic fracture in pediatric and adult trauma patients: Are they different injuries? *J Trauma* 2003;54(6):1146-1151.

8. Chotai N, Alazzawi S, Zehra SS, Barry M: Paediatric pelvic fractures: A review of 2 cohorts over 22 years. *Injury* 2018;49:613-617.

   This is a retrospective review of two separate cohorts of children with PRI (2007-2016 versus 1994-2003) demonstrating an increase in the frequency and severity of injuries and a decrease in mortality from these injuries over time. Level of evidence: III.

9. Kenaway M: Surgical consideration with the operative fixation of unstable pediatric pelvic ring injuries. *Int Orthop* 2017;41(9):1791-1801.

   This is a retrospective review of 29 pediatric patients who underwent surgical fixation by various techniques for their unstable PRI. The authors reported technical challenges to consider in the pediatric patient including reduction of an avulsed iliac apophysis, hardware penetration of sacroiliac screws, and poor purchase of retrograde LC screws. They favored supra-acetabular external fixation for anterior fixation in children. Level of evidence: IV.

10. Oransky M, Arduini M, Tortora M, Zoppi AR: Surgical treatment of unstable pelvic fracture in children: Long term results. *Injury* 2010;41(11):1140-1144.

11. Bucholz RW, Ezaki M, Ogden JA: Injury to the acetabular triradiate physeal cartilage. *J Bone Joint Surg Am* 1982;64(4):600-609.

12. Zwingmann J, Lefering R, Maier D, et al: Pelvic fractures in severely injured children – Results from the TraumaRegister DGU. *Medicine (Baltimore)* 2018;97:(35):e11955.

    This is a prospective multicenter study of the German Trauma Registry analyzing the effect of PRI and mortality in 9,684 pediatric patients of varying age groups. Results show mortality to be associated with the severity of the PRI but lower than the Revised Injury Severity Classification II score prognosis. Level of evidence: III.

13. Gansslen A, Heidari N, Weinberg AM: Fractures of the pelvis in children: A review of the literature. *Eur J Orthop Surg Traumatol* 2013;23(8):847-861.

14. Vitale MG, Kessler MW, Choe JC, Hwang MW, Tolo VT, Skaggs DL: Pelvic fracture in children: An exploration of practice patterns and patient outcomes. *J Pediatr Orthop* 2005;25:581-587.

15. Grisoni N, Connor S, Marsh E, Thompson GH, Cooperman DR, Blakemore LC: Pelvic fractures in a pediatric level 1 trauma center. *J Orthop Trauma* 2002;16(7):458-463.

16. Naqvi G, Johansson G, Yip G, Rehm A, Carrothers A, Stohr K: Mechanisms, patterns and outcomes of paediatric polytrauma in a UK major trauma centre. *Ann R Coll Surg Engl* 2017;99:39-45.

    This is a retrospective review of pediatric trauma admissions at a level I trauma center in the United Kingdom demonstrating a 7% rate of PRIs among pediatric trauma admissions. Level of evidence: IV.

17. Marmor M, Elson J, Mikhail C, Morshed S, Matityahu A: Short-term pelvic fracture outcomes in adolescents differ from children and adults in the National Trauma Data Bank. *J Child Orthop* 2015;9(1):65-75.

18. Zwingmann J, Aghayev E, Sudkamp NP, et al: Pelvic fractures in children results from the German Pelvic Trauma Registry. *Medicine (Baltimore)* 2015;94(51):e2325.

19. de la Calva C, Jover N, Alonso J, Salom M: Pediatric pelvic fractures and differences compared with the adult population. *Pediatr Emerg Care* 2020;36(11):519-522.

    This is a retrospective review of skeletally immature patients with PRI demonstrating that despite having less severe pelvic injury patterns, children sustain PRI after high-energy trauma with a very high rate of associated injuries. Level of evidence: IV.

20. Guerra MRV, Braga SR, Akkari M, Santili C: Pelvic injury in childhood: What is its current importance? *Acta Ortop Bras* 2016;24(3):155-158.

    This is a retrospective review of 25 patients 16 years of age or younger who sustained a PRI with a high reported mortality rate (12%) and rate of associated injuries. Level of evidence: IV.

21. Gansslen A, Hildebrand F, Heidari N, Weinberg AM: Acetabular fractures in children: A review of the literature. *Acta Chir Orthop Traumatol Cech* 2013;80(1):10-14.

22. Leonard M, Ibrahim M, Mckenna P, Boran S, McCormack D: Paediatric pelvic ring fractures and associated injuries. *Injury* 2011;42(10):1027-1030.

23. Galano GJ, Vitale MA, Kessler MW, et al: The most frequent traumatic orthopaedic injuries from a national pediatric inpatient population. *J Pediatr Orthop* 2005;35:39-44.

24. Subasi M, Arslan H, Onen A, Ozen S, Kaya M: Long-term outcomes of conservatively treated paediatric pelvic fractures. *Injury* 2004;35(8):771-781.

25. Smith WR, Oakley M, Morgan SJ: Pediatric pelvic fractures. *J Pediatr Orthop* 2004;24(1):130-135.

26. Tuovinen H, Söderlund T, Lindahl J, Laine T, Åström P, Handolin L: Severe pelvic fracture-related bleeding in pediatric patients: Does it occur? *Eur J Trauma Emerg Surg* 2012;38(2):163-169.

27. Tile M: Acute pelvic fractures: I. Causation and classification. *J Am Acad Orthop Surg* 1996;4:143-151.

28. Torode I, Zieg D: Pelvic fractures in children. *J Pediatr Orthop* 1985;5(1):76-84.

29. Kenaway M: MRI evaluation of the posterior pelvic bony and soft tissues with Tile C displaced pelvic fractures in young children. *J Pediatr Orthop* 2020;40(7):e579-e586.

    This is a retrospective review of eight patients with evidence of iliac apophysis avulsion on MRI. The authors describe the radiographic findings of this pathology including intact attachment of the iliac apopyhsis to the posterior sacroiliac complex with displacement of the bony ilium. This finding must be considered when fixing this injury as the iliac wing must actually be reduced to the apophysis. Level of evidence: IV.

30. Junkins EP, Nelson DS, Carroll KL, Hansen K, Furnival RA: A prospective evaluation of the clinical presentation of pediatric pelvic fractures. *J Trauma* 2001;51:64-68.

31. McAlister DM, Webb HR, Wheeler PD, et al: Pubic symphyseal width in pediatric patients. *J Pediatr Orthop* 2005;25:725-727.

32. Nejad AH, Jamali A, Wooton-Gorges SL, Boakes JL, Ferguson TA: Symphysis pubis width in the pediatric population: A computerized tomography study. *J Trauma Acute Care Surg* 2012;73:923-927.

33. Oetgen ME, Andelman S, Martin BD: Age-based normative measurements of the pediatric pelvis. *J Orthop Trauma* 2017;31:e205-e209.

    This is a retrospective analysis of 821 pelvic CT scans in pediatric patients to establish normative age-based measurements of the widths of the pubic symphysis, sacroiliac joints (SIJs), and TRC demonstrating an age-dependent decrease in the widths of the pubic symphysis and SIJ but not the TRC, which remains relatively stable until its closure. Level of evidence: III.

34. Bayer J, Neubauer J, Saueressig U, Sudkamp NP, Reising K: Radiological evaluation of the posterior pelvic ring in paediatric patients: Results of a retrospective study developing age- and gender-related non-osseous baseline characteristics in paediatric pelvic computed tomography – References for suspected sacroiliac joint injury. *Injury* 2016;47(4):853-858.

    This is a retrospective review of 427 CT scans in pediatric patients to establish age-based and gender-based normative data of the sacroiliac joint width in children demonstrating distinct changes with growth. They recommend considering sacroiliac injury if joint width exceeds the 97th percentile published in their study. Level of evidence: III.

35. Misiura AK, Nanassy AD, Urbine J: Usefulness of pelvic radiographs in the initial trauma evaluation with concurrent CT: Is additional radiation exposure necessary? *Int J Pediatr* 2018;2018:6260954.

    This is a retrospective review of pediatric patients after trauma where 34% of pelvic fractures identified on CT were missed on initial radiographs. The authors suggest that there is no added benefit of pelvic radiograph when concurrent CT is also obtained and should be omitted. Level of evidence: IV.

36. Bent MA, Hennrikus WL, Latorre JE, et al: Role of computed tomography in the classification of pediatric pelvic fracture – Revisited. *J Orthop Trauma* 2017;31:e200-e204.

    This is a retrospective chart review of 30 pediatric patients with pelvic fractures with both CT and radiograph for comparison. The authors found that although CT identified fractures missed on radiographs alone, these findings did not alter management. They recommended selective use of pelvic CT in pediatric trauma patients. Level of evidence: IV.

37. Smith W, Shurnas P, Morgan S, et al: Clinical outcomes of unstable pelvic fractures in skeletally immature patients. *J Bone Joint Surg Am* 2005;87(11):2423-2431.

38. Gardner MJ, Routt C: The anti-shock iliosacral screw. *J Orthop Trauma* 2010;24(10):86-89.

39. Abrassart S, Stern R, Peter R: Unstable pelvic ring injury with hemodynamic instability: What seems the best procedure choice and sequence in the initial management? *Orthop Traumatol Surg Res* 2013;99(2):175-182.

40. Vo NJ, Althoen M, Hippe DS, Prabhu SJ, Valji K, Padia SA: Pediatric abdominal and pelvic trauma: Safety and efficacy of arterial embolization. *J Vasc Interv Radiol* 2014;25(2):215-220.

41. Tanizaki S, Maeda S, Matano H, Sera M, Nagai H, Ishida H: Time to pelvic embolization for hemodynamically unstable pelvic fractures may affect the survival for delays up to 60 min. *Injury* 2014;45(4):738-741.

42. Scolaro JA, Firoozabadi R, Routt MLC: Treatment of pediatric and adolescent pelvic ring injuries with percutaneous screw placement. *J Pediatr Orthop* 2018;38(3):133-137.

    This is a retrospective review of surgically treated PRIs in children. Most of the pediatric PRIs can be treated without surgery. In the setting of instability, percutaneous pelvic screw fixation can be performed safely. Level of evidence: IV.

43. Guimaraes JA, Mendes PH, Vallim FC, et al: Surgical treatment for unstable pelvic fractures in skeletally immature patients. *Injury* 2014;45(suppl 5):S40-S45.

44. Karunakar MA, Goulet JA, Mueller KL, Bedi A, Le TT: Operative treatment of unstable pediatric pelvis and acetabular fractures. *J Pediatr Orthop* 2005;25(1):34-38.

45. Langford JR, Burgess AR, Liporace FA, Haidukewych GJ: Pelvic fractures: Part 2. Contemporary indications and techniques for definitive surgical management. *J Am Acad Orthop Surg* 2013;21:458-468.

46. Whiting PS, Auston D, Avilucea FR, et al: Negative stress examination under anesthesia reliably predicts pelvic ring union without displacement. *J Orthop Trauma* 2017;31(4):189-193.

    This is a retrospective cohort study of 34 adults with closed PRIs that underwent stress EUA to assess the stability of their PRI. A negative EUA accurately predicted pelvic stability and union without displacement after weight bearing as tolerated. Level of evidence: III.

47. Sagi CH, Coniglione F, Stanford JH: Examination under anesthetic for occult pelvic ring instability. *J Orthop Trauma* 2011;25(9):529-536.
48. Baskin KM, Cahill AM, Kaye RD, et al: Closed reduction with CT-guided screw fixation for unstable sacroiliac joint fracture-dislocation. *Pediatr Radiol* 2004;34:963-969.
49. Burn M, Gary JL, Holzman M, et al: Do safe radiographic sacral screw pathways exist in a pediatric patient population and do they change with age? *J Orthop Trauma* 2016;30:41-47.

    This study includes an analysis of pelvic CT in pediatric patients to determine the rate of radiographically safe osseous pathways for iliosacral and transsacral style screws after PRI. The authors found that nearly all patients could accommodate an iliosacral screw in the first sacral segment. The second sacral segment could accommodate transsacral screw in most patients, especially in older children. However, only half of the patients could accommodate a transsacral screw in the second sacral segment. Level of evidence: II.

50. Starr AJ, Ortega G, Reinert CM: Management of an unstable pelvic ring disruption in a 20-month-old-patient. *J Orthop Trauma* 2009;23(2):159-162.
51. Eberbach H, Hohloch L, Feucht MJ, Konstantinidis L, Sudkamp NP, Zwingmann J: Operative versus conservative treatment of apophyseal avulsion fractures of the pelvis in the adolescents: A systematical review with meta-analysis of clinical outcome and return to sports. *BMC Musculoskelet Disord* 2017;18(1):162.

    This is a systematic review and meta-analysis of pelvic apophyseal avulsion fractures. Surgical fixation had better overall outcomes including return to sport compared with nonsurgical management when fracture displaced >15 mm. Level of evidence: II.

52. Sathya C, Alali AS, Wales PW, et al: Mortality among injured children treated at different trauma center types. *JAMA Surg* 2015;150:874-881.
53. Morshed S, Knops S, Jurkovich GJ, Wang J, Mackenzie E, Rivara FP: The impact of trauma-center care on mortality and function following pelvic ring and acetabular injuries. *J Bone Joint Surg Am* 2015;97:265-272.
54. Keshishyan RA, Rozinov VM, Malakohov OA, et al: Pelvic polyfractures in children. Radiographic diagnosis and treatment. *Clin Orthop Relat Res* 1995;320:28-33.
55. Gobba M, Khaled SA, Galal A, Azeem HA: Functional outcome of pelvic fractures in children: Does age affect outcome? *Egypt Orthop J* 2017;52:72-77.

    This is a prospective study of 30 pediatric patients with PRI comparing functional and radiologic outcomes according to treatment and age. Similar results were obtained between surgical and nonsurgical management (although surgical injuries were more severe). Children younger than 7 years had significantly better outcome measures at 6 months. Level of evidence: III.

56. Signorino PR, Densmore J, Werner M, et al: Pediatric pelvic injury: Functional outcome at 6-month follow-up. *J Pediatr Surg* 2005;40(1):107-112.
57. Schwarz N, Posch E, Mayr J, Fischmeister FM, Schwarz AF, Ohner T: Long-term results of unstable pelvic ring fractures in children. *Injury* 1998;29:431-433.
58. McLaren AC, Rorabeck CH, Halpenny J: Long-term pain and disability in relation to residual deformity after displaced pelvic ring fractures. *Can J Surg* 1990;33(6):492-494.
59. Von Heyden J, Hauschild O, Strohm PC, Stuby F, Sudkamp NP, Schmal H: Pediatric acetabular fractures: Data from the German Pelvic Trauma Registry Initiative. *Acta Orthop Belg* 2012;78(5):611-618.
60. Dimeglio A: Growth in pediatric orthopaedics. *J Pediatr Orthop* 2001;21:549-555.
61. Watts HG: Fractures of the pelvis in children. *Orthop Clin North Am* 1976;7:615-624.
62. Letournel É: Acetabulum fractures: Classification and management. *Clin Orthop Relat Res* 1980;151:81-106.
63. Tannast MM, Najibi SS, Matta JM: Two to twenty-year survivorship of the hip in 810 patients with operatively treated acetabular fractures. *J Bone Joint Surg Am* 2012;94(17):1559-1567.
64. Heeg M, de Ridder VA, Tornetta P, de Lange S, Klasen HJ: Acetabular fractures in children and adolescents. *Clin Orthop Relat Res* 2000;375:80-86.
65. Sen MK, Warner SJ, Sama N, et al: Treatment of acetabular fractures in adolescents. *Am J Orthop (Belle Mead NJ)* 2015;44(10):465-470.
66. Shaath MK, Ippolito JA, Adams MR, Sirkin MS, Reilly MC: The role of computed tomographic scan in the diagnosis of acetabular fracture in the immature pelvis. *J Orthop Trauma* 2019;33(2):S32-S36.

    This is a retrospective case series of 16 acetabular fractures identified on CT that were initially missed on plain radiographs in 69% of cases and 91% of cases in children younger than 12 years. The authors recommend obtaining a CT scan in all skeletally immature patients with suspected pelvic injury. Level of evidence: IV.

67. Parvaresh KC, Pennock AT, Bomar JD, Wenger DR, Upasani VV: Analysis of acetabular ossification from the triradiate cartilage and secondary centers. *J Pediatr Orthop* 2018;38(3):e145-e150.

    This is a retrospective analysis of 159 CT scans of children aged 6 to 16 years demonstrating a sequential appearance of the secondary ossification centers of the acetabulum that close before closure of the TRC, generally 2 to 3 years later in boys than in girls. Level of evidence: III.

68. Fabricant PD, Hirsch BP, Holmes I, et al: A radiographic study of the ossification of the posterior wall of the acetabulum: Implications for the diagnosis of pediatric and adolescent hip disorders. *J Bone Joint Surg Am* 2013;95:230-236.

69. Blanchard C, Kushare I, Boyles A, Mundy A, Beebe AC, Klingele KE: Traumatic, posterior pediatric hip dislocations with associated posterior labrum osteochondral avulsion: Recognizing the acetabular "fleck" sign. *J Pediatr Orthop* 2016;36:602-607.

    This is a retrospective case review of 10 patients treated surgically for traumatic posterior hip dislocations and suspected associated labral tears and fractures. The authors describe the fleck sign on CT that coincides with a large posterior ostechondral labral avulsion seen intraoperatively. Level of evidence: IV.

70. Thanacharoenpanich S, Bixby S, Breen MA, Kim YJ: MRI is better than CT Scan for detection of structural pathologies after traumatic posterior hip dislocation in children and adolescents. *J Pediatr Orthop* 2020;40(2):86-92.

    This is a retrospective review of imaging in 27 pediatric patients after traumatic hip dislocation. The authors found MRI to be superior to CT scan for detection of structural injuries. Some of the unique structural injuries including entrapment of posterior labrum and posterior unossified acetabular fractures could be seen only on an MRI, which can impact treatment decision making. Level of evidence: IV.

71. Yee MA, Davis ME, Perdue AM, Hake ME: Examination under anesthesia for evaluation of hip stability in posterior wall acetabulum fractures. *J Orthop Trauma* 2019;33:S19-S21.

    This is a case-based description of the pelvic EUA technique for assessing stability of posterior wall fracture in adults. Level of evidence: V.

72. Ziran N, Soles GLS, Matta JM: Outcomes after surgical treatment of acetabular fractures: A review. *Patient Saf Surg* 2019;13:16.

    This is a literature review summarizing the factors that affect clinical outcomes after surgical treatment of acetabular fractures. The authors highlight the evidence supporting articular reduction as the most influential factor affecting outcomes. Level of evidence: V.

73. Liporace FA, Ong B, Mohaideen A, Ong A, Koval KJ: Development and injury of the triradiate cartilage with its effects on acetabular development: Review of the literature. *J Trauma* 2003;54:1245-1249.

74. Ponseti IV: Growth and development of the acetabulum in the normal child: Anatomical, histological and roentgenographic studies. *J Bone Joint Surg Am* 1978;60:575-585.

75. Trousdale RT, Ganz R: Posttraumatic acetabular dysplasia. *Clin Orthop Relat Res* 1994;305:124-132.

76. Badina A, Vialle R, Fitoussi F, Damsin JP: Case reports: Treatment of traumatic triradiate cartilage epiphysiodesis. *Clin Orthop Relat Res* 2013;471:3701-3705.

77. Herrera-Soto JA, Price CT: Traumatic hip dislocations in children and adolescents: Pitfalls and complications. *J Am Acad Orthop Surg* 2009;17(1):15-21.

78. Vialle R, Odent T, Pannier S, Pauthier F, Laumonier F, Glorion C: Traumatic hip dislocation in childhood. *J Pediatr Orthop* 2005;25(2):138-144.

79. Sulaiman AR, Munajat I, Mohd FE: Outcome of traumatic hip dislocation in children. *J Pediatr Orthop B* 2013;22:557-562.

80. Podeszwa DA, De La Rocha A, Larson AN, Sucato DJ: Surgical hip dislocation is safe and effective following acute traumatic hip instability in the adolescent. *J Pediatr Orthop* 2015;35(5):435-442.

81. Morris AC, Yu JC, Gilbert SR: Arthroscopic treatment of traumatic hip dislocations in children and adolescents: A preliminary study. *J Pediatr Orthop* 2017;37(7):435-439.

    This is a retrospective review of seven patients (ages of 8 to 17 years) who had incongruent reduction of a traumatic hip dislocation. The patients were treated with hip arthroscopy and reduction and/or débridement of impediments to reduction without repair. Osteonecrosis or recurrent instability did not develop in any of the patients. Level of evidence: IV.

82. Mehlman CT, Hubbard GW, Crawford AH, Roy DR, Wall EJ: Traumatic hip dislocation in children. Long-term followup of 42 patients. *Clin Orthop Relat Res* 2000;376:68-79.

83. Manner HM, Mast NH, Ganz R, et al: Potential contribution of femoroacetabular impingement to recurrent traumatic hip dislocation. *J Pediatr Orthop B* 2012;21:574-578.

84. Kutty S, Thornes B, Curtin WA, Gilmore MF: Traumatic posterior dislocation of the hip in children. *Pediatr Emerg Care* 2001;17:32-35.

85. Herrera-Soto JA, Price CT, Reuss BL, Riley P, Kasser JR, Beaty JH: Proximal femoral epiphysiolysis during reduction of hip dislocation in adolescents. *J Pediatr Orthop* 2006;26(3):371-374.

86. Kennon JC, Bohsali KI, Ogden JA, Ogden J, Goney TM: Adolescent hip dislocation combined with proximal femoral physeal fractures and epiphysiolysis. *J Pediatr Orthop* 2016;36:253-261.

    This is a retrospective review of 12 adolescent patients with traumatic hip dislocation and associated proximal femoral epiphysiolysis, three of which occurred iatrogenically in the emergency department under conscious sedation. Nine patients subsequently developed osteonecrosis. The authors recommend performing closed reduction in the operating room with muscle relaxation to prevent iatrogenic injury. Level of evidence: IV.

87. Zupanc O, Krizancic M, Daniel M, et al: Shear stress in epiphyseal growth plate is a risk factor for slipped capital femoral epiphysis. *J Pediatr Orthop* 2008;28:444-451.

88. Shapiro F: Pathophysiologic approaches to growth plate fracture-separations, in *Pediatric Orthopedic Deformities, Volume 1: Pathobiology and Treatment of Dysplasias, Physeal Fractures, Length Discrepancies and Epiphyseal and Joint Disorders.* Switzerland, Springer International Publishing, 2015, pp 526-546.

89. Odent T, Glorion C, Pannier S, Bronfen C, Lagnlais J, Pouliquen JC: Traumatic dislocation of the hip with separation of the capital epiphysis: 5 adolescent patients with 3-9 years of follow-up. *Acta Orthop Scand* 2003;74:49-52.

90. Novais EN, Heare TC, Hill MK, Mayer SW: Surgical hip dislocation for the treatment of intra-articular injuries and hip instability following traumatic posterior dislocation in children and adolescents. *J Pediatr Orthop* 2016;35:673-679.

This is a retrospective review of eight patients with traumatic hip dislocation who underwent SHD for nonconcentric reductions and intra-articular pathology (capsule-labral complex disruptions, posterior wall fractures, and femoral head fractures). The authors propose the SHD as a safe and effective option for these patients with direct access to intra-articular pathology for repair. Level of evidence: IV.

91. Price CT, Pyevich MT, Knapp DR, Phillips JH, Hawker JJ: Traumatic hip dislocation with spontaneous, incomplete reduction: A diagnostic trap. *J Orthop Trauma* 2002;16(10):730-735.

92. Mayer SW, Stewart JR, Fadell MF, Kestel L, Novais EN: MRI as a reliable and accurate method for assessment of posterior hip dislocation in children and adolescents without the risk of radiation exposure. *Pediatr Radiol* 2015;45:1355-1362.

93. Hearty T, Swaroop VT, Gourineni P, Robinson L: Standard radiographs and computed tomographic scan underestimating pediatric acetabular fracture after traumatic hip dislocation: Report of 2 cases. *J Orthop Trauma* 2011;25:e68-e73.

94. Rubel IF, Kloen P, Potter HG, Helfet DL: MRI assessment of the posterior acetabular wall fracture in traumatic dislocation of the hip in children. *Pediatr Radiol* 2002;32:435-439.

95. Vialle R, Pannier S, Odent T, Schmit P, Pauthier F, Glorion C: Imaging of traumatic dislocation of the hip in childhood. *Pediatr Radiol* 2004;34:970-979.

96. Kruppa CG, Sietsema DL, Khoriaty JD, Dudda M, Schildhauer TA, Jones CB: Acetabular fractures in children and adolescents: Comparison of isolated acetabular fractures and acetabular fractures associated with pelvic ring injuries. *J Orthop Trauma* 2018;32(2):e39-e45.

This is a retrospective cohort comparative analysis between isolated acetabular fractures and those associated with PRI. Isolated injuries were most commonly posterior wall fractures, associated with greater displacement and more frequent surgical fixation than those associated PRI. The PRI-associated acetabular fracture patients had higher incidence and severity of associated injuries. Level of evidence: III.

97. McCarthy JC, Noble PC, Schuck MR, Wright J, Lee K: The Otto E. Aufranc Award: The role of labral lesions to the development of early degenerative hip disease. *Clin Orthop Relat Res* 2001;393:25-37.

98. Clement RC, Carpenter DP, Cuomo AV: Spontaneous healing of a bucket-handle posterior labral detachment after hip dislocation in a five-year-old child: A case report. *JBJS Case Connect* 2018;8(2):e28.

This study is a case report of a 20-month-old girl with high-energy trauma and multiple injuries including a hip dislocation. Because of associated injuries, she was unable to undergo surgical fixation of a large labral tear, which was shown to heal spontaneously on a follow-up MRI 2 months after injury. She had an excellent outcome 2.5 years from injury. Level of evidence: V.

99. Banskota AK, Spiegel DA, Shrestha S, Shrestha OP, Rajbhandary T: Open reduction for neglected traumatic hip dislocation in children and adolescents. *J Pediatr Orthop* 2007;27(2):187-191.

100. Kumar S, Jain AK: Neglected traumatic hip dislocation in children. *Clin Orthop Relat Res* 2005;431:9-13.

101. Lark RK, Dial BL, Alman BA: Complications after pediatric hip fractures: Evaluation and management. *J Am Acad Orthop Surg* 2020;28:10-19.

The authors review the literature on the most common complications associated with pediatric femoral neck fractures, including osteonecrosis, nonunion, coxa vara, and premature physeal arrest. A review of management options for each complication is offered. The authors conclude that the best management is initial prevention stressing anatomic reduction and biomechanically stable fixation where warranted. Level of evidence: V.

102. Sankar WN, Mehlman CT: The community orthopaedic surgeon taking trauma call: Pediatric femoral neck fracture pearls and pitfalls. *J Orthop Trauma* 2019;33:S22-S26.

The authors review the pearls and pitfalls of emergent management of this injury, reviewing the Delbet classification and the potential for osteonecrosis. An excellent schematic diagram of the vasculature of the proximal femoral neck and epiphysis is included. Level of evidence: V.

103. Truetta J: The normal vascular anatomy of the human femoral head during growth. *J Bone Joint Surg Br* 1957;39:358-394.

104. Shrader MW, Schwab JH, Shaughnessy WJ, Jacofsky DJ: Pathologic femoral neck fractures in children. *Am J Orthop (Belle Mead NJ)* 2009;38:83-86.

105. Colonna PC: Fracture of the neck of the femur in children. *Am J Surg* 1929;6:793-797.

106. Moon ES, Mehlman CT: Risk factors for avascular necrosis after femoral neck fractures in children: 25 Cincinnati cases and meta-analysis of 360 cases. *J Orthop Trauma* 2006;20(5):323-329.

107. Shrader MW, Jacofsky DJ, Stans AA, Shaughnessy WJ, Haidukewych GJ: Femoral neck fractures in pediatric patients: 30 years experience at a level 1 trauma center. *Clin Orthop Relat Res* 2007;454:169-173.

108. Togrul E, Bayram H, Gulsen M, Kalaci A, Ozbarlas S: Fractures of the femoral neck in children: Long-term follow-up in 62 hip fractures. *Injury* 2005;36(1):123-130.

109. Yeranosian M, Horneff JG, Baldwin K, Hosalkar HS: Factors affecting the outcome of fractures of the femoral neck in children and adolescents. *Bone Joint J* 2013;95-B:135-142.

110. Spence D, DiMauro JP, Miller PE, Glotzbecker MP, Hedequist DJ, Shore BJ: Osteonecrosis after femoral neck fractures in children and adolescents: Analysis of risk factors. *J Pediatr Orthop* 2016;36:111-116.

This is a retrospective review of 70 patients with pediatric femoral neck fractures from one institution. Osteonecrosis developed in 29% of patients. The median time to diagnosis of osteonecrosis was 7.8 months. Predictors of osteonecrosis in their series were initial fracture displacement and Delbet classification. Level of evidence: III.

111. Dial BL, Lark RK: Pediatric proximal femur fractures. *J Orthop* 2018;15:529-535.

This is a review article on pediatric proximal femur fractures. In addition to reviewing the Delbet classification and the complications associated with these fractures, the authors offer a useful review of pediatric femoral neck fracture reduction and fixation techniques. Level of evidence: V.

112. Leadbetter GW: A treatment for fracture of the neck of the femur. Reprinted from *J Bone Joint Surg* 1938;20:108-113. *Clin Orthop Relat Res* 2002;399:4-8.

113. Boardman MJ, Herman MJ, Buck B, Pizzutillo PD: Hip fractures in children. *J Am Acad Orthop Surg* 2009;17(3):162-173.

114. Flynn JM, Wong KL, Yeh GL, Meyer JS, Davidson RS: Displaced fractures of the hip in children. Management by early operation and immobilisation in a hip spica cast. *J Bone Joint Surg Br* 2002;84(1):108-112.

115. Forster NA, Ramseier LE, Exner GU: Undisplaced femoral neck fractures in children have a high risk of secondary displacement. *J Pediatr Orthop B* 2006;15(2):131-133.

116. Patterson JT, Tangtiphaiboontana J, Pandya NK: Management of pediatric femoral neck fracture. *J Am Acad Orthop Surg* 2018;26:411-419.

This is an up-to-date comprehensive review of pediatric femoral neck fractures discussing classification, options for treatment, options for fixation, anticipated outcomes, and a review of potential complications. Level of evidence: V.

117. Molnar RB, Routt ML Jr: Open reduction of intracapsular hip fractures using a modified Smith-Petersen surgical exposure. *J Orthop Trauma* 2007;21:490-494.

118. Swiontkowski MF, Winquist RA: Displaced hip fractures in children and adolescents. *J Trauma* 1986;26(4):384-388.

119. Davison BL, Weinstein SL: Hip fractures in children: A long-term follow-up study. *J Pediatr Orthop* 1992;12(3):355-358.

120. Riley PM Jr, Morscher MA, Gothard MD, Riley PM Sr: Earlier time to reduction did not reduce rates of femoral head osteonecrosis in pediatric hip fractures. *J Orthop Trauma* 2015;29(5):231-238.

121. Stone JD, Hill MK, Pan Z, Novais EN: Open reduction of pediatric femoral neck fractures reduces osteonecrosis risk. *Orthopedics* 2015;38(11):e983-e990.

122. Al Khatib N, Younis MH, Hegazy A, Ibrahim T: Early versus late treatment of pediatric femoral neck fractures: A systematic review and meta-analysis. *Int Orthop* 2019;43:677-685.

The authors conducted a systematic review of the literature and a statistical meta-analysis in the attempt to evaluate if pediatric femoral neck fractures treated early (<24 hours) was associated with a lower rate of osteonecrosis than those treated late (>24 hours). They concluded that the cumulative evidence at present does not indicate an association between time to treatment or method of reduction of femoral neck fractures in children and the risk of osteonecrosis. Level of evidence: III.

123. Herrera-Soto JA, Duffy MF, Birnbaum MA, VanderHave KL: Increased intracapsular pressures after unstable slipped capital femoral epiphysis. *J Pediatr Orthop* 2008;28:723-728.

124. Crepeau A, Birnbaum MA, VanderHave KL, Herrera-Soto JA: Intracapsular pressures after stable slipped capital femoral epiphysis. *J Pediatr Orthop* 2015;35:e90-e92.

125. Nakaniida A, Sakuraba K, Hurwitz EL: Pediatric orthopaedic injuries requiring hospitalization: Epidemiology and economics. *J Orthop Trauma* 2014;28:167-172.

126. Li H, Zhao L, Huang L, Kuo KN: Delayed slipped capital femoral epiphysis after treatment of femoral neck fracture in children. *Clin Orthop Relat Res* 2015;473(8):2712-2717.

127. Kocher MS, Sink EL, Blasier RD, et al: Treatment of pediatric diaphyseal femur fractures. *J Am Acad Orthop Surg* 2009;17(11):718-725.

128. American Academy of Orthopaedic Surgeons: *Treatment of Pediatric Diaphyseal Femur Fractures: Evidence-Based Clinical Practice Guidelines*. 2015. Available at: www.aaos.org/research/guidelines/PDFF. Accessed May 21, 2020.

129. Jevsevar DS, Shea KG, Murray JN, Sevarino KS: AAOS clinical practice guideline on the treatment of pediatric diaphyseal fractures. *J Am Acad Orthop Surg* 2015;23:e101.

130. Oetgen ME, Blatz AM, Matthews A: Impact of clinical practice guideline on the treatment of pediatric femoral fractures in a pediatric hospital. *J Bone Joint Surg Am* 2015;97:1641-1646.

131. Roaten JD, Kelly DM, Yellin JL, et al: Pediatric femoral shaft fractures: A multicenter review of the AAOS clinical practice guidelines before and after 2009. *J Pediatr Orthop* 2019;39:394-399.

To determine if the AAOS clinical practice guidelines (CPG) issued in 2009 changed clinical treatment of pediatric femoral shaft fractures, consecutive series from 2004 to 2013 of pediatric femoral shaft fracture patients from four trauma centers were reviewed. A total of 2,646 fractures were evaluated. The authors found considerable variability among the four centers regarding treatment methods and adherence to AAOS CPG recommendations. Level of evidence: III.

132. Weltsch D, Baldwin KD, Talwar D, Flynn JM: Expert consensus for a principle-based classification for treatment of diaphyseal pediatric femur fractures. *J Pediatr Orthop* 2020;40(8):e669-e675.

Recognizing the deviation from the published AAOS CPG on PDFFs, the authors proposed a principle-based classification scheme to guide treatment. They then retrospectively reviewed 289 consecutive PDFF cases comparing actual treatment with the proposed ideal principle-based treatment. They found more suboptimal clinical results in undertreated fractures, compared with those treated ideally within the principle-based scheme. Overtreated fractures had good clinical results but resulted in increased hospital length of stay and hospital charges. Level of evidence: III.

133. Podeszwa DA, Mooney JF III, Cramer KE, Mendelow MJ: Comparison of Pavlik harness application and immediate spica casting for femur fractures in infants. *J Pediatr Orthop* 2004;24(5):460-462.

134. DiFazio R, Vessey J, Zurakowski D, Hresko MT, Matheney T: Incidence of skin complications and associated charges in children treated with hip spica casts for femur fractures. *J Pediatr Orthop* 2011;31:17-22.

135. Rush JK, Kelly DM, Sawyer JR, Beaty JH, Warner WC: Treatment of pediatric femur fractures with the Pavlik harness: Multiyear clinical and radiographic outcomes. *J Pediatr Orthop* 2013;33:614-617.

136. Blatz AM, Gillespie CW, Katcher A, et al: Factors associated with nonaccidental trauma evaluation among patients below 36 months old presenting with femur fractures at a level-1 pediatric trauma center. *J Pediatr Orthop* 2019;39:175-180.

The authors reviewed 281 children at their institution who were younger than 36 months with femoral shaft fractures. Despite AAOS CPG recommendations, they found that less than half (41%) of the patients younger than 36 months were evaluated for nonaccidental trauma (NAT). Younger patients, patients transferred from other institutions, and patients presenting with concomitant fractures were more likely to undergo NAT evaluation. Level of evidence: III.

137. Flynn JM, Garner MR, Joes KJ, et al: The treatment of low-energy femoral shaft fractures: A prospective study comparing the "walking spica" with the traditional spica cast. *J Bone Joint Surg Am* 2011;93:2196-2202.

138. Leu D, Sargent MC, Ain MC, et al: Spica casting for pediatric femoral fractures: A prospective, randomized controlled study of single leg versus double leg spica casts. *J Bone Joint Surg Am* 2012;94:1259-1264.

139. Mansour AA III, Wilmoth JC, Mansour AS, Lovejoy SA, Mencio GA, Martus JE: Immediate spica casting of pediatric femoral fractures in the operating room versus the emergency department: Comparison of reduction, complications, and hospital charges. *J Pediatr Orthop* 2010;30(8):813-817.

140. Cassinelli EH, Young B, Vogt M, Pierce MC, Deeney VF: Spica cast application in the emergency room for select pediatric femur fractures. *J Orthop Trauma* 2005;19:709-706.

141. Tisherman RT, Hoellwarth JS, Mendelson SA: Systematic review of spica casting for the treatment of pediatric diaphyseal femur fractures. *J Child Orthop* 2018;12:136-144.

The authors performed a systematic review of the literature regarding spica cast treatment of PDFFs. They found spica casting provides a safe, effective means for definitive management of PDFFs. The overall reported complication rate was 19.6%, with most of those being skin compromise. Unacceptable fracture angulation occurred in 4.2% and excessive limb shortening in 1.9% of patients. Level of evidence: II.

142. Nielsen E, Skaggs DL, Ryan D, Andras LM: Molding spica casts to maintain alignment of femur fractures. *J Pediatr Orthop* 2018;38:e267-e270.

The authors reviewed 52 patients treated with spica casting to assess the amount of varus and procurvatum that occurs at the fracture from initial reduction at time of spica cast application to fracture union. They concluded that femur fractures gain 5° of varus and 10° of procurvatum during this time. Surgeons should account for this to avoid angular malunions with this treatment. Level of evidence: IV.

143. Heffernan MJ, Gordon JE, Sabatini CS, et al: Treatment of femur fractures in young children: A multicenter comparison of flexible intramedullary nails to spica casting in young children aged 2 to 6 years. *J Pediatr Orthop* 2015;35(2):126-129.

144. Illing P, Lascombes P: Femur, in Dietz HG, Schmittenbecher PP, Slongo T, Wilkins KE, eds: *Elastic Stable Intramedullary Nailing in Children*. Thieme, 2006, pp 109-141.

145. Green JK, Werner FW, Dhawan R, Evans PJ, Kelley S, Webster DA: A biomechanical study on flexible intramedullary nails used to treat pediatric femoral fractures. *J Orthop Res* 2005;23:1315-1320.

146. Luhmann SJ, Schootman M, Schoenecker PL, Dobbs MB, Gordon JE: Complications of titanium elastic nails for pediatric femoral shaft fractures. *J Pediatr Orthop* 2003;23:443-447.

147. Sagan ML, Datta JC, Olney BW, Lansford TJ, McIff TE: Residual deformity after treatment of pediatric femur fractures with flexible titanium nails. *J Pediatr Orthop* 2010;30(7):638-643.

148. Ho CA, Skaggs DL, Tang CW, Kay RM: Use of flexible intramedullary nails in pediatric femur fractures. *J Pediatr Orthop* 2006;26:497-504.

149. Moroz LA, Launay F, Kocher MS, et al: Titanium elastic nailing of fractures of the femur in children. Predictors of complications and poor outcome. *J Bone Joint Surg Br* 2006;88(10):1361-1366.

150. Sink EL, Gralla J, Repine M: Complications of pediatric femur fractures treated with titanium elastic nails: A comparison of fracture types. *J Pediatr Orthop* 2005;25:577-580.

151. Shaha JS, Cage JM, Black SR, Wimberly RL, Shaha SH, Riccio AI: Redefining optimal nail to medullary canal diameter ratio in stainless steel flexible intramedullary nailing of pediatric femur fractures. *J Pediatr Orthop* 2017;37(7):e398-e402.

The authors retrospectively reviewed 261 children treated at their institution with retrograte stainless steel flexible intramedullary nails. Stainless steel flexible intramedullary nails maintain fracture alignment without an increase in complications at lower summed nail diameter/femoral (isthmus) intramedullary canal diameter ratios than described previously as ideal for titanium flexible nails. Level of evidence: III.

152. Wall EJ, Jain V, Vora V, Mehlman CT, Crawford AH: Complications of titanium and stainless steel elastic nail fixation in pediatric femur fractures. *J Bone Joint Surg Am* 2008;90:1305-1313.

153. Shaha J, Cage JM, Black S, Wimberly RL, Shaha SH, Riccio AI: Flexible intramedullary nails for femur fractures in pediatric patients heavier than 100 pounds. *J Pediatr Orthop* 2018;38:88-93.

The authors reviewed the same cohort as from Ref. 151. In that cohort, they had 24 patients who weighed more than 100 pounds. The size of the nails, insertion technique, and the use of distal eyelet interlocking screws were at the discretion of the treating surgeon. The 24 heaviest patients had similar results with treatment to the 237 patients who weighed less than 100 pounds. Level of evidence: III.

154. Ellis HB, Ho CA, Podeszwa DA, Wilson PL: A comparison of locked versus nonlocked Enders rods for length unstable pediatric femoral shaft fractures. *J Pediatr Orthop* 2011;31:825-833.

155. Rapp M, Gros N, Zachert G, et al: Improving stability of elastic stable intramedullary nailing in a transverse midshaft femur fracture model: Biomechanical analysis of using end caps or a third nail. *J Orthop Surg Res* 2015;10:96.

156. Busch MT, Perkins CA, Nickel BT, Blizzard DJ, Willimon SC: A quartet of elastic stable intramedullary nails for more challenging pediatric femur fractures. *J Pediatr Orthop* 2019;39:e12-e17.

The authors publish a retrospective review of 14 patients who underwent insertion of four elastic intramedullary nails. There were no hardware failures or revision surgeries in the 12 followed to fracture union. Their surgical technique is described. They offer this technique as a way to increase canal fill and construct stiffness in more unstable pediatric femur fracture patterns. Level of evidence: IV.

157. Sink EL, Faro F, Polusky J, Flynn K, Gralla J: Decreased complications of pediatric femur fractures with a change in management. *J Pediatr Orthop* 2010;30:633-637.

158. Kanlic EM, Anglen JO, Smith DG, et al: Advantages of submuscular bridge plating for complex femur fractures. *Clin Orthop Relat Res* 2004;426:244-251.

159. Li Y, Hedequist DJ: Submuscular plating of pediatric femur fracture. *J Am Acad Orthop Surg* 2012;20:596-603.

160. Heyworth BE, Hedequist DJ, Nasreddine AY, Stamoulis C, Hresko MT, Yen YM: Distal femoral valgus deformity following plate fixation of pediatric femoral shaft fractures. *J Bone Joint Surg Am* 2013;95(6):526-533.

161. Pate O, Hedequist D, Leong N, Hresko T: Implant removal after submuscular plating for pediatric femur fractures. *J Pediatr Orthop* 2009;29:709-712.

162. Keeler KA, Dart B, Luhmann SJ, et al: Antegrade intramedullary nailing of pediatric femoral fractures using an interlocking pediatric femoral nail and a lateral trochanteric entry point. *J Pediatr Orthop* 2009;29:345-351.

163. Crosby SN Jr, Kim E, Koehler DM, et al: Twenty-year experience with rigid intramedullary nailing of femoral shaft fractures in skeletally immature patients. *J Bone Joint Surg Am* 2014;96:1080-1089.

164. MacNeil JA, Francis A, El-Hawary R: A systematic review of rigid, locked, intramedullary nail insertion sites and avascular necrosis of the femoral head in the skeletally immature. *J Pediatr Orthop* 2011;31(4):377-380.

165. Gautier E, Ganz K, Krugel N, Gill T, Ganz R: Anatomy of the medial circumflex artery and its surgical implications. *J Bone Joint Surg Br* 2000;82:679-683.

166. Hosalkar HS, Pandya NK, Cho RH, Glaser DA, Moor MA, Herman MJ: Intramedullary nailing of pediatric femoral shaft fracture. *J Am Acad Orthop Surg* 2011;19:472-481.

167. Jeng C, Sponseller PD, Yates A, et al: Subtrochanteric femoral fractures in children. Alignment after 90 degrees-90 degrees traction and cast application. *Clin Orthop Relat Res* 1997;341:170-174.

168. Pombo MW, Shilt JS: The definition and treatment of pediatric subtrochanteric femur fractures with titanium elastic nails. *J Pediatr Orthop* 2006;26:364-370.

169. Xu Y, Bian J, Shen K, Xue B: Titanium elastic nailing versus locking compression plating in school-aged pediatric subtrochanteric femur fractures. *Medicine (Baltimore)* 2018;97(29):e11568.

Titanium elastic nailing and hip plating were both safe and effective methods of treatment for pediatric subtrochanteric femur fractures in this younger and lighter patient population. Nails are minimally invasive with a relatively simple technique, best for lighter and younger patients. Plate fixation should be used for larger children and was associated with a smaller complication rate than that of the TENs. Level of evidence: III.

170. Herrera-Soto JA, Meuret R, Phillips JH, Vogel DJ: The management of pediatric subtrochanteric femur fractures with a statically locked intramedullary nail. *J Orthop Trauma* 2015;29(1):e7-e11.

171. Parikh SN, Nathan ST, Priola MJ, Eismann EA: Elastic nailing for pediatric subtrochanteric and supracondylar femur fractures. *Clin Orthop Relat Res* 2014;472(9):2735-2744.

172. Li Y, Heyworth BE, Glotzbecker M, et al: Comparison of titanium elastic nail and plate fixation of pediatric subtrochanteric femur fractures. *J Pediatr Orthop* 2013;33(3):232-238.

CHAPTER 44

Knee Trauma

SCOTT YANG, MD • MATTHEW F. HALSEY, MD

ABSTRACT

Fractures around the knee joint in children and adolescents are relatively uncommon compared with other pediatric fractures. However, injuries in this location can be associated with major difficulties and complications. Thus, it is critical for the surgeon taking care of these fractures to understand the common fracture types, along with the evaluation, treatment methods, and expected complications.

Keywords: distal femoral physeal injuries; patella sleeve fractures; pediatric knee trauma; proximal tibial physeal injuries; tibial spine fractures; tibial tubercle fractures

INTRODUCTION

Fractures around the knee joint in children and adolescents are relatively uncommon compared with other pediatric fractures. However, the location of the fractures can lead to significant complications. Neurovascular injury and compartment syndrome can occur with these injuries. Clinical suspicion and careful evaluation are paramount in evaluating children with displaced fractures around the knee to avoid these complications. Most fractures around the knee involve a physis of the distal femur or proximal tibia, leading to significant implications for subsequent growth disturbances due to the major contribution of the distal femur and proximal tibia to lower limb growth. Extensor mechanism injuries and those affecting knee stability can also result in diminished knee function and disability if not carefully managed.

Dr. Yang or an immediate family member serves as a board member, owner, officer, or committee member of the Pediatric Orthopaedic Society of North America and the Scoliosis Research Society. Dr. Halsey or an immediate family member serves as a board member, owner, officer, or committee member of the Pediatric Orthopaedic Society of North America and the Scoliosis Research Society.

DISTAL FEMUR PHYSEAL AND CONDYLAR FRACTURES

Epidemiology, Classification, and Mechanism

Injuries to the distal femoral physis are rare, accounting for less than 1% of all fractures in children.[1] Distal femoral physeal fractures are classified with the Salter-Harris classification. Among these fractures, the most common fracture is Salter-Harris type II, accounting for 59% to 70%. Femoral condyle fractures are most often physeal (Salter-Harris type III and IV), which combined represent 6% to 21% of distal femoral physeal fractures.[2,3] Higher energy mechanisms are usually at fault, including motor vehicle accidents and sports-related collisions, such as a football tackle. Medial femoral condyle fractures often occur as a result of a valgus-type stress in which the physis and epiphysis preferentially fracture instead of tearing the medial ligamentous structures.[4] Fractures typically occur in the adolescent or preadolescent age group, though can occur at any age including birth-related trauma.

Growth and Anatomy

The distal femoral physis contributes to nearly 70% of the growth of the femur.[5] Because of the significant growth contribution of the distal femoral physis, fractures in this location can carry significant risk for subsequent limb deformity if complete or partial growth arrest occurs. The anatomy of the distal femoral physis is unique in that it is undulating and irregularly contoured consisting of a central ridge, lateral ridge, and medial peak. The unique undulating contour of the physis contributes to a precise lock-and-key fit, and injury at the physis may lead to more complex shearing physeal injury than other locations, accounting for the propensity of growth arrest in these fractures. These undulations also undergo change with age,[6] and it has been recently proposed that the decreased height in the central ridge with development may contribute to a weaker distal femoral physis during adolescence. The patterns of distal femoral physis closure are not fully understood, although a recent MRI study suggested that the distal femoral physis undergoes maturation and closure in a uniform pattern throughout the medial, central, and lateral portions of the physis,[7] accounting for the relative decreased frequency of Salter-Harris III or IV fractures in the distal femur compared with other locations, such as the distal tibia, where asymmetrical closure occurs.

Initial Evaluation

Initial evaluation should include high-quality biplanar radiographs. If a nondisplaced physeal fracture is suspected based on examination or subtle widening of the physis on radiographs, MRI is useful to confirm the diagnosis and in some instances can demonstrate periosteal entrapment in the physis.[8,9] Stress radiography for suspected physeal fractures should not be performed to prevent unnecessary patient discomfort or inadvertent fracture displacement. Salter-Harris type III and IV injuries require a high index of diagnostic suspicion because 39% were missed on initial presentation.[4] These fractures require advanced three-dimensional CT for both diagnostic aid and quantification of fracture displacement because plain radiographs underestimate displacement.[10] The direction of distal fragment displacement can vary based on the deforming force, although special attention should be given to those with anterior displacement as the neurovascular bundle can become tethered. Critical neurovascular structures reside along the distal femoral region. The popliteus artery traverses distally from the adductor hiatus near the metaphyseal region of the distal femur to the popliteus fossa. The sciatic nerve bifurcates into the common peroneal and tibial nerves proximal to the popliteus fossa. Attention to detail and documentation of the limb neurovascular examination is paramount. Urgent reduction of the fracture should be performed if the limb is dysvascular, with plans for vascular surgery consultation, and careful postoperative neurovascular monitoring is important in these rare but critical scenarios.

Management

Management of the distal femoral physeal fracture often is surgical apart from nondisplaced fractures that can be managed with a long leg cast and frequent radiographic monitoring for displacement. Best possible anatomic reduction should be achieved. Displaced Salter-Harris I fractures are managed with reduction and transphyseal smooth pin fixation, anterograde or retrograde. Often, pin fixation is supplemented with cast immobilization. Retrograde pin fixation theoretically risks intra-articular infection because of pin-site communication with the knee joint. However, a recent series describing retrograde pin fixation of the distal femur in 163 children demonstrated a 6.7% rate of pin tract infection with no patients having a concomitant septic arthritis of the knee.[11] Smooth pin fixation of distal femoral physis can cause a low incidence (7% to 13%) of physeal bar formation in an animal model,[12] although transphyseal smooth pin fixation has not been clearly associated with increased rate of clinical growth arrest.[13] Displaced Salter-Harris II fractures are managed with closed versus open reduction, and if the attached metaphyseal fragment is of sufficient size, partially threaded cannulated screws are placed through the metaphyseal fragment to provide compression at the fracture site (**Figure 1**).

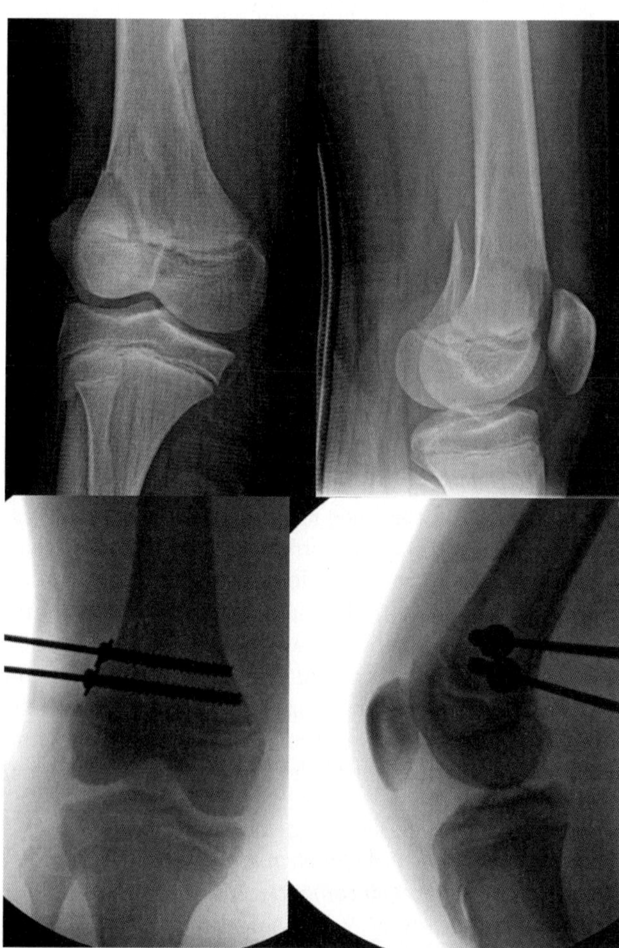

FIGURE 1 Radiographs of the knee of a 13-year-old boy with a right Salter-Harris II distal femur fracture sustained after a football injury. Near-anatomic closed reduction was obtained and stabilized with cannulated screw fixation of the metaphyseal fragment.

Femoral condyle fractures (Salter-Harris type III and IV) require special attention for accurate anatomic reduction of both the joint and physis and often require open reduction. Arthrogram can be difficult to interpret in the distal femur and can lead to malreduction if used as a judge for anatomic reduction. Therefore, the joint surface is visualized via a formal arthrotomy to aid in anatomic reduction, with compression screws placed across fragments. A quality lateral radiograph can aid safe screw placement in the triangle bordered by Blumensaat line, trochlear groove, and distal femoral physis after femoral condyle fracture reduction.[14]

Postoperative care follows a general template in which cast immobilization and pins can generally be discontinued in approximately 4 weeks, with graduated knee range of motion and weight bearing allowed.

Complications

Complications in the management of distal femur physeal fractures include infection, joint stiffness, arthritis from articular malreduction, and most commonly growth arrest. Fractures involving the distal femur often result in partial or complete growth arrest, with incidence up to 52%.[15] All Salter-Harris fracture types, whether displaced or not, can present with subsequent growth arrest. A trend toward increased incidence of growth arrest has been demonstrated for increasing numerical Salter-Harris classification.[3,13] Displaced fractures have also been associated with subsequent growth disturbance more frequently than nondisplaced fractures.[2,3,15] A recent trend toward more frequent surgical management of distal femoral physeal fractures has not proven to decrease the overall complication rate of 40%, most of which consisted of growth arrest.[2] All distal femoral physeal fractures should be monitored for at least 1 year for the development of growth arrest and addressed accordingly. The treatment plan should be tailored to the type of disturbance (ie, partial or complete; central or peripheral) and remaining growth. MRI or CT can help characterize the anatomic location and severity of the physeal bar. If a small peripheral physeal bar forms with incipient angular deformity and more than 2 years of growth remaining, a physeal bar resection may be attempted. Otherwise, a completion epiphysiodesis can be performed to ablate the remnant open physis. For projected limb-length difference >2 cm, contralateral distal femoral epiphysiodesis can be considered. For a large projected difference >4 to 5 cm, femoral lengthening is a reasonable option (**Figure 2**).

PATELLA SLEEVE FRACTURES

Patella fractures are relatively rare in children and adolescents, with patella sleeve fractures accounting for over half of these injuries.[16] The patella begins to ossify around age 3 years, with ossification progressing from the center to the periphery as the child matures.[17] The distal or proximal cartilaginous sleeve can be pulled off the ossified section of the patella with a powerful contraction of the quadriceps against a fixed leg and foot. Because the cartilaginous sleeve of tissue is not ossified, radiographic diagnosis can be difficult, frequently leading to misdiagnosis and diagnostic delay.[18] Patients will have a history of acute knee pain and swelling, often after maximal effort running or jumping similar to tibial tubercle fractures that affect an older age group. The patients will have pain over the patella and may have an extensor lag if the extensor mechanism is completely disrupted. If plain radiographs are not diagnostic, MRI will be, although ultrasonography can also be helpful in confirming the diagnosis at substantially less cost.[19,20] Nondisplaced and minimally displaced fractures can be managed in a cast, but displaced fractures will require surgical repair of the extensor mechanism, using either transosseous suture or suture anchors to repair the cartilaginous avulsion to the ossified patella.[21] Supplemental tension band wiring to protect the repair should be considered.

PEDIATRIC PROXIMAL TIBIA FRACTURES

In general, fractures involving the proximal tibia are unusual as the area is stabilized by the presence of the fibular head laterally and the medial collateral ligament insertion extending onto the metaphysis medially. Interestingly, the site of a fracture in the proximal tibia changes as the skeleton matures: In preschool and early grade school children, the fractures occur in the metaphysis; in preteens, fractures occur in the physis as Salter-Harris I and II fractures; at a slightly older age, tibial tubercle avulsion fractures are more common; and finally, as the proximal tibial physis closes, flexion-type tibial tubercle fractures and Salter-Harris III and IV fractures occur.[22]

TIBIAL SPINE FRACTURES

The anterior tibial spine forms the tibial attachment of the anterior cruciate ligament (ACL). Tibial spine fractures typically occur in children aged 8 to 14 years.[21] The most common mechanism of injury is a noncontact pivot-type rotational sports injury, similar to ACL injuries.[23] It is thought that the incomplete ossification of the tibial spine in this age group leads to its propensity to fracture. The Meyers and McKeever classification system is based on the degree of displacement as judged on the lateral knee radiograph.[24] Type I fractures are nondisplaced, whereas type II are displaced anteriorly but with

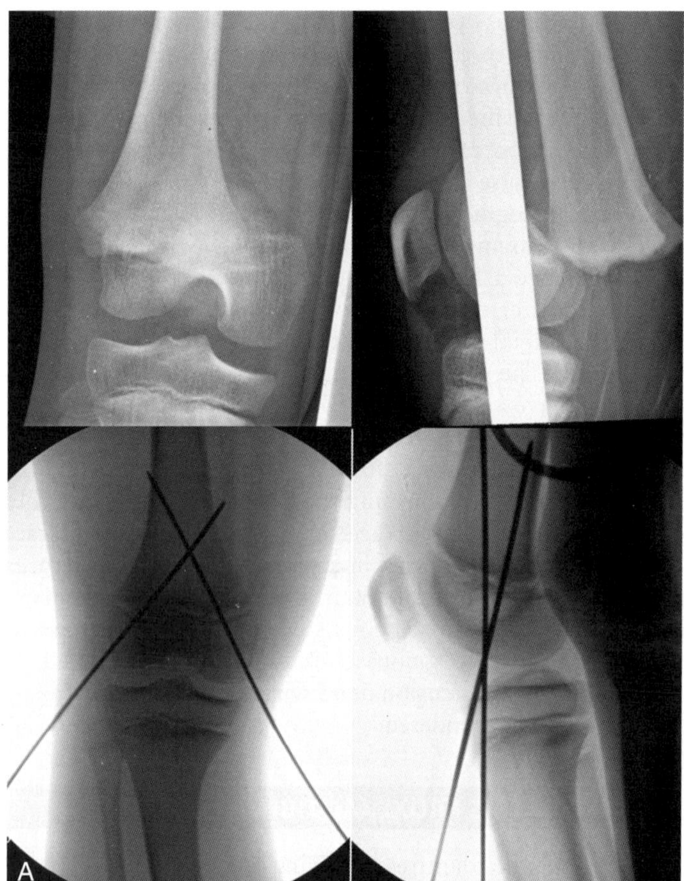

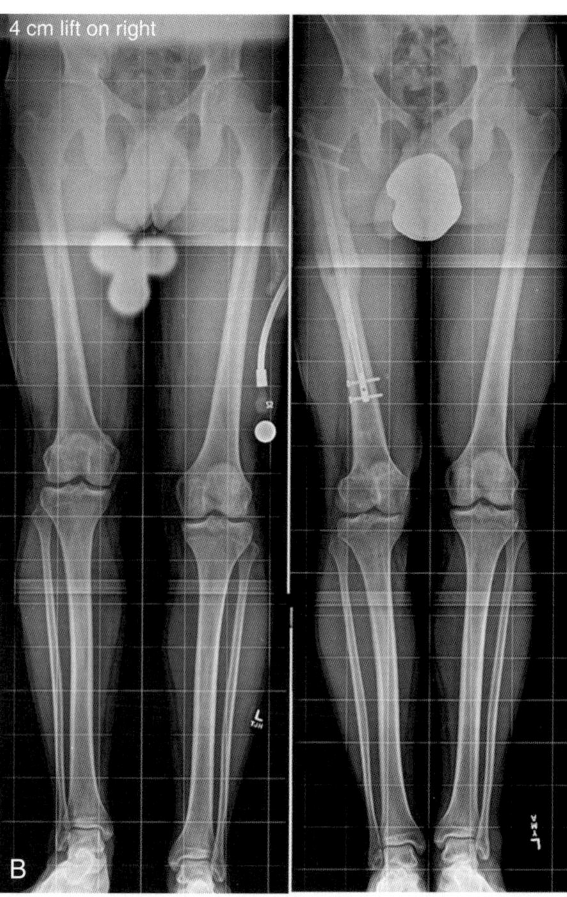

FIGURE 2 A, Radiographic and fluoroscopic images showing a distal femur Salter-Harris I fracture in a 12-year-old boy after a dirt bike accident. Closed reduction with retrograde cross pinning of the fracture was performed. B, Radiographs showing a femoral lengthening procedure to manage the subsequent development of a 4.5-cm growth arrest.

an intact posterior hinge. Type III fractures are completely displaced. These can involve just the anterior spine or the entire intercondylar eminence and can be comminuted.

Patients will typically present with an injury, acute knee pain, and a notable knee hemarthrosis. After identification of the tibial spine fracture on the lateral radiograph, an MRI is indicated.[25] The rate of associated meniscal tears is high.[26,27] Many patients will demonstrate meniscal entrapment at the fracture site blocking reduction. Non-ACL ligamentous injury is seen in approximately one-third of patients.[27] These soft-tissue injuries are more likely in the type II and type III fractures. Initial treatment usually consists of aspiration of the hemarthrosis for symptomatic relief and to aid in fracture reduction. Although the ACL has its least tension in approximately 30° of knee flexion, reduction and immobilization in full extension allow the lateral femoral condyle to assist in reduction of the fracture. Immobilization for 6 weeks with protected weight bearing, followed by progressive rehabilitation, is used to manage fractures that are adequately reduced with closed manipulation.[28,29]

The anterior horn of the medial meniscus was the most common block to anatomic reduction in one study,[30] although the intrameniscal ligament is frequently entrapped in the fracture as well.[27] Arthroscopic reduction and internal fixation techniques have advantages over arthrotomy with lower morbidity and earlier mobilization.[28] Fixation techniques include antegrade screw fixation or anchoring sutures.[31,32] Physeal sparring techniques regardless of fixation are important in patients with notable growth remaining.[29] Residual laxity after fracture repair can occur, with approximately 20% of patients requiring a delayed ACL reconstruction. Arthrofibrosis is a notable complication in 10% of patients, usually related to delayed (>4 weeks) initiation of postoperative range of motion.[33,34]

TIBIAL TUBERCLE FRACTURES

Tibial tubercle fractures account for 0.4% to 2.7% of all physeal injuries.[35,36] A 2016 meta-analysis[37] found that more than 95% of these injuries occur in males at an average age of 14.6 years. Although a quarter of the fractures are associated with a history of Osgood-Schlatter disease, it is not considered an independent risk factor. Generally, tibial tubercle fractures occur during sports activities that require jumping, such as basketball, high jump, and hurdling. The fracture mechanism may be either a concentric or eccentric contraction of the quadriceps during takeoff or landing.

Patients will present with significant swelling, pain, and difficulty with ambulation. Physical examination demonstrates tenderness over the tibial tubercle, and perhaps at the quadriceps insertion into the patella. Active extension of the knee is difficult or impossible and there is an obvious extensor lag.

Typically, the neurovascular examination is normal, but the anterior and lateral compartments may be swollen and tense because the anterior tibial recurrent artery can be injured at the lateral border of the tubercle,[38-41] raising the concern for a concomitant compartment syndrome. Despite the rather innocuous appearance of this type of fracture and the low energy of the typical mechanism, the surgeon should always have a high degree of suspicion for compartment syndrome as it occurs in nearly 1 of 20 patients.[37]

Biplanar radiography of the knee is usually sufficient to establish the diagnosis, although CT may be considered if there is comminution and/or intra-articular extension of the fracture; similarly, MRI may be considered if there is extension of the fracture into the joint to evaluate for intra-articular meniscal or ligament injury.

Several different classification systems for tibial tubercle fractures exist, most based on the anatomic extent of the fracture.[41-44] The tubercle ossifies from proximal to distal; thus, as the skeleton matures, extension of the fracture into the joint becomes less likely. The classification systems do help with treatment decisions as well as determining the clinical course and overall prognosis.

The goal of treatment is to restore the extensor mechanism; further goals include restoring the articular surface and the meniscal anatomy if there is intra-articular extension. Nondisplaced fractures may be managed with a long leg cast in full extension for 4 to 6 weeks. Most tibial tubercle fractures (88%) require open reduction.[37] Adequate access to the fracture can be achieved with an incision centered over the patellar tendon, which allows for removal of any interposed periosteum, hematoma, or small bone fragments. If there is intra-articular extension, visualization of the joint surface can be obtained through a parapatellar arthrotomy or arthroscopic evaluation.

Typically, fracture fixation is obtained with partially threaded cancellous screws placed parallel to the joint surface, into the metaphysis and epiphysis as needed (**Figure 3**). Kirschner wires, suture anchors, or a tension band can be used to achieve fixation as well. Associated soft-tissue injuries, such as patellar or quadriceps tendon ruptures, should be addressed at the time of surgery. As there is a risk of compartment syndrome associated with tibial tubercle fractures, prophylactic anterior compartment fasciotomy and hematoma decompression should be considered.[45]

Postoperatively, the knee should be immobilized in a cast or hinged knee brace, in mild flexion, for 4 to 6 weeks. Toe-touch weight bearing with crutches is encouraged. After the fracture is healed, rehabilitation of the knee, formally or at home, should focus on obtaining full range of motion and re-establishing the strength of the quadriceps. It should be expected that most patients will be able to return to their previous level of sports participation.

Complications associated with tibial tubercles do occur (28%); the most common are bursitis (56%) and pain (18%) associated with the implants used to

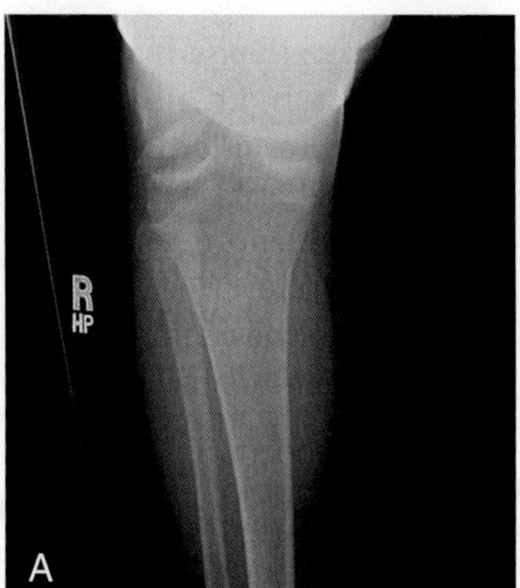

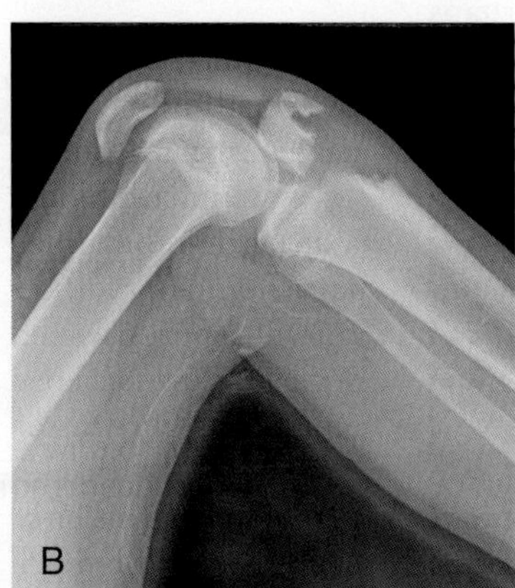

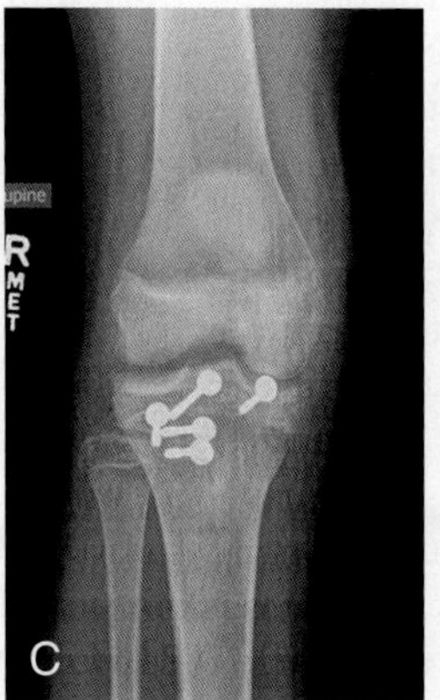

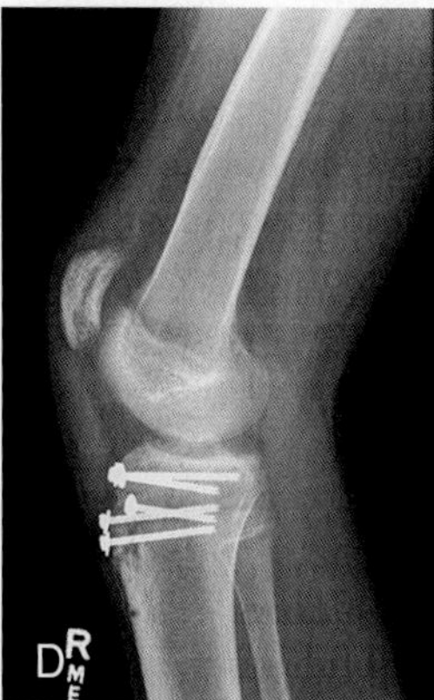

FIGURE 3 Radiographs of the knee of a 15-year-old boy who sustained complex right tibial tuberosity fracture with intra-articular split while landing from a jump during a basketball game. **A** and **B**, Preoperative radiographs. Open reduction, arthrotomy, and internal fixation with multiple partially threaded cannulated screws were performed with satisfactory outcome. **C** and **D**, Follow-up radiographs.

maintain fracture reduction, but others include compartment syndrome and deformity.[37] Removal of the implant is usually sufficient to address any pain associated with the implants. Functionally significant deformity is unusual as these fractures usually occur just as the physis is beginning to close.[40-42,46] Recurvatum occurred in 4% of patients and leg-length discrepancy in 5% of patients included in a recent meta-analysis.[37] Recurvatum was seen only in patients who presented at an age younger than 13 years. Leg-length discrepancy, when it occurred, averaged 1.4 cm (1 to 2 cm) and none met the criteria for surgical intervention to equalize the leg lengths.

PROXIMAL TIBIAL PHYSEAL FRACTURES

Incidence rates for proximal tibial physeal fractures are low (0.4% to 2.0%).[42,47] Salter-Harris I/II fractures generally occur early in the second decade, whereas the Salter-Harris III/IV fractures occur in the midteen years as the physis closes from posteromedial to anterolateral. Usually, physeal fractures will occur either in extension, especially in the 10- to 12-year-old patient, or in flexion in the older patient; coronal plane (varus/valgus) injury can and does happen as well.[22] Extension injuries typically have a higher energy mechanism (eg, bike riding),[22] demonstrate posterior metaphyseal displacement, and have a higher risk of injury to the popliteus artery.[22,48,49] However, the flexion injuries usually occur from low-energy jumping and landing, similar to tibial tubercle fractures.[22,47,50-52] The risk of a flexion-type Salter-Harris fracture is increased if the patient has an increased posterior tibial slope angle.[53] Flexion-type injuries are much more likely to occur in boys than girls.

Patients will present with complaints of pain, swelling, and inability to walk. Examination is remarkable for swelling, tenderness over the proximal tibia, and perhaps some visual deformity. Neurovascular examination is usually normal, but a high degree of suspicion for vascular injury in extension injuries is prudent;[48] determination of ankle-brachial indices would be appropriate in the context of a displaced extension-type proximal tibial physeal fracture. Flexion-type injuries do not typically cause neurologic or vascular injury.[54]

Biplanar radiographs of the knee will usually suffice to demonstrate the fracture; stress radiographs have been described but are not typically performed because of pain and risk of displacement.[55] CT is usually reserved for fractures with intra-articular extension to help determine the fracture pattern and degree of displacement. MRI may be indicated to identify soft-tissue injury, especially for Salter-Harris III/IV fractures.

For any Salter-Harris fracture, nonsurgical management with a long leg cast, for 4 to 6 weeks, would be appropriate for nondisplaced fractures.[22,48,49] Closed reduction, followed by casting, may be appropriate as well if the reduction can be maintained without extreme positioning of the knee in a cast. If the reduction is difficult to maintain, the fracture can be stabilized with crossed percutaneous Kirschner wires placed in the coronal plane.[48] Open treatment is indicated for any fracture that has more than 2 mm of residual displacement; open evaluation allows for the removal of any interposed tissue, such as periosteum, ligament, or pes anserinus. Fracture reduction is usually maintained with crossed Kirschner wires, partially threaded cancellous screws, or a plate and screw construct.[45,55]

Complications associated with proximal tibial physeal fractures include deformity and, in the case of extension injuries, vascular injury. Deformity can occur in as many as 25% of these fractures and can include leg-length discrepancy and angular deformity, especially in those patients who presented at a younger age with a higher energy injury mechanism.[56] Finally, coexistent ligamentous injury can occur as well.[57]

SUMMARY

The management of fractures around the knee depends on the amount of displacement. All displaced fractures require a careful neurovascular examination on initial evaluation. For displaced fractures, management is surgical and special consideration of articular and physeal involvement dictates consideration of future complications. Growth disturbance is a common complication of physeal fractures especially involving the distal femur and requires postinjury surveillance. Tibial spine avulsions are associated with other concomitant soft tissues of the knee that may affect overall management.

KEY STUDY POINTS

- Displaced fractures along the distal femur and proximal tibia can present neurovascular injury, requiring special attention.
- Pediatric knee fractures commonly involve growth centers including the distal femoral physis, proximal tibial physis, or tibial tubercle apophysis.
- Growth arrest frequently occurs after physeal fractures around the knee, especially for the distal femur, which can have profound implications on limb alignment and length.
- Tibial spine fractures are notable knee injuries and may have residual ACL instability even after repair of displaced fractures.

ANNOTATED REFERENCES

1. Mann D, Rajmaira S: Distribution of physeal and nonphyseal fractures in 2,650 long-bone fractures in children aged 0-16 years. *J Pediatr Orthop* 1990;10:713-716.
2. Adams AJ, Mahmoud MAH, Wells L, Flynn JM, Arkader A: Physeal fractures of the distal femur: Does a lower threshold for surgery lead to better outcomes? *J Pediatr Orthop B* 2020;29(1):40-46.

   This is a retrospective review of 70 distal femur physeal fractures managed from 2007 to 2016 and the associated complications. This cohort was compared with a previous cohort from the same institution. Complication rate remains high at 40% in the more recent cohort, with most being distal femoral growth disturbance. Level of evidence: III.
3. Arkader A, Warner WC, Horn BD, et al: Predicting the outcome of physeal fractures of the distal femur. *J Pediatr Orthop* 2007;27(6):703-708.
4. Pennock AT, Ellis HB, Willimon SC, et al: Intra-articular physeal fractures of the distal femur: A frequently missed diagnosis in adolescent athletes. *Orthop J Sports Med* 2017;5(10):2325967117731 56.

   This is a retrospective review of 49 patients intra-articular (Salter-Harris III and IV) distal femoral physeal fractures. About 39% of patients were initially misdiagnosed. Majority of patients returned to sports or prior level of function after surgical management. Of the total, 12% of patients required another procedure for limb-length discrepancy or angular deformity. Level of evidence: IV.
5. Anderson M, Messner MB, Green WT: Distribution of lengths of the normal femur and tibia in children from one to eighteen years of age. *J Bone Joint Surg Am* 1964;46:1197-1202.
6. Liu RW, Armstrong DG, Levine AD, Gilmore A, Thompson GH, Cooperman DR: An anatomic study of the distal femoral epiphysis. *J Pediatr Orthop* 2013;33:743-749.
7. Margalit A, Cottrill E, Nhan D, et al: The spatial order of physeal maturation in the normal human knee using magnetic resonance imaging. *J Pediatr Orthop* 2019;39(4): e318-e322.

   In this study, 165 pediatric knee magnetic resonance images were evaluated specifically for physeal maturation in eight distinct locations. No major difference in age was found for different stages of physeal maturation. This suggests that physeal maturation is potentially uniform in the distal femur, regardless of location along the physis. Level of evidence: III.
8. Chen J, Abel MF, Fox MG: Imaging appearance of entrapped periosteum within a distal femoral Salter-Harris II fracture. *Skeletal Radiol* 2015;44(10):1547-1551.
9. Segal LS, Shrader MW: Periosteal entrapment in distal femoral physeal fractures: Harbinger for premature physeal arrest? *Acta Orthop Belg* 2011;77(5):684-690.
10. Lippert WC, Owens RF, Wall EJ: Salter-Harris type III fractures of the distal femur: Plain radiographs can be deceptive. *J Pediatr Orthop* 2010;30(6):598-605.
11. Murgai RR, Compton E, Illingworth KD, Kay RM: The incidence of pin tract infections and septic arthritis in percutaneous distal femur pinning. *J Pediatr Orthop* 2019;39(6): e462-e466.

    In this study, 163 patients who had retrograde pinning of the distal femur were identified (included both fracture and distal femoral osteotomy cases). Among these, no cases of septic arthritis of the knee were identified. Overall pin-site infection was 6.7%. This study demonstrates that retrograde distal femoral pinning is potentially safe despite theoretical risk of septic arthritis based on intracapsular pin location. Level of evidence: III.
12. Dahl WJ, Silva S, Vanderhave KL: Distal femoral physeal fixation: Are smooth pins really safe? *J Pediatr Orthop* 2014;34(2):134-138.
13. Garrett BR, Hoffman EB, Carrara H: The effect of percutaneous pin fixation in the treatment of distal femoral physeal fractures. *J Bone Joint Surg Br* 2011;93-B: 689-694.
14. Wall EJ, May MM: Growth plate fractures of the distal femur. *J Pediatr Orthop* 2012;32(suppl 1):S40-S46.
15. Basener CJ, Mehlman CT, DiPasquale TG: Growth disturbance after distal femoral growth plate fractures in children: A meta-analysis. *J Orthop Trauma* 2009;23(9):663-667.
16. Ray JM, Hendrix J: Incidence, mechanism of injury, and treatment of fractures of the patella in children. *J Trauma* 1992;32(4):464-467.
17. Skaggs DL: Extra-articular injuries of the knee, in Beaty JH, Kasser JR, eds: *Rockwood and Wilkins' Fractures in Children*, ed 6. Philadelphia, PA, Lippincott Williams & Wilkins, 2006, pp 937-984.
18. Gao GX, Mahadev A, Lee EH: Sleeve fracture of the patella in children. *J Orthop Surg (Hong Kong)* 2008;16(1):43-46.
19. Bates DG, Hresko MT, Jaramillo D: Patellar sleeve fracture: Demonstration with MR imaging. *Radiology* 1994;193(3):825-827.
20. Ditchfield A, Sampson MA, Taylor GR: Case reports. Ultrasound diagnosis of sleeve fracture of the patella. *Clin Radiol* 2000;55(9):721-722.
21. Hunt DM, Somashekar N: A review of sleeve fractures of the patella in children. *Knee* 2005;12(1):3-7.
22. Mubarak SJ, Kim JR, Edmonds EW, et al: Classification of proximal tibial fractures in children. *J Child Orthop* 2009;3(3):191-197.
23. Aderinto J, Walmsley P, Keating JF: Fractures of the tibial spine: Epidemiology and outcome. *Knee* 2008;15(3): 164-167.
24. Meyers MH, McKeever FM: Fracture of the intercondylar eminence of the tibia. *J Bone Joint Surg Am* 1959;41-A:209-220, discussion 220-222.
25. Green D, Tuca M, Luderowski E, Gausden E, Goodbody C, Konin G: A new, MRI-based classification system for tibial spine fractures changes clinical treatment recommendations when compared to Myers and Mckeever. *Knee Surg Sports Traumatol Arthrosc* 2019;27(1):86-92.

Section 7: Trauma

Twenty tibial spine fractures were graded both on plain radiography and MRI using the Meyers and McKeever system. The use of MRI changed the fracture grade and as a result modified the treatment recommendations in 32.5% of cases. Level of evidence: II.

26. Mitchell JJ, Sjostrom R, Mansour AA, et al: Incidence of meniscal injury and chondral pathology in anterior tibial spine fractures of children. *J Pediatr Orthop* 2015;35(2): 130-135.

27. Rhodes JT, Cannamela PC, Cruz AI, et al: Incidence of meniscal entrapment and associated knee injuries in tibial spine avulsions. *J Pediatr Orthop* 2018;38(2):e38-e42.

    In this study, 163 patients with a mean age of 11.8 years with all grades of tibial spine injuries were evaluated. Preoperative MRI was performed in 47% of cases. High percentages of coexistent meniscal injury, osteochondral injury, and non-ACL ligamentous injuries were identified. Meniscal entrapment preventing full reduction of the tibial spine was not seen well on preoperative MRI but was noted intraoperatively in 39.9% of cases. Level of evidence: IV.

28. Coyle C, Jagernauth S, Ramachandran M: Tibial eminence fractures in the paediatric population: A systematic review. *J Child Orthop* 2014;8(2):149-159.

29. Tuca M, Bernal N, Luderowski E, et al: Tibial spine avulsion fractures: Treatment update. *Curr Opin Pediatr* 2019;31(1):103-111.

    This is a review article on the diagnosis, classification, and management of tibial spine avulsion injuries. The authors discuss methods of fixation, including physeal sparing techniques, rehabilitation, and common postoperative complications, seen in these injuries. Level of evidence: V.

30. Kocher MS, Micheli LJ, Gerbino P, et al: Tibial eminence fractures in children: Prevalence of meniscal entrapment. *Am J Sports Med* 2003;31(3):404-407.

31. Seon JK, Park SJ, Lee KB, et al: A clinical comparison of screw and suture fixation of anterior cruciate ligament tibial avulsion fractures. *Am J Sports Med* 2009;37(12): 2334-2339.

32. Bomar JD, Edmonds EW: Surgical reduction and fixation of tibial spine fractures in children: Arthroscopic suture fixation. *JBJS Essent Surg Tech* 2016;6(2):e17.

    This is a surgical technique descriptive paper discussing the authors' preferred steps for arthroscopic suture or screw fixation of tibial spine avulsion fractures. Level of evidence: V.

33. Mitchell JJ, Mayo MH, Axibal DP, et al: Delayed anterior cruciate ligament reconstruction in young patients with previous anterior tibial spine fractures. *Am J Sports Med* 2016;44(8):2047-2056.

    In this study, 101 patients with anterior tibial spine avulsion fractures were followed for at least 2 years to see if they underwent subsequent ACL reconstruction. Nineteen percent of patients required subsequent ACL reconstruction, for which older age was a risk factor. Level of evidence: IV.

34. Patel NM, Park MJ, Sampson NR, Ganley TJ: Tibial eminence fractures in children: Earlier posttreatment mobilization results in improved outcomes. *J Pediatr Orthop* 2012;32(2):139-144.

35. Bolesta MJ, Fitch RD: Tibial tubercle avulsions. *J Pediatr Orthop* 1986;6(2):186-192.

36. Mosier SM, Stanitski CL: Acute tibial tubercle avulsion fractures. *J Pediatr Orthop* 2004;24(2):181-184.

37. Pretell-Mazzini J, Kelly DM, Sawyer JR, et al: Outcomes and complications of tibial tubercle fractures in pediatric patients: A systematic review of the literature. *J Pediatr Orthop* 2016;36(5):440-446.

    The authors performed a meta-analysis of 23 eligible articles covering 336 fractures. The distribution of tibial tubercle fracture types was determined and the rates of complications as well as return to play were evaluated. The authors suggested that longer term follow-up studies would be useful but found that 98% of all patients returned to preinjury activity and range of motion. Level of evidence: III.

38. Brey JM, Conoley J, Canale ST, et al: Tibial tuberosity fractures in adolescents: Is a posterior metaphyseal fracture component a predictor of complications? *J Pediatr Orthop* 2012;32(6):561-566.

39. Wall JJ: Compartment syndrome as a complication of the Hauser procedure. *J Bone Joint Surg Am* 1979;61(2):185-191.

40. Frey S, Hosalkar H, Cameron DB, Heath A, David Horn B, Ganley TJ: Tibial tuberosity fractures in adolescents. *J Child Orthop* 2008;2(6):469-474.

41. Pandya NK, Edmonds EW, Roocroft JH, Mubarak SJ: Tibial tubercle fractures: Complications, classification, and the need for intra-articular assessment. *J Pediatr Orthop* 2012;32(8):749-759.

42. Ogden JA, Tross RB, Murphy MJ: Fractures of the tibial tuberosity in adolescents. *J Bone Joint Surg Am* 1980;62(2):205-215.

43. Ryu RK, Debenham JO: An unusual avulsion fracture of the proximal tibial epiphysis. Case report and proposed addition to the Watson-Jones classification. *Clin Orthop Relat Res* 1985;194:181-184.

44. McKoy BE, Stanitski CL: Acute tibial tubercle avulsion fractures. *Orthop Clin North Am* 2003;34(3):397-403.

45. Pace JL, McCulloch PC, Momoh EO, Nasreddine AY, Kocher MS: Operatively treated type IV tibial tubercle apophyseal fractures. *J Pediatr Orthop* 2013;33(8):791-796.

46. Zrig M, Annabi H, Ammari T, et al: Acute tibial tubercle avulsion fractures in the sporting adolescent. *Arch Orthop Trauma Surg* 2008;128:1437-1442.

47. Burkhart SS, Peterson HA: Fractures of the proximal tibial epiphysis. *J Bone Joint Surg Am* 1979;61(7):996-1002.

48. Zionts LE: Fractures around the knee in children. *J Am Acad Orthop Surg* 2002;10(5):345-355.

49. Vyas S, Ebramzadeh E, Behrend C, Silva M, Zionts LE: Flexion-type fractures of the proximal tibial physis: A report of five cases and review of the literature. *J Pediatr Orthop B* 2010;19(6):492-496.

Section 7: Trauma

50. Aerts BRJ, Ten Brinke B, Jakma TSC, Punt BJ: Classification of proximal tibial epiphysis fractures in children: Four clinical cases. *Injury* 2015;46(8):1680-1683.
51. Blanks RH, Lester DK, Shaw BA: Flexion-type Salter II fracture of the proximal tibia. Proposed mechanism of injury and two case studies. *Clin Orthop Relat Res* 1994;301: 256-259.
52. Noerdlinger MA, Lifrak JT, Cole PA: Proximal tibial physis fractures and the use of noninvasive studies in detecting vascular injury: A case report and literature review. *Am J Orthop (Belle Mead NJ)* 2000;29(11):891-895.
53. Watanabe H, Majima T, Takahashi K, et al: Posterior tibial slope angle is associated with flexion-type Salter-Harris II and Watson-Jones type IV fractures of the proximal tibia. *Knee Surg Sports Traumatol Arthrosc* 2019;27(9):2994-3000.

    Sixteen Salter-Harris II flexion-type injuries in 12 adolescents (mean 14.6 years) were identified. Radiographic analysis of these patients compared with a normal matched cohort demonstrated that those who sustained injuries had a relatively increased posterior tibial slope angle than matched control patients, suggesting a potential anatomic risk factor. Level of evidence: III.
54. Mudgal CS, Popovitz LE, Kasser JR: Flexion-type Salter-Harris I injury of the proximal tibial epiphysis. *J Orthop Trauma* 2000;14(4):302-305.
55. Mayer S, Albright JC, Stoneback JW: Pediatric knee dislocations and physeal fractures about the knee. *J Am Acad Orthop Surg* 2015;23(9):571-580.
56. Gautier E, Ziran BH, Egger B, Slongo T, Jakob RP: Growth disturbances after injuries of the proximal tibial epiphysis. *Arch Orthop Trauma Surg* 1998;118(1-2):37-41.
57. Vrettakos AN, Evaggelidis DC, Kyrkos MJ, et al: Lower limb deformity following proximal tibia physeal injury: Long-term follow-up. *J Orthop Traumatol* 2012;13(1):7-11.

CHAPTER 45

Tibia, Ankle, and Foot Fractures

YING LI, MD • MARK SEELEY, MD, FACS, FAOA

ABSTRACT

Fractures of the tibia, ankle, and foot are common in children and adolescents. It is helpful to be familiar with the characteristics of the most frequent types of fractures, including epidemiology, mechanism of injury, diagnosis, classification, treatment options, and potential complications.

Keywords: foot fracture; proximal tibia fracture; tibial shaft fracture; Tillaux fracture; triplane fracture

INTRODUCTION

Fractures of the tibia, ankle, and foot are common in children and adolescents. The incidence and pattern of each fracture type vary based on the age of the patient, the mechanism of injury, and the anatomic location. Nonsurgical management is successful for many of these fractures. Surgical intervention is reserved for physeal malreductions, articular displacement, and unstable fractures not amenable to closed management. Fractures associated with open wounds will frequently require surgical management as well. Long-term follow-up of physeal fractures in patients who are skeletally immature is required to monitor for growth arrest and resultant deformities.

Dr. Li or an immediate family member serves as a board member, owner, officer, or committee member of the Pediatric Orthopaedic Society of North America and the Scoliosis Research Society. Dr. Seeley or an immediate family member has received royalties from Orthopaediatrics and serves as a paid consultant to or is an employee of Orthopaediatrics.

PROXIMAL TIBIA METAPHYSEAL FRACTURES

Proximal tibia metaphyseal fractures are most common in children 6 years of age and younger.[1,2] These fractures usually result from an extension and/or valgus force. The fibula frequently remains intact. These injuries are increasingly common trampoline injuries and are commonly referred to as trampoline fractures.[3] Most patients can be treated nonsurgically with immobilization with the knee in slight flexion and application of a varus mold. The development of a late valgus deformity after these fractures was first described by the author of a 1953 study.[1] Although this deformity can occur even after a nondisplaced fracture, it occurs more commonly with fractures with a persistent medial metaphyseal gap and in those with an ipsilateral fibula fracture.[4,5] One theory that has been proposed to explain the late valgus deformity is overgrowth secondary to increased vascularity to the medial proximal tibia physis after the fracture.[6,7] This deformity can develop up to 18 months after the injury. Most patients will experience spontaneous improvement of the deformity with excellent long-term outcomes.[1,4,8] Although persistent deformities can be corrected with medial proximal tibia hemiepiphysiodesis,[2] surgical correction of a valgus deformity is rarely necessary.[4]

TIBIAL SHAFT FRACTURES

Tibial shaft fractures account for 15% of all pediatric long bone fractures.[9] The most frequent mechanism of injury is indirect trauma, such as a twisting injury, and the most common resulting fracture pattern is spiral or oblique. Most of these fractures occur in the distal third of the tibia, followed by fractures in the middle third of the tibia.[9,10]

Most tibial shaft fractures can be managed with closed reduction and immobilization. Initial fracture displacement, immediate postreduction fracture malalignment, and presence of a fibula fracture are predictors of loss of reduction.[11,12] Fracture alignment should be closely monitored during the first 3 weeks. Isolated tibial shaft fractures are at risk of varus angulation secondary to deforming forces from the anterior and deep posterior compartment musculature plus the tethering effect of the intact fibula.[10] In contrast, tibial shaft fractures with an associated fibula fracture are more at risk of subsequent valgus angulation. Acceptable fracture alignment is controversial, but general principles are shown in **Table 1**. It is important to assess for apex posterior angulation because this will have the least remodeling potential of all the residual angular deformities.[13] Children with low-energy fractures can be casted with the knee in 10° of flexion and allowed to be weight bearing as tolerated, as this has not been found to affect time to fracture union and fracture alignment and may lead to better short-term functional outcomes.[14]

Indications for surgical management of tibial shaft fractures in the pediatric age group include failure of closed management, open fractures with unstable wounds (typically Gustilo grades II and III), floating knee injuries, coexistent vascular injuries requiring repair, and selected cases of polytrauma. In addition, surgical stabilization of tibial fractures associated with compartment syndrome simplifies subsequent fasciotomy wound management. In the skeletally immature, flexible intramedullary nailing with titanium or stainless steel nails is most commonly performed when surgical stabilization is necessary (**Figure 1**). Flexible intramedullary nailing of tibial shaft fractures has been found to result in a substantially shorter time to union and better functional outcomes compared with external fixation.[15] Flexible intramedullary nailing of displaced tibial shaft fractures with an intact fibula can decrease the duration of immobilization compared with nonsurgical treatment.[16] Increased patient age and weight are not associated with a higher risk of malunion or a longer time to healing after flexible intramedullary nailing of tibial shaft fractures.[17,18] Open reduction and plate osteosynthesis is another option for skeletally immature patients, especially those with fracture patterns not amenable to intramedullary nails. Both flexible intramedullary nailing and plate fixation result in predictable fracture healing. Although plate fixation leads to a shorter period of immobilization, more anatomic reductions, and a lower rate of secondary surgeries compared with flexible intramedullary nailing, surgical time and wound complications may be increased.[19] Adolescents with a closed or closing proximal tibia physis can be treated with standard adult rigid intramedullary nailing techniques, although specific criteria to judge at what degree of skeletal maturity it is safe to violate the proximal tibia physis remain elusive.[20,21]

External fixation was previously considered the standard treatment of pediatric open tibial shaft fractures. However, a high rate of complications with external fixation has been reported, including delayed union, malunion, limb-length discrepancy, and pin tract infections.[22] Although external fixation remains an option for unstable fractures and open fractures with extensive soft-tissue loss, immediate flexible intramedullary nailing of open tibial shaft fractures has not been found to result in increased rates of wound or infectious complications or compartment syndrome compared with closed fractures. Similar to external fixation, patients with Gustilo type II and III fractures treated with immediate flexible intramedullary nailing can experience substantially prolonged bone healing.[23]

Compartment syndrome is a major concern in tibial shaft fractures regardless of treatment technique. Compartment syndrome has been reported in up to 12% of all pediatric tibial shaft fractures, with those older than 13 years and those injured in a motor vehicle accident at highest risk.[24] Incidence of compartment syndrome has been reported to be as high as 20% after flexible intramedullary nailing of tibial shaft fractures.[25] Awareness of and monitoring for compartment syndrome, both at the initial diagnosis and after nonsurgical or surgical intervention, are required.

TABLE 1

Acceptable Alignment for Pediatric Tibial Shaft Fractures

	Age < 8 yr	Age ≥ 8 yr
Valgus	5°	5°
Varus	10°	5°
Anterior angulation	10°	5°
Posterior angulation	5°	0°
Shortening	10 mm	5 mm
Rotation	5°	5°

Reproduced with permission from Heinrich SD, Mooney JF: Fractures of the shaft of the tibia and fibula, in Beaty JH, Kasser JR, eds: *Rockwood and Wilkins' Fractures in Children*, ed 7. Philadelphia, PA, Lippincott Williams & Wilkins, 2010, pp 930-966.

ANKLE FRACTURES

Distal Tibia Physeal Fractures

Ankle fractures account for 5% of all pediatric fractures.[26] Although a 2016 MRI study showed that children much more frequently sustain standard ankle sprains than epiphyseal plate injuries,[27] the physes around the ankle are still susceptible to injury. In comparison with the upper extremity epiphyseal plates, the distal tibia physis has a higher rate of growth arrest after injury, with rates up to 66.7%.[28-30] Fracture morphology depends on the skeletal

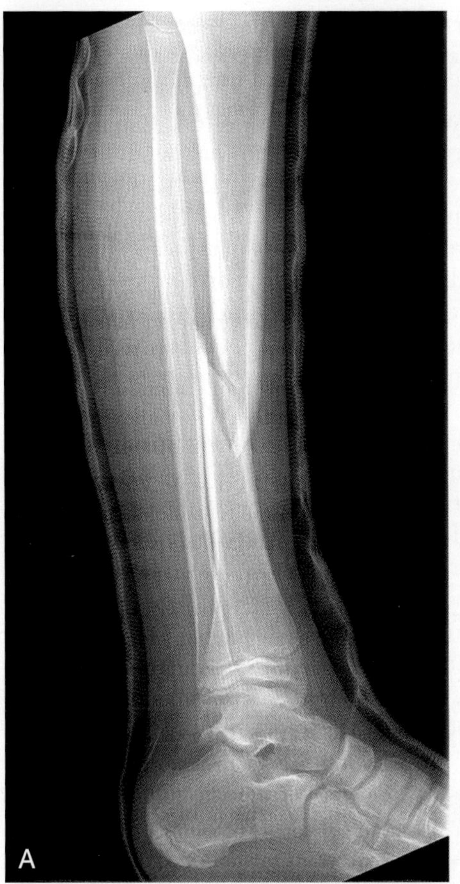

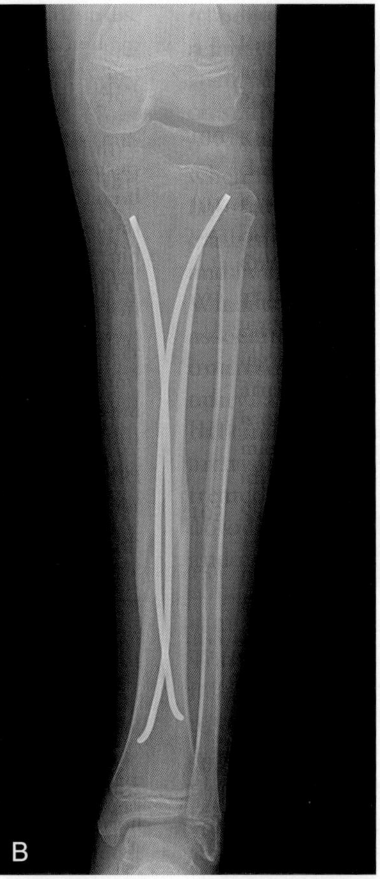

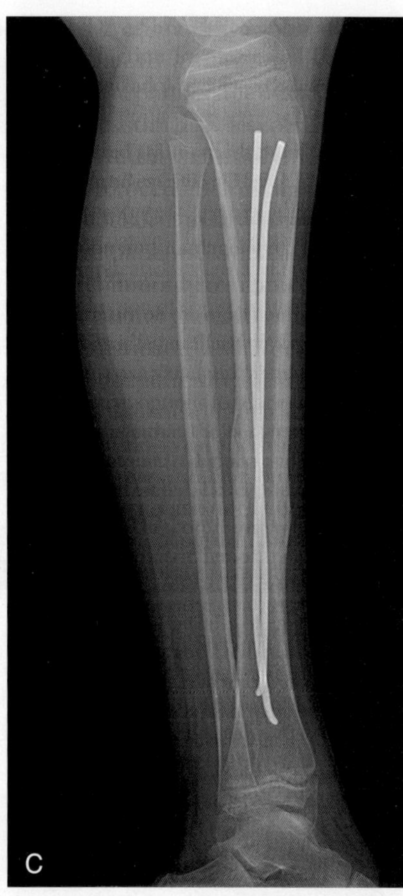

FIGURE 1 Lateral radiograph of a tibial shaft fracture in which apex posterior angulation persisted after attempted closed reduction (**A**). AP (**B**) and lateral (**C**) radiographs after titanium elastic nailing.

maturity of the patient and mechanism of injury.[28] The central-medial portion of the distal tibia physis begins to close at approximately 12 to 15 years of age for girls and 13 to 17 years for boys. Closure occurs over an 18-month period and progresses in a predictable (anteromedial, medial, posterior, anterolateral) fashion.[31]

Classification of distal tibia physeal fractures not only guides treatment but also provides prognostic implications. Most fractures can be classified with the Salter-Harris system. The commonly accepted rule is that severity of physeal fractures increases with Salter-Harris grade and so does the risk for premature physeal closure. The Dias-Tachdjian classification is less commonly used because of its complexity, but this system is based on the position of the foot and the direction of force at the time of the injury.[32] Pronation injuries may have a higher rate of growth arrest than supination-external rotation injuries, thus requiring closer follow-up.[29,33-36] Abduction injuries have a relatively poor prognosis for premature physeal closure regardless of whether closed or open treatment is performed.[29,33,34]

The evaluating physician should have a low threshold for obtaining a CT scan. A CT scan can be a valuable tool to evaluate physeal and intra-articular involvement as well as fracture displacement.[35] The radiation from a standard ankle CT is estimated to be equivalent to the dose received by 0.9 chest radiographs.[37] This information has been shown to change surgical indications as well as surgical strategy.[38-40]

Salter-Harris types I and II fractures can be treated with closed reduction and immobilization. Both fractures can be immobilized for 4 to 6 weeks in a short leg cast. If the fracture is felt to be stable, then a walking boot can be considered. In patients who are approaching skeletal maturity, minimal residual displacement at the physis can be accepted as long as a large procurvatum deformity does not develop, as this would hinder ankle dorsiflexion and predispose the patient to an Achilles contracture.[41] Surgical intervention is recommended for fractures with greater than 2 mm residual displacement, Salter-Harris types III and IV fractures with articular step-off, or external rotation deformity. Persistent gapping of greater than 3 mm suggests interposed periosteum and premature physeal closure has been found to occur in 60% of fractures that do not undergo open reduction.[28,34] Fractures can be stabilized with percutaneous insertion of smooth pins that cross the physis (**Figure 2**) or placement of screws in the epiphysis and metaphysis parallel to the physis. Distal tibia physeal fractures should be followed up for a growth arrest for at least 1 year or until skeletal maturity.[42]

Supination-inversion mechanisms can cause Salter-Harris types III or IV fractures of the medial malleolus. These fractures have a high potential for physeal growth disturbance.[43,44] Nondisplaced fractures can be managed nonsurgically in a cast for 4 to 6 weeks, while surgical intervention should be pursued for articular step-off and displacement greater than 2 mm. Because of the potential for partial growth arrest and subsequent varus deformity, these fractures need to be followed up until physeal growth is ascertained. An oblique Park-Harris line would suggest a partial growth arrest, and management is based on the degree of deformity and growth remaining.

TRANSITIONAL FRACTURES: TILLAUX AND TRIPLANE

Tillaux fractures occur when an external rotational force on the foot or leg leads to avulsion of the anterolateral distal tibia epiphysis by the anterior tibiofibular ligament. These injuries are Salter-Harris type III fractures, and the avulsed portion of the epiphysis is termed the Tillaux fragment. These fractures are considered transitional fractures because they generally occur in adolescents who are within 1 year of completing closure of the distal tibia physis. Standard ankle radiographs are not always diagnostic as the overlap between the distal tibia and fibula on an AP view can be superimposed over the fracture line, and the fracture is not seen on a lateral when there is no sagittal plane displacement. The mortise view increases the sensitivity for identifying this fracture. Because of the patient being near physeal closure, there is little risk for a clinically significant growth arrest. The main goal in treatment is to restore articular congruity. A CT scan is useful to assess articular displacement and fracture morphology and guide surgical fixation[35] (**Figure 3**). Closed or open reduction and fixation with pins or screws is recommended for fractures with greater than 2 mm displacement or articular step-off.[45,46] Most displaced fractures will have a large piece of periosteum that can flip into the fracture site. An open approach allows removal of interposed periosteum that can block the reduction.

Triplane fractures tend to occur earlier in adolescence than Tillaux fractures. They frequently involve more force,

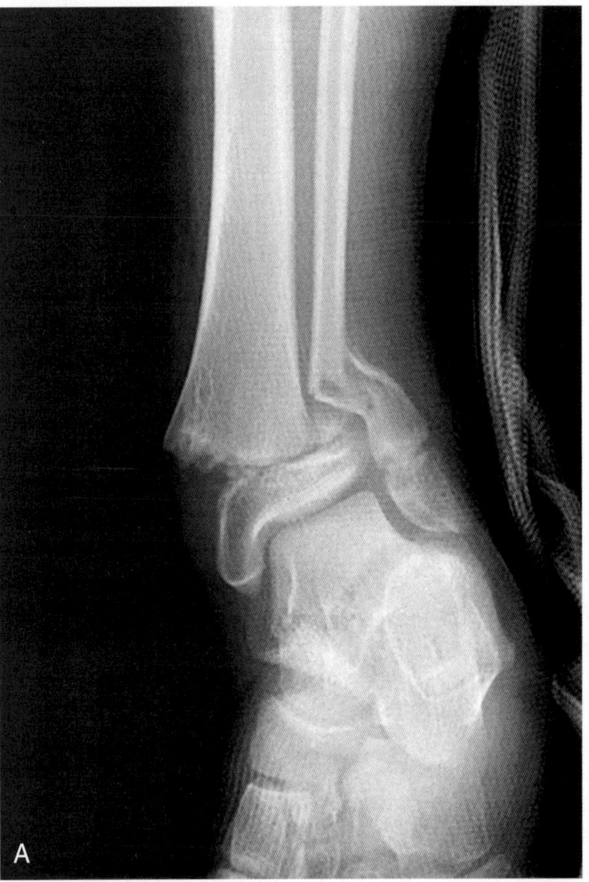

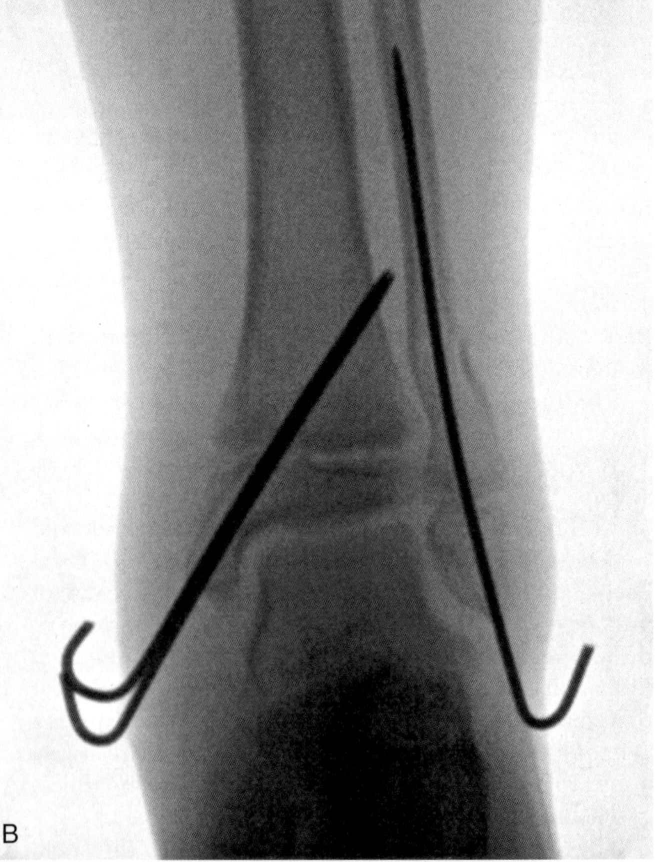

FIGURE 2 AP radiograph of a Salter-Harris type II distal tibia fracture and distal fibula fracture before (**A**) and after (**B**) open reduction and percutaneous pinning. A large flap of interposed periosteum was removed from the distal tibia fracture site.

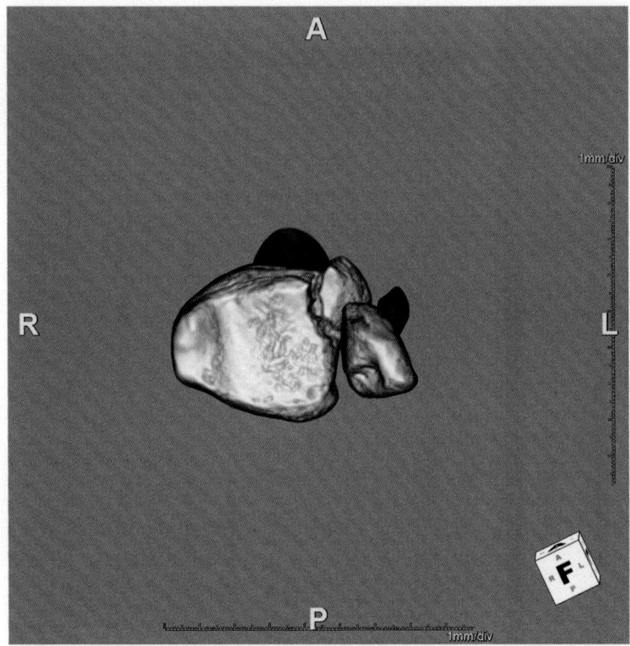

FIGURE 3 Three-dimensional axial image of a Tillaux fracture.

resulting in a complex though predictable Salter IV fracture.[40] Fracture morphology consists of an axial plane fracture through the physis, a sagittal plane fracture through the epiphysis, and a coronal plane fracture through the metaphysis and can consist of multiple parts. Radiographs can be difficult to interpret because of the acute changes in fracture direction, and a CT is recommended for surgical decision making. Two-part and three-part fractures are the most common. A two-part triplane fracture is a Salter-Harris type IV fracture, whereas a three-part triplane fracture is a combined Salter-Harris type II (metaphyseal) and III (epiphyseal) fracture[47] (**Figure 4**). Triplane fractures are intra-articular, and treatment focuses on restoring articular congruity. Closed reduction by internally rotating the foot and immobilization in 30° of knee flexion in a long leg splint can be performed. If surgical treatment is required, percutaneous pins or screws inserted across the differing planes of the fracture and supplemented with postoperative immobilization is a successful technique as long as adequate reduction can be obtained[45,46] (**Figure 5**). As triplane fractures occur more frequently in patients with greater remaining growth potential than Tillaux fractures, postoperative follow-up looking for growth irregularities is recommended.

The risk of concurrent ipsilateral tibial shaft fractures and ankle fractures was recently evaluated in the pediatric population.[48] Patients with a tibial shaft fracture at the junction of the middle and distal thirds and those with oblique and spiral fracture patterns were most at risk. Sixty percent of the concurrent ankle fractures in this study were transitional fractures.

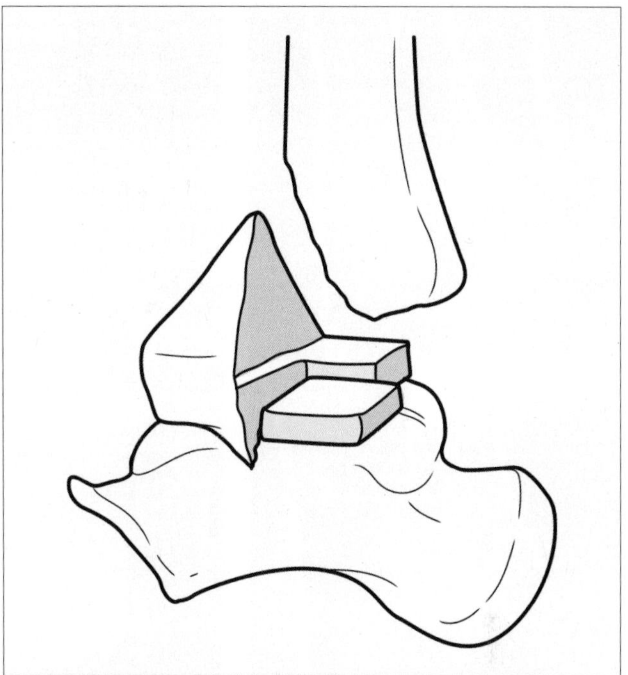

FIGURE 4 Schematic drawing of a three-part triplane fracture, which is a combined Salter-Harris type II and III fracture. The Salter-Harris type III fracture also is known as a Tillaux fragment.

Fibular Fractures

Low-grade inversion injuries can cause isolated Salter-Harris types I and II fractures of the distal fibula. The majority of these fractures can be managed with 3 to 4 weeks of immobilization. When accompanying a distal tibia fracture, surgical treatment for fibula fractures can be considered when establishing length will help facilitate reduction of the tibia or for unstable fractures. The relationship between the fibula and tibia is not static and changes during growth. Therefore, in patients with greater than 3 years of growth remaining, the fibular physis needs to be respected.[49,50] If fixation must cross the epiphyseal plate, smooth Kirschner wires should be used.

FOOT FRACTURES

Calcaneus Fractures

Pediatric calcaneal fractures are rare. They can often be missed as a consequence of their subtle clinical and radiographic presentation.[51] Delay in diagnosis can occur in 30% to 50% of cases.[51,52] Extra-articular fractures are more common than intra-articular fractures in children, and the majority of these fractures can be managed nonsurgically with long-term satisfactory results.[52,53] Plain lateral and axial views of the calcaneus are frequently diagnostic, but CT scan is necessary to assess fracture

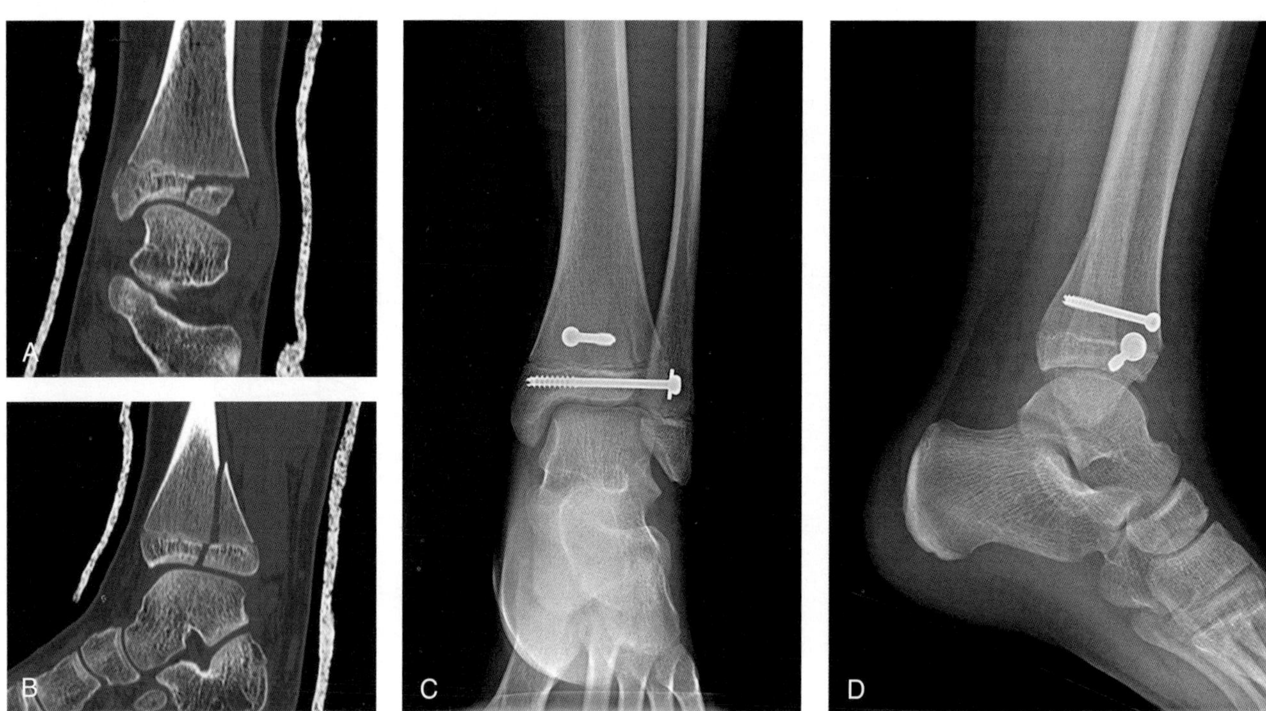

FIGURE 5 Coronal (**A**) and sagittal (**B**) CT scans demonstrating a triplane fracture. AP (**C**) and lateral (**D**) radiographs after screw fixation.

displacement and subtalar joint involvement. In children, remodeling of the height and width of the calcaneus will occur, which makes subtalar joint displacement the primary indication for surgery. When the subtalar joint is involved, it is often impacted into the body of the calcaneus (Essex-Lopresti joint depression) without an intra-articular split. If it is impacted into the calcaneus in such a way that the subtalar joint is no longer congruent, then reduction to reestablish a congruent articulation is indicated. This fracture pattern is very amenable to a minimally invasive (sinus tarsi) approach with percutaneous pinning or screw fixation.[54,55] Adolescents with more adultlike Sanders II and III displaced intra-articular fractures may require open reduction and internal fixation through a more extensile lateral approach.[53,56]

Talus Fractures

Traumatic fractures of the talus can include high-energy talar neck and talar body fractures, but also traumatic osteochondral lesions of the talar dome and fractures of the lateral process. The authors will focus here on the high-energy talar neck and body injuries. Talar neck fractures are classically caused by forced dorsiflexion of the talus into the anterior lip of the distal tibia, although medial, lateral, or rotational movement or positioning during the injury can result in ipsilateral medial or lateral malleolar fractures.[57] In children, the majority of these fractures are of lesser severity and carry a lower risk of osteonecrosis.[58] With increasing age and exposure to motor vehicle accidents, higher rates of displaced talar neck and body fractures are seen. With this, the notable complications of osteonecrosis, posttraumatic arthrosis, nonunion, and residual pain seen in adults can be experienced.[59,60] Displaced fractures should be treated with closed versus open reduction and internal fixation to avoid fracture displacement and promote union. Patients must have weight-bearing restrictions until fracture stability or union has been achieved.

Midfoot Fractures/Dislocations

Cuboid fractures in children most frequently occur with forced abduction of the foot and have been referred to as a nutcracker fracture caused by compression between the calcaneus and the fourth and fifth metatarsals. This is one traumatic cause of an acute limp in the toddler age group. In children younger than 10 years, these injuries are almost always extra-articular and isolated and are treated nonsurgically. In older adolescents, fractures with intra-articular involvement and/or associated additional midfoot injuries are more complex and often require surgical management.[61]

Lisfranc injuries in children and adolescents are most frequently sports-related injuries.[62] Lisfranc injures should be considered when a cuboid fracture is identified in combination with a fracture at the base of the second metatarsal.[63] Although the diagnosis is frequently made on plain and stress (weight-bearing) radiographs,[64] advanced imaging may be required for surgical decision making and preoperative planning. Nonsurgical management may be used in minimally displaced (<2 mm) injuries, comprising a non–weight-bearing cast for 6 weeks followed by protected weight bearing. Traumatic injuries with more displacement will require reduction and fixation, which may need to be staged if the patient's soft-tissue swelling precludes immediate treatment. A number of surgical strategies involving percutaneous pins, screws, plates, and TightRope devices have been described.[65-67] In general, joint preservation as opposed to primary fusion is favored in this age group.

Metatarsal Fractures

Metatarsal fractures are the most common pediatric foot fracture, accounting for 5% to 7% of all pediatric fractures and up to 60% of all pediatric foot fractures.[26,68] Almost all pediatric metatarsal fractures can be managed nonsurgically. In one review of 337 children with metatarsal fractures, only 10 required surgical treatment.[69] Surgical treatment is more likely in patients with multiple metatarsal fractures with increased translation. In patients with multiple metatarsal fractures, patients with extra-articular fractures and less than 75% displacement of the most displaced metatarsal should still be considered for nonsurgical care.[70] Clear indications for surgical reduction and fixation include open fractures and compartment syndrome.

The apophysis at the base of the fifth metatarsal can be confused with an avulsion fracture. This secondary ossification center appears at approximately 8 years of age and fuses by the age of 12 years in girls and 15 years in boys. There are numerous injury patterns to the proximal fifth metatarsal, with some requiring more aggressive treatment. Jones fractures, which occur at the metaphyseal-diaphyseal junction of the fifth metatarsal, are at risk for delayed union or nonunion in an adolescent. Treatment for an acute Jones fracture can include a non–weight-bearing cast for 6 weeks for nondisplaced fractures, advancing weight bearing as radiographic appearance of bone healing appears. Surgical treatment should be considered in high-performance athletes, displaced fractures, and fractures failing an initial trial of nonsurgical management. Many forms of surgical management, from open reduction and internal fixation to intramedullary screw fixation, have been described.[71]

Adolescents performing repetitive impact activities are at risk for stress fractures. Callus formation may be seen on radiographs but not in all cases. MRI can be useful in diagnosing the occult fracture and help guide treatment. The initial treatment of stress fractures is rest in a walking boot. Recurrent stress fractures should prompt an assessment of bone mineral density and an assessment of metabolic and nutritional factors if abnormal. Individual foot anatomic variations and the environment of the repeated activity predisposing to the stress fractures should also be evaluated.

Phalangeal Fractures

Fractures of the phalanges of the lesser toes can occur from direct impact with an object or a crush injury from a falling object. The vast majority of these can be treated nonsurgically with a form of buddy-taping and a protective shoe with rare requirements for percutaneous pinning. Fractures of the hallux may require more aggressive management given its greater role in weight bearing and balance.[72] Intra-articular fractures involving the first metatarsophalangeal joint or interphalangeal joint may require reduction and fixation depending on articular displacement. Fractures that involve more than one-third of the joint surface may result in rotational deformities or joint instability and require stabilization with pins or a small screw.

Seymour fractures, classically described in the hand, will involve the toes as well, especially the hallux. These juxtaepiphyseal fractures of the terminal phalanx[73] are usually open if there is fracture displacement, with a subungual nail bed injury. Most patients will report bleeding around the nail at the time of the injury.[74] Like in the hand, appropriate treatment consists of timely irrigation and débridement, fracture reduction, and antibiotic administration.[75]

These fractures can sometimes present late after provisional care was provided in the emergency department at the time of injury. Radiographs are helpful in evaluating the fracture and the potential presence of osteomyelitis. Persistent drainage or gross purulence warrants surgical drainage and débridement.[76] If the patients received an adequate amount of antibiotics, the fracture and nail bed can be observed. The patient and family should be counseled on the potential for nail bed deformity in the long term.

SUMMARY

Most fractures of the tibia, ankle, and foot in pediatric patients have good clinical and radiographic outcomes with nonsurgical treatment. Anatomic reduction and fixation of physeal fractures, intra-articular fractures, and unstable fractures is generally recommended. Complications such as growth disturbances can occur after certain fractures in skeletally immature patients and should be closely monitored in the short term and potentially long term.

KEY STUDY POINTS

- Physeal fractures can lead to a growth disturbance in skeletally immature patients.
- Compartment syndrome can result after proximal tibia physeal fractures and tibial shaft fractures. Careful initial assessment and monitoring is necessary.
- Closed tibial shaft fractures that fail reduction, open fractures, fractures associated with compartment syndrome, and polytrauma may be indications for surgical treatment.
- Distal tibia physeal fractures with persistent gapping of greater than 3 mm suggests interposed periosteum. These fractures have a high risk of premature physeal closure if open reduction is not performed.
- Tillaux and triplane fractures are intra-articular, and treatment focuses on restoring articular congruity.
- Seymour fractures occur in the foot as well as the hand. Timely irrigation and débridement of the open fractures, with reduction, nail bed repair, and antibiotic management, gives the best results.

ANNOTATED REFERENCES

1. Cozen L: Fracture of the proximal portion of the tibia in children followed by valgus deformity. *Surg Gynecol Obstet* 1953;97(2):183-188.
2. Jordan SE, Alonso JE, Cook FF: The etiology of valgus angulation after metaphyseal fractures of the tibia in children. *J Pediatr Orthop* 1987;7(4):450-457.
3. Cho MJ, Kim J, Kim SJ, et al: Rapidly growing pediatric trampoline-related injuries in korea: A 10 year single center retrospective study. *Korean J Pediatr* 2019;62:90-94.

   This single-center, retrospective study reviewed 178 trampoline-related injuries over a 10-year period. Sixty-seven children (37.6%) had fractures, and proximal tibia fractures were the most common. Fractures were significantly more common in younger children (younger than 6 years). Level of evidence: IV.
4. Yang BW, Shore BJ, Rademacher E, May C, Watkins CJ, Glotzbecker MP: Prevalence of cozen's phenomenon of the proximal tibia. *J Pediatr Orthop* 2019;39(6):e417-e421.

   One hundred eighty-one proximal tibia fractures with an average age of 4.55 years were retrospectively reviewed. One hundred forty patients had initial valgus angulation <4°, of which 20 developed increasing valgus angulation in follow-up (14.3%). Only four of these 20 patients (20%) had persistent valgus angulation with longer follow-up. Risk factors for increasing angulation were persistent medial metaphyseal gap and ipsilateral fibula fracture. The authors suggest that these two groups be followed up for Cozen phenomenon, whereas other proximal tibia fractures do not require such surveillance. Level of evidence: IV.
5. Nenopoulos S, Vrettakos A, Chaftikis N, et al: The effect of proximal tibial fractures on the limb axis in children. *Acta Orthop Belg* 2007;73:345-353.
6. Tuten HR, Keeler KA, Gabos PG, Zionts LE, MacKenzie WG: Posttraumatic tibia valga in children. A long-term follow-up note. *J Bone Joint Surg Am* 1999;81(6):799-810.
7. Zionts LE, MacEwen GD: Spontaneous improvement of post-traumatic tibia valga. *J Bone Joint Surg Am* 1986;68(5):680-687.
8. Robert M, Khouri N, Carlioz H, Alain JL: Fractures of the proximal tibial metaphysis in children: Review of a series of 25 cases. *J Pediatr Orthop* 1987;7(4):444-449.
9. Yang JP, Letts RM: Isolated fractures of the tibia with intact fibula in children: A review of 95 patients. *J Pediatr Orthop* 1997;17(3):347-351.
10. Shannak AO: Tibial fractures in children: Follow-up study. *J Pediatr Orthop* 1988;8(3):306-310.
11. Ho CA, Dammann G, Podeszwa DA, Levy J: Tibial shaft fractures in adolescents: Analysis of cast treatment successes and failures. *J Pediatr Orthop B* 2015;24(2):114-117.
12. Kinney MC, Nagle D, Bastrom T, Linn MS, Schwartz AK, Pennock AT: Operative versus conservative management of displaced tibial shaft fracture in adolescents. *J Pediatr Orthop* 2016;36(7):661-666.

    This retrospective study showed that initial fracture displacement and associated fibula fracture were predictors of failure of closed reduction and casting of closed tibial shaft fractures. Level of evidence: III.
13. Dwyer AJ, John B, Krishen M, Hora R: Remodeling of tibial fractures in children younger than 12 years. *Orthopedics* 2007;30(5):393-396.
14. Silva M, Eagan MJ, Wong MA, Dichter DH, Ebramzadeh E, Zionts LE: A comparison of two approaches for the closed treatment of low-energy tibial fractures in children. *J Bone Joint Surg Am* 2012;94(20):1853-1860.
15. Kubiak EN, Egol KA, Scher D, Wasserman B, Feldman D, Koval KJ: Operative treatment of tibial fractures in children: Are elastic stable intramedullary nails an improvement over external fixation? *J Bone Joint Surg Am* 2005;87(8):1761-1768.
16. Canavese F, Botnari A, Andreacchio A, et al: Displaced tibial shaft fractures with intact fibula in children: Nonoperative management versus operative treatment with elastic stable intramedullary nailing. *J Pediatr Orthop* 2016;36(7):667-672.

    This retrospective study demonstrated similar treatment outcomes between nonoperative management versus operative treatment with elastic stable intramedullary nailing of displaced tibial shaft fractures with an intact fibula in pediatric patients. Patients treated nonoperatively had a longer period of immobilization. Level of evidence: III.
17. Goodbody CM, Lee RJ, Flynn JM, Sankar WN: Titanium elastic nailing for pediatric tibia fractures: Do older, heavier kids do worse? *J Pediatr Orthop* 2016;36(5):472-477.

This retrospective review did not show a difference in time to union or malunion rate based on age or weight in pediatric patients with tibia fractures treated with titanium elastic nailing. Level of evidence: III.

18. Marengo L, Paonessa M, Andreacchio A, Dimeglio A, Potenza A, Canavese F: Displaced tibia shaft fractures in children treated by elastic stable intramedullary nailing: Results and complications in children weighing 50 kg (110 lb) or more. *Eur J Orthop Surg Traumatol* 2016;26(3):311-317.

    This retrospective review did not find poorer outcomes in older or heavier patients with closed displaced tibial shaft fractures treated with elastic stable intramedullary nailing. Level of evidence: IV.

19. Pennock AT, Bastrom TP, Upasani VV: Elastic intramedullary nailing versus open reduction internal fixation of pediatric tibial shaft fractures. *J Pediatr Orthop* 2017;37(7):e403-e408.

    This retrospective study demonstrated predictable healing with elastic intramedullary nailing and open reduction and internal fixation with a plate and screws in patients with unstable tibial shaft fractures. Plate fixation led to a shorter period of immobilization, more anatomic reductions, and a lower rate of secondary surgeries, but there was a trend toward longer surgical times and increased rates of wound-related complications. Level of evidence: III.

20. Court-Brown CM, Byrnes T, McLaughlin G: Intramedullary nailing of tibial diaphyseal fractures in adolescents with open physes. *Injury* 2003;34:781-785.

21. Weltsch D, Baldwin KD: Rigid locked nail fixation for pediatric tibia fractures-where are the data? *World J Orthop* 2019;10:299-303.

    This well-referenced editorial points out the considerable progress that has been made in the field of skeletal maturity estimation in the past decade, but there still remains no benchmark for precise determination of potential growth remaining around the knee for quantifying the risk of damage to the proximal tibia physis.

22. Myers SH, Spiegel D, Flynn JM: External fixation of high-energy tibia fractures. *J Pediatr Orthop* 2007;27(5):537-539.

23. Pandya NK, Edmonds EW: Immediate intramedullary flexible nailing of open pediatric tibial shaft fractures. *J Pediatr Orthop* 2012;32(8):770-776.

24. Shore BJ, Glotzbecker MP, Zurakowski D, Gelbard E, Hedequist DJ, Matheney TH: Acute compartment syndrome in children and teenagers with tibial shaft fractures: Incidence and multivariable risk factors. *J Orthop Trauma* 2013;27(11):616-621.

25. Pandya NK, Edmonds EW, Mubarak SJ: The incidence of compartment syndrome after flexible nailing of pediatric tibial shaft fractures. *J Child Orthop* 2011;5(6):439-447.

26. Landin LA: Epidemiology of children's fractures. *J Pediatr Orthop B* 1997;6(2):79-83.

27. Boutis K, Plint A, Stimec J et al: Radiographic-negative lateral ankle injuries in children: Occult growth plate fracture or sprain? *JAMA Pediatr* 2016:170(1):e154114.

    One hundred thirty-five children with the clinical diagnosis of Salter I distal fibula fracture without plain radiographic abnormalities underwent MRI of both ankles. Only 3% had MRI-confirmed distal fibula physeal injuries, with the majority (80%) having lateral ligamentous injuries. Level of evidence: II.

28. Barmada A, Gaynor T, Mubarak SJ: Premature physeal closure following distal tibia physeal fractures: A new radiographic predictor. *J Pediatr Orthop* 2003;23(6):733-739.

29. Rohmiller MT, Gaynor TP, Pawelek J, Mubarak SJ: Salter-Harris I and II fractures of the distal tibia: Does mechanism of injury relate to premature physeal closure? *J Pediatr Orthop* 2006;26(3):322-328.

30. Nenopoulos SP, Papavasiliou VA, Papavasiliou AV: Outcome of physeal and epiphyseal injuries of the distal tibia with intra-articular involvement. *J Pediatr Orthop* 2005;25(4):518-522.

31. Spiegel PG, Cooperman DR, Laros GS: Epiphyseal fractures of the distal ends of the tibia and fibula. A retrospective study of two hundred and thirty-seven cases in children. *J Bone Joint Surg Am* 1978;60(8):1046-1050.

32. Dias LS, Tachdjian MO: Physeal injuries of the ankle in children: Classification. *Clin Orthop Relat Res* 1978;136:230-233.

33. Russo F, Moor MA, Mubarak SJ, Pennock AT: Salter-Harris II fractures of the distal tibia: Does surgical management reduce the risk of premature physeal closure? *J Pediatr Orthop* 2013;33(5):524-529.

34. Leary JT, Handling M, Talerico M, Yong L, Bowe JA: Physeal Fractures of the distal tibia; predictive factors of premature physeal closure and growth arrest. *J Pediatr Orthop* 2009;29(4):356-361.

35. Nenopoulos A, Beslikas T, Gigis I, Sayegh F, Christoforidis I, Hatzokos I: The role of CT in diagnosis and treatment of distal tibial fractures with intra-articular involvement in children. *Injury* 2015;46(11):2177-2180.

36. Binkley A, Mehlman CT, Freeh E: Salter-Harris II ankle fractures in children: Does fracture pattern matter? *J Orthop Trauma* 2019;33:e190-e195.

    A retrospective review of 141 skeletally immature patients with radiographically confirmed Salter II ankle fractures showed a premature physeal closure rate of 28.8% in pronation-external rotation injuries, 24.1% in supination-plantarflexion injuries, and 11.4% in supination-external rotation injuries. The pronation-external rotation group had a statistically significant higher rate of resultant angular deformity. Level of evidence: III.

37. Biswas D, Bible JE, Bohan M, Simpson AK, Whang PG, Grauer JN: Radiation exposure from musculoskeletal computerized tomorphaic scans. *J Bone Joint Surg Am* 2009;91:1882-1889.

38. Cutler L, Molloy A, Dhukuram V, Bass A: Do CT scans aid assessment of distal tibial physeal fractures? *J Bone Joint Surg Br* 2004;86:239-243.

39. Eismann EA, Stephan ZA, Mehlman T, Denning J, Mehlman T, Parikh SN: Pediatric triplane ankle fractures: Impact of radiographs and computed tomography on fracture classification and treatment planning. *J Bone Joint Surg Am* 2015;97:995-1102.

40. Hadad MT, Sullivan BT, Sponseller PD: Surgically relevant patterns in triplane fractures: A mapping study. *J Bone Joint Surg Am* 2018;100:1039-1046.

Thirty-three cases of triplane fractures were superimposed on unfractured bone templates to generate fracture maps, and areas of fracture frequency were identified. Metaphyseal fractures were consistent across all triplane fractures and manifest as medial-lateral fracture in the posterior metaphysis. Epiphyseal fractures have a common anterior fracture component and then class (# of parts)-dependent posterior fracture patterns.

41. Domzalski ME, Lipton GE, Lee D, Guille JT: Fractures of the distal tibial metaphysis in children: Patterns of injury and results of treatment. *J Pediatr Orthop* 2006;2006(2):171-176.
42. Schurz M, Binder H, Platzer P, Schulz M, Hajdu S, Vecsei V: Physeal injuries of the distal tibia: Long-term results in 376 patients. *Int Orthop* 2010;34(4):547-552.
43. Caterini R, Farsetti P, Ippolito E: Long-term followup of physeal injury to the ankle. *Foot Ankle* 1991;11:372-383.
44. Luhmann SJ, Oda JE, O'Donnell J, Keller KA, Schoenecker PL, Dobbs MB: An analysis of suboptimal outcomes of medial malleolus fractures in skeletally immature children. *AM J Orthop* 2012;41:113-116.
45. Choudhry IK, Wall EJ, Eismann EA, Crawford AH, Wilson L: Functional outcome analysis of triplane and Tillaux fractures after closed reduction and percutaneous fixation. *J Pediatr Orthop* 2014;34(2):139-142.
46. Lurie B, Van Rysselberghe N, Pennock AT, Upasani VV: Functional outcomes of Tillaux and triplane fractures with 2 to 5 millimeters of intra-articular gap. *J Bone Joint Surg Am* 2020;102(8):679-686.

    In this retrospective study, 57 patients with post–closed reduction CT scans demonstrating 2- to 5-mm residual articular step-off were reviewed. Thirty-four patients had triplane fractures, and 23 had Tillaux fractures. Functional outcome scores revealed that patients who were treated nonsurgically and had less than 2.5 mm gap had a significantly higher functional score (90%) than those patients with greater than 2.5 mm gap (75%). Surgical management likely conveys the greatest functional benefit when the intra-articular gap exceeds 2.5 mm. Level of evidence: III.

47. Cooperman DR, Spiegel PG, Laros GS: Tibial fractures involving the ankle in children: The so-called triplane epiphyseal fracture. *J Bone Joint Surg Am* 1978;60(8):1040-1046.
48. Sheffer BW, Villarreal ED, Oschner MG, et al: Concurrent ipsilateral tibial shaft and distal tibia fractures in pediatric patients: Risk factors, frequency, and risk of missed diagnosis. *J Pediatr Orthop* 2020;1:e1-e5.

    A retrospective review of 517 tibial shaft fractures showed 22 (4.3%) had concurrent distal tibia fractures. Patients with concurrent fractures were slightly older (12.7 years) than the remaining cohort (11 years). Patients with a fracture at the junction of the middle and distal thirds and those with spiral or oblique patterns were most at risk. Ankle-specific imaging is recommended in these higher risk patients. Level of evidence: III.

49. Karrholm J, Hansson LI, Selvik G: Changes in tibiofibular relationships due to growth disturbances after ankle fractures in children. *J Bone Joint Surg Am* 1984;66:1198-1210.
50. Chung T, Jaramillo D: Normal maturing distal tibia and fibula: Changes with age at MR imaging. *Radiology* 1995;194:227-232.
51. Inokuchi S, Usami N, Hiraishi E, Hashimoto T: Calcaneal fractures in children. *J Pediatr Orthop* 1998;18(4):469-474.
52. Brunet JA: Calcaneal fractures in children. Long-term results of treatment. *J Bone Joint Surg Br* 2000;82(2):211-216.
53. Petit CJ, Lee BM, Kasser JR, Kocher MS: Operative treatment of intra-articular calcaneal fractures in the pediatric population. *J Pediatr Orthop* 2007;27(8):856-862.
54. Abdelgawad AA, Kanlic E: Minimally invasive (sinus tarsi) approach for open reduction and internal fixation of intra-articular calcaneus fractures in children: Surgical technique and case report of two patients. *J Foot Ankle Surg* 2015;54:135-139.
55. Tong L, Li M, Li F, et al: A minimally invasive (sinus tarsi) approach with percutaneous K-wire fixation for intra-articular calcaneus fractures in children. *J Pediatr Orthop B* 2018;27:556-562.

    Twenty-five cases of calcaneus fractures in children (average age of 9.8 years) treated by sinus tarsi approach and percutaneous Kirschner wire fixation were retrospectively reviewed. The treatment technique resulted in good functional outcomes with minimal wound complications. Level of evidence: IV.

56. Pickle A, Benaroch TE, Guy P, Harvey EJ: Clinical outcome of pediatric calcaneal fractures treated with open reduction and internal fixation. *J Pediatr Orthop* 2004;24:178-180.
57. Jensen I, Wester JU, Rasmussen F, Lindequist S, Schantz K: Prognosis of fracture of the talus in children. *Acta Orthop Scand* 1994;65(4):398-400.
58. Eberl R, Singer G, Schalamon J, et al: Fractures of the talus-differences between children and adults. *J Trauma* 2010;68:126-130.
59. Kruppa C, Snoap T, Siesema DL, Schildhauer TA, Dudda M, Jones CB: Is the midterm progress of pediatric and adolescent talus fractures stratified by age? *J Foot Ankle Surg* 2018;57:471-477.

    This retrospective review of children with talus fractures who were followed up for over 1 year after injury showed that patients between the ages of 16 to 18 years had the worst outcomes, with 75% having residual arthrosis. Level of evidence: IV.

60. Smith JT, Curtis TA, Spencer S, et al: Complications of talus fractures in children. *J Pediatr Orthop* 2010;30:779-784.
61. Ruffing T, Ruckauer T, Bludau F, et al: Cuboid nutcracker fracture in children: Management and results. *Injury* 2019;50:607-612.

    A retrospective review of 16 cuboid fractures with outcome scores showed younger children with isolated, extra-articular fractures did well, but worse results were found in adolescent patients with intra-articular fractures and in those associated with midtarsal disruption. Level of evidence: IV.

62. Hill JF, Heyworth BE, Lierhaus A, Kocher MS, Mahan ST: Lisfranc injuries in children and adolescents. *J Pediatr Orthop B* 2017;26(2):159-163.

This retrospective study of children treated for bony or ligamentous Lisfranc injuries demonstrated that 34% of patients underwent open reduction and internal fixation. Full weight bearing was allowed in the surgical group at a mean of 14.5 weeks compared with 6.5 weeks in the nonsurgical group. Level of evidence: IV.

63. Ribbans WJ, Natarajan R, Alavala S: Pediatric foot fractures. *Clin Orthop Relat Res* 2005;432:107-115.

64. Knijnenberg LM, Dingemans SA, Terra MP, et al: Radiographic anatomy of the pediatric Lisfranc joint. *J Pediatr Orthop* 2018;38:510-513.

    Two hundred forty-three non–weight-bearing pediatric foot radiographs across a range of age groups were reviewed. None of the patients had a traumatic injury. The distance between the base of the first and second metatarsals was always <3 mm. The distance between the medial cuneiform and the proximal second metatarsal was <2 mm after the age of 6 years. Both measurements approached adult valuses at the age of 6 years. Level of evidence: III.

65. Veijola K, Laine HJ, Pajulo O: Lisfranc injury in adolescents. *Eur J Pediatr Surg* 2013;23:297-303.

66. Welck MJ, Zinchenko R, Rudge B: Review: Lisfranc injuries. *Injury* 2015;46:536-541.

67. Tzatzairis T, Firth G, Parker L: Adolescent Lisfranc injury treated with TightRope™: A case report and review of literature. *World J Orthop* 2019;10:115-122.

    The authors describe a case of an 11-year-old patient with a displaced Lisfranc ligament injury repaired with open reduction and a mini TightRope™ device with good results.

68. Crawford HA: Fractures and dislocations of the foot, in Flynn JM, Skaggs DL, Waters PM, eds. *Rockwood and Wilkins' Fractures in Children.* New York, NY, Wolters Kluwer, 2015, pp 1225-1270.

69. Robertson NB, Roocroft JH, Edmonds EW: Childhood metatarsal shaft fractures: Treatment outcomes and relative indications for surgical intervention. *J Child Orthop* 2012;6:125-129.

70. Mahan ST, Lierhaus AM, Spencer SA, Kasser JR: Treatment dilemma in multiple metatarsal fractures: When to operate? *J Pediatr Orthop B* 2016;25:354-360.

    This retrospective study of 98 pediatric patients with multiple metatarsal fractures concluded that younger patients and those with less than 75% displacement should be considered for nonoperative care. Level of evidence: IV.

71. Mahan ST, Hoellwarth JS, Spencer SA, Kramer DE, Hedequist DJ, Kasser JR: Likelihood of surgery in isolated fifth metatarsal fractures. *J Pediatr Orthop* 2015;35(3):296-302.

72. Petnehazy T, Schalamon J, Hartwig C, et al: Fractures of the hallux in children. *Foot Ankle Int* 2015;36:60-63.

73. Seymour N: Juxta-epiphyseal fractures of the terminal phalanx of the finger. *J Bone Joint Surg Br* 1966;48:347-349.

74. Kensinger DR, Guille JT, Horn BD, Herman MJ: The stubbed great toe: Importance of early recognition and treatment of open fractures of the distal phalanx. *J Pediatr Orthop* 2001;21:31-34.

75. Reyes BA, Ho CA: The high risk of infection with delayed treatment of open Seymour fractures: Salter-Harris I/II or Juxta-epiphyseal fractures of the distal phalanx with associated nailbed laceration. *J Pediatr Orthop* 2017;37:247-253.

    Thirty-four patients with 35 Seymour fractures involving the hand were retrospectively studied. Thirty-one percent received acute, appropriate treatment, and their infection rate was zero. Thirty-seven percent received acute, partial treatment, and their infection rate was 15%. Thirty-one percent received delayed treatment, and their infection rate was 45%. The authors concluded that timing and quality of initial treatment significantly influences infection rates. Level of evidence: III.

76. Morris B, Mullen S, Schroeppel P, Vopat B: Open physeal fracture of the distal phalanx of the hallux. *Am J Emerg Med* 2017;35:1035.e1-1035.e3.

    The authors present a case of delayed presentation of a Seymour fracture of the hallux, present the successful surgical treatment of the case, and review the literature on this injury.

CHAPTER 46

Spine Trauma

DANIEL J. HEDEQUIST, MD • MICHAEL P. GLOTZBECKER, MD

ABSTRACT

Unique characteristics in children predispose them to spine injuries that differ from those in adults. The size of children, anatomic differences of the cervical spine, and normal radiographic variants all need to be considered during the initial evaluation of a spine injury. Routine plain radiographs are used in the primary setting of trauma, followed by MRI and CT when indicated. Younger children are predisposed to upper cervical spine injuries, the most common being odontoid fractures. Adolescents generally sustain subaxial cervical spine injuries as well as thoracic and lumbar injuries that are more consistent with adult spine trauma. Spinal cord injuries without radiographic abnormality, Chance fractures, and apophyseal ring injuries are unique to children, given their size and spinal plasticity. The management of individual injuries varies and may range from nonsurgical management with an orthosis to surgical management with instrumented stabilization and fusion.

Keywords: cervical spine; dentocentral synchondrosis; spinal cord injuries without radiographic abnormality (SCIWORA); spine trauma; thoracolumbar spine; vertebral fractures

Dr. Glotzbecker or an immediate family member is a member of a speakers' bureau or has made paid presentations on behalf of Biomet, DePuy, a Johnson & Johnson Company, Medtronic, and NuVasive; serves as a paid consultant to or is an employee of NuVasive; and has received research or institutional support from CSSG, GSSG, and HSG. Neither Dr. Hedequist nor any immediate family member has received anything of value from or has stock or stock options held in a commercial company or institution related directly or indirectly to the subject of this chapter.

INTRODUCTION

Spine fractures represent approximately 1% of all fractures seen in level 1 pediatric trauma centers and are related to the patient's age and size. The anatomic differences in children vary and are deterministic of injury patterns. Younger children have a large head-to-body ratio and, consequently, sustain more upper cervical spine injuries, whereas adolescents sustain the most thoracolumbar injuries. For all children, the most common mechanism of fracture is a motor vehicle crash, with cervical trauma more common in younger children. The second most common cause of injury also is related to age, with falls more common in younger children and sports-related injuries more common in older children and adolescents. In up to 19% of patients, nonaccidental trauma is the cause of spine injuries in toddlers (children younger than 3 years), and it has a 25% mortality rate.[1] Spine trauma also is associated with nonspinal injuries, including head trauma, chest trauma, and abdominal injuries, as well as other noncontiguous spinal injuries.[2]

ANATOMY

Anatomic differences in children predispose each pediatric age group to differing injury patterns. Children younger than 8 years have more horizontally aligned cervical facets, greater ligamentous laxity, and a larger head-to-body ratio, all of which predispose them to upper cervical spine injuries at the cranial-cervical junction and C1-C2. Children younger than 6 years also have open synchondroses (cartilaginous growth centers), the largest of which is at C2 (the dentocentral synchondrosis), which makes odontoid fractures through the physis much more common in younger children. The dentocentral synchondrosis fuses when a child is approximately 6 years of age; before that, younger children are at risk of sustaining an injury at the dens through this growth center (**Figure 1**). Subaxial spine fractures, thoracic burst or compression

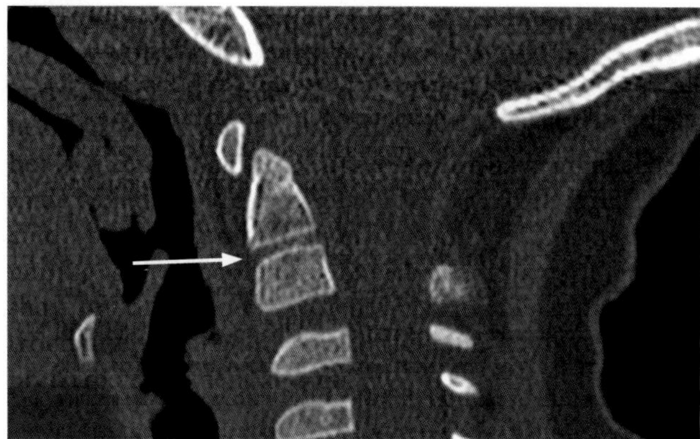

FIGURE 1 Sagittal CT scan of the spine of a 3-year-old patient. The arrow points to the dentocentral synchondrosis.

fractures, and lumbar spine injuries become more common as children develop (older than 10 years) and their anatomy becomes more similar to that of an adult.

INITIAL EVALUATION

The diagnosis, workup, and management of cervical spine trauma in children varies with age.[3] The initial evaluation of a child with suspected spine trauma begins in the field because children pose unique transport challenges related to their small size and anatomic differences. Children must be placed in cervical collars, with increased stability obtained by taping their heads to sandbags or intravenous fluid bags placed on either side of the head to further minimize cervical motion. Compared with adults, children have a larger cranium relative to their body size, and their occiput has a greater posterior offset that predisposes them to inadvertent cervical flexion when lying flat (**Figure 2**). This possible flexion must be counteracted by placing the child on a specialized pediatric backboard with an occipital recess cutout or elevating the child's body with blankets to allow the cranium to translate posteriorly. Generally, this is important in children younger than 8 years and can be assessed clinically by positioning the head so that the pinna is level with or posterior to the shoulder.

The initial physical examination should focus on all body systems. The evaluation of a child with suspected spine trauma should begin after a thorough primary survey because spine trauma often is associated with other injuries. The clinical evaluation of the back includes a standard inspection and palpation of the entire area, with care being taken to log roll the patient while using spinal precautions. A detailed neurologic examination should be performed because spine fractures and instability potentially can be associated with a spinal cord injury. Given the risk of lap-belt injuries in children, inspection and palpation of the anterior abdominal wall and the pelvic

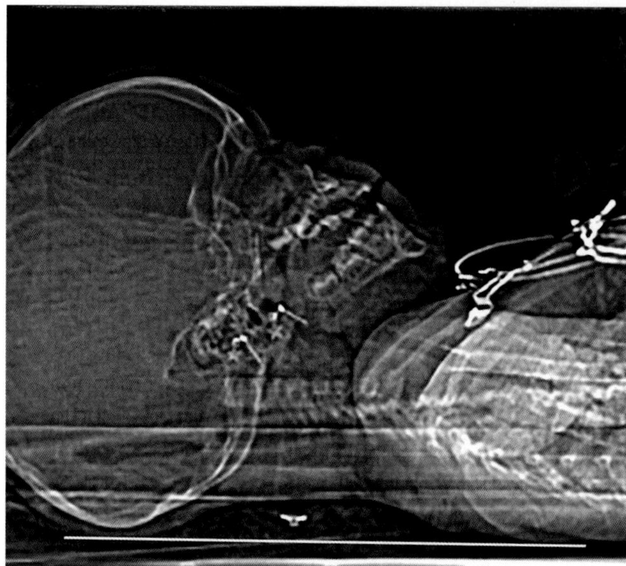

FIGURE 2 Lateral scout view in a CT scan of a 2-year-old patient being evaluated for neck trauma. Note the position of the child's neck in flexion; the white line extending from the back of the occiput to the shoulders at the bottom of the image indicates that no recess was applied to account for the large cranium because the occiput is in line with the thorax, not posterior.

region are paramount in younger children who have been injured in a motor vehicle crash.

RADIOGRAPHIC STUDIES

Standard radiography remains the initial imaging modality of choice for pediatric trauma patients. At a minimum, radiographs should include a cross-table lateral view with an AP view of the cervical spine. In children 3 to 16 years of age, two or more radiographic views detect cervical spine abnormalities with a sensitivity of 90% and a lateral radiograph alone has a 73% sensitivity and 92% sensitivity.[4] Patients with substantial neck pain despite normal-appearing radiographs require further imaging (usually CT). Because of the associated injuries, CT of the cervical spine should be considered for obtunded or uncooperative children with head injuries or facial trauma who will be undergoing CT. Plain radiographs of the thoracic and lumbar spine should be taken in cases of suspected injury indicated by the physical examination findings, associated injuries, or the patient's history. Normal anatomic variation exists for children younger than 8 years and may be mistaken for fractures or a ligamentous injury.[5] Ossification centers (most commonly the dens in children younger than 5 years) can be mistaken for a fracture line. Vertebral height differences as well as differences in morphology may be mistaken for compression fractures. Cervical pseudosubluxation resulting from ligamentous laxity (most commonly C2 on C3), loss of normal cervical lordosis, and increased apparent anterior soft-tissue swelling caused by crying are all examples of normal variants in the pediatric cervical spine. Subtle wedging of thoracic and lumbar vertebra as well as apparent disk irregularities (Schmorl nodes) must all be evaluated in context with the history and physical examination findings, and further imaging should be based on the complete evaluation.

CT is used to evaluate a suspected bony or ligamentous injury. Newer classification systems for spine trauma rely on CT for the anatomic classification of fractures. The increased use of CT for cervical screening has become more commonplace, especially in children who are more severely injured. In some centers, CT has been shown to be as efficacious as MRI in clearing the cervical spine in children who are severely injured to avoid the need for cervical collars and spinal precautions in patients who are obtunded.[6] However, the routine use of CT as a screening tool for cervical injuries is not appropriate because of the radiation dosing required and the ability to diagnose most suspected injuries with plain radiographs and a physical examination. Awake and alert patients with reliable examination findings do not require CT imaging based solely on the mechanism of injury. CT for thoracic and lumbar spine injuries should be limited to studying documented fractures. Before ordering CT, a discussion with the trauma team is warranted regarding the potential need for thoracic or abdominal CT for associated injuries. CT angiography should be considered in a patient with cervical facet fractures, upper cervical spine fractures, or fractures through the foramen because of the potential for vertebral artery injury with these fractures.[7]

In spinal trauma, MRI may be obtained for clearance and for the documentation of known injuries. MRI is an excellent cervical spine screening tool with high sensitivity and specificity when used within the first 48 hours of injury in children who are obtunded.[8] Children with a documented or suspected spine injury with a neurologic deficit should undergo MRI to determine the extent of neurologic injuries and/or compression, which may aid in treatment decisions. When surgical treatment of spine trauma is indicated, MRI and CT of the associated area should be obtained to clearly identify the extent of bony, ligamentous, and neural injuries.

CERVICAL SPINE CLEARANCE

Clearance of the cervical spine of children in the acute setting frequently is the job of the orthopaedic team. Patients requiring clearance may range from evaluation of an apprehensive child in the emergency department to the obtunded child in the intensive care unit setting. The goals of clearance are to provide expeditious diagnosis of injuries, to remove collars in children without injuries, to avoid unnecessary radiation, and to minimize the missing of injuries. These goals are improved when an algorithmic approach is taken by the treating physicians.[9,10] Consultation with the on-call spine team, use of plain radiographs as an initial study, and repeat examination of children the following day are hallmarks of successful spine clearance programs.[11-13] MRI studies have been shown to be sensitive and specific when evaluating the cervical spine in obtunded pediatric patients and are critical for clearance to avoid unnecessary spinal precautions and cervical collars in children who are unable to cooperate given other severe injuries.[8,14]

SPECIFIC INJURIES

Spinal Cord Injuries Without Radiographic Abnormality

Spinal cord injuries without radiographic abnormality (SCIWORA) describes a neurologic injury without apparent radiographic or CT evidence of a bony or ligamentous spinal column injury. The use of MRI has improved understanding of spinal column injuries in patients with apparently normal CT and radiographic findings. SCIWORA is thought to occur because of the plasticity of a child's spine, which allows stretch to occur without bony failure but causes damage to the neural elements that do not tolerate stretch as well. Most cases of SCIWORA occur in younger children secondary to motor vehicle and pedestrian-vehicle crashes. Infants and young children who have an SCIWORA should be screened for nonaccidental trauma. The degree of spinal cord injury ranges from mild and transient to severe and permanent, including profound quadriplegia. MRI evidence of facet and ligamentous injuries may be seen at the same level or even at levels away from the spinal cord injury. Spinal cord injuries seen on MRI range from mild cord contusions to complete disruptions. Treatment involves preventing further neurologic damage by stabilization with bracing treatment and supportive care of the spinal cord injury. Bracing treatment is worthwhile in patients with questionable ligamentous instability; however, if there is no evidence of injury other than neurologic injury, it is unclear if bracing treatment plays any role.[15,16] Neurologic recovery is dependent on the initial degree of spinal cord injury, which was documented in a 2013 multicenter study in which 94% of the patients with SCIWORA and a normal MRI had full recovery compared with only 27% of patients with abnormal MRI findings having full recovery.[17]

Cranial-Cervical Junction Injuries

Injuries to the cranial-vertebral junction include ligament injuries, fractures, and combined injuries. Occipital condyle fractures are more common in the adolescent population and necessitate further evaluation of the supporting ligamentous structures to rule out more substantial injuries. Atlanto-occipital region injuries are high-energy injuries caused by sudden deceleration, with the head moving forward on the cervical spine. These injuries may be subtle and difficult to diagnose or highly unstable, such as atlanto-occipital dissociations. In the past, these injuries have universally been considered fatal injuries; however, improvements in modern emergency medical systems with rapid stabilization and transport have allowed some children to survive such injuries. Modern imaging techniques plus a high degree of suspicion have improved the accuracy of diagnosis, given the challenges in adequately assessing the craniovertebral junction with plain radiographs. Correlation of MRI findings with the degree of injury can be difficult; however, any radiographic evidence of distraction is highly suggestive of an unstable injury, and these patients have some degree of retroclival hematoma and posterior ligamentous signal on MRI. Patients have neck pain and frequently have complete or incomplete spinal cord injuries. Lateral gaze palsy secondary to injury to the sixth cranial nerve may be present. Multisystem injuries are common, including brain, chest, abdominal, and appendicular injuries. In patients with true atlanto-occipital dissociations, an instrumented occiput to cervical fusion is required because halo immobilization is insufficient for these ligamentous injuries.[18] Among survivors of this injury, hydrocephalus and residual neurologic deficits are common.[18]

C1 Fractures

Fractures of the ring of C1 (also known as Jefferson fractures) in children may occur through the synchondroses of C1. These fractures are difficult to diagnose on plain radiographs and may be seen with CT or MRI in a child with a suspected fracture after the physical examination or by knowing the mechanism of injury.[19] The management of a Jefferson fracture is either with an orthosis or with a halo vest. Stability of the fracture is determined by lateral overhang of the lateral mass of C1 on C2, which can best be appreciated with coronal CT reformatted images. Overlap of more than 5 mm on either side is indicative of a transverse atlantal ligament injury, which is best studied with MRI. Because of growth asymmetry, children younger than 7 years may have a pseudospread of the lateral masses in relationship to the dens. Edema seen on MRI or a definitive synchondrosis fracture in these children may help differentiate pseudospread from traumatic overhang. Injuries with greater severity ultimately need proof of ligamentous stability with flexion-extension radiographs after a period of treatment in a halo vest. Early stabilization and fusion are recommended only in cases of substantial displacement and evidence of complete ligamentous disruption.

Odontoid Fractures

Odontoid fractures are the most common pediatric cervical spine fracture. This fracture is commonly seen in children younger than 5 years through the dentocentral synchondrosis. Sudden deceleration with hyperflexion of the head is the mechanism most commonly seen in these patients, usually resulting from a motor vehicle crash. The child usually has substantial cervical apprehension and pain. Radiographs demonstrate the anterior and flexed position of the dens through the dentocentral synchondrosis. CT is usually sufficient to clarify the injury, although MRI also may be used (**Figure 3**). Neurologic function is usually intact, given the ample space available for the spinal cord at that level. Treatment is reduction under anesthesia with translation and hyperextension under fluoroscopy and immobilization in a halo vest for 6 to 8 weeks in a position of hyperextension. These injuries do have potential for remodeling.[20] Nondisplaced fractures could potentially be treated in a noninvasive halo or a Minerva orthosis.

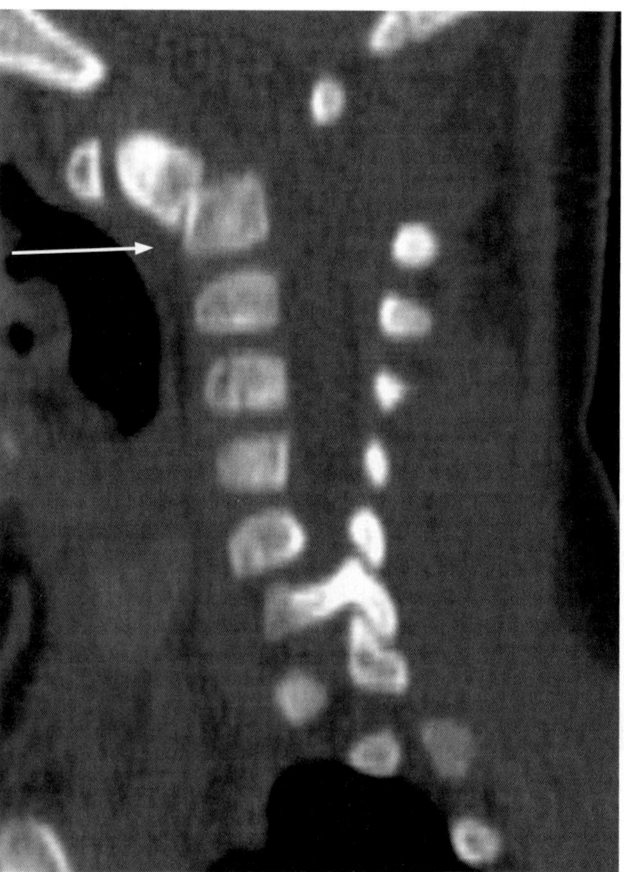

FIGURE 3 Sagittal CT scan of the spine of a 2-year-old child involved in a motor vehicle crash. The arrow points through the flexed odontoid fracture, which is a physeal fracture in a child of this age.

Hangman's Fractures

Hangman's fractures are rare in children and appear as defects in the pars of C2 with spondylolisthesis of C2 on C3. The mechanism of this fracture is thought to be related to forced hyperextension. Patients with acute injuries should be managed with a closed reduction and halo placement for 6 weeks. Occasionally, C2 pars defects may be seen on lateral radiographs in the workup of subacute neck pain. These defects may be differentiated from an acute injury by either the lack of edema on MRI or more sclerotic borders of the fracture edges on CT. Treatment options for subacute C2 pars defects include observation, Minerva-type bracing treatment, and halo placement.[21] Attempts at closed treatment with immobilization are warranted and may result in complete healing of the defects. Persistent nonunions of the C2 pars region may result in instability. If worrisome amounts of translation are seen on flexion-extension radiographs, an instrumented fusion is warranted. Treatment should be individualized based on a variety of factors, including radiographic signs of instability and neurologic status.

Atlantoaxial Rotatory Subluxation

C1-C2 rotatory subluxation may result from an infection, head positioning during surgery, or trauma. Patients have neck pain and spasms, such as holding the head rotated to one side with the chin tilted, and resist attempts at movement secondary to pain. Confirmation of the subluxated C1-C2 complex is done with CT (**Figure 4**). The Fielding-Hawkins classification describes the severity of displacement; however, treatment is usually mandated depending on the physical presentation and the length of symptoms. High-energy mechanisms (such as those resulting from a motor vehicle crash) with acute torticollis deserve further workup with MRI to rule out a traumatic C1-C2 ligamentous injury. Low-energy mechanisms do not require additional imaging and can be managed with a soft collar, NSAIDs, and antispasmodics for the first week. Patients who do not have an initial response after 1 week may need to be admitted and placed in halter or halo traction. Reduction is usually seen with an improvement in pain and return to a normal clinical appearance. Failure of traction to reduce the subluxation then requires reduction by positioning the head in a neutral position under anesthesia with halo vest placement. If surgical repositioning does not reduce the subluxation, a period of halo traction may reduce it. If reduction can be obtained, treatment in a halo vest for 6 weeks will maintain reduction in more than 70% of patients.[22] Failure to obtain a reduction or recurrent subluxation after halo traction are treated with instrumented C1-C2 fusion. Traumatic torticollis with a ligamentous injury visible on MRI frequently requires C1-C2 fusion. However, a trial of halo vest immobilization and subsequent assessment of stability with flexion-extension radiographs is reasonable before proceeding with arthrodesis.

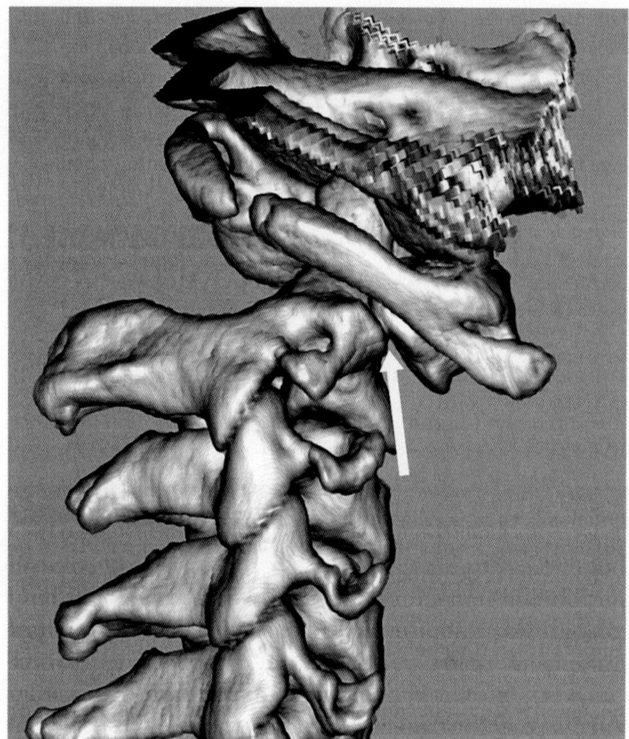

FIGURE 4 Reconstructed three-dimensional CT image from a 12-year-old child with fixed C1-C2 rotatory subluxation. The arrow points to the displacement of the C1 articular surface anteriorly and downward in relationship with the C2 joint surface.

SUBAXIAL CERVICAL INJURIES

Subaxial cervical spine injuries are more common in children older than 10 years and usually are the result of a motor vehicle crash or sport participation. Subaxial cervical injury patterns tend to resemble adult-type injuries because the anatomy of an adolescent has reached a mature state.[23] Injuries include spinous process avulsion fractures; ligamentous injuries (including facet subluxations and dislocations); facet fractures; compression fractures; and burst fractures with multicolumn involvement.

The AOSpine Group developed a working classification for cervical spine injuries in adults, which is transferrable to the adolescent population.[24] This classification describes fracture morphology, with more unstable injuries having posterior ligamentous injuries. Facet alignment, focal kyphosis, translation, and posterior spinous process distraction are factors in determining injury stability. CT and MRI are paramount for decision making. The classification system revolves around the CT findings, with MRI determining the degree of posterior ligamentous injury. Treatment is related to the injury pattern, the potential for stability, and the presence of neurologic deficit or cord compression. Stable injury patterns may be treated with cervical collars, whereas unstable injuries require stabilization and fusion with segmental rigid instrumentation. Facet subluxation or dislocations require MRI evaluation of the disk space before reduction to prevent exacerbation of a traumatic disk herniation. Some injuries, which are deemed stable, may subsequently demonstrate instability secondary to more severe ligamentous injury than was appreciated on imaging and will require stabilization. Flexion-extension radiographs in the nonacute setting ultimately determine cervical stability.

THORACOLUMBAR SPINE TRAUMA

Multiple descriptive classifications for thoracolumbar spine trauma are primarily based on fracture morphology. In an effort to improve communication among treating physicians, provide standardization for research, and aid physicians in determining appropriate treatment, the AOSpine Group developed the thoracolumbar injury classification system. This system considers the bony and ligamentous aspects of injuries as well as the neurologic status of the patient in an attempt to guide treatment.[25] The thoracolumbar injury classification system has been applied to the pediatric population with relatively good specificity and sensitivity for morphology but with poor reliability for predicting treatment.[26] The AOSpine classification currently is being studied in children. The following sections describe the classic fracture patterns according to relative severity.

Thoracic Compression Fractures

Compression fractures are commonly seen in children. They usually occur in the thoracic spine and are contiguous over two or three levels. Frequently, compression fractures are related to a fall or athletic injury with a shock-wave effect through the spine, hence the multilevel nature of the injury. Radiographs will reveal a subtle loss of height over multiple levels, which should correspond to the region of back pain. Normal morphologic variations in children can resemble compression fractures; however, when associated with back pain and localized tenderness, radiographs should be interpreted as suggestive of fracture. If necessary, MRI may be helpful in differentiating true fractures from morphologic variations. Compression fractures are stable injuries, and a thoracic hyperextension-type brace is not required, although it may be useful for improving symptoms. Special mention should be made about patients with painful compression fractures in the absence of an injury. In this scenario, consideration should be given to an underlying bone density problem (such as juvenile osteoporosis) or the potential for malignancy, most notably leukemia, which may include malaise, atraumatic back pain, and compression fractures (**Figure 5**).

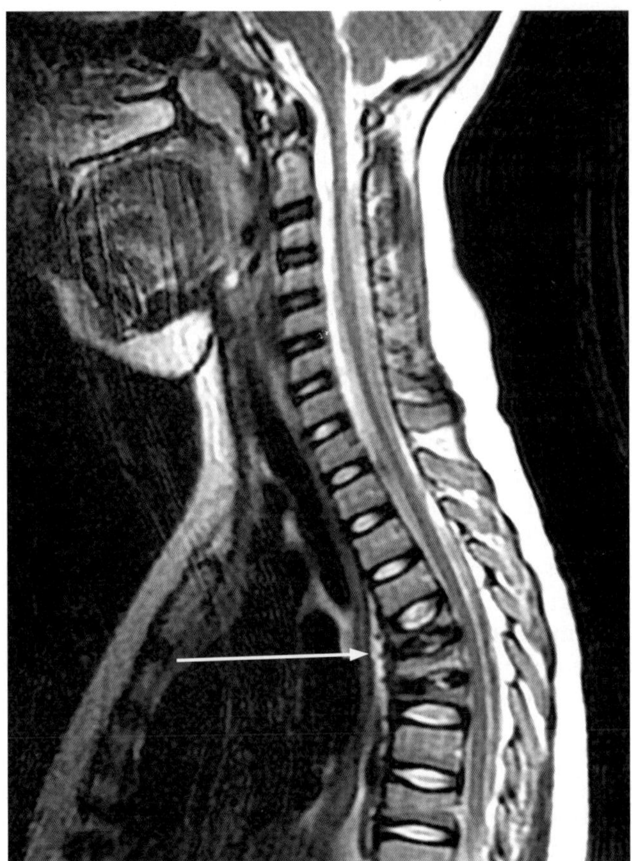

FIGURE 5 Sagittal T2-weighted magnetic resonance image of the spine of a 7-year-old child with gradual onset of upper thoracic back pain. The arrow points to three continuous levels of compression fractures related to pathologic fractures resulting from leukemia.

Burst Fractures

Burst fractures are high-energy injuries seen in older children and adolescents. The mechanisms of injury usually are motor vehicle trauma or high-velocity activities such as skiing, all-terrain vehicle use, or participation in motocross.[27] Although most patients are neurologically intact, some will have partial or incomplete spinal cord injuries. The risk of a spinal cord injury is higher in patients with thoracic burst fractures, and recovery is directly related to the severity of neurologic injury.[28] The degree of neurologic compression can be evaluated by MRI. Burst fractures may have extension to one or both end plates but classically involve the vertebral body, with the fracture extending through the posterior wall of the vertebral body. The presence of a posterior column injury may be difficult to define, but newer classification systems have focused on injuries to the posterior ligamentous complex. MRI evidence of a posterior ligamentous injury and CT scans showing interspinous widening or facet disruption signify a potentially unstable injury that may benefit from surgery. Treatment ranges from bracing treatment with a thoracolumbar spinal orthosis to surgical stabilization and is based on a variety of factors, including canal compromise, loss of vertebral height, the location of the fracture, and the neurologic status of the patient. Most surgeons believe that an absolute indication for surgery is a burst fracture in the setting of an incomplete or a complete neurologic injury. Focal kyphosis with loss of height in the setting of an insufficient posterior ligamentous complex also is suggestive of the need for surgical stabilization. Surgical treatment varies and ranges from anterior decompression with structural support and instrumentation to posterior instrumentation with distraction and realignment (**Figure 6**). Nonsurgical treatment in patients who are neurologically intact is associated with good functional outcomes; however, care must be taken to monitor for progressive focal kyphosis, especially at the level of the thoracolumbar junction, where loss of alignment adversely affects overall sagittal alignment.

Flexion-Distraction Injuries (Chance Fractures)

Chance fractures are flexion-distraction injuries of the thoracolumbar spine and are commonly secondary to a sudden deceleration against a lap belt in a motor vehicle crash. Correct placement of a lap belt is dependent on the size of the child. Inherent to child safety is positioning the belt in contact with the pelvis, which is facilitated by using a booster seat for younger children. Chance fractures in children are a result of a sudden deceleration of the vehicle, with the momentum of a child going forward and flexing over an incorrectly applied lap belt, which is lying at the abdominal/umbilical level. This sudden deceleration results in a flexion injury to the anterior column and distraction of the posterior column. The resulting thoracolumbar injury may be ligamentous, bony, or mixed. Frequently, the diagnosis may be delayed because the association of this fracture with intra-abdominal injuries requiring laparotomy is high. In any patient with

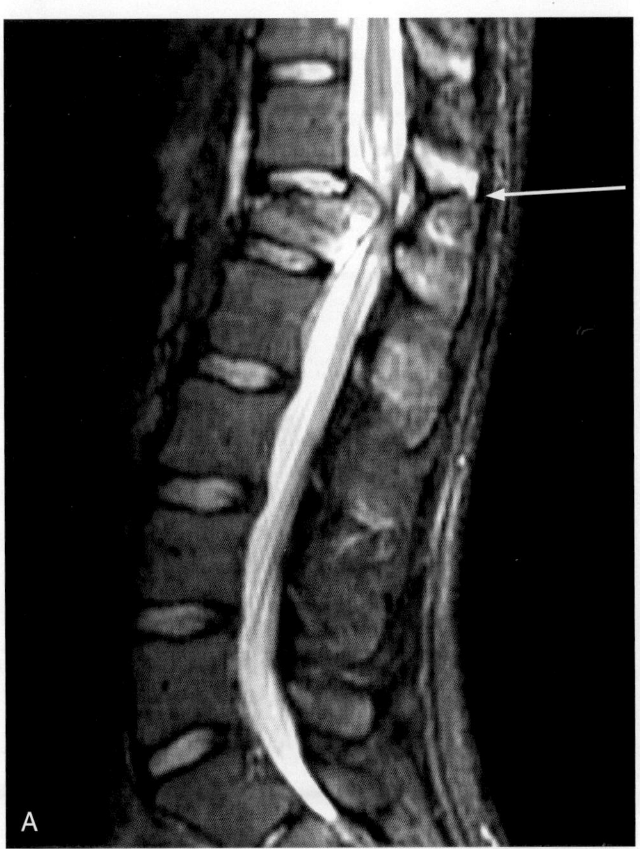

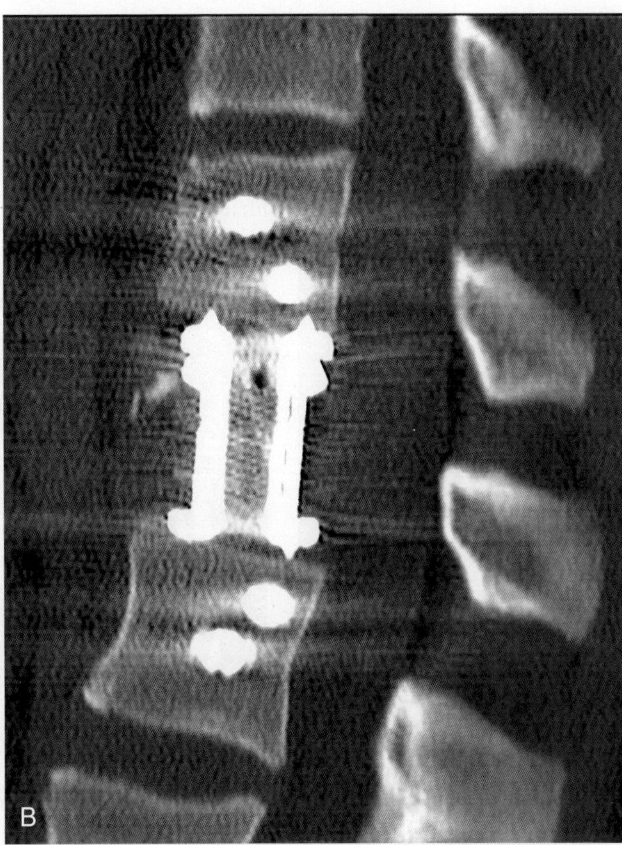

FIGURE 6 **A**, Sagittal T2-weighted MRI scan from a 14-year-old child involved in a high-speed motor vehicle crash. Note the fracture with retropulsion, cord compression, signal changes, and especially the signal change in the interspinous posterior ligamentous complex (as depicted with arrow). All these variables signify a highly unstable fracture. **B**, Postoperative CT scan after corpectomy and anterior plating. Note the restoration of height and the decompressed canal.

a Chance fracture, the trauma team must consider the possibility of intra-abdominal injuries. These injuries frequently occur in children younger than 10 years, with most cases occurring in the upper lumbar spine. These injuries are associated with neurologic deficit in more than 40% of patients.[29] Chance fractures may be treated nonsurgically with hyperextension casting or bracing treatment if the injury is purely bony in nature without substantial kyphosis and in the absence of neurologic injury. A tendency exists for progressive kyphosis with nonsurgical management of this injury, so close follow-up is required. Patients with ligamentous injuries, greater deformity, and neurologic deficits are best treated with reduction and rigid posterior instrumentation and fusion (**Figure 7**).

Apophyseal Ring Injuries

In growing children, the disk attachment to the end plate is an apophysis, which may become avulsed during trauma. Frequently, apophyseal ring injuries occur in adolescents with trauma sustained during athletic events, and evidence of a previous apophysitis is usually present. Injuries are usually at the thoracolumbar junction and may include neurologic deficit if there is retropulsion into the canal. Lumbar apophyseal ring injuries frequently have radiculopathy. If no neurologic deficit is present, treatment usually involves bracing treatment, which is followed by physical therapy. The presence of a motor deficit usually requires surgical treatment, which includes diskectomy and instrumented fusion. The described long-term outcomes after apophyseal ring injuries suggest that most patients do not have a permanent neurologic deficit and return to normal activities.[30] However, among patients managed nonsurgically, resorption of retropulsed bone did not occur, and those with large lesions had a higher frequency of chronic pain with limited activities.[30,31]

SUMMARY

Successful management of pediatric spine trauma begins in the field with appropriate transport and is followed by a thorough assessment in the emergency department. Plain radiographs will document most injuries, with CT and MRI used as adjuncts to further classify injuries. Maintenance of a high degree of suspicion of injury is important in patients who are obtunded or younger children who may be uncooperative during the examination or are noncommunicative. Children younger than 8 years more commonly sustain upper cervical spine trauma, with odontoid fractures being more common in younger patients because of dentocentral synchondrosis. SCIWORA exists because of the plasticity of a young child's spinal column and should be suspected when the neurologic examination does not correlate with normal findings on plain radiographs and/or CT scans. Flexion-distraction injuries are caused by inappropriately applied lap belts, and evaluation of the spine is warranted in a child involved in a motor vehicle crash with a lap-belt sign and concern for an intra-abdominal injury. The treatment of all injuries should consider the age of the child, the alignment and stability of the fracture, and the presence of neurologic injury or compression.

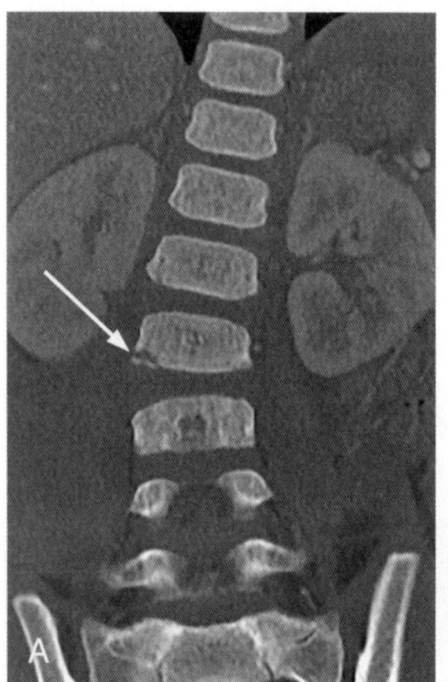

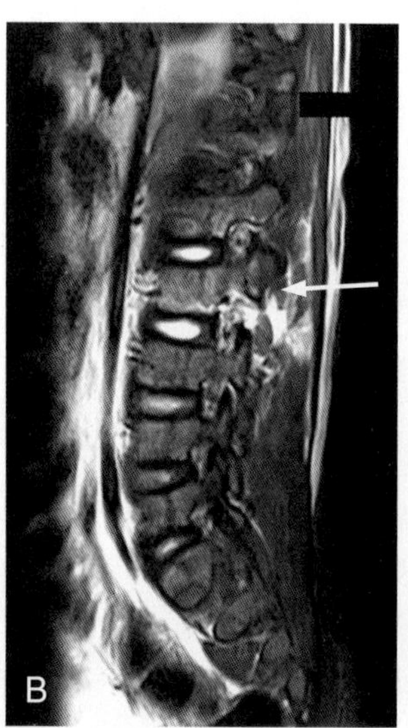

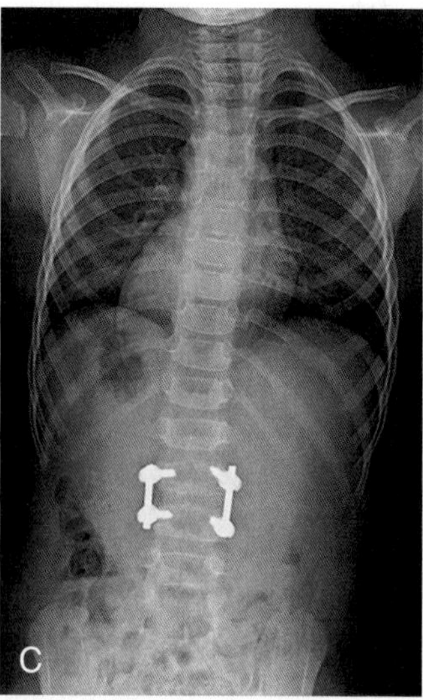

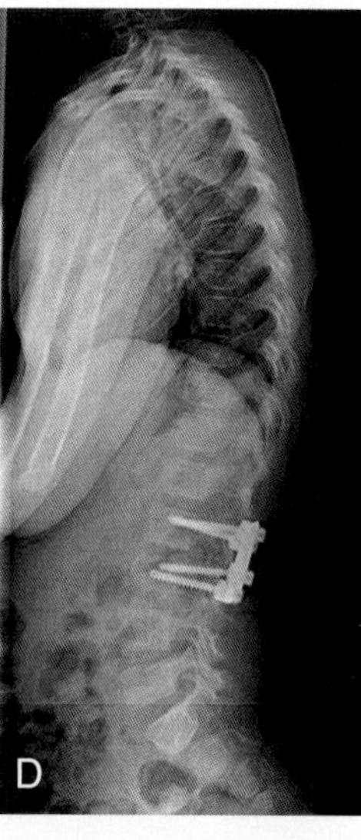

FIGURE 7 **A**, CT scan from a 3-year-old child with a suspected Chance fracture after a seat belt injury in a high-speed motor vehicle crash. The arrow points to the end plate fracture. Note the scoliosis present, which is indicative of a posterior ligament injury with facet subluxation. **B**, T2-weighted MRI scan from the same patient documents signal changes at the facet and posterior ligamentous complex indicative of a mixed bony-ligamentous Chance injury evident at the arrow. PA (**C**) and lateral (**D**) radiographs after reduction and instrumented fusion. At the time of the surgical procedure, the posterior ligaments were completely disrupted with a unilateral facet dislocation.

KEY STUDY POINTS

- Younger children have a larger head-to-body ratio than adults, thus predisposing them to upper cervical spine injuries.
- Chance fractures may be avoided by using booster seats for young children to ensure the correct placement of an automobile lap belt.
- SCIWORA exists in children because of the plasticity of the spine and should be suspected in a child with a neurologic deficit despite normal findings on plain radiographs.
- Normal radiographic variants exist in the pediatric cervical spine and must be considered when evaluating cervical spine imaging in the trauma setting.

ANNOTATED REFERENCES

1. Knox JB, Schneider JE, Cage JM, Wimberly RL, Riccio AI: Spine trauma in very young children: A retrospective study of 206 patients presenting to a level 1 pediatric trauma center. *J Pediatr Orthop* 2014;34(7):698-702.

2. Hofbauer M, Jaindl M, Höchtl LL, Ostermann RC, Kdolsky R, Aldrian S: Spine injuries in polytraumatized pediatric patients: Characteristics and experience from a level I trauma center over two decades. *J Trauma Acute Care Surg* 2012;73(1):156-161.

3. Madura CJ, Johnson JM Jr: Classification and management of pediatric subaxial cervical spine injuries. *Neurosurg Clin N Am* 2017;28:91-102.

   In this review article, the authors discuss injuries to the pediatric cervical spine at levels C3-C7 (the subaxial cervical spine). Anatomic differences that make the pediatric cervical spine more flexible are discussed. The techniques for diagnosis and management of young children (aged 8 years and younger), and how they differ from the treatment of adolescents or adults, are reviewed.

4. Kadom N, Palasis S, Pruthi S, et al: ACR Appropriateness Criteria® suspected spine trauma-child. *J Am Coll Radiol* 2019;55:S286-S299.

   Choosing the appropriate imaging in children with traumatic spine injuries is challenging as recommendations differ from those applied to adults. This article uses most current evidence and a panel of pediatric experts to summarize the best imaging practices for children with accidental spinal trauma.

5. Lustrin ES, Karakas SP, Ortiz AO, et al: Pediatric cervical spine: Normal anatomy, variants, and trauma. *Radiographics* 2003;23(3):539-560.

6. Gargas J, Yaszay B, Kruk P, Bastrom T, Shellington D, Khanna S: An analysis of cervical spine magnetic resonance imaging findings after normal computed tomographic imaging findings in pediatric trauma patients: Ten-year experience of a level I pediatric trauma center. *J Trauma Acute Care Surg* 2013;74(4):1102-1107.

7. Tolhurst SR, Vanderhave KL, Caird MS, et al: Cervical arterial injury after blunt trauma in children: Characterization and advanced imaging. *J Pediatr Orthop* 2013;33(1):37-42.

8. Henry M, Scarlata K, Riesenburger RI, et al: Utility of STIR MRI in pediatric cervical spine clearance after trauma. *J Neurosurg Pediatr* 2013;12(1):30-36.

9. Lee JH, Sung IY, Kang JY, Park SR: Characteristics of pediatric onset spinal cord injury. *Pediatr Int* 2009;51:254-257.

10. Pannu GS, Shah MP, Herman MJ: Cervical spine clearance in pediatric trauma centers: The need for standardization and an evidence-based protocol. *J Pediatr Orthop* 2017;37:e145-e149.

    Twenty-seven surgeons from 25 separate trauma centers were polled regarding cervical spinal injury clearance protocols. Of the 25 hospitals, 21 (84%) were level 1 trauma centers. The survey demonstrated notable variability in which personnel and which imaging modalities were used for cervical spinal clearance. There was also notable variability between the institutions regarding protocols for clearance of potential cervical spinal injuries in children. Level of evidence: IV.

11. Parent S, Mac-Thiong JM, Roy-Beaudry M, Sosa JF, Labelle H: Spinal cord injury in the pediatric population: A systematic review of the literature. *J Neurotrauma* 2011;28:1515-1524.

12. Herman MJ, Brown KO, Sponseller PD, et al: Pediatric cervical spine clearance: A consensus statement and algorithm from the pediatric cervical spine clearance working group. *J Bone Joint Surg Am* 2019;101(1):e1.

    This paper provides a cervical spine algorithm to be used in the acute trauma setting fort clearance of the cervical spine. The study provides for a clinical practice guideline based on the expert opinions of a group of surgeons experienced in taking care of pediatric trauma patients.

13. Kavuri V, Pannu G, Moront M, et al: "Next day" examination reduces radiation exposure in cervical spine clearance at a level 1 pediatric trauma center: Preliminary findings. *J Pediatr Orthop* 2019;39:e339-e342.

    Repeat next day clinical examinations and involving the Spine Service before obtaining a cervical CT scan reduced the number of cervical CT scans done at one trauma center without missing a clinically significant spinal injury or producing an increase in hospital length of stay. It did yield a slight increase in the time to removal of cervical collars. Level of evidence: IV.

14. Frank JB, Lim CK, Flynn JM, Dormans JP: The efficacy of magnetic resonance imaging in pediatric cervical spine clearance. *Spine (Phila Pa 1976)* 2002;27:1176-1179.

15. Launay F, Leet AI, Sponseller PD: Pediatric spinal cord injury without radiographic abnormality: A meta-analysis. *Clin Orthop Relat Res* 2005;433:166-170.

16. Bosch PP, Vogt MT, Ward WT: Pediatric spinal cord injury without radiographic abnormality (SCIWORA): The absence of occult instability and lack of indication for bracing. *Spine (Phila Pa 1976)* 2002;27(24):2788-2800.

17. Mahajan P, Jaffe DM, Olsen CS, et al: Spinal cord injury without radiologic abnormality in children imaged with magnetic resonance imaging. *J Trauma Acute Care Surg* 2013;75(5):843-847.

18. Astur N, Klimo P Jr, Sawyer JR, Kelly DM, Muhlbauer MS, Warner WC Jr: Traumatic atlanto-occipital dislocation in children: Evaluation, treatment, and outcomes. *J Bone Joint Surg Am* 2013;95(24):e194.
19. AuYong N, Piatt J Jr: Jefferson fractures of the immature spine. Report of 3 cases. *J Neurosurg Pediatr* 2009;3(1):15-19.
20. Razii N, Sharma A, Ahuja S: Complete remodeling of a displaced odontoid synchondrosis fracture managed conservatively: A case report. *J Pediatr Orthop B* 2019;28:411-414.

    The authors present an interesting case of an angulated C2 synchondrosis fracture that presented late and could not be reduced. It was treated conservatively, and an MRI 7 years post injury showed complete healing and substantial remodeling of the dens.
21. Pizzutillo PD, Rocha EF, D'Astous J, Kling TF Jr, McCarthy RE: Bilateral fracture of the pedicle of the second cervical vertebra in the young child. *J Bone Joint Surg Am* 1986;68(6):892-896.
22. Glotzbecker MP, Wasser AM, Hresko MT, Karlin LI, Emans JB, Hedequist DJ: Efficacy of nonfusion treatment for subacute and chronic atlanto-axial rotatory fixation in children. *J Pediatr Orthop* 2014;34(5):490-495.
23. Murphy RF, Davidson AR, Kelly DM, Warner WC Jr, Sawyer JR: Subaxial cervical spine injuries in children and adolescents. *J Pediatr Orthop* 2015;35(2):136-139.
24. Vaccaro AR, Koerner JD, Radcliff KE, et al: AOSpine subaxial cervical spine injury classification system. *Eur Spine J* 2015;25(7):2173-2184.
25. Vaccaro AR, Oner C, Kepler CK, et al, for the AOSpine Spinal Cord Injury & Trauma Knowledge Forum: AOSpine thoracolumbar spine injury classification system: Fracture description, neurological status, and key modifiers. *Spine (Phila Pa 1976)* 2013;38(23):2028-2037.
26. Savage JW, Moore TA, Arnold PM, et al: The reliability and validity of the thoracolumbar injury classification system in pediatric spine trauma. *Spine (Phila Pa 1976)* 2015;40(18):E1014-E1018.
27. Sawyer JR, Beebe M, Creek AT, Yantis M, Kelly DM, Warner WC Jr: Age-related patterns of spine injury in children involved in all-terrain vehicle accidents. *J Pediatr Orthop* 2012;32(5):435-439.
28. Vander Have KL, Caird MS, Gross S, et al: Burst fractures of the thoracic and lumbar spine in children and adolescents. *J Pediatr Orthop* 2009;29(7):713-719.
29. Arkader A, Warner WC Jr, Tolo VT, Sponseller PD, Skaggs DL: Pediatric Chance fractures: A multicenter perspective. *J Pediatr Orthop* 2011;31(7):741-744.
30. Higashino K, Sairyo K, Katoh S, Takao S, Kosaka H, Yasui N: Long-term outcomes of lumbar posterior apophyseal endplate lesions in children and adolescents. *J Bone Joint Surg Am* 2012;94(11):e74.
31. Chang CH, Lee ZL, Chen WJ, Tan CF, Chen LH: Clinical significance of ring apophysis fracture in adolescent lumbar disc herniation. *Spine (Phila Pa 1976)* 2008;33(16):1750-1754.

CHAPTER 47

Disaster and Mass Casualty Preparedness

MARK R. SINCLAIR, MD, FAAOS • SUSAN A. SCHERL, MD

ABSTRACT

Each department of a hospital is tasked by The Joint Commission to create a department-specific mass casualty plan that fully integrates with its hospital and community plan of disaster management. Although pediatric orthopaedic departments are integral members of trauma programs at the hospitals, this component of trauma care is frequently overlooked. Lessons learned from war injuries, terrorist attacks, and numerous natural disasters over the past 20 years can increase physician and hospital resilience when a similar event affects their community. Some events, such as earthquakes, mass shootings, and terrorist bombings, can be particularly impactful to a pediatric orthopaedic service. Providing aid when disaster occurs internationally adds complexity to already difficult circumstances.

Keywords: children and adolescents; disaster; mass casualty; preparedness

INTRODUCTION

"If the hospital experiences an actual emergency, the hospital implements its response procedures related to care, treatment, and services for its patients."[1] This is a quote from the 2019 Joint Commission Standards and Elements of Performance. Now substitute orthopaedic department for hospital in the previous sentence. Is the department ready? And is it specifically ready for the pediatric and adolescent population that will be affected?

In 2018, there were 73.4 million children (ages 0 to 17 years) in the United States, making up 22% of the population.[2] Despite this, planning for pediatric care in mass casualty incidents is regularly overlooked.[3] Pediatricians and parents are aware that different age groups bring different challenges. This will remain true in a mass casualty incident. To safely manage children in the 0 to 5 years age group, numbering 23.8 million in the 2018 US population, unique medical equipment and age-specific knowledge and skills are required. Children in the 6 to 11 years age group, numbering 24.6 million, still require downsized equipment, although the physiologic responses are maturing. Children in the 12 to 17 years age group, although becoming adult-like in size and physiology, are still minors with consent and disposition issues after treatment that can complicate care. The National Commission on Children and Disasters was charged by the President of the United States and Congress to undertake a comprehensive review of disaster laws, programs, and policies to assess the gaps in plans for children, and it presented its report in 2010.[4] Although there has been progress, in 2015, the organization Save the Children issued the National Report Card on Protecting Children in Disasters and found that 79% of the National Commission's recommendations remained unfulfilled.[5]

PRINCIPLES OF DISASTER RESPONSE

Mitigation, preparedness, response, and recovery are the four phases of emergency management. Mitigation and preparedness need to occur before the emergency happens. Response is where the clinician is most significantly involved, and the area for which she or he needs to be most prepared. Recovery followed by adequate debriefing will improve subsequent performance and provide stress counseling to staff.

Dr. Sinclair or an immediate family member serves as a board member, owner, officer, or committee member of Pediatric Orthopaedic Society of North America. Dr. Scherl or an immediate family member serves as a board member, owner, officer, or committee member of the American Academy of Orthopaedic Surgeons, the American Academy of Pediatrics, the American Orthopaedic Association, and the Pediatric Orthopaedic Society of North America.

As part of disaster planning, hospitals arrange an Incident Command System to provide structure and leadership. This will likely follow the structure of the National Incident Management System because that is required of hospitals receiving certain federal funds for emergency preparedness. The orthopaedic department can and must dovetail into this structure with its department-specific plan.[6] An example of this is outlined in **Figure 1**. This department plan, just like the overall hospital plan, must be reviewed and updated at least annually.[1] Specific orthopaedic supplies and inventory should also be reviewed and updated at least annually.

Although an orthopaedic surgeon will not be in charge of triage in a disaster situation, the orthopaedic surgeon on call will need to be available to assist with triage and with prioritization of surgical cases. Although there are numerous triage systems that may each have specific benefits,[7,8] a basic understanding of the START (simple triage and rapid treatment) system is helpful. The START method separates patients into four basic categories to streamline treatment (**Figure 2**). Patients requiring emergent care for survival are labeled immediate/red. Patients requiring care but whose survival does not depend on it occurring emergently are labeled delayed/yellow. The walking wounded who may or may not require care are labeled minor/green. Patients who are not expected to survive even with emergent care are labeled expectant/black. During a disaster, patients will need reevaluation and may shift between categories based on the evolving medical condition and the available resources.

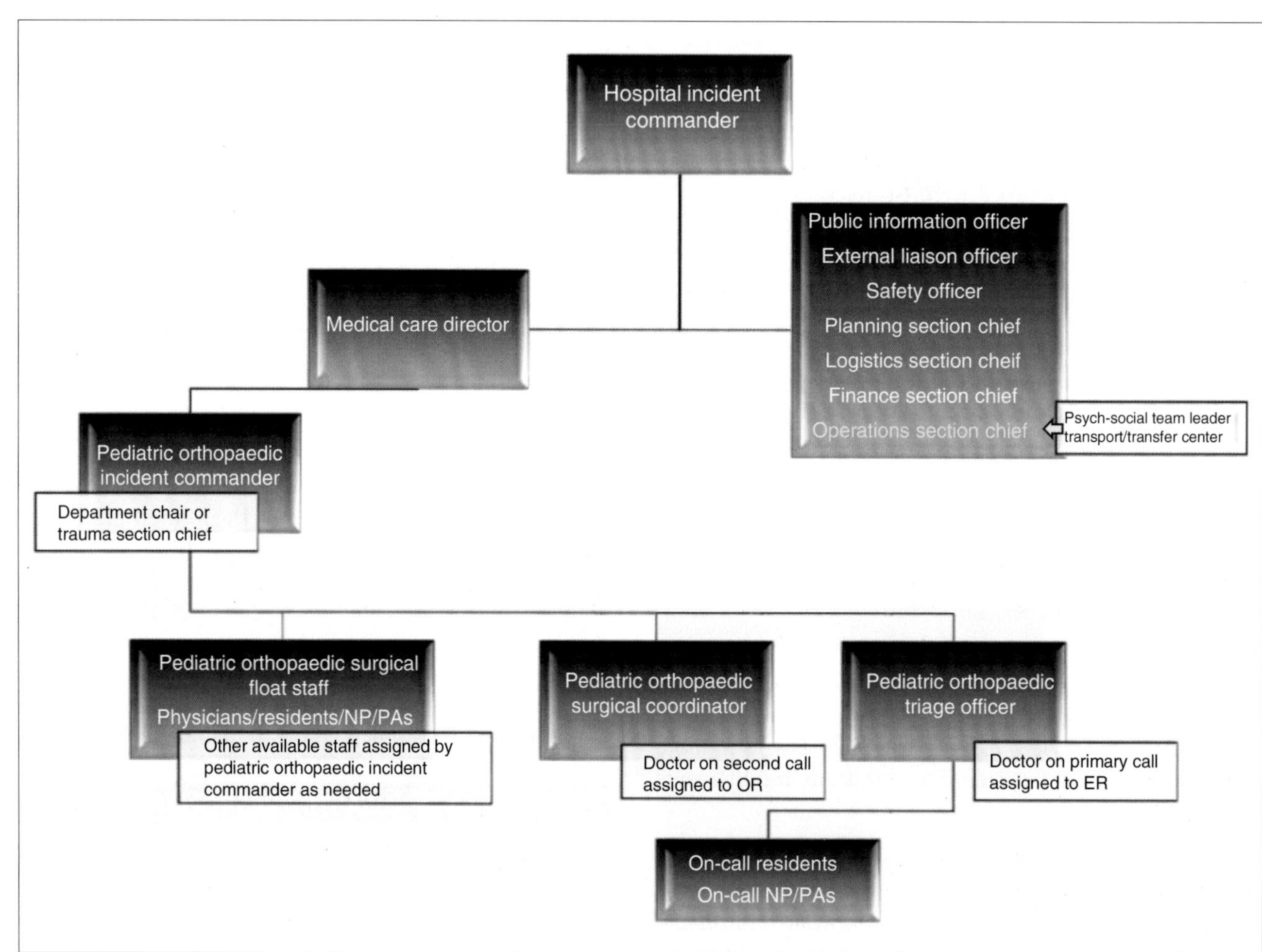

FIGURE 1 A schematic drawing of a pediatric orthopaedic hierarchy that can be rapidly used when needed. It uses individuals who are on call and supplements them with available department members. This system is designed to merge into the overall hospital Incident Command System. If the disaster response continues for an extended time, a rotation of providers needs to be developed by the pediatric orthopaedic incident commander. ER = emergency room, NP = nurse practitioner, OR = operating room, PA = physician assistant.

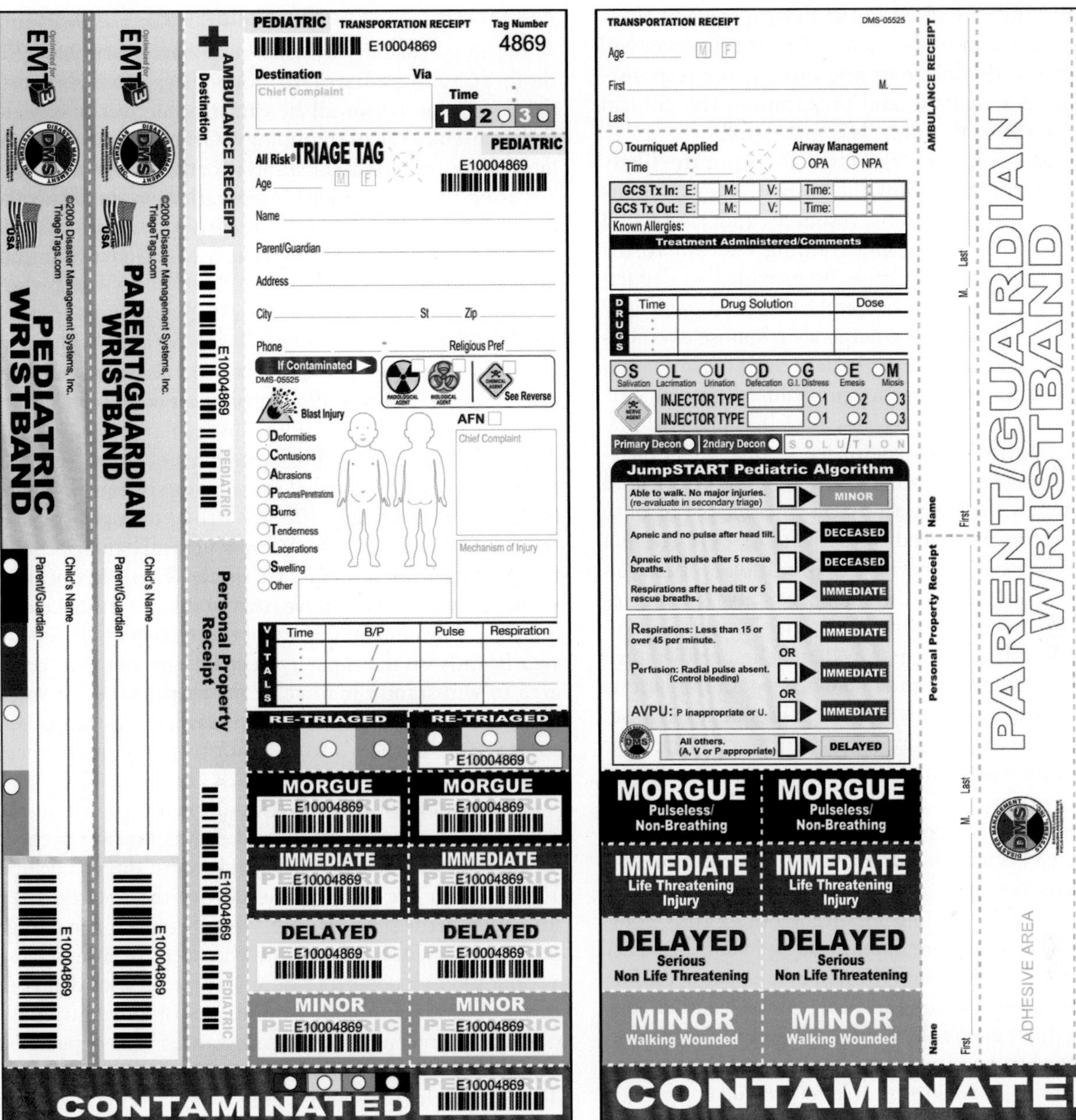

FIGURE 2 **A** and **B**, Photographs of the front and back of a pediatric triage tag. There are detachable wristbands to link the pediatric patient with the parent/guardian. There is room to record basic vital signs and personal information. There are also the red/yellow/green/black triage color receipts and a brief schematic chart explaining how to quickly classify each patient on presentation. (© Disaster Management Systems, Inc. Rancho Cucamonga, CA 91730 USA, TriageTags.com.)

MEETING REGULATORY REQUIREMENTS

Hospitals conduct a hazard vulnerability analysis to identify potential emergent situations that could affect demand for the hospital's services, its ability to provide those services, the likelihood of those events occurring, and the consequences of those events.[1] This is required for compliance with The Joint Commission Standards and Elements of Performance. All hospitals have a written Emergency Operations Plan (EOP) to manage an emergency surge that suddenly increases demand for the hospital's services. This EOP also plans for a disaster that, because of its scope or duration, requires outside assistance to sustain the hospital's patient care and security functions. Because compliance with these requirements is mostly an administrative task, the clinician may not have been significantly involved in the development of these plans. But should an actual event occur, the clinician will need to step to the forefront and provide the response. Without proper training and preparation, the clinical execution of the EOP will be less successful.

Emergency response exercises incorporate likely disaster scenarios that allow the hospital to evaluate its handling of communications, resources and assets, and patients.[1] Initial and ongoing training relevant to the emergency response roles must be provided to department staff. In addition, the hospital has to modify its EOP based on its evaluation of emergency response exercises and responses to actual emergencies.[1] Staff must demonstrate knowledge of emergency procedures through participation in drills and exercises, as well as posttraining tests, participation in instructor-led feedback (eg, questions and answers), or other methods determined and documented by the hospital.[1] As an emergency response exercise, the hospital needs to activate its EOP twice a year at each site included in the overall plan. Tabletop discussions, though useful, are not acceptable substitutes for these exercises. To satisfy the twice-a-year requirement, the hospital must first evaluate the performance of the previous exercise and make needed modifications to the EOP before conducting the subsequent exercise. At least one of the hospital's two emergency response exercises should include an influx of simulated patients.[1]

For individuals in a department leadership position, how will staff be notified that emergency response procedures have been initiated? How will information and instructions continue to be communicated to staff? Answers to these questions are needed to be fully compliant with The Joint Commission requirements.[1] As part of the communication plan, the names and contact information for the physicians and staff, as well as other contacts with other hospitals, need to be maintained should patients need to be transferred or accepted in transfer.[1] The department needs to be able to provide emergency response without outside help for at least 96 hours.[1] This will require plans for succession and duty delegation in addition to communication. Although not specifically required by The Joint Commission, emergency communication information with equipment suppliers is part of a thoughtful plan for orthopaedic surgery departments.

Another point of stress of regulatory agencies is avoiding lapses of routine care during times of emergency. That care needs to continue to be provided by the hospital during the emergency, or alternative sites of care, treatment, and services need to be identified.[1] It is not uncommon for outside doctors or providers to want to volunteer to assist other department or hospital in its ongoing disaster response. There are regulations affecting that as well.[1]

Preparation for Specific Incidents

Many mass casualty/disaster response efforts have little to do with pediatric orthopaedics. Power failures, fires, and floods can all be catastrophic, yet may yield little musculoskeletal pathology. Other scenarios (listed later) may require a substantial orthopaedic response. Focusing the department's preparation on these specific scenarios, while still being receptive to an all-hazards approach, is the most appropriate use of department time and resources.

Earthquake

Earthquakes have the capacity to cause large-scale, sudden-onset disasters. Earthquakes are constantly occurring because the tectonic plates in the Earth's crust shift. Approximately 500,000 earthquakes occur worldwide each year, with 100,000 of these being strong enough to be felt. Approximately 100 are strong enough to cause structural damage (0.1%). With structural damage comes the potential for human casualties. When this occurs, many survivors will have sustained musculoskeletal injuries.[9] The clinical impact of these events will depend significantly on the capacity of structures in the affected area to withstand the force of the earthquake. As such, an earthquate of similar strength may have less impact in some regions of the world and catastrophic consequences in others.[10,11]

The rapidity of orthopaedic surgical response in the setting of catastrophic earthquakes is significant because the need for orthopaedic care will be substantial. The first 10 days after the earthquake will see the greatest need for orthopaedic surgical care.[12] A substantial percentage of fractures will be open, and the need for amputation as opposed to reconstruction will increase with delays in care.[13] The fracture and wound care of extremity injuries in children in these circumstances will depend on resources available. An initial damage-control orthopaedics approach to pediatric care using casting, external fixation, and percutaneous pinning is appropriate in situations where sterility is challenged and supplies and radiologic capabilities are limited. In such situations, early damage-control orthopaedics response anticipating subsequent referral or more definitive care in follow-up as infrastructure recovers is the most appropriate plan to salvage as much life and limb as possible.[11] This will be a substantial deviation from standard practice for most responding pediatric orthopaedic surgeons, but must be anticipated for an effective and helpful disaster response.

Terrorist Bombing

The terrorist bombings of Oklahoma City and the Boston Marathon were very different, but both yielded notable civilian casualties, including children. The bombing of the Alfred P. Murrah Federal Building in Oklahoma City occurred shortly after 9 AM on a workday. There were 816 casualties, of which 92% were adults. Of the 66 children injured, there were 19 deaths. This mortality rate was higher than that for adults (29% versus 20%). Of significance, among pediatric casualties aged 6 months to 5 years, the death rate was 71% (15 of 21). Injuries were most often caused by flying glass and other debris, as well as collapsing ceilings causing crush and head injuries.[14] As was the case in the World Trade Center attack, structural collapse was the most important factor for fatality in the Oklahoma City bombing.[15]

The Boston Marathon bombing occurred near the finish line of the race, which was crowded with spectators. Because the bombing occurred outdoors and the bombs were placed at ground level, the death toll was relatively low (3), but the number of wounded was substantial, and most (66% of victims) had lower extremity injuries. There were 278 wounded, of which 124 were treated at local trauma centers.[16] Numerous patients were treated with extremity tourniquets applied at the scene, and then transported quickly. No victims who arrived alive at Boston's trauma centers died.[17] It has been demonstrated that tourniquet application before the onset of hemorrhagic shock notably improves survival among battlefield casualties.[18] It is questionable, however, if civilian-improvised tourniquets were all that effective for the victims of the Boston Marathon bombing. It has been recognized that commercial, purpose-designed limb tourniquets are more effective and should be made more available for usage among first responders.[19]

School and Other Civilian Mass Shootings

From Columbine (1999) to Parkland (2018), a lot has been learned about appropriate tactics for law enforcement to limit casualties, and what clinicians can expect when casualties arrive. The shooters at Columbine High School were active for 49 minutes. After that event, law enforcement changed its tactics from surround and contain to immediate action and rapid deployment. This was done to limit the time of exposure of civilians to active shooters. The benefits of such tactics were most recently witnessed in the Dayton mass shooting (2019), in which the shooter was active for less than 1 minute before being neutralized by law enforcement.

The victims of these shootings often die from hemorrhage, either internal or external. After the Sandy Hook shooting in 2012, the American College of Surgeons created a study group to enhance survivability of mass shootings. The recommendations of this group are referred to as the Hartford Consensus.[20] The THREAT mnemonic (**Figure 3**) was created to provide an integrated response that would maximize survivability. In addition,

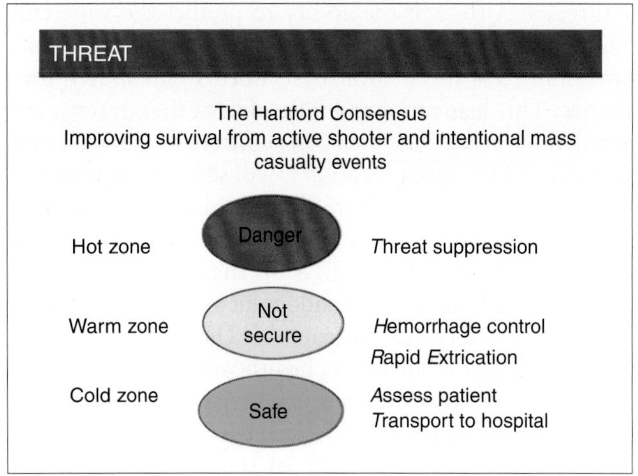

FIGURE 3 The THREAT mnemonic demonstrating the integrated response from rapid responders most likely to improve the survival rates of victims involved in active shooter and other intentional mass casualty events. (Obtained from https://www.stopthebleed.org/resources-poster-booklet. © American College of Surgeons.)

the use of Tactical Combat Casualty Care programs successfully developed by the military to reduce preventable deaths among soldiers was translated into the Stop the Bleed educational program for civilians.[21,22]

Although orthopaedic surgeons are no strangers to extremity injuries from penetrating trauma, most of these injuries are from low-velocity firearms. The weapon of choice in mass shootings is frequently the semiautomatic civilian AR-15 rifle. This weapon fires smaller bullets at medium to high velocity (>2,000 feet/s), which notably increases the wounding potential. Surviving victims with high-velocity extremity injuries will require serial surgical débridement with delayed wound closure. Fractures in this setting require prompt administration of first-generation cephalosporins and continued treatment for 24 to 72 hours.[23] A thorough evaluation for neurologic and vascular injuries followed by a span-scan-plan approach to the initial musculoskeletal management is prudent. Transfusion requirements for pediatric victims with smaller blood volumes should not be underestimated. Massive transfusions (>1 total blood volume within 24 hours) should be performed via a blood bank–based pediatric massive transfusion protocol designed to conserve blood products and achieve balanced red blood cell to fresh frozen plasma ratio deployment to avoid coagulopathy and other transfusion-related complications.[24]

Severe Weather Outbreak

Tornadoes are more common in the United States than anywhere else in the world. During the early spring and summer, the Midwest and Southeastern regions of the United States are particularly vulnerable to tornado outbreaks. Although the ability to predict the supercell thunderstorms that give rise to severe tornadoes is excellent, only 10% to 20% of these storms will spawn tornadoes. This leads to many false alarms that desensitize populations in endemic areas. In addition, the severity of a tornado and the exact location it will start are impossible to predict accurately. Therefore, despite improvements in modern tornado forecasting, the casualties seen with severe tornadoes (EF4 or EF5 on the Enhanced Fujita Scale) remain high if the tornadoes hit a population center that is not sheltered underground.[25] Damage to community infrastructure, including healthcare facilities, should be anticipated in storms of this severity.

Pediatric casualties in this scenario are typically representative of the percentage of the involved population. Head injuries are the most problematic injury,[26] but extremity wounds and fractures, in addition to spinal injuries from structural collapse, are frequently seen.[27] Penetrating trauma from windblown debris should be anticipated, as should fungal and mycoplasma infections that occur when dirt deep to the topsoil becomes aerosolized and is sprayed on traumatic wounds.[28] Some injuries in pediatric patients can yield developmental deformities with continued growth (**Figure 4**).

International Disaster Response

Many pediatric orthopaedic surgeons are familiar with doing work in foreign countries on medical/surgical missions. The level of surgical care that can be successfully achieved on such missions depends on the supporting infrastructure available. In a disaster response, devastated or crippled medical and civilian infrastructure should be anticipated. Security may also be a concern, turning disaster responders into potential victims. Surgical concepts of "keep it simple, keep it sterile," helpful in medical missions, will hold true in ground zero international disaster response. The damage-control orthopaedics concepts mentioned previously that guide earthquake response give the responding surgeon a base from which to start.

The Office of US Foreign Disaster Assistance, under the umbrella of the United States Agency for International Development, is responsible for coordinating the US government's response to international disasters. The organization also partners with many humanitarian organizations with previous experience in the affected country. Prospective orthopaedic surgical volunteers are strongly encouraged not to go to disaster sites alone, but to contact an agency or organization that is working on the ground and has authorization from the government to bring in personnel. The International Medical Corps is one such organization that has partnered with the American Academy of Orthopaedic Surgeons in providing disaster response internationally. One can become an American Academy of Orthopaedic Surgeons–registered disaster response volunteer by participating in a Disaster Response Course, developed by the Society of Military Orthopaedic Surgeons and cosponsored by the American Academy of Orthopaedic Surgeons, Orthopaedic Trauma Association, and Pediatric Orthopaedic Society of North America.[29] More information is available by contacting disasterprep@aaos.org.

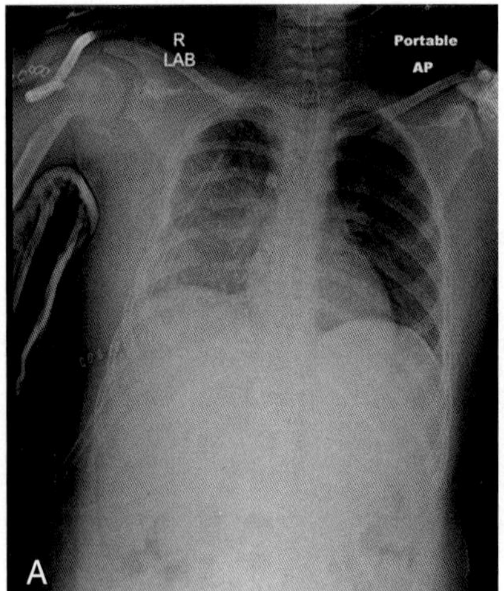

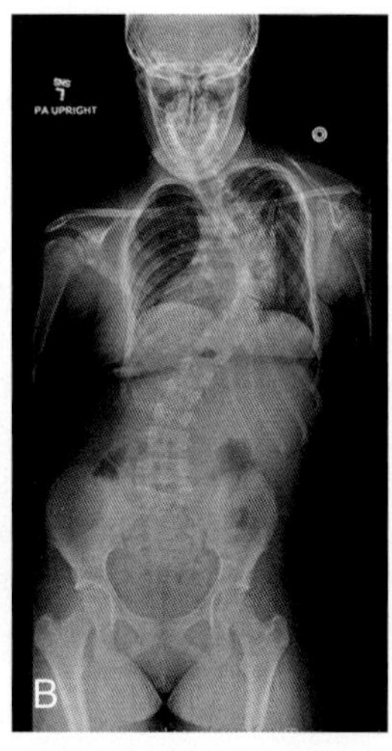

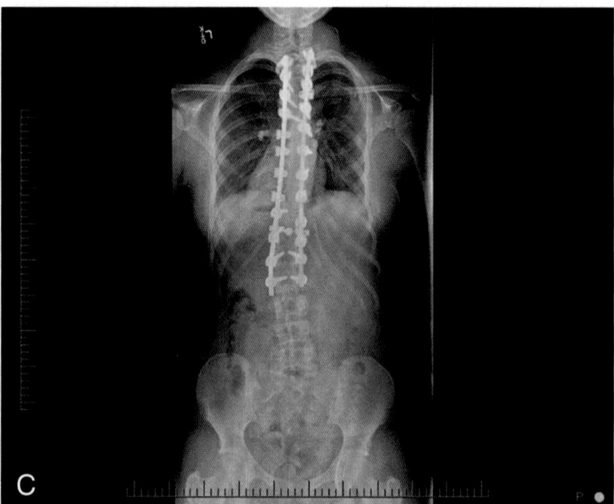

FIGURE 4 **A**, An AP radiograph of the chest of a 10-year-old girl depicting an open right proximal humerus fracture and a significant right chest wall injury from a rebar projectile caused by an EF5 tornado. **B**, A standing PA scoliosis radiograph of the same patient 2.5 years later after the development of significant thoracogenic scoliosis. **C**, A standing PA scoliosis radiograph 7 years after injury following posterior spinal fusion with instrumentation.

SUMMARY

Although there will never be a perfect disaster response, clinical training and planning will improve the capacity and resilience of the clinician responders. Regulatory bodies have come to understand the importance of this and now require hospitals and the individual departments to prepare for such events. Although an all-hazards approach to disaster planning is required, pediatric orthopaedic departments would be wise to specifically focus on scenarios that are likely to tax specific personnel and resources. Communication between providers and between facilities is best arranged before the disaster occurrence. Although US disasters require individual hospital and department planning, responding to an international disaster is best done under the umbrella of a State Department–approved agency that can facilitate a volunteer's ability to be effective in an austere and foreign environment.

KEY STUDY POINTS

- Specific planning for pediatric and adolescent patients in a disaster response is necessary because this age group makes up 22% of the population and has age-specific medical needs.
- Mitigation, preparedness, response, and recovery are the four phases of disaster management, but the clinician is most significantly responsible for the response phase.
- Preparation, planning, and practice are most important for an effective disaster response. Hospital regulatory agencies understand this and are demanding more specific action in these areas.
- Although an all-hazards approach is required of the hospital, it is prudent for orthopaedic departments to focus on the disasters that will affect them the most.

ANNOTATED REFERENCES

1. Comparison of Medicare Hospital Requirements to 2019 Joint Commission Hospital Standards. March 21, 2019. Available at https://www.jointcommission.org/standards/. Accessed October 15, 2020.

   This is a 2019 publication from The Joint Commission comparing disaster preparedness requirements for hospitals from the Centers of Medicare and Medicaid Services with those of The Joint Commission, facilitating compliance with the directives of both agencies.

2. America's Children: Key National Indicators of Well-Being, 2019: *Demographic Background*. ChildStats.gov. Available at: https://www.childstats.gov/pdf/ac2019/ac_19.pdf. Accessed October 15, 2020.

   The Federal Interagency Forum on Child and Family Statistics (Forum) is a collection of 23 federal government agencies involved in research and activities related to children and families. The Forum's annual report, *America's Children: Key National Indicators of Well-Being*, provides a summary of national indicators of child well-being and monitors changes in these indicators over time.

3. Lozon MM, Bradin S: Pediatric disaster preparedness. *Pediatr Clin North Am* 2018;65:1205-1220.

   The authors review the unique challenges that are present when providing care for children during a disaster response. This includes the unique physiologic, developmental, and social needs of children in these situations. Level of evidence: V.

4. National Commission on Children and Disasters: *2010 Report to the President and Congress*. AHRQ Publication No. 10-M037. Rockville, MD, Agency for Healthcare Research and Quality, October 2010.

5. Save the Children: *Children Still at Risk: U.S. Children 10 Years After Hurricane Katrina*. 2015 National Report Card on Protecting Children in Disasters, 2015. https://www.savethechildren.org/content/dam/usa/reports/emergency-prep/disaster-report-2015.pdf.

6. Born CT, Mamczak C, Pagenkopf E, et al: Disaster management response guidelines for Departments of Orthopaedic Surgery. *JBJS Rev* 2016;4(1):e1.

   The authors of this review article discuss how to develop an orthopaedic department–specific disaster response plan, and how to dovetail that into the overall hospital response plan. This article gives specific and concrete information about communication in a disaster, personnel hierarchy during the response, and disaster recovery phase. Level of evidence: V.

7. Toida C, Muguruma T, Abe T, et al: Introduction of pediatric physiological and anatomical triage score in mass-casualty incident. *Prehosp Disaster Med* 2018;33(2):147-152.

   The authors explore the use of the Pediatric Physiological and Anatomical Triage Score in evaluating 137 patients younger than 16 years. The authors showed a significant association between the Pediatric Physiological and Anatomical Triage Score and the predicted mortality rate, mechanical ventilation time, intensive care unit stay, and hospital stay. The authors concluded that the Pediatric Physiological and Anatomical Triage Score was superior to other methods of secondary triage in the age group studied. Level of evidence: III.

8. Wallis LA, Carley S: Comparison of paediatric major incident primary triage tools. *Emerg Med J* 2006;23:475-478.

9. Moitinho de Almeida M, van Loenhout JAF, Thapa SS, et al: Clinical and demographic profile of admitted victims in a tertiary hospital after the 2015 earthquake in Nepal. *PLoS One* 2019;14(7):e0220016.

   The authors studied 501 patients admitted to their hospital after the 2015 earthquake in Nepal. Nearly 89% were admitted for injuries, mostly of the lower extremities, and 66% of all injuries were fractures. About 69% of patients underwent surgery. The authors concluded that tertiary hospitals should

Section 7: Trauma

have preparedness plans to cope with a large influx of injured patients, many of whom will require orthopaedic surgical services. Level of evidence: IV.

10. Zhang L, Zhao M, Fu W, et al: Epidemiological analysis of trauma patients following the Lushan earthquake. *PLoS One* 2014;9(5):e97416.
11. Bar-On E, Lebel E, Kreiss Y, et al: Orthopaedic management in a mega mass casualty situation. The Israel Defense Forces Field Hospital in Haiti following the January 2010 earthquake. *Injury* 2011;42:1053-1059.
12. Gamulin A, Armenter-Duran J, Assal M, et al: Conditions found among pediatric survivors during the early response to natural disaster: A prospective case study. *J Pediatr Orthop* 2012;32:327-333.
13. Bar-On E, Lebel E, Blumberg N, et al: Pediatric orthopaedic injuries following an earthquake: Experience in an acute phase field hospital. *J Trauma Acute Care Surg* 2013;74(2): 617-621.
14. Mallonee S, Shariat S, Stennies G, et al: Physical injuries and fatalities resulting from the Oklahoma City bombing. *J Am Med Assoc* 1996;276(5):382-387.
15. Glenshaw MT, Vernick JS, Li G, et al: Preventing fatalities in building bombings: What can we learn from the Oklahoma City bombing? *Disaster Med Public Health Prep* 2007;1(1):27-31.
16. Tolbert D, von Keudell A, Rodriguez EK: Lessons from the Boston marathon bombing: An orthopaedic perspective on preparing for high volume trauma in an Urban Academic Center. *J Orthop Trauma* 2015;29:S7-S10.
17. Boston Trauma Center Chiefs' Collaborative: Boston Marathon bombings: An after-action review. *J Trauma Acute Care Surg* 2014;77(3):501-503.
18. Kragh JF Jr, Littrel ML, Jones JA, et al: Battle casualty survival with emergent tourniquet use to stop limb bleeding. *J Emerg Med* 2011;41(6):590-597.
19. King DR, Larentzakis A, Ramly EP, et al: Tourniquet use at the Boston Marathon bombing: Lost in translation. *J Trauma Acute Care Surg* 2015;78(3):594-599.
20. Jacobs LM, Carmona R, Butler F, et al: The Hartford Consensus IV: A call for increased national resilience. *Bull Am Coll Surg* 2016;101(3):17-24.

    The overarching principle of the Hartford Consensus is that no one should die from uncontrolled bleeding. In the fourth consensus statement, the ACS Joint Committee to Create a National Policy to Enhance Survivability from Intentional Mass Casualty and Active Shooter Events focused on the implementation of strategies to empower lay bystanders (immediate responders) to help victims of mass casualty events. The curriculum for a public Stop the Bleed training program was recommended. Level of evidence: V.
21. Butler FK: Two decades of saving lives on the battlefield: Tactical Combat Casualty Care turns 20. *J Spec Oper Med* 2017;17:166-172.

    The original Tactical Combat Casualty Care article is more than 20 years old. In the ensuing decades since its original publication, the author discusses the changes in the program because more evidence became available and feedback from user medics was obtained. The best practice concepts subsequently developed in battlefield trauma care have been translated to civilian prehospital trauma care, resulting in potential lives saved in the civilian trauma sector. Level of evidence: V.
22. Lei R, Swartz MD, Harvin JA, et al: Stop the bleed training empowers learners to act to prevent unnecessary hemorrhagic death. *Am J Surg* 2018;217:368-372.

    The authors evaluated a Stop the Bleed curriculum received by third-year medical students, school nurses, health profession students who were not trained to be doctors or nurses, and non–healthcare-related community members. Although all were willing to intervene in helping a stranger with life-threatening external hemorrhage, all groups thought ill-prepared to do so. After the curriculum, all groups showed a significant improvement in knowledge of hemorrhage control techniques. In addition, all groups showed increased willingness and preparedness to intervene in providing initial treatment to a stranger with severe bleeding. Level of evidence: II.
23. Hospenthal DR, Murray CK, Andersen RC, et al: Guidelines for the prevention of infections associated with combat-related injuries. 2011 update: Endorsed by the Infectious Disease Society of America and the Surgical Infection Society. *J Trauma* 2011;71:S210-S234.
24. Kamyszek RW, Leraas HJ, Reed C, et al: Massive transfusion in the pediatric population: A systemic review and summary of best-evidence practice strategies. *J Trauma Acute Care Surg* 2019;86:744-754.

    Children requiring massive blood product transfusion have a historically high mortality (33% to 50%). In this 2019 review, the authors evaluate the current literature of massive transfusion protocols in the pediatric cohort and review their own institution's protocol. In aggregating the reviewed studies, the authors found that implementation of a massive transfusion protocol did not significantly reduce mortality or major morbidity, which is counter to the adult experience. Further research is necessary in the pediatric cohort to bring pediatric massive transfusion protocols up to adult standards. Level of evidence: IV and V.
25. Chiu CH, Schnall AH, Mertzlufft CE, et al: Mortality from a tornado outbreak, Alabama, April 27, 2011. *Am J Public Health* 2013;103:e52-e58.
26. Chern JJ, Miller JH, Tubbs RS, et al: Massive pediatric neurosurgical injuries and lessons learned following a tornado disaster in Alabama. *J Neurosurg Pediatr* 2011;8:588-592.
27. Hartmann EH, Creel N, Lepard J, Maxwell RA: Mass casualty following unprecedented tornadic events in the southeast: Natural disaster outcomes at a level 1 trauma center. *Am Surg* 2012;78:770-773.
28. Benedict K, Park BJ: Invasive fungal infections after natural disasters. *Emerg Infect Dis* 2014;20:349-355.
29. Kelly DM, Heyworth BE, Kruse RW, et al: Current state of pediatric orthopaedic disaster response. *J Pediatr Orthop* 2014;34:231-238.

SECTION 8

Sports-Related Topics

Section Editor:

Jennifer M. Weiss, MD, FAAOS

CHAPTER 48

Ligamentous Knee Injuries

CORDELIA W. CARTER, MD • MELINDA S. SHARKEY, MD

ABSTRACT

Sports-related ligamentous injuries of the knee have become increasingly common in skeletally immature patients. Despite concerns for physeal injury, clinical and functional outcomes for patients with complete anterior cruciate ligament tears are generally better with early surgical treatment than with delayed or nonsurgical care. Reinjury of the anterior cruciate ligament graft following surgical reconstruction remains a significant complication, and outcomes of revision anterior cruciate ligament surgery are not as reliable. Our understanding of the incidence, natural history, and appropriate treatment algorithm for other ligamentous injuries of the knee in the pediatric population, including multiligamentous knee injury patterns, continues to evolve. When surgery is indicated for treatment of a ligamentous knee injury, careful preoperative evaluation of each patient's physiologic and skeletal maturity is necessary to determine the optimal surgical technique.

Keywords: ACL avulsion; anterior cruciate ligament (ACL) tear; pediatric sports; physeal injury; tibial eminence fracture; tibial spine fracture

Dr. Carter or an immediate family member serves as a board member, owner, officer, or committee member of the American Academy of Orthopaedic Surgeons and the Pediatric Orthopaedic Society of North America. Dr. Sharkey or an immediate family member serves as a board member, owner, officer, or committee member of the Pediatric Orthopaedic Society of North America.

INTRODUCTION

There has been a recent shift in how children are coached and trained in youth sports programs. Early specialization in one sport has become commonplace, with athletes being asked to perform at increasingly higher levels from increasingly younger ages. In parallel with this increase in intensity in youth sports, the incidence of sports-related injuries in the skeletally immature population has risen, with injury involving the anterior cruciate ligament (ACL) as one notable example.[1,2] The clinical presentation, methods of evaluation, recommended treatments, functional outcomes, and common complications for young athletes who sustain injuries of the primary ligaments of the knee, with particular focus on injuries of the ACL and the tibial spine, have been reviewed.

ACL INJURIES

Midsubstance ACL injuries were historically thought to be rare in the pediatric population; however, several studies have reported increasing rates of ACL injury and subsequent surgical ACL reconstruction for pediatric and adolescent patients.[2,3] A 2016 study reported that the nationwide increase in ACL injuries in children 10 to 14 years of age was 18.9% between 2007 and 2011; a concomitant increase in the rate of ACL reconstructions of 27.6% was reported for the years studied.[2] Proposed reasons for this increase include both enhanced awareness of the possibility of midsubstance ACL tears in the pediatric cohort and a true increase in the rate of ACL injuries as more children participate in sports in a systematic, specialized fashion.

Multiple risk factors for ACL injury in the pediatric athlete have been identified, including intrinsic anatomic factors, such as increased posterior tibial slope,[4,5] increased Q angle, and decreased width of the intercondylar notch.[6] Commonly identified mechanical and neuromuscular risk factors for ACL injury include reduced knee flexion angles, high quadriceps forces (increased quadriceps to hamstring strength ratio), and increased internal hip rotation and dynamic valgus landing postures.[7] A combination of these known risk factors has likely contributed to a higher incidence of ACL tears in young female athletes compared with the male peers. One study reported an adjusted relative risk for female athletes of 2.10, although the absolute number of ACL tears in young male athletes remains high.[8,9] Extrinsic risk factors that have been identified for ACL tears in the adolescent population include the level of competition and the sport played. Specifically, collegiate athletes have been shown to have higher rates of ACL tears than high school athletes.[8] In addition, athletes participating in sports, such as football, soccer, rugby, lacrosse, and basketball, are at highest risk for ACL injury.[8,9]

Because ACL injuries are so common and devastating to a young athlete, various ACL injury prevention programs have been created. In a systematic review of the literature on neuromuscular training intervention programs, the Prevent Injury and Enhance Performance program, the Knee Injury Prevention Program, and the Sportsmetrics program were each found to successfully reduce the rate of noncontact ACL injuries in adolescent female athletes. A range of 70 to 98 athletes needed to be trained to prevent one ACL injury.[7] A cost analysis of screening and prevention programs for ACL injuries in young athletes found that the introduction of neuromuscular prevention programs universally would be more cost effective than screening for and training only at-risk athletes.[10]

Evaluation

After a noncontact, twisting-type injury, young athletes with ACL tears frequently report the sudden onset of knee pain that may be accompanied by a popping sensation. Difficulty bearing weight and hemarthrosis are commonly present. The initial evaluation includes inspecting the soft tissues; performing passive motion of the ipsilateral hip, knee, and ankle; carefully palpating the entire affected limb; and assessing neurovascular status. Clinical tests for ACL deficiency include the Lachman, anterior drawer, and pivot shift tests. Because these tests may be difficult to perform and/or interpret in a young, anxious patient, results should be compared with similar tests performed on the contralateral, unaffected knee and may need to be repeated.

The presence of associated injuries of the menisci may be established by evaluating for tenderness of the joint line; decreased passive knee motion also may indicate a meniscal injury with displacement. Injuries of the collateral ligaments may be evaluated by varus and valgus stress testing of the knee performed at 0° and 30° of flexion. Specialized maneuvers such as the dial test and posterior drawer test also can be performed to evaluate other structures of the knee, including the posterolateral corner and posterior cruciate ligament, respectively. If ACL injury in a skeletally immature patient is suspected, limb alignment and lengths are assessed clinically. In addition, the patient's degree of physiologic maturity may be gauged by use of Tanner staging of sexual maturation.

Orthogonal radiographs of the affected knee should be obtained, with additional radiographs obtained as suggested by the physical examination findings. MRI of the knee is helpful for confirming an ACL tear (95% sensitivity and 88% specificity),[6] elucidating additional injuries, and assessing physeal patency (**Figure 1**). Before surgical treatment, a bone age study (a PA radiograph of the left hand, which is then compared with the Greulich and Pyle atlas of normal standards) is generally performed for skeletally immature patients to estimate the amount of remaining skeletal growth. Standing hip-to-ankle alignment radiographs may be obtained to evaluate for preexisting angular deformity or limb-length discrepancy of the lower limbs before surgical intervention.

Management

Partial tears of the ACL may occur in pediatric patients. The limited available data suggest that nonsurgical treatment may be successful in some patients with partial ACL

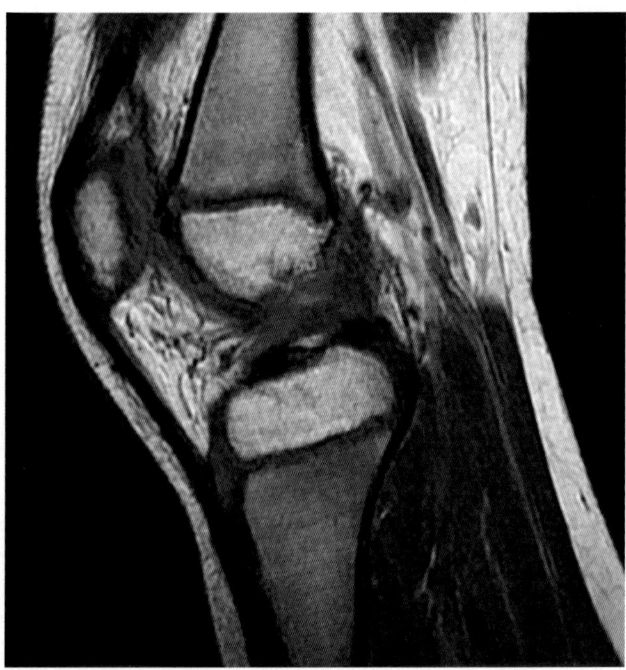

FIGURE 1 Sagittal T1-weighted magnetic resonance image through the knee of a 9-year-old skeletally immature boy shows a complete midsubstance anterior cruciate ligament tear.

tears.[11,12] In a prospective, cohort study of 45 skeletally immature patients with partial ACL tears, the authors reported that only one-third of the patients required surgical reconstruction for symptomatic instability. Tears involving more than 50% of the ACL fibers and predominantly the posterolateral bundle were more likely to require reconstruction. Similarly, nonsurgical treatment was more likely to be unsuccessful in patients older than 14 years and in those with objective signs of knee instability on clinical tests (eg, the pivot shift test).[11]

Although most of the current literature is focused on surgical reconstruction of the torn ligament, several authors have recently reported on arthroscopic-assisted repair performed in the specific instance of proximal femoral ACL avulsion injuries. This injury pattern is fundamentally different from the more common midsubstance ligament injury, in that most ACL fibers remain in continuity because the site of failure is the proximal insertion on the lateral femoral condyle. For patients with this injury pattern, primary repair of the ligament back to its native femoral footprint using suture anchors and/or transosseous tunnels offers potential advantages over ligament reconstruction, such as preservation of proprioceptive function and avoidance of morbidity from autograft harvest. This technique has gained popularity recently in the adult population[13] and has also been described for use in children: The authors of a 2017 study reported on the results of five pediatric patients (average age = 9.2 years) who had undergone arthroscopic-assisted proximal ACL repair using bioabsorbable suture anchors. These authors found that at an average follow-up of 43.4 months, all patients had a clinically stable knee, MRI-demonstrated healing, and improved outcomes scores and had returned to their previous level of activity without evidence of physeal injury.[14] Historically, full-thickness ACL tears in skeletally immature patients were treated with nonsurgical measures, including bracing treatment, physical therapy, and activity modification, until children reached skeletal maturity, and a standard ACL reconstruction could be performed without risking injury to the physes. Although nonsurgical treatment should remain part of the discussion regarding the treatment of children with ACL injuries, there is mounting evidence that delayed surgical reconstruction is associated with worse outcomes in this population. A 2014 meta-analysis of studies examining nonsurgical versus surgical treatment of children and adolescents with ACL tears found that patients treated surgically had substantially less knee instability and pathologic laxity, substantially higher rates of return to activity, substantially lower rates of symptomatic posttreatment medial meniscus tears, and higher functional outcomes scores.[15]

Efforts have been made to clarify the relationship between delayed surgical reconstruction in this population and the presence of associated intra-articular injuries of cartilage and menisci.[16-19] One retrospective chart review evaluated 70 patients, 14 years or younger, who had undergone ACL reconstruction. The authors reported that increased time to surgery was independently associated with the presence of medial meniscal tears and chondral injuries of both medial and lateral compartments. In addition, patients who had undergone surgical stabilization more than 12 weeks after injury had substantially higher rates of severe or irreparable medial meniscal tears and lateral chondral injuries. Subjective knee instability was also associated with higher rates of meniscal tears in this study.[16] A second retrospective chart review of 370 pediatric patients who underwent ACL reconstruction found that patients treated more than 150 days after injury had substantially higher rates of medial meniscal tears than those treated sooner; when present, meniscal tears were significantly associated with chondral injury in the same compartment.[17] Two prospective cohort studies also examined this question. A substantial association was found between self-reported episodes of instability and the presence of medial meniscal tears and chondral injuries. Increased time to surgery was also associated with the increasing severity of concomitant injures.[18,19] It is now widely accepted that patients with ACL injury who undergo delayed reconstruction may experience additional episodes of knee instability; this in turn puts them at risk for sustaining further injuries of the meniscus and cartilage, which may be more severe and ultimately irreparable. The authors of a recent study investigated insurance status as a possible cause of delayed presentation for care of an ACL injury: a retrospective analysis of 119 pediatric patients treated surgically for an ACL and/or meniscus injury at a single institution revealed that patients with public insurance were significantly more likely than those with private insurance to experience a delay in presentation for specialized care.[20]

After the decision to proceed with surgical reconstruction of the ACL is made, the next step in the treatment algorithm is choosing an appropriate surgical technique. Traditional ACL reconstruction techniques involve the creation of tunnels in the distal femur and proximal tibia that would directly violate the open physes in a skeletally immature individual. Substantial work has been done to quantify the amount of physeal injury that reliably results in physeal arrest. Studies previously performed in animal models suggest that when less than 5% of the cross-sectional area of the physis is violated, growth arrest does not occur; however, when more than 7% to 9% of the physis is violated, growth disturbance—with resultant limb-length discrepancy and/or angular deformity—is possible. Growth disturbance may also result from placement of a bone block (eg, a bone–patellar tendon–bone graft) across an open physis and from peripheral physeal disruption, which is often attributed to overzealous dissection near the perichondrial ring of LaCroix and/or fixation devices placed in close proximity to the physes.[6,21]

Two studies have used computer modeling to generate three-dimensional MRI reconstructions of a skeletally immature knee and simulate transphyseal tunnels that would be made at the time of ACL reconstruction.[22,23] One study, using 8-mm tunnels and optimal trajectory angles for tunnel placement, determined that, in the 31 knees studied (patients age 10 to 15 years), 2.4% of the distal femoral physis and 2.5% of the proximal tibial physis were affected, on average, by tunnel drilling.[22] It was also determined that increasing the graft diameter by 1 mm resulted in an average 1.1% increase in the physeal volume affected. Changing the drill angle to achieve a more vertical tunnel had a much smaller effect, with a calculated decrease of 0.2% in the volume of injured physis for every 5° increase in the angle of the drill tunnel.

In a similar study, the volumetric injury produced by computer-generated creation of transphyseal tunnels in 10 children aged 5 to 10 years was investigated.[23] The authors reported that drill holes measuring up to 9 mm in diameter resulted in an average physeal volume affected of less than 3.8% for the tibia and 5.4% for the femur, with the individual maximum percentage of volume removed remaining less than 9%, even with 9-mm drill holes placed across the physes of a 5-year-old child.[23]

Physeal-sparing ACL Reconstruction

Despite data supporting the use of transphyseal tunnels for ACL reconstruction in skeletally immature patients, physeal injury and subsequent growth disturbance remain important concerns. To address this issue, several physeal-sparing ACL reconstruction techniques have been developed. The two primary techniques are (1) the combined intra-articular and extra-articular extraphyseal technique in which no tunnels are drilled and fixation of the autograft iliotibial band (ITB) on both the femoral and tibial sides is achieved using sutures securing the graft to the periosteum[24,25] (**Figure 2**); and (2) the ACL reconstruction techniques in which tunnels are drilled in an all-epiphyseal fashion.[26] A variety of fixation methods for all-epiphyseal ACL reconstruction techniques exist, including suspensory fixation, epiphyseal interference screws, and/or a metaphyseal post[6] (**Figure 3**).

A 2014 study evaluated the risk of MRI-documented physeal injury after ACL reconstruction using an all-epiphyseal technique performed in 15 skeletally immature patients.[27] The authors reported that, on average, 2.1% of the total tibial physeal area was compromised using this technique; however, no femoral physeal disturbance was noted. At an average follow-up of 18 months after surgery, there were no cases of growth arrest or resultant limb deformity.

Considerable attention has been paid to evaluating the biomechanics of nontraditional ACL reconstruction techniques.[28-30] A 2011 study evaluated six adult cadaver knees in the intact state after ACL disruption and after ACL reconstruction using all-epiphyseal and ITB physeal-sparing techniques and a hybrid method involving the creation of a transtibial tunnel coupled with an over-the-top (physeal-sparing) femoral technique. The authors reported that all three reconstruction techniques improved knee stability; the ITB method best restored both translational and rotational control, although it overconstrained the knee to rotational forces at some flexion angles.[28] In a follow-up study investigating pivot-shift kinematics, all three techniques improved knee stability. The ITB technique allowed for less translation and rotation than the normal ACL–intact state, and the all-epiphyseal technique was reported to achieve the best restoration of normal knee kinematics.[29]

Outcomes for patients undergoing physeal-sparing ACL reconstruction are generally good.[24,26,31-33] In a study in which the ITB physeal-sparing ACL reconstruction technique was used to treat 44 skeletally immature prepubescent patients (average age = 10.3 years), clinical (Lachman and pivot shift tests) and functional (International Knee Documentation Committee and Lysholm scores) outcome measures at the 5-year follow-up showed good results; only 2 patients required revision surgery. A clinically important growth disturbance did not develop in any of the patients, despite average patient growth of 21.5 cm.[24] The authors of a recent study reported on a single institution's experience with the ITB physeal-sparing ACL reconstruction over a 23-year period. In a cohort of 237 patients treated at an average age of 11.2 years, it was found that greater than 96% had clinically stable knees at an average follow-up of 25 months. At an average follow-up of 6.2 years, patient-reported outcomes were excellent, graft rupture rate was 6.6%, and no significant growth disturbance was noted.[34] The authors of a smaller case series described their experience with 21 male patients (average age = 11.8 years) followed up for 3 years after ACL reconstruction using the ITB technique. Similarly good results were found. The authors reported a 14% rate of revision ACL surgery; for the patients not requiring revision, the clinical and functional outcomes were excellent, and no growth disturbances were detected.[31]

Reported outcomes in two early studies of all-epiphyseal ACL reconstruction also have been favorable, although the number of patients studied in each series was small.[26,32] A recent retrospective analysis of 103

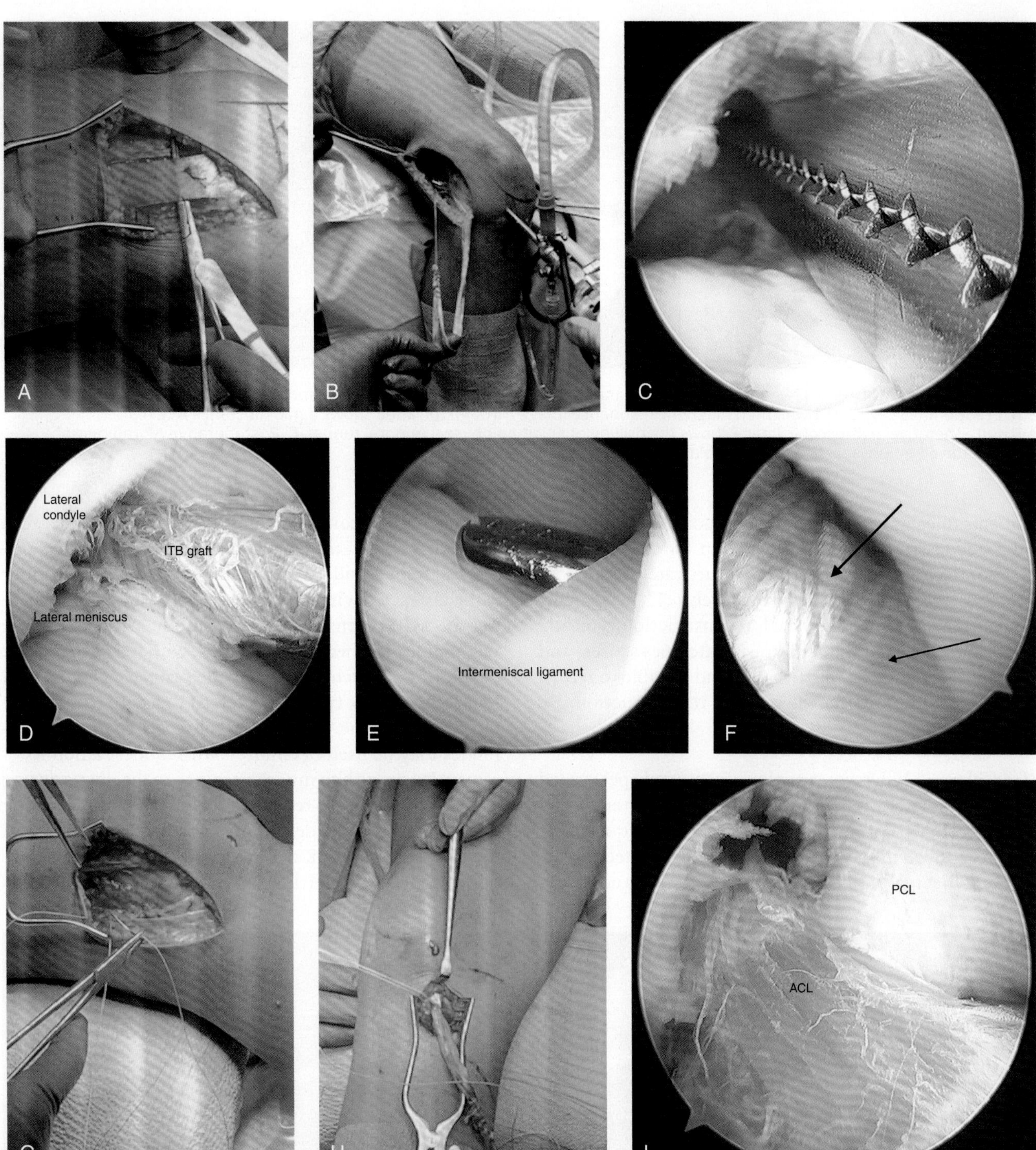

FIGURE 2 Intraoperative photographs and arthroscopic images demonstrating the physeal-sparing ACL reconstruction using autograft iliotibial band. **A**, Harvest of the central iliotibial band. **B**, After detachment of the graft proximally, the end is brought into the lateral wound and whip stitched. Its distal attachment at Gerdy tubercle is left intact. **C**, Under arthroscopic guidance, a curved clamp is brought into the knee and used to pierce the lateral capsule in the over-the-top position. **D**, The graft is retrieved and shuttled into the knee. **E**, A small incision is made on the proximal leg (distal to the tibial physis and medial to the apophysis) and a clamp is placed from this wound under the intermeniscal ligament and into the knee under arthroscopic guidance. **F**, After preparation of the proximal tibia with a small rasp, the graft (large arrow) is retrieved and shuttled under the intermeniscal ligament (small arrow). **G**, The graft is sutured to the lateral femoral condyle. **H**, The graft is sutured to the periosteum of the proximal tibia. **I**, Final intra-articular appearance. ACL = anterior cruciate ligament, IBT = internal bone transport, PCL = posterior cruciate ligament

Section 8: Sports-Related Topics

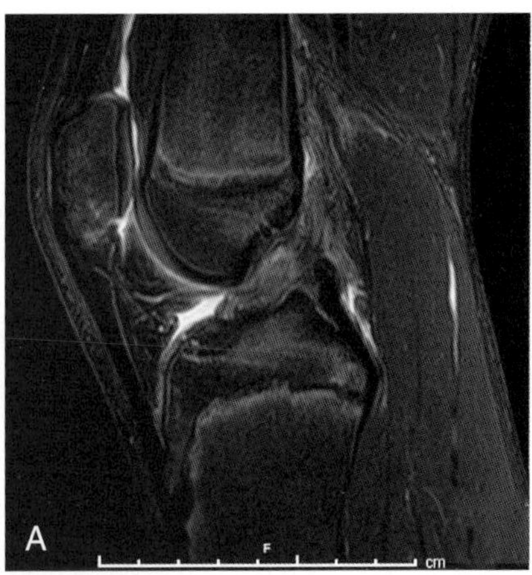

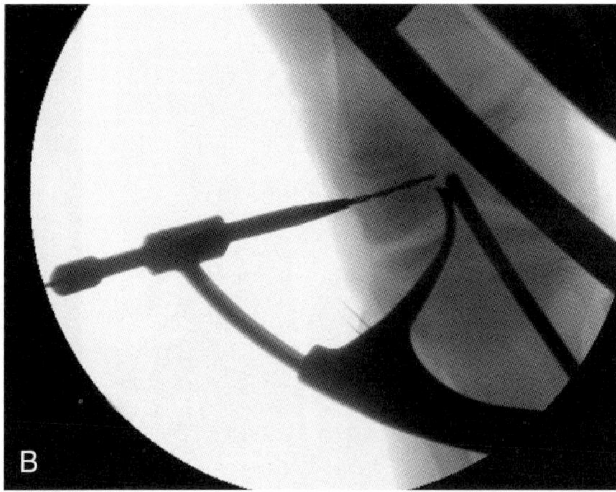

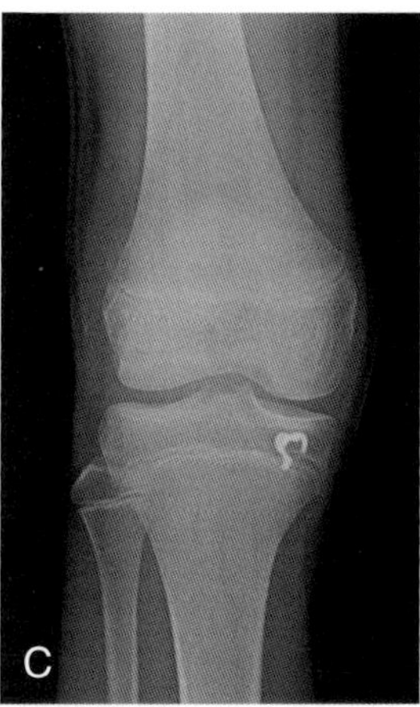

FIGURE 3 Images from a 12-year-old boy with an anterior cruciate ligament (ACL) injury and substantial remaining growth. **A**, Preoperative sagittal T2-weighted magnetic resonance image through the knee shows a midsubstance ACL tear. **B**, Intraoperative arthroscopic image shows the drilling of an all-epiphyseal femoral tunnel. **C**, Postoperative AP radiograph shows the all-epiphyseal femoral and tibial tunnels.

patients (mean age 12.1 years) undergoing all-epiphyseal ACL reconstruction and followed up for an average of 21 months found that the graft rupture rate was 10.7%, and growth disturbance occurred rarely (<1%).[33] Patients undergoing all-epiphyseal ACL reconstruction typically have stable knees, high functional outcomes scores, and a small risk of growth disturbance and are able to return to sports activities after the surgical reconstruction.

Transphyseal ACL Reconstruction

Transphyseal ACL reconstruction is commonly performed in patients with a modest amount of growth remaining (**Figure 4**). Variations in transphyseal techniques have been described in the literature. In one hybrid technique, patients deemed at risk for growth disturbance from a transphyseal tunnel created in the femur undergo a physeal-sparing technique on the femoral side, with transphyseal tunnel drilling on the tibial side. (The distal femur is the fastest growing physis in the body, and tunnel drilling for ACL reconstruction potentially affects the more vulnerable periphery of this physis, with the potential for resultant distal femoral valgus deformity.) This type of hybrid method is typically referred to as a partial transphyseal technique. In addition, physeal-respecting techniques may be used in children with modest amounts of remaining growth to minimize injury to the physis during a transphyseal ACL reconstruction. Physeal-respecting techniques can include the use of soft-tissue grafts and metaphyseal fixation, avoidance of dissection near the perichondrial ring of LaCroix, optimization of tunnel

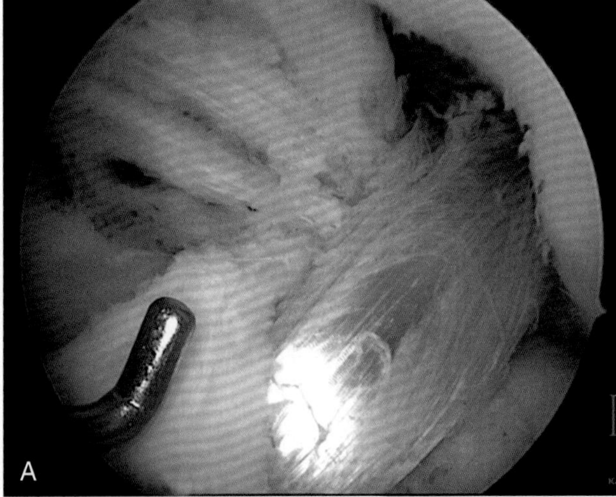

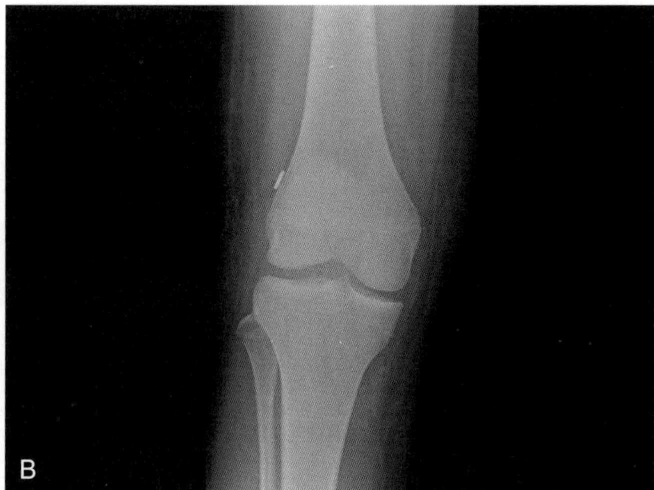

FIGURE 4 **A**, Arthroscopic image of the intra-articular appearance of the newly reconstructed anterior cruciate ligament (ACL) in a 14-year-old girl approaching skeletal maturity. ACL reconstruction was performed using a transphyseal technique. **B**, Postoperative AP radiograph shows placement of the transphyseal tunnels.

Section 8: Sports-Related Topics

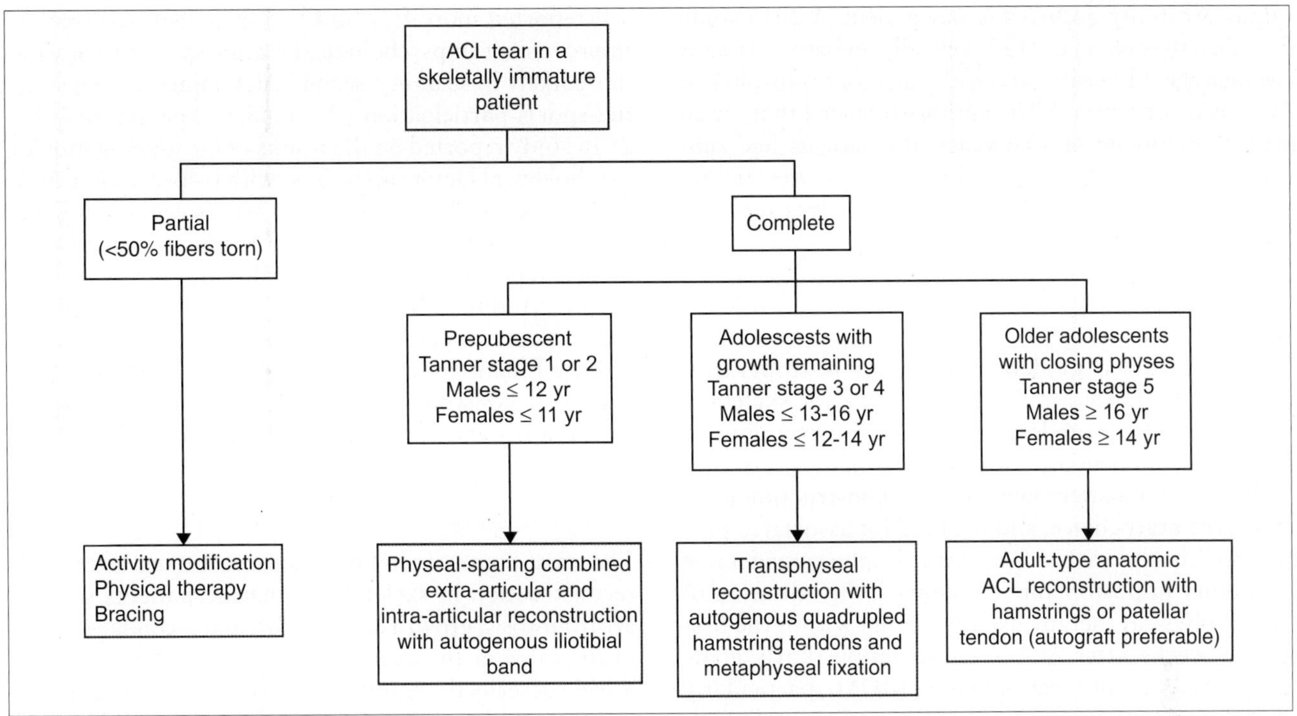

FIGURE 5 A treatment algorithm for the surgical management of complete anterior cruciate ligament injuries in skeletally immature patients. ACL = anterior cruciate ligament. (Reproduced from Frank JS, Gambacorta PL: Anterior cruciate ligament injuries in the skeletally immature athlete: Diagnosis and management. *J Am Acad Orthop Surg* 2013;21[2]:78-87. © 2013 by American Academy of Orthopaedic Surgeons.)

size (as previously discussed, larger tunnels are associated with greater amounts of physeal disturbance), and the use of vertical tunnels. An algorithm for the surgical treatment of ACL injuries in skeletally immature patients is presented in **Figure 5**.

In terms of graft choice for ACL reconstruction, soft-tissue grafts are generally used in skeletally immature patients to minimize the risk of iatrogenic growth disturbance that accompanies placement of a bone plug across an open physis. Traditionally, this has been a quadrupled hamstring tendon graft, although recent interest has been focused on the use of autograft quadriceps tendon graft in this population. Similar to hamstring autograft, the quadriceps tendon may be harvested as an all–soft tissue graft, thus minimizing the risk of physeal arrest when placed across the epiphyseal plates. Early outcomes with use of quadriceps tendon for pediatric ACL reconstruction are encouraging: a recent retrospective analysis of 83 patients who had undergone primary transphyseal ACL reconstruction with soft-tissue autograft and followed up for a minimum of 2 years found that the patients who had a quadriceps tendon graft had significantly larger grafts than patients who had hamstring tendon grafts (9.6 mm versus 7.8 mm, $P < 0.001$). Additionally, patients with quadriceps tendon grafts were significantly less likely to sustain a tear of the ACL graft ($P < 0.05$).[35]

When selecting a graft for use in pediatric ACL reconstruction, it is important to remember that data support the routine use of autograft tissue in this population. A case-control study of 73 pediatric patients (average age = 15 years) undergoing ACL reconstruction with either autograft or allograft tendon reported a more than fourfold greater risk of revision surgery for patients treated with allograft tendon.[36]

Reported outcomes of patients treated with transphyseal ACL reconstruction are generally good.[37-40] At an average follow-up of 3.6 years, a low rate of revision (3%), high functional outcomes scores, and no clinically detectable growth disturbance were reported in 59 patients (average age = 14.7 years) who had undergone transphyseal ACL reconstruction with soft-tissue autograft and metaphyseal fixation.[37] A 2013 study reported on the outcomes of 32 skeletally immature patients (average age = 11.3 years) treated with ACL reconstruction using a variation of the transphyseal technique in which the tibial and femoral tunnels were drilled comparatively vertical and a hamstring allograft was used for the reconstruction.[38] Fixation was kept far from the physes (screw and washer on the tibial side and an Endobutton [Smith & Nephew] on the femoral side). At a follow-up of 6 years, the functional outcomes measures of all of the patients had improved; one rerupture had occurred; and no limb-length discrepancy was noted, although valgus deformity occurred in one patient. A 2015 study described the outcomes of 27 skeletally immature patients (average age = 13 years) who had undergone transphyseal ACL reconstruction.[39] The authors reported that, at an average follow-up of 10.6 years, the patients had substantially improved functional outcomes scores and no detectable growth arrest; graft rerupture was reported in 3 of 27 patients (11%).

Postoperative Care, Rehabilitation, and Return to Play

No standardized guidelines exist for postoperative care, rehabilitation, and return to play for skeletally immature patients undergoing ACL reconstruction. As a result, recommendations vary based on the preference of the surgeon, patient factors, the reconstruction technique, the graft choice, and the need for associated procedures (such as meniscal repair). Despite considerable variability in postoperative regimens, the initiation of formal physical therapy usually occurs within the first several weeks after ACL reconstruction. Early goals include recovery of range of motion (ROM), particularly the achievement of terminal knee extension and patellar mobility, and isometric strengthening. Athletes are gradually advanced in weight bearing, ROM, strengthening, and endurance; sport-specific skills are introduced in a supervised setting after more basic skills have been mastered.

Numerous factors may contribute to the decision to allow an athlete to return to play, including recovery of quadriceps strength (as measured by muscle girth). Perhaps, the most important indicator is the patient's ability to demonstrate functional readiness, which is typically assessed by performance on various testing measures (eg, the single-leg hop, triple-hop distance, crossover hop, Y balance, and step-down tests). Although patients were traditionally cleared for return to play after a safe amount of time had elapsed (generally 6 to 9 months), a recent study found that even 9 months after ACL reconstruction, many adolescent patients do not demonstrate adequate functional movement patterns to allow safe return to sport.[41] It has been suggested that maturity-specific rehabilitation strategies may be needed to optimally prepare young athletes for return to play.

Although a young athlete's physical preparedness is a crucial component of return-to-sport assessment, a significant amount of attention has been placed recently on psychological readiness for ensuring a safe return to sport. Using the ACL–Return to Sport after Injury scale, the authors of a 2019 study analyzed the psychological readiness of 115 patients younger than 20 years who had undergone ACL reconstruction and subsequently returned to sport. Significantly, patients who self-reported more fear and had demonstrated smaller improvement in psychological readiness over time were more likely to sustain a second ACL injury after resuming sports participation ($P < 0.05$).[42] The authors of a 2016 study reported on the results of the investigation of psychological factors associated with recovery after ACL reconstruction. It was found that self-esteem was significantly associated with return to sport, as well as with patient-reported measures of health and physical functioning. Additionally, patients who reported an internal locus of control performed better on objective measures of knee function such as the single-leg hop test.[43] These studies demonstrate that a young athlete's psychological state is a key and potentially modifiable, factor affecting outcomes following ACL surgery.

Complications

The most common complications occurring after ACL reconstruction in skeletally immature patients include arthrofibrosis, growth disturbance, and secondary injury of the same or the contralateral ACL. Arthrofibrosis is a well-described complication after adult ACL reconstruction and has been shown to occur in children and adolescents. A retrospective case series described a single institution's experience with 902 young patients treated with ACL reconstruction.[44] An overall incidence of arthrofibrosis of 8.3% was reported in this cohort (average age = 15 years), with female sex, older age, the use of bone–patellar tendon–bone autograft, and concomitant meniscal repair being additional risk factors for arthrofibrosis.

Growth arrest sometimes occurs after ACL reconstruction in skeletally immature patients despite efforts to avoid this complication. One recent case series reported on four patients (average age = 14.2 years) in whom clinically important growth disturbances, including tibial recurvatum and genu valgum, developed after transphyseal ACL reconstruction using physeal-respecting techniques (eg, soft-tissue autograft, metaphyseal fixation on the femur).[45] Another group of researchers retrospectively reviewed the postoperative MRIs of 43 patients (average age = 14.8 years) who had undergone transphyseal ACL reconstruction using soft-tissue graft.[46] The authors found that the average bone tunnel to epiphyseal plate cross-sectional area ratios were 2.6% for the proximal tibia and 2.3% for the distal femur. Despite this, focal physeal bone bridges were noted in five knees, although no patient had resultant limb deformity. Growth disturbance also has been reported with physeal-sparing techniques, with one patient in a recent series of all-epiphyseal ACL reconstructions developing clinically significant growth arrest[33] (**Figure 6**).

Secondary ACL injury in either the ipsilateral or contralateral knee has been reported to occur with alarming

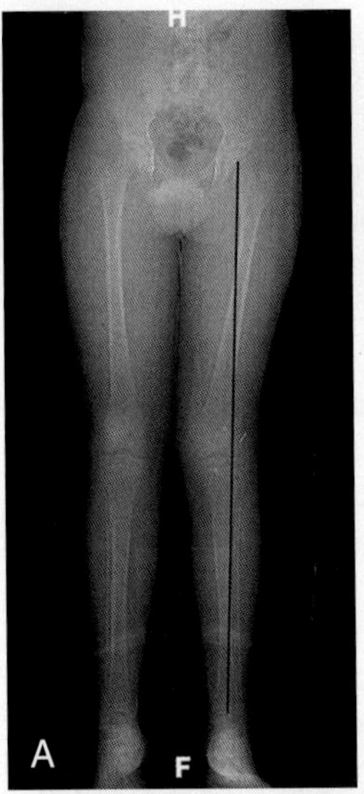

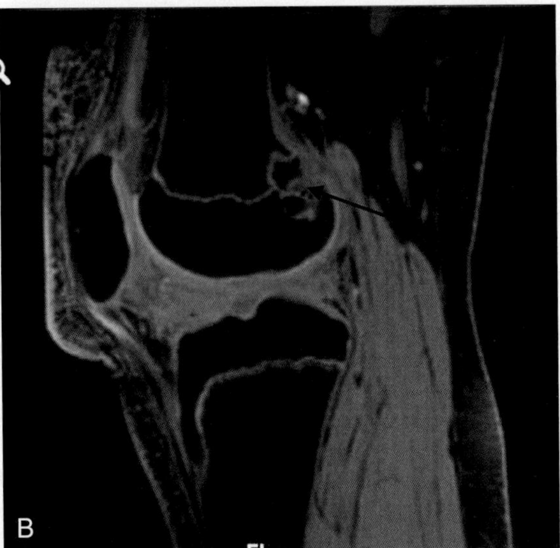

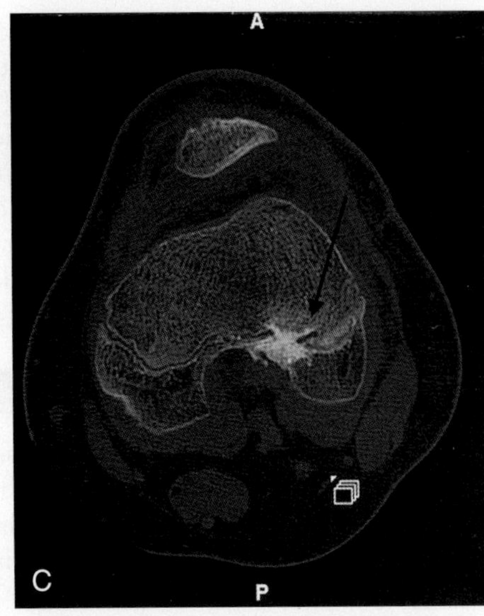

FIGURE 6 Diagnostic imaging of a 13-year-old boy who presented with gradual loss of knee extension and increasing limb deformity 1 year after undergoing an ACL reconstruction using all-epiphyseal bone tunnels. **A**, Three-joint limb alignment radiograph demonstrating asymmetric valgus malalignment of the knee. **B**, Sagittal magnetic resonance image demonstrates disturbance of the posterolateral aspect of the distal femoral physis. **C**, Axial CT scan of the knee demonstrates the presence of a bony bar with premature arrest at the posterolateral femoral physis. Black arrows identify the area of localized physeal injury resulting in the formation of a physeal bar.

frequency. In a 2014 cohort study, the incidence of second ACL injury in young athletes (average age = 17 years) within 2 years of the index surgery was reported.[47] The authors found that the overall incidence of a second injury in this cohort of young patients who had returned to sports was more than five times greater than that of healthy control athletes. Nearly 30% of athletes sustained a second ACL injury within 24 months of return to sports, with approximately one-third of the injuries occurring in the ipsilateral knee and two-thirds in the contralateral knee.[47] A 2014 case-control study found that patients younger than 20 years at the time of ACL reconstruction had a 29% chance of sustaining a second ACL injury (either knee) within 5 years of the index surgery; a return to cutting and pivoting sports increased the odds of injury.[48] Another group of authors recently analyzed a continuous cohort of 85 patients younger than 18 years who underwent primary ACL reconstruction with autograft and were followed up for a minimum of 2 years. The authors reported a very high return to sport among these athletes (91%). However, 32% of the overall cohort sustained a second ACL injury; later return to sport was protective against new ACL injury.[49] Finally, a recent systematic review and meta-analysis of the existing literature confirmed that younger patients returning to high-level sporting activities were at greatest risk for subsequent knee injury.[50] The authors found that athletes younger than 25 years who return to sports had a secondary rate of ACL injury (ipsilateral or contralateral knee) of 23%.[50]

Revision ACL Reconstruction

Several recent studies have reported on the outcomes of revision ACL reconstruction in the pediatric population. One retrospective case series included 90 patients with an average age of 16.6 years who sustained ACL graft rupture at an average of 1.28 years after the initial surgery. Following revision ACL reconstruction, 20% of these patients went on to sustain a new graft rupture, 20% sustained a contralateral ACL tear, and only 55% were able to return to sport at preinjury level of play.[51] Another group of authors compared the outcomes of pediatric patients who underwent revision ACL reconstruction with those of patients who underwent primary ACL surgery and reported similar results. Specifically, patients who required revision ACL reconstruction were significantly more likely to have concomitant injuries and to have graft failure; additionally, patient-reported outcomes scores were lower and the patients were less likely to return to sport ($P < 0.05$).[52]

Future Directions

Reconstruction of the injured ligament remains the clear standard of care for surgical management of a symptomatic ACL rupture in young athletes. However, one new area of research in the field of pediatric ACL surgery bears mention—the bridge-enhanced anterior cruciate ligament repair procedure. Early clinical outcomes of this procedure have recently been published: 10 patients who underwent ACL reconstruction with autograft hamstring tendon were compared with 10 patients who had undergone the bridge-enhanced anterior cruciate ligament repair procedure and were followed up for 24 months. There were no failures noted in either group; additionally, there were no significant differences between the groups with regard to clinical outcomes scores, physical functioning, and instrumented laxity.[53] Although enhanced ligament repair is a promising area of active research, there are not enough data at this point to support its routine use.

TIBIAL SPINE FRACTURES

Avulsion fractures of the tibial spine, also known as tibial eminence fractures, are uncommon injuries, with an annual incidence previously estimated to be 3 per 100,000 children and adolescents.[54] This injury is often referred to as the childhood equivalent of an ACL injury, with failure occurring through the bone-ligament interface rather than through the substance of the ligament itself. As tensile forces are initially applied to the knee, the ACL stretches, with resultant permanent plastic deformation of the ligament. Increased tensile load ultimately leads to failure of the incompletely ossified tibial plateau at the insertion of the ACL, resulting in a tibial spine avulsion fracture.[55]

Skeletally immature patients presenting with this injury are typically aged 8 to 14 years and commonly report a sports-related injury mechanism. Pedestrians struck by motor vehicles and bicyclists who sustain a fall also may have tibial spine fractures.[56]

Evaluation

Patients with tibial spine fractures report the acute onset of knee pain, which is often accompanied by swelling, decreased motion, and the inability to ambulate. The physical examination and the initial radiographic assessment are similar to those previously described for ACL tears.

The modified Myers and McKeever classification system is most commonly used to describe tibial spine fractures. Type I fractures are minimally displaced; type II fractures are displaced anteriorly with an intact posterior bony hinge; type III fractures are completely displaced from the fracture bed (**Figure 7, A**); and type IV fractures are displaced and comminuted.[56]

Additional imaging studies, such as CT and MRI, may be useful for identifying associated intra-articular injuries of the meniscus and chondral surface that commonly occur in the setting of a tibial spine fracture. One retrospective evaluation of 20 patients with tibial eminence fractures who underwent preoperative MRI evaluation revealed that 90% of the patients had bone contusions similar to those seen in patients with midsubstance ACL tears; meniscal tears were present in 40% of these patients.[57]

Although a 2003 study demonstrated a 3.8% rate of associated meniscal tears,[58] other studies have shown the rate of concomitant intra-articular pathology to be as high as 30%.[54,59] In a retrospective review of 58 patients with anterior tibial spine fractures, the authors reported meniscal tears in 33% of the patients with type II fractures and 12% of those with type III fractures.[59] When present, meniscal tears most commonly affected the anterior horn of the medial meniscus and the posterior horn of the lateral meniscus (**Figure 7, C**). Chondral injury was identified in 7% of the patients.

Advanced imaging studies, such as MRI, may be useful for identifying potential blocks to fracture reduction. The anterior horn of the medial meniscus and the intermeniscal ligament are the two structures most frequently

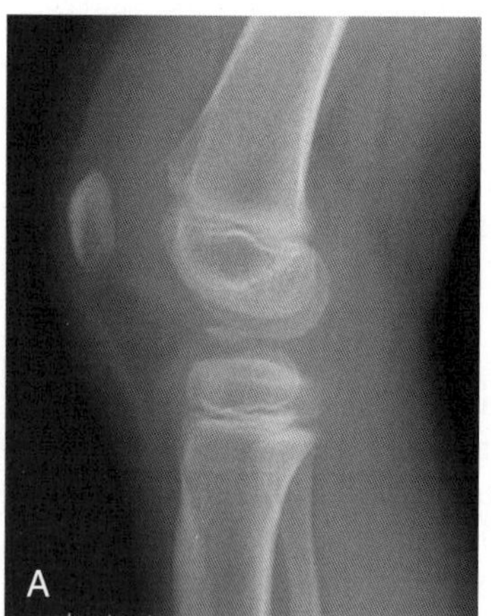

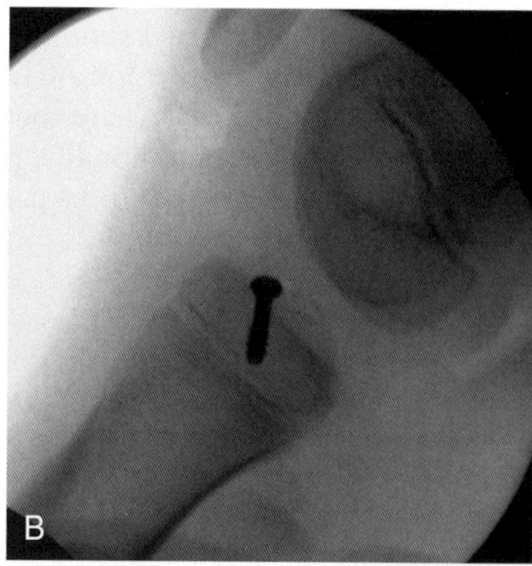

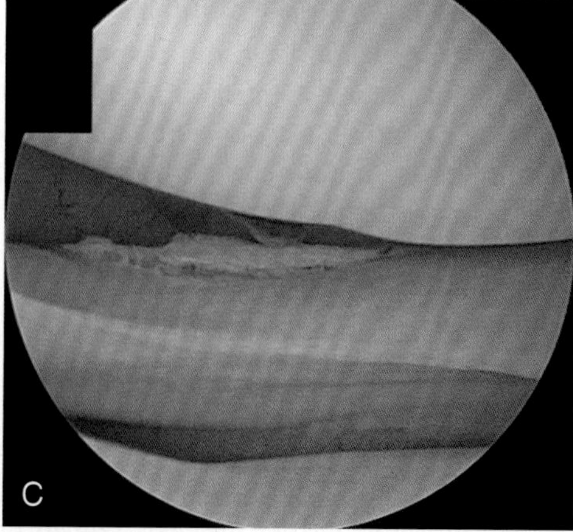

FIGURE 7 **A**, Preoperative lateral radiograph of the knee of a 7-year-old girl shows a type III tibial spine fracture. **B**, Intraoperative lateral fluoroscopic image of the knee of the patient in part **A** after arthroscopically assisted reduction and fixation using a cannulated, all-epiphyseal screw. **C**, Arthroscopic image shows a concomitant vertical tear of the posterior horn of the lateral meniscus.

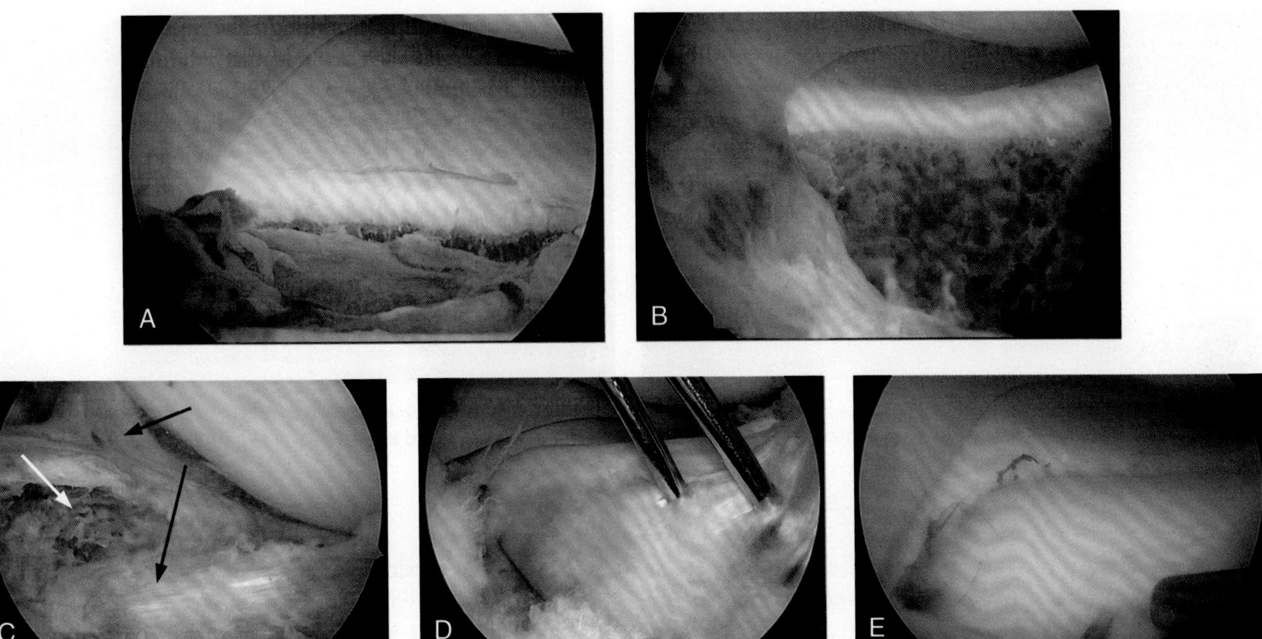

FIGURE 8 Arthroscopic images of the knee of a 13-year-old boy with a type III tibial spine fracture. **A**, Entrapment of the anterior horn of the medial meniscus in the fracture site. **B**, Following removal of the entrapped meniscus. **C**, Interposition of the intermeniscal ligament within the fracture bed. **D**, Following reduction and provisional fixation with Kirschner wires. **E**, Final fracture alignment after cannulated screw fixation. Short black arrow identifies the ACL; white arrow identifies the displaced fracture fragment (with ACL attached); long black arrow points to the intermeniscal ligament displaced into the fracture site where it may act as a mechanical block to reduction.

interposed in the fracture bed[58-60] (**Figure 8**). Soft-tissue impediments to fracture reduction are extremely common in the setting of displaced tibial spine fractures, with one study reporting a rate of soft-tissue entrapment to be as high as 65% for type III fractures.[58] A 2015 study reported a similarly high rate of meniscal entrapment, with 48% of the patients with type III fractures having entrapment of the meniscus within the fracture bed.[59]

Treatment

Patients with type I fractures are routinely treated with immobilization in a long leg cast. The position of the knee remains a subject of debate, with arguments made for placing the knee in either full extension (this theoretically allows the lateral femoral condyle to physically maintain fracture reduction) or in slight flexion (theoretically preventing elongation of the ACL during terminal extension).[61]

Closed reduction followed by radiographic confirmation of adequate alignment is the chosen treatment for most patients with type II fractures. A 2015 study suggested that less than 5 mm of displacement may be acceptable, with greater initial displacement correlating with a high rate of subsequent surgery to address late instability and impingement resulting from fracture malunion.[62] Patients with type II fractures in which acceptable reduction cannot be achieved by closed means and fractures that are completely displaced (types III and IV) are candidates for surgical treatment.

Surgical treatment of displaced tibial spine fractures has traditionally consisted of open reduction and internal fixation via arthrotomy, although arthroscopically assisted reduction and internal fixation procedures have become increasingly commonplace. Concomitant intra-articular pathology, including meniscal tears and chondral injuries, is treated at the time of the index procedure. After surgical reduction and stabilization, patients are generally immobilized in a long leg cast or a hinged knee brace for a short period before knee ROM exercises are begun.

Many methods of fixation have been described, with the two most common being (1) screw fixation, which typically involves the use of a self-tapping cannulated screw placed across the fracture fragments in an all-epiphyseal fashion, and (2) suture fixation, in which sutures are placed through the substance of the ACL, shuttled through small tunnels in the tibia, and tied over a bony bridge on the anterior tibial cortex[56] (**Figure 9**). A proposed advantage of screw fixation is the relative ease of the technique. Advantages of suture fixation include avoiding the possibility of subsequent hardware removal and the ability to fix comminuted fractures. Numerous variations of these techniques have been described, including the use of both absorbable and nonabsorbable suture materials, suture anchors, bioabsorbable implants (including nails and screws), and suture buttons.

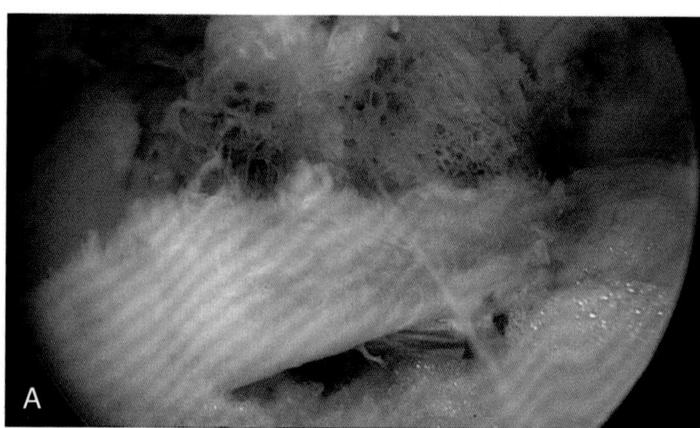

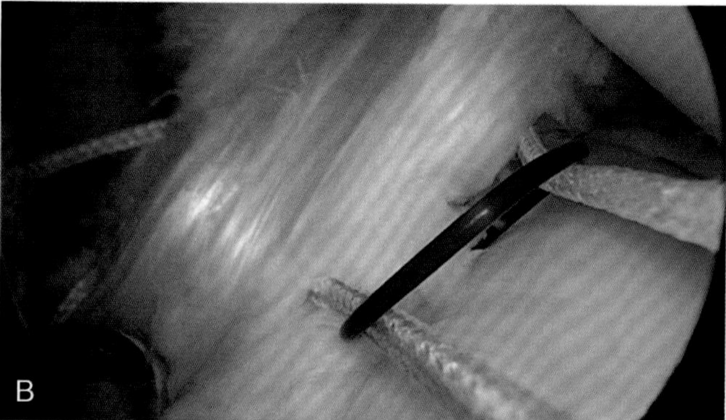

FIGURE 9 Arthroscopic images of a 13-year-old girl with a type IV tibial spine fracture treated with arthroscopically assisted reduction and suture fixation. **A**, The displaced fracture fragment, with the interposed intermeniscal ligament. **B**, Preparation for suture shuttling after fracture reduction.

Several attempts have been made to elucidate a difference in patient outcomes based on the surgical technique used. Two retrospective patient chart reviews have recently been published, each describing the authors' institutional experience in managing displaced tibial spine fractures.[62,63] In one study, the authors reviewed the charts of 31 patients, 13 of whom had been treated with open reduction and internal fixation and 18 of whom had undergone arthroscopically assisted reduction and internal fixation.[63] Patient sex, age, fracture type, fixation method (both screw and suture constructs were used), and length of postoperative immobilization were similar between the groups. The authors found that postoperative arthrofibrosis was more likely to develop in patients who waited longer for surgery (>7-day delay from injury to surgery) and those who had longer surgical times (>120 minutes). The authors concluded that the method of surgery used should be the method that could be performed with the most efficiency.

The authors of a 2015 study reported on their institution's experience managing displaced tibial spine fractures using closed, open, and arthroscopic techniques.[62] In their review of 76 patients, it was found that open and arthroscopic methods of treatment achieved a similar amount of fracture reduction and comparable rates of complications, including arthrofibrosis (11% in the group treated with open reduction and internal fixation and 12.5% in the arthroscopic group). In addition, no substantial difference in functional outcomes as assessed by Lysholm scores was found between the two surgical groups. Although the closed management (casting) group had approximately 50% less initial displacement of the fracture than the surgically treated group, this group had higher rates of revision for symptomatic loose bodies, instability, and impingement. Because of this, the authors concluded that surgical management should be considered for tibial spine fractures with displacement greater than 5 mm. The study authors also suggest that surgeon comfort with the procedure should guide the choice between open and arthroscopic surgical techniques.

A 2014 systematic review of the literature regarding the treatment of tibial eminence fractures reported that the available level of evidence to support clinical decision-making in this setting is quite low (all studies were level III or IV).[64] The authors concluded that neither an open nor an arthroscopic method of fixation was demonstrated to be superior. The authors similarly noted that neither a screw nor a suture fixation technique demonstrated a clear superiority over the other, with appreciable healing noted in patients treated with each method. The need for higher quality research in this area was recognized.

Mixed results have been reported from biomechanical studies performed to determine the optimal fixation techniques for patients with displaced tibial spine fractures. A 2007 study reported on 64 skeletally immature porcine knees in which tibial eminence fractures were created and then fixed with one screw, two screws, or nonabsorbable sutures.[65] In the laboratory, the construct using a commercially available ultra-high–molecular-weight polyethylene (UHMWPE) suture provided more fixation strength than a screw. It also was noted that the addition of a second screw did not enhance the construct strength. A 2005 study that used human cadaver knees reported similar findings, with UHMWPE suture fixation achieving greater ultimate strength than screw fixation.[66] However, the authors of a 2008 biomechanical study using immature bovine knees found no significant mechanical difference when comparing four methods of tibial spine fracture fixation (nonabsorbable suture, three bioabsorbable nails, one resorbable screw, and one metal screw).[67] The authors noted that the specimens repaired with a single metal screw demonstrated the greatest initial stiffness and failure force and the least amount of deformation. The suture and resorbable screw constructs demonstrated the highest levels of deformation at the fracture site during cyclic loading conditions.

Although suture and screw constructs have traditionally been used for fixation of tibial spine fractures, many other fixation methods exist. This heterogeneity is likely due, at least in part, to the fact that no single fixation method has been proved superior. Another cadaver biomechanical study compared four different methods of physeal-sparing fixation: (1) UHMWPE suture plus suture button, (2) suture anchors, (3) polydioxanone suture plus suture button, and (4) screw fixation.[68] After performing both load-to-failure and cyclic testing of the specimens in each group, the authors concluded that the UHMWPE suture plus button construct was biomechanically superior at the time of surgery. In addition, the suture anchor construct demonstrated the most variability in its ability to supply stable fixation for these fractures.

Complications

Residual laxity of the knee may be noted after treatment of a tibial spine fracture and usually is the result of plastic deformation of the ACL occurring at the time of initial injury. Although ACL laxity may be demonstrated objectively, clinical knee instability is rarely present after fracture fixation.[56] Commonly reported complications reported after treatment of tibial spine fractures include fracture malunion, fracture nonunion, hardware prominence, loss of fixation, and knee stiffness.

Arthrofibrosis is a well-documented complication of the surgical treatment of pediatric tibial spine fractures. In a study of 205 pediatric patients treated surgically for a displaced tibial spine fracture, arthrofibrosis (defined as 10° extension loss and/or less than 90° flexion at 3 months postoperatively) developed in 20 patients (10%).[69] The average time to surgery for these patients was 8.1 days, and postoperative immobilization was generally 4 to 6 weeks. The patients were treated with a second surgical procedure, which usually involved a combination of arthroscopic lysis of adhesions followed by manipulation under anesthesia. Of eight patients treated with manipulation under anesthesia alone, three sustained an intraoperative distal femoral physeal fracture. Isolated manipulation under anesthesia for postoperative arthrofibrosis in the skeletally immature knee, if performed, should be undertaken with extreme caution because of the documented risk of physeal injury.

In a 2012 study, the results of a retrospective chart review were reported for 40 patients treated surgically for a displaced tibial spine fracture. Arthrofibrosis developed in 7 of the 40 patients (17.5%), necessitating a second surgery.[70] Interestingly, the authors found that patients who had begun ROM therapy within 4 weeks of surgery had substantially faster return to full activity and were less likely to experience the development of arthrofibrosis than patients for whom ROM rehabilitation was initiated after 4 weeks. The goal of surgical treatment of these injuries is to achieve adequate fracture reduction in a timely fashion, with secure fracture fixation that will allow for early postoperative mobilization.

Although reinjury has not been reported widely in the literature, a recent study investigated the rate of subsequent ACL injury in pediatric patients who had been treated for a tibial spine fracture. The authors of this retrospective case series of 101 patients reported that 19% of patients who sustain a tibial spine fracture went on to have a second ACL-related injury of the knee, with older children being most at risk.[71]

SUMMARY

Sport-related ligamentous injuries of the knee have become increasingly common in skeletally immature patients. Clinical and functional outcomes for patients with complete ACL tears and displaced tibial spine fractures are generally better with early surgery than with delayed or nonsurgical care. Careful preoperative evaluation of the physes in these patients is important for determining the optimal surgical technique. Knowledge of potential complications after surgical treatment of these injuries, including growth arrest and reinjury, is crucial so that patients and their families may be counseled appropriately and complications can be recognized and addressed in a timely manner.

KEY STUDY POINTS

- Various physeal-sparing and physeal-respecting ACL reconstruction techniques have been developed for the skeletally immature knee.
- Growth disturbances related to physeal injury have been reported in a small number of skeletally immature patients after ACL reconstruction.
- Secondary ACL injury occurs commonly (both contralateral ACL tear and ipsilateral ACL graft rupture), and *early return to sport* and *low psychological readiness* are risk factors.
- Arthrofibrosis can commonly result after surgical fixation of tibial spine fractures, so secure fixation and early mobilization is paramount.
- Older children treated for a tibial spine fracture are at risk for future ACL injury.

ANNOTATED REFERENCES

1. Carter CW, Micheli LJ: Training the child athlete for prevention, health promotion, and performance: How much is enough, how much is too much? *Clin Sports Med* 2011;30(4):679-690.
2. Werner BC, Yang S, Looney AM, Gwathmey FW Jr: Trends in pediatric and adolescent anterior cruciate ligament injury and reconstruction. *J Pediatr Orthop* 2016;36(5):447-452.

   The authors of this retrospective cohort study evaluated the rates of ACL injury, ACL reconstruction, and associated surgical procedures in the pediatric cohort from 2007 to 2011 and found substantial increases in each rate compared with adult rates during the same period. Level of evidence: III.
3. Dodwell ER, Lamont LE, Green DW, Pan TJ, Marx RG, Lyman S: 20 years of pediatric anterior cruciate ligament reconstruction in New York State. *Am J Sports Med* 2014;42(3):675-680.
4. O'Malley MP, Milewski MD, Solomito MJ, Erwteman AS, Nissen CW: The association of tibial slope and anterior cruciate ligament rupture in skeletally immature patients. *Arthroscopy* 2015;31(1):77-82.
5. Dare DM, Fabricant PD, McCarthy MM, et al: Increased lateral tibial slope is a risk factor for pediatric anterior cruciate ligament injury: An MRI-based case-control study of 152 patients. *Am J Sports Med* 2015;43(7):1632-1639.
6. Fabricant PD, Jones KJ, Delos D, et al: Reconstruction of the anterior cruciate ligament in the skeletally immature athlete: A review of current concepts. AAOS exhibit selection. *J Bone Joint Surg Am* 2013;95(5):e28.
7. Noyes FR, Barber-Westin SD: Neuromuscular retraining intervention programs: Do they reduce noncontact anterior cruciate ligament injury rates in adolescent female athletes? *Arthroscopy* 2014;30(2):245-255.
8. Beynnon BD, Vacek PM, Newell MK, et al: The effects of level of competition, sport, and sex on the incidence of first-time noncontact anterior cruciate ligament injury. *Am J Sports Med* 2014;42(8):1806-1812.
9. Gornitzky AL, Lott A, Yellin JL, Fabricant PD, Lawrence JT, Ganley TJ: Sport-specific yearly risk and incidence of anterior cruciate ligament tears in high school athletes. *Am J Sports Med* 2016;44(1):2716-2723.

   The authors of this meta-analysis of the literature regarding ACL injury in high-school athletes concluded that females had a 1.57-fold greater rate of injury than males; female soccer players and male football players were at highest risk for ACL injury. Level of evidence: II.
10. Swart E, Redler L, Fabricant PD, Mandelbaum BR, Ahmad CS, Wang YC: Prevention and screening programs for anterior cruciate ligament injuries in young athletes: A cost-effectiveness analysis. *J Bone Joint Surg Am* 2014;96(9):705-711.
11. Kocher MS, Micheli LJ, Zurakowski D, Luke A: Partial tears of the anterior cruciate ligament in children and adolescents. *Am J Sports Med* 2002;30(5):697-703.
12. Busch MT, Fernandez MD, Aarons C: Partial tears of the anterior cruciate ligament in children and adolescents. *Clin Sports Med* 2011;30(4):743-750.
13. DiFelice GS, van der List JP: Clinical outcomes of arthroscopic primary repair of proximal anterior cruciate ligament tears are maintained at mid-term follow-up. *Arthroscopy* 2018;34(4):1085-1093.

    Ten patients with proximal ACL avulsion injuries treated with arthroscopic suture anchor repair were evaluated at 6 years postoperatively and found to have good motion, high self-reported outcome scores, clinically stable knees, and low rates of revision surgery. Level of evidence: IV.
14. Bioni M, Gaddi D, Gorla M, et al: Arthroscopic anterior cruciate ligament repair for proximal anterior cruciate ligament tears in skeletally immature patients: Surgical technique and preliminary results. *Knee* 2017;24(1):40-48.

    The authors of this retrospective review of five children (average age = 9.2 years, follow-up = 43.4 months) who underwent arthroscopic suture anchor repair of a proximal ACL avulsion reported 100% return to activity, high patient-reported International Knee Documentation Committee and Lysholm scores, and no iatrogenic physeal injury. Level of evidence: IV.
15. Ramski DE, Kanj WW, Franklin CC, Baldwin KD, Ganley TJ: Anterior cruciate ligament tears in children and adolescents: A meta-analysis of nonoperative versus operative treatment. *Am J Sports Med* 2014;42(11):2769-2776.
16. Lawrence JT, Argawal N, Ganley TJ: Degeneration of the knee joint in skeletally immature patients with a diagnosis of an anterior cruciate ligament tear: Is there harm in delay of treatment? *Am J Sports Med* 2011;39(12):2582-2587.
17. Dumont GD, Hogue GD, Padalecki JR, Okoro N, Wilson PL: Meniscal and chondral injuries associated with pediatric anterior cruciate ligament tears: Relationship of treatment time and patient-specific factors. *Am J Sports Med* 2012;40(9):2128-2133.
18. Anderson AF, Anderson CN: Correlation of meniscal and articular cartilage injuries in children and adolescents with timing of anterior cruciate ligament reconstruction. *Am J Sports Med* 2015;43(2):275-281.
19. Newman JT, Carry PM, Terhune EB, et al: Factors predictive of concomitant injuries among children and adolescents undergoing anterior cruciate ligament surgery. *Am J Sports Med* 2015;43(2):282-288.
20. Williams AA, Mancini NS, Solomito MJ, Nissen CW, Milewski MD: Chondral injuries and irreparable meniscal tears among adolescents with anterior cruciate ligament or meniscal tears are more common in patients with public insurance. *Am J Sports Med* 2017;45(9):2111-2115.

    The authors performed a retrospective review of pediatric patients undergoing ACL and/or meniscal surgery at their institution between 2013 and 2016 and analyzed the type and severity of injuries as a function of insurance type. Patients with public insurance were significantly more likely to experience a delay in presentation for care and to have more severe injuries of the cartilage and meniscus, $P < 0.05$. Level of evidence: III.

21. Frank JS, Gambacorta PL: Anterior cruciate ligament injuries in the skeletally immature athlete: Diagnosis and management. *J Am Acad Orthop Surg* 2013;21(2):78-87.

22. Kercher J, Xerogeanes J, Tannenbaum A, Al-Hakim R, Black JC, Zhao J: Anterior cruciate ligament reconstruction in the skeletally immature: An anatomical study utilizing 3-dimensional magnetic resonance imaging reconstructions. *J Pediatr Orthop* 2009;29(2):124-129.

23. Shea KG, Belzer J, Apel PJ, Nilsson K, Grimm NL, Pfeiffer RP: Volumetric injury of the physis during single-bundle anterior cruciate ligament reconstruction in children: A 3-dimensional study using magnetic resonance imaging. *Arthroscopy* 2009;25(12):1415-1422.

24. Kocher MS, Garg S, Micheli LJ: Physeal sparing reconstruction of the anterior cruciate ligament in skeletally immature prepubescent children and adolescents. *J Bone Joint Surg Am* 2005;87(11):2371-2379.

25. Kocher MS, Garg S, Micheli LJ: Physeal sparing reconstruction of the anterior cruciate ligament in skeletally immature prepubescent children and adolescents: Surgical technique. *J Bone Joint Surg Am* 2006;88(1 suppl 2):283-293.

26. Anderson AF: Transepiphyseal replacement of the anterior cruciate ligament using quadruple hamstring grafts in skeletally immature patients. *J Bone Joint Surg Am* 2004;86(1 suppl 2):201-209.

27. Nawabi DH, Jones KJ, Lurie B, Potter HG, Green DW, Cordasco FA: All-inside, physeal-sparing anterior cruciate ligament reconstruction does not significantly compromise the physis in skeletally immature athletes: A postoperative physeal magnetic resonance imaging analysis. *Am J Sports Med* 2014;42(12):2933-2940.

28. Kennedy A, Coughlin DG, Metzger MF, et al: Biomechanical evaluation of pediatric anterior cruciate ligament reconstruction techniques. *Am J Sports Med* 2011;39(5):964-971.

29. Sena M, Chen J, Dellamaggioria R, Coughlin DG, Lotz JC, Feeley BT: Dynamic evaluation of pivot-shift kinematics in physeal-sparing pediatric anterior cruciate ligament reconstruction techniques. *Am J Sports Med* 2013;41(4):826-834.

30. McCarthy MM, Tucker S, Nguyen JT, Green DW, Imhauser CW, Cordasco FA: Contact stress and kinematic analysis of all-epiphyseal and over-the-top pediatric reconstruction techniques for the anterior cruciate ligament. *Am J Sports Med* 2013;41(6):1330-1339.

31. Willimon SC, Jones CR, Herzog MM, May KH, Leake MJ, Busch MT: Micheli anterior cruciate ligament reconstruction in skeletally immature youths: A retrospective case series with a mean 3-year follow up. *Am J Sports Med* 2015;43(12):2974-2981.

32. Lawrence JT, Bowers AL, Belding J, Cody SR, Ganley TJ: All-epiphyseal anterior cruciate ligament reconstruction in skeletally immature patients. *Clin Orthop Relat Res* 2010;468(7):1971-1977.

33. Cruz AI, Fabricant PD, McGraw M, Rozell JC, Ganley TJ, Wells L: All-epiphyseal ACL reconstruction in children: Review of safety and early complications. *J Pediatr Orthop* 2017;37(3):204-209.

    The authors performed a retrospective analysis of 103 patients (mean age, 12.1 years) who had undergone physeal-sparing ACL reconstruction using all-epiphyseal bone tunnels between 2007 and 2013 and were followed up for a minimum of 6 months. Graft rupture was the most common complication (10.7%). Clinically significant growth disturbance and arthrofibrosis were less common (1% and 2% of the cohort, respectively). Contralateral ACL tear and ipsilateral meniscal tears were also reported, at rates of 2% and 3%. Level of evidence: IV.

34. Kocher MS, Heyworth BE, Fabricant PD, Tepolt FA, Micheli LJ: Outcomes of physeal-sparing ACL reconstruction with iliotibial band autograft in skeletally immature prepubescent children. *J Bone Joint Surg Am* 2018;100:1087-1094.

    These authors report on a single institution's clinical experience with physeal-sparing ACL reconstruction using iliotibial autograft over a 23-year period. About 237 prepubescent patients (mean age 11.2 years) were identified for study inclusion, representing 240 knees. Physical examination data were available for 225 of the 240 knees at average follow-up of 25 months; 96.8% had grade A Lachman testing and 98.8% were grade A on pivot-shift testing. Patient-reported outcomes were available for 137 (57%) of the knees at average follow-up of 6.2 years, which were excellent. Graft rupture rate was 6.6%. No significant growth disturbance was noted. Level of evidence: IV.

35. Pennock AT, Johnson KP, Turk RD, et al: Transphyseal anterior cruciate ligament reconstruction in the skeletally immature: Quadriceps tendon autograft versus hamstring tendon autograft. *Orthop J Sports Med* 2019;7(9). doi:10.1177/2325967119872450.

    The authors performed a retrospective review of 83 skeletally immature patients who underwent primary ACL reconstruction and were followed up for a minimum of 2 years. Twenty-seven patients had quadriceps tendon and 56 had hamstring tendon autografts used. When the groups were compared, there were no significant differences in patient-reported outcomes measures. However, the hamstring tendon grafts were significantly smaller than the quadriceps tendon grafts and patients with hamstring tendon were more likely to sustain a graft rupture ($P < 0.05$). Level of evidence: III.

36. Engelman GH, Carry PM, Hitt KG, Polousky JD, Vidal AF: Comparison of allograft versus autograft anterior cruciate ligament reconstruction graft survival in an active adolescent cohort. *Am J Sports Med* 2014;42(10):2311-2318.

37. Kocher MS, Smith JT, Zoric BJ, Lee B, Micheli LJ: Transphyseal anterior cruciate ligament reconstruction in skeletally immature pubescent adolescents. *J Bone Joint Surg Am* 2007;89(12):2632-2639.

38. Kumar S, Ahearne D, Hunt DM: Transphyseal anterior cruciate ligament reconstruction in the skeletally immature: Follow-up to a minimum of sixteen years of age. *J Bone Joint Surg Am* 2013;95(1):e1.

39. Calvo R, Figueroa D, Gili F, et al: Transphyseal anterior cruciate ligament reconstruction in patients with open physes: 10-year follow-up study. *Am J Sports Med* 2015;43(2):289-294.

40. Hui C, Roe J, Ferguson D, Waller A, Salmon L, Pinczewski L: Outcome of anatomic transphyseal anterior cruciate ligament reconstruction in Tanner stage 1 and 2 patients with open physes. *Am J Sports Med* 2012;40(5):1093-1098.

41. Boyle MJ, Butler RJ, Queen RM: Functional movement competency and dynamic balance after anterior cruciate ligament reconstruction in adolescent patients. *J Pediatr Orthop* 2016;36(1):36-41.

    This retrospective cohort study compared skeletally immature adolescents, skeletally mature adolescents, and adult patients who had undergone ACL reconstruction. At 9 months after surgery, all groups had deficits on functional movement screening, with unique deficits in the adolescent cohorts. Level of evidence: IV.

42. McPherson AL, Feller JA, Hewett TE, Webster KE: Smaller change in psychological readiness to return to sport is associated with second anterior cruciate ligament injury among younger patients. *Am J Sports Med* 2019;47(5):1209-1215.

    The authors analyzed the psychological readiness of 115 patients younger than 20 years who had undergone ACL reconstruction and subsequently returned to sport using the ACL–Return to Sport after Injury scale. Young athletes who reported more fear and demonstrated smaller improvements in their psychological readiness were significantly more likely to sustain a second ACL injury, $P < 0.05$. Level of evidence: II.

43. Christino MA, Fleming BC, Machan JT, Shalvoy RM: Psychological factors associated with anterior cruciate ligament reconstruction recovery. *Orthop J Sports Med* 2016;4(3). doi:10.1177/2325967116638341.

    In this study of 27 young adult patients following ACL reconstruction, the authors note that psychological factors including self-esteem and an internal locus of control were significantly associated with surgical outcomes including return-to-sport rates and patient-reported measures including the International Knee Documentation Committee, 36-Item Short Form, and Knee injury and Osteoarthritis Outcome Score–Quality of Life subscale. Level of evidence: III.

44. Nwachukwu BU, McFeely ED, Nasreddine A, et al: Arthrofibrosis after anterior cruciate ligament reconstruction in children and adolescents. *J Pediatr Orthop* 2011;31(8):811-817.

45. Shifflett GD, Green DW, Widmann RF, Marx RG: Growth arrest following ACL reconstruction with hamstring autograft in skeletally immature patients: A review of 4 cases. *J Pediatr Orthop* 2016;36(4):355-361.

    The authors of this retrospective case series detailed the evaluation, treatment, and clinical outcomes of four skeletally immature patients (average age = 14.2 years) in whom growth disturbance occurred (recurvatum, genu valgum) after transphyseal ACL reconstruction. Level of evidence: IV.

46. Yoo WJ, Kocher MS, Micheli LJ: Growth plate disturbance after transphyseal reconstruction of the anterior cruciate ligament in skeletally immature adolescent patients: An MR imaging study. *J Pediatr Orthop* 2011;31(6):691-696.

47. Paterno MV, Rauh MJ, Schmitt LC, Ford KR, Hewett TE: Incidence of second ACL injuries 2 years after primary ACL reconstruction and return to sport. *Am J Sports Med* 2014;42(7):1567-1573.

48. Webster KE, Feller JA, Leigh WB, Richmond AK: Younger patients are at increased risk for graft rupture and contralateral injury after anterior cruciate ligament reconstruction. *Am J Sports Med* 2014;42(3):641-647.

49. Dekker TJ, Godin JA, Dale KM, Garrett WE, Taylor DC, Riboh JC: Return to sport after pediatric anterior cruciate ligament reconstruction and its effect on subsequent anterior cruciate ligament injury. *J Bone Joint Surg Am* 2017;99:987-904.

    The authors analyzed a continuous cohort of patients <18 years who underwent primary ACL reconstruction with autograft and were followed up for a minimum of 2 years. Of the 112 patients, 85 eligible patients with average age of 13.9 years were included in final analysis. Return-to-sport rate was 91%, with 84% returning to same sport. Rate of a second ACL injury was 32% (19% with graft tear, 13% with contralateral ACL tear). Timing of return to sport was only significant predictor of second injury, with slower return being protective, $P < 0.05$. Level of evidence: IV.

50. Wiggins AJ, Grandhi RK, Schneider DK, Stanfield D, Webster KE, Myer GD: Risk of secondary injury in younger athletes after anterior cruciate ligament reconstruction: A systematic review and meta-analysis. *Am J Sports Med* 2016;44(7):1861-1876.

    The authors of this systematic review found the rate of secondary ACL injury was 15% for patients who had undergone ACL reconstruction. Factors that increased the risk of reinjury included young age (<25 years) and return to sport (combined risk, 23%). Level of evidence: II.

51. Christino MA, Tepolt FA, Sugimoto D, Micheli LJ, Kocher MS: Revision ACL reconstruction in children and adolescents. *J Pediatr Orthop* 2020;40(3):129-134. doi:10.1097/BPO.0000000000001155.

    This retrospective case series reports on a single-institution experience with ACL revision reconstruction over a 16-year period. Ninety knees were included in analysis, with average patient age of 16.6 years, 28.8% of whom had open physes, and an average time to failure of 1.28 years. Patients who underwent revision reconstruction had a 20% graft reinjury rate and 25% required additional surgical procedures. Additionally, 20% sustained contralateral ACL injuries. Only 55% of patients reported the ability to return to sport at the preinjury level. Level of evidence: IV.

52. Ouillette R, Edmonds E, Chambers H, Bastrom T, Pennock A: Outcomes of revision anterior cruciate ligament surgery in adolescents. *Am J Sports Med* 2019;47(6):1346-1352.

    The authors performed a retrospective review of pediatric patients undergoing revision ACL reconstruction between 2009 and 2017 and followed up for a minimum of 2 years. Patient outcomes were compared with those who had undergone primary reconstruction. Sixty eligible knees were identified, 48 of whom (84%) were included in final analysis.

Compared with patients undergoing primary ACL surgery, those undergoing revision had more concomitant injuries, lower patient-reported scores, lower return-to-sport rates, and higher rates of graft failure ($P < 0.05$). Level of evidence: IV.

53. Murray MM, Kalish LA, Fleming BC, et al: Bridge-enhanced anterior cruciate ligament repair: Two-year results of a first-in-human study. *Orthop J Sports Med* 2019;7(3). doi:10.1177/2325967118824356.

    The authors report on the early clinical outcomes of 10 patients who underwent the bridge-enhanced anterior cruciate ligament repair procedure compared with a control group of 10 patients who underwent standard ACL reconstruction with quadrupled autograft hamstring tendon. There were no failures in the first 24 months postoperative for either group; there were no differences in clinical outcomes scores, laxity, or hop testing. Bridge-enhanced anterior cruciate ligament repair patients had significantly greater hamstring strength. Level of evidence: II.

54. Johnson AC, Wyatt JD, Treme G, Veitch AJ: Incidence of associated knee injury in pediatric tibial eminence fractures. *J Knee Surg* 2014;27(3):215-219.
55. Anderson CN, Anderson AF: Tibial eminence fractures. *Clin Sports Med* 2011;30(4):727-742.
56. Herman MJ, Martinek MA, Abzug JM: Complications of tibial eminence and diaphyseal fractures in children: Prevention and treatment. *J Am Acad Orthop Surg* 2014;22(11):730-741.
57. Shea KG, Grimm NL, Laor T, Wall E: Bone bruises and meniscal tears on MRI in skeletally immature children with tibial eminence fractures. *J Pediatr Orthop* 2011;31(2):150-152.
58. Kocher MS, Micheli LJ, Gerbino P, Hresko MT: Tibial eminence fractures in children: Prevalence of meniscal entrapment. *Am J Sports Med* 2003;31(3):404-407.
59. Mitchell JJ, Sjostrom R, Mansour AA, et al: Incidence of meniscal injury and chondral pathology in anterior tibial spine fractures of children. *J Pediatr Orthop* 2015;35(2):130-135.
60. Archibald-Seiffer N, Jacobs J Jr, Zbojniewicz A, Shea K: Incarceration of the intermeniscal ligament in tibial eminence injury: A block to closed reduction identified using MRI. *Skeletal Radiol* 2015;44(5):717-721.
61. Shin YW, Uppstrom TJ, Haskel JD, Green DW: The tibial eminence fracture in skeletally immature patients. *Curr Opin Pediatr* 2015;27(1):50-57.
62. Edmonds EW, Fornari ED, Dashe J, Roocroft JH, King MM, Pennock AT: Results of displaced pediatric tibial spine fractures: A comparison between open, arthroscopic, and closed management. *J Pediatr Orthop* 2015;35(7):651-656.
63. Watts CD, Larson AN, Milbrandt TA: Open versus arthroscopic reduction for tibial eminence fracture fixation in children. *J Pediatr Orthop* 2016;36(5):437-439.

    This retrospective chart review of 31 patients treated surgically for displaced tibial eminence fractures demonstrated that a delay in time to surgery (>7 days from injury) and longer surgical times (>120 minutes) were associated with higher rates of postoperative arthrofibrosis. Level of evidence: III.

64. Gans I, Baldwin KD, Ganley TJ: Treatment and management outcomes of tibial eminence fractures in pediatric patients. *Am J Sports Med* 2014;42(7):1743-1750.
65. Eggers AK, Becker C, Weimann A, et al: Biomechanical evaluation of different fixation methods for tibial eminence fractures. *Am J Sports Med* 2007;35(3):404-410.
66. Bong MR, Romero A, Kubiak E, et al: Suture versus screw fixation of displaced tibial eminence fractures: A biomechanical comparison. *Arthroscopy* 2005;21(10):1172-1176.
67. Mahar AT, Duncan D, Oka R, Lowry A, Gillingham B, Chambers H: Biomechanical comparison of four different fixation techniques for pediatric tibial eminence avulsion fractures. *J Pediatr Orthop* 2008;28(2):159-162.
68. Anderson CN, Nyman JS, McCullough KA, et al: Biomechanical evaluation of physeal-sparing fixation methods in tibial eminence fractures. *Am J Sports Med* 2013;41(7):1586-1594.
69. Vander Have KL, Ganley TJ, Kocher MS, Price CT, Herrera-Soto JA: Arthrofibrosis after surgical fixation of tibial eminence fractures in children and adolescents. *Am J Sports Med* 2010;38(2):298-301.
70. Patel NM, Park MJ, Sampson NR, Ganley TJ: Tibial eminence fractures in children: Earlier posttreatment mobilization results in improved outcomes. *J Pediatr Orthop* 2012;32(2):139-144.
71. Mitchell JJ, Mayo MH, Axibal DP, et al: Delayed anterior cruciate ligament reconstruction in young patients with previous anterior tibial spine fractures. *Am J Sports Med* 2016;44(8):2047-2056.

    The authors of this retrospective case series investigated the rate of subsequent ACL injury and surgery for 101 pediatric patients who had previously sustained a tibial spine fracture and were followed up for a minimum of 2 years. Nineteen percent of patients with a previous tibial spine fracture sustained an ipsilateral ACL injury requiring ACL reconstruction. The odds ratio for ACL reconstruction increased with age, by a factor of 1.3 per annum. Level of evidence: IV.

CHAPTER 49

Meniscal Tears in Children and Adolescents

MELINDA S. SHARKEY, MD • CORDELIA W. CARTER, MD

ABSTRACT

The diagnosis and management of pediatric and adolescent meniscal injury is an evolving area of pediatric sports medicine practice. A growing body of literature is contributing to an evidence base for informing treatment decisions for different types of traumatic meniscal tears as well as the symptomatic discoid meniscus.

Keywords: discoid meniscus; meniscus injury; meniscus surgery; pediatric meniscus

INTRODUCTION

Meniscal tear rates are increasing in children and adolescents, partly because of increasing participation in organized sports and partly because of increased recognition of these injuries.[1,2] The menisci perform the critical functions of load distribution across the knee joint, shock absorption, and proprioception and also contribute to knee stability.[1-3] At birth, the menisci are completely vascularized and composed of cells with a large cytoplasm to nucleus ratio. By 10 years of age, the menisci have adultlike characteristics, with only the peripheral one-third of the meniscus having a direct blood supply and the tissue largely composed of collagen fibers arranged circumferentially.[1-3]

Dr. Sharkey or an immediate family member serves as a board member, owner, officer, or committee member of the Pediatric Orthopaedic Society of North America. Dr. Carter or an immediate family member serves as a board member, owner, officer, or committee member of the American Academy of Orthopaedic Surgeons and the Pediatric Orthopaedic Society of North America.

TRAUMATIC MENISCAL TEARS

Evaluation

Most meniscal tears result from a noncontact, twisting injury that is frequently related to a sports activity. On presentation, patients generally report pain and may note mechanical symptoms, such as locking, catching, and giving way. Physical examination may show knee effusion and joint line tenderness. If tolerated, meniscal compression tests may elicit pain. Because of the common association of meniscal tears with ligamentous injuries, an examination for knee stability is important. Plain radiographs of the knee should be obtained to evaluate for fractures, loose bodies, and osteochondritis dissecans lesions; however, results will often be negative in a patient with a meniscus injury. MRI is the study of choice (**Figure 1**). A 2015 study reported that MRI had high diagnostic accuracy for assessing knee disorders in children and adolescents, although lateral meniscus tears were one of the most frequently missed pathologies on MRI (18.8%) that were later identified at the time of arthroscopy.[4]

In addition to the known association between tears of the anterior cruciate ligament and the menisci, two reports have described a similarly high rate of meniscal injury in the setting of tibial eminence fractures in children.[5,6] The authors of a 2015 study found an overall 21% meniscal tear rate, with a 33% tear rate in children with type II tibial spine fractures.[5] A 2011 study reported a 40% rate of meniscal tears in 20 children with tibial spine fractures.[6]

The authors of a 2018 study highlighted the potential for a greater prevalence of meniscal root tears than previously reported[7] (**Figure 2**). Of 314 knee scopes performed for meniscal injury with and without ligamentous injury in patients with a mean age of 16 years, a total of 18.5% or 58/314 knees demonstrated a complete posterior meniscal root tear, most associated with concomitant anterior cruciate ligament injury. Because meniscal root

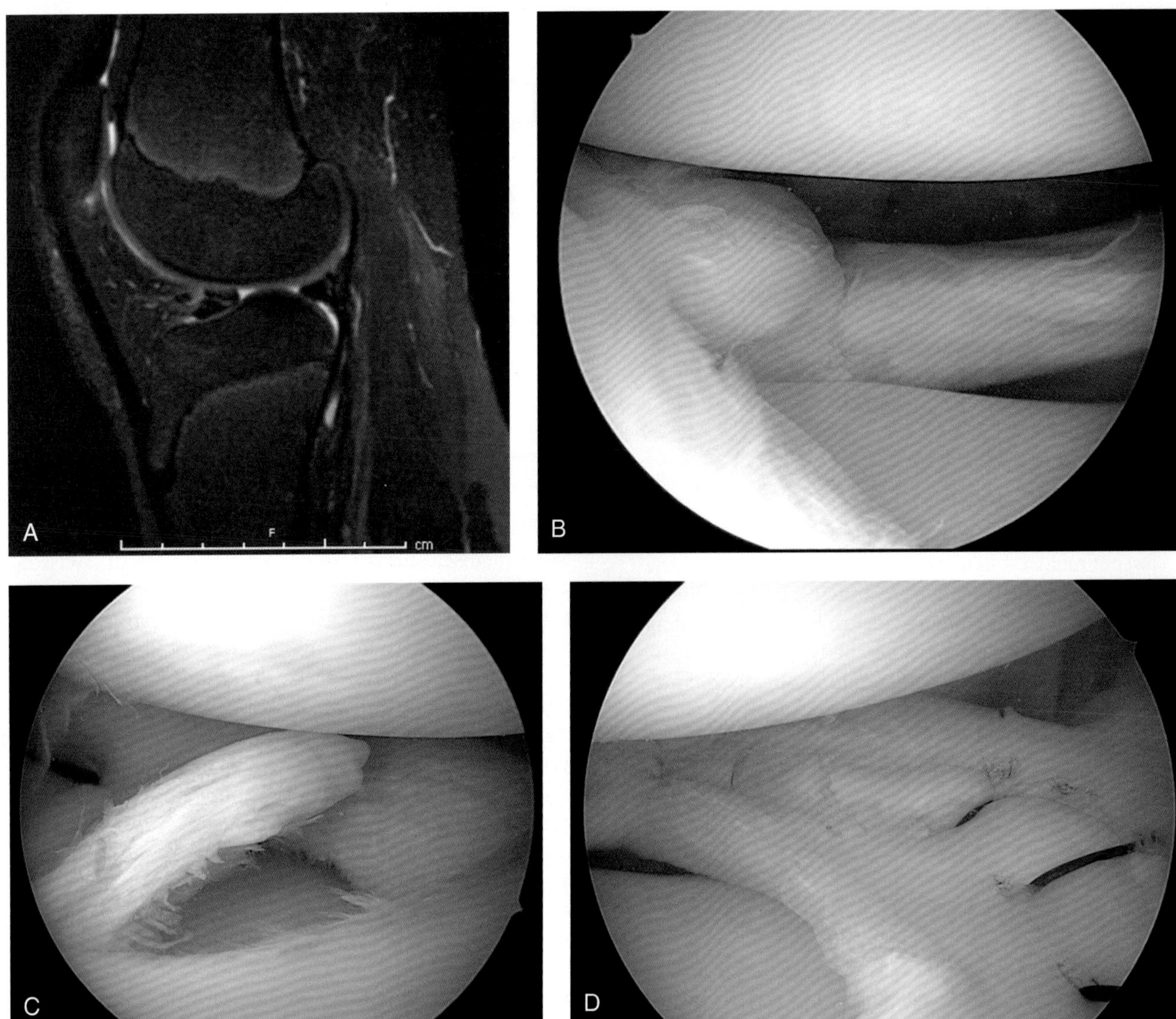

FIGURE 1 **A**, Sagittal T2-weighted magnetic resonance image of the knee of a 13-year-old girl shows an anteriorly displaced bucket-handle tear of the posterior horn of the lateral meniscus. Arthroscopic images show the displaced tear (**B**), reduction of the tear (**C**), and final meniscal repair (**D**).

tears have been shown to be biomechanically equivalent to total meniscal loss, it is important surgeons recognize and are prepared to manage these tears.

Management

Some pediatric meniscal tears, such as partial thickness tears comprising less than 50% of the total meniscal thickness, may be suitable for nonsurgical management. An attempt at nonsurgical treatment also may be made for patients with small (<1 cm), stable, longitudinal tears in the peripheral red-red zone. These tears are generally found at the time of diagnostic arthroscopy in the setting of ligamentous injury. Most symptomatic meniscal tears require surgical management (**Figure 1**). Management includes arthroscopic evaluation of the knee and débridement and/or repair of the meniscal tear or tears.

If surgery is indicated, an attempt should be made to repair meniscal tears in pediatric patients whenever possible. Tear patterns that are generally considered amenable to repair are similar in children and adults and include longitudinal, vertical, and bucket-handle tear morphologies. Attempts are typically made to repair radial tears, especially if the tear extends to the periphery of the meniscus. Oblique and horizontal tear configurations are less amenable to repair. Meniscal tears that are complex in nature, with extensive tissue maceration or degeneration, may be irreparable.

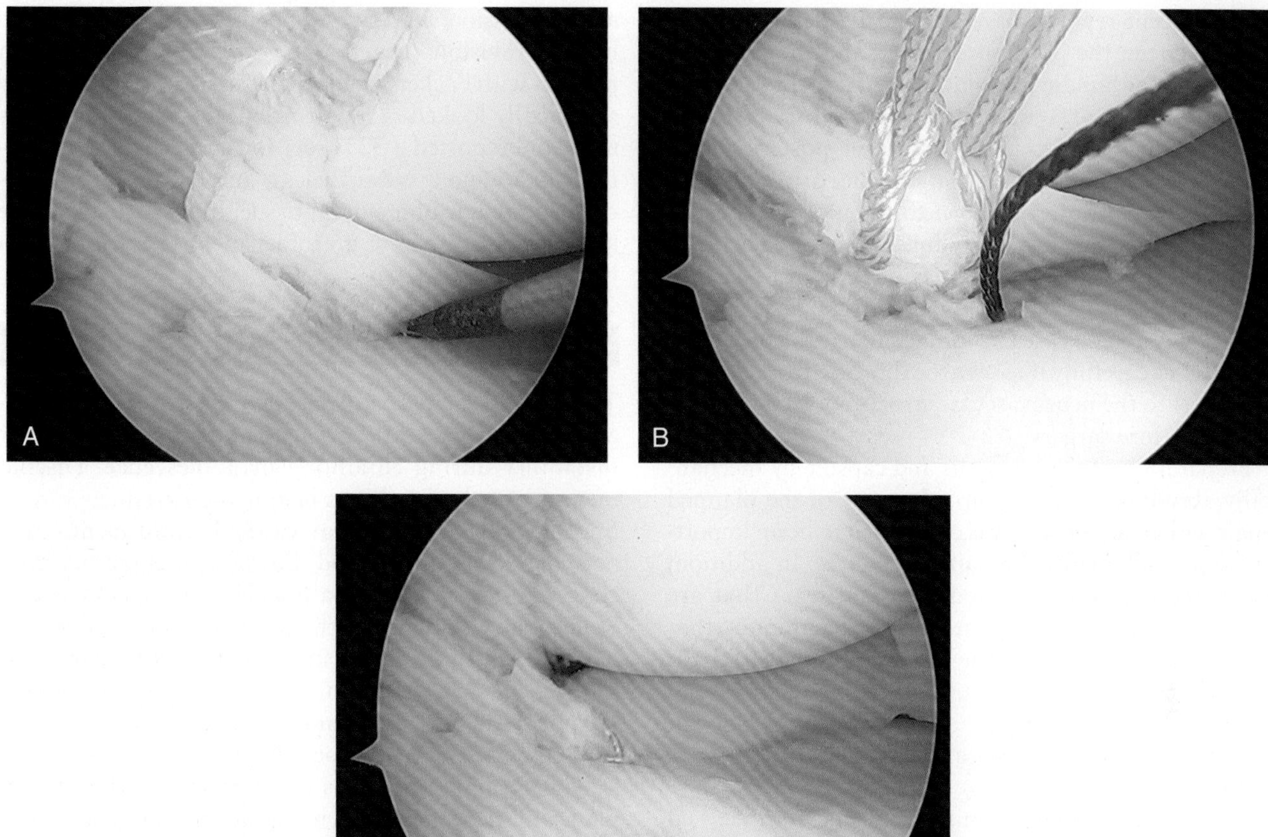

FIGURE 2 Arthroscopic image demonstrating a **(A)** complete meniscal root tear of the medial meniscus in a child with a congenital anterior cruciate ligament deficiency. **B**, Appearance of tear after sutures have been placed through meniscal root and before being shuttled through a tibial tunnel and tied over a button on the anterior tibia. **C**, Arthroscopic image of final repair.

As in adults, tears in the peripheral red-red zone in children are considered most likely to heal because of the robust blood supply. Surgical repair of tears in the more central zones of the meniscus, especially in younger children, may be attempted because of the perceived potential for healing in children and the known importance of an intact meniscus for long-term knee health.

Tears that are deemed irreparable by virtue of poor tissue quality, poor vascular supply, or some combination of factors are best treated by partial meniscectomy, which may be performed using a combination of meniscal biters and/or punches and a small arthroscopic shaver. In this situation, the objective is to leave as much stable meniscal tissue as possible, with the goal of minimizing both the risk of recurrent meniscal tearing and that of future arthritic degeneration.

Meniscal allograft transplant is being performed as a salvage option for children and adolescents with symptomatic meniscus-deficient knees. Short-term and midterm outcomes of these procedures are being reported in small series of patients and show improvements in patient-reported knee function.[8,9]

Viable methods of meniscal repair include all-inside, inside-out, and outside-in techniques, with the choice of technique depending on the location and morphology of the tear, the size of the patient, and the preference and comfort of the surgeon. Hybrid repairs, which include a combination of repair techniques, also may be performed. Typically, anterior horn tears are repaired in an outside-in fashion with monofilament suture. Tears of the body and posterior horn may be repaired with an all-inside fixation system or an inside-out technique with the sutures tied just outside the joint capsule. It is generally recommended to avoid an all-inside repair technique in younger children because the smaller distances from the meniscal anchors placed through the joint capsule and the popliteus neurovascular bundle may put the bundle at increased risk for direct injury.

Two recent reports more specifically define the distance between the posterior menisci and the popliteus neurovascular bundle in children aged 2 to 18 years.[10,11] Both studies, a cadaver study and an MRI study, found the popliteus artery to be closest to the posterior horn of the lateral meniscus and that distances from various locations at the posterior horn to the artery increased with increasing age in a fairly linear fashion. The measurements from these studies may be fairly conservative because these were all performed with the knees in full extension. Surgeons are encouraged to use the preoperative MRI to carefully measure the distance from the tear of interest to the neurovascular structures on individual patients before surgery.

Preparation of the meniscus and capsule by mechanically abrading the tissue on either side of the planned repair with a rasp or shaver is considered to be an important step in all meniscal repair procedures. In addition, young patients with isolated meniscal tears that are chronic in nature may benefit from techniques that are intended to optimize the vascularity of the repair. Trephination, injection of autologous blood clots, and microfracture of the notch at the level of the posterior cruciate ligament have all been described for this purpose.[1]

A 2013 study reported on the frequency of meniscal tear patterns in relation to skeletal maturity.[3] In 293 patients aged 10 to 19 years who underwent arthroscopy for a meniscal injury, 67% of the tears involved the lateral meniscus, 22% involved the medial meniscus, and 11% involved both menisci. The most frequent tear patterns were complex (28%), vertical (16%), discoid (14%), and bucket-handle (14%).

Outcomes

Two recent articles highlight the lack of high-quality outcome studies for pediatric and adolescent meniscus surgery.[12,13] After reviewing thousands of articles on meniscus tears, one group found that high-quality data do not exist on the natural history of untreated meniscus tears nor whether management of meniscus tears alters the natural history of knee function and health.[12] The other group found meniscal outcomes studies in pediatric patients undergoing surgery that met the criteria, but all studies were at best case series with no comparative studies and no consistent preoperative and postoperative patient-reported outcomes.[13]

Single-center series of pediatric and adolescent patients undergoing meniscus surgery generally show favorable outcomes and return to activity, although revision surgery rates for meniscal repair is higher than for partial meniscectomy.[14-16] General revision surgery rates after meniscal repair range from 4% to 18%, with the most recent and largest series (907 patients) reporting a 13% revision surgery rate for meniscal repairs.[14] The highest revision surgery rates are generally noted in patients with bucket-handle meniscus tears. A 2019 study specifically looked at repair of bucket-handle meniscus tears and reported a 32% revision surgery rate at short-term follow-up.[17] Nevertheless, authors uniformly recommend repair of meniscal tissue, if possible, given the known importance of an intact menisci for long-term joint health.

DISCOID MENISCUS

The discoid meniscus is an uncommon meniscal variant that may present with symptomatic tearing and/or instability during childhood or adolescence. Discoid menisci are almost always lateral and extremely rare to find medially. The etiology of the discoid meniscus is not completely understood; however, it is considered a congenital anomaly with a possible genetic component. Studies have shown that the normal meniscus does not have a discoid precursor. Estimates of incidence vary, with a lower incidence (0.4% to 5.2%) in those of Western European descent and a much higher incidence (up to 17%) reported in Asian countries.[2,18,19]

The normal meniscus is wedge shaped in the coronal plane and crescent shaped in the axial plane. The central area of a discoid meniscus, however, is partially or completely filled in and may lack normal attachments to the surrounding capsule, distal femur, and proximal tibia. In addition to an anomalous discoid shape, the thickness of the meniscus may be abnormally increased, resulting in a block of abnormal tissue (**Figure 3**). This variation may be responsible, at least in part, for the pathognomonic snapping of the knee because it is brought passively into flexion and extension. Increased meniscal thickness is one of the most difficult problems to correct surgically.[2,18,19]

Although the abnormal macromorphology of a discoid meniscus is generally the most striking feature, investigation into the histopathology of the discoid meniscus shows a disorganization of the circumferential collagen network at a molecular level. These structural abnormalities compromise the ability of the discoid meniscus to withstand normal stresses across the knee and predispose it to tears. The mechanical dysfunction of the discoid meniscus is further demonstrated by its association with the relatively rare lateral femoral condyle osteochondritis dissecans lesion.

The traditional Watanabe classification system consists of three types of discoid meniscus variants: type I, complete discoid shape; type II, incomplete discoid shape; and type III, Wrisberg variant. The Wrisberg variant is described as a more normally shaped meniscus, but it lacks normal peripheral attachments (except the ligament of Wrisberg).[1,18,19] A contemporary classification

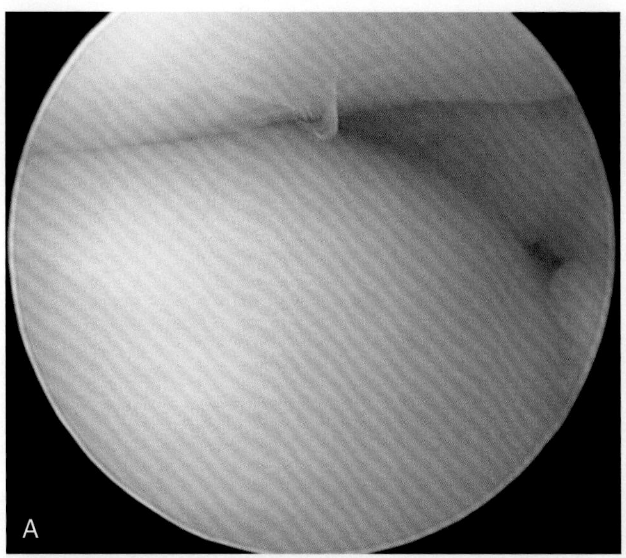

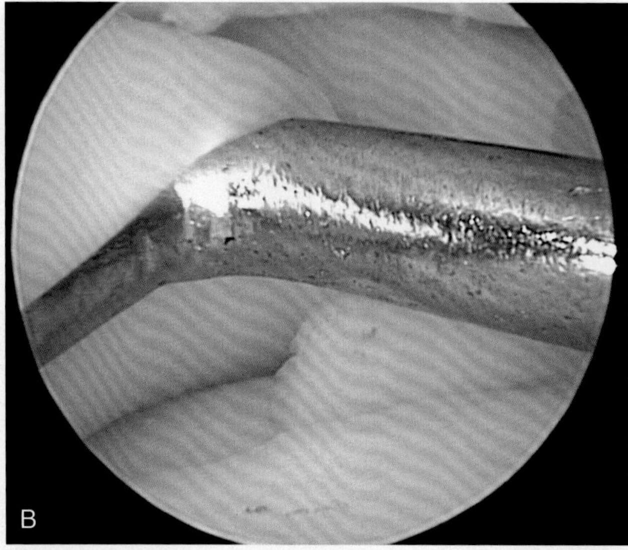

FIGURE 3 Arthroscopic images show a complete blocklike discoid lateral meniscus in a 4-year-old boy. **A**, Native appearance of the discoid meniscus, with complete obstruction of the lateral tibial plateau. **B**, The arthroscopic probe is displacing the meniscus superiorly, revealing the tibial plateau beneath.

system, which may be more clinically and surgically relevant, incorporates peripheral stability patterns.[18] Discoid menisci may be classified as complete or incomplete; stable or unstable, based on the presence or absence of peripheral attachments; and intact or torn, based on the presence or absence of a meniscal tear.[20] Peripheral instability may be present at any location along the meniscal margin and may be an important, although less obvious, contributing factor to symptomatology in the setting of a discoid meniscus.

Evaluation

Presenting symptoms in patients with a symptomatic discoid meniscus can include palpable and/or audible snapping, locking, pain, limited extension, quadriceps atrophy, giving way, effusion, and/or the inability to bear weight. Younger children tend to present with symptoms related to limited knee range of motion,[21] and a young child with a new onset flexion contracture should be assumed to have a torn discoid meniscus until proven otherwise. Older children tend to present more acutely with symptoms related to an acute tear through the abnormal meniscal tissue. In fact, children with isolated and symptomatic lateral meniscus pathology are commonly found to have a discoid meniscus. A recent study reported that of 261 knee arthroscopies performed for isolated lateral meniscus pathology in children, 97% of children younger than 13 years had a discoid meniscus and 59% of those aged 14 to 16 years had a discoid meniscus.[21]

The physical examination may demonstrate lateral joint line tenderness, possible snapping of the knee with flexion and extension, pain with meniscal compression tests (McMurray, Apley, and Thessaly tests), limited motion, and/or effusion. New or asymmetric flexion contracture of the knee in a young patient may indicate a torn and/or displaced discoid lateral meniscus.

Radiographs of the knee with a discoid lateral meniscus may show subtle differences compared with a nondiscoid knee. A recent comparison of radiographs of the knees of children with symptomatic discoid lateral menisci with those of age-matched control subjects found differences in the mean height of the lateral tibial spine, the lateral joint space distance, the height of the fibular head, and the obliquity of the lateral tibial plateau.[22]

MRI remains the modality of choice for making the diagnosis of a discoid meniscus (**Figure 4**). In a recent study, the performance of MRI and preoperative physical examination findings in the diagnosis of intra-articular pathology of the knee in children and adolescents was evaluated.[4] The overall diagnostic accuracy was 92.7% for MRI and 95.3% for preoperative clinical examination. Despite this accuracy, the most common pathology missed on MRI but found at the time of diagnostic arthroscopy was the presence of a discoid lateral meniscus (26.7% of cases).[19] Incomplete and Wrisberg variant discoid menisci may be particularly likely to be missed on MRI. A 2017 study found that MRI criteria for discoid meniscus (three or more contiguous 5 mm sagittal cuts showing continuity between anterior and posterior horn or the meniscus extending past the midline of the lateral compartment on the coronal cuts) were unreliable after age 13 years, but more accurate in younger children.[21]

A 2018 study reported on the ability of the preoperative history, physical examination, and MRI to predict

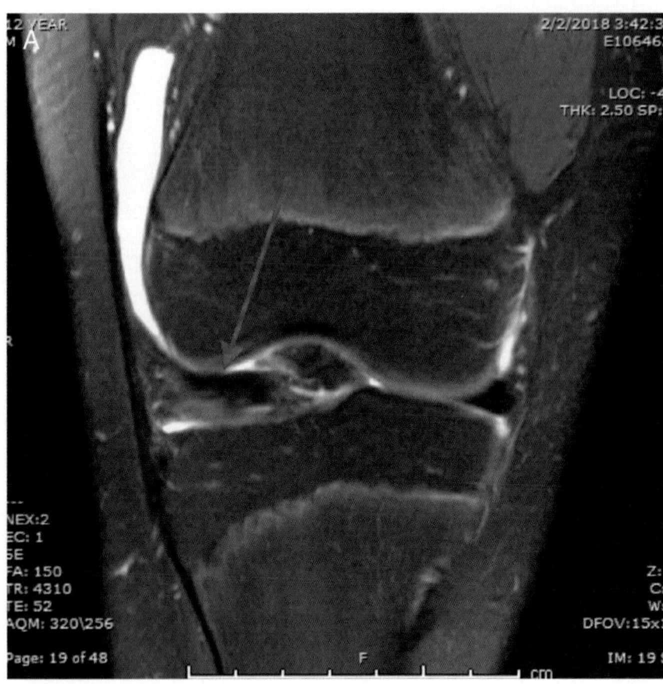

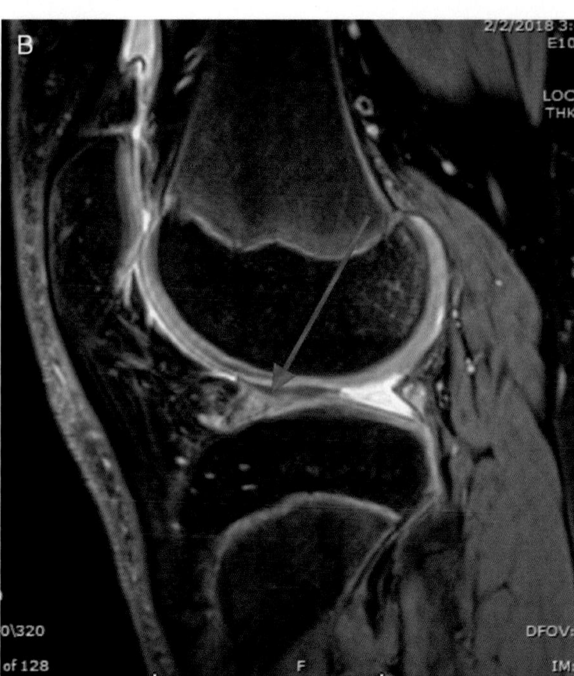

FIGURE 4 Coronal (**A**) and sagittal (**B**) magnetic resonance images show a torn, displaced discoid lateral meniscus in a symptomatic 12-year-old girl.

concomitant articular cartilage lesions in patients having a symptomatic discoid meniscus as associated articular cartilage injuries because these injuries may portend poorer outcomes.[23] Of 34 patients studied, 14 had associated chondral injury and the presence of symptoms for more than 6 months and an extension block were the most sensitive and specific for predicting these injuries.

Treatment

Surgical treatment may be beneficial for young patients with symptoms related to a discoid meniscus (pain, effusion, limited range of motion, mechanical symptoms, and associated activity restrictions). Surgical treatment of a symptomatic discoid meniscus has evolved over time. Previously, complete or subtotal meniscectomy was performed for a symptomatic discoid meniscus. Variable long-term outcomes have been reported for total meniscectomy, with some studies showing excellent results with no evidence of degenerative changes and other studies demonstrating poor function, osteoarthritis, pain, instability, and even the development of osteochondritis dissecans lesions associated with the discoid lateral meniscus.[18]

Currently, surgical treatment includes arthroscopic saucerization of the symptomatic discoid meniscus, with the goal of leaving a peripheral rim with a width of approximately 6 to 8 mm. Saucerization includes removal of abnormal, redundant central meniscal tissue, until normal morphology is achieved. Debulking an abnormally thick discoid lateral meniscus may be particularly difficult. After partial meniscectomy is completed, the remaining tissue is inspected for tearing and/or peripheral instability. Meniscal tears are repaired using the techniques described previously. Unstable menisci are stabilized by suturing them to the adjacent capsule (**Figure 5**). Menisci that have extensive complex tearing and tissue maceration may not be candidates for these techniques; patients with this type of unsalvageable meniscal tearing commonly undergo subtotal meniscectomy.

A 2016 study warns of an easily missed bucket-handle–like tear pattern that can be seen in discoid menisci: the inverted discoid meniscus segment.[24] A total of 19/121 retrospectively reviewed surgeries for symptomatic discoid meniscus showed this tear pattern, which the authors note can be missed because the tear occurs more centrally in the discoid meniscus and leaves more meniscal rim.

Outcomes

Short-term and midterm outcomes have been reported for contemporary management of the discoid meniscus, and the results have generally been good, whether peripheral rim instability was present and needed to be managed.[25,26]

Few long-term outcome studies of arthroscopic saucerization exist, and the surgical management methods used are variable. One long-term outcome study (8- to 14-year

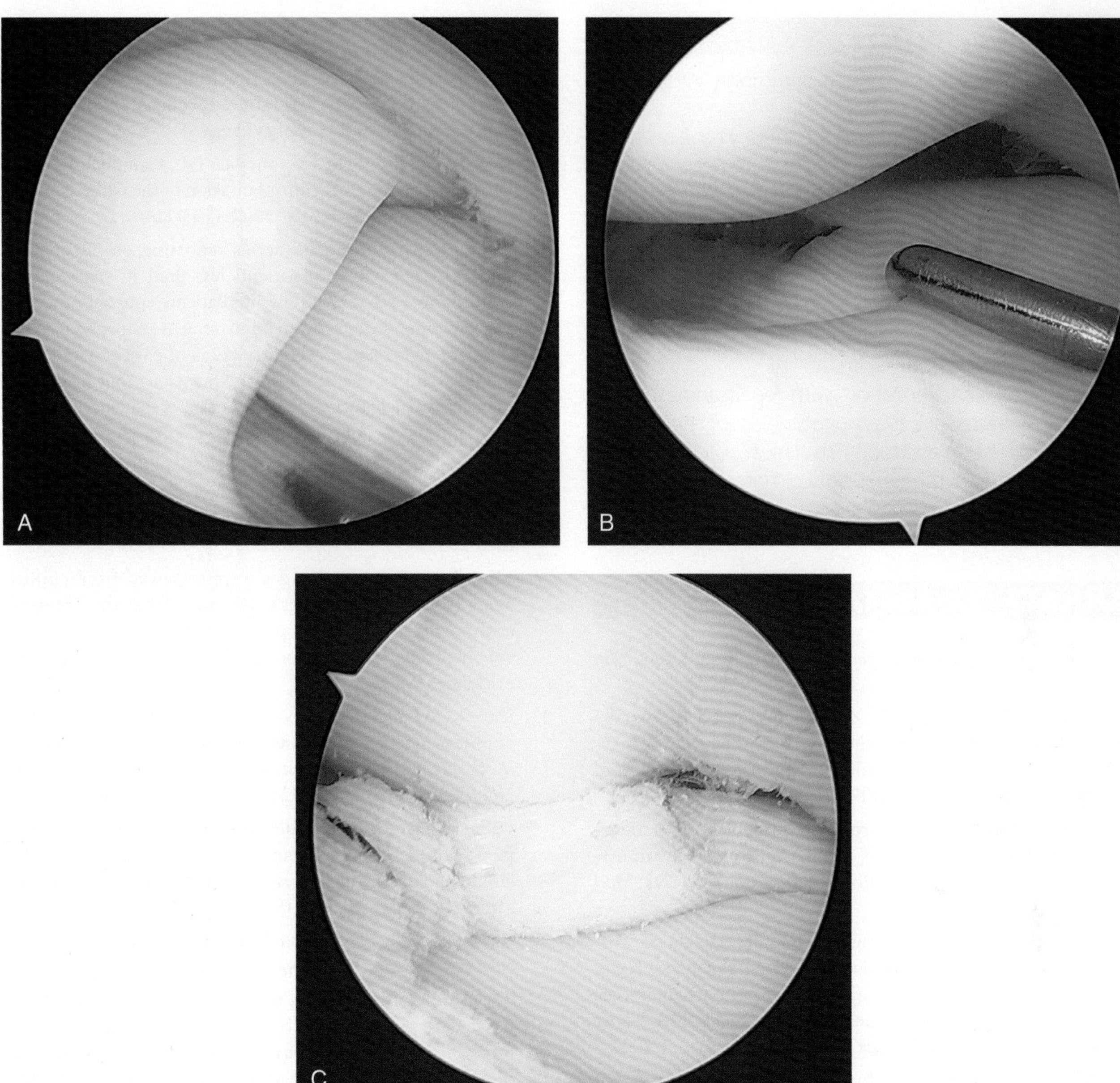

FIGURE 5 Arthroscopic images showing the (**A**) initial view and (**B**) complex tear of a complete and unstable discoid meniscus. **C**, Arthroscopic image after saucerization and repair of meniscal tear and stabilization of meniscus to capsule.

follow-up) described patient-reported function and radiographic changes after arthroscopic reshaping of a discoid meniscus.[27] A total of 48 knees in 38 children (mean age, 9.9 years) were included. Whether treated with partial meniscectomy or some type of repair or subtotal meniscectomy, 94% of knees were rated as good or excellent despite significant degenerative changes on radiographs, particularly in meniscectomy group. However, two other recent studies report that clinical outcomes deteriorate after surgical management of discoid menisci because patients are followed up for longer periods.[28,29] These studies highlight the need for management of discoid menisci to continue to evolve and improve.

SUMMARY

As increasing numbers of young children and adolescents participate in organized sports, meniscal injury rates have continued to increase. A growing body of literature is informing the evaluation and treatment of these injuries in children and adolescents, although higher evidence level comparative studies are not yet available. Short-term and midterm outcomes are generally quite good for young patients with meniscal pathology that is treated using contemporary surgical methods, although retearing of the meniscus requiring additional surgical procedures remains a concern.

KEY STUDY POINTS

- The lateral meniscus is most commonly injured in children and adolescents.
- Skeletally immature patients frequently have an isolated meniscal injury; skeletally mature patients are more likely to sustain meniscal injury in the setting of a ligamentous injury of the knee.
- Bucket-handle meniscal tears have the highest rates of surgical revision after meniscal repair.
- In addition to anomalous macromorphology and microarchitecture, discoid lateral menisci commonly demonstrate peripheral instability.
- Arthroscopic saucerization, with repair and stabilization as necessary, is a procedure associated with good short-term and midterm clinical outcomes for patients with a symptomatic discoid lateral meniscus.

ANNOTATED REFERENCES

1. Carter CW, Kocher MS: Meniscus repair in children. *Clin Sports Med* 2012;31(1):135-154.
2. Francavilla ML, Restrepo R, Zamora KW, Sarode V, Swirsky SM, Mintz D: Meniscal pathology in children: Differences and similarities with the adult meniscus. *Pediatr Radiol* 2014;44(8):910-925, quiz 907-919.
3. Shieh A, Bastrom T, Roocroft J, Edmonds EW, Pennock AT: Meniscus tear patterns in relation to skeletal immaturity: Children versus adolescents. *Am J Sports Med* 2013;41(12):2779-2783.
4. Gans I, Bedoya MA, Ho-Fung V, Ganley TJ: Diagnostic performance of magnetic resonance imaging and pre-surgical evaluation in the assessment of traumatic intra-articular knee disorders in children and adolescents: What conditions still pose diagnostic challenges? *Pediatr Radiol* 2015;45(2):194-202.
5. Mitchell JJ, Sjostrom R, Mansour AA, et al: Incidence of meniscal injury and chondral pathology in anterior tibial spine fractures of children. *J Pediatr Orthop* 2015;35(2):130-135.
6. Shea KG, Grimm NL, Laor T, Wall E: Bone bruises and meniscal tears on MRI in skeletally immature children with tibial eminence fractures. *J Pediatr Orthop* 2011;31(2):150-152.
7. Wilson PL, Wyatt CW, Romero J, Sabatino MJ, Ellis HB: Incidence, presentation, and treatment of pediatric and adolescent meniscal root injuries. *Orthop J Sports Med* 2018;6(11). doi:10.1177/2325967118803888.

   A total of 18.5% of 314 knee arthroscopies in children and adolescents demonstrated a complete meniscal root tear, a much higher incidence than previously noted. Level of evidence: IV.
8. Middleton S, Asplin L, Stevenson C, Thompson P, Spalding T: Meniscal allograft transplantation in the paediatric population: Early referral is justified. *Knee Surg Sports Traumatol Arthrosc* 2019;27(6):1908-1913.

   A single surgeon case series of 23 meniscal allograft transplants in patients primarily teenage patients. Scores for multiple patient-reported knee function questionnaires were improved and no allograft failures occurred. Follow-up was short to mid-term. Level of evidence: IV.
9. Riboh JC, Tilton AK, Cvetanovich GL, Campbell KA, Cole BJ: Meniscal allograft transplantation in the adolescent population. *Arthroscopy* 2016;32(6):1133-1140.e1.

   A single institution case series reporting on 32 meniscal allograft transplants in patients less than 17 years old and a minimum of 2-year follow-up. Patient-reported functional outcomes measures showed improvement. Most repeat operations were for chondral injury (22% of patients) and 6% of patients had re-operation on the meniscus, but no revision meniscal transplants were done. Level of evidence: IV.
10. Schachne JM, Heath MR, Yen YM, Shea KG, Green DW, Fabricant PD: The safe distance to the popliteal neurovascular bundle in pediatric knee arthroscopic surgery: An age-based magnetic resonance imaging anatomic study. *Orthop J Sports Med* 2019;7(7). doi:10.1177/2325967119855027.

    Magnetic resonance images were reviewed from children aged 10 to 18 years for the distance from the anterolateral portal line to the neurovascular bundle from different meniscus locations on the lateral meniscus. Level of evidence: IV.
11. Shea KG, Dingel AB, Styhl A, et al: The position of the popliteal artery and peroneal nerve relative to the menisci in children: A cadaveric study. *Orthop J Sports Med* 2019;7(6). doi:10.1177/2325967119842843.

    Cadaver knees from children aged 2 to 11 years were examined with CT scans to identify the most posterior extent of lateral and medial meniscus and the distance to the popliteus artery. Level of evidence: IV.
12. Chambers HG, Chambers RC: The natural history of meniscus tears. *J Pediatr Orthop* 2019;39(6 suppl 1):S53-S55.

    Thousands of articles on meniscal tears were searched to try to determine the understanding of the natural history of meniscal tears and whether treatment for meniscal tears alters the natural history. Very little definitive data were found. Level of evidence: IV.
13. Liechti DJ, Constantinescu DS, Ridley TJ, Chahla J, Mitchell JJ, Vap AR: Meniscal repair in pediatric populations: A systematic review of outcomes. *Orthop J Sports Med* 2019;7(5). doi:10.1177/2325967119843355.

    A total of eight studies met inclusion criteria for this systematic review. There were no comparative studies, so it was not possible to provide strong recommendations regarding surgical treatment for pediatric meniscus tears. Level of evidence: IV.
14. Patel NM, Mundluru SN, Beck NA, Ganley TJ: Which factors increase the risk of reoperation after meniscal surgery in children? *Orthop J Sports Med* 2019;7(5). doi:10.1177/2325967119842885.

    A large single-center series of 907 knee surgeries for meniscal injury looked at revision surgery rates for partial meniscectomy versus repair. Level of evidence: IV.

15. Shieh AK, Edmonds EW, Pennock AT: Revision meniscal surgery in children and adolescents: Risk factors and mechanisms for failure and subsequent management. *Am J Sports Med* 2016;44(4):838-843.

At a single center, 293 patients younger than 20 years with 324 meniscal surgeries (including 46 discoid meniscus surgeries) were evaluated at a mean follow-up of 40 months. Overall, 13% of the patients required revision surgery. Level of evidence: III.

16. Vanderhave KL, Moravek JE, Sekiya JK, Wojtys EM: Meniscus tears in the young athlete: Results of arthroscopic repair. *J Pediatr Orthop* 2011;31(5):496-500.

17. Kramer DE, Kalish LA, Martin DJ, et al: Outcomes after the operative treatment of bucket-handle meniscal tears in children and adolescents. *Orthop J Sports Med* 2019;7(1). doi:10.1177/2325967118820305.

A case series of 185 surgeries for bucket-handle meniscus tears in patients younger than 19 years with at least 6-month follow-up showed a 24% revision surgery rate. Level of evidence: IV.

18. Kushare I, Klingele K, Samora W: Discoid meniscus: Diagnosis and management. *Orthop Clin North Am* 2015;46(4):533-540.

19. McKay S, Chen C, Rosenfeld S: Orthopedic perspective on selected pediatric and adolescent knee conditions. *Pediatr Radiol* 2013;43(suppl 1):S99-S106.

20. Klingele KE, Kocher MS, Hresko MT, Gerbino P, Micheli LJ: Discoid lateral meniscus: Prevalence of peripheral rim instability. *J Pediatr Orthop* 2004;24(1):79-82.

21. Ellis HB Jr, Wise K, LaMont L, Copley L, Wilson P: Prevalence of discoid meniscus during arthroscopy for isolated lateral meniscal pathology in the pediatric population. *J Pediatr Orthop* 2017;37(4):285-292.

Of 261 knee arthroscopies performed for isolated lateral meniscus pathology, 75% demonstrated discoid morphology and 25% demonstrated tears of a normally shaped meniscus. Level of evidence: IV.

22. Choi SH, Ahn JH, Kim KI, et al: Do the radiographic findings of symptomatic discoid lateral meniscus in children differ from normal control subjects? *Knee Surg Sports Traumatol Arthrosc* 2015;23(4):1128-1134.

23. Lau BC, Vashon T, Janghala A, Pandya NK: The sensitivity and specificity of preoperative history, physical examination, and magnetic resonance imaging to predict articular cartilage injuries in symptomatic discoid lateral meniscus. *J Pediatr Orthop* 2018;38(9):e501-e506.

The patient history was most sensitive and specific for diagnosing associated chondral injury when a discoid meniscus was present, particularly a report of symptoms for more than 6 months and an extension block. Level of evidence: II.

24. LaMont L, Ellis H, Wise K, Wilson P: The inverted discoid meniscus segment: Clinical, radiographic, and arthroscopic description of a hidden tear pattern. *Am J Sports Med* 2016;44(6):1534-1539.

Of 121 discoid meniscus surgeries, 19 menisci demonstrated an inverted/flipped meniscus segment that could be easily missed. Level of evidence: III.

25. Carter CW, Hoellwarth J, Weiss JM: Clinical outcomes as a function of meniscal stability in the discoid meniscus: A preliminary report. *J Pediatr Orthop* 2012;32(1):9-14.

26. Yoo WJ, Jang WY, Park MS, et al: Arthroscopic treatment for symptomatic discoid meniscus in children: Midterm outcomes and prognostic factors. *Arthroscopy* 2015;31(12):2327-2334.

27. Ahn JH, Kim KI, Wang JH, Jeon JW, Cho YC, Lee SH: Long-term results of arthroscopic reshaping for symptomatic discoid lateral meniscus in children. *Arthroscopy* 2015;31(5):867-873.

28. Haskel JD, Uppstrom TJ, Dare DM, Rodeo SA, Green DW: Decline in clinical scores at long-term follow-up of arthroscopically treated discoid lateral meniscus in children. *Knee Surg Sports Traumatol Arthrosc* 2018;26(10):2906-2911.

At an average follow-up of 11 years, 21 patients who had previously undergone discoid meniscus saucerization surgery reported functional outcomes. Compared to the 2-year postoperative function in this same group, patient-reported functional outcomes scores declined as time from surgery increased. Level of evidence: IV.

29. Lee CR, Bin SI, Kim JM, Lee BS, Kim NK: Arthroscopic partial meniscectomy in young patients with symptomatic discoid lateral meniscus: An average 10-year follow-up study. *Arch Orthop Trauma Surg* 2018;138(3):369-376.

A total of 66 patients (73 knees) who had previously undergone partial meniscectomy for discoid lateral meniscus were studied a mean of 10 years after surgery. Over 30% of patients had unfavorable clinical outcomes and these outcomes were related to duration of symptoms prior to surgery as well as limb alignment at latest follow-up. MRI studies showed progression degenerative changes of the cartilage and the residual meniscus in most patients. Level of evidence: IV.

CHAPTER 50

Patellar Instability

CORINNA C.D. FRANKLIN, MD

ABSTRACT

Patellar instability refers to subluxation or dislocation of the patella out of the trochlear groove, usually laterally. This condition is thought to be more common in adolescent girls. The medial patellofemoral ligament is the key medial structure resisting lateral subluxation of the patella dynamically, and the vastus medialis obliquus is the main muscular contributor to patellar stability. Important radiographic measurements are patellar height, patellar tilt, sulcus angle, and the tibial tubercle-trochlear groove distance. No preferred method exists for the management of patellar instability. Patients with a first-time patellar dislocation may be treated with measures such as physical therapy to strengthen the vastus medialis obliquus, core, and gluteal musculature. Current surgical management typically involves reconstruction of the medial patellofemoral ligament, with correction of underlying anatomic factors if necessary.

Keywords: patellar instability; patellofemoral instability; pediatric knee; pediatric sports

INTRODUCTION

Patellar instability refers to subluxation or dislocation of the patella out of the trochlear groove of the femur, usually laterally. Acute, traumatic patellar dislocations are the most common acute knee disorder in adolescent athletes.[1] Atraumatic patellar instability is also possible, particularly in patients with ligamentous laxity.

EPIDEMIOLOGY

An often-cited 1994 study from Finland reported the incidence of acute patellar dislocation in children younger than 16 years to be 0.04% (43 per 100,000 children).[2] A 2004 study reported the highest incidence of patellar instability in girls between the ages of 10 and 17 years.[3] In 2012, a longitudinal epidemiologic study of emergency department visits for patellar dislocation reported the annual overall rate to be 2.29 per 100,000 individuals.[4] The highest incidence occurred in individuals between the ages of 15 and 19 years; sex was not an important differentiating factor. Half of patellar dislocations occurred during sports participation. The estimates for recurrence rates have ranged from 15% to 44%.[1]

A 2015 study specifically evaluating patellofemoral instability in high school athletes found that, for comparable sports, girls had higher rates of patellar instability than boys.[5] Injury rates were higher in competition than in practice, and physical contact was a common injury mechanism.

Reported risk factors for patellar instability include female sex, race (black or white being at higher risk than Hispanic individuals), sports participation, anatomic factors, and a personal or family history of patellar instability.[3,4,6] Ligamentous laxity may also play a role; patients should be examined for generalized laxity or hypermobility, with referral to a geneticist if Ehlers-Danlos syndrome is suspected.[7] A 2013 study found trochlear dysplasia to be an important risk factor for recurrent patellar instability, particularly in skeletally immature patients.[6]

The natural history of patellar instability has not been fully characterized. Limited high-level data exist, and comparing studies is difficult, in part because of the wide variety of reconstruction procedures and treatment options.

Dr. Franklin or an immediate family member serves as a board member, owner, officer, or committee member of the American Academy of Orthopaedic Surgeons, the Pediatric Orthopaedic Society of North America, the Pediatric Research in Sports Medicine, and the Ruth Jackson Orthopaedic Society.

ANATOMY AND PATHOANATOMY

The medial patellofemoral ligament (MPFL) is thought to be the most important restraint in preventing lateral subluxation and dislocation of the patella, particularly from full extension to 30° of flexion, and it is most taut at full extension.[1,8] The MPFL is approximately 55 mm long and variably thick (ranging in thickness from 3 to 30 mm).[8] Studies seem to agree that its insertion is along the superomedial aspect of the patella,[8,9] although the MPFL insertion is more variable in skeletally immature patients[10] (**Figure 1**). The origin of the MPFL is more controversial. Using a radiographic method, authors found the MPFL origin to be just proximal to the femoral physis.[11] However, a later anatomic study reported that the MPFL originates at or below the physis in children.[12] A radiographic method has been described for placing the origin of the MPFL. On a lateral radiograph of the knee, with the posterior condylar margin overlapped, the origin should be 1.3 mm anterior to the posterior cortex extension and 2.5 mm distal to the posterior origin of the medial femoral condyle, just proximal to the level of the posterior point of Blumensaat line[13] (**Figure 2**). In agreement with these findings, the authors of a 2011 study used a radiographic method to determine that the MPFL originates just distal to the femoral physis.[14]

After the patella is engaged, at approximately 20° of flexion, the trochlear groove provides stability. As a result, trochlear dysplasia can contribute to patellar instability. A 2011 study described the relationship between trochlear dysplasia (a morphologically abnormal and/or shallow trochlea) and recurrent patellar dislocations. However, it is unknown whether the dysplasia is congenital or a result of recurrent dislocations.[15] Data from a 2010 case-controlled study found trochlear dysplasia to be more common in women with patellar dislocations.[16]

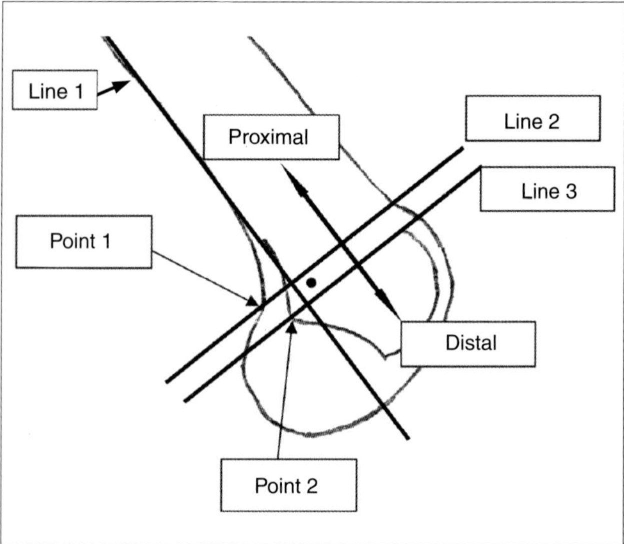

FIGURE 2 Illustration showing the femoral origin of the medial patellofemoral ligament, which is just anterior (1.3 mm) to the posterior cortex extension (line 1), just distal (2.5 mm) to the posterior origin of the medial femoral condyle (point 1/line 2), and just proximal to the level of the posterior point of the Blumensaat line on a lateral radiograph (point 2/line 3). (Adapted with permission from Schöttle PB, Schmeling A, Rosenstiel N, Weiler A: Radiographic landmarks for femoral tunnel placement in medial patellofemoral ligament reconstruction. *Am J Sports Med* 2007;3[5]:801-804.)

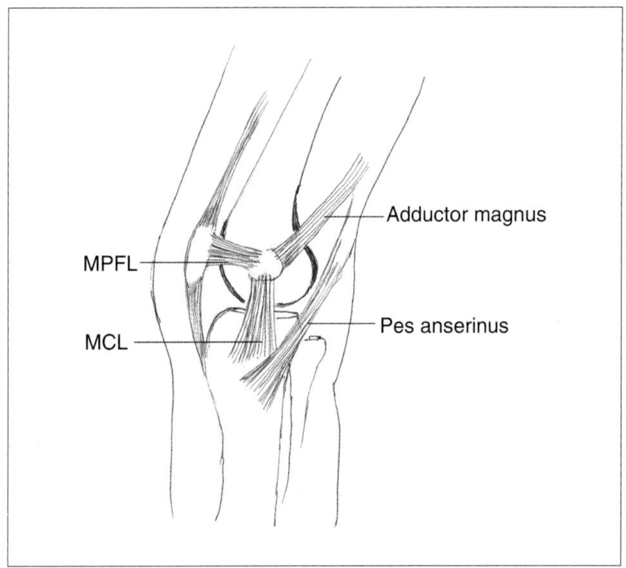

FIGURE 1 Illustration of the anatomy of the lateral aspect of the knee showing the insertion of the medial patellofemoral ligament (MPFL) on the patella. MCL = medial collateral ligament. (Reproduced with permission from Hennrikus W, Pylawka T: Patellofemoral instability in skeletally immature athletes, In Lieberman JR, Khanuja HS: *Instructional Course Lectures*. Woltkers Kluwer, 2013, vol 62, pp 445-453.)

The main contributor to dynamic stability of the patella is the vastus medialis obliquus, which exerts a medial and posterior force that opposes lateral patellar instability.[17] Alignment of the lower limb is also an important factor. A higher quadriceps (Q) angle indicates a more lateral pull of the quadriceps on the patella, potentially increasing the risk of subluxation or dislocation.[17] Internal femoral rotation and/or external tibial rotation also may be predisposing factors to patellar instability; these factors may be dynamically worsened by hip or core weakness.[17]

The position of the patella also contributes to its stability. In patella alta, the knee must flex further for the patella to engage with the trochlea, allowing a greater range for instability before attaining the bony stability of the trochlea.

A 2017 MRI study compared skeletally immature patients with first-time traumatic patellar dislocations with similarly aged control subjects. The authors found that the patients with patellar instability differed from the control subjects in each measure studied, including measures of trochlear dysplasia (trochlear depth, sulcus angle), patella alta, and tibial tuberosity to trochlear groove (TT-TG) distance. Trochlear dysplasia and lateral patellar tilt together had the strongest association with having had a patellar dislocation.[18] Another 2017 study evaluating predictors of recurrent patellar instability determined that trochlear dysplasia, skeletal immaturity, and patella alta were all risk factors for recurrence in patients with first-time patellar dislocations.[19]

IMAGING

When evaluating patients with patellar instability, plain radiographs of the knee (AP, lateral, and Merchant views) should be obtained. MRI is also often helpful. Relevant measurements on plain radiographs are the sulcus angle (normal = 138°, with 6° SD)[20] (**Figure 3, A**); patellar tilt (>5° is abnormal)[21] (**Figure 3, B**); and patellar height. Several indices can be used to determine patella height, including the Insall-Salvati ratio, which is the ratio of the diagonal length of the patella to the length of the patellar tendon (normal is 0.8 to 1.2)[22] (**Figure 3, C**); the Blackburne-Peel ratio, which is the ratio of the height of the articular surface of the patella from the plateau to the length of the articular surface of the patella (>1 suggests patella alta)[23] (**Figure 3, D**); and the Caton-Deschamps index, which is the ratio between the articular facet length of the patella and the distance between the articular facet of the patella and the anterior corner of the superior tibial epiphysis (normal = 0.6 to 1.3)[24] (**Figure 3, E**). A 2011 study found the Caton-Deschamps index to be a useful measurement in children and adolescents.[25]

Rupture of the MPFL may be seen on MRI, and it is best seen on T2-weighted images. In addition, osteochondral damage may be noted, and the patella may remain tilted or subluxated[26] (**Figure 4**). Importantly, MRI allows for the measurement of the distance between the tibial tubercle and the trochlear groove, known as the TT-TG distance. If the tibial tubercle is positioned directly under the trochlear groove, there will be a direct line of pull keeping the patella aligned; however, if the tibial tubercle is lateral to the trochlea, the resultant force will

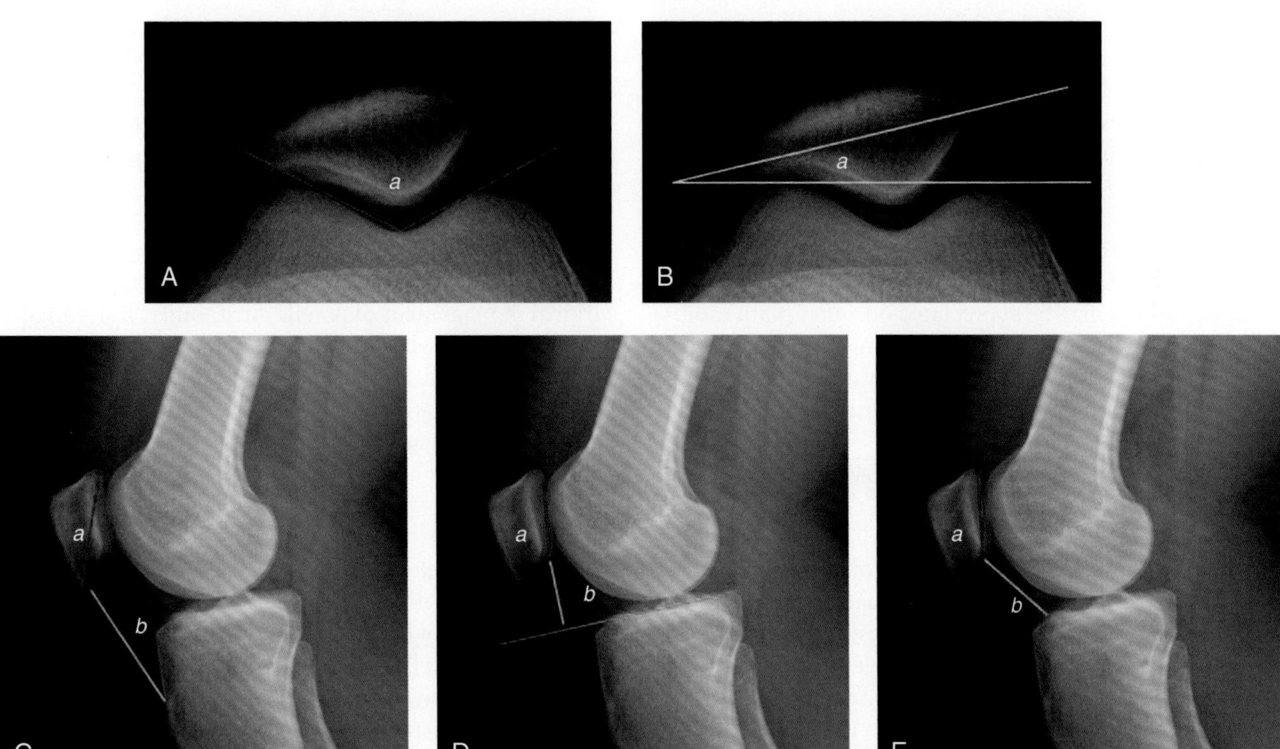

FIGURE 3 Measurements on plain radiographs can be used to evaluate patellar instability. **A**, A normal sulcus angle (a) is 138° with 6° SD. **B**, Patellar tilt (*a*) greater than 5° is abnormal. **C**, The Insall-Salvati ratio (*b*/*a*) is the ratio of the length of the patellar tendon (blue line) to the diagonal length of the patella (red line); normal is 0.8-1.2. **D**, The Blackburne-Peel ratio (*b*/*a*) is the height of the articular surface of the patella from the plateau (blue line) to the length of the articular surface of the patella (red line); greater than 1 suggests patella alta. **E**, The Caton-Deschamps index (*b*/*a*) is the distance between the articular facet of the patella and the anterior corner of the superior tibial epiphysis (blue line) and the articular facet length of the patella (red line); normal is 0.6-1.3.

Section 8: Sports-related Topics

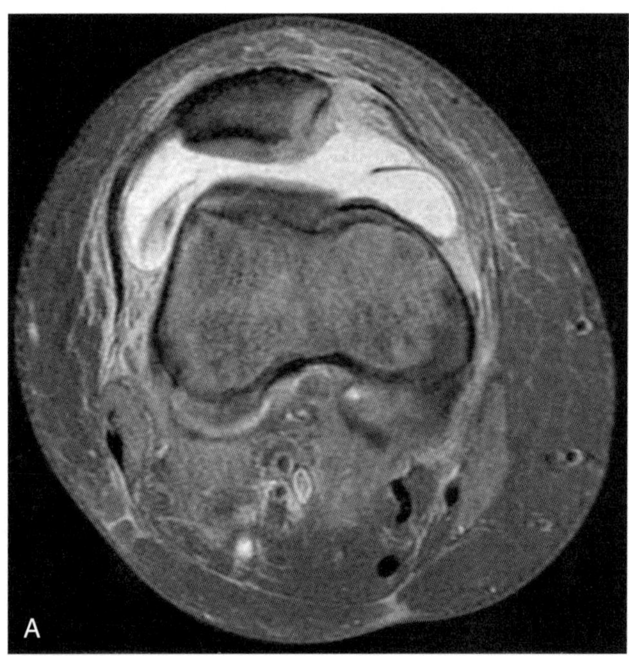

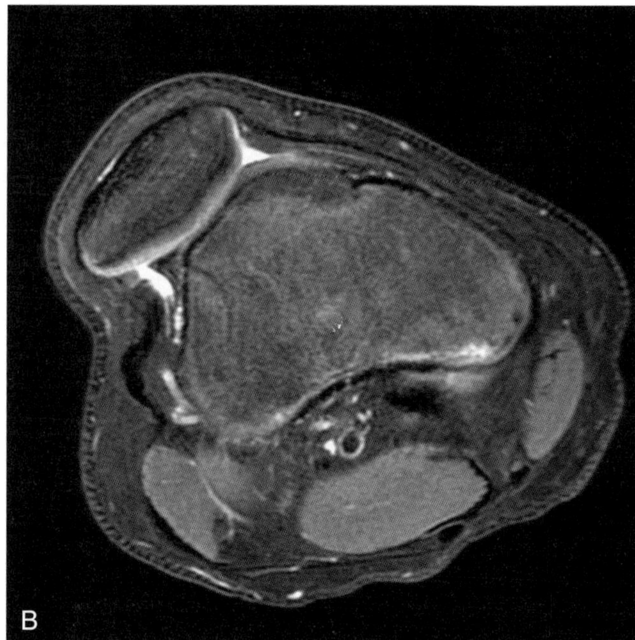

FIGURE 4 **A**, Magnetic resonance image shows rupture of the medial patellofemoral ligament and osteochondral damage to the patella with a loose body. **B**, Magnetic resonance image shows a patellar dislocation.

tend to pull the patella laterally, which can contribute to instability. This can be assessed by measuring the medial/lateral distance between the tibial tubercle and trochlear grove on successive MRIs or CTs. A TT-TG distance less than 15 mm is normal, whereas a TT-TG distance greater than 20 mm is excessive.[26] A 2013 comparison study reported that MRI may underestimate the TT-TG distance compared with measurements determined with CT; this should be considered in surgical planning.[27]

Loose bodies may be appreciated on either plain radiographs or MRIs. The use of MRI may help to better localize the location of the loose body and determine its origin; this may help in surgical planning.

MANAGEMENT

There is currently no preferred method for the management of patellar instability, and only limited high-level data are available to guide treatment decisions. The authors of a 2015 systematic review were unable to determine whether surgical management of primary patellar dislocation was indicated because of insufficient data.[28] Nonsurgical measures are often used, particularly in patients with first-time dislocations or those with instability without frank dislocation.

Physical Therapy

Physical therapy for patellar instability generally focuses on strengthening the vastus medialis obliquus and the gluteal and core musculature.[1] Weak gluteal muscles can cause adduction and internal rotation of the femur, which exacerbates patellar instability.[29] Closed kinetic chain exercises are likely a more effective therapy for patellar instability.[30,31] Bracing treatment or taping to assist with patellar tracking and prevent lateral subluxation may also be helpful.[29,32]

Surgical Care

More than 100 procedures have been described for the surgical management of patellar instability. Relevant criteria to consider when deciding on a particular procedure should include the age and skeletal maturity of the patient, the underlying pathoanatomy (patella alta, femoral and tibial rotation, patellar tilt, and Q angle), the condition of the cartilage, and associated injuries.

Lateral Release

Isolated lateral release is no longer recommended for the treatment of patellar instability.[1] It may be appropriate in combination with other procedures, particularly in the setting of patellar tilt but should be used judiciously, because if excessive or not indicated, lateral release can lead to medial instability.[33]

Primary Repair and Medial Reefing

A 2008 randomized controlled trial examined whether primary repair of the medial structures in patients with acute patellar dislocation improved outcomes compared with nonsurgical management.[34] The authors reported that the rate of recurrent dislocation and long-term outcomes did not differ substantially, and they did not advocate primary repair. In patients with recurrent patellar instability and normal anatomy, medial reefing without lateral release was shown to be an effective treatment in a 2014 case series.[35]

Proximal Realignment

The author of a 1979 study described a proximal realignment involving a lateral release and a long, open medial tightening.[36] However, this procedure has been reported to exacerbate patellofemoral arthritis.[37]

Distal Realignment

For patients with an increased TT-TG distance, the tibial tubercle may be osteotomized and moved anteromedially to correct malalignment of the extensor mechanism. In patients with patella alta, some distalization also can be performed. A 2015 cadaver study demonstrated that lateralizing the tibial tubercle increased patellar tilt and decreased patellar stability, whereas the reverse was the case for medializing the tibial tubercle.[38] Another 2013 cadaver study found that 3.5-mm screws were adequate for fixation of the tibial tubercle, and their use may reduce screw irritation.[39] Tibial tubercle transfer may be combined with other reconstruction procedures; a 2015 case series reported good results when combining MPFL reconstruction with tibial tubercle transfer.[40] This procedure has limited application in skeletally immature patients because of the open tibial apophysis.

Several additional distal soft-tissue procedures have been described, including transfer of the patellar tendon medially (whole or in part) or transfer of the semitendinosus muscle to the patella.[1] A modification of the Roux-Goldthwait technique has been described in which the patellar tendon is split and the lateral half is detached distally and then passed under the medial half and sewn to the insertion of the sartorius.[41] A lateral release also is performed with this modified technique.

MPFL Reconstruction

Most recently, the main focus of surgical management of patellar instability has been reconstruction of the MPFL using tendon graft to restore medial resistance to lateral subluxation and dislocation. Many different options have been described for graft choice, the fixation method, the location of fixation, the appropriate position for fixation, and graft tension. A 2017 systematic review reported no difference in recurrent instability with the use of allografts versus autografts; however, this study included only level IV evidence.[42]

A 2012 case series described a representative technique using ipsilateral semitendinosus autograft. This is looped and fixed through a patellar tunnel with a cortical suspensory system, and a femoral tunnel with an interference screw. Placement of the femoral tunnel is based both on radiographic landmarks and checking the isometry of the graft in tension between 0° and 30° of knee flexion.[43]

A 2013 study described a technique for MPFL reconstruction in patients with open epiphyseal plates using gracilis autograft.[44] Two tunnels are made in the proximal two-thirds of the patella, and both ends of the whipstitched graft are fixed into the patella. Using the method described by the authors of a 2007 study,[13] a guide pin is placed at the MPFL origin and drilled across to the lateral side, using fluoroscopy to avoid the physis. This is overdrilled to produce a tunnel, and the looped graft is inserted with a suture and fixed with an interference screw at 30° of knee flexion (**Figures 5** and **6**). The vastus medialis obliquus aponeurosis is sutured back over to the patella.

A method of MPFL reconstruction using the medial portion of the quadriceps tendon has been described.[45] This portion of the quadriceps tendon is amputated proximally (but remains attached at the patella) and is turned down and oversewn. The free portion is sewn under the medial retinaculum to the medial intermuscular septum or fixed in place with a suture anchor. This technique is particularly useful in very young patients, because it can be performed without drilling near the physis.

A 2019 study reported on a technique for congenital and obligatory patellar dislocations in children. The authors' technique includes splitting the fascia lata, realigning the extensor mechanism proximally and a portion of the patellar tendon distally, and plicating

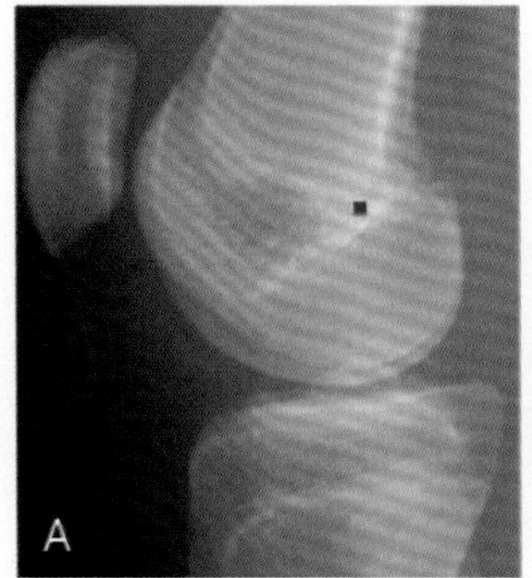

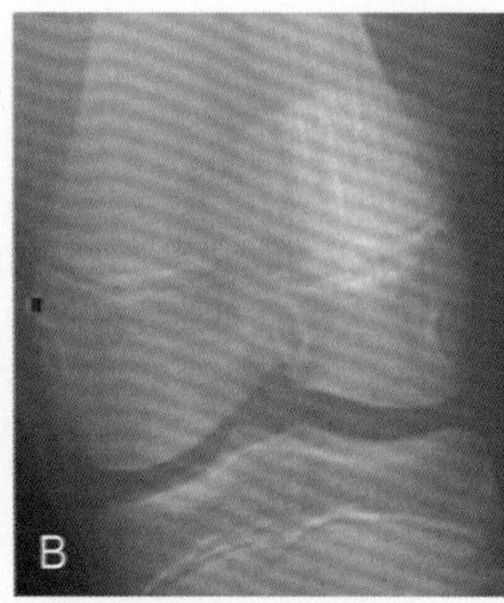

FIGURE 5 Cross-reference of the physis on a lateral radiographic view is made onto an AP radiographic view. This technique was used to demonstrate that the same point (dot) that is projected on or proximal to the physis on the lateral radiographic view is distal to the physis on the AP view. (Reproduced with permission from Nelitz M, Dreyhaupt J, Reichel H, Woelfle J, Lippacher S: Anatomic reconstruction of the medial patellofemoral ligament in children and adolescents with open growth plates: Surgical technique and outcome. *Am J Sports Med* 2013;41[1]:58-63.)

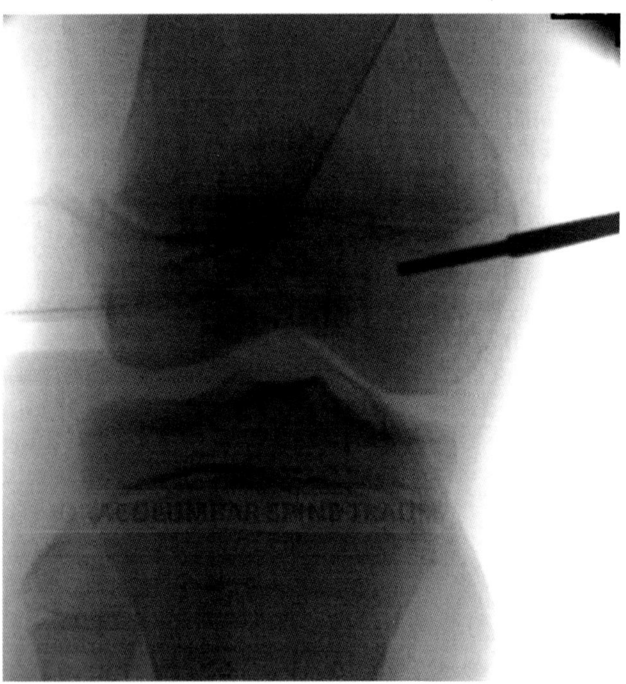

FIGURE 6 Radiograph shows a bioresorbable interference screw used to secure the graft, with the medial condyle tunnel distal to the physis. Graft placement distal to the physis is demonstrated. (Reproduced with permission from Nelitz M, Dreyhaupt J, Reichel H, Woelfle J, Lippacher S: Anatomic reconstruction of the medial patellofemoral ligament in children and adolescents with open growth plates: Surgical technique and outcome. *Am J Sports Med* 2013;41[1]:58-63.)

the medial capsule over the patella. Their study group included patients with Down syndrome and Larsen syndrome, and they reported overall promising results, with 11 of 12 patients maintaining a stable patella.[46]

A systematic review analyzed the existing literature to report on complications and determine the use of various methods. Notably, the authors found a dearth of high-level studies, with no level I studies and only two level II studies. Among the studies included in the analysis, the overall complication rate was 26.1%. Complications included continued apprehension, persistent instability, stiffness, patellar fracture, and pain. Clear conclusions about the superiority of one procedure over the others were not possible.[47]

Guided Growth

A 2015 study described hemiepiphysiodesis to correct genu valgum in patients with patellar instability.[48] Improvements in the anatomic lateral distal femoral angle and symptoms were reported. Hemiepiphysiodesis may be considered for skeletally immature patients with patellar instability and genu valgum.

Trochleoplasty

Trochlear dysplasia is a significant contributor to patellar instability; a 2016 study found that trochlear dysplasia affected the outcome of soft-tissue-only surgery for patellar instability.[49] To that end, there has been a recent increase in interest in trochleoplasty as an addition to the surgical arsenal in the management of patellar instability. Several case series have reported good midterm results with trochleoplasty for patients with severe trochlear dysplasia.[50-52] Trochleoplasty is often combined with other procedures such as MPFL reconstruction. A recent technique article detailed surgical procedure for patellar instability comprising a lateral release, MPFL reconstruction with allograft, and thin-flap, groove-deepening trochleoplasty. The authors advocate this procedure in the setting of patellar instability and a lateral trochlear inclination of 0° or less on axial MRI.[53] Two recent case series examined the use of trochleoplasty in adolescents and reported it to be effective in the absence of severe torsional or axial deformity and safe regarding growth disturbance in patients with less than 2 years of growth remaining.[54,55]

RETURN TO SPORTS

Limited data exist on return to sports after surgical management of patellar instability. A 2010 systematic review was unable to draw conclusions on return to sports efficacy after MPFL reconstruction because of the quality of the reviewed studies.[56] However, a 2013 case series reported that 100% of patients returned to sports after MPFL reconstruction, but only approximately 50% were able to participate at their prior level or a higher level.[57] A 2013 study suggested that skeletally immature athletes may return to sports participation 4 to 6 months after surgery for patellofemoral instability.[58]

A 2018 systematic review found that most studies used time-based criteria in deciding when patients could return to play after MPFL reconstruction/repair.[59] A 2018 study did report on strength and functional testing of patients at 6 months after patellar realignment surgery and found that in some patients, deficits remained at that time, particularly in those who had tibial tubercle osteotomies.[60] A 2019 Delphi method consensus article suggested eight criteria for return to play after surgery for patellar instability: negative apprehension; bone healing (if there was a bony procedure); knee stability via functional tests; lower extremity strength via functional tests; lower extremity power via hop test; comparable range of motion to contralateral side; adequate score on knee-specific patient-reported outcome measure; and gait normalization.[61]

SUMMARY

No preferred method exists for the management of patellar instability; additional high-level studies are needed to better clarify appropriate treatment strategies. Current treatment generally involves nonsurgical management for primary dislocations and subluxation in the absence of a loose fragment in the joint. Physical therapy is used to strengthen the vastus medialis obliquus, core, and gluteal musculature. Current surgical management typically involves reconstruction of the MPFL, with correction of underlying anatomic factors if necessary.

KEY STUDY POINTS

- The MPFL is the primary restraint to lateral subluxation of the patella from 0° to 30° of knee flexion.
- Patella alta, femoral anteversion, and external tibial torsion can contribute to patellar instability.
- An abnormal TT-TG distance (>20 mm) can predispose an individual to patellar instability.
- Physical therapy for patellar instability includes strengthening of the vastus medialis obliquus, core, and gluteal musculature.
- Lateral release in isolation is not recommended for treatment of patellar instability.
- Current surgical management of patellar instability often includes MPFL reconstruction with correction of anatomic parameters if indicated.
- Trochleoplasty is gaining acceptance in the management of patellar instability with trochlear dysplasia

ANNOTATED REFERENCES

1. Hennrikus W, Pylawka T: Patellofemoral instability in skeletally immature athletes. *Instr Course Lect* 2013;62(2):445-453.
2. Nietosvaara Y, Aalto K, Kallio PE: Acute patellar dislocation in children: Incidence and associated osteochondral fractures. *J Pediatr Orthop* 1994;14(4):513-515.
3. Fithian DC, Paxton EW, Stone ML, et al: Epidemiology and natural history of acute patellar dislocation. *Am J Sports Med* 2004;32(5):1114-1121.
4. Waterman BR, Belmont PJ Jr, Owens BD: Patellar dislocation in the United States: Role of sex, age, race, and athletic participation. *J Knee Surg* 2012;25(1):51-57.
5. Mitchell J, Magnussen RA, Collins CL, et al: Epidemiology of patellofemoral instability injuries among high school athletes in the United States. *Am J Sports Med* 2015;43(7):1676-1682.
6. Lewallen LW, McIntosh AL, Dahm DL: Predictors of recurrent instability after acute patellofemoral dislocation in pediatric and adolescent patients. *Am J Sports Med* 2013;41(3):575-581.
7. Hinton RY, Sharma KM: Acute and recurrent patellar instability in the young athlete. *Orthop Clin North Am* 2003;34(3):385-396.
8. Amis AA, Firer P, Mountney J, Senavongse W, Thomas NP: Anatomy and biomechanics of the medial patellofemoral ligament. *Knee* 2003;10(3):215-220.
9. Smirk C, Morris H: The anatomy and reconstruction of the medial patellofemoral ligament. *Knee* 2003;10(3):221-227.
10. Shea KG, Polousky JD, Jacobs JC Jr, et al: The patellar insertion of the medial patellofemoral ligament in children: A cadaveric study. *J Pediatr Orthop* 2015;35(4):e31-e35.
11. Shea KG, Grimm NL, Belzer J, Burks RT, Pfeiffer R: The relation of the femoral physis and the medial patellofemoral ligament. *Arthroscopy* 2010;26(8):1083-1087.
12. Shea KG, Polousky JD, Jacobs JC Jr, et al: The relationship of the femoral physis and the medial patellofemoral ligament in children: A cadaveric study. *J Pediatr Orthop* 2014;34(8):808-813.
13. Schöttle PB, Schmeling A, Rosenstiel N, Weiler A: Radiographic landmarks for femoral tunnel placement in medial patellofemoral ligament reconstruction. *Am J Sports Med* 2007;35(5):801-804.
14. Nelitz M, Dornacher D, Dreyhaupt J, Reichel H, Lippacher S: The relation of the distal femoral physis and the medial patellofemoral ligament. *Knee Surg Sports Traumatol Arthrosc* 2011;19(12):2067-2071.
15. Bollier M, Fulkerson JP: The role of trochlear dysplasia in patellofemoral instability. *J Am Acad Orthop Surg* 2011;19(1):8-16.
16. Balcarek P, Jung K, Ammon J, et al: Anatomy of lateral patellar instability: Trochlear dysplasia and tibial tubercle-trochlear groove distance is more pronounced in women who dislocate the patella. *Am J Sports Med* 2010;38(11):2320-2327.
17. Greiwe RM, Saifi C, Ahmad CS, Gardner TR: Anatomy and biomechanics of patellar instability. *Oper Tech Sports Med* 2010;18(2):62-67.
18. Askenberger M, Janarv P-M, Finnbogason T, Arendt EA: Morphology and anatomic patellar instability risk factors in first-time traumatic lateral patellar dislocations: A prospective magnetic resonance imaging study in skeletally immature children. *Am J Sports Med* 2017;45(1):50-58.

    This cross-sectional study examined patellofemoral joint morphology and anatomic patellar instability risk factors in children with and without a primary patellar dislocation and found that there was a significant difference for the mean value of all anatomic risk factors (trochlear dysplasia, patellar tilt, TT-TG distance, and patella alta) between children who did and did not have a patellar dislocation. Trochlear dysplasia and patellar tilt had the strongest association with patellar dislocations. Level of evidence: III.
19. Jaquith BP, Parikh SN: Predictors of recurrent patellar instability in children and adolescents after first-time dislocation. *J Pediatr Orthop* 2017;37(7):484-490.

This retrospective review of first-time patellar dislocators found that trochlear dysplasia, skeletal immaturity, patella alta (Caton-Deschamps Index >1.45), and contralateral patellar instability were predictors of repeat dislocation. Level of evidence: IV.

20. Merchant AC, Mercer RL, Jacobsen RH, Cool CR: Roentgenographic analysis of patellofemoral congruence. *J Bone Joint Surg Am* 1974;56(7):1391-1396.
21. Grelsamer RP, Bazos AN, Proctor CS: Radiographic analysis of patellar tilt. *J Bone Joint Surg Br* 1993;75(5):822-824.
22. Insall J, Salvati E: Patella position in the normal knee joint. *Radiology* 1971;101(1):101-104.
23. Blackburne JS, Peel TE: A new method of measuring patellar height. *J Bone Joint Surg Br* 1977;59(2):241-242.
24. Phillips CL, Silver DA, Schranz PJ, Mandalia V: The measurement of patellar height: A review of the methods of imaging. *J Bone Joint Surg Br* 2010;92(8):1045-1053.
25. Thévenin-Lemoine C, Ferrand M, Courvoisier A, Damsin J-P, Ducou le Pointe H, Vialle R: Is the Caton-Deschamps index a valuable ratio to investigate patellar height in children? *J Bone Joint Surg Am* 2011;93(8):e35.
26. Diederichs G, Issever AS, Scheffler S: MR imaging of patellar instability: Injury patterns and assessment of risk factors. *Radiographics* 2010;30(4):961-981.
27. Camp CL, Stuart MJ, Krych AJ, et al: CT and MRI measurements of tibial tubercle-trochlear groove distances are not equivalent in patients with patellar instability. *Am J Sports Med* 2013;41(8):1835-1840.
28. Magnussen RA, Duffee AR, Kalu D, Flanigan DC: Does early operative treatment improve outcomes of primary patellar dislocation? A systematic review. *Curr Orthop Pract* 2015;26(3):281-286.
29. Colvin AC, West RV: Patellar instability. *J Bone Joint Surg Am* 2008;90(12):2751-2762.
30. Stensdotter AK, Hodges PW, Mellor R, Sundelin G, Häger-Ross C: Quadriceps activation in closed and in open kinetic chain exercise. *Med Sci Sports Exerc* 2003;35(12):2043-2047.
31. Escamilla RF, Fleisig GS, Zheng N, Barrentine SW, Wilk KE, Andrews JR: Biomechanics of the knee during closed kinetic chain and open kinetic chain exercises. *Med Sci Sports Exerc* 1998;30(4):556-569.
32. Cowan SM, Bennell KL, Hodges PW: Therapeutic patellar taping changes the timing of vasti muscle activation in people with patellofemoral pain syndrome. *Clin J Sport Med* 2002;12(6):339-347.
33. Song G-Y, Hong L, Zhang H, Zhang J, Li Y, Feng H: Iatrogenic medial patellar instability following lateral retinacular release of the knee joint. *Knee Surg Sports Traumatol Arthrosc* 2016;24(9):2825-2830.

    A review of multiple existing studies concluded that aggressive or inappropriate lateral retinacular release of the knee joint leads to medial instability. Level of evidence: IV.
34. Palmu S, Kallio PE, Donell ST, Helenius I, Nietosvaara Y: Acute patellar dislocation in children and adolescents: A randomized clinical trial. *J Bone Joint Surg Am* 2008;90(3):463-470.
35. Boddula MR, Adamson GJ, Pink MM: Medial reefing without lateral release for recurrent patellar instability: Midterm and long-term outcomes. *Am J Sports Med* 2014;42(1):216-224.
36. Insall J, Bullough PG, Burstein AH: Proximal "tube" realignment of the patella for chondromalacia patellae. *Clin Orthop Relat Res* 1979;144:63-69.
37. Schüttler KF, Struewer J, Roessler PP, et al: Patellofemoral osteoarthritis after Insall's proximal realignment for recurrent patellar dislocation. *Knee Surg Sports Traumatol Arthrosc* 2014;22(11):2623-2628.
38. Stephen JM, Lumpaopong P, Dodds AL, Williams A, Amis AA: The effect of tibial tuberosity medialization and lateralization on patellofemoral joint kinematics, contact mechanics, and stability. *Am J Sports Med* 2015;43(1):186-194.
39. Warner BT, Kamath GV, Spang JT, Weinhold PS, Creighton RA: Comparison of fixation methods after anteromedialization osteotomy of the tibial tubercle for patellar instability. *Arthroscopy* 2013;29(10):1628-1634.
40. Ahmad R, Calciu M, Jayasekera N, Schranz P, Mandalia V: Combined medial patellofemoral ligament reconstruction and tibial tubercle osteotomy: Results at a mean follow-up of two years. *Bone Joint J* 2015;97-B(suppl 10):8.
41. Marsh JS, Daigneault JP, Sethi P, Polzhofer GK: Treatment of recurrent patellar instability with a modification of the Roux-Goldthwait technique. *J Pediatr Orthop* 2006;26(4):461-465.
42. Weinberger JM, Fabricant PD, Taylor SA, Mei JY, Jones KJ: Influence of graft source and configuration on revision rate and patient-reported outcomes after MPFL reconstruction: A systematic review and meta-analysis. *Knee Surg Sports Traumatol Arthrosc* 2017;25(8):2511-2519.

    The authors of this systematic review examined the influence of the graft source (allograft versus autograft) and the configuration (single-limbed versus double-limbed) on the failure rate and outcomes of MPFL reconstruction. No difference was found between graft sources with regard to revision rates; however, it was concluded that a double-limbed configuration should be used. Level of evidence: IV.
43. Howells NR, Barnett AJ, Ahearn N, Ansari A, Eldridge JD: Medial patellofemoral ligament reconstruction: A prospective outcome assessment of a large single centre series. *J Bone Joint Surg Br* 2012;94(9):1202-1208.
44. Nelitz M, Dreyhaupt J, Reichel H, Woelfle J, Lippacher S: Anatomic reconstruction of the medial patellofemoral ligament in children and adolescents with open growth plates: Surgical technique and clinical outcome. *Am J Sports Med* 2013;41(1):58-63.
45. Noyes FR, Albright JC: Reconstruction of the medial patellofemoral ligament with autologous quadriceps tendon. *Arthroscopy* 2006;22(8):904.e1-904.e7.
46. Sever R, Fishkin M, Hemo Y, Wientroub S, Yaniv M: Surgical treatment of congenital and obligatory dislocation of the patella in children. *J Pediatr Orthop* 2019;39(8):436-440.

    This case series evaluated a procedure for fixed and obligatory patellar dislocation in children, comprising quadriceps realignment, medial plication, and patellar tendon splitting, and found it to be successful in 11 of 12 patients. Level of evidence: IV.

47. Shah JN, Howard JS, Flanigan DC, Brophy RH, Carey JL, Lattermann C: A systematic review of complications and failures associated with medial patellofemoral ligament reconstruction for recurrent patellar dislocation. *Am J Sports Med* 2012;40(8):1916-1923.
48. Kearney SP, Mosca VS: Selective hemiepiphyseodesis for patellar instability with associated genu valgum. *J Orthop* 2015;12(1):17-22.
49. Hiemstra LA, Kerslake S, Loewen M, Lafave M: Effect of trochlear dysplasia on outcomes after isolated soft tissue stabilization for patellar instability. *Am J Sports Med* 2016;44(6):1515-1523.

    This case series found that trochlear dysplasia, when significant, correlated negatively with outcomes after soft-tissue procedures for patellar instability. Level of evidence: IV.
50. McNamara I, Bua N, Smith TO, Ali K, Donell ST: Deepening trochleoplasty with a thick osteochondral flap for patellar instability: Clinical and functional outcomes at a mean 6-year follow-up. *Am J Sports Med* 2015;43(11):2706-2713.
51. Ntagiopoulos PG, Byn P, Dejour D: Midterm results of comprehensive surgical reconstruction including sulcus-deepening trochleoplasty in recurrent patellar dislocations with high-grade trochlear dysplasia. *Am J Sports Med* 2013;41(5):998-1004.
52. Nelitz M, Dreyhaupt J, Lippacher S: Combined trochleoplasty and medial patellofemoral ligament reconstruction for recurrent patellar dislocations in severe trochlear dysplasia: A minimum 2-year follow-up study. *Am J Sports Med* 2013;41(5):1005-1012.
53. Vogel LA, Pace JL: Trochleoplasty, medial patellofemoral ligament reconstruction, and open lateral lengthening for patellar instability in the setting of high-grade trochlear dysplasia. *Arthrosc Tech* 2019;8(9):e961-e967.

    This paper describes a technique for groove-deepening trochleoplasty along with MPFL reconstruction for patellar instability. Level of evidence: V.
54. Camathias C, Studer K, Kiapour A, Rutz E, Vavken P: Trochleoplasty as a solitary treatment for recurrent patellar dislocation results in good clinical outcome in adolescents. *Am J Sport Med* 2016;44(11):2855-2863.

    This case series in young patients found good outcomes for solitary trochleoplasty as a surgical treatment for patellar instability in the setting of trochlear dysplasia, without torsional or axial severe malalignment. Level of evidence: V.
55. Nelitz M, Dreyhaupt J, Williams SRM: No growth disturbance after trochleoplasty for recurrent patellar dislocation in adolescents with open growth plates. *Am J Sports Med* 2018;46(13):3209-3216.

    This case series found that adolescents with 2 years or less of growth remaining and high-grade trochlear dysplasia could have a trochleoplasty without deleterious effects on growth. Level of evidence: IV.
56. Fisher B, Nyland J, Brand E, Curtin B: Medial patellofemoral ligament reconstruction for recurrent patellar dislocation: A systematic review including rehabilitation and return-to-sports efficacy. *Arthroscopy* 2010;26(10): 1384-1394.
57. Lippacher S, Dreyhaupt J, Williams SR, Reichel H, Nelitz M: Reconstruction of the medial patellofemoral ligament: Clinical outcomes and return to sports. *Am J Sports Med* 2014;42(7):1661-1668.
58. Hennrikus W, Pylawka T: Patellofemoral instability in skeletally immature athletes. *J Bone Joint Surg Am* 2013;95(2):176-183.
59. Zaman S, White A, Shi WJ, Freedman KB, Dodson CC: Return-to-play guidelines after medial patellofemoral ligament surgery for recurrent patellar instability: A systematic review. *Am J Sports Med* 2018;46(10):2530-2539.

    This systematic review included 53 studies and found that most used time-based criteria with fewer using objective or subjective patient-centered criteria; they concluded that further study was needed.
60. Krych AJ, O'Malley MP, Johnson NR, et al: Functional testing and return to sport following stabilization surgery for recurrent lateral patellar instability in competitive athletes. *Knee Surg Sports Traumatol Arthrosc* 2018;26(3):711-718.

    The authors of this case series evaluated the performance of athletes who underwent patellar stabilization surgery 6 months postoperatively and found that strength deficits persisted, particularly after tibial tubercle osteotomy. Level of evidence: IV.
61. White AE, Chatterji R, Zaman SU, et al: Development of a return to play checklist following patellar instability surgery: A Delphi-based consensus. *Knee Surg Sports Traumatol Arthrosc* 2020;28(3):806-815.

    The authors of this study used a Delphi method to develop a list of eight return to sports criteria following patellar instability surgery. Level of evidence: V.

CHAPTER 51

Osteochondritis Dissecans of the Knee and Elbow

MARC TOMPKINS, MD • RYAN P. COENE, MS • MIKHAIL A. KLIMSTRA, MD
MATTHEW D. MILEWSKI, MD

ABSTRACT

Osteochondritis dissecans can commonly affect the knee and elbow, particularly in a young athletic cohort. An understanding of the epidemiology, pathophysiology, clinical presentation, diagnostic imaging characteristics, and nonsurgical and surgical treatment options is important to optimize patient outcomes.

Keywords: capitellum; cartilage repair; elbow; knee; osteoarthritis; osteochondritis dissecans (OCD); osteochondrosis

INTRODUCTION

Osteochondritis dissecans (OCD) continues to be an idiopathic disease process that challenges surgeons, clinicians, patients, and their families. A current working definition of OCD states that it is a focal, idiopathic alteration of subchondral bone with risk for instability and disruption of adjacent articular cartilage that may result in premature osteoarthritis.[1] Despite its relatively low incidence, it is encountered in most orthopaedic and sports medicine clinics, and the American Academy of Orthopaedic Surgeons has produced a set of clinical practice guidelines for the diagnosis and management of OCD of the knee.[2] Although many of these clinical practice guideline recommendations lack strong evidence from the literature, these recommendations have helped guide future research efforts for this vexing condition.

Dr. Tompkins or an immediate family member has received non-income support (such as equipment or services), commercially derived honoraria, or other non–research-related funding (such as paid travel) from Allosource–ROCK Group and Vericel–ROCK Group and serves as a board member, owner, officer, or committee member of the American Orthopaedic Society for Sports Medicine, the Pediatric Research in Sports Medicine Society, and ROCK. None of the following authors or any immediate family member has received anything of value from or has stock or stock options held in a commercial company or institution related directly or indirectly to the subject of this chapter: Dr. Coene, Dr. Klimstra, and Dr. Milewski.

OCD OF THE KNEE

Epidemiology

Data from a large US managed care system have estimated the incidence of OCD of the knee in patients aged between 6 and 19 years as 9.5 per 100,000 children.[3] In that cohort, there was a 3.3 times increased risk of OCD in patients of age 12 to 19 years compared with a younger group aged between 6 and 11 years, with male children having a 3.8 times greater risk of OCD compared with females. This study suggested a bilaterality rate of 7%, but the rate of bilaterality has been suggested as high as 29% with 40% of the bilateral lesions being asymptomatic at the time of presentation for the contralateral lesion.[4] Within the knee, the authors of a 2014 study found the incidence of lesions to be 64% medial femoral condyle lesions; 32% lateral femoral condyle lesions; and the patella, trochlear groove, and tibial plateau making up less than 4% of the cases.[3] Despite lesions of the trochlea and patella being rare, reports suggest that 38% of the trochlear lesions are unstable and 24% had additional OCD lesions.[5] Another 2014 report found that in patients with multifocal lesions of the knee, 74% of the lesions require surgical treatment.[6] An epidemiologic study in adults found that in adults with

This chapter is adapted from Milewski MD, Tompkins MA, Shea KF, Ganley TJ: Osteochondritis dissecans of the knee and elbow, in Martus JE, ed: *Orthopaedic Knowledge Update®: Pediatrics*, ed 5. Rosemont, IL, American Academy of Orthopaedic Surgeons, 2016, pp 555-565.

OCD lesions, the lesions were more likely to be identified in the ankle, rather than the knee; the study also found that the incidence of OCD in adults was higher in men than in women.[7] One unique aspect of epidemiology of OCD in the knee is the association between discoid lateral meniscus and lateral femoral condyle OCD. The authors of a 2018 study[8] found that, over a 15-year period, nearly 15% of patients with symptomatic discoid lateral meniscus also had lateral femoral condyle OCD.

Pathophysiology

OCD was originally thought to be due to inflammation, but this has since been disproved. A variety of etiologies is theorized to cause OCD lesions including trauma, repetitive injury, overload due to malalignment, and genetic predispositions. There has been research examining potential genetic links for OCD, which has identified potential loci associated with OCD.[9] In a cohort study of patients with OCD, the family history of OCD was 14%, which is higher than the general cohort, further supporting a genetic component to this disease. Some authors have recently proposed links to vitamin D insufficiency and fluoroquinolone use.[10]

OCD is referred to as osteochondrosis in the veterinary literature and has caprine, porcine, bovine, and equine models.[11,12] Osteochondrosis is the leading cause of lameness in horses and leg weakness in pigs with PTH1R being identified as a strong candidate gene in equine and bovine models.[13] These animal models have also been used to reexamine the potential vascular etiology of OCD lesions, and CT and MRI coupled with histologic sectioning have confirmed an area of subchondral vascular failure in a porcine model.[11,14] Continued animal research will shed further light on potential vascular etiologies and genetic predisposition for OCD in humans.

More studies in humans are now teaching us about the development of OCD. Using pediatric cadaver knees, the authors of a 2018 study[15] found changes identical to osteochondrosis in animals, and these changes were associated with failure of the epiphyseal cartilage blood supply.

Mechanisms that affect development of OCD are also further illustrated in the literature. The authors of a 2017 study found that in patients with OCD, there was a larger tibial spine than in patients without OCD. They concluded that larger medial tibial spines may lead to impingement, increased contact pressures, and repetitive microtrauma to the medial femoral condyle, serving as a potential predisposing factor for developing OCD.[16] The authors of a 2020 study found an association between basketball and soccer athletes and the incidence of OCD.[17] In another 2018 study, the authors found a difference in presentation of OCD in catchers suggesting that frequent time spent in a catcher's position influences the location and onset of OCD.[18] The authors of a 2016 study also found that there was a more distal origin of the posterior cruciate ligament in patients with medial femoral condyle OCD and hypothesize that this could have an effect on the development of OCD in this location.[19]

History and Physical Examination

OCD of the knee can present with a wide range of symptoms that often can be quite benign for a long period. Occasional activity-related pain without swelling is noted early and often only progress to limping and swelling with mechanical symptoms in advanced lesions.

Physical examination findings can be quite subtle unless unstable advanced lesions are present. Mild effusion or tenderness to palpation over the lesion site may be noted. In particular for medial femoral condyle lesions, Wilson sign may elicit pain with internal tibial rotation as the knee is extended but has been found to be positive in only 25% of cases with a known OCD lesion.[20]

Imaging

Radiographic evaluation of an adolescent with knee pain is essential to making the diagnosis of an OCD lesion because of the often benign and nondescript physical examination findings. Radiographs should include an AP, lateral, sunrise, and notch views. The notch view aids in better visualization of more posteriorly located femoral condylar lesions that may not be seen on standard coronal views. As the most common lesion location is the posterolateral medial femoral condyle, most advocate for obtaining a notch view. Similarly, patellofemoral lesions may be missed without an appropriate sunrise view. Bilateral radiographs have been advocated because the rate of bilateral lesions has been reported to be 29%[4] (**Figure 1**). Standing alignment radiographs or left hand radiographs for bone age determinations may also be necessary if surgical intervention is being considered.[21]

A multicenter research group identified important radiographic features including location, epiphyseal plate maturity, size, fragmentation, displacement, boundary, central radiodensity, and contour.[22] The same group was able to demonstrate that using specific criteria, it was possible to reliably evaluate OCD healing.[23] The authors of a 2016 study found that a smaller notch width index was associated with knees having a medial femoral condyle OCD lesion.[24] This anatomic risk factor could contribute to tibial eminence impingement. The authors of a 2015 study found greater medial and posterior tibial slope in knees with medial femoral condyle OCD lesions.[25] The authors of a 2010 study[21] found an association between medial OCD lesions and varus alignment along with lateral OCD lesions and valgus

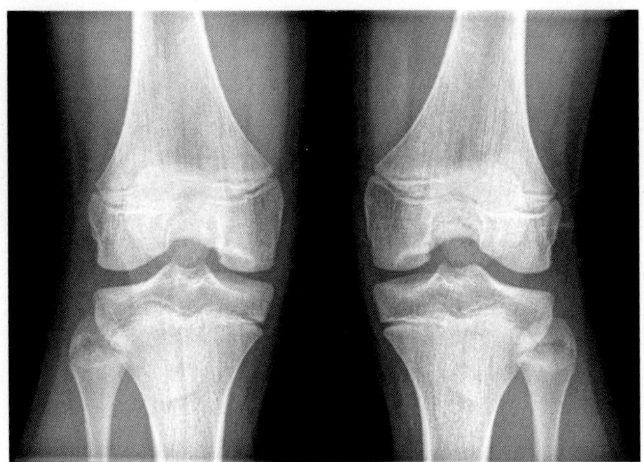

FIGURE 1 Notch radiograph of the knees of a 13-year-old boy with bilateral knee pain shows evidence of bilateral lesions of the medial femoral condyle. (Courtesy of Kevin G. Shea, MD, Stanford University Center.)

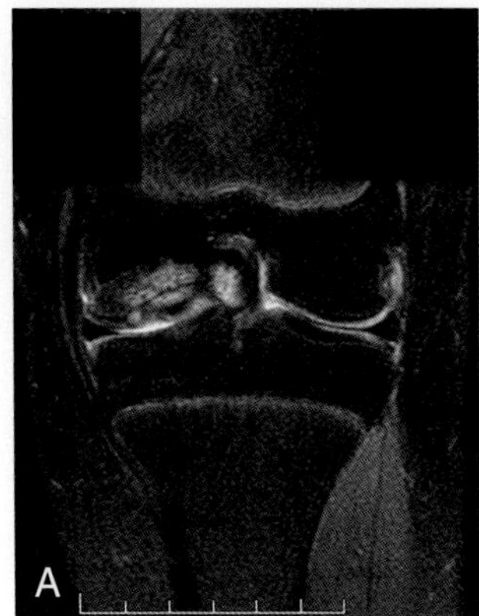

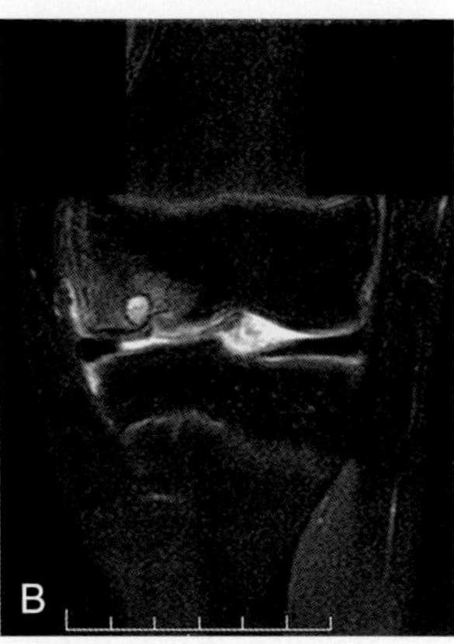

FIGURE 2 Magnetic resonance image of the knees of a 13-year-old girl with an osteochondritis dissecans lesion of the medial femoral condyle (**A**); note the cystlike structure (**B**). (Reproduced with permission from Milewski MD, Nissen CW, Shea K: Treatment of juvenile osteochondritis dissecans of the knee, in Diduch D, Bedi A: *Insall and Scott: Surgery of the Knee*, ed 6. Philadelphia, PA, Elsevier, 2017.)

alignment. Further studies will need to define the most reliable specific radiographic features that correlate with prognosis and healing.

Bone scan and CT scans have been largely replaced by MRI in regard to initial assessment of OCD articular cartilage integrity, subchondral bone status, and instability. A study on MRI and classification of OCD lesion stability has demonstrated limitations of historical MRI classification systems.[26] MRI criteria for instability of OCD lesions in adults include a hyperintense signal seen on T2 sequences at the fragment-femur interface, adjacent focal cystic (high signal intensity) areas, a focal defect in articular cartilage (>5 mm), and a hyperintense signal line equal to fluid that traverses both articular cartilage and subchondral bone.[27] These were refined for juvenile patients to the following criteria: a rimlike hyperintense signal equal to joint fluid plus a second deeper linear margin of low signal plus multiple sites of discontinuity of subchondral bone.[28] These criteria were 100% sensitive and specific for instability in this younger cohort (**Figure 2**). It was also found that multiple cystlike foci or a single cystlike focus greater than 5 mm in size was highly specific for instability (100%) but had low sensitivity (25% to 38%). Three-dimensional gradient-recalled echo T1-weighted MRI combined with routine sequences also showed exceptional sensitivity, specificity, and accuracy in detection of OCD instability in juveniles with OCD lesions.[29] A study on ultrasonography has suggested that ultrasonography can be used for screening and monitoring of OCD.[30]

Management

Management of knee OCD lesions in young patients can vary depending on the patient's age, location, size, and stability of the lesion. Goals of treatment, especially in young patients, include saving the native progeny fragment if possible and hopefully preventing osteoarthritis through early detection and prompt treatment.

Nonsurgical Management

Younger patients particularly those with wide open physes have a greater propensity to heal OCD lesions with nonsurgical management. Initial conservative treatment is recommended in patients with open physes, minimal symptoms, and stable lesions on initial imaging. Age, lesion size, and the presence or absence of mechanical symptoms play a role in the predictability of healing as described in the nomogram developed by the authors of a 2008 study.[31] The authors of a 2013 study[32] also developed a nomogram to predict healing including age, normalized lesion size, and the size of cystlike lesions on MRI. The authors of a 2016 study[33] demonstrated that these nomograms have high interrater and intrarater reliability for predicting healing of juvenile OCD lesions. Unfortunately, healing may take 6 to 12 months with activity restrictions, bracing treatment, and/or casting. There remains no consensus on the exact methods for nonsurgical treatment.

The authors of a 2018 study found that, using the International Cartilage Repair Society classification, grade I-II lesions were managed successfully 78% of the time, but the risk of failure in grade III-IV lesions was high with conservative management.[34] A database review from a large health system suggested that at least 33.5% of pediatric patients with knee OCD progressed to surgery.[35] Another report found that in patients with multifocal lesions, 74% required surgery.[6] Of patients treated nonsurgically, approximately 30% are likely to develop arthritis at 35 years after diagnosis.[36]

Surgical Management

For lesions that fail conservative management or those lesions thought to be unstable at the time of initial diagnosis, surgical management is the recommended form of management. A variety of surgical options are available depending on the size, instability of the lesion, age of the patient, and need for salvage due to nonviable progeny. In general, surgical management begins with arthroscopic assessment of stability. Multiple prior grading classifications have been described but lacked rigorous assessment of interrater and intrarater reliability.[37] A multicenter OCD research group has developed and validated a new arthroscopic classification system to help better assess lesion instability[38] (**Figure 3**).

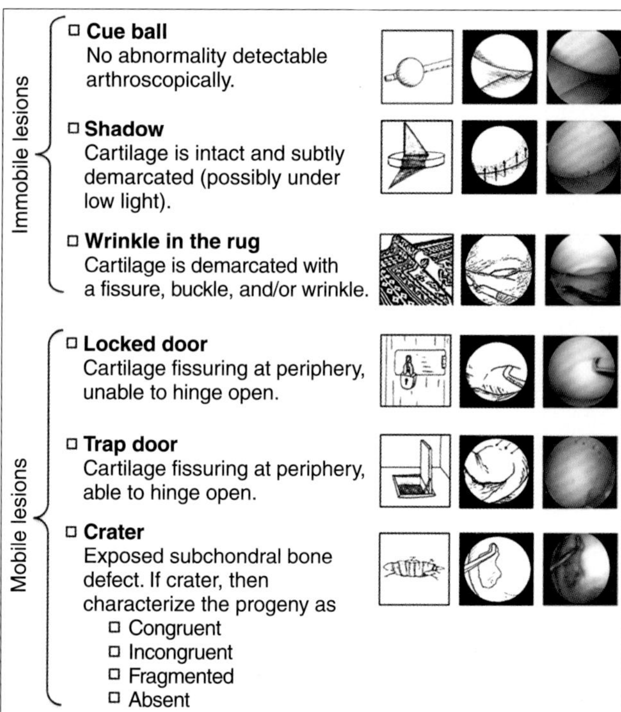

FIGURE 3 Illustration depicts the Research on Osteochondritis Dissecans of the Knee Arthroscopy Classification System to better assess the stability of osteochondritis dissecans lesions. (Reproduced with permission from Carey JL, Wall EJ, Grimm NL, et al: Novel arthroscopic classification of osteochondritis dissecans of the knee: A multicenter reliability study. *Am J Sports Med* 2016;44[7]:1694-1698.)

Although many different surgical techniques and hardware are available for lesion stabilization, the goals of treatment of OCD are fairly simple. These goals include drilling to stimulate or incite a vascular healing response to the avascular subchondral bone; fixation to stabilize loose subchondral bone and articular cartilage; bone grafting when needed to support articular cartilage contour, stability and vascularity; and when needed, salvage of the articular cartilage and subchondral bone with biologic replacements. Surgical excision of the OCD lesion, without a salvage procedure, has been shown to portend worse outcomes and higher risk for osteoarthritis.[39] Similarly, untreated OCD lesions or those that fail to heal despite treatment have been shown to carry a higher likelihood of subsequent osteoarthritis.

Drilling of the subchondral bone adjacent to an OCD lesion aims to stimulate a vascular healing response by disrupting the sclerotic margin and introducing biologic factors from adjacent healthier cancellous bone.[40] A variety of drilling techniques has been described, but the two main techniques can be divided into transarticular (or through the articular cartilage into the subchondral bone) and retroarticular (or from behind the lesion through the subchondral bone into the lesion but not through the articular cartilage; **Figure 4**).[40,41] Intercondylar notch drilling along with retroarticular drilling with bone grafting have also been described.[42] No studies have shown superiority based on technique, and reported outcomes from properly chosen younger patients with fairly stable lesions have been good.

Fixation of unstable OCD lesions as demonstrated on preoperative imaging and/or confirmed at the time of arthroscopy can be performed with a variety of fixation devices.[43] It has long been thought that the healing of these lesions is better in skeletally immature patients, but no difference has been found between skeletally immature and mature patients.[44] Fixation with metal screws (headed or headless), bioabsorbable screws or implants, and biologic fixation have been described.[45] Metal screws offer the advantage of rigid fixation without a potential synovitic response to a bioabsorbable device but come with the potential need for hardware removal and can also complicate follow-up MRI. Bioabsorbable screws and implants offer the advantage of not needing hardware removal and not impeding postoperative MRI but have the potential for hardware failure and synovitis-type reactions.[46] Biologic fixation with small osteochondral allograft transplantation system (OATS) plugs has also been described along with a hybrid technique combining metal screw fixation and OATS plug fixation.[47] Future prospective studies will need to determine if there is any advantage to specific fixation devices over others (**Table 1**).

Salvage procedures should be considered when lesions have failed fixation or previous excision. Marrow stimulation procedures have been used in the management of OCD lesions, but the additional subchondral bone loss associated with OCD lesions makes marrow stimulation techniques challenging in these patients. Microfracture has been shown to produce inferior results to other techniques such as OATS.[48] Different osteochondral scaffolds are now being used and results are promising.[49,50]

Biologic restoration of both the subchondral bone and the articular cartilage surface is an advantage of OATS both in terms of lesion fixation and during lesion salvage.[47]

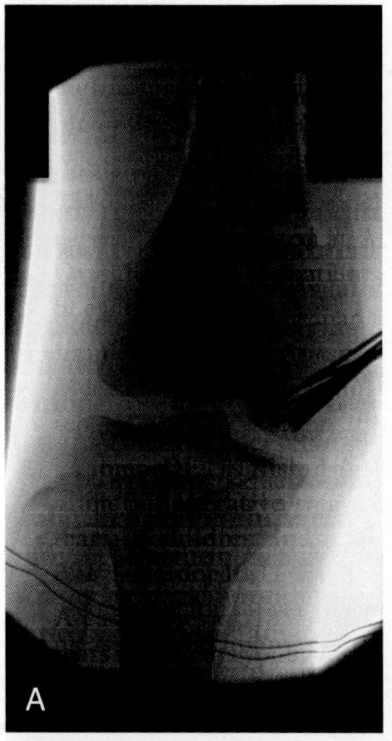
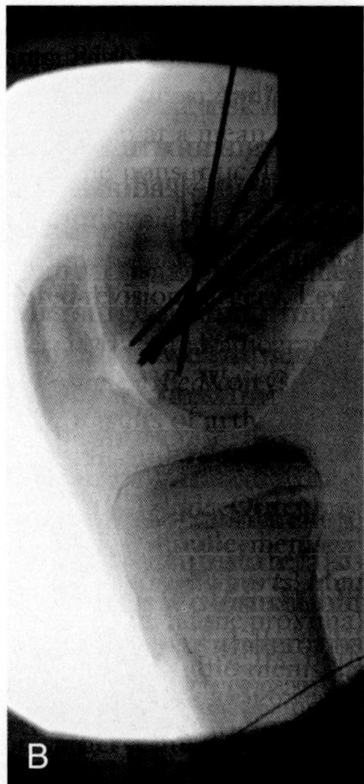

FIGURE 4 AP (**A**) and lateral (**B**) fluoroscopic images of the knee of a 12-year-old girl with an osteochondritis dissecans lesion of the medial femoral condyle. After nonsurgical treatment failed, the patient underwent arthroscopy. The lesion was found to be stable and the lesion was treated with retroarticular drilling of the subchondral bone. (Reproduced with permission from Milewski MD, Nissen CW, Shea K: Treatment of juvenile osteochondritis dissecans of the knee, in Diduch D, Bedi A: *Insall and Scott: Surgery of the Knee*, ed 6. Philadelphia, PA, Elsevier, 2017.)

Limitations to OATS include lesion size and donor site morbidity. Donor site morbidity, however, from OATS harvest has been reported to be less significant in younger patients.[51] At short-term follow-up, mosaicplasty was found to restore the joint surface and produce satisfactory functional results.[52] Hybrid fixation with fixation of a portion of the OCD lesion and the remainder filled in with osteochondral grafting has demonstrated good longer term results of healing and subjective outcomes.[53]

Fresh frozen ostechondral allografts can address some of these limitations and have been used to treat large OCD lesions.[54-56] There is no donor site morbidity, and ostechondral allografts can address much larger defects. Disadvantages include concerns about lack of bone integration between graft and host, host immune response, and chondrocyte viability after transplantation. The authors of a 2007 study showed 5-year survivorship to be 91%.[54] Midterm viability of these grafts as salvage for large OCD lesions and functional outcomes have been good.[57,58]

Autologous chondrocyte implantation (ACI) is another technique that can be used to salvage OCD of the knee. With long-term results showing good survivorship and clinical outcomes for osteochondral defect treatment, it provides the advantage of using the patient's own chondrocytes. Disadvantages for the management of OCD of the knee with ACI include cost of the second procedure along with the fact that ACI does not necessarily address the subchondral bone deficiency associated with OCD lesions. Midterm to long-term results have been promising for the use of ACI with bone grafting in the management of OCD of the knee.[59,60] Long-term studies will be needed to examine other newer generation cartilage regeneration options such as minced juvenile cartilage in the management and salvage of OCD of the knee.

OSTEOCHONDRITIS DISSECANS OF THE ELBOW

Epidemiology and Pathophysiology

The incidence of OCD of the elbow has recently been estimated to be 2.2 per 100,000, but seven times higher in males than females[61] and three times higher in obese patients.[62] Although the condition is rare, a prevalence between 2% to 3% has been documented in young athletes in certain sports, particularly baseball.[63-65] Elbow OCD lesions represented 12% of all OCDs presenting in the Kaiser Permanente system.[35] Participants in baseball,

TABLE 1

Bioabsorbable Versus Metal Implants for Osteochondritis Dissecans Fixation

Implant	Advantages	Disadvantages
Bioabsorbable	Removal may not be necessary Does not produce substantial artifact with MRI	Concerns about strength and implant failure Incomplete absorption Backing out from bone May result in substantial cyst formation around implants
Metal	Does not leave cystic lesions during screw absorption Titanium screws may induce less MRI artifact	May produce substantial artifact on MRI studies Removal may be necessary if close to cartilage surface and not recessed within stable bone Backing out from bone

gymnastics, and other overhead sports are at relatively high risk for this condition.[63,64] Those who begin to play at a young age, play for longer periods, or experience elbow pain have a higher risk for OCD.[63] In many athletes, the cause of OCD is thought to be related to overload of the lateral compartment of the elbow[66] and perhaps limitations in elbow vascularity. The possible vascular etiology for elbow OCD is thought to be caused by a vascular watershed area in the location of an OCD lesion.[64] Secondary overload in these areas may also enhance the risk of development and/or progression of the condition.[67]

OCD of the elbow and Panner disease may represent different stages of a related condition. Historically, Panner disease has been described in patients younger than 10 years; in many patients, the condition will resolve with time.[68] OCD of the elbow is thought to arise in older patients and, in many patients, these lesions do not heal.[69]

History and Physical Examination

Many young patients with OCD of the elbow have relatively minor symptoms, including occasional mechanical symptoms, minimal loss of motion, and occasional effusion.[70] In some patients, the only notable physical examination finding may be a 5° to 10° loss of full extension compared with the contralateral elbow. Advanced OCD lesions have been correlated with longer symptom duration.[71]

Radiographic Evaluation

Most OCD lesions of the elbow can be seen on plain radiographs. In particular, an AP with the elbow in 45° of flexion can identify more anterior lesions, which are more common in baseball players.[72] However, certain aspects of the lesions may be better seen with MRI, such as surrounding bone edema, cystic change, loose bodies, or more subtle lesions not fully appreciated on radiographs[73] (**Figures 5** and **6**). Some of these findings can affect clinical decision making for specific treatments. The authors of a 2018 study recently showed radial head lesions or changes in 30% of patients with capitellar OCD lesions,[74] especially those with more advanced lesions. Conversely, the authors of a 2016 study also showed a greater incidence of capitellar OCD lesions in patients with chronic radial head subluxation/dislocation indicating that changes on either side of the radiocapitellar joint will affect the opposite side.[75] Newer techniques of cartilage evaluation, including those with ultrasound which has been useful in identifying unstable lesions and also screening high-risk populations, may complement other forms of advanced imaging in the future.[76]

Nonsurgical Management

Younger patients with substantial growth remaining may respond well to activity modifications. In some patients, both rest and short periods of immobilization may be beneficial. For throwing athletes, switching to another position may be valuable, such as having a pitcher play as a first baseman. The authors of a 2018 study found that over half of stable capitellar OCD lesions, particularly smaller lesions and those without cystlike lesions, were able to heal with nonsurgical treatment.[77] The authors of a 2019 study have shown that radial head enlargement and advanced skeletal age of the affected elbow compared with the contralateral elbow were predictors of lack of healing with conservative treatment.[78]

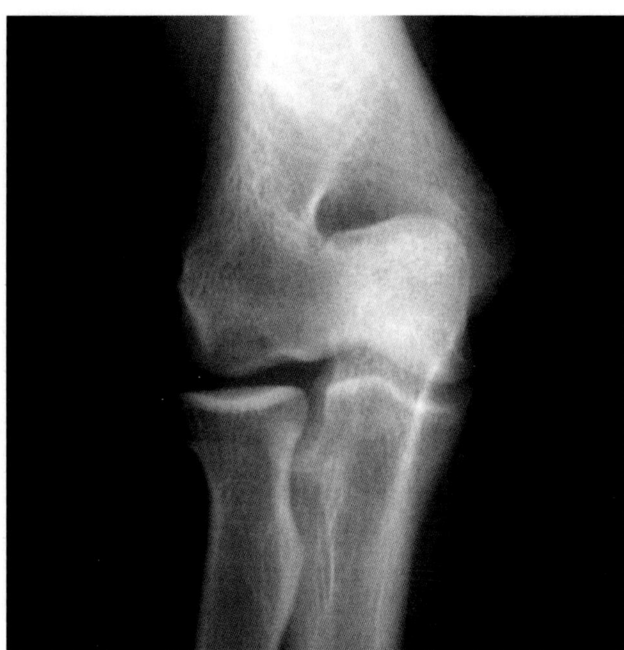

FIGURE 5 AP radiograph shows an osteochondritis dissecans lesion of the elbow. (Courtesy of Kevin G. Shea, MD, Stanford University Center.)

Surgical Management

For patients who do not respond to activity modifications and/or restrictions, surgical intervention may be necessary.[79,80] Larger lesions, including those that expand to involve the lateral wall and those with intra-articular loose bodies, may progress to surgery more frequently than small lesions (**Figure 7**). The authors of a 2011 study developed a staging system that may be helpful for the evaluation and management of this condition.[81] Most of the published series on OCD of the elbow represent level IV evidence, so surgical treatment recommendations must be understood in that context.[79,82]

Arthroscopic débridement with and without drilling has shown reasonable outcomes in shorter term follow-ups with this approach showing better outcomes for smaller lesions.[80,83-85] The authors of a 2017

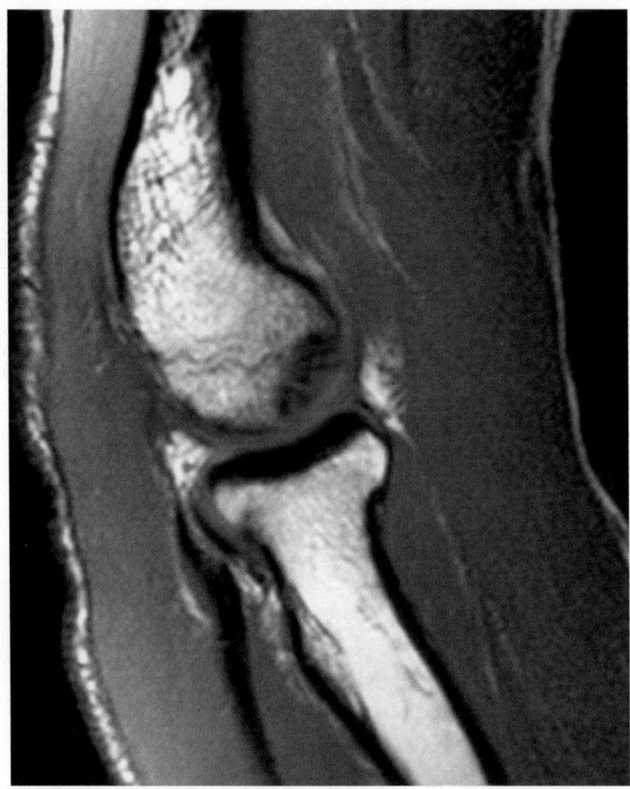

FIGURE 6 Sagittal magnetic resonance image shows osteochondritis dissecans of the elbow. (Courtesy of Kevin G. Shea, MD, Stanford University Center.)

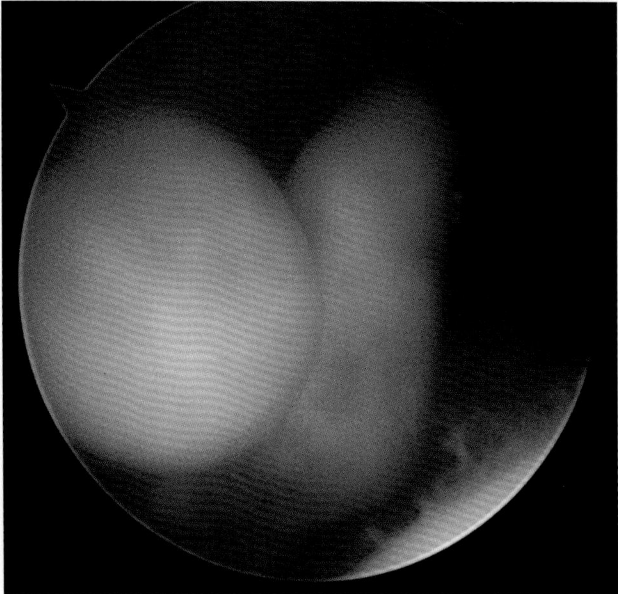

FIGURE 7 Arthroscopic view depicts osteochondritis dissecans of the elbow with intra-articular free bodies. (Courtesy of Kevin G. Shea, MD, Stanford University Center.)

study showed good short-term results, but only 62% returned to sports.[86] Larger, lateral, or uncontained lesions may have a worse prognosis than contained lesions.[70,87,88] Lesion fixation has been advocated for larger, unstable in situ lesions, with good short-term outcomes demonstrated.[89,90] Fixation can be performed using several different fixation devices through an arthroscopic or mini-open approach, depending on surgeon preference. To address large uncontained lesions, the harvest of osteochondral autografts from the knee and mosaicplasty procedures have been reported and shown a high rate of return to play (94%).[91-94] In addition, the authors of a 2018 study recently showed excellent clinical outcomes and return to sport using a costal (rib) osteochondral autograft reconstruction technique.[95] Accessing the joint to treat certain size lesions at some locations can be technically challenging, so novel techniques, including the use of oblique grafts, have been developed to address challenges with joint access.[96]

In addition, some investigators have looked for more localized areas within the elbow for local transplantation or osteochondral allograft[97] as opposed to distant sites such as the knee or rib[98-100] to avoid donor site morbidity.

SUMMARY

OCD of the knee and elbow continues to be a challenging disease process in regard to diagnosis, prognosis, and treatment. The goals of treatment, whether surgical or nonsurgical, are to resolve symptoms and retain as much normal bone and cartilage as possible at the lesion site. Multicenter prospective studies are needed to assess optimal outcomes and refine treatment algorithms.

KEY STUDY POINTS

- Radiographic evaluations are essential when diagnosing an OCD lesion of the knee and elbow; however, important aspects of the OCD lesions may be better seen with MRI. Diagnostic imaging modalities continue to evolve.
- Assessing the potential instability of an OCD lesion is key to early treatment.
- Surgical intervention should be considered for patients having unstable OCD lesions of the knee and elbow and/or OCD lesions that do not heal with nonsurgical treatment such as activity modification.
- Surgical management of OCD of the knee and elbow can involve drilling, fixation, or salvage techniques depending on the stability of the native fragment.

ANNOTATED REFERENCES

1. Edmonds EW, Shea KG: Osteochondritis dissecans: Editorial comment. *Clin Orthop Relat Res* 2013;471(4):1105-1106.
2. Chambers HG, Shea KG, Anderson AF, et al: American Academy of Orthopaedic Surgeons Clinical Practice Guideline on: The diagnosis and treatment of osteochondritis dissecans. *J Bone Joint Surg Am* 2012;94(14):1322-1324.
3. Kessler JI, Nikizad H, Shea KG, Jacobs JC Jr, Bebchuk JD, Weiss JM: The demographics and epidemiology of osteochondritis dissecans of the knee in children and adolescents. *Am J Sports Med* 2014;42(2):320-326.
4. Cooper T, Boyles A, Samora WP, Klingele KE: Prevalence of bilateral JOCD of the knee and associated risk factors. *J Pediatr Orthop* 2015;35(5):507-510.
5. Wall EJ, Heyworth BE, Shea KG, et al: Trochlear groove osteochondritis dissecans of the knee patellofemoral joint. *J Pediatr Orthop* 2014;34(6):625-630.
6. Backes JR, Durbin TC, Bentley JC, Klingele KE: Multifocal juvenile osteochondritis dissecans of the knee: A case series. *J Pediatr Orthop* 2014;34(4):453-458.
7. Weiss JM, Shea KG, Jacobs JC Jr, et al: Incidence of osteochondritis dissecans in adults. *Am J Sports Med* 2018;46(7):1592-1595.

   In this large epidemiologic study of OCD lesions in adults, the most common location for lesions was the ankle rather than the knee. Men had a higher incidence of lesions than women and were more likely to have a lateral femoral condyle lesion. Level of evidence: IV.
8. Takigami J, Hashimoto Y, Tomihara T, et al: Predictive factors for osteochondritis dissecans of the lateral femoral condyle concurrent with a discoid lateral meniscus. *Knee Surg Sports Traumatol Arthrosc* 2018;26(3):799-805.

   The authors report over a 15-year study period, 14.5% of patients with symptomatic discoid lateral meniscus also had a lateral femoral condyle OCD lesion. Males, younger patients (age 5 to 11 years), and type C meniscal shifts seen on MRI were risk factors for lateral condyle OCD. Level of evidence: III.
9. Yellin JL, Trocle A, Grant SF, Hakonarson H, Shea KG, Ganley TJ: Candidate loci are revealed by an initial genome-wide association study of juvenile osteochondritis dissecans. *J Pediatr Orthop* 2017;37(1):e32-e36.

   In this study, the authors found that multiple single-nucleotide polymorphisms may be associated with a genetic basis for OCD. Level of evidence: III.
10. Bruns J, Werner M, Soyka M: Is vitamin D insufficiency or deficiency related to the development of osteochondritis dissecans? *Knee Surg Sports Traumatol Arthrosc* 2016;24(5):1575-1579.

    In this review of mostly an adult population with OCD lesions, vitamin D_3 deficiency was associated with high-grade OCD lesions. Level of evidence: IV.
11. Olstad K, Ekman S, Carlson CS: An update on the pathogenesis of osteochondrosis. *Vet Pathol* 2015;52(5):785-802.
12. Toth F, Nissi MJ, Wang L, Ellermann JM, Carlson CS: Surgical induction, histological evaluation, and MRI identification of cartilage necrosis in the distal femur in goats to model early lesions of osteochondrosis. *Osteoarthritis Cartilage* 2015;23(2):300-307.
13. Bates JT, Jacobs JC Jr, Shea KG, Oxford JT: Emerging genetic basis of osteochondritis dissecans. *Clin Sports Med* 2014;33(2):199-220.
14. Toth F, Nissi MJ, Ellermann JM, et al: Novel application of magnetic resonance imaging demonstrates characteristic differences in vasculature at predilection sites of osteochondritis dissecans. *Am J Sports Med* 2015;43(10):2522-2527.
15. Olstad K, Shea KG, Cannamela PC, et al: Juvenile osteochondritis dissecans of the knee is a result of failure of the blood supply to growth cartilage and osteochondrosis. *Osteoarthritis Cartilage* 2018;26(12):1691-1698.

    Twenty-three pediatric cadaver knee specimens were evaluated using CT imaging and histologic analysis. Histologic changes in detected lesions were identical to osteochondrosis seen in animals and represented failure of epiphyseal cartilage canal blood supply with ischemic chondronecrosis. Level of evidence: V.
16. Cavaignac E, Perroncel G, Thepaut M, Vial J, Accadbled F, De Gauzy JS: Relationship between tibial spine size and the occurrence of osteochondritis dissecans: An argument in favour of the impingement theory. *Knee Surg Sports Traumatol Arthrosc* 2017;25(8):2442-2446.

    Patients 8 to 17 years of age with OCD were matched to a control group, and magnetic resonance comparative analysis of tibial spine and intercondylar notch heights was performed. Authors found that patients with OCD had larger tibial spines, whereas intercondylar height was not statistically different from that in control group. Level of evidence: IV.
17. Price MJ, Tuca M, Nguyen J, et al: Juvenile osteochondritis dissecans of the trochlea: A cohort study of 34 trochlear lesions associated with sporting activities that load the patellofemoral joint. *J Pediatr Orthop* 2020;40(3):103-109.

    In a case-controlled comparison, the authors demonstrated that playing either basketball or soccer was statistically significant for the presence of a trochlear OCD lesion, suggesting repetitive patellofemoral loading may play a role in disease pathogenesis. Level of evidence: III.
18. McElroy MJ, Riley PM, Tepolt FA, Nasreddine AY, Kocher MS: Catcher's knee: Posterior femoral condyle juvenile osteochondritis dissecans in children and adolescents. *J Pediatr Orthop* 2018;38(8):410-417.

    The authors report in this case-control study, when comparing children and adolescent baseball/softball catchers with position players with OCD lesions, catchers presented at an earlier age and had more posterior femoral condylar involvement compared with noncatchers. Level of evidence: III.
19. Ishikawa M, Adachi N, Yoshikawa M, et al: Unique anatomic feature of the posterior cruciate ligament in knees associated with osteochondritis dissecans. *Orthop J Sports Med* 2016;4(5):2325967116648138.

This retrospective case-control study investigated the position of posterior cruciate ligament attachment and its relation to medial femoral condylar OCD lesions and found that on MRI, the posterior cruciate ligament footprint was more distal in patients with medial femoral condylar OCD. Level of evidence: III.

20. Conrad JM, Stanitski CL: Osteochondritis dissecans: Wilson's sign revisited. *Am J Sports Med* 2003;31(5):777-778.
21. Jacobi M, Wahl P, Bouaicha S, Jakob RP, Gautier E: Association between mechanical axis of the leg and osteochondritis dissecans of the knee: Radiographic study on 103 knees. *Am J Sports Med* 2010;38(7):1425-1428.
22. Wall EJ, Polousky JD, Shea KG, et al: Novel radiographic feature classification of knee osteochondritis dissecans: A multicenter reliability study. *Am J Sports Med* 2015;43(2):303-309.
23. Wall EJ, Milewski MD, Carey JL, et al: The reliability of assessing radiographic healing of osteochondritis dissecans of the knee. *Am J Sports Med* 2017;45(6):1370-1375.

    This multicenter study demonstrated excellent interrater and intrarater reliability when judging both overall healing of femoral condylar OCD lesions and on five specific features of healing (OCD boundary, sclerosis, size, shape, and ossification). Level of evidence: III.

24. Chow RM, Guzman MS, Dao Q: Intercondylar notch width as a risk factor for medial femoral condyle osteochondritis dissecans in skeletally immature patients. *J Pediatr Orthop* 2016;36(6):640-644.

    Thirty-five patients with medial femoral condyle OCD lesions were compared with matched control subjects. The authors found a substantially smaller notch width index in patients with OCD lesions. Level of evidence: III.

25. Wechter JF, Sikka RS, Alwan M, Nelson BJ, Tompkins M: Proximal tibial morphology and its correlation with osteochondritis dissecans of the knee. *Knee Surg Sports Traumatol Arthrosc* 2015;23(12):3717-3722.
26. Ellermann JM, Donald B, Rohr S, et al: Magnetic resonance imaging of osteochondritis dissecans: Validation study for the ICRS classification system. *Acad Radiol* 2016;23(6):724-729.

    In this retrospective case series, the authors show current limitations of the International Cartilage Repair Society classification system in predicting OCD lesion stability when comparing radiologist interpretation of stability and arthroscopic findings. They report a sensitivity, specificity, and accuracy of 70%, 81%, and 76%, respectively, with high interreader variability. Level of evidence: IV.

27. De Smet AA, Ilahi OA, Graf BK: Reassessment of the MR criteria for stability of osteochondritis dissecans in the knee and ankle. *Skeletal Radiol* 1996;25(2):159-163.
28. Kijowski R, Blankenbaker DG, Shinki K, Fine JP, Graf BK, De Smet AA: Juvenile versus adult osteochondritis dissecans of the knee: Appropriate MR imaging criteria for instability. *Radiology* 2008;248(2):571-578.
29. Chen CH, Liu YS, Chou PH, Hsieh CC, Wang CK: MR grading system of osteochondritis dissecans lesions: Comparison with arthroscopy. *Eur J Radiol* 2013;82(3):518-525.
30. Jungesblut OD, Berger-Groch J, Meenen NM, Stuecker R, Rupprecht M: Validity of ultrasound compared with magnetic resonance imaging in evaluation of osteochondritis dissecans of the distal femur in children. *Cartilage* 2019:1947603519828434.

    The authors demonstrate that ultrasonography can be an effective and less expensive technique for detecting and monitoring stage II to IV OCD lesions, but it has limitations of detecting stage I lesions as well as those close to the intercondylar notch or of the far posterior condyles. Level of evidence: V.

31. Wall EJ, Vourazeris J, Myer GD, et al: The healing potential of stable juvenile osteochondritis dissecans knee lesions. *J Bone Joint Surg Am* 2008;90(12):2655-2664.
32. Krause M, Hapfelmeier A, Moller M, Amling M, Bohndorf K, Meenen NM: Healing predictors of stable juvenile osteochondritis dissecans knee lesions after 6 and 12 months of nonoperative treatment. *Am J Sports Med* 2013;41(10):2384-2391.
33. Uppstrom TJ, Haskel JD, Gausden EB, et al: Reliability of predictive models for non-operative healing potential of stable juvenile osteochondritis dissecans knee lesions. *Knee* 2016;23(4):698-701.

    This study evaluated the reliability of predictive models for healing of stable juvenile OCD lesions with nonsurgical treatment. They demonstrated high interrater and intrarater reliability for both systems for lesion healing. Level of evidence: III.

34. Ananthaharan A, Randsborg PH: Epidemiology and patient-reported outcome after juvenile osteochondritis dissecans in the knee. *Knee* 2018;25(4):595-601.

    This retrospective review reported successful nonsurgical treatment of patients with grade I and II OCD lesions, whereas those with grade III and IV lesions had a fivefold increased risk of failing conservative management. Level of evidence: III.

35. Weiss JM, Nikizad H, Shea KG, et al: The incidence of surgery in osteochondritis dissecans in children and adolescents. *Orthop J Sports Med* 2016;4(3):2325967116635515.

    This database review from a large health system described that knees represented 58.5% of all joints requiring surgery for OCD lesion. They report 35.3% of all OCD lesions progressed to surgery. Patients aged 12 to 19 years with OCD lesions of the knee, elbow, and ankle were significantly at higher risk of progression to surgery compared with patients aged 6 to 11 years. Level of evidence: III.

36. Sanders TL, Pareek A, Johnson NR, et al: Nonoperative management of osteochondritis dissecans of the knee: Progression to osteoarthritis and arthroplasty at mean 13-year follow-up. *Orthop J Sports Med* 2017;5(7):2325967117704644.

    The authors report 15% of patients in this case series developed arthritis at an average 13 years from diagnosis, corresponding to a cumulative incidence of 30% at 35 years. Rate of arthroplasty was low, with a cumulative incidence of 8% at 35 years. Risk factors for developing arthritis included body mass index >25 kg/m^2 at time of diagnosis, patellar OCD lesion, and diagnosis as an adult. Level of evidence: IV.

37. Jacobs JC Jr, Archibald-Seiffer N, Grimm NL, Carey JL, Shea KG: A review of arthroscopic classification systems for osteochondritis dissecans of the knee. *Orthop Clin North Am* 2015;46(1):133-139.
38. Carey JL, Wall EJ, Grimm NL, et al, Research in OsteoChondritis of the Knee (ROCK) Group: Novel arthroscopic classification of osteochondritis dissecans of the knee: A multicenter reliability study. *Am J Sports Med* 2016;44(7):1694-1698.

    This multicenter study found excellent intraobserver and interobserver reliability for the Research in Osteochondritis of the Knee OCD knee arthroscopy classification system, a novel system used to assess lesion instability. Level of evidence: III.
39. Sanders TL, Pareek A, Obey MR, et al: High rate of osteoarthritis after osteochondritis dissecans fragment excision compared with surgical restoration at a mean 16-year follow-up. *Am J Sports Med* 2017;45(8):1799-1805.

    This retrospective cohort study looked at the rates of developing arthritis and need for arthroplasty in patients who underwent fragment excision, fragment preservation, or chondral defect grafting for femoral condylar OCD lesions. Mean follow-up was 16 years. The calculated cumulative incidence of arthritis at 30 years was 70% and 51% for fragment excision and preservation, respectively. The cumulative incidence of arthroplasty at 30 years was 32% and 11% for fragment excision and preservation, respectively. Body mass index >25 kg/m^2, older age at diagnosis, and fragment excision were predictive of osteoarthritis. Level of evidence: III.
40. Heyworth BE, Edmonds EW, Murnaghan ML, Kocher MS: Drilling techniques for osteochondritis dissecans. *Clin Sports Med* 2014;33(2):305-312.
41. Lee CS, Larsen CG, Marchwiany DA, Chudik SC: Extra-articular, intraepiphyseal drilling for osteochondritis dissecans of the knee: Characterization of a safe and reproducible surgical approach. *Orthop J Sports Med* 2019;7(2):2325967119830397.

    The authors of this descriptive anatomic characterization study describe two safe and reproducible tunnel approaches (one anterior and one posterior to the medial collateral ligament) for extra-articular, intraepiphyseal OCD drilling. Level of evidence: V.
42. Lykissas MG, Wall EJ, Nathan S: Retro-articular drilling and bone grafting of juvenile knee osteochondritis dissecans: A technical description. *Knee Surg Sports Traumatol Arthrosc* 2014;22(2):274-278.
43. Grimm NL, Ewing CK, Ganley TJ: The knee: Internal fixation techniques for osteochondritis dissecans. *Clin Sports Med* 2014;33(2):313-319.
44. Wu IT, Custers RJH, Desai VS, et al: Internal fixation of unstable osteochondritis dissecans: Do open growth plates improve healing rate? *Am J Sports Med* 2018;46(10):2394-2401.

    This multicenter, retrospective cohort study reports skeletally immature and mature patients heal at comparable rates after internal fixation for unstable OCD lesions, with comparable functional and subjective improvement postoperatively. They reported 76% of lesions healed at >2 years postoperatively. Lateral femoral condyle lesions were an independent risk factor for failure. Level of evidence: III.
45. Webb JE, Lewallen LW, Christophersen C, Krych AJ, McIntosh AL: Clinical outcome of internal fixation of unstable juvenile osteochondritis dissecans lesions of the knee. *Orthopedics* 2013;36(11):e1444-1449.
46. Camathias C, Gogus U, Hirschmann MT, et al: Implant failure after biodegradable screw fixation in osteochondritis dissecans of the knee in skeletally immature patients. *Arthroscopy* 2015;31(3):410-415.
47. Lintz F, Pujol N, Pandeirada C, Boisrenoult P, Beaufils P: Hybrid fixation: Evaluation of a novel technique in adult osteochondritis dissecans of the knee. *Knee Surg Sports Traumatol Arthrosc* 2011;19(4):568-571.
48. Gudas R, Kalesinskas RJ, Kimtys V, et al: A prospective randomized clinical study of mosaic osteochondral autologous transplantation versus microfracture for the treatment of osteochondral defects in the knee joint in young athletes. *Arthroscopy* 2005;21(9):1066-1075.
49. Perdisa F, Kon E, Sessa A, et al: Treatment of knee osteochondritis dissecans with a cell-free biomimetic osteochondral scaffold: Clinical and imaging findings at midterm follow-up. *Am J Sports Med* 2018;46(2):314-321.

    This case series demonstrates promising results in managing grade III to IV knee OCD lesions with cell-free osteochondral scaffold implantation, based on good functional and subjective scores, as well as with favorable MRI follow-up at 2 and 5 years postoperatively. Level of evidence: IV.
50. Gabusi E, Paolella F, Manferdini C, et al: Cartilage and bone serum biomarkers as novel tools for monitoring knee osteochondritis dissecans treated with osteochondral scaffold. *Biomed Res Int* 2018;2018:9275102.

    The authors followed serum biomarkers for cartilage and bone turnover in patients after implantation of biomimetic osteochondral scaffolds for knee OCD. They demonstrated increased cartilage and bone synthetic biomarkers postoperatively, which at 1 year were comparable to those of healthy subjects. The authors concluded that serum biomarkers can serve as a useful tool for monitoring OCD patients in follow up. Level of evidence: IV.
51. Nishimura A, Morita A, Fukuda A, Kato K, Sudo A: Functional recovery of the donor knee after autologous osteochondral transplantation for capitellar osteochondritis dissecans. *Am J Sports Med* 2011;39(4):838-842.
52. Chadli L, Cottalorda J, Delpont M, Mazeau P, Thouvenin Y, Louahem D: Autologous osteochondral mosaicplasty in osteochondritis dissecans of the patella in adolescents. *Int Orthop* 2017;41(1):197-202.

    Eight patellar OCD lesions were managed with autologous osteochondral mosaicplasty and produced significantly improved International Knee Documentation Committee, Lysholm, and Tegner activity scores with radiographic and

MRI findings demonstrating complete graft integration at an average follow-up of 28.6 months. Level of evidence: IV.

53. Chadli L, Steltzlen C, Beaufils P, Toanen C, Pujol N: Neither significant osteoarthritic changes nor deteriorating subjective outcomes occur after hybrid fixation of osteochondritis dissecans in the young adult. *Knee Surg Sports Traumatol Arthrosc* 2019;27(3):740-744.

    The authors of this case series demonstrate favorable mid-term results with hybrid (screw plus osteochondral graft) fixation, with all fragments stable at time of screw removal 3 months after surgery, good functional scores, and no significant osteoarthritic changes at mean 10-year follow-up. Level of evidence: IV.

54. Emmerson BC, Gortz S, Jamali AA, Chung C, Amiel D, Bugbee WD: Fresh osteochondral allografting in the treatment of osteochondritis dissecans of the femoral condyle. *Am J Sports Med* 2007;35(6):907-914.

55. Lyon R, Nissen C, Liu XC, Curtin B: Can fresh osteochondral allografts restore function in juveniles with osteochondritis dissecans of the knee? *Clin Orthop Relat Res* 2013;471(4):1166-1173.

56. Filardo G, Andriolo L, Soler F, et al: Treatment of unstable knee osteochondritis dissecans in the young adult: Results and limitations of surgical strategies–The advantages of allografts to address an osteochondral challenge. *Knee Surg Sports Traumatol Arthrosc* 2019;27(6):1726-1738.

    In this review, the authors summarize results and limitations of surgical strategies for treatment of unstable knee OCD lesions. Level of evidence: V.

57. Sadr KN, Pulido PA, McCauley JC, Bugbee WD: Osteochondral allograft transplantation in patients with osteochondritis dissecans of the knee. *Am J Sports Med* 2016;44(11):2870-2875.

    Osteochondral allograft transplantation was performed in 149 knees for type III or IV OCD lesions and demonstrated 95% and 93% OCA survivorship at 5 and 10 years, respectively. Twenty-three percent of patients underwent revision surgery, and graft failure occurred in 8% of patients. Level of evidence: IV.

58. Cotter EJ, Frank RM, Wang KC, et al: Clinical outcomes of osteochondral allograft transplantation for secondary treatment of osteochondritis dissecans of the knee in skeletally mature patients. *Arthroscopy* 2018;34(4):1105-1112.

    The authors of this case series report outcomes in 37 patients who underwent osteochondral allograft transplantation with an average of 7.29 years' follow-up. They demonstrate significant improvement in patient reported outcome measures, 81.8% return-to-sport rate, 5.1% failure rate, and 35.9% reoperation rate. Level of evidence: IV.

59. Roffi A, Andriolo L, Di Martino A, et al: Long-term results of matrix-assisted autologous chondrocyte transplantation combined with autologous bone grafting for the treatment of juvenile osteochondritis dissecans. *J Pediatr Orthop* 2020;40(2):e115-e121.

    The authors report significant improvement in clinical scores 10 years following matrix-assisted autologous chondrocyte transplantation combined with autologous bone grafting. They report a 16% failure rate, all occurring by 12 months postoperatively, with lesion size >3.5 cm and female sex being risk factors for failure. Level of evidence: IV.

60. Beck JJ, Sugimoto D, Micheli L: Sustained results in long-term follow-up of autologous chondrocyte implantation (ACI) for distal femur juvenile osteochondritis dissecans (JOCD). *Adv Orthop* 2018;2018:7912975.

    Ten patients underwent ACI for distal femoral OCD at an average age of 18 years, with average lesion size of 9 cm^2. Patient-reported outcomes at 12 years were favorable. The authors note treatment for knee symptoms was required for all patients at some point after ACI. Level of evidence: IV.

61. Kessler JI, Jacobs JC Jr, Cannamela PC, Weiss JM, Shea KG: Demographics and epidemiology of osteochondritis dissecans of the elbow among children and adolescents. *Orthop J Sports Med* 2018;6(12):2325967118815846.

    In this review of the Kaiser Permanente database, 37 pediatric patients with elbow OCD were studied. Males had 7 times risk of elbow OCD compared with females, and the older adolescents (12 to 19 years old) had 22 times the risk of elbow OCD compared with younger patients. Level of evidence: III.

62. Kessler JI, Jacobs JC Jr, Cannamela PC, Shea KG, Weiss JM: Childhood obesity is associated with osteochondritis dissecans of the knee, ankle, and elbow in children and adolescents. *J Pediatr Orthop* 2018;38(5):e296-e299.

    In this review of the Kaiser Permanente database, 269 pediatric patients with OCD were reviewed. Extreme obesity based on body mass index for age was strongly associated with an increased risk of OCD of the elbow and ankle. Level of evidence: IV.

63. Kida Y, Morihara T, Kotoura Y, et al: Prevalence and clinical characteristics of osteochondritis dissecans of the humeral capitellum among adolescent baseball players. *Am J Sports Med* 2014;42(8):1963-1971.

64. Dexel J, Marschner K, Beck H, et al: Comparative study of elbow disorders in young high-performance gymnasts. *Int J Sports Med* 2014;35(11):960-965.

65. Matsuura T, Iwame T, Suzue N, et al: Cumulative incidence of osteochondritis dissecans of the capitellum in preadolescent baseball players. *Arthroscopy* 2019;35(1):60-66.

    In this Japanese study, 1,275 pediatric baseball players were screened over 1 year to determine the incidence of capitellar OCD. The cumulative incidence of capitellar OCD was 1.8%, and players aged 10 to 11 years were almost four times more likely to have a capitellar OCD than younger players (6- to 9-year-olds). Level of evidence: III.

66. van den Ende KI, McIntosh AL, Adams JE, Steinmann SP: Osteochondritis dissecans of the capitellum: A review of the literature and a distal ulnar portal. *Arthroscopy* 2011;27(1):122-128.

67. Nissen CW: Osteochondritis dissecans of the elbow. *Clin Sports Med* 2014;33(2):251-265.

68. Claessen FM, Louwerens JK, Doornberg JN, van Dijk CN, Eygendaal D, van den Bekerom MP: Panner's disease: Literature review and treatment recommendations. *J Child Orthop* 2015;9(1):9-17.

69. Ruchelsman DE, Hall MP, Youm T: Osteochondritis dissecans of the capitellum: Current concepts. *J Am Acad Orthop Surg* 2010;18(9):557-567.

70. Shi LL, Bae DS, Kocher MS, Micheli LJ, Waters PM: Contained versus uncontained lesions in juvenile elbow osteochondritis dissecans. *J Pediatr Orthop* 2012;32(3):221-225.

71. Cheng C, Milewski MD, Nepple JJ, Reuman HS, Nissen CW: Predictive role of symptom duration before the initial clinical presentation of adolescents with capitellar osteochondritis dissecans on preoperative and postoperative measures: A systematic review. *Orthop J Sports Med* 2019;7(2):2325967118825059.

In this systematic review of the literature, the effects of symptom duration before presentation were analyzed in elbow OCD. Advanced OCD lesions were observed in patients with a longer symptom duration. Level of evidence: IV.

72. Kajiyama S, Muroi S, Sugaya H, et al: Osteochondritis dissecans of the humeral capitellum in young athletes: Comparison between baseball players and gymnasts. *Orthop J Sports Med* 2017;5(3):2325967117692513.

In this study, capitellar OCD radiographic characteristics were compared between baseball players and gymnasts. Baseball players had more anteriorly located lesions than gymnasts. The AP radiograph with the elbow in 45° of flexion was thought to be most appropriate for baseball players. Level of evidence: III.

73. Zbojniewicz AM, Laor T: Imaging of osteochondritis dissecans. *Clin Sports Med* 2014;33(2):221-250.

74. Wu M, Eisenberg K, Williams K, Bae DS: Radial head changes in osteochondritis dissecans of the humeral capitellum. *Orthop J Sports Med* 2018;6(4):2325967118769059.

In this study from Boston Children's Hospital, radial head lesions were seen in 30% of elbows with capitellar OCD. The lesions were in the anterior aspect of the radial head predominately in patients with more advanced capitellar lesions. Level of evidence: II.

75. Jarrett DY, Walters MM, Kleinman PK: Prevalence of capitellar osteochondritis dissecans in children with chronic radial head subluxation and dislocation. *AJR Am J Roentgenol* 2016;206(6):1329-1334.

This study examines the prevalence of OCD in patients with chronic radial head subluxation/dislocation and found a much higher percentage of patients with radial head subluxation having a capitellar OCD (33.3%) versus 1.6% in patients with dislocation. Level of evidence: III.

76. Yang TH, Lee YY, Huang CC, et al: Effectiveness of ultrasonography screening and risk factor analysis of capitellar osteochondritis dissecans in adolescent baseball players. *J Shoulder Elbow Surg* 2018;27(11):2038-2044.

This study examines the effectiveness of ultrasonography versus MRI to detect capitellar OCD lesions in adolescent baseball players in Taiwan. Ultrasonography was most useful for stage 2 and higher stage OCD lesions. Resting elbow pain, lower body height, and age at introduction to baseball were predictors of capitellar OCD prevalence. Level of evidence: III.

77. Niu EL, Tepolt FA, Bae DS, Lebrun DG, Kocher MS: Nonoperative management of stable pediatric osteochondritis dissecans of the capitellum: Predictors of treatment success. *J Shoulder Elbow Surg* 2018;27(11):2030-2037.

In this study of stable OCD lesions of the capitellum, the authors find that smaller lesions, Hefti stage I lesions, and those without a cystlike lesion were more likely to heal with conservative treatment. Level of evidence: II.

78. Funakoshi T, Furushima K, Miyamoto A, Kusano H, Horiuchi Y, Itoh Y: Predictors of unsuccessful nonoperative management of capitellar osteochondritis dissecans. *Am J Sports Med* 2019;47(11):2691-2698.

In this Japanese study, 22 mosaicplasty for capitellar OCD cases were reviewed and compared between centrally and laterally located lesions. Lateral lesions were larger than central lesions and had more radial head changes. Clinical outcomes were satisfactory for both locations. Level of evidence: II.

79. de Graaff F, Krijnen MR, Poolman RW, Willems WJ: Arthroscopic surgery in athletes with osteochondritis dissecans of the elbow. *Arthroscopy* 2011;27(7):986-993.

80. Lewine EB, Miller PE, Micheli LJ, Waters PM, Bae DS: Early results of drilling and/or microfracture for grade IV osteochondritis dissecans of the capitellum. *J Pediatr Orthop* 2016;36(8):803-809.

At a minimum follow-up of 2 years, approximately 70% of patients who underwent fragment removal and microfracture for grade IV capitellar OCD lesions demonstrated improvement, which was identified as no further tenderness in the joint or resolution of bony edema on MRI. Level of evidence: IV.

81. Ahmad CS, Vitale MA, ElAttrache NS: Elbow arthroscopy: Capitellar osteochondritis dissecans and radiocapitellar plica. *Instr Course Lect* 2011;60:181-190.

82. Chen NC: Osteochondritis dissecans of the elbow. *J Hand Surg Am* 2010;35(7):1188-1189.

83. Arai Y, Hara K, Fujiwara H, Minami G, Nakagawa S, Kubo T: A new arthroscopic-assisted drilling method through the radius in a distal-to-proximal direction for osteochondritis dissecans of the elbow. *Arthroscopy* 2008;24(2):237.e1-237.e4.

84. Ueda Y, Sugaya H, Takahashi N, et al: Arthroscopic fragment resection for capitellar osteochondritis dissecans in adolescent athletes: 5- to 12-year follow-up. *Orthop J Sports Med* 2017;5(12):2325967117744537.

In this case series, midterm to long-term functional outcomes and radiographic changes of 38 patients with skeletally immature elbows who underwent arthroscopic resection for capitellar OCD were observed. Clinical outcomes were excellent in elbows with small lesions and acceptable in elbows with larger lesions. Level of evidence: IV.

85. Bexkens R, van Bergen CJA, van den Bekerom MPJ, Kerkhoffs G, Eygendaal D: Decreased defect size and partial restoration of subchondral bone on computed tomography after arthroscopic debridement and microfracture for osteochondritis dissecans of the capitellum. *Am J Sports Med* 2018;46(12):2954-2959.

    In this case series, defect size changes and subchondral bone healing were analyzed with CT in 67 patients who underwent arthroscopic débridement and microfracture for advanced capitellar OCD. This surgical technique improved defect size at a mean follow-up of 29 months. However, imaging findings did not correlate with clinical outcomes. Level of evidence: IV.

86. Bexkens R, van den Ende KIM, Ogink PT, van Bergen CJA, van den Bekerom MPJ, Eygendaal D: Clinical outcome after arthroscopic debridement and microfracture for osteochondritis dissecans of the capitellum. *Am J Sports Med* 2017;45(10):2312-2318.

    In this study, the clinical outcomes of 77 patients who underwent arthroscopic débridement and microfracture, and loose body removal if needed, for advanced capitellar OCD were evaluated. This surgical technique provided good clinical results, particularly in patients with shorter duration of symptoms, open epiphyseal plates, and loose body removal. Level of evidence: IV.

87. Yamagami N, Yamamoto S, Aoki A, Ito S, Uchio Y: Outcomes of surgical treatment for osteochondritis dissecans of the elbow: Evaluation by lesion location. *J Shoulder Elbow Surg* 2018;27(12):2262-2270.

    In this Japanese study, 30 male athletes who underwent surgical treatment for advanced elbow OCD were observed for over a year. Osteochondral autograft transplantation demonstrated favorable outcomes in central and lateral localized elbow OCD lesions. Level of evidence: III.

88. Matsuura T, Hashimoto Y, Nishino K, Nishida Y, Takahashi S, Shimada N: Comparison of clinical and radiographic outcomes between central and lateral lesions after osteochondral autograft transplantation for osteochondritis dissecans of the humeral capitellum. *Am J Sports Med* 2017;45(14):3331-3339.

    This retrospective cohort study compared the clinical outcomes of 87 patients who underwent osteochondral autograft transplantation (OAT) for either lateral or central elbow OCD lesions. Clinical and radiographic outcomes were superior in patients who underwent OAT for central lesions. However, satisfactory outcomes were seen in lateral lesions. Level of evidence: III.

89. Hennrikus WP, Miller PE, Micheli LJ, et al: Internal fixation of unstable in situ osteochondritis dissecans lesions of the capitellum. *J Pediatr Orthop* 2015;35:467-473.

90. Uchida S, Utsunomiya H, Taketa T, et al: Arthroscopic fragment fixation using hydroxyapatite/poly-L-lactate acid thread pins for treating elbow osteochondritis dissecans. *Am J Sports Med* 2015;43(5):1057-1065.

91. Iwasaki N, Kato H, Ishikawa J, Masuko T, Funakoshi T, Minami A: Autologous osteochondral mosaicplasty for osteochondritis dissecans of the elbow in teenage athletes. *J Bone Joint Surg Am* 2009;91(10):2359-2366.

92. Lyons ML, Werner BC, Gluck JS, et al: Osteochondral autograft plug transfer for treatment of osteochondritis dissecans of the capitellum in adolescent athletes. *J Shoulder Elbow Surg* 2015;24(7):1098-1105.

93. Bae DS, Ingall EM, Miller PE, Eisenberg K: Early results of single-plug autologous osteochondral grafting for osteochondritis dissecans of the capitellum in adolescents. *J Pediatr Orthop* 2020;40(2):78-85.

    This case series evaluated 28 patients with unstable elbow OCD who were surgically treated with single-plug OATS. This surgical technique is safe and effective in improving elbow function and pain with a high rate of return to sports and minimal donor site morbidity. Level of evidence: IV.

94. Funakoshi T, Momma D, Matsui Y, et al: Autologous osteochondral mosaicplasty for centrally and laterally located, advanced capitellar osteochondritis dissecans in teenage athletes: Clinical outcomes, radiography, and magnetic resonance imaging findings. *Am J Sports Med* 2018;46(8):1943-1951.

    This case series evaluated the efficacy of mosaicplasty in 22 teenage athletes through the use of clinical scores and imaging. Postoperative clinical scores improved significantly from preoperative scores. Radiography demonstrated complete graft incorporation and absence of severe osteoarthritic changes in all cases. Mosaicplasty resulted in satisfactory clinical and imaging outcomes in teenage athletes with OCD of the humeral capitellum. Level of evidence: IV.

95. Sato K, Iwamoto T, Matsumura N, et al: Costal osteochondral autograft for advanced osteochondritis dissecans of the humeral capitellum in adolescent and young adult athletes: Clinical outcomes with a mean follow-up of 4.8 years. *J Bone Joint Surg Am* 2018;100(11):903-913.

    This study examined long-term clinical outcomes in 72 patients who underwent costal osteochondral grafting for treatment of severe capitellum OCD. This technique efficaciously achieved anatomic and biologic reconstruction in management of capitellum OCD. Level of evidence: IV.

96. Miyamoto W, Yamamoto S, Kii R, Uchio Y: Oblique osteochondral plugs transplantation technique for osteochondritis dissecans of the elbow joint. *Knee Surg Sports Traumatol Arthrosc* 2009;17(2):204-208.

97. Mirzayan R, Lim MJ: Fresh osteochondral allograft transplantation for osteochondritis dissecans of the capitellum in baseball players. *J Shoulder Elbow Surg* 2016;25(11):1839-1847.

    The authors described fresh osteochondral allograft transplantation to manage capitellum OCD in nine male baseball players. All nine players returned to playing baseball following surgery. Fresh osteochondral allograft transplantation for capitellum OCD is a viable treatment option that restores function and improves pain in throwers. Level of evidence: IV.

98. Bexkens R, van den Bekerom MPJ, Eygendaal D, Oh LS, Doornberg JN: Topographic analysis of 2 alternative donor sites of the ipsilateral elbow in the treatment of capitellar osteochondritis dissecans. *Arthroscopy* 2018;34(7):2087-2093.

This retrospective study investigated the use of two alternative donor sites: the nonarticulating part of the radial head and the lateral olecranon tip, of the ipsilateral elbow for capitellar autologous transplantation. There is a less than a 0.2 mm difference in the topographic subchondral bone match between the four common lesion locations and the two proposed alternative donor sites. This suggests that the proposed donor sites may have potential as a donor source in the management of capitellar OCD. Level of evidence: III.

99. Shimada K, Temporin K, Oura K, Tanaka H, Noguchi R: Anconeus muscle-pedicle bone graft with periosteal coverage for osteochondritis dissecans of the humeral capitellum. *Orthop J Sports Med* 2017;5(9):2325967117727531.

In this case series, a treatment algorithm for advanced osteochondritis dissecans was established by determining the utilization of and problems associated with anconeus muscle–pedicle bone graft with periosteal coverage (ABGP). Sixteen patients with moderately sized capitellar OCD lesions were treated with ABGP. All but one patient had improvement within 6 months after undergoing ABGP. This surgical procedure is a useful treatment option for moderately sized capitellar OCD lesions. Level of evidence: IV.

100. Oshiba H, Itsubo T, Ikegami S, Nakamura K, Uchiyama S, Kato H: Results of bone peg grafting for capitellar osteochondritis dissecans in adolescent baseball players. *Am J Sports Med* 2016;44(12):3171-3178.

This study investigated the use of bone peg grafting in 11 male baseball players with early stage capitellar OCD lesions. Ninety-one percent of the patients returned to preoperative baseball ability levels within 12 months after undergoing bone peg grafting. Level of evidence: IV.

CHAPTER 52

Shoulder Injuries

NATASHA TRENTACOSTA, MD • J. LEE PACE, MD

ABSTRACT

With increasing participation of children and adolescents in organized sports and early specialization in a single sport, the risk of shoulder injuries in young athletes will continue to increase. Children and adolescents experience acute traumatic injuries to the shoulder during practice and competition, and chronic overuse injuries occur secondary to the repetitive shoulder motions required in sports, such as baseball, swimming, and racquet sports. The unique nature of the pediatric shoulder requires a different diagnostic, prognostic, and treatment approach to shoulder injuries than that needed in adult patients.

Keywords: overuse injuries; shoulder injuries; shoulder trauma; sports injuries

INTRODUCTION

Shoulder injuries in athletic children and adolescents are likely to continue to increase as this population increases their participation in organized sports, focuses on a single sport throughout the year without cross training, and achieves higher levels of competitive play. Although lower extremity injuries are seen more commonly, children involved in sports, such as tennis, baseball, judo, gymnastics, and snowboarding, are more likely to sustain upper extremity injuries.[1] A 2014 study found 2.15 shoulder injuries per 10,000 athlete exposures in high school students, with the highest rates seen in football, wrestling, and baseball.[2] An investigation using a national emergency department database found shoulder injuries to encompass 16.2% of all injuries presenting in the past 10 years.[3] The shoulders of children and adolescents are subject to acute traumatic athletic injuries as well as chronic overuse injuries resulting from participation in overhead sports. Some injury patterns are different than that seen in their adult counterparts, whereas others can be similar. Early recognition of these injuries and proper management may help avoid long-term disability.

Dr. Pace or an immediate family member is a member of a speakers' bureau or has made paid presentations on behalf of Arthrex, Inc.; serves as a paid consultant to or is an employee of Arthrex, Inc. and Grand Rounds, Inc.; has received research or institutional support from Arthrex, Inc.; and serves as a board member, owner, officer, or committee member of the American Orthopaedic Society for Sports Medicine, the Pediatric Orthopaedic Society of North America, and the Pediatric Research in Sports Medicine. Neither Dr. Trentacosta nor any immediate family member has received anything of value from or has stock or stock options held in a commercial company or institution related directly or indirectly to the subject of this chapter.

SHOULDER ANATOMY

The shoulder complex encompasses a group of joints that act in concert to provide mobility and function to the upper extremity. The four joints that work in a coordinated manner are the glenohumeral, sternoclavicular, acromioclavicular, and scapulothoracic joints. Although not a true joint, the scapulothoracic articulation results from the concave nature of the anterior scapula gliding over the convex posterior thorax to provide stability and motion to the shoulder complex, and this articulation is an important component in the propagation of the kinetic chain of energy.

The presence of epiphyseal plates and the altered collagen composition of the shoulder ligaments and tendons define the pediatric shoulder and predispose it to injury patterns dissimilar to those seen in adults. The three main ossification centers in the proximal humeral epiphysis are the humeral head, the greater tuberosity, and the lesser tuberosity (**Figure 1**). The tuberosities fuse to the

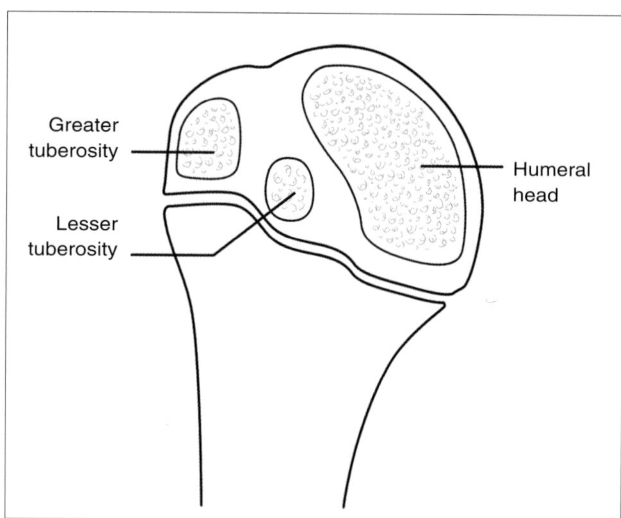

FIGURE 1 Illustration demonstrating the centers of ossification in the proximal humerus. The ossification center of the humeral head is typically identified after age 6 months. The ossification centers of the greater tuberosity and lesser tuberosity are identified by age 7 months to 3 years and by age 2 to 5 years, respectively.

humeral head at approximately 13 years of age, whereas the humeral epiphysis fuses to the diaphysis near the age of 17 years.[4] The three ossification centers of the clavicle are the lateral epiphysis, the medial epiphysis, and the diaphysis. The clavicle is unique in that the epiphyses both ossify and fuse very late in adolescence. The lateral epiphysis often appears at approximately 18 years of age and rapidly fuses within 1 year. The medial epiphysis also appears near the age of 18 years, but it may not completely fuse until 25 years of age. The cartilage of the physis represents a weak link that makes it susceptible to injury, particularly just before skeletal maturity.[5]

Much of the stability of the shoulder complex arises from the soft-tissue structures. The glenohumeral joint has both static and dynamic stabilizers. The static stabilizers include the glenohumeral capsule, labrum, and glenohumeral ligaments. The dynamic stabilizers include the rotator cuff muscles, the long head of the biceps, the deltoid muscle, and the other scapulothoracic muscles. The sternoclavicular joint is stabilized by the anterior and posterior sternoclavicular ligaments, the costoclavicular ligament, and the interclavicular ligament. The acromioclavicular joint is predominantly stabilized by the coracoclavicular ligaments, with contributions from the joint capsule and acromioclavicular ligament.

KINETIC CHAIN MECHANICS

Overhead sports, including baseball, swimming, racquet sports, and volleyball, rely on the coordinated generation and transfer of energy from the lower extremities through the hips, torso, and upper extremities. The kinetic chain is a sophisticated chain of muscle contractions that allows for efficient energy transfer and prepares the body to withstand the muscle imbalances generated by the act of the overhead motion. The kinetic chain generates tremendous force and control during various athletic overhead motions. The disruption of any part of this mechanism can lead to poor performance and may ultimately predispose the athlete to injury. Knowledge and evaluation of the kinetic chain in the overhead athlete will aid in the diagnosis and management of many shoulder injuries. Typically, an abnormality in the chain results in either a slower velocity at the distal end of the mechanism or an overcompensation of the distal segment in an attempt to maintain a certain velocity despite a disruption earlier in the chain. The area that overcompensates is often the area that becomes injured because excessive forces are concentrated in that area.

PATIENT EVALUATION

History

As with any injury presentation, a thorough history and physical examination are imperative to the diagnosis and treatment of shoulder injuries in a young athlete. The athlete's sport and position as well as the mechanism of injury are important considerations. Most injuries sustained to the shoulder during football are a result of direct trauma. Because spearing has been outlawed in football, more shoulder injuries are possible as more focus has been placed on shoulder-body contact for tackling. Judo has a substantially higher proportion of shoulder injuries caused by throwing, flipping, and falling compared with other martial arts disciplines, such as karate and taekwondo.[6] Higher injury rates are seen with higher levels of contact and, interestingly, the amount of protective equipment worn in male athletes playing hockey and lacrosse.[7] Among high school baseball players, especially pitchers, the shoulder is the most common site of injury, with muscle strains being the most predominant injury.[8,9]

Knowledge of an athlete's training is helpful because unsound practices and abrupt changes may lead to overuse injuries. For throwing athletes, knowledge of the number and types of pitches per week is important. The patient's growth history should be assessed because peak growth velocity is a risk factor for injury. The passive elongation of soft tissues over actively elongating bone leads to temporary inflexibility, muscle imbalance, and an increased risk of injury. A history of joint laxity should be ascertained in patients presenting with instability symptoms.

Physical Examination

A focused musculoskeletal examination can provide more objective measures to aid in the diagnosis of shoulder pain. The range of motion should be assessed in overhead athletes and a comparison made with the contralateral side to check for differences. Stability should be assessed in both traumatic and atraumatic situations. Muscle atrophy may be a sign of nerve impingement disorders. Provocative impingement tests are important to assess for subacromial bursitis and impingement as well as rotator cuff strength. Biceps strength and irritability could indicate superior labral pathology. Dynamic examination of the scapula is also imperative when evaluating scapular dyskinesis or winging.

Given the proximity of neurovascular structures to many of the bony structures of the shoulder girdle, a careful examination of neurovascular status is warranted in all patients with suspected fractures and brachial plexus injuries. Traction to the brachial plexus can produce radicular pain into the arm and hand after a shoulder tackle in football. Open fractures and those that could cause neurovascular injury should be attended to immediately.

Imaging

Appropriate imaging is undertaken after the history is obtained and the physical examination is completed. When dealing with traumatic bony injuries to the shoulder, radiography often reveals the pathology. Pathologic bone lesions may be found incidentally in patients who have a fracture through a weak bone lesion. Advanced imaging techniques, such as MRI, are usually needed to detect soft-tissue injuries and often an MRI arthrogram is needed to detect subtle labral pathology. These imaging modalities are typically reserved for patients with suspected surgical pathology or pain that does not resolve with a course of conservative management. A CT scan of the sternoclavicular joint is important when a dislocation of the sternoclavicular joint is suspected.

TRAUMATIC SHOULDER INJURIES

Patients with a traumatic shoulder injury often report a single event or an acute event superimposed on a history of overuse. These injuries often occur in contact sports, such as football, basketball, hockey, and wrestling.

Sprains and Strains

Sprains and strains account for approximately 38% of all shoulder injuries seen in high school athletes.[2] Injuries may occur to the acromioclavicular joint, the sternoclavicular joint, or about the glenohumeral joint as a result of direct trauma or a fall onto an outstretched arm, which often leads to bony injuries in younger adolescent athletes and sprains in older adolescent athletes.

Injuries to the acromioclavicular joint may involve a sprain to the supporting ligaments or result in a distal clavicle fracture. For diagnosis and treatment, radiographic evaluation, including standard shoulder views as well as Zanca views, is needed. Most acromioclavicular injuries are successfully managed with nonsurgical methods, with the arm placed in a sling followed by physical therapy. Surgical intervention is reserved for patients with advanced injuries.

Similarly, trauma to the sternoclavicular joint can cause ligamentous injury or, in severe cases, the medial clavicle may dislocate or fracture through the physis. Dislocations can be either anterior or posterior, depending on the mechanism of injury. These injuries should be suspected in children with trauma to the chest region so that a posterior dislocation or physeal injury is not missed; a serendipity radiographic view (40° cephalic tilt view of sternoclavicular joint) or CT scan is often required to make the diagnosis. Closed management of anterior dislocations can often achieve success without complications. Historically, posterior sternoclavicular dislocations have been thought to be stable following closed reduction, requiring surgical intervention only for recurrent or symptomatic dislocations. The authors of a 2014 study reported more failed closed reductions with sternoclavicular joint dislocations versus physeal fractures.[10] It was also found that posterior sternoclavicular joint dislocation and medial clavicular physeal fractures occur with nearly equivalent frequency in patients with open medial physes, although differentiation of such is often unreliable based on radiography and CT because of the late ossification and fusion of the medial clavicle epiphysis. Open stabilization procedures with consultation of a thoracic surgeon are currently being advocated because of this increased recognition of recurrent instability, difficulty of differentiation from physeal fractures, increased reports of mediastinal complications, and consistently good surgical outcomes.

Insertional Injuries and Avulsion Fractures

Acute fractures to the shoulder are uncommon in the pediatric and adolescent cohorts, with the exception of midshaft clavicle fractures. Participation in certain sports predisposes participants to fractures of the shoulder. A large number of fractures occur in children who are horseback riders, with nearly two-thirds of these fractures occurring in the upper extremity (particularly the proximal humerus).[11] In martial arts, nearly 50% of the injuries seen in the shoulder region are fractures.[6]

An increasing number of insertional injuries and avulsion fractures are occurring as the result of poor training techniques. During puberty, the development of muscle mass increases in adolescents, whereas tendon and bony insertions remain weak and unable to absorb generated loads. Avulsion injuries can result from this developmental imbalance.

Subscapularis avulsion of the lesser tuberosity is an uncommon injury; however, several reports of acute and missed chronic cases exist in the literature.[12-20] The diagnosis of an avulsion of the lesser tuberosity may often be delayed because symptoms overlap those of other shoulder injuries, such as instability, physeal injury, or muscle strain. Clinical awareness of this condition will help ensure that a proper physical examination is performed and that radiographs are carefully evaluated to avoid missing an avulsion of the lesser tuberosity and preventing its potential sequelae of malunion, nonunion, impingement, instability, pain, or weakness. Although the size of a bony avulsion may vary, this injury is treated with surgical repair of the fragment and the subscapularis to the humerus.

Similarly, the coracoid is vulnerable to avulsion before fusion of the physis.[21] This injury often results from collisions in football. Given the amount of force required to sustain this type of injury, concurrent injuries may be seen. Treatment is often successful with nonsurgical measures.

Shoulder Instability

Shoulder instability includes the spectrum of injury ranging from subluxation to frank dislocations of the glenohumeral joint. The prevalence of glenohumeral dislocations in patients younger than 18 years is 31.0 per 100,000 person-years for males and 8.2 per 100,000 person-years for females.[22] These dislocations account for approximately 0.01% of all injuries in children, with most occurring in patients 10 years and older.[22-24] Similar to their adult counterparts, approximately 90% of shoulder dislocations are anterior traumatic dislocations that result from a fall onto an abducted, externally rotated arm.[25] Nearly 30% of upper extremity injuries involving the shoulder, mostly consisting of shoulder dislocations or sprains, result from skiing injuries.[26]

An accurate diagnosis and prompt treatment is necessary to identify any bony or labral pathology requiring surgical management and allow a quick return to play. MRI arthrogram is the preferred modality for identifying the hallmark imaging findings of a Hill-Sachs humeral impaction fracture and a Bankart lesion of the anterior inferior glenoid rim. Initial management of acute shoulder dislocations includes closed reduction under conscious sedation followed by postreduction immobilization.

The natural history of traumatic shoulder dislocation in patients younger than 20 years follows a course of recurrent instability and dislocation. Recurrent instability produces persistent symptoms that can interfere with sports participation and activities of daily living and may damage the articular cartilage of the glenoid fossa and humeral head. The rate of recurrent dislocation in patients with open physes varies widely in the literature, with reported rates ranging from 40% to 100%.[24,27-37]

A 2015 study examined a focused cohort of 10- to 16-year-old patients with shoulder dislocations and found that recurrent dislocation was substantially greater in those aged 14 to 16 years than in those 13 years or younger.[38] Similar results of lower dislocation rates in patients younger than 13 years were reported in an early study.[24] It has been hypothesized that the inherent laxity of the shoulder in children imparts more resiliency to structural damage than that seen in the shoulders of adolescents and adults.[24] The difference in recurrence rates may also be a reflection of the variation in the type of sport played and lower participation rates of children in contact sports. Those at risk for subsequent dislocations include adolescent boys and those participating in contact sports.[38-40]

It is important to differentiate whether a patient is able to voluntarily sublux or dislocate one or both shoulders in the absence of structural defects. Voluntary shoulder instability, though rare, may be seen in pediatric or adolescent athletes and accompanied with psychiatric comorbidities, as this unique ability may be used for secondary gain. Patients can use selective muscle contraction and relaxation to sublux or dislocate the shoulder. Treatment for voluntary shoulder instability is nonoperative consisting of skillful neglect along with a prolonged course of physical therapy working on core and periscapular strengthening. Any underlying psychiatric issues should be addressed as well through referral to psychiatry in order to be appropriately treated.

Definitive management for pediatric shoulder dislocations is controversial. Although many physicians choose definitive treatment with immobilization and physical therapy for adolescents older than 13 years with first-time dislocations, the higher rates of recurrent shoulder dislocations in this cohort warrant consideration of early surgical stabilization.[38,41,42] In a comparison of early arthroscopic intervention with nonsurgical treatment followed by delayed arthroscopic treatment in a pediatric cohort, the authors found that early surgical intervention was beneficial.[43] In clinical studies looking at shoulder dislocations in pediatric patients, up to 44% of the patients required surgical intervention.[22,31,44,45] Conversely, a high percentage of high school athletes with shoulder instability have been shown to achieve successful return to sport without missing any additional time for shoulder injury. In a recent series of 129 scholastic athletes, in which 97 athletes underwent nonsurgical management, 85% of athletes with shoulder instability were able to return to the same sport without injury for at least one full season.[46]

When surgery is necessary, arthroscopic treatment with little to no modification from adult techniques has become the standard treatment.[32] In a study of anterior surgical shoulder stabilization in high school and collegiate athletes, the authors reported an 11% dislocation rate in patients younger than 20 years.[47] In a 2010 study, no recurrences were reported in five of six patients between the ages of 11 and 15 years, who underwent surgical stabilization for posttraumatic shoulder instability.[48] A 2012 study of adolescents who underwent arthroscopic shoulder stabilization found that 81% of the patients returned to their preinjury sport; however, a 21% dislocation recurrence rate was reported, with higher rates seen in water polo and rugby players.[49] In young patients, risk factors for postsurgical failure include multiple preoperative dislocations, presence of a Hill-Sachs lesion, and glenoid bone loss greater than 13.5%.[50,51]

Multidirectional Instability

Multidirectional instability of the shoulder, which is characterized by involuntary or voluntary subluxation in any combination of anterior, inferior, and posterior directions, is a complex entity seen in a variety of young patients and is often characterized by pain. This pathologic laxity may result from repetitive microtrauma to the static stabilizers of the shoulder that create a large patulous inferior capsular pouch with a widened rotator interval, usually in conjunction with some predisposing laxity. The quality and quantity of collagen in patients with multidirectional instability has been shown to be reduced compared with those without this condition.[52] The physical examination may reveal hyperlaxity in other joints of the body and scapulothoracic dyskinesis.

A regimented rehabilitation program that focuses on strengthening the dynamic stabilizers of the shoulder is successful in more than 80% of these patients by compensating for the lack of passive stability and assists in active control of the shoulder.[53,54] Strengthening exercises start with the scapular stabilizers which are key in placing the glenohumeral joint in space and avoiding instability. Rotator cuff strengthening exercises are added to compensate for any neuromuscular control deficiency or asynchronous firing of the rotator cuff musculature. If pain and instability persists despite increasing core and periscapular strength testing after a least 6 months of regimented rehabilitation, arthroscopic management with capsulolabral shift with or without rotator interval closure may lead to improved outcomes.[55-59]

CHRONIC OVERUSE INJURIES

Overhead athletes involved in throwing, swimming, volleyball, gymnastics, and racquet sports often present with chronic shoulder pain secondary to repetitive microtrauma, which is generally referred to as an overuse injury. These injuries occur when training demands exceed the physiologic ability of an individual's body to compensate as submaximal forces are repetitively loaded on tissue causing microscopic tissue damage.[60,61] Children are at particular risk for overuse injuries because of their weaker physes and muscle imbalance. The adolescent growth spurt is a unique time in development that can make pediatric patients more susceptible to such injury. During the growth spurt, bone tends to be weaker because of slower bone mineralization compared with the rate of linear bone growth, the physeal cartilage tends to be weaker in general, the musculotendinous junction tightens as lengthening bones impart more tension, and coordination is lacking.[62-64]

Throwing athletes produce high levels of force throughout the upper extremity that lead to overuse of the stabilizing structures in an attempt to create a stable shoulder joint during the arc of motion. This force increases during the midteen to late teen years because of the increase in muscle development. Poor biomechanics and scapular dyskinesis along with excessive throwing contribute to the development of these common maladies. Overuse and noncontact injuries account for most shoulder injuries in baseball.[3]

Proper biomechanics, particularly core activation in the initiation of kinetic chain events, is important in preventing overuse injuries. A coordinated approach is needed among trainers, therapists, and physicians in assessing pitching mechanics in pediatric athletes. Since the mid 1990s, efforts have been undertaken to decrease the number of overuse injuries in pediatric throwing athletes by limiting pitch counts and mandating rest days between pitching appearances. Muscle fatigue from overuse can lead to poor dynamic stability and subsequent injury. Cross training in different seasons is also encouraged because it allows the body time to recover, which is not possible if a single sport is played throughout the year. A 2012 study found that youth league baseball coaches had poor knowledge of the current recommendations to prevent overuse injuries in pediatric pitchers.[65]

Little Leaguer's Shoulder

Commonly seen in pediatric baseball pitchers, Little Leaguer's shoulder (LLS) is considered a chronic torsional injury of the proximal humeral physis that can, in severe cases, resemble a Salter-Harris I injury. Poor throwing mechanics can produce a high level of external rotational torque on the proximal humeral physis. Almost one-third of patients with LLS have glenohumeral internal rotation deficit (GIRD), characterized by an altered glenohumeral rotational profile compared with the contralateral side.[66] LLS typically manifests as insidious shoulder pain (particularly in the follow-through phase of throwing) and limited range of motion. It is often seen in male pitchers between 11 and 13 years of age because this is the period of maximal physeal growth resulting in relatively weak physes. Those who throw curve balls, continue throwing through fatigue, are overweight, lift weights, and play on multiple teams are at increased risk for this overuse condition.[67] The repetitive stress of throwing produces radiographic physeal widening of the proximal humeral physis compared with the contralateral side. In patients with severe, untreated LLS, premature closure of the epiphyseal plate may occur and can lead to angular deformity. The diagnosis of this condition relies mainly on clinical assessment and can be supported by radiographic widening (**Figure 2**). Magnetic resonance image, although rarely needed in making the diagnosis, may show widening and edema within the proximal humeral physis.

The rehabilitation regimen for LLS is cessation of throwing activities for a minimum of 8 to 12 weeks followed by gradual rehabilitation of the shoulder and return to play. There is a graduated program that progresses from range of motion through strengthening, endurance, and speed, with stress on the importance of control and proper biomechanics. Prevention of injury is paramount and requires adherence to recommendations on pitch counts and rest days as well as maintenance of proper pitching biomechanics. An undiagnosed overuse injury can lead to chronic pain with throwing, shoulder instability, and degenerative arthritis.[68]

Glenohumeral Internal Rotation Deficit and Rotator Cuff Injury

GIRD is a shoulder syndrome commonly seen in pitchers and overhead athletes, such as swimmers and tennis players. It is defined by the objective loss of internal rotation compared with the contralateral side and results from derangements of the dynamic shoulder restraints. Repetitive microtrauma to the posterior capsule leads to scarring and contracture of the posteroinferior capsule with corresponding stretching of the anterior capsular structures resulting in a posterosuperior translation of the humeral head on the glenoid with combined external rotation and abduction of the shoulder. This can result in structural injury to the labrum or rotator cuff tendons. The changes in range of motion and resulting torsional stresses of overhead activities can lead to bony adaptations in the humerus, such as increased humeral head retroversion and, ultimately, alteration of the normal scapular and shoulder biomechanics. It may also lead to calcification or ossification of the joint capsule insertion on the posterior glenoid, known as a Bennett lesion, which may be asymptomatic or cause pain with throwing.

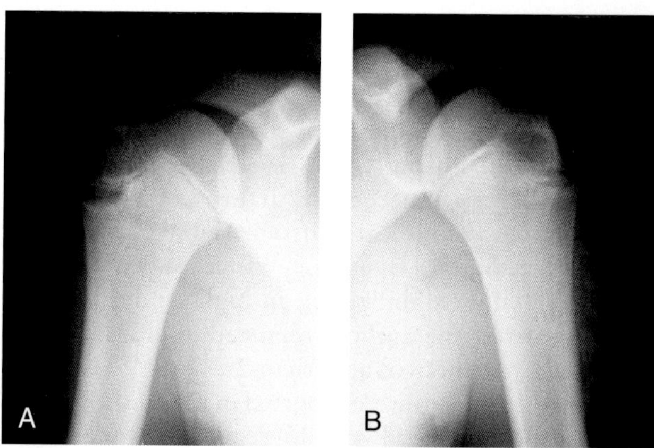

FIGURE 2 **A** and **B**, Comparison radiographs of Little Leaguer's shoulder and contralateral shoulder. External rotation AP comparison radiographs of the proximal humerus. Note the widening of the proximal humeral physis.

Posterior capsule stretching to decrease pain and the adaptive changes seen in throwing are integral to the treatment and prevention of GIRD. A strengthening program that focuses on the posterior shoulder muscles to counterbalance the stronger internal rotators of the shoulder helps treat and prevent shoulder pain in throwing athletes with GIRD. Often Bennett lesions are asymptomatic and treated conservatively, although large, painful lesions may require surgical débridement.

In children and adolescents, rotator cuff injury tends to be rare when compared with such injuries in adults, but rotator cuff tendinitis has been increasingly described in the adolescent population, particularly in swimmers, throwers, and racquetball and tennis players, and it often occurs with other intra-articular pathology, especially labral tears.[25,69-71] GIRD can lead to internal impingement of the rotator cuff tendon and subsequent rotator cuff injury. With internal impingement, the rotator cuff, labrum, and joint capsule are repetitively pinched between the greater tuberosity and superior glenoid rim at the extremes of abduction and external rotation, which occurs multiple times in overhead sports. It has been reported that frank tears of the rotator cuff, which were thought to occur only in adults, also exist in the pediatric population[72,73] (**Figure 3**).

High-performance swimmers experience high repetitive forces across the shoulder as a result of the multiple shoulder revolutions needed to propel their bodies long

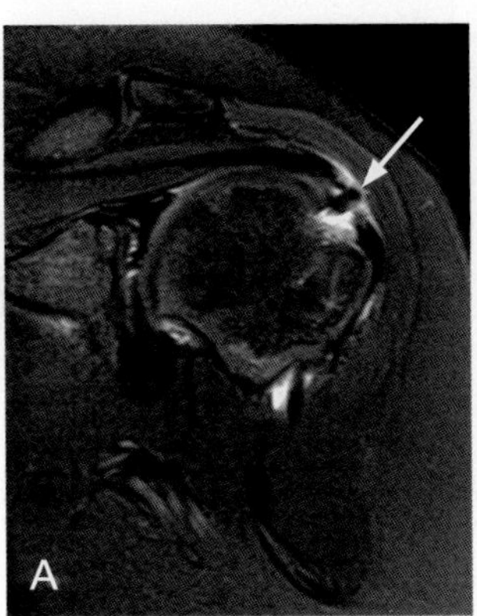

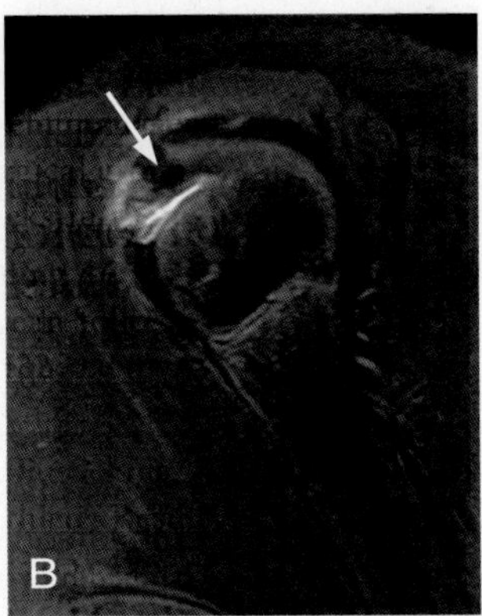

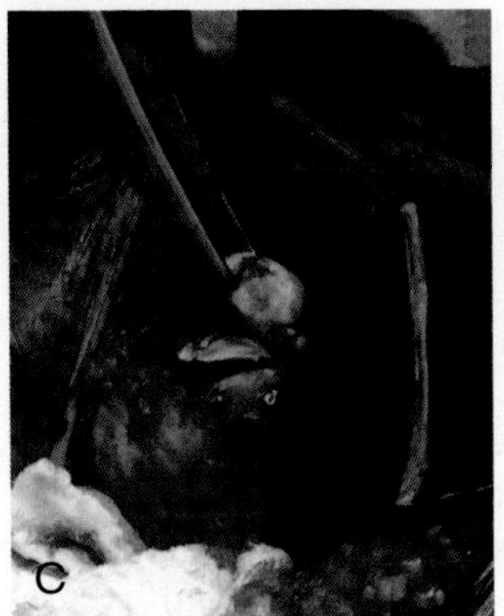

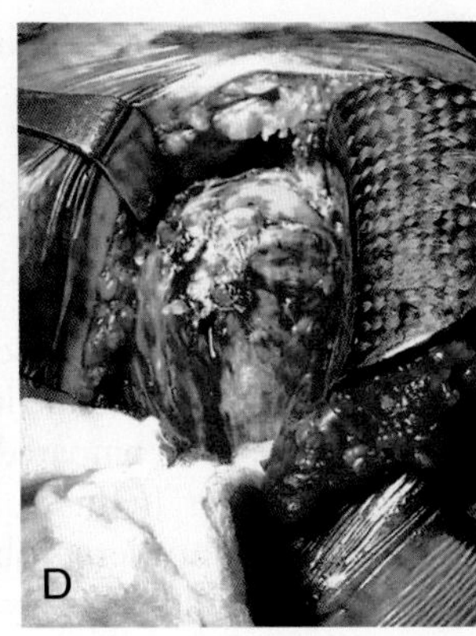

FIGURE 3 Magnetic resonance images and intraoperative photographs from a 12-year-old boy with rotator cuff tear. Four weeks after falling off a cargo net in gym class, he presented to the orthopaedic offices with an inability to lift his left arm. With normal radiograph, he was sent for an MRI of the left shoulder. Coronal T2-weighted (**A**) and sagittal T2-weighted (**B**) magnetic resonance images show a periosteal avulsion of the supraspinatus footprint in a patient with open epiphyseal plates. **C**, Through a deltopectoral approach, the avulsion of the supraspinatus footprint was identified with no bony component. **D**, An open rotator cuff repair with medial row fixation using suture anchors and lateral row soft-tissue fixation was accomplished. (Courtesy of Micah Lissy, MD, UHS Sports Medicine, Binghamton, NY.)

distances in the water. An increase in overuse shoulder injuries occurs in these swimmers, usually after the age of 10 years. A condition called swimmer's shoulder often develops in these athletes. This condition is an ill-defined overuse injury of the shoulder synonymous with rotator cuff tendinitis and impingement syndrome. It results in pain from impingement of the humeral head and rotator cuff on the coracoacromial ligament. Gymnasts also experience rotator cuff tendinitis, predominantly in the supraspinatus tendons.[74]

The treatment options for rotator cuff pathology tend to involve nonsurgical modalities, relying on a course of physical therapy. Surgical intervention may be considered if nonsurgical management is unsuccessful and symptoms and the presence of some degree of rotator cuff tear and/or persistent impingement persist; however, the results of surgical treatment are largely undetermined in the pediatric population.[70,75]

Superior Labrum Anterior and Posterior Tears

Although uncommon, superior labrum anterior and posterior (SLAP) tears can occur in the pediatric overhead athlete and cause insidious nonspecific shoulder pain during overhead activities.[76] The etiology is thought to be the peel-back phenomenon that results in a more vertical and posterior force vector on the biceps tendon in the abducted and externally rotated position. There should be a high suspicion for SLAP tears in throwing athletes who have refractory pain; MRI may be needed to aid in making the diagnosis.

Initial management should consist of nonsurgical measures, including rest and physical therapy. The role for surgical treatment of SLAP tears remains controversial. The authors of a 2000 study[77] suggest arthroscopic treatment of SLAP tears if there is no improvement after rest, NSAID administration, and physical therapy for young overhead athletes.

Gymnast Shoulder

Gymnasts tend to experience sustained forces rather than the repetitive torsional stresses seen in other overhead athletes. This type of stress produces a benign cortical hypertrophy (known as a ringman's shoulder lesion) at the insertion of the pectoralis major muscle at the anterolateral aspect of the proximal humerus.[78] The lesion, which is asymptomatic, is thought to occur exclusively in gymnasts and does not warrant intervention. Awareness of the imaging findings in these athletes may allow for accurate diagnosis and avoid unnecessary imaging and biopsy.

Snapping Scapula Syndrome

Snapping scapula syndrome is an uncommon condition typically due to an inflamed and painful bursa at the superior and medial aspect of the scapula. Overuse is thought to be the most likely factor contributing to snapping scapula syndrome in this population and is associated with scapular dyskinesis. The authors of a 2015 study reported that 75% of the patients with this syndrome were able to return to sports after treatment with nonsurgical measures that focused on physical therapy, with strengthening of the rhomboids and trapezius muscles and stretching of the pectoralis muscles.[79] If nonsurgical measures are unsuccessful in relieving symptoms, further workup is indicated, including CT to assess for structural causes such as osteochondromas or anatomic anomalies in angulation of the scapula.

This information will aid in surgical planning should a structural lesion, hooked superomedial border, or anterior angulation be found requiring mass excision or superomedial border excision.

Scapular Dyskinesis

An increased incidence of scapular dyskinesis and shoulder injury rates were found in adolescents who participate in throwing sports compared with preadolescent overhead throwing athletes. In these patients, the dyskinesis is often secondary to another problem, such as glenohumeral instability, impingement syndrome, rotator cuff weakness, or labral injury. Management consists of scapular stabilization rehabilitation focusing on strengthening and stretching of the scapular muscles to regain control of scapular protraction, retraction, depression, elevation, and rotation, along with treatment of any underlying pathology.

Osteolysis of the Distal Clavicle

Stress osteolysis of the distal clavicle is rare in adolescent athletes but can be seen in those who participate in overhead athletics weight lifting. It results in a decrease in mineralization of the distal clavicle and causes resorption of the distal tip of the clavicle.[80] Although most patients improve within 3 to 6 months with nonsurgical measures including modification of weight-training techniques, NSAIDs, and icing, a small percentage may require distal clavicle excision to continue overhead and weight-lifting activities.

OTHER CAUSES OF SHOULDER PAIN

Less common causes of shoulder pain include quadrilateral space syndrome, suprascapular nerve entrapment, axillary artery occlusion, axillary vein thrombosis, posterior capsule laxity, and glenoid spurs. These alternative diagnoses should be considered when evaluating pediatric patients with shoulder pain.

SUMMARY

The participation of children and adolescents in organized sports and the early specialization of these individuals in a single sport have led to an increasing rate of injuries in pediatric shoulders. Acute traumatic injuries to the shoulder can result in sprains, strains, fractures, and dislocations. Chronic overuse injuries also occur in pediatric patients. The presence of open physes and differences in collagen composition in pediatric shoulder tissue compared with the adult shoulder create a unique environment for injury and require special treatment considerations.

KEY STUDY POINTS

- Shoulder injuries in pediatric athletes continue to rise with increasing sports participation and specialization.
- The adolescent growth spurt is a unique time in development and can make older children more susceptible to shoulder injury.
- Knowledge of the kinetic chain of energy generation in the overhead athlete is important for understanding injury treatment and prevention.
- Acute traumatic events during practice or, more likely, competition can lead to sprains, strains, dislocations, or fractures of the structures that encompass the shoulder region.
- Overhead athletes are susceptible to overuse injuries in the shoulder because of repetitive motions across the joint.

ANNOTATED REFERENCES

1. Caine D, Caine C, Maffulli N: Incidence and distribution of pediatric sport-related injuries. *Clin J Sport Med* 2006;16(6):500-513.
2. Robinson TW, Corlette J, Collins CL, Comstock RD: Shoulder injuries among US high school athletes, 2005/2006-2011/2012. *Pediatrics* 2014;133(2):272-279.
3. Trofa DP, Obana KK, Swindell HW, et al: Increasing burden of youth baseball elbow injuries in US emergency departments. *Orthop J Sports Med* 2019;7(5):2325967119845636.

   The number of injuries sustained by youth baseball players is overall decreasing, except with respect to elbow injuries. Shoulder injuries have seen a declining prevalence in presentation to the emergency department, with 16.2% of injuries being sustained in the shoulder. Level of evidence: IV.
4. Zember JS, Rosenberg ZS, Kwong S, Kothary SP, Bedoya MA: Normal skeletal maturation and imaging pitfalls in the pediatric shoulder. *Musculoskelet Imaging* 2015;35(4):1108-1122.
5. Peterson CA, Peterson HA: Analysis of the incidence of injuries to the epiphyseal growth plate. *J Trauma* 1972;12(4):275-281.
6. Yard EE, Knox CL, Smith GA, Comstock RD: Pediatric martial arts injuries presenting to emergency departments, United States 1990-2003. *J Sci Med Sport* 2007;10(4):219-226.
7. Yard EE, Comstock RD: Injuries sustained by pediatric ice hockey, lacrosse, and field hockey athletes presenting to United States emergency departments, 1990-2003. *J Athl Train* 2006;41(4):441-449.
8. Collins CL, Comstock RD: Epidemiological features of high school baseball injuries in the United States, 2005-2007. *Pediatrics* 2008;121(6):1181-1187.
9. Krajnik S, Fogarty KJ, Yard EE, Comstock RD: Shoulder injuries in US high school baseball and softball athletes, 2005-2008. *Pediatrics* 2010;125(3):497-501.

10. Lee JT, Nasreddine AY, Black EM, Bae DS, Kocher MS: Posterior sternoclavicular joint injuries in skeletally immature patients. *J Pediatr Orthop* 2014;34(4):369-375.
11. Landin LA: Fracture patterns in children: Analysis of 8,682 fractures with special reference to incidence, etiology and secular changes in a Swedish urban population 1950-1979. *Acta Orthop Scand Suppl* 1983;202:1-109.
12. Garrigues GE, Warnick DE, Busch MT: Subscapularis avulsion of the lesser tuberosity in adolescents. *J Pediatr Orthop* 2013;33(1):8-13.
13. Provance AJ, Polousky JD: Isolated avulsion fracture of the subscapularis tendon with medial dislocation and tear of biceps tendon in a skeletally immature athlete: A case report. *Curr Opin Pediatr* 2010;22(3):366-368.
14. LaMont LE, Green DW, Altchek DW, Warren RF, Wickiewicz TL: Subscapularis tears and lesser tuberosity avulsion fractures in the pediatric patient. *Sports Health* 2015;7(2):110-114.
15. Klasson SC, Vander Schilden JL, Park JP: Late effect of isolated avulsion fractures of the lesser tubercle of the humerus in children: Report of two cases. *J Bone Joint Surg Am* 1993;75(11):1691-1694.
16. Paschal SO, Hutton KS, Weatherall PT: Isolated avulsion fracture of the lesser tuberosity of the humerus in adolescents: A report of two cases. *J Bone Joint Surg Am* 1995;77(9):1427-1430.
17. Kowalsky MS, Bell JE, Ahmad CS: Arthroscopic treatment of subcoracoid impingement caused by lesser tuberosity malunion: A case report and review of the literature. *J Shoulder Elbow Surg* 2007;16(6):e10-e14.
18. Coates MH, Breidahl W: Humeral avulsion of the anterior band of the inferior glenohumeral ligament with associated subscapularis bony avulsion in skeletally immature patients. *Skeletal Radiol* 2001;30(12):661-666.
19. Levine B, Pereira D, Rosen J: Avulsion fractures of the lesser tuberosity of the humerus in adolescents: Review of the literature and case report. *J Orthop Trauma* 2005;19(5):349-352.
20. Shibuya S, Ogawa K: Isolated avulsion fracture of the lesser tuberosity of the humerus: A case report. *Clin Orthop Relat Res* 1986;211:215-218.
21. Asbury S, Tennent TD: Avulsion fracture of the coracoid process: A case report. *Injury* 2005;36(4):567-568.
22. Lawton RL, Choudhury S, Mansat P, Cofield RH, Stans AA: Pediatric shoulder instability: Presentation, findings, treatment, and outcomes. *J Pediatr Orthop* 2002;22(1):52-61.
23. Zacchilli MA, Owens BD: Epidemiology of shoulder dislocations presenting to emergency departments in the United States. *J Bone Joint Surg Am* 2010;92(3):542-549.
24. Postacchini F, Gumina S, Cinotti G: Anterior shoulder dislocation in adolescents. *J Shoulder Elbow Surg* 2000;9(6):470-474.
25. Edmonds EW, Roocroft JH, Parikh SN: Spectrum of operative childhood intra-articular shoulder pathology. *J Child Orthop* 2014;8(4):337-340.
26. Carr D, Johnson RJ, Pope MH: Upper extremity injuries in skiing. *Am J Sports Med* 1981;9(6):378-383.
27. Deitch J, Mehlman CT, Foad SL, Obbehat A, Mallory M: Traumatic anterior shoulder dislocation in adolescents. *Am J Sports Med* 2003;31(5):758-763.
28. Hovelius L: Anterior dislocation of the shoulder in teen-agers and young adults: Five-year prognosis. *J Bone Joint Surg Am* 1987;69(3):393-399.
29. Hovelius L: The natural history of primary anterior dislocation of the shoulder in the young. *J Orthop Sci* 1999;4(4):307-317.
30. Hovelius L, Augustini BG, Fredin H, Johansson O, Norlin R, Thorling J: Primary anterior dislocation of the shoulder in young patients: A ten-year prospective study. *J Bone Joint Surg Am* 1996;78(11):1677-1684.
31. Hovelius L, Eriksson K, Fredin H, et al: Recurrences after initial dislocation of the shoulder: Results of a prospective study of treatment. *J Bone Joint Surg Am* 1983;65(3):343-349.
32. Jakobsen BW, Johannsen HV, Suder P, Søjbjerg JO: Primary repair versus conservative treatment of first-time traumatic anterior dislocation of the shoulder: A randomized study with 10-year follow-up. *Arthroscopy* 2007;23(2):118-123.
33. Marans HJ, Angel KR, Schemitsch EH, Wedge JH: The fate of traumatic anterior dislocation of the shoulder in children. *J Bone Joint Surg Am* 1992;74(8):1242-1244.
34. Robinson CM, Howes J, Murdoch H, Will E, Graham C: Functional outcome and risk of recurrent instability after primary traumatic anterior shoulder dislocation in young patients. *J Bone Joint Surg Am* 2006;88(11):2326-2336.
35. Rowe CR: Prognosis in dislocations of the shoulder. *J Bone Joint Surg Am* 1956;38(5):957-977.
36. Rowe CR, Sakellarides HT: Factors related to recurrences of anterior dislocations of the shoulder. *Clin Orthop* 1961;20:40-48.
37. Wagner KT Jr, Lyne ED: Adolescent traumatic dislocations of the shoulder with open epiphyses. *J Pediatr Orthop* 1983;3(1):61-62.
38. Leroux T, Ogilvie-Harris D, Veillette C, et al: The epidemiology of primary anterior shoulder dislocations in patients aged 10 to 16 years. *Am J Sports Med* 2015;43(9):2111-2117.
39. Leroux T, Wasserstein D, Veillette C, et al: Epidemiology of primary anterior shoulder dislocation requiring closed reduction in Ontario, Canada. *Am J Sports Med* 2014;42(2):442-450.
40. Robinson CM, Dobson RJ: Anterior instability of the shoulder after trauma. *J Bone Joint Surg Br* 2004;86(4):469-479.
41. Li X, Ma R, Nielsen NM, Gulotta LV, Dines JS, Owens BD: Management of shoulder instability in the skeletally immature patient. *J Am Acad Orthop Surg* 2013;21(9):529-537.
42. Franklin CC, Weiss JM: The natural history of pediatric and adolescent shoulder dislocation. *J Pediatr Orthop* 2019;6(suppl 1):S50-S52.

    Most studies of pediatric and adolescent shoulder instability agree that recurrent anterior shoulder instability is likely in young patients. Some authors advocate for consideration of early surgery in this high-risk population. Level of evidence: V.
43. Jones KJ, Wiesel B, Ganley TJ, Wells L: Functional outcomes of early arthroscopic Bankart repair in adolescents aged 11 to 18 years. *J Pediatr Orthop* 2007;27(2):209-213.

44. Simonet WT, Cofield RH: Prognosis in anterior shoulder dislocation. *Am J Sports Med* 1984;12(1):19-24.

45. Hovelius L, Lind B, Thorling J: Primary dislocation of the shoulder: Factors affecting the two-year prognosis. *Clin Orthop Relat Res* 1983;176:181-185.

46. Shanley E, Thigpen C, Brooks J, et al: Return to sport as an outcome measure for shoulder instability: Surprising findings in nonoperative management in a high school athlete population. *Am J Sports Med* 2019;47(5):1062-1067.

A high percentage of high school athletes with shoulder instability achieved successful return to sport without missing any additional time for shoulder injury. Those with shoulder subluxations were at an almost three times the odds of a successful return compared with those sustaining a dislocation. Level of evidence: II.

47. Mazzocca AD, Brown FM Jr, Carreira DS, Hayden J, Romeo AA: Arthroscopic anterior shoulder stabilization of collision and contact athletes. *Am J Sports Med* 2005;33(1):52-60.

48. Kraus R, Pavlidis T, Heiss C, Kilian O, Schnettler R: Arthroscopic treatment of post-traumatic shoulder instability in children and adolescents. *Knee Surg Sports Traumatol Arthrosc* 2010;18(12):1738-1741.

49. Castagna A, Delle Rose G, Borroni M, et al: Arthroscopic stabilization of the shoulder in adolescent athletes participating in overhead or contact sports. *Arthroscopy* 2012;28(3):309-315.

50. Dickens JF, Owens BD, Cameron KL, et al: The effect of subcritical bone loss and exposure on recurrent instability after arthroscopic Bankart repair in intercollegiate American football. *Am J Sports Med* 2017;45(8):1769-1775.

Arthroscopic stabilization of anterior shoulder instability in American football players with <13.5% glenoid bone loss provides reliable outcomes and low recurrence rates. Level of evidence: III.

51. Ozturk BY, Maak TG, Fabricant MP, et al: Return to sports after arthroscopic anterior stabilization in patients younger than 25 years. *Arthroscopy* 2013;29(12):1922-1931.

52. Rodeo SA, Suzuki K, Yamauchi M, Bhargava M, Warren RF: Analysis of collagen and elastic fibers in shoulder capsule in patients with shoulder instability. *Am J Sports Med* 1998;26(5):634-643.

53. Burkhead WZ Jr, Rockwood CA Jr: Treatment of instability of the shoulder with an exercise program. *J Bone Joint Surg Am* 1992;74(6):890-896.

54. Kuroda S, Sumiyoshi T, Moriishi J, Maruta K, Ishige N: The natural course of atraumatic shoulder instability. *J Shoulder Elbow Surg* 2001;10(2):100-104.

55. Kim SH, Kim HK, Sun JI, Park JS, Oh I: Arthroscopic capsulolabroplasty for posteroinferior multidirectional instability of the shoulder. *Am J Sports Med* 2004;32(3):594-607.

56. McIntyre LF, Caspari RB, Savoie FH III: The arthroscopic treatment of multidirectional shoulder instability: Two-year results of a multiple suture technique. *Arthroscopy* 1997;13(4):418-425.

57. Treacy SH, Savoie FH III, Field LD: Arthroscopic treatment of multidirectional instability. *J Shoulder Elbow Surg* 1999;8(4):345-350.

58. Gartsman GM, Roddey TS, Hammerman SM: Arthroscopic treatment of multidirectional glenohumeral instability: 2- to 5-year follow-up. *Arthroscopy* 2001;17(3):236-243.

59. Baker CL III, Mascarenhas R, Kline AJ, Chhabra A, Pombo MW, Bradley JP: Arthroscopic treatment of multidirectional shoulder instability in athletes: A retrospective analysis of 2- to 5-year clinical outcomes. *Am J Sports Med* 2009;37(9):1712-1720.

60. Lord J, Winell JJ: Overuse injuries in pediatric athletes. *Curr Opin Pediatr* 2004;16(1):47-50.

61. Marsh JS, Daigneault JP: The young athlete. *Curr Opin Pediatr* 1999;11(1):84-88.

62. Micheli LJ: Overuse injuries in children's sports: The growth factor. *Orthop Clin North Am* 1983;14(2):337-360.

63. Caine D, Maffulli N, Caine C: Epidemiology of injury in child and adolescent sports: Injury rates, risk factors, and prevention. *Clin Sports Med* 2008;27(1):19-50, vii.

64. Bright RW, Burstein AH, Elmore SM: Epiphyseal-plate cartilage: A biomechanical and histological analysis of failure modes. *J Bone Joint Surg Am* 1974;56(4):688-703.

65. Fazarale JJ, Magnussen RA, Pedroza AD, Kaeding CC, Best TM, Classie J: Knowledge of and compliance with pitch count recommendations: A survey of youth baseball coaches. *Sports Health* 2012;4(3):202-204.

66. Heyworth BE, Kramer DE, Martin DJ, Micheli LJ, Kocher MS, Bae DS: Trends in presentation, management and outcomes of little league shoulder. *Am J Sports Med* 2016;44(6):1431-1438.

LLS is being diagnosed with increased frequency. Concomitant elbow pain may be seen in up to 13% of LLS patients. Almost one-third of LLS patients had GIRD. Level of evidence: IV.

67. Lyman S, Fleisig GS, Waterbor JW, et al: Longitudinal study of elbow and shoulder pain in youth baseball pitchers. *Med Sci Sports Exerc* 2001;33(11):1803-1810.

68. Sabick MB, Kim YK, Torry MR, Keirns MA, Hawkins RJ: Biomechanics of the shoulder in youth baseball pitchers: Implications for the development of proximal humeral epiphysiolysis and humeral retrotorsion. *Am J Sports Med* 2005;33(11):1716-1722.

69. Drakos MC, Rudzki JR, Allen AA, Potter HG, Altchek DW: Internal impingement of the shoulder in the overhead athlete. *J Bone Joint Surg Am* 2009;91(11):2719-2728.

70. Kibler WB, Dome D: Internal impingement: Concurrent superior labral and rotator cuff injuries. *Sports Med Arthrosc* 2012;20(1):30-33.

71. Eisner EA, Roocroft JH, Edmonds EW: Underestimation of labral pathology in adolescents with anterior shoulder instability. *J Pediatr Orthop* 2012;32(1):42-47.

72. Ryu RK, Fan RS: Adolescent and pediatric sports injuries. *Pediatr Clin North Am* 1998;45(6):1601-1635, x.

73. Ireland ML, Andrews JR: Shoulder and elbow injuries in the young athlete. *Clin Sports Med* 1988;7(3):473-494.

74. Snook GA: A review of women's collegiate gymnastics. *Clin Sports Med* 1985;4(1):31-37.

75. Kibler WB: Rehabilitation of rotator cuff tendinopathy. *Clin Sports Med* 2003;22(4):837-847.

76. Bedi A, Dodson C, Altchek DW: Symptomatic SLAP tear and paralabral cyst in a pediatric athlete: A case report. *J Bone Joint Surg Am* 2010;92(3):721-725.

77. Kocher MS, Waters PM, Micheli LJ: Upper extremity injuries in the paediatric athlete. *Sports Med* 2000;30(2):117-135.

78. Fulton MN, Albright JP, El-Khoury GY: Cortical desmoid-like lesion of the proximal humerus and its occurrence in gymnasts (ringman's shoulder lesion). *Am J Sports Med* 1979;7(1):57-61.

79. Haus B, Nasreddine AY, Suppan C, Kocher MS: Treatment of snapping scapula syndrome in children and adolescents. *J Pediatr Orthop* 2016;36(5):541-547.

    Although most patients with snapping scapula syndrome can be treated successfully with nonsurgical measures, those that do not respond well require a further workup to look for possible structural components to the syndrome. These patients often obtain relief from surgical intervention. Level of evidence: IV.

80. Auringer ST, Anthony EY: Common pediatric sports injuries. *Semin Musculoskelet Radiol* 1999;3(3):247-256.

CHAPTER 53

Ankle Injuries

DEEPAK RAMANATHAN, MD • JOEL KOLMODIN, MD • PAUL M. SALUAN, MD

ABSTRACT

Ankle injuries are exceedingly common in pediatric athletes and represent a leading cause of missed athletic participation. The incidence of acute ankle injuries may be increased in patients with underlying abnormalities, such as tarsal coalition or Achilles tendon contracture. Acute ankle injuries, such as ankle sprains and peroneal tendon injuries, generally can be treated nonsurgically with a short period of immobilization and limited weight bearing followed by focused rehabilitation. Chronic ankle pain, often the result of repetitive ankle trauma, is typically caused by abnormalities such as talar osteochondral lesions, ankle tendon instability, and peroneal tendon pathology. Surgical management is sometimes indicated for the management of chronic ankle pathologies.

Keywords: peroneal tendon; sprain; syndesmosis; talar osteochondritis dissecans (OCD); talus

Dr. Saluan or an immediate family member is a member of a speakers' bureau or has made paid presentations on behalf of Arthrex, Inc.; serves as an unpaid consultant to Equalizer, LLC and Middle Path Innovations, LLC; has stock or stock options held in Equalizer, LLC and Middle Path Innovations, LLC; and serves as a board member, owner, officer, or committee member of the Pediatric Orthopaedic Society of North America. Neither of the following authors nor any immediate family member has received anything of value from or has stock or stock options held in a commercial company or institution related directly or indirectly to the subject of this chapter: Dr. Ramanathan and Dr. Kolmodin.

INTRODUCTION

Ankle injuries are exceedingly common in pediatric athletes and are a leading cause of missed athletic participation. Such injuries are expected to increase as the rate of athletic participation increases and sports participation begins at younger ages. A thorough understanding of ankle anatomy and pathology is needed to accurately diagnose and treat pediatric patients who have ankle pain. Athletic injuries, such as a distal fibular physeal fracture, a lateral process talus fracture, peroneal tendon injuries, osteochondral defects of the talus, and sequelae of tarsal coalition, can be very subtle on imaging and at the physical examination and often are misdiagnosed. Diagnostic and treatment considerations when treating commonly encountered ankle injuries in pediatric athletes are highlighted.

LOW ANKLE SPRAIN

Ankle sprains—90% of which are low ankle sprains—represent the most common reason for missed athletic participation in adolescent athletes, and they may result in long-term dysfunction if not treated appropriately. The classic low ankle sprain is defined as a sprain that results in an injury to the lateral ligamentous structures of the ankle, which occur below the level of the distal tibiofibular syndesmosis. These sprains are typically inversion injuries, and the position of the foot during inversion determines the location of the lateral ankle ligamentous injury. Excessive inversion of the plantarflexed foot leads to injury to the anterior talofibular ligament (ATFL), the most common ligament injured by an ankle sprain. Excessive inversion of the dorsiflexed foot causes injury to the calcaneofibular ligament and, less commonly, the posterior talofibular ligament. An increased propensity

This chapter is adapted from Kolmodin J, Saluan PM: Ankle injuries, in Martus JE, ed: *Orthopaedic Knowledge Update®: Pediatrics*, ed 5. Rosemont, IL, American Academy of Orthopaedic Surgeons, 2016, pp 579-589.

for these inversion injuries is known to occur in conjunction with obvious cavovarus foot deformity as well as in conjunction with subtle cavovarus foot deformity.[1]

Acute low ankle sprains typically manifest by a large amount of lateral ankle swelling, pain with weight bearing, and pain in the lateral ankle. The physical examination characteristically shows focal tenderness to palpation over the involved lateral ankle ligamentous structures. The patient may have pain with resisted eversion of the foot, a sign of peroneal tendon injury during the inversion episode. In patients with a history of numerous ankle sprains, the anterior drawer test may be positive. This test involves anterior translation of the slightly plantarflexed foot; excessive anterior translation represents chronic laxity of the injured ATFL. In addition, inversion stress testing of the neutral foot may demonstrate increased laxity, such as in the setting of an attritional calcaneofibular ligament.

The Ottawa Ankle Rules have been proven as a reliable tool for determining when radiography is necessary in the evaluation of an acute ankle sprain.[2,3] In this case, a fracture is suspected when there is (1) difficulty with weight bearing, (2) tenderness to palpation over the medial or lateral malleolus, (3) tenderness over the navicular, or (4) tenderness over the base of the fifth metatarsal. A lower threshold for obtaining radiographs exists after a patient referral in the outpatient setting, because referrals are often made in situations of more severe injury or chronic symptoms. An alternate proposed guideline known as the Low Risk Ankle Rules consider ankle radiographs unnecessary if there is tenderness and swelling isolated to the distal fibula and/or adjacent lateral ligaments distal to the tibial anterior joint line.[4] A 2017 retrospective comparison of the Ottawa Ankle Rules and the Low Risk Ankle Rules found that the former demonstrated 100% sensitivity in the pediatric emergency department.[4] When radiographs are necessary, weight-bearing AP, lateral, and mortise views are recommended. Varus stress views can be used to evaluate for excessive talar tilt in the setting of ATFL laxity. External rotation stress views should be obtained to rule out a syndesmotic injury, which is characteristic of a high ankle sprain. MRI is rarely warranted, except in the setting of prolonged pain or instability. In this case, MRI is performed to evaluate for associated injuries such as peroneal tendon pathology, talar osteochondral lesions, fractures of the anterior calcaneal process, or fractures of the lateral talar process. Lateral process talar fractures are especially important to consider in the differential diagnosis; a 2016 study demonstrated that as many as 42% of these injuries are initially misdiagnosed as ankle sprains.[5] Even talar body and neck fractures can occasionally be overlooked in low-energy trauma patients thought to have minor ankle injuries.[6]

The treatment of an acute low ankle sprain includes rest, ice, compression, and elevation. After the acute phase of injury has resolved, physical therapy is recommended, focusing on peroneal strength and proprioceptive training.[7] Return to play is most efficient when early functional rehabilitation occurs.[8] Bracing treatment also is used to prevent recurrent ligament sprains, and bracing treatment has proved to be a far more reliable method for ankle stabilization during athletic participation than rehabilitation alone.[9]

Surgical management is recommended when patients demonstrate persistent pain and instability despite aggressive nonsurgical treatment. The most common surgical technique is the anatomic technique developed by the author of a 1966 study[10] and later modified by the authors of a 1980 study.[11] This technique involves shortening and reattaching the ATFL and the calcaneofibular ligament to the distal fibula followed by reinforcement with the extensor retinaculum. Various studies have demonstrated good to excellent results in 90% of patients using this technique.[12,13] Alternative reconstruction methods exist, such as peroneal tenodesis to augment the lax lateral ligaments, but these are not typically used in the pediatric population because of their nonanatomic nature and propensity to produce subtalar stiffness.

HIGH ANKLE SPRAIN

The classic high ankle sprain is an injury to the distal tibiofibular syndesmosis. A much less common variant than a low ankle sprain, high ankle sprains represent less than 10% of all ankle sprains, although this incidence is higher in collision sports. These injuries are invariably rotational injuries, usually caused by external rotation of the foot relative to the leg. Such excessive external rotation causes the talus to drive the distal tibia and fibula apart, leading to a failure of the ligaments that normally maintain their position relative to one another. Associated injuries are quite common, including Weber type B and C ankle fractures, osteochondral defects, and peroneal tendon injuries.

The distal tibiofibular syndesmosis is a complex arrangement of ligaments whose purpose is to maintain the relationship between the distal tibia and the fibula. The ligamentous complex primarily acts to control translational and rotational forces, while allowing small amounts of physiologic motion. The most important ligaments of the syndesmosis include the anterior-inferior tibiofibular ligament, the posterior-inferior tibiofibular ligament, the transverse tibiofibular ligament, and the interosseous ligament. The deltoid ligament also contributes to syndesmotic stability; it prevents lateral translation of the talus. The anterior-inferior tibiofibular ligament originates from the anterior distal tibia (Chaput tubercle) and inserts into the anterior aspect of the distal fibula (Wagstaffe tubercle). The posterior-inferior tibiofibular ligament, which originates from the posterior distal tibia (Volkmann tubercle) and inserts into the posterior aspect of the lateral malleolus, is the strongest component of the syndesmosis. The interosseous ligament represents a distal thickening of the interosseous membrane, transversely connecting the tibia and the fibula.

Patients with high ankle sprains often report pain slightly above the ankle joint. They are frequently unable to bear weight on the injured limb, a factor that distinguishes the high ankle sprain from the classic low ankle sprain. Patients typically demonstrate tenderness to palpation over the distal tibial syndesmosis anterolaterally, which can extend up the leg. In fact, the level of the proximal tenderness (the tenderness length) has been shown to correlate with return to play time. Patients also may demonstrate medial ankle pain in situations in which the deltoid ligament is injured; deltoid injury signifies increased instability of the ankle joint.

Various provocative tests are used to diagnose a high ankle sprain. The Hopkin squeeze test is performed by applying compressive pressure to the midcalf level; the response is considered positive if pain is elicited during the maneuver. The external rotation test is performed by dorsiflexing and externally rotating the foot—essentially re-creating the forces that caused the injury. The test is positive if pain is elicited.

As with low ankle sprains, radiographic evaluation of suspected high ankle sprains includes AP, lateral, and mortise views of the ankle (**Figure 1**). Decreased tibiofibular overlap on the AP view and increased tibiofibular clear space on the mortise view are suggestive of a syndesmotic injury, which can be confirmed with external rotation stress and gravity stress views. Because Tillaux fractures can be misdiagnosed by those who have limited knowledge of the distal tibial physeal closure pattern, careful attention must be paid to ankle radiographs of skeletally immature patients. Advanced imaging is rarely indicated, although MRI can be used when there is a high suspicion of injury in a patient with negative radiographic findings. MRI is highly sensitive and specific for syndesmotic injury.[14]

The management of distal tibiofibular syndesmotic injuries varies depending on the nature and the severity of the injury. Syndesmotic sprains with no evidence of tibiofibular diastasis can be treated with a short non–weight-bearing period. Weight bearing is then gradually reinstituted, and bracing treatment with a rigid orthosis is used to prevent external rotation forces at the ankle. Patients should be counseled regarding the prolonged recovery time after a high ankle sprain. Patients also should be observed closely after nonsurgical treatment, because a known complication of a high ankle sprain is distal tibiofibular synostosis, which is rarely symptomatic but can require surgical excision if it is excessively painful.

Surgical indications for syndesmotic injuries include failed nonsurgical treatment, evidence of instability on stress radiographs, and an associated fracture. The surgical treatment of these injuries has evolved. Traditional management included reduction and screw fixation of the syndesmosis, and screw fixation was attained by capturing either three or four cortices. Excellent results

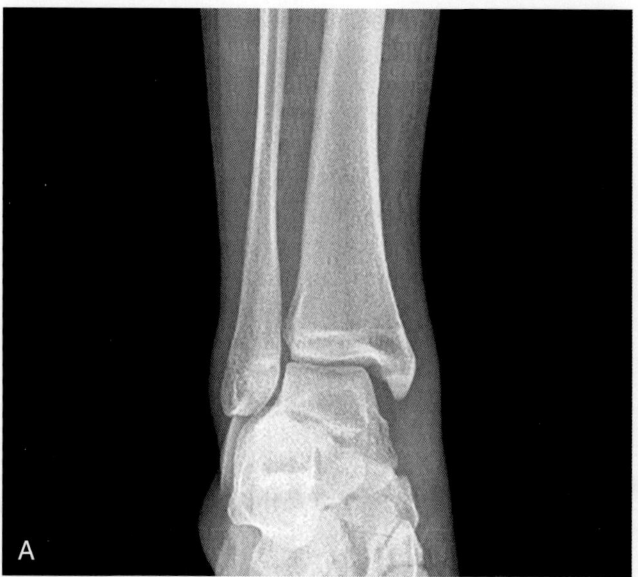

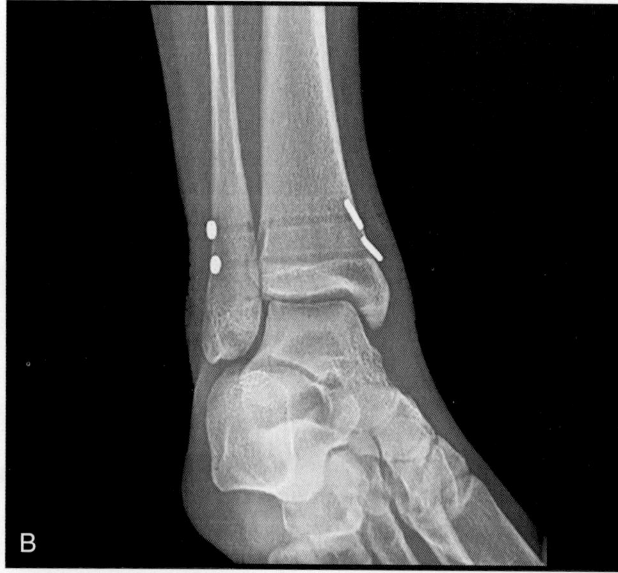

FIGURE 1 **A**, AP stress radiograph of the ankle of an adolescent athlete shows an isolated syndesmotic sprain. **B**, Mortise radiograph after fixation of the syndesmosis with a suture-button.

have been reported when the syndesmosis was accurately reduced.[15] However, the use of a syndesmotic screw requires eventual screw removal and adds risk for screw breakage and other complications if it is left in place too long.[16] To address these shortcomings, suture-button fixation recently has been advocated. Theoretically, suture-button fixation allows a small amount of physiologic motion at the syndesmosis, which may prevent subtle, inaccurate reduction.[17] In addition, the suture-button device does not require removal. Early results using the suture-button technique have been very encouraging, showing comparable outcomes and a faster return to activity.[16,17] A recent meta-analysis of seven randomized controlled trials determined that dynamic stabilization of the syndesmosis was associated with a lower rate of complications (especially malreduction and clinical instability) and revision surgeries when compared with screw fixation.[18]

ANKLE SPRAIN EQUIVALENT FRACTURES

Ankle injuries can vary greatly depending on the skeletal status of the patient. For the patient who is skeletally immature, ankle fractures are more common than ankle sprains. In fact, fractures of the distal tibia and fibula are second only to fractures of the distal radius as the most common physeal fractures in children. Classically, the distal fibular physeal fracture has been considered the equivalent injury to the low ankle sprain in the athlete who is skeletally immature. Thus, a patient with normal radiographs and symptoms of an ankle sprain with focal tenderness over the distal fibular physis is presumed to have a physeal fracture, because the cartilage of the epiphyseal plate is biomechanically weaker than the neighboring lateral ankle ligaments. However, subsequent studies have demonstrated that this is not always the case. Two studies, in 2008 and 2001, found that the incidence of a distal fibular physeal fracture in a patient who is skeletally immature and has lateral ankle pain and negative radiographs is rather low, ranging from 14% to 18%.[19,20] Furthermore, a 2015 study found that unrecognized ATFL avulsion fractures occur in up to 26% of skeletally immature patients with a presumed ankle sprain.[21] These three studies demonstrate that ligamentous injuries of the ankle do occur in patients who are skeletally immature, despite the presence of open physes. Thus, the accurate diagnosis of ankle injuries can be challenging in the pediatric population.

Equivalent injuries to the high ankle sprain in the patient who is skeletally immature are the Tillaux fracture (**Figure 2**) and the triplane fracture. It has been established that distal tibial physeal closure occurs in a characteristic central-to-medial-to-lateral fashion, which means that the anterolateral portion of the physis is the last to close. This process occurs during an 18-month window for adolescents aged 13 to 16 years, during which time transitional fractures such as these occur.[22] Because the anterolateral tibial epiphysis is the site of distal tibiofibular ligament attachment, this area is the most susceptible to fracture during rotational ankle injuries. Transitional fractures with more than 2 mm of displacement should undergo CT scan for preoperative planning and fixation.[23] The Tillaux fracture is a Salter-Harris type III fracture that involves fracture in the sagittal and axial planes within the epiphysis only. The triplane fracture is a Salter-Harris type IV fracture that includes a coronal fracture that extends into the distal tibial metaphysis.

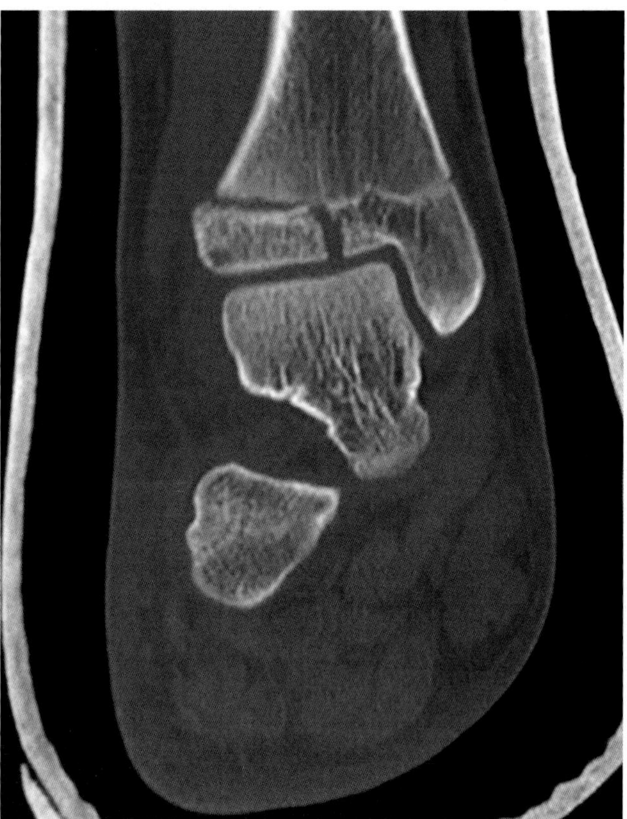

FIGURE 2 Coronal slice CT image from an adolescent athlete shows a Tillaux fracture with 4 mm of displacement at the articular surface.

For the patient with a Tillaux or triplane fracture, closed reduction with or without fixation is the standard treatment. An internal rotation reduction maneuver is used to achieve reduction (**Figure 3**); if the fracture is displaced, fixation is typically performed with cannulated screws in the epiphysis and/or the metaphysis, depending on the nature of the fracture. Postreduction CT scans are recommended in cases when a nonanatomic reduction is obtained. A 2014 study demonstrated that good long-term outcomes could be achieved with residual fracture displacement up to 2.5 mm after reduction.[24] Larger

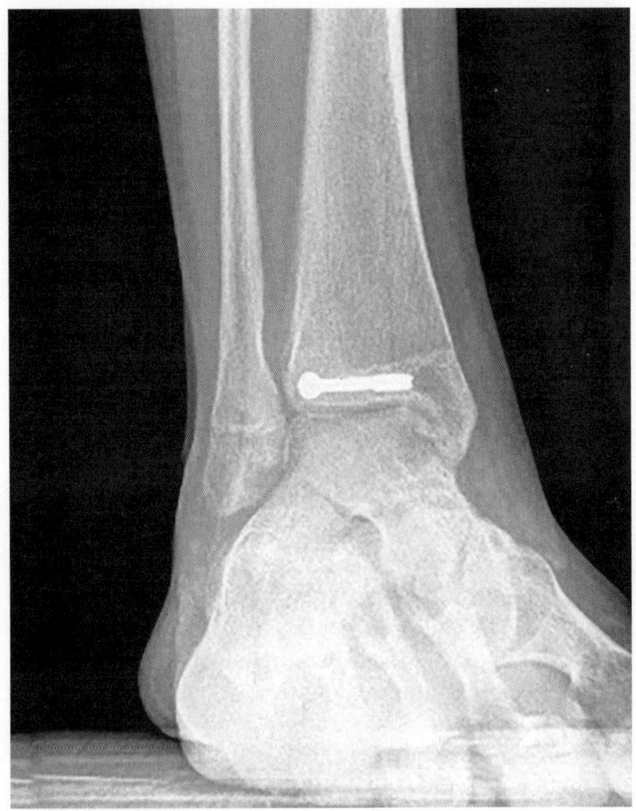

FIGURE 3 Mortise radiograph of the ankle of the patient shown in **Figure 2** after open reduction and internal fixation through the distal tibial epiphysis.

amounts of displacement necessitate open, anatomic reduction and internal fixation. Reduction often can be obtained in a closed manner, and internal fixation is typically accomplished with two anterior-to-posterior screws through the epiphysis (Tillaux fracture) or metaphysis (triplane fracture). Because the fracture is transitional in nature, expeditious physeal closure is expected, and angular deformity is rarely a concern.

PERONEAL TENDON INJURIES

Peroneal tendon injuries—both acute and chronic—are uncommon in the young, athletic population, although they remain an overlooked cause of lateral ankle pain. Peroneal tendon pathology takes many forms, including tenosynovitis, a tendon tear, and tendon instability. These injuries often are observed in the setting of lateral ankle ligamentous instability. Anatomic studies have demonstrated that the tendons are perched along the distal fibula at 15° to 25° of plantar flexion, making them susceptible to inversion injury at this position. Thus, peroneal tendon injury occurs when there is rapid dorsiflexion of the inverted foot. This rapid movement causes reflexive contraction of the peroneus brevis and longus, which can lead to frank tendon injury or injury to the superior peroneal retinaculum (SPR).[25] Chronic symptoms can develop when the tendons are not anatomically located in their retromalleolar position and subsequently subluxate abnormally with ankle motion. In cases in which the SPR is disrupted, the peroneal tendons will subluxate repeatedly, which often leads to longitudinal tears, most frequently in the peroneus brevis where it runs within the fibular groove. Peroneal tendon injuries at the level of the ankle should be differentiated from Iselin disease, which is a traction apophysitis seen in the pediatric population and results from repetitive traction of the peroneus brevis at its attachment at the base of the fifth metatarsal. Differential diagnosis of lateral fifth metatarsal pain in the pediatric population also includes symptomatic os vesalianum, a rare accessory bone adjacent to the fifth metatarsal in the substance of the peroneus brevis tendon.[26]

The peroneal tendons include the peroneus brevis and peroneus longus. The peroneus brevis originates from the distal half of the lateral fibula and inserts into the base of the fifth metatarsal, making it a strong evertor and plantar flexor of the foot. The peroneus longus originates more proximally on the lateral fibula and inserts into the medial cuneiform and the first metatarsal base, thus allowing it to assist in foot eversion and plantar flexion. Together, the peroneal tendons provide supplemental lateral ankle stability. Both the peroneus brevis and peroneus longus run posterior to the lateral malleolus in the retromalleolar sulcus. This sulcus is deepened by a fibrocartilaginous rim, which provides moderate inherent stability to the tendons as they course through the region. Within the sulcus, the peroneus longus is found posterior to the peroneus brevis; the brevis can be easily identified further by its low-lying muscle belly, which typically terminates approximately 3 cm from the tip of the fibula. The SPR, which runs from the posterolateral ridge of the fibula to the lateral calcaneus, is essential to the proper function of the peroneal tendon complex. This retinacular structure functions as the primary restraint to peroneal tendon subluxation within the retromalleolar sulcus.

Young patients with peroneal tendon pathology often report an acute injury, usually accompanied by a popping sound or sensation. They typically experience localized pain posterior to the lateral malleolus, with symptoms of clicking and popping with ankle motion, signifying either peroneal tendon instability or tendinopathy. The physical examination will exhibit tenderness to palpation in this region, as well as pain elicited with dorsiflexion and eversion against resistance. In some instances, patients may be able to voluntarily subluxate the tendons with eversion of the foot.

Plain radiographs are used in the initial evaluation of suspected peroneal tendon injuries, including weight-bearing foot and ankle radiographs. Occasionally, a cortical avulsion of the SPR can be seen, which is classically termed a rim fracture. It can be seen on a mortise view of the ankle, which brings the distal fibula into profile as the leg is internally rotated. CT can be used to assess the osseous anatomy of the lateral ankle, specifically the convexity of the retromalleolar sulcus. MRI often is useful in identifying specific peroneal tendon pathology, such as an SPR tear, a pathologic low-lying peroneus brevis muscle belly, the presence of an anomalous peroneus quartus muscle, and tendon tears.

SPR injuries are characterized according to the Ogden classification.[25] Grade I injuries are characterized by partial avulsion of the SPR from the distal fibula, allowing subluxation of the tendons. Grade II injuries involve separation of the SPR from the distal fibrocartilaginous rim; in this case, the tendons pass between the SPR and the rim. In grade III injuries, there is a frank cortical avulsion of the SPR from the distal fibula, forming the classic rim fracture. Grade IV injuries are characterized by SPR failure at the calcaneus instead of the fibula.

Acute peroneal tendon injuries in the pediatric population should initially be treated nonsurgically with rest, ice, and NSAIDs. Physical therapy and ankle bracing treatment can be effective in preventing further ankle instability episodes. In more severe cases where SPR injury and peroneal tendon subluxation are suspected, immobilization in a short leg cast and protected weight bearing for 4 to 6 weeks is advocated. Care should be taken to make sure that the peroneal tendons are appropriately reduced in the retromalleolar sulcus during casting; slight ankle plantar flexion during casting is sometimes necessary and is well tolerated in the pediatric population.

Acute repair of the SPR is rarely indicated, except in a serious athlete. With acute repair, the torn retinaculum or the cortical avulsion can be directly repaired to its fibular origin with excellent success and quick return to function. Both traditional open and newer endoscopic techniques have been described in SPR repair.[27] Chronic peroneal tendon injuries, such as a chronically lax SPR or a peroneal tendon tear, frequently require surgical management; prior studies have demonstrated success rates of less than 50% with the nonsurgical treatment of chronic disorders.[25]

The management of chronic peroneal subluxation or dislocation focuses on reestablishing a competent SPR and retromalleolar sulcus. SPR repair is typically performed by detaching and reattaching the retinacular tissue in a pants-over-vest manner, allowing the redundant SPR tissue to reinforce the repair. This construct can be augmented by local tissue, such as local Achilles tendon tissue or the plantaris tendon. In cases of a dysplastic, shallow retromalleolar sulcus, a groove-deepening procedure may be indicated to enhance the stability of the tendons.[28] Current techniques involve removal of the subcortical bone of the posterior lateral malleolus and subsequent impaction of the thin cortical rim of bone that remains. These techniques produce a deepened sulcus that is characterized by a smooth remaining floor. Systematic reviews of the surgical procedures addressing peroneal tendon dislocation demonstrate good patient-reported outcomes, high satisfaction scores, and a quick return to play with superior results in those patients who underwent groove deepening and SPR repair.[29]

Peroneal tendon tears are uncommon in the pediatric athlete, although they can occur as the result of repetitive tendon subluxation. When present, tears are usually longitudinal and involve the peroneus brevis. This tendon is prone to injury from the sharp posterolateral ridge of the distal fibula.

Tears of the peroneus longus are far less common. When present, these tears are frequently seen in conjunction with peroneus brevis tears and occur distal to the tip of the fibula. Nonsurgical management of peroneal tendon tears has poor outcomes, so surgical management often is indicated. The standard repair of longitudinal tears involves débridement, repair, and tubularization of the tendon using a small monofilament suture.[30] Peroneus brevis tenodesis is a reliable method to manage chronic tears,[31] but this procedure is not routinely performed in the pediatric population.

Intrasheath subluxation of the uninjured peroneal tendons within the peroneal groove has also been described.[32] This intrasheath subluxation usually occurs as painful snapping due to relative switching of the anatomic alignment of both peroneal tendons. An uncommon variant of such intrasheath subluxation involves a longitudinal split within the peroneus brevis tendon through which the peroneus longus tendon subluxates.[32] Dynamic ultrasonography is a useful diagnostic tool because subluxation is often not appreciated on physical examination and the SPR is generally intact in this population.[32]

TALAR OSTEOCHONDRITIS DISSECANS

In the pediatric population, talar osteochondritis dissecans (OCD) occurs infrequently. Originally thought to be the result of an avascular process, OCD is now thought to be caused by acute or repetitive microtrauma. The talus is the third most common joint at which to find evidence of OCD, behind only the knee and the capitellum. OCD is 1.5 times more frequent in females than males, and it is 7 times more likely to occur in adolescents than in younger children.[33] Talar OCD occurs almost exclusively in the talar dome, although it has been reported in the talar head.[34] For OCD involving the talar dome, lesions on the medial and lateral aspects of the talar dome occur at approximately equal rates, although a slight trend is toward an increased prevalence of medial lesions.[35] Numerous studies have demonstrated distinct differences between medial and lateral talar OCD lesions. Lateral lesions are invariably associated with a history of trauma, and they tend to be smaller and more superficial. Medial lesions are less frequently associated with trauma (64% to 82%) but tend to be larger and deeper.[36,37]

The talus articulates with the tibia, the fibula, the navicular, and the calcaneus. The talar dome, which articulates with the tibial plafond, is trapezoidal in shape—narrower posteriorly than anteriorly. The talus has no tendinous attachments and is mostly covered by cartilage. Thus, its blood supply is provided by a limited number of small branches of the dorsalis pedis, peroneal, and posterior tibial arteries. Blood supply to the talar dome occurs in a retrograde fashion. Because of the relatively limited vascularity of the talar dome and the inherent avascularity of its articular cartilage, talar OCD lesions have limited capacity for spontaneous healing. In addition, talar OCD lesion healing is inhibited by the fact that the tibiotalar joint is subjected to a tremendous amount of force—more per unit area than any other joint in the body.

Patients with talar OCD report a history of prolonged ankle pain, usually following a traumatic episode or a series of traumatic episodes. They often experience mechanical symptoms, such as catching and grinding, which may signal the presence of a loose body or an unstable cartilage flap. Because it is an intra-articular process, most patients also report swelling and ankle stiffness. These patients may be referred to an orthopaedic surgeon after a prolonged period of unsuccessful nonsurgical management. Evaluation often demonstrates swelling and diffuse ankle pain, with restricted range of motion. Because these lesions are associated with recurrent trauma, instability testing is vital in patients with suspected talar OCD, including anterior drawer and inversion/eversion testing.

Radiographic evaluation begins with standard ankle radiographs, including weight-bearing AP, lateral, and mortise views. However, many talar OCD lesions, particularly low-grade lesions, are not visible on plain radiographs. CT can be used for evaluation (**Figure 4**), but it is successful only in evaluating the integrity of subchondral bone; it is not effective in the diagnosis and characterization of lesions that are purely cartilaginous. Thus, MRI is recommended for further evaluation of all known or suspected talar OCD lesions. MRI also is useful for evaluating the integrity of articular cartilage, bone edema, and surrounding soft-tissue pathology. Recently, there has been interest in evaluating these lesions with single photon emission computed tomography-CT (SPECT-CT). It is reported that this advanced imaging modality allows a three-dimensional localization of scintigraphic osteoblastic activity in the lesion area, which can provide valuable information about the subchondral plate.[38,39]

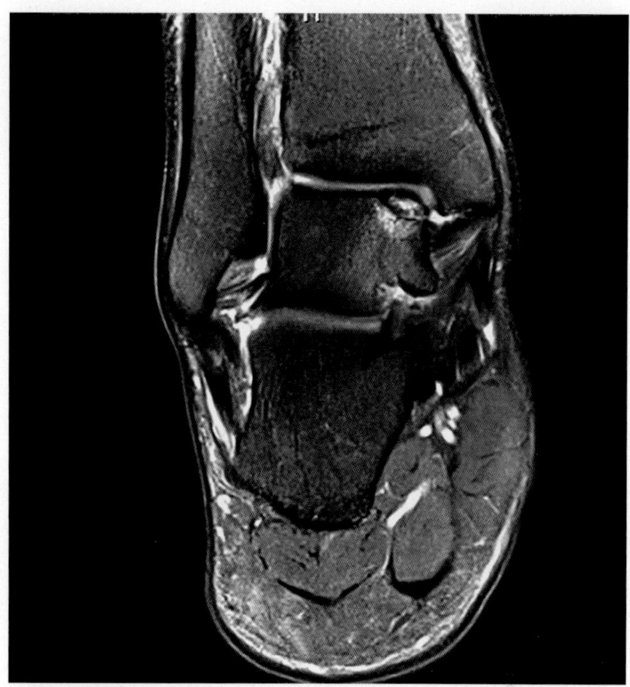

FIGURE 4 Coronal slice CT of the ankle of an adolescent athlete shows a posteromedial talar osteochondritis dissecans lesion.

Various classifications exist for talar OCD lesions. The best recognized system is the Berndt and Harty classification,[35] which characterizes lesions based on plain radiography. Stage I lesions are those with an area of subchondral compression; stage II lesions are those with a partially detached osteochondral fragment; stage III lesions are those with a fully detached osteochondral fragment; and stage IV lesions are those with a visible loose body. A second frequently used classification system is the Hepple staging system, which is based on MRI findings.[40] This staging system is very useful for surgical planning, because MRI has been found to correlate closely with arthroscopic findings.[41]

Nonsurgical management typically involves immobilization and strict adherence to a non–weight-bearing period for 6 to 9 weeks, which is followed by gradual transition to full weight bearing and physical therapy. This treatment is routinely recommended for Berndt and Harty grade I and II lesions, although the original article (1959) reported overall poor outcomes in 75% of the talar OCD lesions treated nonsurgically.[35] A systematic review in 2003 supported these findings, demonstrating a success rate of only 45% with nonsurgical management based on radiographic and clinical outcomes.[42] The treating surgeon should be aware, however, that the patient who responds well to nonsurgical management may demonstrate persistent radiographic evidence of disease despite having no symptoms.[34]

Surgery is generally indicated for patients with symptomatic OCD lesions if radiographs do not demonstrate radiographic healing or if there is no improvement in symptoms despite nonsurgical management. In contrast with OCD lesions of the knee and elbow in which skeletal maturity and larger lesion size clearly have a negative effect on healing potential and outcomes with nonsurgical management, outcomes of nonsurgical and surgical management of OCD lesions of the talus do not appear to be directly related to lesion size or skeletal status.[43] This finding may suggest that there is less overall functional healing capacity for OCD lesions in the ankle compared with those of the knee and elbow, even in skeletally immature patients with small lesions. Thus, prolonged nonsurgical management of small lesions in skeletally immature patients may not be beneficial, and surgical intervention may be indicated in these patients.

Numerous surgical strategies for the management of talar OCD lesions are available. Regardless of the treatment, the goal is to restore the anatomy of the talar dome, thus reestablishing normal joint reactive forces within the ankle joint. The broad categories of surgical management are as follows: repair of the lesion, débridement and stimulation of the lesion, and transplantation to fill the lesion.[44] Current trends favor arthroscopic management over open treatment, although open measures in the form of an arthrotomy and a medial malleolar osteotomy may be needed for surgical therapies that are more aggressive[45] (**Figure 5**).

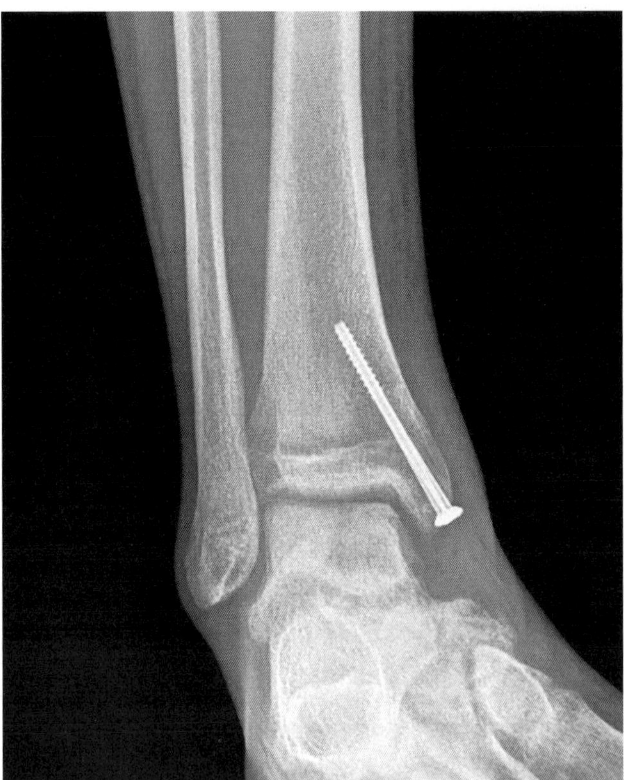

FIGURE 5 Mortise radiograph of the patient shown in **Figure 4** after medial malleolar osteotomy and osteochondral autograft from the ipsilateral knee.

In patients in whom the cartilage surface is intact and stable, as with grade I lesions, antegrade or retrograde drilling may be used. This drilling stimulates healing by opening the sclerotic subchondral bone and allowing bleeding into the defect. Antegrade drilling occurs through the intact cartilage of the OCD lesion. It is accomplished arthroscopically and is the most accurate way to confirm penetration of the subchondral bone. Retrograde drilling is accomplished by inserting 0.062-inch Kirschner wires into the defect through the tarsal sinus laterally or the talar body medially; image guidance is used to triangulate the defect. Prior studies have shown up to 91% fair or good outcomes with antegrade and retrograde techniques.[46]

In cases of grade II lesions with relatively normal cartilage and adequate attached subchondral bone, simple fragment fixation is recommended. Fixation can occur with either screws or bioabsorbable devices. It is important to débride the back side of the fragment and remove any loose tissue before fixation of the fragment. Lesions that are located anteriorly may be amenable to arthroscopic fixation. However, lesions that are focused on the posterior talar dome are difficult to access with appropriate instrumentation. In these cases, a medial malleolar osteotomy (for medial lesions) or an anterolateral tibial osteotomy (for lesions located further laterally) may be indicated. Because of the inherently congruent nature of the ankle joint, accessing the talar lesion is often technically challenging. In a recently conducted anatomic study, maximal dorsiflexion of the tibiotalar joint during posterior ankle arthroscopy possibly provided superior access than neutral flexion or noninvasive distraction.[47] Recently, some authors have advocated lesion salvage procedures, such as drilling or fixation, whenever possible, because they yield reliable results in most patients. Lesion salvage procedures have been shown, however, to have slightly higher revision rates compared with techniques that are more aggressive, such as microfracture or osteochondral transfer techniques.[43]

The most common surgical intervention for grade III and IV lesions involves the removal of loose bodies, aggressive débridement, and drilling of the subchondral bone (microfracture). This process allows for the release of marrow elements into the defect, resulting in the formation of fibrocartilage in the cartilage gap. Débridement and microfracture have produced reliable results in recent studies.[43,45,48] In the largest systematic review to date, a group of researchers found good or excellent results in 85% of patients who were treated with débridement and microfracture; most of these patients had lesions of grade III or higher.[49]

Débridement and microfracture have produced reliable results, although these techniques are limited by their inability to address large defects and provide hyaline cartilage within the defect. It also is unclear how well these techniques can address an uncontained OCD lesion, a lesion that includes the lateral or medial shoulder of the talus. A 2015 large study of talar OCD in the adolescent population found a high revision rate of 27% for patients who had undergone drilling, fragment fixation, or microfracture.[43] Thus, recent research has sought to determine the optimal surgical strategy based on the characteristics of a given lesion. Newer strategies have been developed to address situations in which drilling, fragment fixation, or microfracture may not be effective options and include osteochondral transfer (autograft or allograft) and autologous chondrocyte implantation.

Within the pediatric population, the most frequently used technique is osteochondral autograft transfer. This procedure involves the harvest of circular osteochondral plugs from a patient donor site (typically the ipsilateral knee) and insertion into the talar defect in a side-by-side manner, frequently through a tibial osteotomy. The largest series using this technique was published in 2008 and reported good to excellent results in 93% of the patients, with only 3% of the patients exhibiting donor site knee pain.[50] Subsequent studies have shown high rates of return to sport, although many patients modify their sporting activities.[51] In a recent 5- to 24-year follow-up study, 76% of patients returned to sport after undergoing arthroscopic débridement and bone marrow stimulation of osteochondral talus defects.[52] For uncontained defects, small, circular osteochondral plugs may not be able to effectively re-create the shoulder of the talus, leading to excessive shear forces at the site and premature graft failure. Thus, some authors advocate using large (partial talar body) allograft transfer in this case. This is an area of active research, however, because outcomes studies in this particular clinical situation are lacking. A recent systematic review of 21 studies found that there was no clearly superior surgical salvage option after failure of primary surgery for the talar OCD lesion.[53]

SUMMARY

Ankle injuries are commonly seen in the pediatric population and often are the cause of missed athletic participation. Subtle pediatric ankle injuries, such as physeal fractures, peroneal tendon injuries, and osteochondral injuries, commonly go unnoticed at the initial evaluation by primary care providers. Accurate diagnosis by the orthopaedic provider requires knowledge of pediatric ankle anatomy and injury patterns, which are different from those in the adult athlete. Indications for the nonsurgical management of ankle injuries are expanded in the pediatric athlete compared with their adult counterparts. Surgical intervention for various pathologies can be effective when used for the correct indication.

KEY STUDY POINTS

- Ankle injuries can vary depending on the skeletal status of a patient. Distal fibula fractures are common in patients who are skeletally immature, although purely ligamentous injuries and ATFL avulsion fractures occur regularly.
- Syndesmotic reduction with screw or suture-button fixation yields reliable results. Suture-button fixation, however, has been shown to produce a lower rate of malreduction and rarely requires a second surgery for removal.
- Poor outcomes are seen with nonsurgical management of talar OCD lesions. Surgical options vary depending on lesion characteristics. In the pediatric population, first-line management typically entails osteochondral fragment salvage procedures, such as drilling or fragment fixation whenever possible.

ANNOTATED REFERENCES

1. Fortin PT, Guettler J, Manoli A II: Idiopathic cavovarus and lateral ankle instability: Recognition and treatment implications relating to ankle arthritis. *Foot Ankle Int* 2002;23(11):1031-1037.

2. David S, Gray K, Russell JA, Starkey C: Validation of the Ottawa Ankle Rules for acute foot and ankle injuries. *J Sport Rehabil* 2016;25(1):48-51.

   This review of strictly applying the Ottawa Ankle Rules in 124 consecutive high school and college athletes within 1 hour after injury resulted in no missed fractures but overestimated the need for radiographs. Level of evidence: III.

3. Plint AC, Bulloch B, Osmond MH, et al: Validation of the Ottawa Ankle Rules in children with ankle injuries. *Acad Emerg Med* 1999;6(10):1005-1009.

4. Ellenbogen AL, Rice AL, Vyas P: Retrospective comparison of the low risk ankle rules and the Ottawa Ankle Rules in a pediatric population. *Am J Emerg Med* 2017;35(9):1262-1265. doi:10.1016/j.ajem.2017.03.058.

   This study is a retrospective review of 980 patients at a children's hospital, which determined that Low Risk Ankle Rules are not sensitive enough for use in the emergency department setting. However, the Ottawa Ankle Rules demonstrated 100% sensitivity. Level of evidence: IV.

5. Wu Y, Jiang H, Wang B, Miao W: Fracture of the lateral process of the talus in children: A kind of ankle injury with frequently missed diagnosis. *J Pediatr Orthop* 2016;36(3):289-293.

A review of 12 consecutive children who had treatment for a lateral process talus fracture at one institution demonstrated that five fractures (42%) were missed at the initial visit to the emergency department. Nonetheless, outcomes were good or excellent in 11 of the 12 patients. Level of evidence: IV.

6. Young KW, Park YU, Kim JS, Cho HK, Choo HS, Park JH: Misdiagnosis of talar body or neck fractures as ankle sprains in low energy traumas. *Clin Orthop Surg* 2016;8(3):303-309. doi:10.4055/cios.2016.8.3.303.

   This study is a retrospective review of seven patients with three talar neck fractures and four talar body fractures. All injuries were sustained during low-energy trauma episodes. Therefore, the authors recommend including talar fractures in the differential diagnosis of patients with ankle pain after a seemingly minor ankle injury. Level of evidence: IV.

7. Hupperets MD, Verhagen EA, van Mechelen W: Effect of unsupervised home based proprioceptive training on recurrences of ankle sprain: Randomised controlled trial. *Br Med J* 2009;339:b2684.

8. Maffulli N, Ferran NA: Management of acute and chronic ankle instability. *J Am Acad Orthop Surg* 2008;16(10):608-615.

9. Janssen KW, van Mechelen W, Verhagen EA: Bracing superior to neuromuscular training for the prevention of self-reported recurrent ankle sprains: A three-arm randomised controlled trial. *Br J Sports Med* 2014;48(16):1235-1239.

10. Broström L: Sprained ankles. VI. Surgical treatment of "chronic" ligament ruptures. *Acta Chir Scand* 1966;132(5):551-565.

11. Gould N, Seligson D, Gassman J: Early and late repair of lateral ligament of the ankle. *Foot Ankle* 1980;1(2): 84-89.

12. Cho BK, Kim YM, Kim DS, Choi ES, Shon HC, Park KJ: Outcomes of the modified Brostrom procedure using suture anchors for chronic lateral ankle instability: A prospective, randomized comparison between single and double suture anchors. *J Foot Ankle Surg* 2013;52(1):9-15.

13. Petrera M, Dwyer T, Theodoropoulos JS, Ogilvie-Harris DJ: Short- to medium-term outcomes after a modified Broström repair for lateral ankle instability with immediate postoperative weightbearing. *Am J Sports Med* 2014;42(7):1542-1548.

14. Sikka RS, Fetzer GB, Sugarman E, et al: Correlating MRI findings with disability in syndesmotic sprains of NFL players. *Foot Ankle Int* 2012;33(5):371-378.

15. Schepers T: Acute distal tibiofibular syndesmosis injury: A systematic review of suture-button versus syndesmotic screw repair. *Int Orthop* 2012;36(6):1199-1206.

16. Schepers T, Van Lieshout EM, de Vries MR, Van der Elst M: Complications of syndesmotic screw removal. *Foot Ankle Int* 2011;32(11):1040-1044.

17. Naqvi GA, Cunningham P, Lynch B, Galvin R, Awan N: Fixation of ankle syndesmotic injuries: Comparison of tightrope fixation and syndesmotic screw fixation for accuracy of syndesmotic reduction. *Am J Sports Med* 2012;40(12):2828-2835.

18. Grassi A, Samuelsson K, D'Hooghe P, et al: Dynamic stabilization of syndesmosis injuries reduces complications and reoperations as compared with screw fixation: A meta-analysis of randomized controlled trials. *Am J Sports Med* 2020;48(4):1000-1013. doi:10.1177/0363546519849909.

    This is a meta-analysis of randomized controlled trials, which demonstrated that dynamic fixation of syndesmotic injuries was superior to static screw fixation at 2-year follow-up. Outcomes were especially superior for dynamic fixation with regard to malreduction, clinical instability, and revision surgery. Level of evidence: I.

19. Sankar WN, Chen J, Kay RM, Skaggs DL: Incidence of occult fracture in children with acute ankle injuries. *J Pediatr Orthop* 2008;28(5):500-501.

20. Farley FA, Kuhns L, Jacobson JA, DiPietro M: Ultrasound examination of ankle injuries in children. *J Pediatr Orthop* 2001;21(5):604-607.

21. Kwak YH, Lim JY, Oh MK, Kim WJ, Park KB: Radiographic diagnosis of occult distal fibular avulsion fracture in children with acute lateral ankle sprain. *J Pediatr Orthop* 2015;35(4):352-357.

22. Kleiger B, Mankin HJ: Fracture of the lateral portion of the distal tibial epiphysis. *J Bone Joint Surg Am* 1964;46:25-32.

23. Parikh SN, Mehlman CT: The community orthopaedic surgeon taking trauma call: Pediatric ankle fracture pearls and pitfalls. *J Orthop Trauma* 2017;31 suppl 6:S27-S31. doi:10.1097/BOT.0000000000001014.

    This study is a review of the existing literature on paediatric ankle fractures which emphasizes the use of CT and a physeal-respecting approach to fracture management in this age group. Level of evidence: V.

24. Choudhry IK, Wall EJ, Eismann EA, Crawford AH, Wilson L: Functional outcome analysis of triplane and tillaux fractures after closed reduction and percutaneous fixation. *J Pediatr Orthop* 2014;34(2):139-143.

25. Philbin TM, Landis GS, Smith B: Peroneal tendon injuries. *J Am Acad Orthop Surg* 2009;17(5):306-317.

26. Forrester RA, Eyre-Brook AI, Mannan K: Iselin's disease: A systematic review. *J Foot Ankle Surg* 2017;56(5):1065-1069. doi:10.1053/j.jfas.2017.04.030.

    Iselin disease is described in this case report as a traction apophysitis of the fifth metatarsal base which is an uncommon finding in adolescents. Level of evidence: IV.

27. Hau WWS, Lui TH, Ngai WK: Endoscopic superior peroneal retinaculum reconstruction. *Arthrosc Tech* 2017;7(1):e45-e51. doi:10.1016/j.eats.2017.08.050. eCollection 2018 January.

    This is a technical note article that describes endoscopic superior peroneal retinaculum reconstruction as a useful tool that is both minimally invasive and comprehensive in treating peroneal retinaculum injury. Level of evidence: V.

28. Walther M, Morrison R, Mayer B: Retromalleolar groove impaction for the treatment of unstable peroneal tendons. *Am J Sports Med* 2009;37(1):191-194.

29. Van Dijk PA, Gianakos AL, Kerkhoffs GM, Kennedy JG: Return to sports and clinical outcomes in patients treated for peroneal tendon dislocation: A systematic review. *Knee Surg Sports Traumatol Arthrosc* 2016;24(4):1155-1164. doi:10.1007/s00167-015-3833-z.

    This systematic review found that surgical treatment of peroneal tendon dislocation provides significantly higher rates of return to sports. Based on their review of existing literature, the authors recommend surgical management should include groove deepening of the superior peroneal tunnel and tendon stabilization via superior peroneal retinaculum repair. Level of evidence: IV.

30. Steel MW, DeOrio JK: Peroneal tendon tears: Return to sports after operative treatment. *Foot Ankle Int* 2007;28(1):49-54.
31. Heckman DS, Reddy S, Pedowitz D, Wapner KL, Parekh SG: Operative treatment for peroneal tendon disorders. *J Bone Joint Surg Am* 2008;90(2):404-418.
32. Raikin SM: Intrasheath subluxation of the peroneal tendons. Surgical technique. *J Bone Joint Surg Am* 2009;91(suppl 2, pt 1):146-155. doi:10.2106/JBJS.H.01356.
33. Kessler JI, Weiss JM, Nikizad H, et al: Osteochondritis dissecans of the ankle in children and adolescents: Demographics and epidemiology. *Am J Sports Med* 2014;42(9):2165-2171.
34. Thacker MM, Dabney KW, Mackenzie WG: Osteochondritis dissecans of the talar head: Natural history and review of literature. *J Pediatr Orthop B* 2012;21(4):373-376.
35. Berndt AL, Harty M: Transchondral fractures (osteochondritis dissecans) of the talus. *J Bone Joint Surg Am* 1959;41:988-1020.
36. Canale ST, Belding RH: Osteochondral lesions of the talus. *J Bone Joint Surg Am* 1980;62(1):97-102.
37. Flick AB, Gould N: Osteochondritis dissecans of the talus (transchondral fractures of the talus): Review of the literature and new surgical approach for medial dome lesions. *Foot Ankle* 1985;5(4):165-185.
38. Tamam C, Tamam MO, Yildirim D, Mulazimoglu M: Diagnostic value of single-photon emission computed tomography combined with computed tomography in relation to MRI on osteochondral lesions of the talus. *Nucl Med Commun* 2015;36(8):808-814. doi:10.1097/MNM.0000000000000323.
39. Leumann A, Valderrabano V, Plaass C, et al: A novel imaging method for osteochondral lesions of the talus – Comparison of SPECT-CT with MRI. *Am J Sports Med* 2011;39(5):1095-1101. doi:10.1177/0363546510392709.
40. Hepple S, Winson IG, Glew D: Osteochondral lesions of the talus: A revised classification. *Foot Ankle Int* 1999;20(12):789-793.
41. Mintz DN, Tashjian GS, Connell DA, Deland JT, O'Malley M, Potter HG: Osteochondral lesions of the talus: A new magnetic resonance grading system with arthroscopic correlation. *Arthroscopy* 2003;19(4):353-359.
42. Verhagen RA, Struijs PA, Bossuyt PM, van Dijk CN: Systematic review of treatment strategies for osteochondral defects of the talar dome. *Foot Ankle Clin* 2003;8(2):233-242, viii-ix.
43. Kramer DE, Glotzbecker MP, Shore BJ, et al: Results of surgical management of osteochondritis dissecans of the ankle in the pediatric and adolescent population. *J Pediatr Orthop* 2015;35(7):725-733.
44. Murawski CD, Kennedy JG: Operative treatment of osteochondral lesions of the talus. *J Bone Joint Surg Am* 2013;95(11):1045-1054.
45. Goh GS, Bin Abd Razak HR, Mitra AK: Outcomes are favorable after arthroscopic treatment of osteochondritis dissecans of the talus. *J Foot Ankle Surg* 2015;54(1):57-60.
46. Kumai T, Takakura Y, Higashiyama I, Tamai S: Arthroscopic drilling for the treatment of osteochondral lesions of the talus. *J Bone Joint Surg Am* 1999;81(9):1229-1235.
47. Hirtler L, Schellander K, Schuh R: Accessibility to talar dome in neutral position, dorsiflexion, or noninvasive distraction in posterior ankle arthroscopy. *Foot Ankle Int* 2019;40(8):978-986. doi:10.1177/1071100719847134.

    This is a cadaver study of 20 matched pairs of anatomic ankle specimens, which concluded that accessibility of the talar dome is best in maximal dorsiflexion. This finding is relevant for surgical technique and planning in arthroscopic treatment of osteochondral lesions of the talus. Level of evidence: V.

48. Barnes CJ, Ferkel RD: Arthroscopic debridement and drilling of osteochondral lesions of the talus. *Foot Ankle Clin* 2003;8(2):243-257.
49. Zengerink M, Struijs PA, Tol JL, van Dijk CN: Treatment of osteochondral lesions of the talus: A systematic review. *Knee Surg Sports Traumatol Arthrosc* 2010;18(2):238-246.
50. Hangody L, Vásárhelyi G, Hangody LR, et al: Autologous osteochondral grafting: Technique and long-term results. *Injury* 2008;39(suppl 1):S32-S39.
51. Paul J, Sagstetter M, Lämmle L, et al: Sports activity after osteochondral transplantation of the talus. *Am J Sports Med* 2012;40(4):870-874.
52. Van Eekeren IC, van Bergen CJ, Sierevelt IN, Reilingh ML, van Dijk CN: Return to sports after arthroscopic debridement and bone marrow stimulation of osteochondral talar defects: A 5- to 24-year follow-up study. *Knee Surg Sports Traumatol Arthrosc* 2016;24(4):1311-1315. doi:10.1007/s00167-016-3992-6.

    This is a retrospective review of 93 patients who underwent arthroscopic debridement and bone marrow stimulation of osteochondral lesions of the talus. Of these, 76% of patients returned to sports at long-term follow-up. However, the long-term activity level after these procedures never reached preinjury baselines. Level of evidence: IV.

53. Lambers KTA, Dahmen J, Reilingh ML, van Bergen CJA, Stufkens SAS, Kerkhoffs GMMJ: No superior surgical treatment for secondary osteochondral defects of the talus. *Knee Surg Sports Traumatol Arthrosc* 2018;26(7):2158-2170. doi:10.1007/s00167-017-4629-0.

    This is a systematic review of 21 studies that described surgical treatment for talar osteochondral defects after failed primary surgery. No significant difference between various treatments could be identified due to the low levels of evidence and the limited numbers of patients in these studies. Level of evidence: IV.

CHAPTER 54

Overuse Conditions

PAMELA J. LANG, MD • RICHARD E. BOWEN, MD • JENNIFER J. BECK, MD

ABSTRACT

Promoting safe, well-rounded participation in youth athletics can help develop a lifetime of physical activity and healthy habits while decreasing the risk of injuries. It has become clear that current training regimens of early sport specialization, year-round activity participation, and training of increasing intensity are leading to an increase in overtraining and burnout in young athletes. Although the medical community has a clear understanding of the problem of overuse and burnout, further research is needed on the efficacy of prevention programs, the management of overuse injuries, and the appropriate timing of return to sports after an injury.

Keywords: burnout; chronic pain; overtraining; overuse; young athletes

INTRODUCTION

According to the National Federation of State High School Associations, participation in high school athletics has increased dramatically from approximately 4 million participants in 1971 to approximately 8 million participants in 2014.[1] Along with this increase in sports participation, the intensity and time requirements of competition and training have amplified. With an increase in the popularity of club sports participation, many children are now playing a single sport throughout the year, without periods of rest and recovery. Consequently, there are increasing numbers of overuse conditions being diagnosed in children. Currently, approximately 50% of childhood sports-related injuries are attributed to overuse.[2-8]

Overuse injuries are caused by repetitive submaximal loading with inadequate rest, resulting in the inability for structural repair and adaptation.[2,3,9] For the purpose of research, an overuse injury has been defined as "a condition to which no identifiable single external transfer of energy could be associated but that led to the athlete being unable to take full part in athletics training."[10] The four stages of overuse are (1) pain after activity, (2) pain during activity but without hindering performance, (3) pain during activity leading to detrimental effects on performance, and (4) unrelenting pain, even at rest.[11] The loss of practice and competition time would be expected for injuries that progress to stages three or four.

Recent research has focused on understanding the etiology and epidemiology of pediatric overuse injuries, describing overuse injuries in pediatric-specific subpopulations and sports, determining risk factors associated with pediatric overuse injuries, and defining prevention strategies for coaches, parents, and medical providers.[2-4,12-15] The treatment of pediatric overuse injuries has received little attention because the traditional treatment modalities of rest, anti-inflammatory medications, physical therapy, and bracing treatment still apply for most patients. For example, a 12-year-old runner with heel pain secondary to Sever apophysitis can be successfully managed with activity modification and stretching.

EPIDEMIOLOGY AND RISK FACTORS

Overuse injuries make up at least 50% of the sports-related injuries that occur during childhood.[2,8,14] Approximately 50% of overuse injuries in high school athletes result in

Dr. Bowen or an immediate family member serves as an unpaid consultant to Imagen. Dr. Beck or an immediate family member serves as a board member, owner, officer, or committee member of the Pediatric Orthopaedic Society of North America and the Pediatric Research in Sports Medicine. Neither Dr. Lang nor any immediate family member has received anything of value from or has stock or stock options held in a commercial company or institution related directly or indirectly to the subject of this chapter.

loss of play time or sports participation of more than 1 week.[3] A 2015 study reported that 7.7% of chronic or overuse injuries in high school athletes resulted in more than 21 days of lost competition time, and 2.5% of the athletes required surgical intervention to treat cartilage and disk injuries, tendinosis, tendinitis, or muscle strain.[2] Stress fractures were the most common season-ending overuse injury.[2] Two studies found that the most common site of an overuse injury is the lower leg, with approximately 70% of overuse injuries in high school athletes involving the leg.[2,3]

Girls have a higher rate of overuse injuries than boys (13.3% versus 5.5%, respectively), and these injuries occur early during the high school years (30.7% of overuse injuries occurred during the ninth grade).[3] The same sex prevalence was found in high school and collegiate athletes.[2] The lower leg, knee, and ankle, in particular, are the areas that are more commonly affected in girls compared with boys. In a report on high school distance runners, tibial stress injuries were found in 41% of the girls and 34% of the boys, and patellofemoral pain occurred in 21% of the girls and 16% of the boys.[5] The authors of a 2015 study reported that the variability in body mass index (BMI) and sport characteristics between sexes is responsible for approximately 50% of the increased risks of overuse injuries in girls, with the other 50% attributable to biologic differences.[16]

Risk factors for overuse injury can be categorized as either intrinsic or extrinsic.[13,17] Intrinsic risk factors are those that are unique to an individual. Some intrinsic risk factors are not modifiable, including sex and maturation status. Factors such as BMI, biomechanical movement patterns, and anatomic alignment are potentially modifiable intrinsic risk factors.[17] Skeletally immature athletes with joint hypermobility, muscle weakness, and muscle tightness are at increased risk for overuse injury.[9]

Extrinsic risk factors include environment, equipment, and (probably most importantly) training regimens.[17] The authors of an investigation of extrinsic risk factors involved in overuse injury described three scenarios in which these factors play a role in the development of overuse injury.[18] These scenarios involved (1) a rapid increase in training load after a period of decreased activity, (2) participation at an athletic level that exceeds an individual's skill or fitness level, and (3) continuous participation at a high level of athletics or in a single activity or sport.[18]

PHYSIOLOGIC CONSIDERATIONS IN THE GROWING ATHLETE

Skeletally immature athletes have areas of rapidly growing cartilage, physes, and apophyses, with decreased tensile strength compared with that of surrounding bone and up to five times less tensile strength than surrounding ligaments and tendons.[9,19] The hypertrophic zone, including the zone of provisional calcification, is the weakest portion of the physis; this increases its propensity to injury during phases of rapid growth.[9,20] In addition, muscle and tendon adaptations lag behind longitudinal bone growth, which results in the need for a greater percentage of muscle force to perform the same movements.[19] This increased relative muscle contraction force leads to increased forces transferred to the apophysis and makes the physis and apophysis more vulnerable to injury.[19] The apophysis itself is subject to twice the tensile force as the adjacent tendon, making it a particularly vulnerable area in children.[19]

Repetitive stress on the apophysis or physis can result in apophysitis or epiphysiolysis, respectively. Apophysitis is a common cause of pain in the knee, foot and pelvis.[21] Epiphysiolysis due to chronic stress on the physis can result in physeal widening, early calcification, and physeal bar formation, which ultimately lead to growth disturbances such as premature distal radius physeal closure in the wrists of gymnasts.[20,22-25] Growth disturbances related to physeal stress injury also have been documented in the proximal humerus, distal femur, and proximal tibia.[13,22,26,27] One theory is that repetitive stress leads to a disruption of the metaphyseal blood supply, altered endochondral ossification of the physis, and physeal widening caused by chondrocyte accumulation in the proliferative zone.[20]

Not only is there greater stress on the physis and apophysis of bone during periods of growth, but also the mechanical structure of the bone itself may not be able to withstand the demands of high-level, continuous competition. Muscle adaptation and bone mineralization in skeletally immature individuals lags behind linear bone growth.[22,28] Measurements of bone mineral density in a group of boys and girls during the adolescent growth period found that bone mass decreased relative to bone size just before the time of peak height velocity.[29] Following this drop in bone mineral density, a continuous increase occurred until approximately 4 years after peak height velocity.[29] These findings imply that the risk of osseous overuse injury may be highest during the period just before peak height velocity growth.

OVERTRAINING, SPECIALIZATION, AND BURNOUT

Burnout, which also is known as overtraining syndrome or nonfunctional overreaching, is a maladaptive process resulting from excessive exercise and inadequate rest.[9] It may be caused by an increased training load with inadequate recovery, monotony of training, or overscheduling. Ultimately, burnout increases an athlete's risk for an overuse injury.[9] A 2011 study surveyed 360 pediatric athletes aged 6 to 18 years presenting to sports medicine clinics for injury evaluation. The authors found a substantial association between an athlete's or parent's perception of too much training or competitive play without enough rest between scheduled activities and the time immediately leading up to the onset of symptoms.[15]

The pathophysiology behind burnout is a systemic inflammatory response, affecting the neurohormonal axis (hypothalamus, pituitary, and end organs such as the thyroid, the gonad, and the adrenal glands).[9] As a result, there are detrimental effects on immunity and mood in addition to a decreased level of athletic performance.[9] A survey of 376 English athletes found a lack of confidence and bad feelings in athletes with burnout when their level of performance did not meet their expectations.[30] Diagnostic criteria of burnout include a persistent decrease in performance even after weeks to months of rest, along with mood disturbances that cannot be attributed to other causes.[31] Burnout in a child has been described as decreased enthusiasm to participate in practices or games, chronic muscle or joint pain, an elevated resting heart rate, personality changes, and difficulty in successfully completing familiar routines.[11]

Overtraining and burnout in athletes are becoming more common or, at least, are more widely recognized. At least one occurrence of overtraining was reported by 110 of the 376 athletes (29%) in a survey of English athletes.[30] Women, elite athletes, and participants in sports with low physical demands were more likely to report overtraining.[30] In a recent study of socioeconomic status and training, athletes with high socioeconomic status reported more hours per week in organized sports, increased specialization, and more overuse injuries compared with those with lower socioeconomic status.[32] A survey of athletes with overtraining syndrome found they were more likely to rate their sport as their most important activity, and they spent a limited amount of time engaged in other hobbies, suggesting that specialization in a single sport may increase the risk of burnout by encouraging an individual to focus all of his or her energy on one sport.[30]

Efforts to combat early sports specialization have grown with additional evidence that it does not provide benefits and may in fact be detrimental.[33] In a 2015 study where specialization was defined as "year-round intensive training in a single sport at the exclusion of other sports," specialization was found to be an independent risk factor for overuse and serious overuse injuries, even when accounting for patient age and hours spent participating in that sport.[12] In addition, a dose-response relationship between the degree of specialization and the severity of the overuse injury was found, with a serious overuse injury more likely to develop in the youth athletes who were the most specialized.[12] The modest association between sports specialization and overuse injury reported in a 2016 review of three retrospective studies was further supported in a 2018 meta-analysis which found a relationship between overuse injury and the level of specialization.[34,35] The association between specialization and injury may depend on the sport. A 2017 case-control study found that those who specialized in individual sports did so at younger ages, reported higher training volumes, and sustained more overuse injuries that young athletes who specialized in team sports.[36]

PREVENTION

In response to the rising concern about overuse injuries in youth athletes, the STOP Sports Injuries campaign was initiated in 2007 by the American Orthopaedic Society for Sports Medicine. It is estimated that approximately 50% of overuse injuries in children and adolescents may be preventable.[24] It is believed that prevention of overuse injuries during childhood may be important in preventing chronic overuse conditions later in life and promoting lifelong activity and sports participation.[2,7,13,37] The prevention of overuse injury is a multidisciplinary undertaking and involves improved injury surveillance, identification of risk factors, thorough preparticipation physical examinations, proper supervision and education of coaches and medical staff, improved training and conditioning, sport alterations, and delayed specialization.[13,24,38]

A detailed patient history is important in screening for overuse injury or burnout. The history should include assessment of the athlete's attitude and level of fatigue, parental pressure, and coach involvement. To determine an athlete's training workload, an assessment should be made regarding the number of hours per week of participation in a structured sport along with sport-specific measures such as pitch counts, miles run per week, and the number of team memberships, conditioning or strength training sessions, and days off per week.[9,13] The physical examination should include methods to screen for joint hypermobility (such as the Beighton and Horan Joint Mobility Index) and muscle tightness or imbalances (such as the Ober test, the Thomas test, and evaluation of the popliteal angle, the degree of ankle dorsiflexion, and the glenohumeral internal rotation deficit).[9]

Prevention programs should be aimed at encouraging an appropriate training progression. Training and prevention programs should ultimately strive to help young athletes improve their ability to dampen forces applied to their body.[17] The American Academy of Pediatrics Council on Sports Medicine and Fitness released recommendations aimed at reducing overuse injuries and overtraining in skeletally immature individuals.[11,39] It was suggested that the amount of time in any single sporting activity be limited to a maximum of 5 d/wk, with at least 1 day off from any organized physical activity each week.[11,39] The recommendations also include allowing 2 to 3 months away from any particular sport each year.[11,39] In addition, children and adolescents should get at least 7 hours of sleep per night to decrease chronic fatigue and reduce the injury rate.[15,40] In 2015, the International Olympic Committee published their consensus statement on youth athletic development[41] (**Table 1**).

UPDATE ON COMMON OVERUSE INJURIES

Common pediatric overuse injuries of the upper extremity, lower extremity, and spine are listed in **Table 2**.

Elbow Injuries in Young Throwers

With more than 5 million children participating in baseball, rates of elbow injuries seem to be increasing in throwing athletes despite regulations and safety measures implemented by organizational leagues.[42,43] The diagnosis and treatment of pediatric elbow overuse injuries warrants attention.

In the past, elbow pain was described by the general term Little Leaguer's elbow; however, it is now understood that multiple etiologies contribute to elbow pain in young, throwing athletes. Ulnar collateral ligament injuries, olecranon stress fractures, capitellar osteochondritis dissecans, medial epicondyle apophysitis, and fractures commonly occur in throwing athletes. An increased risk of pitching-related arm pain has been shown in young athletes who pitch on consecutive days, pitch on multiple teams with overlapping seasons, and pitch multiple games per day.[42-44] Throwing curveballs is associated with a 1.66-fold increased risk of pitching-related injuries in athletes aged 9 to 18 years, whereas those who pitch with arm tiredness and pain have more than a 7-fold greater risk of pitching-related injury.[44]

In response to the increasing incidence of pediatric elbow injuries in throwing athletes, a set of guidelines for youth pitchers based on established guidelines and clinical experience was proposed in 2012[43] (**Table 3**); however, despite these guidelines, elbow injuries continue to occur. The treatment of these elbow injuries often

TABLE 1

International Olympic Committee Consensus Statement on Youth Athletic Development

General Principles	Conditioning for Injury Prevention	Coaching	Nutrition, Hydration, Heat	Sports Medicine Governing Bodies
Allow for a wider definition of sport success Commit to psychologic development of resilient and adaptable athletes Use an evidence-based framework for athlete development and coaching Encourage unstructured play Promote safety, health, and respect for rules, athletes, and the game Assist athletes with sport-life balance	Encourage varied strength and conditioning programs Develop programs with diversity and variability of athletic exposure Promote injury prevention programs, protective equipment legislation, and rule changes No youth athlete should compete, train, or practice in a way that loads the affected injured area or interferes with or delays recovery when in pain or not completely rehabilitated and recovered from an illness or injury	Provide a challenging and enjoyable environment Use research-based techniques that promote innovation and proper technique Encourage athlete intrapersonal and interpersonal skill development Seek interdisciplinary support and guidance	Provide dietary education on a healthy, balanced diet Provide education on risks associated with dietary supplements and energy drinks Mitigate risks of energy deficiency in athletes Educate and train on heat-related illness Create a written emergency plan for treating medical emergencies	Protect the health and well-being of youth in sports with education and safeguards Diversification and variability of athletic exposure should be encouraged Competitions should be age and skill appropriate, with sufficient rest and recovery

TABLE 2

Common Overuse Injuries in Pediatric Patients

Location	Conditions
Upper extremity	Distal clavicle osteolysis
	Proximal humeral physeal separation
	Rotator cuff tendinitis
	Olecranon stress fractures
	Capitellum osteochondritis dissecans
	Ulnar collateral ligament strain/tear
	Medial epicondyle apophysitis/fracture
	Chronic exertional compartment syndrome
	Gymnast wrist
Lower extremity	Femoral/tibial/metatarsal stress fracture
	Femoroacetabular impingement
	Medial tibial stress syndrome
	Chronic exertional compartment syndrome
	Patellofemoral syndrome
	Iliotibial band friction syndrome
	Osteochondritis dissecans
	Osgood-Schlatter disease
	Sinding-Larsen-Johansson disease
	Patellar tendinitis
	Symptomatic plica
	Hoffa fat pad syndrome
	Sever disease
	Symptomatic accessory navicular bone
	Symptomatic os trigonum
Spine	Posture-related back pain
	Spondylolysis and spondylolisthesis

includes temporary cessation of pitching and overhead activities, the administration of anti-inflammatory medications, icing of the elbow, and the implementation of physical therapy that focuses on core strengthening along with shoulder and elbow flexibility and strengthening. Proper instruction on performing the sleeper stretch for the shoulder is an important part of the physical therapy program. Young athletes with elbow injuries may require individual coaching or performance evaluations to improve their technique and decrease the risk for future injury. Surgical intervention is rarely required, and it is typically reserved for patients in whom an extensive period of nonsurgical management has been unsuccessful.

TABLE 3

Guidelines for Young Throwing Athletes

- Watch and respond to signs of fatigue; rest for any symptoms
- Minimum 2-3 mo of rest per year, with 4 mo preferred
- Do not pitch >100 game innings in any calendar year
- Follow limits for pitch counts and days of rest
- Avoid pitching on multiple teams with overlapping seasons
- Learn proper throwing mechanics with gradual progression
- Avoid using radar guns
- A pitcher should not also be a catcher
- Any elbow or shoulder pain should initiate a sports medicine referral
- Encourage athletes' involvement in various activities in which they show interest and enthusiasm

Anterior Knee Pain

Patellofemoral pain or patellofemoral stress syndrome is the most common overuse injury in runners and those who participate in running sports such as basketball and soccer. This syndrome has been termed runner's knee and is described as peripatellar knee pain that increases with activities such as running, jumping, stair climbing, squatting, and sitting with the knees flexed for a prolonged time.[17] Specific causes of anterior knee pain unique among young athletes include the apophyseal conditions Sinding-Larsen-Johansson (SLJ) apophysitis and Osgood-Schlatter (OS) apophysitis. SLJ and OS apohysitis are two of the three most common overuse conditions in young athletes.[45] OS disease is caused by chronic tensile stresses of the patellar tendon on the tibial tubercle apophysis. It presents as a prominent and tender tibial tubercle, and patients may have decreased knee motion (flexion). Radiographically, it can result in widening or even fragmentation of the tibial tubercle apophysis (**Figure 1**). Although less common than OS, SLJ is also a cause of chronic anterior knee pain in active adolescents and is a result of chronic tensile stress of the patellar tendon on the inferior pole of the patella. Patients with SLJ have tenderness over the inferior pole of the patella and proximal patellar tendon and may have fragmentation of the inferior pole of the patella seen on the lateral knee radiograph (**Figure 2**). Specialization in a single sport incurs a 1.5-fold increased relative risk of anterior knee pain in adolescent female athletes and a 4-fold increase in SLJ disease, patellar tendinopathy, and OS apophysitis.[46] A 2018 study evaluated the patellar

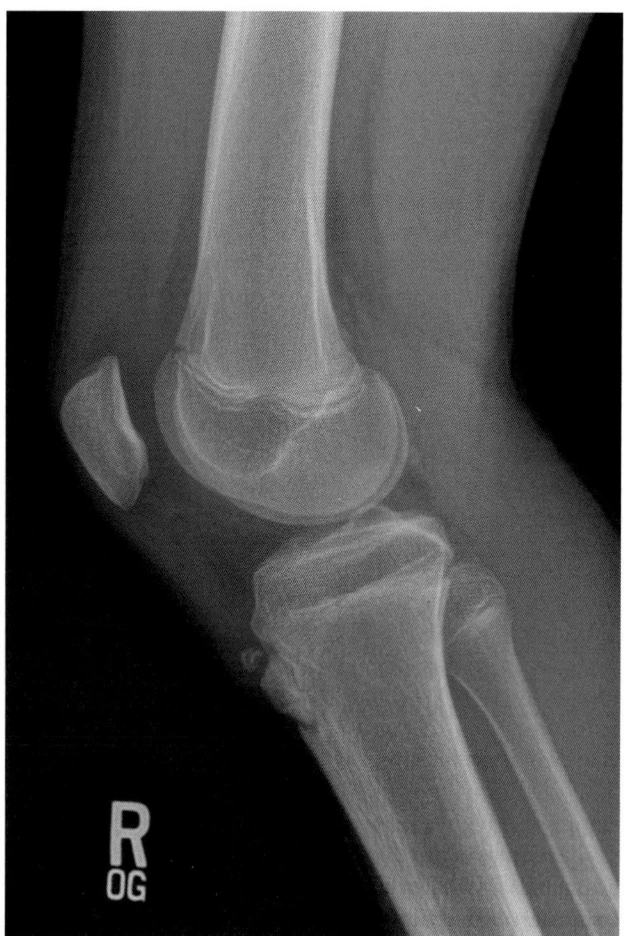

FIGURE 1 Lateral radiograph showing fragmentation of the tibial tubercle consistent with history of Osgood-Schlatter apophysitis.

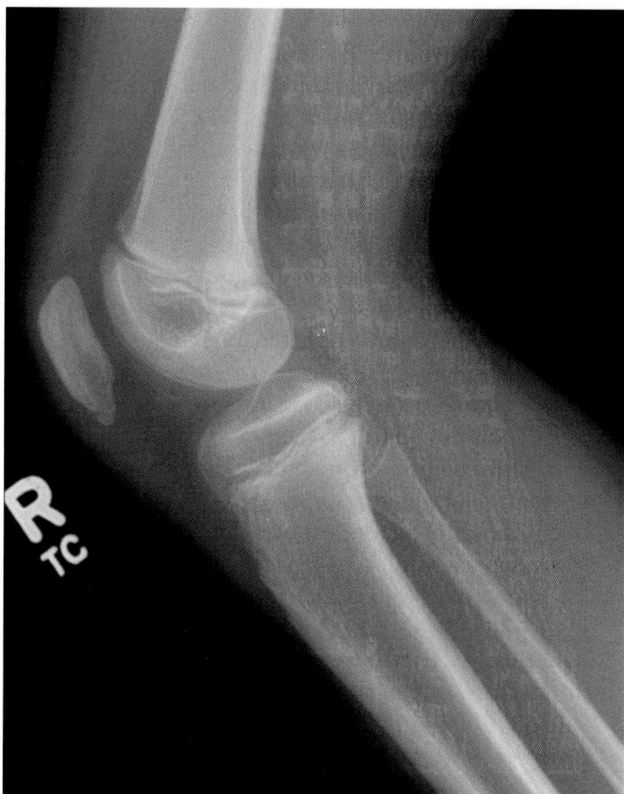

FIGURE 2 Lateral knee radiograph showing fragmentation of the inferior pole of the patella as seen in Sinding-Larsen-Johansson apophysitis.

tendon clinically and by ultrasonography in adolescents, finding patellar tendinopathy in 13% of the 4% of the nonathletes.[47]

Plica syndrome is another cause of anterior knee pain in young athletes. Once termed breast stroker's knee, it is the result of inflammation and fibrosis of a persistent synovial fold, most commonly in the anteromedial capsule.[48,49] It has been associated with lateral maltracking of the patella, a tight lateral retinaculum, and chondral changes of the medial femoral condyle.[49] Patients with a painful synovial plica typically have tenderness over a palpable synovial fold, and symptoms may worsen with sports participation, climbing stairs, or doing squats and lunges.

Treatment of anterior knee pain regardless of specific cause follows a similar protocol. A 2017 meta-analysis summarized the treatment of overuse anterior knee pain, which generally includes improving flexibility and addressing strength deficits.[45] Addressing biomechanical etiologies that may play a role in the development of patellofemoral stress syndrome has become common.[17,50-52] Improving proximal muscle strength and activation has become an important component of the treatment for patellofemoral pain as hip weakness is thought to increase loads across the patellofemoral joint and increase the functional quadriceps angle.[50-52] In addition to proximal stability, excessive or mistimed pronation is thought to alter transverse and frontal plane mechanics at the patellofemoral joint, thereby increasing patellofemoral joint compression forces.[50,51] Proper shoes, the addition of foot orthoses, or gait training may improve foot biomechanics while running.

Another component of the treatment of overuse conditions of the knee is rest. Although there is agreement that athletes should not fully return to sports until symptoms have resolved, a 2017 review noted that there is no consensus on the amount of rest young athletes require with half of the articles recommending 3 to 5 months of active rest, whereas another 21% suggest sports participation can continue as symptoms allow.[45]

Surgical interventions, such as diagnostic arthroscopy, isolated lateral release, and/or plica excision, have been performed with inconsistent results, with less than 40% of patients reporting pain-free outcomes after surgery.[48]

These poor surgical results reinforce the importance of multimodal nonsurgical management for anterior knee pain, including multiple pain management strategies, bracing treatment, physical therapy, coaching on proper techniques, and performance evaluations.

Tibial Stress Injury

Tibial stress injury represents a spectrum of overuse injuries ranging from medial tibial stress syndrome (MTSS), also known as shin splints, to a radiographically evident stress fracture. Leg pain caused by tibial stress injury is common in runners and athletes who participate in running sports. In a survey of high school cross-country runners, 68% of the girls and 59% of the boys had some lower extremity overuse injury or chronic injury in their lifetimes.[5] In an investigation of risk factors associated with chronic exercise-related leg pain in a group of high school cross-country athletes, it was found that 82.4% of athletes had experienced exercise-related leg pain at some time, with 48% experiencing pain during the current season.[7] More than 50% of the athletes who participated in cross-country running experienced leg pain related to running, and 58.4% reported that the pain had interfered with participation in their sport.[7] Most of those who experienced pain during the current season (97.8%) also had similar symptoms in the past.[7] This finding suggests that a history of running-related leg pain is a risk factor for recurrence of symptoms. In high school athletes, a higher weekly mileage total is associated with overuse injury in boys but not in girls. This finding suggests that other factors, such as mechanical alignment or biomechanics, may play a role in the development of overuse injuries.[5] No associations between running-related leg pain and training distance, sex, BMI, foot type, years of running, or age were found.[7]

MTSS is defined as an exercise-induced, localized pain along the distal two-thirds of the posteromedial tibia.[17,53] MTSS is more common in girls than in boys. Risk factors include a lack of running experience, a history of MTSS, and an increased BMI. It is unclear whether overpronation is associated with MTSS.[17,53] A retrospective study of adults showed decreased plantar flexor strength in runners with MTSS, which suggests that decreased plantar flexor muscle endurance may also be a risk for MTSS in younger athletes.[54] The treatment of MTSS is nonsurgical and includes foot orthoses, leg taping and bracing treatment, anti-inflammatory medications, icing, physical therapy to address muscle imbalance and weakness, and running analyses to improve foot strike forces and body position.

Tibial stress fractures occur in healthy bone when repetitive loading surpasses the bone's ability to remodel, resulting in the accumulation of microinjury within the bone.[17,55] Fatigue stress fractures are the more common type of stress fracture in pediatric athletes. In contrast, insufficiency stress fractures occur under normal loading conditions in the setting of pathologic bone.[17]

A stress fracture in a juvenile or an adolescent girl should raise suspicion that the patient may be affected by the female athlete triad. These patients should be assessed for amenorrhea and decreased bone mineral density. More recently, the term relative energy deficiency in sport has replaced female athlete triad to address the increasing rate of male patients with this metabolic abnormality.[56] The definition has been broadened to include dysfunction of metabolism, menses, bone health, immunity, protein synthesis, and cardiovascular health. Because pain associated with an osseous injury is often the presenting symptom, orthopaedic surgeons should be aware of the proper workup and referral for these patients. Confirmation of the diagnosis may include laboratory blood tests, bone mineralization tests, and nutritional and psychological evaluations. Although the multidisciplinary treatment plan is often best coordinated by a primary care physician who is knowledgeable about relative energy deficiency in sport, it is often initiated by an orthopaedic surgeon.

Overuse Conditions of the Foot and Ankle

The most common overuse injury of the foot and ankle in children is Sever apophysitis, which is an apophysitis at the calcaneal tubercle due to traction from the Achilles tendon.[21] Sever apophysitis presents as heel pain in skeletally immature athletes, 8 to 15 years of age, and resolves with fusion of the apophysis. Up to 60% of children have bilateral symptoms. Children may also have pain in the associated tendon, consistent with Achilles tendinitis. Lateral calcaneal radiographs are warranted in unilateral heel pain to rule out calcaneus tumors. Treatment of Sever apophysitis and Achilles tendinitis may include rest, Achilles stretching, eccentric strengthening, anti-inflammatory medications, heel cups or orthotics, and immobilization. A 2015 trial compared a wait-and-see approach, heel lifts, and a structured eccentric strengthening program for the treatment of Sever apophysitis, finding that they each improved patients' symptoms, without significant differences between treatment regimens.[57] Young patients with Achilles tendon pain do not seem to have tendon changes of tendinopathy associated with their pain. The same study that evaluated the patellar tendon in adolescents found signs of Achilles tendinopathy on clinical and ultrasonography evaluation in just 1% of the athletes and none of the nonathletes.[47]

More rare than Sever apophysitis is Iselin apophysitis, which is apophysitis at the base of the fifth metatarsal due to traction of the peroneus brevis tendon. Iselin disease is seen in young athletes participating in sports with recurrent running, cutting, jumping, and inversion stresses.[58] It can be mistaken for an avulsion injury, but is differentiated from a fracture by history and by the longitudinal orientation of the apophysis in contrast to a more transverse fracture line.[58] A 2015 case series reported relief of symptoms after about 4 weeks of treatment and average return to sport after about 5 weeks using a variety of nonsurgical treatments.[58]

SUMMARY

Promoting safe, well-rounded participation in youth athletics can help develop a lifetime of physical activity and healthy habits while decreasing the risk for injuries. It has become increasingly clear that current training regimens of early sport specialization, year-round activity participation, and increasingly intense training are leading to the increase in overtraining and burnout in youth athletes. Although the medical community has a clear understanding of the problems of overuse injuries and burnout, further research is needed on the efficacy of prevention programs, the treatment of overuse injuries, and the appropriate amount of time needed before return to sports after an injury.

KEY STUDY POINTS

- Approximately 50% of sports-related injuries in pediatric patients are overuse injuries.
- The education of parents, coaches, and medical providers can help prevent overuse injuries.
- Early specialization in a single sport increases the risk of overuse injuries in pediatric patients.
- Evaluation for the female athlete triad, now known as relative energy deficiency in sport, should be considered in any female athlete with a stress fracture.

ANNOTATED REFERENCES

1. National Federation of State High School Associations: *2013-14 High School Athletics Participation Survey.* 2014, pp 53-71. Available at: http://www.nfhs.org/participationstatistics/participationstatistics/. Accessed January 1, 2015.
2. Roos KG, Marshall SW, Kerr ZY, et al: Epidemiology of overuse injuries in collegiate and high school athletics in the United States. *Am J Sports Med* 2015;43(7):1790-1797. doi:10.1177/0363546515580790.
3. Schroeder AN, Comstock RD, Collins CL, Everhart J, Flanigan D, Best TM: Epidemiology of overuse injuries among high-school athletes in the United States. *J Pediatr* 2015;166(3):600-606. doi:10.1016/j.jpeds.2014.09.037.
4. Hoang QB, Mortazavi M: Pediatric overuse injuries in sports. *Adv Pediatr* 2012;59(1):359-383. doi:10.1016/j.yapd.2012.04.005.
5. Tenforde AS, Sayres LC, McCurdy ML, Collado H, Sainani KL, Fredericson M: Overuse injuries in high school runners: Lifetime prevalence and prevention strategies. *PM R* 2011;3(2):125-131. doi:10.1016/j.pmrj.2010.09.009.
6. Hjelm N, Werner S, Renstrom P: Injury profile in junior tennis players: A prospective two year study. *Knee Surg Sports Traumatol Arthrosc* 2010;18(6):845-850. doi:10.1007/s00167-010-1094-4.
7. Reinking MF, Austin TM, Hayes AM: Risk factors for self-reported exercise-related leg pain in high school cross-country athletes. *J Athl Train* 2010;45(1):51-57. doi:10.4085/1062-6050-45.1.51.
8. Bonza JE, Fields SK, Yard EE, Comstock RD: Shoulder injuries among United States high school athletes during the 2005-2006 and 2006-2007 school years. *J Athl Train* 2009;44(1):76-83. doi:10.4085/1062-6050-44.1.76.
9. Smucny M, Parikh SN, Pandya NK: Consequences of single sport specialization in the pediatric and adolescent athlete. *Orthop Clin North Am* 2015;46(2):249-258. doi:10.1016/j.ocl.2014.11.004.
10. Timpka T, Jacobsson J, Dahlström Ö, et al: The psychological factor "self-blame" predicts overuse injury among top-level Swedish track and field athletes: A 12-month cohort study. *Br J Sports Med* 2015;49(22):1472-1477. doi:10.1136/bjsports-2015-094622.
11. Brenner JS: Overuse injuries, overtraining, and burnout in child and adolescent athletes. *Pediatrics* 2007;119(6):1242-1245. doi:10.1542/peds.2007-0887.
12. Jayanthi NA, LaBella CR, Fischer D, Pasulka J, Dugas LR: Sports-specialized intensive training and the risk of injury in young athletes: A clinical case-control study. *Am J Sports Med* 2015;43(4):794-801. doi:10.1177/0363546514567298.
13. Difiori JP, Benjamin HJ, Brenner J, et al: Overuse injuries and burnout in youth sports: A position statement from the American Medical Society for Sports Medicine. *Clin J Sport Med* 2014;24(1):3-20. doi:10.1097/JSM.0000000000000060.
14. Franklin CC, Weiss JM: Stopping sports injuries in kids: An overview of the last year in publications. *Curr Opin Pediatr* 2012;24(1):64-67. doi:10.1097/MOP.0b013e32834ec618.
15. Luke A, Lazaro RM, Bergeron MF, et al: Sports-related injuries in youth athletes: Is overscheduling a risk factor? *Clin J Sport Med* 2011;21(4):307-314. doi:10.1097/JSM.0b013e3182218f71.
16. Stracciolini A, Casciano R, Friedman HL, Meehan WP III, Micheli LJ: A closer look at overuse injuries in the pediatric athlete. *Clin J Sport Med* 2015;25(1):30-35. doi:10.1097/jsm.0000000000000105.
17. Paterno MV, Taylor-Haas JA, Myer GD, Hewett TE: Prevention of overuse sports injuries in the young athlete. *Orthop Clin North Am* 2013;44(4):553-564. doi:10.1016/j.ocl.2013.06.009.
18. Hogan KA, Gross RH: Overuse injuries in pediatric athletes. *Orthop Clin North Am* 2003;34(3):405-415. doi:10.1016/S0030-5898(03)00006-3.

19. Hawkins D, Metheny J: Overuse injuries in youth sports: Biomechanical considerations. *Med Sci Sports Exerc* 2001;33(10):1701-1707. doi:10.1097/00005768-200110000-00014.

20. Paz DA, Chang GH, Yetto JM Jr, Dwek JR, Chung CB: Upper extremity overuse injuries in pediatric athletes: Clinical presentation, imaging findings, and treatment. *J Clin Imaging* 2015;39(6):954-964. doi:10.1016/j.clinimag.2015.07.028.

21. Achar S, Yamanaka J: Apophysitis and osteochondrosis: Common causes of pain in growing bones. *Am Fam Physician* 2019;99(10):610-618.

Apophysitis and osteochondrosis are common causes of pain in growing bones but have differing etiologies and required management.

22. Caine D, Purcell L, Maffulli N: The child and adolescent athlete: A review of three potentially serious injuries. *BMC Sports Sci Med Rehabil* 2014;6(1):22. doi:10.1186/2052-1847-6-22.

23. De Smet L, Claessens A, Lefevre J, Beunen G: Gymnast wrist: An epidemiologic survey of ulnar variance and stress changes of the radial physis in elite female gymnasts. *Am J Sports Med* 1994;22(6):846-850. doi:10.1177/036354659402200618.

24. Valovich McLeod TC, Decoster LC, Loud KJ, et al: National Athletic Trainers' Association position statement: Prevention of pediatric overuse injuries. *J Athl Train* 2011;46(2):206-220. doi:10.4085/1062-6050-46.2.206.

25. Difiori JP: Overuse injury and the young athlete: The case of chronic wrist pain in gymnasts. *Curr Sports Med Rep* 2006;5:165-167.

26. Blatnik TR, Briskin S: Bilateral knee pain in a high-level gymnast. *Clin J Sport Med* 2013;23:77-79. doi:10.1097/JSM.0b013e31825c464d.

27. Laor T, Wall EJ, Vu LP: Physeal widening in the knee due to stress injury in child athletes. *AJR Am J Roentgenol* 2006;186(5):1260-1264. doi:10.2214/AJR.04.1606.

28. Cuff S, Loud K, O'Riordan MA: Overuse injuries in high school athletes. *Clin Pediatr (Phila)* 2010;49(8):731-736. doi:10.1177/0009922810363154.

29. Faulkner RA, Davison KS, Bailey DA, Mirwald RL, Baxter-Jones AD: Size-corrected BMD decreases during peak linear growth: Implications for fracture incidence during adolescence. *J Bone Miner Res* 2006;21(12):1864-1870. doi:10.1359/jbmr.060907.

30. Matos NF, Winsley RJ, Williams CA: Prevalence of nonfunctional overreaching/overtraining in young English athletes. *Med Sci Sports Exerc* 2011;43(7):1287-1294. doi:10.1249/MSS.0b013e318207f87b.

31. Kreher JB, Schwartz JB: Overtraining syndrome: A practical guide. *Sports Health* 2012;4(2):128-138. doi:10.1177/1941738111434406.

32. Jayanthi NA, Holt DB, LaBella CR, Dugas LR: Socioeconomic factors for sports specialization and injury in youth athletes. *Sports Health* 2018;10(4):303-310. doi:10.1177/1941738118778510.

High single sport specialization athletes reported more serious overuse injuries than low single sport specialization athletes, potentially due to higher rates of sports specialization, more hours per week playing organized sports, higher ratio of weekly hours in organized sports to free play, and greater participation in individual sports. Level of evidence: III.

33. Laprade RF, Agel J, Baker J, et al: AOSSM early sport specialization consensus statement. *Orthop J Sports Med* 2016;4(4):2325967116644241. doi:10.1177/2325967116644241.

Youth advocates, parents, clinicians, and coaches need to work together with the sport governing bodies to ensure healthy environments for play and competition that do not create long-term health issues yet support athletic competition at the highest level desired. Level of evidence: V.

34. Fabricant PD, Lakomkin N, Sugimoto D, Tepolt FA, Stracciolini A, Kocher MS: Youth sports specialization and musculoskeletal injury: A systematic review of the literature. *Phys Sportsmed* 2016;44(3):257-262. doi:10.1080/00913847.2016.1177476.

Further prospective research into the relationship between injury and sport specialization is warranted as the primary evidence that currently exists with regard to early sport specialization is scarce, retrospective, and shows only modest associations between early sports specialization and overuse injury. Level of evidence: III.

35. Bell DR, Post EG, Biese K, Bay C, Valovich McLeod T: Sport specialization and risk of overuse injuries: A systematic review with meta-analysis. *Pediatrics* 2018;142(3):e20180657. Available at: www.aappublications.org/news.

Single sport specialization is associated with an increased risk of overuse musculoskeletal injuries. Level of evidence: IV.

36. Pasulka J, Jayanthi N, McCann A, Dugas LR, LaBella C: Specialization patterns across various youth sports and relationship to injury risk. *Phys Sportsmed* 2017;45(3):344-352. doi:10.1080/00913847.2017.1313077.

Youth athletes in individual sports reported higher levels of single sport specialization, higher training volumes, and greater rates of overuse injuries than team sport athletes. Level of evidence: III.

37. Maffulli N, Longo UG, Gougoulias N, Loppini M, Denaro V: Long-term health outcomes of youth sports injuries. *Br J Sports Med* 2010;44(1):21-25. doi:10.1136/bjsm.2009.069526.

38. Hill DE, Andrews JR: Stopping sports injuries in young athletes. *Clin Sports Med* 2011;30(4):841-849. doi:10.1016/j.csm.2011.07.003.

39. Village G: Intensive training and sports specialization in young athletes. American Academy of Pediatrics. Committee on Sports Medicine and Fitness. *Pediatrics* 2000;106:154-157. doi:10.1542/peds.106.1.154.

40. Milewski MD, Skaggs DL, Bishop GA, et al: Chronic lack of sleep is associated with increased sports injuries in adolescent athletes. *J Pediatr Orthop* 2014;34(2):129-133. doi:10.1097/BPO.0000000000000151.

41. Bergeron M, Mountjoy M, Armstrong N, et al: International Olympic Committee consensus statement on youth athletic development. *Br J Sports Med* 2015;49(13):843-851.

42. Popchak A, Burnett T, Weber N, Boninger M: Factors related to injury in youth and adolescent baseball pitching, with an eye toward prevention. *Am J Phys Med Rehabil* 2015;94(5):395-409. doi:10.1097/PHM.0000000000000184.
43. Fleisig GS, Weber A, Hassell N, Andrews JR: Prevention of elbow injuries in youth baseball pitchers. *Curr Sports Med Rep* 2009;8:250-254. doi:10.1249/JSR.0b013e3181b7ee5f.
44. Yang J, Mann BJ, Guettler JH, et al: Risk-prone pitching activities and injuries in youth baseball: Findings from a national sample. *Am J Sports Med* 2014;42(6):1456-1463. doi:10.1177/0363546514524699.
45. Arnold A, Thigpen CA, Beattie PF, Kissenberth MJ, Shanley E: Overuse physeal injuries in youth athletes: Risk factors, prevention, and treatment strategies. *Sports Health* 2017;9(2):139-147. doi:10.1177/1941738117690847.

    Injury prevention programs that focus on flexibility, strength, and training volume will address risk factors for overuse injury, which include periods of accelerated growth, chronological age, body size, training volume, and previous injury. Level of evidence: III.
46. Hall R, Barber Foss K, Hewett TE, Myer GD: Sports specialization is associated with an increased risk of developing anterior knee pain in adolescent female athletes. *J Sport Rehabil* 2015;24(1):31-35. doi:10.1123/jsr.2013-0101.
47. Cassel M, Risch L, Intziegianni K, et al: Incidence of Achilles and patellar tendinopathy in adolescent elite athletes. *Int J Sports Med* 2018;39(9):726-732. doi:10.1055/a-0633-9098.

    The 3-years incidence of Achilles tendinopathy (1%) in adolescent elite athletes is low while patellar tendinopathy is more common (13%). Level of evidence: III.
48. Kramer DE, Kalish LA, Abola MV, et al: The effects of medial synovial plica excision with and without lateral retinacular release on adolescents with anterior knee pain. *J Child Orthop* 2016;10(2):155-162. doi:10.1007/s11832-016-0724-x.

    Although most patients were satisfied and able to return to sports following plica excision with or without lateral release, residual symptoms were common. Level of evidence: IV.
49. Lyu SR, Hsu CC: Medial plicae and degeneration of the medial femoral condyle. *Arthroscopy* 2006;22(1):17-26. doi:0.1016/j.arthro.2005.08.039.
50. Earl JE, Hoch AZ: A proximal strengthening program improves pain, function, and biomechanics in women with patellofemoral pain syndrome. *Am J Sports Med* 2011;39(1):154-163. doi:10.1177/0363546510379967.
51. Powers CM: The influence of altered lower-extremity kinematics on patellofemoral joint dysfunction: A theoretical perspective. *J Orthop Sports Phys Ther* 2003;33(11):639-646. doi:10.2519/jospt.2003.33.11.639.
52. Zazulak BT, Hewett TE, Reeves NP, Goldberg B, Cholewicki J: Deficits in neuromuscular control of the trunk predict knee injury risk: A prospective biomechanical-epidemiologic study. *Am J Sports Med* 2007;35(7):1123-1130. doi:10.1177/0363546507301585.
53. Hubbard TJ, Mullis Carpenter E, Cordova ML: Contributing factors to medial tibial stress syndrome: A prospective investigation. *Med Sci Sports Exerc* 2009;41(3):490-496. doi:10.1249/MSS.0b013e31818b98e6.
54. Madeley LT, Munteanu SE, Bonanno DR: Endurance of the ankle joint plantar flexor muscles in athletes with medial tibial stress syndrome: A case-control study. *J Sci Med Sport* 2007;10:356-362. doi:10.1016/j.jsams.2006.12.115.
55. Pepper M, Akuthota V, Mccarty EC: The pathophysiology of stress fractures. *Clin Sports Med* 2006;25(1):1-16. doi:10.1016/j.csm.2005.08.010.
56. Mountjoy M, Sundgot-Borgen J, Burke L, et al: The IOC consensus statement: Beyond the female athlete triad—Relative Energy Deficiency in Sport (RED-S). *Br J Sports Med* 2014;48(7):491-497. doi:10.1136/bjsports-2014-093502.
57. Wiegerinck JI, Zwiers R, Sierevelt IN, van Weert HCPM, van Dijk CN, Struijs PAA: Treatment of calcaneal apophysitis: Wait and see versus orthotic device versus physical therapy. A pragmatic therapeutic randomized clinical trial. *J Pediatr Orthop* 2016;36(2):152-157. Available at: www.pedorthopaedics.com.

    Treatment with wait and see, a heel raise inlay, or physical therapy each resulted in a clinically relevant and statistically significant reduction of heel pain due to calcaneal apophysitis without significant difference in heel pain between individual treatment regimes. Level of evidence: I.
58. Sylvester JE, Hennrikus WL: Treatment outcomes of adolescents with Iselin's apophysitis. *J Pediatr Orthop B* 2015;24(4):362-365. doi:10.1097/BPB.0000000000000157.

CHAPTER 55

Pediatric and Adolescent Athletes: Special Considerations

ANDREW J.M. GREGORY, MD, FAAP, FACSM, FAMSSM

ABSTRACT

The care of young athletes involves special considerations. Those caring for these young patients should be aware of sport-related concussion, exertional heat illness, the female athlete triad, sudden cardiac arrest, and other medical conditions affecting sports participation. Familiarity with preparticipation screening, the benefits of strength training, and the potential harm of performance-enhancing supplements will assist caregivers in preventing injuries and providing the best possible care when injury occurs.

Keywords: concussion; heat illness; preparticipation physical; supplements

INTRODUCTION

Children are participating in organized sports at younger ages than in past decades. Physicians who care for young athletes should be aware of considerations that are unique to patients in this age group. Although young athletes generally heal faster from injury than older athletes, certain conditions such as concussion may take longer to heal. Congenital conditions such as Marfan syndrome or hypertrophic cardiomyopathy that preclude sports participation may occur in childhood and should be recognized early to prevent poor outcomes. Other conditions such as heat illness may be more common in children, because young athletes and coaches may not recognize early symptoms. Many infections that commonly occur in children also can affect sports participation.

SPORT-RELATED CONCUSSION

Young athletes are at increased risk for concussion sustained during sports participation.[1] The incidence of concussion varies widely across different sporting disciplines. For athletes younger than 18 years, the sports with the highest incidence rates of concussion per athletic exposure are rugby, hockey, and American football at 4.18 per 1,000, 1.20 per 1,000, and 0.53 per 1,000, respectively. The sports with the lowest incidence rates of concussion are volleyball, baseball, and cheerleading at 0.03 per 1,000, 0.06 per 1,000, and 0.07 per 1,000, respectively.[2] Because athletes may not report symptoms of concussion, a high index of suspicion must be maintained when any young athlete sustains a blow to the head/neck area. A child-specific symptom checklist for athletes, parents, and teachers is recommended for use in children younger than 12 years. Although not yet validated, the Child-SCAT5, introduced in 2016 by the Concussion in Sport Consensus Group, is a standardized concussion assessment tool for use in children aged 5 to 12 years.[3] A helpful checklist of concussion symptoms is available from the Centers for Disease Control and Prevention.[4]

Based on comparative studies, it appears that recovery from concussion is somewhat slower (by a few days) in adolescent athletes than in their adult counterparts.[5] Data are not available for young athletes for comparison with data from high school and college athletes. Although management of concussion in younger athletes is similar to that of adults, a more conservative approach is warranted regarding return

Dr. Gregory or an immediate family member serves as a board member, owner, officer, or committee member of the Pediatric Research in Sports Medicine.

to play for younger athletes with sport-related concussion. Management of concussion includes avoidance of any triggers that worsen symptoms, treatment of headache, rehabilitation for neck pain, and cognitive or vestibular therapy if indicated. Strict rest is not recommended, because this has been shown to increase the number of symptoms and extend the duration of symptoms.[6] There is some newer evidence that aerobic activity may actually improve concussion recovery.[7] Return to play should be considered only when the athlete is symptom free. The return to play protocol includes graded increases in exertion before return to full activity. A minimum of 24 hours is recommended between each stage, and progression to the next stage is allowed only if no symptoms are present at the previous stage. The stages are (1) light activity such as jogging or biking, (2) moderate activity such as sprinting or jumping, (3) intense activity such as sports-specific activity or ball kicking or shooting baskets, (4) sports practice without contact, and (5) sports practice with full contact.

STRENGTH TRAINING IN CHILDREN

Although participation in strength training historically has been considered unsafe for children, it has since proven to be a safe activity for young athletes when simple guidelines are followed. The guidelines of the American Academy of Pediatrics for strength training in children include recommendations to avoid power lifting, bodybuilding, and maximal lifts until physical and skeletal maturity is reached. Adequate fluid and nutritional intake, inclusion of aerobic conditioning, warm-up and cooldown periods, the initial learning of exercises with no weights, the gradual increase in weight if proper form is maintained, and addressing all major muscle groups also are recommended. The guidelines also include recommendations for a preparticipation physical examination, evaluation of any illness or injury before resumption of strength training, and appropriate adult supervision.[8]

In addition to being a safe activity for children, strength training may actually prevent injury during sports participation as well as improve overall body composition. Injury prevention programs have been shown to substantially reduce injury rates in adolescent athletes.[9] The specific reason for their efficacy is unknown; however, it may be related to program content and improvements in muscle strength, proprioceptive balance, and flexibility. Strength training can make positive alterations in overall body composition while reducing body fat, improving insulin sensitivity in adolescents who are overweight, and enhancing cardiac function in children who are obese.[10]

PERFORMANCE-ENHANCING SUPPLEMENTS

Performance-enhancing supplements are used by young athletes beginning as early as middle school. Most young athletes do not have the ideal diet and hydration for sports performance and do not understand the potential harm that these supplements can cause. Supplements by their definition are not drugs and do not have to undergo the same rigorous testing and regulation as drugs. Consequently, supplements may not contain the ingredients shown on their labels and may contain undesirable impurities. Common supplements used by young athletes include creatine, anabolic steroids, human growth hormone, stimulants, and amino acids and other proteins. Few studies exist on the safety of supplement use in adults, and no studies exist regarding the safety of supplements for children.

Creatine is used by young athletes trying to gain muscle, usually in the setting of strength training. Studies of creatine use in adults have demonstrated a positive effect in repeated short bouts of intense activity, but no effects in single sprints or endurance activities. These results have not been replicated in children, and no studies exist on competitive benefits. Weight gain is the most common adverse effect of creatine use. Athletes who consume meat as a regular part of their diet are unlikely to require a creatine supplement. The intake of creatine and other protein should be limited in any athlete with kidney disease.

Anabolic steroids have been shown to have ergogenic effects in adult athletes, but they also cause serious adverse effects in multiple body systems. Of chief concern in young athletes is the effect that anabolic steroids have on early closure of the physes of the long bones. In addition, there appears to be a clear relationship between steroid use and abuse of illegal substances and other risk-taking behaviors in adolescents. Anabolic steroids should only be prescribed for children by endocrinologists in the setting of a growth hormone deficiency. Little information is available about human growth hormone use in young athletes.

Stimulants are commonly used by athletes to maintain a high level of alertness during a sports activity and for performance enhancement. Common stimulants include caffeine, ephedrine, synephrine, and amphetamine. Stimulants have been extensively studied for treatment of attention-deficit hyperactivity disorder in children but not for effects on sports performance. Commonly reported adverse effects include increased pulse rate and palpitations, restlessness, and difficulty sleeping.[11] Potential other adverse effects include addiction, hypertension, arrhythmia, and increased susceptibility to heat-related illness.

Because new supplements are continually introduced in the marketplace, it is difficult for efficacy studies to keep pace. Many new products contain either anabolic steroids or stimulants in different or undetectable forms. Some recently introduced supplements such as products containing beet juice have a high nitrate content. Recent studies of nitrate supplementation revealed either a minor positive effect or no systematic effect on exercise performance. The sugar content of whole beetroot juice might have a slightly more pronounced effect on athletic performance. Although reasonable intake of nitrate supplements (<1 g/d) has no detrimental effect on kidney function, the risk and benefit of higher nitrate intake is unknown.[12]

The continued use of performance-enhancing supplements by young athletes is concerning. Education of athletes by their coaches may reduce the intention to use supplements. Efforts should concentrate on the education of coaches regarding performance-enhancing supplements.

FEMALE ATHLETE TRIAD

In 1992, the female athlete triad was defined as having the following components: an eating disorder, amenorrhea, and osteoporosis. Over time, it was realized that athletes who did not meet the strict definition of the female athlete triad were still experiencing higher rates of sports injuries. In 2007, the American College of Sports Medicine updated the diagnostic guidelines, and the female athlete triad was redefined as a spectrum of abnormalities in energy availability, menstrual function, and bone mineral density.[13] The new definition is less restrictive and allows for the presence of only one or two components to make a diagnosis; therefore, this condition also can apply to male athletes.

Low energy availability is defined as a body mass index less than 17.5 kg/m^2 or less than 85% of expected body weight in adolescents.[14] Other methods for assessing energy availability, dietary intake, and energy expenditure are imprecise. An experienced sports dietitian or an exercise physiologist can provide assistance with these assessments. Athletes with primary or secondary amenorrhea (less than six menses over 12 months) should be evaluated to rule out pregnancy, systemic diseases, and endocrinopathies. The diagnosis of functional hypothalamic amenorrhea in athletes secondary to low energy availability is a diagnosis of exclusion. Screening for low bone mineral density should be done if an athlete has at least one high-risk factor or at least two moderate-risk factors as defined by the Female Athlete Triad Coalition Consensus Statement[14] (**Table 1**).

All adolescent female athletes should be screened for symptoms of the female athlete triad during a preparticipation physical examination. Particular attention should be given to athletes participating in high-risk sports such as gymnastics, cheerleading, dancing, ice skating, cross-country running, and wrestling. An athlete with an abnormality in any of the three components should be educated on injury risks (particularly stress fractures) and the importance of proper nutrition and exercise modifications. The use of oral contraceptives for return of menses without proper nutrition and exercise modification is less desirable. Increased energy availability should allow for return of normal menses and improved bone health. For athletes who do not respond to education alone, treatment by a multidisciplinary team, including a physician, a mental health counselor, and a sports nutritionist, is recommended.

TABLE 1

Risk Factors for Low Bone Mineral Density

Risk Factors
High-risk Factors
History of a DSM-V-diagnosed eating disorder
BMI <17.5 kg/m^2, <85% expected body weight, or recent weight loss of ≥10% in 1 mo
Menarche at 16 yr of age or older
Currently experiencing or has a history of less than six menses over 12 mo
Two prior stress reactions or stress fractures, one high-risk stress reaction or stress fracture, or one low-energy nontraumatic fracture
Prior *Z*-score of less than −2.0 SD (after at least 1 yr from baseline DEXA)
Moderate-risk Factors
Currently experiencing or has a history of disordered eating for 6 mo or more
BMI between 17.5 and 18.5 kg/m^2, 85%-90% expected body weight, or recent weight loss of 5%-10% in 1 mo
Menarche between 15 and 16 yr of age
Currently experiencing or has a history of six to eight menses over 12 mo
One prior stress reaction or stress fracture
Prior *Z*-score between −1.0 and −2.0 SD (after at least a 1-yr interval from baseline DEXA)

BMI = body mass index, DEXA = dual-energy X-ray absorptiometry, DSM-V = Diagnostic and Statistical Manual of Mental Disorders, Fifth Edition

Adapted by permission from BMJ Publishing Group Limited. De Souza MJ, Nattiv A, Joy E, et al: 2014 Female Athlete Triad Coalition consensus statement on treatment and return to play of the female athlete triad: 1st International Conference held in San Francisco, California, May 2012 and 2nd International Conference held in Indianapolis, Indiana, May 2013. *Br J Sports Med* 2014;48:289.

EXERTIONAL HEAT ILLNESS

Exertional heat illness occurs in children and adolescents just as it does in adults. It is no longer believed that children are at greater risk than adults; however, heat-related deaths occur almost yearly in children who play high school football.[15] With appropriate preparation, activity modifications, and monitoring, most healthy children and adolescents can safely participate in outdoor sports and other physical activities in warm to hot climatic conditions.[16] Personnel capable of treating all forms of heat illness, especially exertional heatstroke, by rapidly lowering core body temperature, should be on-site during youth athletic events and community programs involving vigorous physical activity in warm or hot weather conditions. Children and adolescents should be educated on the importance of proper preparation, hydration, reporting of symptoms, and effectively managing recovery and rest, which directly affect exercise heat tolerance and safety.

A core body temperature measurement should be obtained for a young athlete who exhibits signs or symptoms of exertional heat illness, which include fatigue, weakness, lightheadedness, and muscle cramps. The most accurate measurement of core body temperature is with a rectal, not an oral, thermometer.[17] An athlete with acute mental status change and core body temperature greater than 104°F should undergo rapid cooling treatment. Ice-water or cold-water immersion provides the most efficient cooling treatment for exercise-induced hyperthermia and is recommended as the definitive treatment of exertional heatstroke.[18] Heatstroke can be distinguished from heat exhaustion by the presence of an altered mental status (such as hysteria, combativeness, or delirium), syncope, paralysis, ataxia, seizure, and coma. If immersion treatment is not available, continual dousing of the patient with water combined with fanning or continually rotating cold, wet towels are alternatives. Because morbidity is directly related to the duration of the high body temperature, it is important to **cool first and transport second**.

SUDDEN CARDIAC DEATH AND PREPARTICIPATION SCREENING

There is general agreement that young athletes should undergo preparticipation screening before participation in athletic events. Controversy exists regarding when to begin screening, how often to screen, and the best screening methods. The American Heart Association recommends screening that includes a targeted personal history, a family history, and a physical examination. Some key elements of screening are a history of elevated systemic blood pressure, knowledge of certain cardiac conditions in family members, and the presence of a heart murmur. The identification of these elements is designed to identify or at least raise suspicion of cardiovascular diseases. Athletes with positive findings of cardiovascular disease should be referred for further evaluation and testing.[19] Recent studies have supported the use of electrocardiography for screening for potentially lethal cardiac disorders in athletes. Electrocardiography is 5 times more sensitive than a patient history and 10 times more sensitive than a physical examination in detecting cardiac disorders and has a higher positive likelihood ratio, a lower negative likelihood ratio, and a lower false-positive rate than a history or examination.[20] Electrocardiographic screening is currently being used by many major sporting organizations, but it is not widely used in most youth sports organizations.

Every organization that sponsors athletic activities should have a written, structured emergency action plan that includes instructions, preparations, and expectations for the athletes, parents or guardians, coaches, strength and conditioning trainers, athletic directors, and healthcare professionals who provide medical care during practices and games. Precise injury prevention, recognition, treatment, and return to play policies for the common causes of sudden death in athletes also are needed. The emergency action plan should be developed and coordinated with local emergency medical services staff, school public safety officials, on-site first responders, school medical staff, and school administrators. The plan should be specific to each athletic venue and should be practiced at least annually with all involved personnel.[21]

GENERAL MEDICAL CONDITIONS

Certain medical conditions can affect a child's ability to participate in sports. The American Academy of Pediatrics Council of Sports Medicine Fitness has prepared a list of medical conditions that affect sports participation.[22] These conditions range from congenital absence of organs to infections and illnesses. It is recommended that children born with a single eye, kidney, or testicle protect the solitary organ with approved polycarbonate eyewear, a flak jacket, or an athletic cup, respectively, as required. Children with a transplanted kidney may require a specially made abdominal pad for protection. Children with medical illnesses such as diabetes mellitus and epilepsy can participate safely in sports with proper medication and monitoring.

In general, if an illness keeps a child from attending school, he or she should not participate in sports activities. Athletes with a fever (temperature >101°F) should avoid participation in hot and humid environments, because an increased body temperature is a predisposing factor for heat illness. Athletes with diarrhea or nausea should avoid participation because of the risk for dehydration and the possibility of infecting other athletes. Skin rashes should be evaluated by a physician before allowing athletic participation, because several skin infections can be transmitted via skin-to-skin contact. Athletes with herpes, staphylococcal, streptococcal, tinea, or molluscum skin infections should not participate until the infection is treated and the lesions are healed. Covering skin lesions is no longer considered sufficient to prevent transmission.

Universal precautions should be used when handling blood or body fluids in the athletic environment in the same manner as in a hospital or clinic.

Infectious mononucleosis from an Epstein-Barr viral infection is a unique situation, because the spleen may be enlarged and consequently at risk for rupture. Although rupture is quite rare, death may occur. Most documented spleen ruptures have occurred within the first 3 weeks of the illness and were atraumatic, so a minimum of 3 weeks of rest from all physical activities starting from the first day of onset of illness is recommended.[23] Manual palpation of the spleen is known to be unreliable, and imaging of the spleen is challenging to interpret, because the baseline size differs in individuals.

SUMMARY

Young athletes are unique and should be treated differently than adults. Because an increasing number of children are participating in organized sports at younger ages, care providers should be aware of sports-related health concerns, including concussion, the use of performance-enhancing supplements, the female athlete triad, exertional heat illness, and sudden cardiac death. Care providers should keep their Basic Life Support training current if providing sideline coverage for sporting events. Strength training programs; early recognition of factors that predispose a young athlete to injury; the development of a written emergency action plan that is practiced yearly with staff at each specific venue; and the education of athletes, parents, and coaches will aid in ensuring the safety of young athletes and encouraging a lifetime of sports participation.

KEY STUDY POINTS

- Although management of concussion in young athletes is similar to that of adults, a more conservative approach is warranted regarding return to play for younger athletes.
- In addition to being a safe activity for children, strength training may actually prevent injury during sports participation and improve overall body composition.
- Continued use of performance-enhancing supplements by young athletes is a cause for concern. Education of athletes by their coaches reduces the intention to use supplements.
- Adolescent female athletes should be screened for symptoms of the female athlete triad during the preparticipation physical examination. Those with abnormalities in any of the three components should be educated on injury risks, proper nutrition, and exercise modifications.
- A core body temperature measurement with a rectal thermometer should be obtained for a young athlete who exhibits signs or symptoms of exertional heat illness. An athlete with an acute mental status change and core body temperature greater than 104°F should undergo a rapid cooling treatment with ice-water or cold-water immersion.
- Every organization that sponsors athletic activities should have a written, structured emergency action plan that includes instruction, preparation, and expectations for those who provide medical care during practices and games. In addition, precise prevention, recognition, treatment, and return to play policies for the common causes of sudden death in athletes are needed.

ANNOTATED REFERENCES

1. Halstead ME, Walter KD, Moffat K, Council on Sports Medicine and Fitness: American Academy of Pediatrics: Clinical report. Sport-related concussion in children and adolescents. *Pediatrics* 2018;142(6):e20183074.

   This is a literature review of the current state of sport-related concussion knowledge, diagnosis, and management in children and adolescents. Level of evidence: V.

2. Pfister T, Pfister K, Hagel B, Ghali WA, Ronksley PE: The incidence of concussion in youth sports: A systematic review and meta-analysis. *Br J Sports Med* 2016;50(5):292-297.

   Sports with a high degree of physical contact had the highest estimated incidence of concussion, including rugby, American football, and hockey. Level of evidence: II.

3. McCrory P, Meeuwisse WH, Dvorak J, et al: Consensus statement on concussion in sport – The 5th international conference on concussion in sport held in Berlin, October 2016. *Br J Sports Med* 2017;51(11):838-847.

   The authors described the consensus-based recommendations for clinicians caring for athletes with concussions. Management and return to play decisions should be based on clinical judgment and on an individualized basis. Level of evidence: V.

4. Heads Up to Clinicians: Addressing Concussion in Sports Among Kids and Teens. *Concussion Symptom Checklist.* Centers for Disease Control and Prevention. Available at: http://www.cdc.gov/concussion/headsup/clinicians/resource_center/pdfs/Concussion_Symptoms_Checklist.pdf. Accessed June 27, 2016.

   The somatic, cognitive, affective, and sleep symptoms of concussion are presented. Level of evidence: V.

5. Foley C, Gregory A, Solomon G: Young age as a modifying factor in sports concussion management: What is the evidence? *Curr Sports Med Rep* 2014;13(6):390-394.

6. Thomas D, Apps J, Hoffman R: Benefits of strict rest after acute concussion: A randomized controlled trial. *Pediatrics* 2015;13(2):213-223.

7. Leddy JJ, Haider MN, Ellis MJ, et al: Early subthreshold aerobic exercise for sport-related concussion: A randomized clinical trial. *JAMA Pediatr* 2019;173(4):319-325.

   Aerobic exercise programs reduced concussion recovery from 17 to 13 days. Level of evidence: I.

8. McCambridge TM, Stricker PR, American Academy of Pediatrics Council on Sports Medicine and Fitness: Strength training by children and adolescents. *Pediatrics* 2008;121(4):835-840.

9. Soomro N, Sanders R, Hackett D, et al: The efficacy of injury prevention programs in adolescent team sports: A meta-analysis. *Am J Sports Med* 2016;44(9):2415-2424.

   Injury prevention programs resulted in a total injury risk reduction of approximately 40% in adolescents participating in team sports. Level of evidence: I.

10. Lloyd RS, Faigenbaum AD, Stone MH, et al: Position statement on youth resistance training: The 2014 International Consensus. *Br J Sports Med* 2014;48(7):498-505.

11. Stephens MB, Attipoe S, Jones D, Ledford CJ, Deuster PA: Energy drink and energy shot use in the military. *Nutr Rev* 2014;72(suppl 1):72-77.

12. Poortmans JR, Gualano B, Carpentier A: Nitrate supplementation and human exercise performance: Too much of a good thing? *Curr Opin Clin Nutr Metab Care* 2015;18(6):599-604.

13. Matzkin E, Curry EJ, Whitlock K: Female athlete triad: Past, present, and future. *J Am Acad Orthop Surg* 2015;23(7):424-432.

14. Joy E, De Souza MJ, Nattiv A, et al: 2014 female athlete triad coalition consensus statement on treatment and return to play of the female athlete triad. *Curr Sports Med Rep* 2014;13(4):219-232.

15. Kucera KL, Klossner D, Colgate B, Cantu RC: *Annual Survey of Football Injury Research.* National Center for Catastrophic Sport Injury Research, 2018. Available at: https://nccsir.unc.edu/files/2019/02/Annual-Football-2018-Fatalities-FINAL.pdf. Accessed November 10, 2019.

    Nine direct and indirect fatalities were recorded for the 2018 football season (0.21 per 100,000 football participants). There were two fatalities directly related to football during the 2018 football season: both were in high school football, one head and one neck injury. Level of evidence: IV.

16. Bergeron MF, Devore C, Rice SG, Council on Sports Medicine and Fitness and Council on School Health; American Academy of Pediatrics: Policy statement – Climatic heat stress and exercising children and adolescents. *Pediatrics* 2011;128(3):e741-e747.

17. Mazerolle SM, Ganio MS, Casa DJ, Vingren J, Klau J: Is oral temperature an accurate measurement of deep body temperature? A systematic review. *J Athl Train* 2011;46(5):566-573.

18. McDermott BP, Casa DJ, Ganio MS, et al: Acute whole-body cooling for exercise-induced hyperthermia: A systematic review. *J Athl Train* 2009;44(1):84-93.

19. American Heart Association/American Stroke Association: *Preparticipation Cardiovascular Screening of Young Competitive Athletes: Policy Guidance.* Washington, DC, American Heart Association, 2012. Available at: https://www.heart.org/idc/groups/ahaecc-public/@wcm/@adv/documents/downloadable/ucm_443945.pdf. Accessed June 9, 2016.

20. Harmon KG, Zigman M, Drezner JA: The effectiveness of screening history, physical exam, and ECG to detect potentially lethal cardiac disorders in athletes: A systematic review/meta-analysis. *J Electrocardiol* 2015;48(3):329-338.

21. Casa DJ, Guskiewicz KM, Anderson SA, et al: National Athletic Trainers' Association position statement: Preventing sudden death in sports. *J Athl Train* 2012;47(1):96-118.

22. Rice SG, American Academy of Pediatrics Council on Sports Medicine and Fitness: Medical conditions affecting sports participation. *Pediatrics* 2008;121(4):841-848.

23. Putukian M, O'Connor FG, Stricker P, et al: Mononucleosis and athletic participation: An evidence-based subject review. *Clin J Sport Med* 2008;18(4):309-315.

Index

Note: Page numbers followed by "*f*" indicate figures and "*t*" indicate tables.

A

B

C

D

E

F

G

H

N

O

P

Q

R

S

T

U

V

W

X

Z